PAIN MEDICINE

A Comprehensive Review

PAIN MEDICINE

A Comprehensive Review

P. Prithvi Raj, M.D.
Professor of Clinical Anesthesiology,
Academic Director of Pain Medicine,
UCLA School of Medicine,
Los Angeles, California

with 245 illustrations

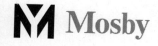
Mosby

St. Louis Baltimore Boston Carlsbad Chicago Naples New York Philadelphia Portland
London Madrid Mexico City Singapore Sydney Tokyo Toronto Wiesbaden

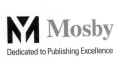

Mosby
Dedicated to Publishing Excellence

A Times Mirror
Company

Editor-in-Chief: Susan M. Gay
Developmental Editor: Sandra Clark Brown
Project Manager: Carol Sullivan Weis
Production Editor: Rick Dudley
Book Designer: Sheilah Barrett
Manufacturing Manager: Dave Graybill

Printed in the United States of America
Composition by The Clarinda Company
Illustration preparation by Top Graphics
Printing/binding by Maple-Vail Book Manufacturing Group

Mosby-Year Book, Inc.
11830 Westline Industrial Drive
St. Louis, MO 63146

International Standard Book Number ISBN 0-8016-7998-2

95 96 97 98 99 / 9 8 7 6 5 4 3 2 1

CONTRIBUTORS

A. ELIZABETH ANSEL, RN

Nurse Administrator,
Pain Control Consultants,
Westerville, Ohio

JEFF M. ARTHUR, MD

Assistant Professor,
Department of Anesthesiology,
Texas Tech University Health Sciences Center,
Lubbock, Texas

HONORIO T. BENZON, MD

Professor of Anesthesia,
Northwestern University Medical School;
Chief, Pain Management Service,
Northwestern Memorial Hospital,
Chicago, Illinois

ROBERT J. BURTON, Jr., MD

Director of Anesthesia,
Paulding-Promina Hospital,
Dallas, Georgia

TERRENCE M. CALDER, MD

Clinical Assistant Professor,
National Naval Medical Center,
Bethesda, Maryland

DONALD D. DENSON, PhD

Associate Professor of Anesthesia,
Department of Anesthesiology,
Emory University School of Medicine,
Atlanta, Georgia

JOELLE F. DESPARMET, MD

Assistant Professor,
McGill University;
Department of Anesthesia,
Montreal Children's Hospital,
Quebec, Canada

RICHARD HAROLD DOCHERTY, MB, ChB

Pain Consultant,
St. Mary's Hospital,
Long Beach, California

JAMES C. EISENACH, MD

Professor,
Department of Anesthesia,
Bowman Gray School of Medicine,
Wake Forest University,
Winston-Salem, North Carolina

DAVID EVANS, MD, FRCPC

Associate Professor,
Department of Anaesthesia,
The Toronto Hospital,
Toronto Western Division,
Toronto, Ontario, Canada

J. DAVID HADDOX, DDS, MD, FACPM

The Center for Pain Medicine,
The Emory Clinic,
Atlanta, Georgia

JAMES E. HEAVNER, DVM, PhD

Professor,
Department of Anesthesiology and Physiology,
Director, Anesthesia Research,
Texas Tech University Health Sciences Center,
Lubbock, Texas

ALLEN H. HORD, MD

Assistant Professor of Anesthesiology,
Director, Division of Pain Medicine,
Anesthesia Department,
Emory University School of Medicine,
Atlanta, Georgia

SHELDON A. ISAACSON, MD

Assistant Professor of Anesthesiology,
University of Rochester,
School of Medicine and Dentistry,
Rochester, New York

GARY W. JAY, MD

Medical Director,
The Headache and Neurological Rehabilitation Institute
  of Colorado,
Northglen, Colorado

JEFFREY A. KATZ, MD

Assistant Professor of Anesthesia,
Associate Medical Director, Pain Center,
Department of Anesthesia,
University of Cincinnati,
Cincinnati, Ohio

Licensed Clinical Psychologist,
The Atlanta Center for Behavioral Medicine,
Atlanta, Georgia

L. DOUGLAS KENNEDY, MD, FACPM
Past Fellow,
Cleveland Clinic Foundation,
Cleveland, Ohio;
Pain Consultants of Lexington,
Lexington, Kentucky

DONALD L. KRAMER, MD
Assistant Professor,
Department of Anesthesiology,
Texas Tech University Health Sciences Center,
Lubbock, Texas

MARGARET P. KRENGEL, OT, CHT
Director, Occupational Therapy Services,
Hand Institute of Georgia,
Division of Workplace Medical Solutions,
Atlanta, Georgia

W. DAVID LEAK, MD
Diplomat, American Board of Pain Management,
Medical Director,
Pain Control Consultants, Inc,
Westerville, Ohio

CHRISTOPHER M. LOAR, MD
Clinical Assistant Professor of Neurology
    and Anesthesiology,
Departments of Neurology and Anesthesiology,
University of Texas Health Science Center at Houston,
Houston, Texas

DAVID R. LONGMIRE, MD
Clinical Assistant Professor of Internal Medicine,
The University of Alabama School of Medicine,
Program at Huntsville;
Adjunct Staff, Pain Management Center,
Department of Anesthesiology,
Cleveland Clinic Foundation,
Cleveland, Ohio

LAURENCE E. MATHER, PhD
Professor,
Department of Anaesthesia and Pain Management,
University of Sydney,
Royal North Shore Hospital,
St. Leonards, Australia

MONICA M. NEUMANN, MD
Assistant Professor,
Department of Anesthesiology,
Loma Linda University School of Medicine,
Loma Linda, California

CARL E. NOE, MD
Medical Director,
Baylor Center for Pain Management,
Baylor Medical Center,
Dallas, Texas

UNIVERSITY PROFESSOR DR. Med. HANS NOLTE
Klinikum Minden,
Institut fur Anaesthesiologie,
Friedrichstrabe, Minden, Germany

RICHARD B. PATT, MD
Associate Professor of Anesthesiology and
    Neuro-Oncology,
Deputy Chief, Pain & Symptom Management Section,
University of Texas,
M.D. Anderson Cancer Center,
Houston, Texas

RONALD P. PAWL, MD
Associate Professor of Neurosurgery,
University of Illinois at Chicago;
Director,
Center for Rehabilitation,
Lake Forest Hospital,
Lake Forest, Illinois

JAMES C. PHERO, DMD
Professor of Clinical Anesthesia,
University of Cincinnati Medical Center,
Cincinnati, Ohio

RICARDO S. PLANCARTE, MD
Chairman, Anesthesiology,
Critical Care and Pain Management,
Instituto Nacional de Cancerologia,
Mexico City, Mexico

GABOR B. RACZ, MB, ChB
Professor and Chairman,
Department of Anesthesiology,
Director of Institute of Pain Management,
Texas Tech University Health Sciences Center,
Lubbock, Texas

P. PRITHVI RAJ, MD
Professor of Clinical Anesthesiology,
Academic Director of Pain Medicine,
UCLA School of Medicine,
Los Angeles, California

SOMAYAJI RAMAMURTHY, MD
Professor of Anesthesiology,
Chief, Pain Management Center,
University of Texas Health Science Center,
San Antonio, Texas

RICHARD L. RAUCK, MD

Director, Pain Control Center,
Associate Professor of Anesthesia,
Department of Anesthesia,
Bowman Gray School of Medicine,
Winston-Salem, North Carolina

JOHN C. ROWLINGSON, MD

Professor of Anesthesiology,
Director, Pain Management Center,
University of Virginia Health Sciences Center,
Charlottesville, Virginia

MICHAEL STANTON-HICKS, MB, BS, Dr. Med.

Director, Pain Management Center,
Cleveland Clinic Foundation,
Cleveland, Ohio

ELISE A. TRUMBLE, PT, MS

Clinical Director,
Physiotherapy Associates,
Marietta, Georgia

MARC A. VALLEY, MD, Major USAF MC

Chief of the Medical Staff,
509th Medical Group,
Whiteman AFB, Missouri

STEVEN D. WALDMAN, MD, MBA

Director, Pain Consortium of Greater Kansas City;
Clinical Professor of Anesthesiology,
University of Missouri at Kansas City,
School of Medicine,
Kansas City, Missouri

NICOLAS E. WALSH, MD

Professor and Chairman,
Department of Rehabilitation Medicine,
University of Texas Health Science Center,
San Antonio, Texas

MARK J. WILLIAMS, MD

Staff Anesthesiologist,
Longview Regional Hospital,
Longview, Texas

To my family, friends and future pain specialists.

PREFACE

Pain medicine is rapidly approaching the period of responsibility and recognition. This has come about because of the significant influence of pain societies in the last 20 years. It is not uncommon today for pain physicians to be consulted for difficult and complex pain syndromes when conventional therapeutic techniques have been unsuccessful. It is certainly time that pain medicine should be recognized as a speciality.

Efforts of certain pain societies to obtain recognition by the American Board of Medical Specialties (ABMS) were partially successful when the American Board of Anesthesiologists (ABA) was granted the authority to award a certificate of added qualification in Pain Management to ABA members upon satisfactory completion of the examination process. This, however, still does not allow pain physicians of other specialties to obtain recognition by the ABMS. The American Board of Pain Medicine (ABPM) took a giant leap toward recognition of pain as a speciality when it started examining only qualified ABMS members for certification in pain medicine. Efforts are also being made by some other pain societies to obtain speciality recognition outside the ABMS.

Even though progress has been spectacular in the United States in terms of recognizing pain as a speciality, the rest of the world, including Europe, is lagging behind. This needs to be remedied. There should be, and will be, increasing awareness of the practice of pain medicine in developing and underdeveloped countries in the twenty-first century. It is our obligation, then, as pain specialists to focus our efforts toward setting guidelines for standards of practice, appropriate training programs, and an examination process to qualify eligible candidates as pain specialists all over the world.

This book has been conceived to fill the void for a comprehensive review of the theoretical knowledge and scope of pain medicine. Even though the information provided is obtainable in other major texts already in print, the format, style, and clarity of illustrations should make easy reading for the physician. Information provided is based on usual clinical practice rather than experimental data only.

The table of contents leads the reader gently from general issues to specifics of pain syndromes and their management. Wherever possible, mechanisms are described and appendixes are provided to further emphasize to the reader the knowledge base required for each syndrome. A special feature of the book is a series of questions provided at the end of each chapter. These, we hope, help the reader to review the subject matter quickly and reliably. For those who wish to enter the examination process in pain medicine, test banks are provided to help with review and preparation for the examination.

The editor and the publisher sincerely hope that the reader will find this book comprehensive.

ACKNOWLEDGMENTS

This book would not have been possible without the tireless, unfailing support of Susan Raj. I expressly thank Marilyn Schwiers for her hard work in copy editing and Sonora Hudson for her manuscript editing. I am grateful to the authors for their preparation of manuscripts. I also take this opportunity to thank all editors and publishers who have given permission for publication of their works in this book.

P. Prithvi Raj

CONTENTS

PART FIVE   PAIN SYNDROMES

SECTION I   ACUTE PAIN SYNDROMES

SECTION II   CHRONIC PAIN SYNDROMES:
A.   NOCICEPTIVE PAIN SYNDROMES

B.   NEUROPATHIC PAIN SYNDROMES

SECTION III   OTHER PAIN SYNDROMES

PART SIX   TEST BANKS

PAIN MEDICINE
A Comprehensive Review

PART ONE

Overview

1 History of Pain Medicine

P. Prithvi Raj

If one assumes that early humans had basically the same anatomy and behavior as their twentieth century counterparts, with perhaps a few external changes, it seems equally safe to assume that experiencing pain has always been a reality for humans, and seeking relief from that pain has always been a natural response.

Evidence suggesting the nature of some of early humankind's ailments does exist: human bones dating from prehistoric times have revealed decalcification, overgrowth, and thickening; and lesions suggestive of tuberculosis of the spine have been observed in the remains of a Neolithic man, who may have lived as long ago as 7000 B.C.[1] Cave art and sculpture depict physical states such as pregnancy, death, childbirth, and the undoubtedly acute pain of injury sustained in battle with beasts or other humans.

Modern-day observation of primitive societies provides some clues about prehistoric humankind's reaction to pain. In these primitive societies, religion, magic, and medical treatment are inseparable for the treatment of ailments. Primitive peoples seem to be psychologically prepared for the effectiveness of magic as a healing force, even when modern medicine is introduced into their society.[1] These and other observations indicate that in prehistoric times treatment of both the physical and spiritual aspects of pain and illness might have included ritual activity, medicinal plants, physical manipulation, and the application of heat, cold, or friction.

ANCIENT CIVILIZATIONS
Early Mesopotamian period

In about 3000 B.C. people living in Mesopotamia, the area that is now Iraq, began to build cities and develop a system of writing. The *asu* was one of several practitioners to whom the populace might have turned for pain relief. His colleagues could have included a priest-physician and an exorcist. The asu used drugs and surgery to attain results.[1,2] An eighth century B.C. Assyrian alabaster relief depicting a priest carrying *opium* poppies during a ceremony involving the sacrifice of a gazelle indicates that opium was one of the drugs used. The earliest known quality assurance in the practice of medicine is found in the code of Hammurabi, written in approximately 1700 B.C. The section regarding disciplinary action includes "If a doctor has treated a man with a metal knife for a severe wound, and has caused the man to die, or has opened a man's tumor with a metal knife and destroyed the man's eye, his (the physician's) hands shall be cut off."[1]

In the early Mesopotamian civilizations, peoples such as the Babylonians and, subsequently, the neighboring Hebrews considered suffering to be a punishment from the gods, possibly an explanation for distressing situations for which they had few solutions. The Hebrews recorded their understanding of the pain of childbirth in the Hebrew Bible, which is thought to have originated during a period extending from the twelfth to the second centuries B.C.[3] In the Book of Genesis God punishes Eve by telling her, "I will greatly multiply thy sorrow . . . in sorrow thou shalt bring forth children. . . ."[4] These notions regarding illness and suffering carried over into medieval Christianity and beyond, well into the nineteenth century.

Egypt

Pain is a frequent topic in the written legacy of the early Egyptians. Evidence of a variety of painful conditions has been found by examining Egyptian mummies. Apparently, Egyptians suffered, among other diseases, tuberculosis, dental caries and abscesses, atherosclerosis, and urinary stones. Pain was considered the result of spirits of the dead entering an individual's body through an ear or nostril.[5] The goal of treatment was to purge the body of this influence, but, apparently, some interim analgesia was also offered. In the Hearst papyrus, circa 1550 B.C., clinicians treating pain are advised to prescribe the drinking of a mixture of beer, juniper, and yeast, to be swallowed by the patient over a period of four days.[6] The medical papyruses reveal substantial use of *hyoscyamus, scopolamine,* and the *opium poppy,* along with ritual and mechanical procedures. This extensive Egyptian pharmacopoeia later influenced Greek, Roman, Hebrew, and Arabic practice.

India

At about the same time in history as the writing of the Hearst papyrus, the original inhabitants of ancient India were invaded by Aryan peoples from the North. The new arrivals brought with them the beginnings of the ancient Hindu scripture, called the *Veda.* Passed on in the oral tradition, it formed the basis for traditional Indian medical practice. Later additions included the teachings of physicians such as Charaka, Sushruta, and Vagbhata. A quotation from Charaka (circa 1000 B.C.) reveals insight into the importance of both spiritual and practical approaches to illness or injury:

Medicines are of three kinds . . .
First, Mantras (magic formulas) and religious acts;
Second, dieting and drugs;
Third, the subjugation of the mind by withdrawing it
from every kind of injurious or harmful act.[2]

Hinduism incorporated many gods. Among them was the powerful god Shiva, who could not only conquer death but also turn into the god Rudra, who shot arrows to produce pain and illness.[1] The heart was thought to be the origin of pain.[5]

The broad pharmacopoeia and wide range of surgical tools in use in ancient India suggest that pain was treated when possible. Certainly, disfigurement was treated by plastic surgeons, who employed techniques still in use today to reconstruct noses cut off as a punishment for adultery (Fig. 1-1). When Indian medical teaching was translated into Persian and Arabic during the eleventh century A.D., it became part of the general Arabic influence on the culture of the Middle Ages.[1]

China

In China medical practice was based primarily on the work of emperor Shen Nung (2800 B.C.), who was an authority on the medical use of herbs,[1] and Huang Ti (2600 B.C.), who is generally credited as having originated the *Nei Ching,*[2] the body of medical knowledge describing *acupuncture.* Virtually every illness, sign, symptom, or pain was thought to be amenable to correction by acupuncture, which allowed the practitioner to correct the imbalance of yang or yin by inserting needles into any of the 355 points along 12 meridians that traverse the body.[1,5] Each of the insertion points affected a particular organ.[2] The influence of Chinese medicine spread to Korea and Japan in the tenth century and to Europe at the end of the seventeenth century.[1]

In the second century the Chinese surgeon Hua T'o reported that when acupuncture failed to relieve pain, he resorted to a concoction made up of wine and an anesthetic, effervescent powder, which apparently caused intoxication and complete insensibility in the patient, allowing the physician to perform surgery.[1]

The vast Chinese pharmacopoeia included *ephedrine; ginseng,* administered to sedate overwrought people; the *willow* plant, containing salicylic acid, helpful for rheumatic pain; and the *Siberian wort,* an antispasmodic, which was used to relieve back pain. Opium was apparently not used until much later in Chinese history.[2]

Greece

The famous healer Asclepios was mentioned in Homer's *Iliad.* He may have been an actual person who, over time, became deified. According to myth, Asclepios had three sons: Machaon, the surgeon; Podalirios, the physician; and Telesphorus, representing convalescence. Asclepios' wife, Epione, soothed pain, and, among his daughters, Hygeia guided health prevention, while Panacea influenced treatment.[1] This multimodal therapy group demonstrates the way in which the Greeks mingled the spiritual and the practical when approaching the mysteries of illness and suffering.

A further reference to pain relief is found in Homer's *Odyssey,* in which Helen of Troy provides Ulysses and his companions with a drug to lull pain and anger, and bring forgetfulness to every sorrow.[7] Since archaeologic evidence exists that strongly indicates the use of the opium poppy at the time of the Trojan Wars (circa 1220 B.C.),[8] it is safe to speculate that Helen's soothing potion contained opium.[2] Opium would have been part of an array of drugs collectively known as Pharmaka. The spectrum of drugs included medications applied locally to soothe pain, dry secretions, and hasten healing.[1]

At the same time, the populace subscribed to the theory that disease and the frailty of old age were the result of arrows shot from the gods Apollo and Artemis,[1] and philosophers disagreed about whether pain was sensed by the heart or the brain.[5]

Temples of healing dedicated to Asclepias were built on many sites, with priests assuming the power of the god Asclepias. If cures were effected, they were probably the result of autosuggestion. Certainly, the temples represented a last resort for patients with conditions not amenable to the treatment offered by physicians using the rational, nonreli-

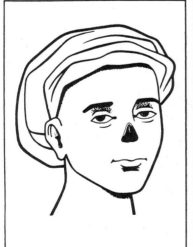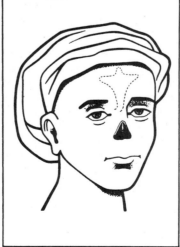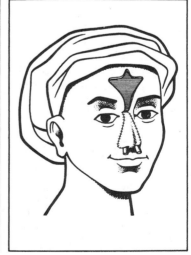

Fig. 1-1 Reconstruction of the nose as described by Sushruta. (From Majno G: *The Healing Hand and Wound in the Ancient World,* Cambridge, Mass, Harvard University Press, 1975.)

gious methods of the time. A parallel might be made between this situation and the modern dilemma faced by sufferers of chronic pain who turn to quackery after receiving little help from the medical establishment.

Despite this strong spiritual component in medicine, Greeks recognized natural causes for disease, and rational methods for healing were important. The teachings of *Hippocrates* have long symbolized the rational yet compassionate approach to diagnosis and treatment. His injunction to study the patient rather than the disease[2] is but one of many approaches still useful today and an essential part of assessing the chronic-pain patient.

The philosopher Plato, a contemporary of Hippocrates, predicted the social welfare state by expecting the ideal state to provide for the health of its citizens and prevent poverty and overpopulation.[2]

The frustrations of dealing with prolonged, incurable pain were recorded for posterity in the writings of physician/philosopher Areteus (circa 100 to 200 A.D.)[9], who is also known for his description of migraine headaches.[1] He instructed the physician to use compassion when caring for the hopelessly ill: "When he can render no further aid, the physician alone can still mourn as a man with his incurable patient. This is the physician's sad lot."[1]

Rome

When Rome replaced Greece as the center of power in the Mediterranean, Roman physicians were strongly influenced by Greek medicine and philosophy, which thrived in the great center of learning at Alexandria (circa 331 B.C. to 290 A.D.).[2,10]

Perhaps the most influential figure in the practice of pain relief and medicine in the first century and beyond was *Galen*. He classified dispositions according to his interpretation of the Greek theory of humors. Patients were considered phlegmatic, sanguine, choleric, and melancholic, terms which are still in use today and which still frequently color our first impressions of patients suffering chronic pain. Galen's extensive use of medication was also profoundly influential. He increased the ingredient list of theriaca, an ancient antidote and panacea, to over 70. The compound was used for 1800 years, well into the nineteenth century, by which time the ingredients numbered over 100. Along with snake venom, opium was among its ingredients, which might have accounted for its popularity and endurance for many centuries.[1]

THE DARK AGES AND THE MIDDLE AGES

During the aptly named "Age of Superstition,"[10] miracles and faith healing were relied upon, rather than known remedies. War and disease made life extremely hard. Epidemics raged through Europe, unchecked by the medical knowledge of the time. People lost faith in medicine, in a response not unlike that of discouraged patients today, and there was a tendency to focus on the life hereafter rather than on life on earth.[11] The mystical element of Christianity was on the rise; and faith, more than reason, influenced the practice of medicine. The sick made pilgrimages to the shrines of saints such as Cosmas and Damian, whose miraculous cures had become part of legend.[2]

During the first five centuries A.D., the early Christians destroyed many classic Greek and Roman texts, perceiving them to be heretical.[1] Some elements of medical practice from these times endured, however, such as the theory of humors. The most serious damage was the suppression of scientific inquiry and experimentation. Because of the political and social atmosphere in the Dark Ages, the rational approach to medicine was not employed until the emergence of the universities in the early Middle Ages.

Fortunately, the classical ideas were kept alive and used as a basis for further scientific endeavor by the Arabists, a term that describes thinkers such as Persians, Christians, Jews, and others who lived in Muslim countries.[7] Their name derives from the fact that not only did they write in Arabic, but they also embraced the Islamic philosophy of the time, which encouraged the preservation of all learning.[2,11]

Among their writings, a concoction named jabrol is recommended as an analgesic. It was a drink containing mandrogorine, which is thought to have been a mixture of atropine and hyoscyamine.[12] A "spongia somnifera," soaked with mandrogorine and many other herbs, is also described.[10] Both of these remedies were part of the Arabists' highly developed understanding of pharmacy and chemistry, which enabled them to develop techniques for drug preparation that are still in use today. They also pioneered the development of efficiently run hospitals in which the terminally ill, elderly, or merely unwanted were cared for.[1]

Among the Arabists, Avicenna (980-1037)[10] stands out as an influential teacher and physician. He attempted to codify all medical knowledge in his *Canon Medicinae*. This text was still in use 600 years later in seventeenth century medical schools, including those of England.[2]

When the Western world began to emerge from the Dark Ages during the twelfth century, the Greek tradition of medicine, enriched by Islamic thought, was yielded back to the West.[11] Possibly as a result of fewer wars and an economic and intellectual revival, this period in history gave rise to a change in the attitude of scholars. First in monasteries, and then in secular universities, the classical writers were studied once more, and the contributions of the Arabists were translated into Latin.[13] Once the classic texts of Galen and Hippocrates entered the universities, they unfortunately came to be regarded as the final medical authority.[13] It took the challenge of the *Renaissance* to unseat them.

RENAISSANCE

By the middle of the fifteenth century rational thought and the notions of personal worth and individuality heralded the start of the Renaissance. The invention of the moveable-type printing press further enhanced the spread of knowledge.

The universities had begun to emerge as centers of learning in Europe, and the unquestioned adherence to the medical practice of ancient Greece and Rome was challenged by individuals such as *Paracelsus,* the controversial medical practitioner, healer, and mystic.[9] Not only did he challenge the absolute authority of Galen and Hippocrates, he also had the audacity to teach in German instead of Latin.[1]

Two hundred years before their use was accepted, he advocated a new class of chemical agents as opposed to the popular galenics of the time, which consisted of plant matter. An avid chemist, Paracelsus described the action of ether on chickens, reporting that this substance "quiets all sufferings, and relieves all pain." Unfortunately this discovery was not followed by the clinical application of ether until well into the nineteenth century.[10]

During the Renaissance the seats of learning embraced the scientific method once more. Although the understanding of physiology outstripped the development of treatment during this period,[5] it becomes more instructive, for the purposes of this review, to shift from studying periods in history to engaging in a chronologic study of diverse methods for managing pain.

DEVELOPMENT OF PAIN MANAGEMENT METHODS
Compression anesthesia

During the sixteenth century, the French surgeon Ambroise Paré was searching for a way to reduce the pain of surgery. He reported that when a firm ligation was made above the seat of the operation, bleeding would be better controlled, and pain would be greatly diminished.[14] His method was not improved upon until the next century when, in 1784, James Moore described his technique in *A Method of Preventing or Diminishing Pain in Several Operations of Surgery*. His compression apparatus employed a vice that screwed down on a limb, exerting pressure on the main nerves.[10] In 1873 Johannes Esmarch refined the method further by substituting a bandage of rubber wound around the proximal portion of the limb. The practitioners of the day were undecided about whether nerve compression or relative ischemia rendered the limb insensible. In 1898 Heinrich Braun established that it was the compression of the nerves that resulted in anesthesia. He declared, however, that this method of anesthesia belonged to history.[14] Cocaine was in widespread use by this time, providing Braun and his colleagues with an alternative not available to earlier generations of surgeons.

Refrigeration anesthesia

Among his writings, Avicenna described the range of analgesics available at the time: "The most powerful of narcotics is opium . . . and the less powerful are snow and ice water."[14] Refrigeration anesthesia was also appreciated in Saxon England at about the same time; a leech book compiled in 1050 described the use of cold water to deaden the pain of draining an abscess.[10]

In 1661 Thomas Bartholin devoted part of a chapter in his medical textbook, *De Nivis Usu Medico,* to reporting on Severino of Naples' technique of rubbing snow and ice on the site of surgical incisions. Bartholin cautioned against gangrene, however, and recommended that ice be applied under narrow parallel bandages only for a quarter of an hour. Apparently the psychologic aspect of pain management was not overlooked in Naples, since Bartholin wrote of Severino's practice: "When he wishes to conceal the nature of the treatment, in order to make the results seem more astonishing, the aforesaid Severino dyes the snow with ground ultramarine or some other colouring matter."[10]

In 1807 Dominique-Jean Larrey, Napoleon's surgeon general, recorded in his memoirs that the $-19°$ F weather allowed him to perform painless amputations on the battlefield.[14]

In the middle of the 1800s, when the marvels of ether and, subsequently, chloroform appeared to be flawed, James Arnott advocated a return to refrigeration techniques. In his 1854 booklet advocating the use of "benumbing cold," he described using a pig's bladder filled with water and ice.[15] His methods achieved limited success, but they were no substitute for general anesthesia or more powerful pain relievers such as morphine.

Morphine

Opium's power to relieve pain was widely recognized by the time of the Renaissance. Paracelsus took the most common forms of opium (powder and a black, sticky gum) and combined them with alcohol to form laudanum.[16] Although this combination might have made the substance easier to take and its action more powerful, there still existed the problem of predicting the effect a given amount of opium might have. This problem was not resolved until the nineteenth century.

In 1803 Prussian pharmacist F.W.A. Sertürner began work on isolating the active ingredient in opium, hoping to establish a dosage scale. By 1817 he had narrowed his search down to morphine. In order to test his hypothesis, he gradually administered morphine to himself and three others, starting at half a grain and repeating this dose until he had reached 1½ grains. At this point he and his companions passed into a markedly depressed, yet dreamy, narcotic state.[16]

The management of pain with morphine was somewhat limited, however, until the developments of the hypodermic syringe and hollow needle. By 1853 these developments had been accomplished by Rynd[16] in Ireland and Pravaz in France.[17]

Until ether was recognized as an effective general anesthetic in 1846 and cocaine found to be a potent local anesthetic in 1884, physicians in Europe and America attempting to relieve their patients' pain had to rely on morphine, alcohol, opiates, and plant matter such as *Hyoscyamus* and *Mandragora*. Consequently, there was a renewed interest in the previous century's fascination with mesmerism and similar methods of dealing with the pain of surgery. Advocates of these measures achieved limited success, however, and ran the high risk of loss of reputation.[1]

Surgery, of necessity, had to be hurried if carried out at all.[1] One can only imagine the courage of Ephraim McDowell's patient who in 1809 underwent removal of a 22½ lb ovarian tumor without a general anesthetic.[10]

General Anesthesia

Even though chloroform, nitrous oxide, and ether had all been discovered by 1831 and were used as intoxicants, they were not used as general anesthetics.[1] In 1846, however, Boston dentist William T.G. Morton made a dramatic public demonstration of ether inhalation's effectiveness as a general anesthetic that could permit surgery without pain. In Germany, Diffenbach, a plastic surgeon, wrote of ether, "The wonderful dream that pain has been taken away from us has become a reality. Pain . . . must bow before the power of the human mind, before the power of ether vapor."[1]

Before long, however, ether fell out of favor because of its irritating properties and long induction period. In 1847 James Simpson pioneered the use of chloroform as a substitute for ether. When announcing his successful use of chloroform in obstetrical procedures, Simpson declared it to be far more pleasant for the patient and more controllable than ether.[11]

Calvinist church leaders opposed the use of any general anesthetic during childbirth, however, clinging to the Biblical imperative that women should bring forth children in sorrow. This opposition lasted until John Snow administered chloroform to Queen Victoria herself during childbirth. The clergy then became reconciled to a more humane point of view.[16]

Chloroform replaced ether as the agent of choice until it became associated with long-term liver damage and sudden death.[1,15] Simpson himself continued to search for alternatives to general anesthesia, trying local application of the vapors of chloroform, ether, carbon disulfide, and hydrocyanic acid, all with poor results.[1]

Some of the difficulties with chloroform were overcome, however, by J.N. von Nussbaum in 1864; he was able to reduce the amount of chloroform administered by using morphine as a preoperative agent. In 1868 J. Harley began giving atropine in response to bradycardia during chloroform anesthesia; by 1880 physicians in England and France were combining the two agents in a combination of doses similar to that used in current practice.[10]

The fact that painless surgery was then possible allowed physicians to use surgery itself to deal with the cause of chronic pain. The outcome of this type of surgery dramatically improved after the acceptance of Joseph Lister's antiseptic technique, first introduced in 1867.[10]

Surgery

As soon as it became possible to operate without the fear of infection, a number of surgeons throughout the world began to attack pain by a new method: the permanent interruption of the central nervous system's afferent pathways.

Among those physicians who pioneered surgery for pain was Hersley of England, who originated the operation for trigeminal neuralgia. The Americans Abbe, the originator of posterior rhizotomy; Spiller and Frazier, who introduced retrogasserian neurectomy and cordotomy; and Harvey Cushing made outstanding contributions to surgical treatment of pain. Chappault, Jaubolay, Sicard, and Leriche developed the French school of neurosurgery and introduced the new concept of ablating the sympathetic nervous system in the management of pain. The Italian Ruggi proposed sympathectomy for visceral pain. Durante, Van Gehuchten, and de Beule of Belgium contributed toward the surgical management of neuralgia; and Jonnesco and Gomolu of Romania performed the first sympathectomy for angina pectoris.[18]

Generally speaking, however, because of the problems

connected with chloroform and ether, the next great advance in the management of pain came with the advent of effective regional anesthesia.

Regional anesthesia

On September 15, 1884, a dramatic report was made on behalf of Carl Koller at the German Ophthalmological Society's meeting in Heidelberg. Koller had been working with colleague Sigmund Freud on the use of cocaine as a treatment for morphine addiction. When Koller learned of the numbing effect of cocaine on the tongue, it occurred to him that he had found the ideal local anesthetic for ophthalmology. This regional anesthetic technique took the world by storm, and, by the year's end, cocaine was providing effective anesthesia not only in ophthalmology, but also in otology, rhinolaryngology, pharyngology, urology, gynecology, and general surgery. Subsequent applications introduced the technique of nerve blocks and spinal, epidural, and caudal anesthesia. The new techniques were further expanded for acute-pain and chronic-pain relief.[1,19]

As surgeons increased their use of regional anesthesia at the beginning of the twentieth century, they became aware of the toxic and addictive effects of cocaine and the need for alternative agents for local anesthesia, substances that could be less dangerous and still have a therapeutic effect.[20]

In 1903 Heinrich Braun pioneered the use of vasoconstrictors with cocaine, finding that adrenaline acted as a chemical tourniquet.[21] He worked to reduce the dosage of both cocaine and adrenaline as much as possible while prolonging the local anesthetic action of the cocaine.

Radiotherapy

At the turn of the twentieth century, radiotherapy became an important tool for managing pain, adding a dramatic new dimension to treatment. The report by Wilhelm Röntgen on Dec. 28, 1895, of a new kind of "ray" can be considered a great milestone in the management of pain.[9] Soon after, roentgen rays were employed in the treatment of many conditions that are accompanied by severe and persistent pain. After the original phase of enthusiasm and the subsequent phase of pessimism had passed, roentgen therapy became an accepted modality in the management of pain.

Physical therapy

Physical medicine may have actually started with the ancient Egyptians' use of electric fish over painful wounds.[5] Within more recent history, the rapid emergence of physical measures, starting in the nineteenth century, included light therapy, electrotherapy, hydrotherapy, thermotherapy, and mechanotherapy.[22] These measures combined with existing techniques to relieve pain and ensured that physical therapy would maintain a prominent place in pain management strategy in the future.

EVOLUTION OF PAIN CENTERS
Early developments

Between 1930 and 1945 significant developments occurred in pain management. The French surgeon Leriche was the first person to identify chronic pain as a disease state.[18] In the early 1930s his classic medical publication, *The Sur-*

gery of Pain, described the treatment of causalgia and reflex sympathetic dystrophy. In 1943 Livingston published a memorable book[23] in which he explained pain mechanisms in causalgia and their related states. These writings stimulated the study of the diagnosis and relief of pain; and sympathetic-block anesthesia became a popular treatment of pain involving known nerve tracts and pain of obscure origin. Woodbridge,[24] Ruth,[25] Mandle,[26] Rovenstine and Wertheim,[27] and many other anesthesiologists popularized diagnostic and therapeutic nerve-block techniques in pain control.

Origin of the pain clinic concept during World War II

During World War II Beecher made some important observations on pain in men wounded in battle.[28] His publications persuaded the medical community that the experience of pain is not always proportional to tissue damage and that many other factors modify pain. During the war Bonica[29] and Alexander[30] developed broad views of pain and its management. They were the first physicians to appreciate the difficult problems presented by chronic-pain patients. They saw that persistent pain is further complicated by increased suffering, depression, psychologic problems, and drug abuse. They also realized that the solution of complex pain problems requires vast knowledge and clinical experience, more than one individual could possess. Both Bonica and Alexander felt that patients with chronic pain could be best managed by a *team* of organized specialists representing different disciplines who are knowledgeable and interested. Evaluations by the members of such a team and integration of their efforts in a true *interdisciplinary* manner could lead to accurate diagnosis and prompt treatment. Bonica attempted to implement this approach during a short experience in treating military personnel with a variety of pain problems at Madigan Army Hospital in Tacoma, Washington, during the war.

Postwar development of nerve-block clinics and pain clinics

After World War II many pain clinic facilities in the United States were organized by anesthesiologists, who predominantly used nerve-block techniques for pain control. Many of these clinics were known as nerve-block clinics, although some were known as pain clinics. Hersey, Rovenstine[31] and Apgar[32] described their nerve-block clinics in detail as early as 1944 and 1948, respectively. Ruben established a pain clinic at the Philadelphia General Hospital in September 1948 and published his "Experience with a pain clinic" in 1951.[33] The popularity of pain clinic activity during the postwar period is shown by Dittrick's 1950 editorial,[34] which suggested that pain clinics offered an opportunity for expansion for anesthesiologists. He especially recognized the model pain clinics run by Stubbs at Doctors' Hospital in Washington, D.C., and by Haugen in Portland, Oregon. Neurosurgeons were recognized as necessary members of these clinics.

At the end of his military duty in late 1946, Bonica implemented the concept of a *team approach* to the management of chronic-pain patients in Tacoma General Hospital, Tacoma, Washington, drawing on the resources of a number

of specialties. In 1947 Alexander, who also independently developed the same concept, initiated a *multidisciplinary* diagnostic and therapeutic pain program at Veterans Administration Hospital in McKinney, Texas.[35] Bonica documented his efforts to organize the joint-team pain clinic in 1951[36] and 1952[37] and then in his monumental textbook on pain, *The Management of Pain,* which was published in 1953.[38] Over the years Bonica continued to succinctly describe his pain clinic concepts and experiences in many subsequent publications.[39-41]

Development of pain centers in the United States

Even though Bonica introduced the idea of a team approach in the early 1950s, it was not until 1960 that he (together with White, a neurosurgeon, and Crowley, a member of the faculty of the University of Washington School of Nursing) developed one of the first multidisciplinary pain centers at the University of Washington in Seattle. This clinic has served as a prototype for hundreds of such clinics in the United States and abroad.

Other pain clinics were launched in the early 1960s, and their contributions to our knowledge of chronic-pain management must be recognized. Among them were the pain clinics affiliated with the University of Southern California School of Medicine in Los Angeles; with Crue at the City of Hope in Duarte, California; with Long in Minneapolis; with Brena in Atlanta; with Seres and Newman in Portland, Oregon; with Hillister and Aronoff in Boston; and with Stieg in Boulder, Colorado.[42] Pain clinic facilities were not developed in other medical centers until the late 1960s and early 1970s.

Growth of pain clinics around the world

In 1976 *Medical World News* listed only 17 pain clinics in the United States. In 1977 a pain clinic directory published by the American Society of Anesthesiologists (ASA) listed over 300 pain-control facilities.[43] In 1979 an ASA committee chaired by Carron conducted a second survey and subsequently published the *International Directory of Pain Clinics/Centers.*[44] As per Bonica's suggestions to the ASA committee, pain centers were classified as (1) major comprehensive pain centers, (2) comprehensive pain centers, (3) syndrome-oriented pain centers, and (4) modality-oriented pain centers. Brena analyzed the data in a 1979 directory[45] and noted that, of the 428 facilities, 278 (65%) were in the United States, 27 (6%) were in Canada, 20 (5%) were in Japan, 18 (4%) were in Britain, and the remainder were in other countries. Only 12% of the facilities surveyed were major comprehensive pain centers, 28% were comprehensive pain centers, 39% were modality-oriented pain centers, and 21% were syndrome-oriented pain centers.

According to Bonica,[29] in 1987 there were between 1800 and 2000 pain facilities in some 36 countries. Of these, 1000 to 1200 were in the United States, 200 to 225 were in Western Europe, 75 were in Canada, 80 were in Asia or Australia, and the remaining countries had between 2 and 20 facilities. A directory recently published by the American Pain Society and American Academy of Pain Medicine[46] lists 240 pain clinics in the United States whose directors are members of these pain organizations.

The rise in the number of pain treatment centers in the United States reflects increasing awareness of chronic pain and its impact on our society. The growth of organizations also confirms the concern health professionals share in managing this difficult and multifaceted problem. Unfortunately, growth has allowed some unprofessional operations run by unqualified physicians to flourish in many parts of the country. These individuals exploit the genuine need for pain clinics for their own financial considerations, enhancing the bases of their practices rather than offering true interdisciplinary service to patients with chronic pain.

PAIN SOCIETIES

Several organizations whose primary purpose is to educate pain management professionals have developed in the past two decades. The International Association for Study of Pain (IASP) was incorporated in 1974. Its goals are to foster and encourage pain research, promote education and training, facilitate dissemination of information, encourage adoption of uniform nomenclature and classification, encourage education in the public regarding pain issues, encourage development of an extensive data bank, and advise on standards of pain treatment.

Soon after its formation the IASP sponsored the scientific journal *Pain,* the first journal specifically devoted to scientific and clinical issues regarding pain. Recently several special interest groups have been developed within the IASP to allow clinicians and researchers a forum to discuss highly specific issues in depth. These special interest groups have access to the IASP's administrative services and can organize scientific sessions at the time of the triennial IASP World Congress.

The IASP presently has over 3600 members from 63 countries. Its members come from virtually every medical specialty, as well as such diverse fields as psychology, medical electronics, physical therapy, pharmacy, psychophysics, orthotics, nursing, and music therapy. It has organized the formation of 19 national chapters, and an additional six provisional chapters are in the formative process.

In an effort to provide a forum for a wider range of professionals involved in pain management, several regional sections of the IAPS were organized. At present, these include the Eastern Pain Association, the Midwest Pain Society, the New England Pain Association, the Southern Pain Society, and the Western USA Pain Society. These organizations hold annual clinical and scientific sessions that allow participation of a substantial segment of their membership.

The American Society of Regional Anesthesia (ASRA), as it presently exists, was organized in 1976. (The initial organization bearing that name was founded in 1923 by Gaston Labat.) The purpose of this resurrected society is to promote the use of regional anesthetic techniques for surgery, obstetrics, and pain management; to stimulate research on regional anesthesia and local anesthetic pharmacology; to provide an educational forum; and to stimulate publication of scientific and educational material related to these topics. Membership now totals over 5000. Pain control has become a major area of interest of the society.

The American Academy of Pain Medicine (AAPM) was organized in 1983 as the American Academy of Algology.

It is made up only of physicians. The all-physician membership is required of any organization that seeks a seat in the ASA House of Delegates, a status that was accorded to the organization in 1989. Having acquired that status, the AAPM has moved forward a process for certification of physicians whose primary activity involves the treatment of pain patients. While some of its goals are clearly political, education of physicians who care for pain patients is a major function of the organization. The *Clinical Journal of Pain,* a previously freestanding publication devoted to the management of clinical pain problems, has become the official journal of the organization.

REFERENCES

1. Lyons AS, Petrucelli JR: *Medicine, an Illustrated History.* New York, Harry N Abrams, 1978.
2. Majno G: *The Healing Hand and Wound in the Ancient World.* Cambridge, Mass, Harvard University Press, 1975.
3. Sandmel S, editor: *The New English Bible, Oxford University Press.* New York, Oxford University Press, 1976.
4. *Holy Bible, King James Version.* New York, Oxford University Press, Gen. 3:16, 1976.
5. Warfield CA: A history of pain relief. *Hospital Practice* 23:121-122, 1988.
6. Leake CD: *The Old Egyptian Medical Papyri.* Lawrence, Kan, University of Kansas Press, 1952.
7. Homer: *The Odyssey,* Cambridge, Houghton Mifflin, 1929 (Translated by GH Palmer).
8. Boardman J: *The Oxford History of the Classical World.* New York, Oxford University Press, 1986.
9. Clendening L: *Source Book of Medical History.* Mineola, NY, Dover Publications, 1960.
10. Armstrong-Davison MH: *The Evolution of Anaesthesia.* Altrincham, UK, John Sherratt & Son, 1965.
11. Margotta R: *An Illustrated History of Medicine.* Feltham, UK, Hamlyn Publishing, 1968 (Translated by S Richards).
12. Potter SO: *Materia Medica, Pharmacy, and Therapeutics.* Philadelphia, Blakiston's Son & Co, 1906.
13. Barber R: *The Penguin Guide to Medieval Europe.* Middlesex, UK, Penguin, 1984.
14. Liljestrand G: The historical development of anesthesia, Section 8: *Local Anesthetics, vol 1.* In Bovet, editor: *International Encyclopedia of Pharmacology and Therapeutics.* Oxford, Pergamon Press, 1971.
15. Sykes WS: *Essays on the First Hundred Years of Anesthesia, vol 2.* Edinburgh, UK, E & S Livingstone, 1961.
16. Clendening L: *Behind the Doctor.* New York, Alfred A Knopf, 1933.
17. Wall PD: To what would Gaston Labat be attending today? *Reg Anaesth* 14:261-264, 1989.
18. Leriche R: *The Surgery of Pain.* Baltimore, Williams & Wilkins, 1939.
19. Wyklicky H, Skopec M: Carl Koller (1857-1944) and his time in Vienna. In Scott DB, McClure J, Wildsmith JAW, editors: *Proceedings of the Centennial Meeting of European Society of Regional Anaesthesia (1984).* Södertälje, Sweden, Information Consulting Medical, 1984.
20. Lassner J: Local anaesthesia—early history. In Scott DB, McClure J, Wildsmith JAW, editors: *Proceedings of the Centennial Meeting of European Society of Regional Anaesthesia (1984).* Sweden, Information Consulting Medical, 1984.
21. Röse W: Heinrich Braun's contribution to the development of local anaesthesia. In Scott DB, McClure J, Wildsmith JAW, editors: *Proceedings of the Centennial Meeting of European Society of Regional Anaesthesia (1984).* Södertälje, Sweden, Information Consulting Medical, 1984.
22. Krusen FH: *Physical Medicine.* Philadelphia, WB Saunders, 1940.
23. Livingston WK: Pain mechanisms: Physiologic interpretation of causalgia and its related states. New York, Macmillan, 1943.
24. Woodbridge PD: Therapeutic nerve block with procaine and alcohol. *Am J Surg* 9:278-288, 1930.

25. Ruth H: Diagnostic, prognostic and therapeutic block. *JAMA* 102:419, 1934.
26. Mandle F: *Di paravertebrale blockade*. Vienna, Springer-Verlag, 1938.
27. Rovenstine EA, Wertheim HM: Therapeutic nerve block. *JAMA* 117:1599-1603, 1941.
28. Beecher HK: Pain in men wounded in battle. *Ann Surg* 123:96-105, 1946.
29. Bonica JJ: Evolution of multidisciplinary/interdisciplinary pain programs. In Aronoff GM, editor: *Pain Centers: A Revolution in Health Care*. New York, Raven Press, 1988.
30. Alexander FAD: The control of pain. In Hale DE, editor: *Anesthesiology*. Philadelphia, FA Davis, 1954.
31. Rovenstine EA, Hersey SG: Therapeutic and diagnostic nerve blocking: A plan for organization. *Anesthesiology* 5:574-582, 1944.
32. Apgar V: A nerve block clinic. *Anesth Analg* 1:49-54, 1948.
33. Ruben JE: Experience with a pain clinic. *Anesthesiology* 12:601-603, 1951.
34. Dittrick H: The pain clinic. *Current Research in Anesthesia and Analgesia* 29:60, 1950 (editorial).
35. Alexander FAD: The genesis of the pain clinic. In *Pain Abstracts, vol 1*, Second World Congress on Pain, International Association for the Study of Pain, Seattle, 1978.
36. Bonica JJ: The role of the anaesthesiologist in the management of intractable pain. *Can Med Assoc J* 65:103-107, 1951.
37. Bonica JJ: Management of intractable pain with analgesic blocks, *JAMA* 150:1581-1586, 1952.
38. Bonica JJ: *The Management of Pain*. Philadelphia, Lea & Febiger, 1953.
39. Bonica JJ: Organization and function of a pain clinic. In Bonica JJ, editor: *Advances in Neurology, vol 4*. New York, Raven Press, 1974.
40. Bonica JJ, Benedetti C, Murphy TM: Functions of pain clinics and pain centers. In Swerdlow M, editor: *Relief of Intractable Pain, ed 3*. Amsterdam, Elsevier, 1983.
41. Bonica JJ: Evolution of pain concepts and pain clinics. *Clinics in Anaesthesiology* 3:1-16, 1983.
42. Crue BL Jr: Historical perspectives. In Ghia JN, editor: *Multidisciplinary Pain Center: Organization and Personnel Functions for Pain Management*. Boston, Kluwer Academic Publishers, 1988.
43. American Society of Anesthesiologists: *Directory of Pain Clinics*. Park Ridge, Ill, The Society, 1977.
44. American Society of Anesthesiologists: *Pain Centers/Clinic Directory*. Park Ridge, Ill, The Society, 1979.
45. Brena SF: Pain control facilities: Patterns of operation and problems of organization in the USA. *Clinics in Anaesthesiology* 3:183-195, 1985.
46. American Pain Society, American Academy of Pain Medicine: *Directory of Pain Management Facilities*. Chicago, The Society, The Academy, 1989.

QUESTIONS: HISTORY OF PAIN MEDICINE

1. In this ancient country pain was considered the result of spirits of the dead entering an individual's body through an ear or nostril.
   A. India
   B. Egypt
   C. Greece
   D. China
2. In about 1000 B.C. this physician wrote:
   Medicine are of three kinds . . .
   First, Mantras and religious acts;
   Second, dieting and drugs;
   Third, the subjugation of the mind by withdrawing it from every kind of injurious or harmful act.
   A. Sushruta
   B. Charaka
   C. Huang Ti
   D. Asclepios
3. Which one of the following drugs was not included in the early Chinese pharmacopeia?
   A. Ephedrine
   B. Ginseng
   C. Siberian wort (antispasmodic)
   D. Opium
4. The practice of acupuncture was first described in:
   A. *Canon Medicinae*
   B. *Nei Ching*
   C. *Veda*
   D. *Iliad*
5. The credit of classifying the humors into phlegmatic, sanguine, choleric, and melancholic is given to which one of the following?
   A. Asclepios
   B. Galen
   C. Plato
   D. Hippocrates

ANSWERS

1. B
2. B
3. D
4. B
5. B

2 Pain Mechanisms

P. Prithvi Raj

Tissue damage caused by injury, disease, or inflammation releases endogenous chemicals, called algogenic, algesic, or pain-producing substances, into the extracellular fluid that surrounds the nociceptors. These substances include H^+, K^+, serotonin, histamine, prostaglandins, bradykinin, substance P (sP), and many others. They play a causal role in pain associated with inflammation, trauma, bone tumors, ischemia, and a variety of other pathophysiologic conditions. In addition to direct excitatory action on the membrane of nociceptors, these agents may have an indirect excitatory action by altering the local microcirculation. The algesic substance can cause increased capillary permeability and either vasoconstriction or vasodilation.

LOCATION OF ALGESIC SUBSTANCES

Serotonin, histamine, K^+, H^+, prostaglandins, and other members of the arachidonic acid cascade are located in tissues; kinins are in plasma; and sP is in nerve terminals. Histamine is found in platelets, basophils, and the granules of mast cells; serotonin is present in mast cells and platelets.[1] Release of these amines may be induced by mechanical injury, noxious heat, radiation, and certain by-products of tissue damage, most notably neutrophil lysosomal materials, thrombin collagen, and epinephrine. Tissue damage also induces release of lipidic acids of the arachidonic acid cascade, such as the leukotrienes, the prostaglandins, and the slow reacting substance of anaphylaxis (SRS-A) (Fig. 2-1).

Bradykinin

Bradykinin is a byproduct of the cascade that is triggered by the activation of factor XII of the Hageman clotting system by exposure to negatively charged surfaces such as collagen. This activation results in the conversion of the enzyme prekallikrein to kallikrein, which then acts on the bradykinin precursor kininogen, resulting in the release of bradykinin into the tissues. Bradykinin produces increased vascular permeability, promotes vasodilation, produces leukocyte chemotaxis, and activates nociceptors. That action of bradykinin on *nociceptors* is potentiated by *prostaglandins* present in the injured tissue compartment.

Prostanoids

The prostaglandins are biosynthesized in the body from certain polyunsaturated essential fatty acids, among which is the abundant arachidonic acid. Arachidonic acid is the precursor of leukotrienes and thromboxanes, which are qualitatively and quantitatively important prostanoids.[2] Precursor fatty acid normally does not occur free in the cell; it is esterized to phospholipids. Conversion into prostaglandins and release of the related substances thus starts with the liberation of the fatty acid by the action of a phospholipase A, which releases the cell-membrane–derived arachidonic acid. A number of stimuli are known to lead to the activation of phospholipase and thus to increased prostaglandin synthesis. These stimuli include norepinephrine and dopamine, which stimulate synthesis of the cellular phospholipids, in part by releasing the nonesterified free fatty acid precursors. Lipooxygenase or cyclooxygenase, both of which are membrane-bound enzymes, act as substrates to synthesize leukotrienes and prostaglandins. Agents such as acetylsalicylic acid and indomethacin inhibit cyclooxygenase and thus deplete these lipidic acids, resulting in relief of pain. Significantly, in damaged skin there is a marked elevation of prostanoid level, which is blocked by cyclooxygenase inhibitors.[3]

PERIPHERAL NOCICEPTOR SYSTEM
Somatic structures

Tissue damage activates distinct types of receptors, called nociceptors, which are at the termination of free nerve endings of A-delta and C afferents, located in various body tissues. The skin is supplied by A-delta high-threshold mechanoreceptors (HTMs) activated by mechanical noxious stimuli; by A-delta myelinated mechanothermal nociceptors (MMTNs) activated by noxious heat and noxious mechanical stimuli; by C polymodal nociceptors (CPNs) activated by mechanical, thermal, and chemical noxious stimuli; and by a miscellaneous group consisting of C mechanical nociceptors and cold nociceptors. Muscles, joints, fasciae, and other deep somatic structures are supplied by C (group IV) and also probably by A-delta (group III) fibers (Figs. 2-2 and 2-3).

Visceral structures

Viscera are also supplied by C afferent fibers, and some also by A-delta afferents, which are activated by disease, inflammation, contraction under isometric conditions, ischemia, rapid distention, and other "adequate" visceral nociceptive stimuli. These nociceptors, activated by noxious stimuli and endogenous algogenic substances, transduce the stimuli into nociceptive impulses that are transmitted to the dorsal horn of the spinal cord or the medulla. The amount of neural activity in nociceptive afferents is influenced not only by the intensity and duration of stimulation but also by the microenvironment of the nociceptors and other factors.

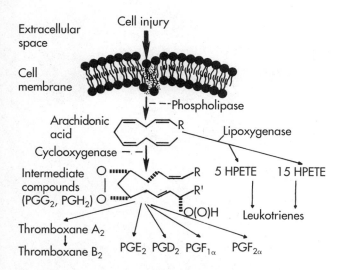

Fig. 2-1 After cell injury the cascade of events leading to synthesis of prostaglandins, thromboxanes, and leukotrienes from arachio-donic acid.

Augmentation of nociceptors

Nociceptive input from the periphery can be enhanced by several factors, including:

· Sensitization of nociceptors by repeated noxious stimuli
· Lowering of the nociceptors' threshold by pain-producing substances
· Segmental reflex responses provoked by tissue injury

Factors that produce inhibition include various forms of counterirritation in the skin, such as rubbing, vibration, and the more sophisticated and expensive methods that use electrical stimulators or acupuncture.

SENSITIZATION

Sensory end organs are assumed to have certain thresholds that remain constant despite changes in conditions and states. With repeated stimulation, however, most sensory organs (including low-threshold C fibers) become fatigued and less responsive. Perl demonstrated that high-threshold polymodal C fibers involved in nociception show the opposite response. With repeated stimulation, these nerve endings displayed enhanced sensitivity, lowered threshold to stimulation, and prolonged and enhanced response to the stimulation (afterdischarge). This phenomenon is called *sensitization.* Tissue damage caused by injury or disease produces a similar type of sensitization at the site of injury, called *primary hyperalgesia,* that is also characterized by a lowered pain threshold, increased sensitivity to suprathreshold stimuli, and spontaneous pain.

After the injury a much larger area of hyperalgesia and allodynia that surrounds the site of injury develops, called *secondary hyperalgesia.* The mechanisms of primary hyperalgesia and secondary hyperalgesia after injury or inflammation are probably similar and involve endogenous biochemical agents.

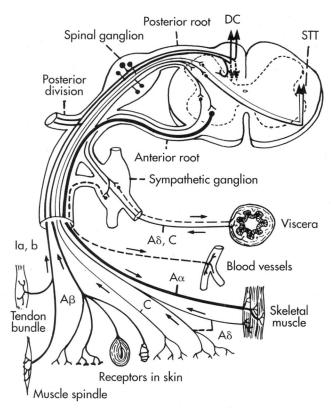

Fig. 2-2 A graphic illustration of a mixed spinal nerve connecting receptors from the periphery to the spinal cord. Note the different types of fibers in the nerve. (From Bonica JJ: *Management of Pain,* ed 2, Philadelphia, 1990, Lea & Febiger.)

TRANSDUCTION OF PAINFUL STIMULI

Although the precise mechanism by which endogenous chemicals participate in peripheral transduction of nociceptive stimuli into nociceptive impulses is not known, these substances may initiate three mechanisms[1]: (1) those that activate nociceptive afferent fibers and produce pain by local application (e.g., bradykinin, acetylcholine, and potassium); (2) those that facilitate the pain evoked by chemicals and physical stimuli by sensitization of nociceptors but are ineffective in evoking pain themselves (e.g., the prostaglandins); and (3) those that produce local extravasation (e.g., sP). In addition to these mediators from extraneural sources, sP and other peptides may have a role in influencing the milieu of the peripheral afferent terminals and thus, indirectly, in the transduction of nociceptive information.

TRANSMISSION OF PAINFUL IMPULSE

Peripheral transmission. The activation of nociceptors results in generalized activity in finely myelinated A-delta and unmyelinated C fibers that project to the dorsal horn of the spinal cord (periphery) or to the medulla (cranial). Peptides such as sP and calcitonin-gene–related peptide (CGRP) have been strongly implicated as neurotransmitters of primary nociceptive afferents (Table 2-1).

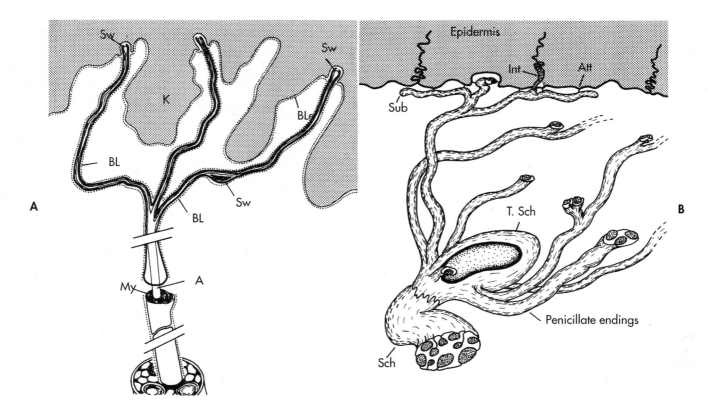

Fig. 2-3 A, Single thin myelinated fiber in the skin. *A,* Site of branching from the nerve bundle; *My,* myelin covering; *BL,* basal lamina; *BLe,* basal lamina of the epidermis; *SW,* Schwann cell; *K,* epidermis. (From Monetray in Perl ER: Characteristics of nociceptors and their activation of neurons in the spinal dorsal horn. In Kruger EL, Liebeskind JC, editors: *Advances in Pain and Research and Therapy, vol 6.* 1984, New York, Raven Press.) **B,** Termination of unmyelinated nerve fibers in the skin. *Sch,* Schwann cell; *T.Sch,* Termination of Schwann cell; *Sub,* Subepidermal zone of the corium; *Att,* Attachment between basal lamina and epidermis; *Int,* Intradermal. (From Cauna N: The morphological characteristics and microtopography of the human digital skin and free nerve endings. *Anal Res* 198:643, 1980.)

Table 2-1 Classification of fibers in peripheral nerves

Fiber group	Innervation	Mean diameter, μm (range)	Mean conduction velocity, m/sec (range)
Erlanger/Gasser classification (afferents and efferents)			
A alpha	Primary muscle spindle motor to skeletal muscles	15(12-20)	100(70-120)
beta	Cutaneous touch and pressure afferents	8(5-15)	50(30-70)
gamma	Motor to muscle spindle	6(6-8)	20(15-30)
delta	Mechanoreceptors, nociceptors	<3(1-4)	15(12-30)
B	Sympathetic preganglionic	3(1-3)	7(3-15)
C	Mechanoreceptors, nociceptors, sympathetic post-ganglionic	1(0.5-1.5)	1(0.5-2)
Lloyd/Hunt classification (muscle afferents only)			
Ia	Annulo spiral ending of muscle spindle	13(11-20)	75(70-120)
b	Neurotendinous spindle		
II	Flower spray ending of neuromuscular spindle	9(4-12)	55(25-70)
III	Pressure sensor in muscle nociceptors	3(1-4)	11(10-25)
IV	Unmyelinated C fibers, mechanical nociceptors	1(0.5-1.5)	1(0.5-2)

Substance P

Neurochemistry. This undecapeptide was first identified in 1931 and named substance P (sP) by von Euler and Gaddum.[4] Some two decades later Lembeck[5] associated this peptide with sensory transmission and probable vasodilation. Since then a great deal of information has been acquired about sP, which is found in unmyelinated primary neurons and their terminals.[6] Like other peptides, sP is synthesized in the cell bodies of small cells (type B) of spinal ganglia and the gasserian ganglion. These cell bodies are transported to the peripheral and central terminals, where they are stored in vesicles in a form amenable to release upon proper stimulus. Approximately four times as much sP is transported peripherally as centrally.[7]

Location

Soma. sP has been demonstrated in the peripheral terminals of unmyelinated primary afferents, which supply the human skin, sweat glands, glands of the nasal mucosa, small blood vessels in the skin and the pulmonary circuit, coronary and cerebral vessels, tooth pulp, and the eye.[6] Stimulation of spinal nerves and the trigeminal nerve have been shown to release sP from skin and tooth pulp, respectively.

Viscera. Visceral and autonomic terminals possess stores of sP that are associated with primary afferents. Sensory fibers containing sP supply the gastrointestinal tract, the ureters, and the trigone and neck of the urinary bladder. These fibers may be responsible for conveying nociceptive information from the viscera; they might also act locally in inducing vasodilation.[6] sP immunoreactive fibers have also been found in the prevertebral ganglia, which contain the sensory fibers that pass to the ganglia through the lumbar splanchnic nerves and may be involved in somatovisceral reflexes and referred pain.

Physiology. The role of these peripheral terminals in nociceptive transmission is uncertain, but sP has been shown not to be algogenic when administered locally to cutaneous terminals and does not activate peripheral nociceptive afferents.[8,9] Antidromic nerve stimulation produces flare and sensitization in the region of skin innervated by the stimulated sensory nerve. The basis for hypothesizing sP as a likely mediator for the neurogenically evoked increase in capillary wall permeability are the following observations: (1) exogenously administered sP induces plasma extravasation in normal and in denervated skin[10]; (2) other peptides, such as vasoactive intestinal peptide (VIP), do not produce such extravasation[11]; (3) capsaicin depletes sP content in skin,[11] and this depletion is accompanied by a loss of the ability of peripheral nerve stimulation to produce extravasation.[12]

NOCICEPTIVE AFFERENTS AND THE DORSAL HORN

Nociceptive afferents contact second order neurons in the dorsal horn of the spinal cord or medulla. Inhibitory interneurons are present in the dorsal horn; they play an important role in modulating the effectiveness of nociceptive afferent input from the periphery.

C polymodal nociceptive afferents synapse exclusively in laminae I, IIo, and V of the dorsal horn; A-delta nociceptors terminate in laminae I and IIo but also penetrate deeper to end in laminae V and X. The synaptic endings of primary afferents in the dorsal horn contain various types of vesicles and excitatory neurotransmitters.

Dorsal horn of the spinal cord

Morphology, physiology, and biochemistry. The dorsal horn, long considered a simple relay station, is now known to contain an incredibly complex circuitry including numerous varieties of neurons and synaptic arrangements and a rich biochemistry that permits not only reception and transmission of nociceptive input but a high degree of sensory processing. These include local abstraction, integration, selection, and appropriate dispersion of sensory impulses. The complex circuitry is activated through the phenomena of central convergence and central summation and through excitatory and inhibitory influences coming from the periphery, from local interneurons, and from the brainstem and cortex. The morphology and biochemistry of the spinal dorsal horn is similar to that of the medullary dorsal horn (trigeminal subnucleus caudalis) (Fig. 2-4).

Nociceptive specific neurons exist in high concentration in lamina I, but some are also found in lamina V (Fig. 2-5). These neurons, which receive exclusive excitatory effects from impulses in slowly conducting primary afferents, including MMTNs and C polymodal nociceptive afferents have small receptive fields and are somatotypically organized within the marginal layer. Wide dynamic-range (WDR) neurons exist in high concentration in lamina V of the dorsal horn, although a few exist in other dorsal horn laminae. The WDR neurons have input from primary afferents that supply skin, subcutaneous tissue, muscle, and viscera. Substantia gelatinosa (SG) neurons in lamina IIo respond to inputs from high threshold and thermoreceptive primary afferents, whereas neurons in lamina IIi respond only to inputs from low-threshold mechanoreceptive primary afferents. Of the various cells in the SG, stalked cells and islet cells are the most important for nociception. It has been proposed that most of the stalked cells are excitatory and that the islet cells are inhibitory neurons (Fig. 2-6).

Neurotransmitters. There are many types of neurotransmitters in the central terminals of primary afferents. The most important of them are excitatory amino acids such as glutamate and aspartate. They are found in large cells of dorsal root ganglion (DRG). A number of other neurotransmitters are found in small cells of the DRG, such as fluoride-resistant acid phosphatase (FRAP), sP, vasoactive intestinal polypeptide (VIP), somatostatin, cholecystokinin (CCK), gastrin-releasing peptide (GRP), angiotensin II, calcitonin-gene–related peptide (CGRP), leuenkephalin (ENK), and dynorphin (DYN).[12-16]

It is important to know that primary afferents contain more than one neurotransmitter in their terminals. They are located either in dense-core vesicles or smaller, clear-core vesicles of the terminal.[9] It has been shown that some presynaptic terminals of the second order neurons contain dense-core vesicles that react with sP antisera. In the same terminals there are small clear-core vesicles that are characteristic of amino acids but do not possess sP immunoreactivity. This situation suggests that certain afferent neurotransmitter systems may co-contain multiple neurotransmitters.[13]

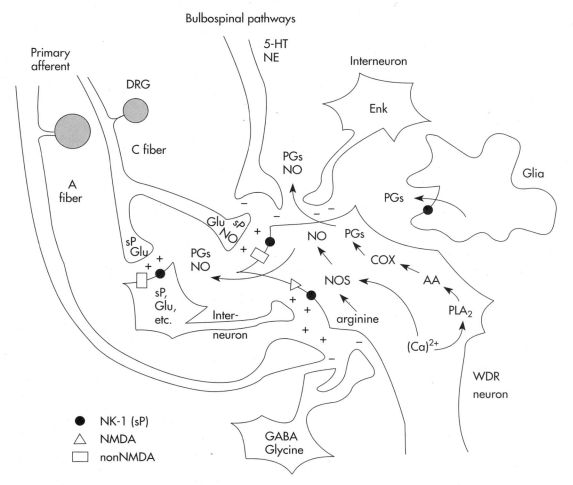

Fig. 2-4 Functional organization of the dorsal horn depicting the process of afferent input: (1) Primary afferent C fiber releases both peptides (sP, CGRP) and excitatory amino acid (glutamate). (2) Dorsal root ganglion cells contain NO synthase and thus are able to synthesize NO. (3) Peptides and EAA evoke excitation in second order neurons (for glutamate it is by non-NMDA receptors). (4) Under appropriate conditions there is excitation of NMDA receptors, leading to an increase in intracellular Ca^{2+} and activation of kinases and phosphorylating enzymes. In this set-up cyclo-oxygenase products (COX) (P9s) and NO are formed. These products move out extracellularly and facilitate transmitter release from primary and nonprimary afferent terminals. (5) Excitatory effects of large afferents are under GABA/glycine control, removal of which results in allodynia. (6) Interneurons contain enkephalin, norepinephrine, and serotonin, reflexly exerting a modulatory control and acting postsynaptically. (Modified from Yaksh TL, Malmberg: Central pharmacology of nociceptive transmission. In Wall PD, Melzack R, editors: *Textbook of Pain,* ed 3. Edinburgh, Churchill Livingstone, 1994.)

For instance, a coexistence of CCK and sP is very common.

sP facilitates the response of cells activated by noxious cutaneous stimuli. Other neurotransmitters such as glutamate, CCK, and VIP appear to be less selective. They produce excitatory and facilitatory effects on neurons that respond to a wide variety of stimuli. Thus there appears to be a correlation between the ability of sP to evoke a progressive depolarization in dorsal horn neurons and the existence of an afferent drive from small fibers. This correlation suggests that there are distinct small primary afferents that release excitatory neurotransmitters (glutamate, CCK, and VIP) in a stimulus-dependent fashion. They exert a powerful postsynaptic action. Furthermore, the postsynaptic

event appears to involve more than one neurotransmitter.

After being subjected to these modulating influences in the dorsal horn, some nociceptive impulses pass directly through interneurons to the anterior and anterolateral horn cells, where they simulate respective neurons. The anterolateral neurons provoke autonomic segmental nocifensive reflex responses. Other nociceptive impulses are transmitted to neurons, the axons of which make up ascending systems, and are thus conveyed to the brainstem and the brain.

ASCENDING PAIN PATHWAYS

In humans, the ascending pathways in the ventrolateral quadrant (spinothalamic tract [STT], the spinoreticular tract

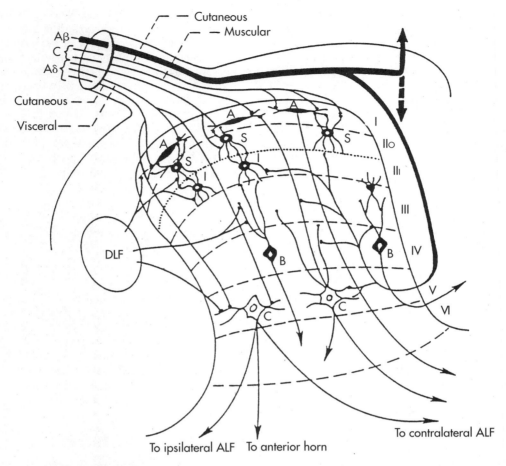

Fig. 2-5 Cross-section of dorsal horn showing input and output, interneurons, and axon terminals of the descending control system. *A,* large marginal neuron that connects to anterolateral funiculus (ALF). *S,* Stalk cell; *I,* islet cell; *B,* antenna cell; *C,* wide dynamic range neurons; *DLF,* dorsolateral funiculus containing descending axons of cells in the brainstem that are inhibitory (off cells) or facilitary (on cells). (From Bonica JJ: *Management of Pain,* ed 2. Philadelphia, 1990, Lea & Febiger.)

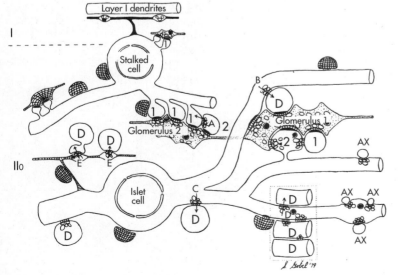

Fig. 2-6 Synaptic connections of lamina IIo islet cells and stalked cells. *I,* Lamina 1; *IIo,* Lamina 2 (outer layer); *D,* dendritic shafts; *Ax,* axonal shafts. The potential sites where layer IIo islet cells could synapse on stalked cell dendrites include dendodendritic synapses on type 1 spines *(arrow A),* dendritic shafts *(arrow B)* inside the glomeruli, and on dendritic shafts outside of the glomeruli *(arrow C),* as well as at axodendritic synapses *(arrow E).* (From Gobel S: An EM analysis of the synaptic connections of horseradish peroxidase filled stalked cells and islet cells in the substantia gelatinosa of adult cat spinal cord. *J Comp Neurol* 194:786, 1980.)

[SRT], and spinomesencephalic tract [SMT]) are the primary pathways for transmission of nociceptive information from the body to the brain (Fig. 2-7). The laterally projecting part of the STT, often called the neospinothalamic tract (nSTT), is much larger in humans than in monkeys and less developed animals. The nSTT is composed of neurons with cell bodies located in laminae I and V and long, fairly large myelinated axons that pass cephalad to the ventroposterolateral thalamic nucleus (VPL). In the VPL, the axons synapse with a third relay of fibers that project to the somatosensory cortex. The SRT, SMT, and the medial part of the STT, often called the paleospinothalamic tract (pSTT), have

cell bodies in the deeper layer of the spinal gray and thin fibers, some long and some short that project to the reticular formation, periaqueductal gray (PAG), hypothalamus, and medial and intralaminar thalamic nuclei. These fibers then make contact with neurons that connect with limbic forebrain structures and diffuse projections to many other parts of the brain. The trigeminal system has similar anatomic and physiologic characteristics, the neotrigeminothalamic tract (nTTT) projecting to the ventroposteromedial thalamic nucleus (VPM) and the paleotrigeminothalamic tract (pTTT) and the trigeminoreticulomesencephalic tract (TRMT) projecting to the same medial thalamic nuclei,

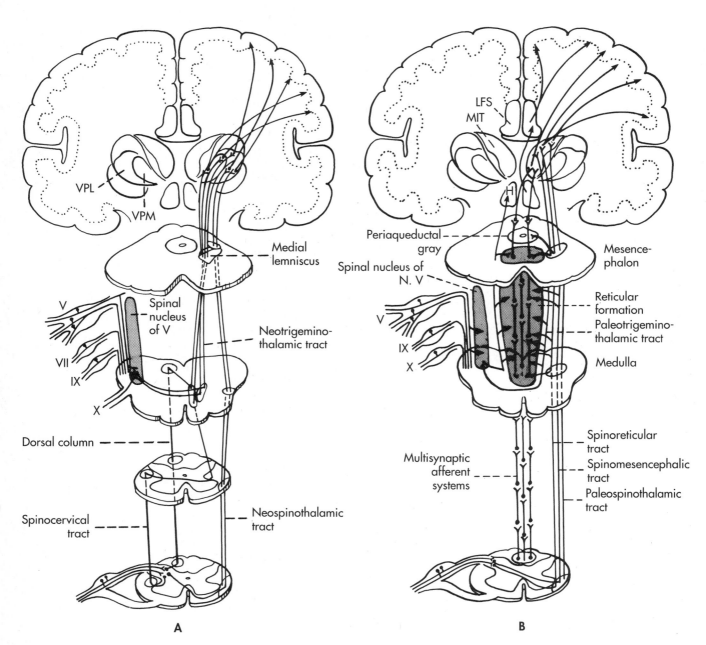

Fig. 2-7 The origin and course of the lateral system (**A**) and the medial system (**B**). (From Bonica JJ: *Management of Pain,* ed 2. Philadelphia, 1990, Lea & Febiger.)

where they make contact with neurons that project to limbic forebrain structures and have diffuse projections to other parts of the brain.

In addition to transmitting nociceptive impulses, these tracts also transmit other sensory information. There is evidence that the dorsal column tract (DCT), dorsal column postsynaptic system (DCPS), spinocervical tract (SCT), and multisynaptic (propriospinal) ascending systems (MAS) may also have a role in nociception. All of the ascending tracts are considered parts of two major systems: the lateral, or lemniscal, system, and the medial, or nonlemniscal, system.[14,17,18]

The lateral system includes the nSTT, nTTP, DCT, DCPS, and SCT. These tracts are composed of long, relatively thick fibers that conduct rapidly, have a discrete somatotopic organization, and make connection with the ventrobasal thalamus and thence with the somatosensory cortex. The evidence suggests that the lateral system is concerned with rapid transmission of phasic discriminative information about the onset of injury, its precise location, and its intensity and duration, and can quickly bring about response that prevents further damage. It has been suggested that these fast nociceptive pathways represent different sensory channels that are individually inhibited or facilitated, depending on the ongoing behavior or behavioral state of the organism.[18]

The medial system is composed of the phylogenetically older pathways—the pSTT, SRT, SMT, and MAS, which transmit nociception from the body, and the nTTT, pTTT, and TRMT for the head. Because of the thinness of these fibers, their multisynaptic nature, and the lack of somatotopic organization, impulses passing through the medial system are much slower in reaching the brain than those in the lateral system and are said to transmit tonic information about the state of the organism.[18] Thus an important, although perhaps not exclusive, role of these medial tracts may be to signal the actual presence of peripheral damage and continue to send messages as long as the wound is susceptible to reinjury. In this way the slow nociceptive pathways may in part determine the level of arousal or the general behavior state necessary to prevent further damage and to foster rest, protection, and care of the damaged area, thereby promoting healing and recuperative processes.

SUPRASPINAL MECHANISMS

Acute pain is a multidimensional experience that includes somatic sensory events in terms of space, time, intensity, and submodality and is associated with aversive motivational-emotional mechanisms leading to escape and other forms of aversive behavior. This complex multidimensional aspect of pain was described in the Melzack-Wall theory of pain[19] and later expanded by Melzack and Casey.[17] They suggested there are three major psychologic dimensions of pain: sensory-discriminative, motivational-affective, and cognitive-evaluative. They believe that these dimensions are subserved by physiologically specialized systems in the neuraxis. Although the Melzack-Casey[17] conceptual model of pain leaves important questions unanswered, it is the best model published to date.

There is evidence that the ventrobasal thalamus and the

somatosensory cortex, which receive input from the rapidly conducting lateral ascending pathways, have anatomic and physiologic characteristics that permit processing of sensory discriminative information (Fig. 2-8). Moreover, the reticular formation (hypothalamus, medial thalamus, and limbic systems) is involved in motivational and affective features of pain. These structures respond differentially to noxious stimuli and are not organized to provide discriminative information. They are strategically connected to activate and influence hypothalamic and limbic forebrain systems responsible for the activation of supraspinal autonomic reflex responses concerned with ventilation, circulation, neuroendocrine function, and the powerful motivational drive that triggers the organism into action. Although the Melzack-Casey model[17] suggests that the sensory-discriminative and

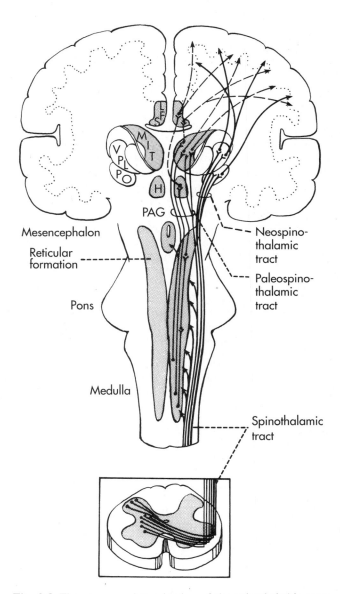

Fig. 2-8 The course and termination of the spinothalamic tract. (From Bonica JJ: *Management of Pain,* ed 2. Philadelphia, 1990, Lea & Febiger.)

motivational-affective dimensions are subserved by two parallel but separate systems, each one of them also influences neural systems that produce aversive, arousal, and motor reactions, and vice versa.

It has long been appreciated that anxiety, fear, apprehension, motivation, and other emotional reactions can markedly influence the pain experience. These emotional states and mental activities influence pain through the corticofugal and subcortical descending influences. These powerful descending influences may affect the sensory-discriminative dimension or the motivational-affective dimension of pain or both. Cognitive functions are then able to act selectively on sensory processing or motivational mechanisms. The powerful descending inhibitory influences exerted on dorsal horn cells can modulate input before it is transmitted to the discriminative and motivational systems. This modulation implies that the sensory input may be localized and defined in terms of its physical properties, evaluated in terms of past experience, and modified before it initiates the descending control system and activates discriminative and/or motivational systems.

The neural system that performs these complex functions of identification, evaluation, and selective input modulation must conduct rapidly to the cortex so that the somatosensory information has the opportunity to undergo further analysis, interact with sensory inputs, and activate memory stores and preset response strategies. Evidence suggests that the lateral ascending systems have the capacity to carry precise information about the nature and location of the stimulus, adapt quickly to give precedence to phasic stimulus changes rather than prolonged tonic activity, and conduct rapidly to the cortex so that ascending impulses can begin activation of central control processes.[18] These rapidly conducting ascending and descending systems can account for the fact that psychologic processes play a powerful role in determining the quality and intensity of pain.[19]

The frontal cortex probably plays a particularly significant role in mediating between cognitive activities and motivational-affective features of pain because it receives information via intracortical fiber systems from virtually all sensory and associated cortical areas and projects strongly to the reticular formation and limbic structures. These developments make possible mobilization of all sorts of associations based on past experience, judgments, and emotions that are involved in evaluation of the sensation. The frontal cortex appears essential in maintaining the negative affective and aversive motivational dimensions of pain. Neocortical processes subserve cognition and psychologic factors including early experience, prior conditioning, anxiety, attention, suggestion, cultural background, and evaluation of the meaning of the pain-producing situation (Fig. 2-9).

A complex interaction of sensory, motivational, and cognitive processes determines the complex sequence of behavior that characterizes pain by acting on mechanisms concerned with integrated motor responses. These mechanisms include all of the brain areas that contribute to overt behavioral response patterns, including the motor cortex, basal ganglia, and response-producing mechanisms in the hypothalamus, brainstem, and ventral horn.

DESCENDING PAIN CONTROL SYSTEM

During the past several years a great deal of new information has been acquired about the anatomy and neurochemical mechanisms of the descending pain control systems.

The models of the descending inhibitory systems have evolved in four regions of the central nervous system (CNS):

· Cortical and diencephalic systems
· Mesencephalic system—PAG and periventricular gray (PVG)
· Parts of the rostroventral medulla (nucleus raphe magnus [NRM] and adjacent nuclei); NRM receives excitatory input from PAG and sends serotonergic and noradrenergic fibers via the dorsolateral funiculus in the medullary dorsal horn
· The spinal and medullary dorsal horn, which receive terminals of axons from the NRM and adjacent nuclei

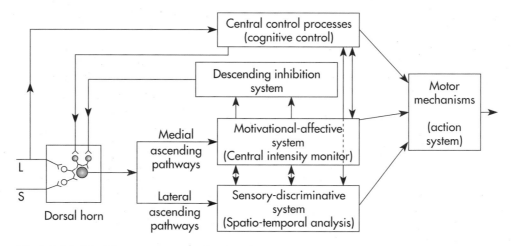

Fig. 2-9 Model of the sensory, motivational, and central control determinants according to Melzack and Casey. (From Melzack R, Casey KL: Sensory, motivational and central control determinants of pain. In Kenshalo DR Jr, editor: *The Skin Senses.* Springfield, Ill, 1986, Charles C Thomas.)

These descending fibers are serotonergic and terminate among nociceptive transmission cells in laminae I, IIo, and V, and thus selectively inhibit nociceptor neurons, including interneurons and the rostrally projecting STT, SRT, and SMT. There is also evidence that norepinephrine-containing neurons originating in the locus coeruleus and other brainstem sites contribute to this endogenous pain system.

NEUROCHEMISTRY OF THE ENDOGENOUS OPIATE SYSTEM
Endorphins

The discovery by Hughes and collaborators[20] of the two amino acid peptides, leuenkephalin and metenkephalin, gave rise to the suggestion that these ligands, found in high concentration at the spinal and medullary dorsal horn and in various other parts of the CNS, might be the agents that are released to act on intrinsic opioid systems. β-endorphin was later isolated from the periphery, and in 1979 the discovery of dynorphin and related opioid peptides was reported.[21] As a result of the discoveries of propeptides, three classes of opioids are currently known: the *enkephalins, dynorphins,* and *β-endorphins,* representing three distinct families of opioid peptides, each class cleaved from a different precursor and each having a distinct anatomic distribution.[22]

Opiate receptors

The opiate-binding sites relevant to analgesia are found throughout primary afferents and the neuraxis; they are stereospecific and of high affinity. Martin and his group[23] initially recognized the μ receptor for morphine as a classic opiate receptor. However, subsequently recognizing that certain benzomorphan analogues showed activity that was qualitatively different from those of morphine-like substances, they introduced two more receptors: κ (for ketocyclazocine) and σ (for Smith-Kline-French [SKF]).[16,22]

Table 2-2 lists the typical actions elicited through these three receptors. Since the opioid peptides did not fit into the system entirely, a δ receptor was introduced for the enkephalins along with a ε receptor that has a selectivity for β-endorphin. A tentative classification of the opioid receptors and their natural ligands is given in Table 2-3.[22] These peptides show considerable overlap between receptors. For example, the enkephalins bind to μ receptors as well as to δ receptors.

The μ receptor is abundant in central areas of pain control, especially in PAG matter in the brainstem and dorsal spinal cord. It is also present in the limbic system. κ receptors are also present in these areas and in deeper layers of the cerebral cortex. δ receptors are distributed generally throughout the neuraxis. Multiple-opioid receptors exist in many parts of the CNS.[22]

Enkephalin. Although enkephalins have a wide distribution throughout the CNS, several regions are consistent with their contribution to pain-control mechanisms.[1,24-29] The most important and clinically relevant location is the dorsal horn, where there are opiate-binding sites in central terminals of primary afferents and dorsal horn neurons. Enkephalin is also found in the PAG and in the raphe magnus, the globus pallidus, and the adjacent nucleus reticularis paragigantocellularis.[30] It is of interest to note that neurons containing serotonin (5-hydroxytryptamine [5-HT]) in these regions also contain enkephalin, and enkephalin and dynorphin coexist in some raphe and dorsal horn neurons.[30]

Dynorphin. Dynorphin and α-neoendorphin are cleaved from proenkephalin B. Dynorphin is found in the hypothalamus, PAG, mesencephalic reticular formation, and spinal and medullary dorsal horns.[31] After its discovery, it was shown that although intracerebral injection of dynorphin does not produce analgesia, intrathecal injection generates a profound and prolonged analgesia. Dynorphin cells are located in laminae I and V of the medullary and spinal dorsal horns at the level of the sacral cord.

β-Endorphins. Proopiomelanocortin (POMC) is the precursor for β-endorphin, adrenocorticotropic hormone (ACTH), and melanocyte-stimulating hormone (MSH).[27] Unlike the enkephalins and dynorphin, which are widely distributed in the neuraxis, POMC neurons are concentrated in the basal hypothalamus with their axons extending rostrally to the limbic system or caudally along the wall of the third ventricle toward the midbrain, PAG, and locus coeruleus. The fact that hypophysectomy can interfere with certain forms of stress-induced analgesia (SIA) indicates that pituitary endorphins may contribute to pain control.

NONOPIATE ENDOGENOUS INHIBITORY SYSTEM

The agents and terminals of descending systems that originate in raphe nuclei and medulla are primarily monoaminergic and release serotonin (5-HT), norepinephrine (NE), and, of course, less importantly, enkephalin and other peptides.

Serotonin. The cell bodies of 5-HT are in the nucleus raphe magnus (NRM), n. raphe obscuras (NRO), n. raphe pallidus (NRP), n. raphe dorsalis (NRD), and other nuclei in the medulla and pons (B_1-B_3, B_7, and B_9 cell groups). NRM—5-HT neurons project their axons through the dorsolateral funiculus to terminate predominantly in laminae I, IIo, IV, and V of the spinal dorsal horn and near the central canal.[13] A similar termination is seen in the medullary dorsal horn. The axons of 5-HT neurons located in NRO and NRP project near the ventral funiculus to the ventral horn. The 5-HT neurons of the NRM and other nuclei provide the serotonergic link in the controls exerted from most rostral sites in the diencephalon and forebrain. The analgesic action of systemic opiates can be blocked by depletion of 5-HT by inhibiting its synthesis with parachlorophenylalenine (pCPA) or by neurotoxic destruction of spinal 5-HT terminals with 5-7 dihydroxytryptamine or lesion of medullary 5-HT cells.

Location of norepinephrine-producing neurons. A second neurochemically distinct monoamine descending system involves noradrenergic neurons whose cell bodies are in A_5, A_6, and A_7 cell groups and whose axons descend in dorsolateral, ventrolateral, and ventral funiculi to end in all of the laminae of the spinal cord.[13] The A_6 and A_7 subgroups project most densely in the ventral horn, especially to motor neurons, but they also contribute afferents to laminae I, IIo, IV to VI, and X. Neurons within A_6 (n. locus

Table 2-2 Opiate receptor classification and action

	Pupil	Respiratory rate	Heart rate	Body temperature	Affect	Nociceptor flexor reflex
μ (mu)	Miosis	Stimulation → depression	Bradycardia	Hypothermia	Indifference	Decrease
κ (kappa)	Miosis	—	—	—	Sedation	Decrease
σ (sigma)	Mydriasis	Stimulation	Tachycardia	—	Delirium	Modest decrease

Adapted from Iwamoto E, Martin WR: Multiple opioid receptors. *Med Res Rev* 1:411, 1981.

Table 2-3 Natural ligands and naloxone sensitivity of opioid receptors

Receptor	Natural ligand prohormone	Naloxone sensitivity
μ (mu)	Methorphamide (Pro ENK A)	Strong
κ (kappa)	Dynorphin (Pro ENK B)	Intermediate
δ (delta)	Enkephalin (Pro ENK A)	Weak
ε (epsilon)	β-Endorphin (propriomelano cortin)	Weak

Modified from Terenius L: Families of opioid peptides and classes of opioid receptors. In Fields HL, Dubner R, Cervero F, editors: *Advances in Pain Research and Therapy, vol 9,* New York, Raven Press, 1985.

coeruleus) have dense projections to the parasympathetic preganglionic cell column in the sacral cord, whereas the neurons in A_7 (n. subcoeruleus) and medial parabrachial nucleus contribute axons to sympathetic preganglionic neurons in the intermediolateral cell column in T_1-L_2 spinal cord.[13,32] Studies have shown that a descending norepinephrine system mediates analgesia and dorsal horn inhibition and that the NE descending system appears to be critical for opiate-induced analgesia.[15,33]

Intrathecal phentolamine, an adrenergic blocker, attenuates the analgesia produced by systematic morphine administration or microinjection of morphine into the PAG. Intrathecal phenoxybenzamine, another α-adrenergic antagonist, blocks behavioral analgesia produced by morphine injected into the magnocellular tegmental field, and intrathecal phentolamine attenuates analgesia induced by electrical stimulation of the same region.[33]

Neurotensin. Neurotensin may be another important agent that contributes to pain-control mechanisms. Intracisternal neurotensin produces profound analgesia, possibly by direct action of the raphe-spinal inhibitory neurons.[28] This action has been confirmed by the demonstration that neurotensin-immunoreactive cells of the PAG project to the rostro ventral medulla (RVM) and that neurotensive input to the RVM also derives from the dorsolateral pons and from the ventral lateral medulla in the region corresponding to the chain of catecholamine cell groups A_1 to A_5.[27]

Modulation of pain transmission. In stark contrast to the concept of a simple straight-through system that transmits information with little information, there is an aston-

ishing degree of modulation at every level of the nervous system. Its almost incredible complexity is exemplified at the level of the dorsal horn where four functional components—*central terminals of primary afferents, neurons of ascending systems, local-circuit interneurons, and axonal terminals of descending systems*—appear to utilize an increasing number of neuroregulators.

Since there is no demonstration of direct primary afferent sP input to projection neurons, it is likely that there is a relay via an excitatory interneuron in the SG. Primary afferents containing sP have been shown to synapse with spinal enkephalin-containing neurons. This arrangement of sP-containing afferents probably exerts subtle controls that adjust the level of impulse transmission to the ascending projecting neurons. It obviously influences the primary afferent input and the interneurons. Basbaum has suggested that the peptidergic components of the bulbospinal inhibitory system provide the fine tuning of descending control.

There are now new concepts of neuronal conductivity for transmission of information from one neuron to another.[13-16] The investigators noted that the multiplicity of action by a neurotransmitter can be explained by the following principles: (a) a neuron may receive input from many neurotransmitters; (b) each neurotransmitter may have multiple actions in a given region; and (c) multiple neurotransmitters may exist in a single neuron.

The thalamic projecting neurons in laminae I and V receive ENK, 5-HT, sP, NE, and other unidentified neurotransmitters, which illustrates that a neuron may receive input from many neurotransmitters. The second principle, that each neurotransmitter may have multiple actions in a given region, is demonstrated by sP, which has been found present in primary afferent terminals and in descending axons. Both inputs may influence the same cell. The third principle, that the same morphologic subtype of neuron may contain different neurotransmitters and provide excitatory or inhibitory input, is illustrated by the fact that different stalked cells contain ENK or γ-aminobutyric acid (GABA) or may contain an unknown excitatory transmitter. Similarly, different islet cells contain ENK, GABA, or neurotensin.

Segmental analgesia

The ENK-containing neurons in lamina I and the stalked cell in lamina II combine to produce strong inhibition on lamina I thalamic projecting neurons. This inhibition may possibly be the mechanism of segmental analgesia achieved by intense transcutaneous or peripheral nerve stimulation. GABA-containing neurons in laminae I and II may produce similar segmental inhibitory effects. Analgesia achieved by stimulation of low-threshold mechanoreceptors, which end in laminae IIi, III, and IV, may be due to the stimulation of lamina IIi islet cells that contain ENK or GABA.

Global modulation

Descending 5-HT and NE-containing axons from the brainstem distribute to widespread regions of the medullary and spinal dorsal horns and give off an enormous number of boutons en passant along their paths. Some authors suggest that the multitargeted effects of these neurons provide a global modulation that enables dorsal horns to respond more effectively to incoming sensory information. Such mechanisms probably form the neural basis of animal and human behavior in the face of pain transmission as we presently know it.

REFERENCES

1. Yaksh TL, Hammond DL: Peripheral and central substrates in the rostral transmission of nociceptive information. *Pain* 13:1, 1982.
2. Granström E: Biochemistry of the prostaglandins, thromboxanes, and leukotrienes. In Bonica JJ, Lindblom U, Iggo A, editors: *Advances in Pain Research and Therapy, Vol 5*. New York, Raven Press, 1983.
3. Winkelmann RK: Kinins from human skin. In Kenshalo DR, editor: *The Skin Senses*. Springfield, Ill, Charles C Thomas, 1968.
4. von Euler US, Gaddum JH: An unidentified depressive substance in certain tissue extracts. *J Physiol* 72:74, 1931.
5. Lembeck F: 5-hydroxytryptamine in a carcinoid tumor. *Nature* 172:910, 1953.
6. Cuello AC, Matthews MR: Peptides in peripheral sensory nerve fibers. In Wall PD, Melzack R, editors: *Textbook of Pain*. Edinburgh, Churchill Livingstone, 1984.
7. Brimijoin S et al: Axonal transport of substance P in the vagus and sciatic nerves of the guinea pig. *Brain Res* 191:443, 1980.
8. Juan H, Lembeck F: Release of prostaglandins from the isolated perfused rabbit ear by bradykinin and acetylcholine. *Agents Actions* 6:642, 1976.
9. Hökfelt T et al: Neuropeptides and pain pathways. In Bonica JJ, Lindblom U, Iggo A, editors: *Advances in Pain Research and Therapy, vol 5*. New York, Raven Press, 1983.
10. Lembeck F, Gamse R, Juan H: Substance P and sensory nerve endings. In Von Euler US, Pernow B, editors: *Substance P*. New York, Raven Press, 1977.
11. Gamse R et al: Capsaicin applied to peripheral nerve inhibits axoplasmic transport of substance P and somatostatin. *Brain Res* 239:447, 1982.
12. Jansco N, Jancso-Gabor A, Szolcsanyi J: Direct evidence of neurogenic inflammation and its prevention by denervation and by pretreatment with capsaicin. *Br J Pharmacol Chemother* 31:138, 1967.
13. Ruda MA, Bennett GJ, Dubner R: Neurochemistry and neurocircuitry in the dorsal horn. *Progr Brain Res* 66:219, 1986.
14. Dubner R: Specialization in nociceptive pathways: Sensory discrimination, sensory modulation, and neural connectivity. In Fields HL, Dubner R, Cervero F, editors: *Advances in Pain Research and Therapy, vol 9*. New York, Raven Press, 1985.
15. Dubner R, Bennett GJ: Spinal and trigeminal mechanisms of nociception. *Ann Rev Neurosci* 6:381, 1983.
16. Dubner R et al: Neural circuitry mediating nociception in the medullary and spinal dorsal horn. In Kruger L, Liebeskind JC, editors: *Advances in Pain Research and Therapy, vol 6*. New York, Raven Press, 1984.
17. Melzack R, Casey KL: Sensory, motivational and central control determinants of pain. In Kenshalo DR Jr, editor: *The Skin Senses*. Springfield, Ill, Charles C Thomas, 1968.
18. Dennis SG, Melzack R: Pain signaling systems in the dorsal and ventral spinal cord. *Pain* 4:97, 1977.
19. Melzack R, Wall PD: Pain mechanisms: A new theory. *Science* 150:971, 1965.
20. Hughes J et al: Identification of two related pentapeptides from the brain with potent opiate, agonist activity. *Nature* 258:577, 1975.
21. Goldstein A et al: Dynorphin-(1-13), an extraordinarily potent opioid peptide. *Proc Natl Acad Sci USA* 76:6666, 1979.
22. Terenius L: Families of opioid peptides and classes of opioid receptors. In Fields HL, Dubner R, Cervero F, editors: *Advances in Pain Research and Therapy, vol 9*. New York, Raven Press, 1985.
23. Martin WR et al: The effects of morphine- and nalorphine-like drugs in the nondependent and morphine-dependent chronic spinal dog. *J Pharmacol Exp Ther* 197:517, 1976.
24. Yaksh TL, Noueihed R: The physiology and pharmacology of spinal opiates. *Ann Rev Pharmacol Toxicol* 25:433, 1985.
25. Basbaum AI: (a) Functional analysis of the cytochemistry of the spinal dorsal horn. In Fields HL, Dubner R, Cervero F, editors: *Advances in Pain Research and Therapy, vol 9*. New York, Raven Press, 1985; (b) Anatomical substrates of pain and pain modulation and their relation to analgesic drug action. In Kuhar M, Pasternak G, editors: *Analgesics: Neurochemical, Behavioral and Clinical Perspectives*. New York, Raven Press, 1984.
26. Basbaum AI, Fields HL: Endogenous pain control mechanisms: Review and hypothesis. *Ann Rev Physiol* 4:451, 1978.
27. Fields HL, Basbaum AI: Brain stem control mechanisms: Review and hypothesis. *Ann Neurol* 40:193, 1978.
28. Basbaum AI, Fields HL: Endogenous pain control systems: Brain stem spinal pathways and endorphin circuitry. *Ann Rev Neurosci* 7:309, 1984.
29. Snyder SH: Brain peptides as neurotransmitters. *Science* 209:976, 1980.
30. Glazer EJ et al: Serotonin neurons in nucleus raphe dorsalis and paragigantocellularis of the cat contain enkephalin. *J Physiol (Paris)* 77:241, 1981.
31. Cruz L, Basbaum AI: Multiple opioid peptides and the modulation of pain: Immunohistochemical analysis of dynorphin and enkephalin in the trigeminal nucleus caudalis and spinal cord of the cat. *J Comp Neurol* 240;4:331, 1985.
32. Westlund KN, Coulter JD: Descending projections of the locus coeruleus and subcoeruleus/medial parabrachial nuclei in monkey: Axonal transport studies and dopamine-beta-hydroxylase immunocytochemistry. *Brain Res Rev* 2:235, 1980.
33. Hammond DL: Pharmacology of central pain-modulating networks (biogenic amines and nonopioid analgesics). In Fields HL, Dubner R, Cervero F, editors: *Advances in Pain Research and Therapy, vol 9*. New York, Raven Press, 1985.

APPENDIX

HUMAN PERIPHERAL RECEPTORS

Receptors	Best stimulus	Velocity (m/sec)
1. Cutaneous mechanoreceptors		
Type I	Skin indentation	60
Type II	Skin deformation	45
Meissner Corpuscle	Skin indentation	55 (velocity)
Pacinian Corpuscle	Pressure changes	50 (vibration)
Warm	Increased temperature	0.5 (warming)
2. Cutaneous nociceptors		
C Polymodal	Noxious heat, mechanical damage	1
C Mechanical	Algesic chemicals	
C Cold	Extreme cold	
A-delta	Mechanical noxious heat	—
A-delta Cold	Algesic chemicals	

CLASSIFICATION OF DORSAL HORN INTERNEURONS

Lamina	Afferent fibers	Stimuli
I	Mainly A-delta and C	Innocuous, mechanical, thermal, polymodal, noxious
IV	A alpha beta, A-delta, and C	Innocuous, mechanical, wide dynamic range
V	A, C cutaneous, Group III muscle	Intense, mechanical, wide dynamic range
VI	A, C, Group I muscle	Proprioceptive, wide dynamic range

NEUROCHEMICAL SYSTEMS
Monoamine systems (MAS)

1. MAS mechanisms are initiated supraspinally but exert antinociceptive action at the spinal cord level via descending pathways.
2. 5-HT cell bodies in the nucleus raphe magnus descend via the DLF to end in 5-HT fields in the rexed laminae of the spinal cord. Release of 5-HT inhibits neurons specifically excited by noxious input.
3. A similar NEP system exists (from the locus ceruleus). Its spinal effect is dose dependent, α-receptor mediated, and separate from opioid mechanisms or vasoconstrictive effect.
4. SPA in the nucleus raphe magnus or local CNS opioid injection can activate the MAS.
5. Morphine analgesia prevented by reserpine induces monoamine depletion.
6. Interaction with the opioid system occurs both supraspinally and in the dorsal horn of the SC.
7. Positive correlation of brain dopamine and SPA from PAG
   a. 5-HT has similar correlation
   b. With NEP spinal and supraspinal mechanisms appear to be opposite in effect

Endogenous opiate system (EOS)

1. Three families of endogenous opiate peptides
   a. β-endorphin/corticotropin family
      precursor: proopiomelanocortin sequence β-endorphin, ACTH, and melanotropin
   b. Enkephalin family
      precursor: proenkephalin
      7 sequences each: 6 met and 1 leuenkephalin
   c. Dynorphin/neoendorphin family
      precursor: prodynorphin
      3 opioid peptide sequences, with leuenkephalin core
2. Generally, dynorphin and enkephalin occur in many of the same areas, including caudate, amygdala, PAG, locus coeruleus and spinal cord.
3. Dynorphin is a relatively poor analgesic.
4. Four subtypes of opiate receptors
   a. Mu (μ): possibly the most potent in inducing analgesia
      i. Classical opioid agonists and antagonists have preference for the μ receptor
      ii. Agonists are more effective with tests of noxious heat
   b. Kappa (κ): predominantly in the spinal cord
      i. Active opiates are analgesics with low potential for development of tolerance or dependency in monkeys
      ii. Agonists have increased potency on tests of nociception using mechanical stimuli
   c. Delta (Δ): predominantly supraspinal
   d. Sigma (δ)

QUESTIONS: PAIN MECHANISMS

1. Tissue damage causes inflammation, which releases chemical substances at the site of injury. Which of the following chemical substances causes pain?
   A. Enkephline
   B. Prostaglandins
   C. Na
   D. Ca

2. The site of substance P in the peripheral tissues is:
   A. Plasma
   B. Vascular endothelium
   C. Nerve terminals
   D. Mast cells

3. For transduction of painful stimuli into nociceptive impulse this condition is necessary:
   A. Local decrease in bradykinin
   B. Inhibition of prostaglandin synthesis
   C. Local extravasation of substance P
   D. Local increase of encephalins

4. The mean conduction velocity (m/sec) of A-delta afferents that transmit nociceptive impulse is:
   A. Greater than 15 m/sec
   B. Greater than 8 m/sec
   C. Greater than 3 m/sec
   D. Less than 3 m/sec

5. In the normal functioning of the dorsal horn this process occurs:
   A. Afferent C fiber inhibits substance P release.
   B. Under appropriate conditions, NMDA receptor can excite.
   C. Excitatory amino acids inhibit secondary neurons.
   D. Interneurons (e.g., contain encephalins, norepinephrine, serotonin) act presynaptically.

ANSWERS

1. B
2. C
3. C
4. C
5. B

3 Evaluation of the Pain Patient

David R. Longmire

During the past two decades much attention has been given to the development of pain management as a clinical specialty.[1-3] New collaboration between basic scientists and medical specialists has improved understanding of many pain mechanisms. However, most of the clinical contributions to pain medicine are still based upon physicians' interpretation of patients' symptoms and physical signs.

In the field such clinical data are of utmost importance, since one major difference between algology and other branches of medicine is that the assessment of pain is expected to include more detailed symptom analysis and documentation than is ordinarily required for many general illnesses. One of the purposes of this chapter is to emphasize those methodological differences that exist between the diagnosis of general health problems and the more specific techniques used in the medical evaluation of pain. In order to encourage standardization of methods that can be used for treatment outcome monitoring, additional emphasis will be placed upon the theory and style of how such examinations should be conducted and recorded.

A significant portion of this chapter is dedicated to the technique of performing the medical history because the importance of adequately documenting the patient's subjective experience cannot be overstated. Indeed, more attention is given to data acquisition than interpretation for the simple reason that interpretation cannot be taught without bias. The analysis of medical information can only be learned through the synthesis of core content provided by (a) sources in the scientific literature,[4-6] (b) attentive clinical experience, and (c) the application of outcome studies as a form of feedback to improve the quality of care. Therefore, while learning to use a standard assessment method for pain, data may be collected, but the acquisition of interpretive skills should be based on a personally designed curriculum.

With limitations of the task better defined, it may be beneficial to consider the definition for the universal experience of pain adopted by the International Association for the Study of Pain.[7] The committee responsible for this effort addressed the physical and psychologic components of this unpleasant subjective experience, i.e., it did not emphasize one aspect over the other. In practice this suggests that, regardless of how extreme pain behavior may seem in an individual patient, all efforts should be made to assess both psychologic and medical conditions that could represent any organic cause for the pain. Therefore, from the outset of the pain consultation, the physician must become the algologic equivalent of the forensic specialist whose task is to find those long-hidden pieces of the medical puzzle through the pain evaluation, using whichever style best suits the complexity of the problem, the rules of the institution, or the personal choice of the investigator.

BASIC ELEMENTS OF THE GENERAL MEDICAL EVALUATION

In general medicine, the initial clinical evaluation of any symptom complex should include a detailed medical history, a general physical examination, appropriate radiologic and laboratory tests, and a differential diagnosis on which a plan of treatment may be founded.[8,9] In theory this could be interpreted to mean that an equally detailed assessment would be required not only for the pain caused by the symptoms and signs of a suspected occult malignancy but also for a minor skin abrasion. In medical practice, a system of triage has evolved where the physician's interpretation of the initial symptoms and signs is used to select subsequent assessment and treatment methods. The choice to proceed with a diagnostic workup is then based on the severity of illness and the complexity of care that will be required for that patient. Within this staged system, there are four styles of history taking; any can be applied to pain medicine. The general styles are syndromic, chronologic, classical, and in its own category, the medical pain history.

Limited data collection: diagnosis by syndrome

If an experienced practitioner collects very basic data from the history consistent with certain positive findings upon examination that match a pattern indicative of a specific syndrome, then a putative diagnosis may be reached and medical treatment can be initiated. This type of therapeutic trial may be used in general medicine and, if successful, may not require further expensive or invasive tests. If the treatment is not effective within a reasonable number of days, then consultation or diagnostic tests can be ordered.

Until the past few decades, syndrome recognition[10] has been the most simple and inexpensive method of providing a primary medical diagnosis. Unfortunately, in the field of pain medicine this style is most susceptible to error through omission of valuable clinical details. Specifically, if a patient with acute pain was inaccurately diagnosed based on etiology or severity, that individual might receive only partial treatment. If the acute processes are inadequately treated, the potential exists for conversion of the symptom production into a chronic pain syndrome.[11,12]

Detailed data collection: chronologic history

At the opposite end of the medical-record spectrum is the chronologic health assessment system. Upon first inspection this appears to be no more than a paper or electronic list of all health care problems, physician visits, and medical and surgical treatments from birth to death in a given patient. Instead, this system of basic questions provides a universal, expandable survey of normal landmarks of growth, development, and aging, plus vital health statistics that are invaluable in epidemiologic research and pain treatment outcome studies. Unfortunately, its application is time intensive, and it is not often used as a first-line method in clinical medicine. The exception is its application in pediatrics, where the health records are developed over a smaller sample time. As interactive computer database and word processing programs become more widely applied in clinical medicine, the chronologic history method may become a viable alternative for universal health record keeping.

Classical form of medical history

The classical method for collecting data during medical evaluation tends to be very goal oriented. Physicians choose this popular method to obtain a regional, anatomic, etiologic, pathologic, and functional diagnosis. The focus of this evaluation begins with the recording of the symptom that is of greatest importance to the patient. This is known as the "chief complaint," since it is usually the one to which the physician is first directed by the affected individual. The somatic distribution of that symptom, the details of where, when, and how the condition began, and any factors that describe the natural course of its development are then recorded as the history of the present illness. Next, details of any previous health problems may be noted as the past medical history, which should include comments regarding early childhood illnesses, trauma, hospitalizations, and surgeries and their respective outcomes. This is generally followed by a review of early and current pharmacologic treatment (medication history), with particular notation of any adverse reactions (allergy history). Often the next portion is comprised of data regarding the health of the patient's blood relatives (family history), support systems, and personal habits such as alcohol or tobacco use (social history). Interaction between each patient's health and their disability or active participation in the work force are then recorded (occupational history). To avoid omissions and document essential negative health problems, a general survey of body functions (review of systems) is conducted using a direct question and answer format.

The classical method of collecting data is widely accepted, and occasionally must be followed by policy, not by preference, in certain institutions. Techniques and subtle nuances associated with the administration and interpretation of this form of medical history may be found in several excellent medical textbooks and in specific articles on this aspect of medical assessment for pain.[13-16]

MEDICAL PAIN HISTORY: PRACTICE GUIDELINES

The style for a single universal medical history for pain is still being developed. To the untrained observer the interim methods used for this type of history may appear to differ only slightly from the more traditional style described in the preceding section. However, in order to increase consistency within the data collection phase, the following suggestions are offered.

First, the terminology in the medical pain history should be compatible with the terminology in the classical form because of its widespread acceptability. The only significant exception to this is to use the term "history of the presenting complaint" instead of "history of the present illness." In the application of this section to clinical pain, the physician should document all features of the complaint as a symptom complex, not as an illness or disease.

Second, there should be no attempt to force the patient who has two or three major symptoms to limit data presentation to only the "chief complaint." For example, the patient who has moderately intense pain in the neck and shoulder but who also has dense upper extremity weakness may be more afraid of permanent paralysis than of suffering. The motor deficit therefore becomes the chief complaint, but the characteristics of the pain symptoms may provide the information necessary to make the diagnosis. Therefore, add a section called "secondary complaints" to the medical pain history to accommodate a list of other symptoms.

A third important difference is the sequence of data presentation within each section. The order in the medical pain history has been modified so that it reflects (a) the major symptoms; (b) all details of the specific symptom complex; (c) a survey of the current health status of the remaining body systems; (d) the perspective of present health compared to past medical, surgical, or traumatic disorders; (e) overview of medications and medication allergies; (f) any genetic contributions to the patient's health; (g) effects of social stressors and support systems on the patient; and (h) disability from, or effective transactions within, the workplace.

Chief complaint and secondary complaints

The chief and secondary complaints are of greatest importance at the first patient-physician visit where all relevant communication begins when patients state their symptoms. Since the content of this statement is usually subjective, it is only fair to record this personal impression by using the patient's own words. More importantly, the physician should avoid the temptation of translating the patient's personal words into medical jargon.

History of the presenting complaint

In pain evaluation, the detailed description and specific features of the chief complaint are known as the "history of the presenting complaint." In assessing the pain history, essential symptom characteristics should be detailed and recorded using the following sequence:

1. Date and time of pain onset. The date and time of pain onset are usually remembered clearly by patients whose symptoms began as a result of trauma. Pain that began insidiously is much more difficult to date. In either situation, the temporal characteristics of pain onset should be recorded using standardized phrases such as ". . . the symptoms began suddenly, fairly rapidly, or gradually . . ." This should be followed by an estimate of the total time that passed between

the pain onset and the date of the initial visit, e.g., ". . . approximately x years ago . . .," with specific details included such as the closest clock time and calendar date recalled.

2. Conditions at the time of onset of pain. Conditions at the onset of pain are most important when there is an acute precipitating event. In cases of motor vehicle accidents or work-related injuries, the patient's activities, mood, and attitude before the onset of pain should be noted in the chart. Subsequently the position (sitting, standing, reclining) and movement (lifting, turning, bending) of the head, trunk, spine, or limbs should be described for both the time of impact and the onset of symptoms. Record this in the chart so that there is a clear verbal picture of any mechanical displacement that could cause a painful injury.[17]

3. Spatial characteristics of clinical pain. There are several pain types that change locations or encompass a greater area with time or increasing intensity. This means that the only time that the true center of a pain field can be identified is shortly after the onset of symptoms. When the pain spreads as time passes, the direction of its spread (proximal to distal or vice versa) may provide helpful diagnostic clues. Once the pain becomes stable, the region to which the pain is finally limited may have a characteristic shape, e.g., dermatomal, radicular, Head's zones, or sympathetic sclerotome.[18,19] When the localization process includes topographic analysis of associated (nonpainful) symptoms, e.g., numbness or cutaneous neurovascular dysfunction, anatomic diagnostic accuracy becomes markedly improved.

Although most of this section relates to verbal descriptors, standard body maps like those found in the McGill Pain Questionnaire,[20] pain drawing instruments,[21] or classic anatomic drawings have become extremely helpful in pain diagnosis. It is, therefore, very useful to include in the medical chart preprinted body diagrams so that patients may draw or shade the distribution of their pains.

4. Qualitative descriptors of pain. The words patients use to describe the quality of their pain experiences often guide physicians to one or more possible etiologies.[22] For example, pain that is described as "throbbing" or "pounding" at a rate similar to the patient's heartbeat suggests involvement of vascular spasm, occlusion, or partial stenosis. Abdominal pain that comes "in waves" every few minutes or the rhythmic pains of labor are more indicative of contractions of a hollow viscus against an obstruction (C.B. Mueller, unpublished data, 1979) which can cause colicky pain. Many other qualitative descriptors were studied, analyzed, and multiply validated within the McGill Pain Questionnaire, so that such words can now be used to differentiate the sensory/affective and emotional components of pain.

5. Timing and persistence of pain. The temporal factors relating to the speed of onset of pain (sudden, gradual) have been mentioned previously. Once the initial (acute) pain has begun, however, there are several changes that can occur. The pain that begins suddenly, with or without apparent injury, is often expected to persist for hours or days. Even without medical treatment, the body's cellular defense mechanisms institute a process of damage containment and repair. When this process is successful, the pain begins to resolve over time and finally returns to the premorbid state. In documenting that type of single event, the characteristics should include the speed of onset, the duration of peak pain levels, and the time course or duration of pain resolution and recovery.

There has been sufficient evidence from studies on postoperative and other forms of acute pain to suggest that inadequate treatment of acute pain can lead to persistent or chronic pain. This pain can become sustained through reverberatory neural loops, sympathetically maintained, or independently established through structural or biochemical aberrations of the healing process.

In the histories of such patients, one can find patterns of pain that persist at levels close to the initial intensity, are continuous but fluctuate widely in intensity, or seem to respond to treatment or otherwise disappear, only to return repeatedly. Each of these patterns must be documented, with additional reference to frequency and duration of exacerbations.[23]

6. Provocative factors. There are relatively few direct questions that must be asked regarding factors that make the pain more severe, since patients generally volunteer this information early. One possible reason to address this topic before the physical examination is to help the patient avoid any additional pain caused by the manipulations of an uninformed examiner.

Factors that increase pain can be classified as direct (mechanical, postural, activity related); indirect (stress, emotional upset, depression); biochemical (catamenial, dietary, glucose/electrolyte); and environmental (temperature, barometric pressure).

7. Palliative factors. Considering any factor that reduces or palliates the symptoms is as important in differentiating the etiology as it is in selecting possible pain treatments. If the pain is reduced by the application of heat, cold, rest, or controlled exercise, then physical therapy may aid in treating inflammatory mechanical pain mechanisms. If the patient states that certain medications blocked the intense pain while others did not, then analysis of the pharmacologic classes that were effective may be helpful in reaching a pathophysiologic diagnosis.

During this section of the patient's pain history, questions may be asked about the palliative effects of earlier medications that were used for the current condition. If the patient supports a verbal list of failed treatments by presenting medication bottles, record the method of prescribing from each individual label. Most importantly, directly assess the manner in which the patient actually took a particular medication, so that the true palliative effect might be estimated.

8. Severity of the pain symptoms. The global pain experience is so tortuous in its path through nociception,

transmission, attention, affect, and verbal/behavioral response that any attempts to quantify a single component by using a unidirectional measurement are tenuous at best.[24] However, in clinical medicine the physician must make other similar judgments on a daily basis using assessment techniques that are even less scientific and equally subjective. In all cases of clinical pain, therefore, attempting to quantify pain intensity for the medical record is an expected element in each patient's pain history. Several methods have been developed for evaluating the patient's subjective report of pain intensity,[25] and comparative reviews have been performed to test the relative validity of each technique. The most logical method for evaluating pain is the Visual Analogue Scale (VAS), where the patient is asked to place a mark on a 10-cm horizontal line that is anchored on the far left by the words "no pain whatsoever" and on the extreme right by the phrase "the worst pain imaginable." The true form of this scale contains no vertical graticules and no list of verbal cues to indicate mild, moderate, or severe pain.[26] Although this test has been validated in numerous studies as part of the McGill Pain Questionnaire, it requires sufficient insight and basic motor skills to complete.

A simpler method used widely in North America is to ask the patient to verbally report the pain intensity level. The usual method preferred by patients is the Numeric Rating Scale (NRS-11), which requires the patient to select a number from 0 (no pain) to 10 (the worst pain imaginable). The patients should use either the VAS or the NRS-11 to report their pain intensity for the medical record.

9. Associated symptoms. As noted previously, many nonpainful symptoms can accompany painful disorders. The loss of range of motion caused by a painful injury to an extremity may appear to create a paresis when in actuality the only motor deficit is due to guarding against pain. Similarly, hyperesthesia to point stimulation or to the surface application of cold can accompany regional pain. In conditions where certain sensory nerves are injured, normal sensation may be markedly reduced or absent, while the only remaining neural activity creates spontaneous pain. Hence, patients with chief complaints of pain of this type may have associated symptoms of reduced sensation in a similar geographic area.

Other nonpainful symptoms to document are shifts in the perceived temperature of one or both hands or feet, or the sensation of swelling in a similar distribution.

Systems review

In the systems review section, the patient is asked questions about symptoms that are ordinarily associated with dysfunction in different somatic systems. Any positive responses currently experienced by the patient are documented and added to the section "History of the Presenting Complaint." Together, these results provide the physician with a clearer understanding of the relationship between the chief complaint and the patient's overall current health status.

Past medical history

During the systems review, it is common for patients to discuss current symptoms that began months or years ago but still persist. To acquire an even better perspective of an individual's health, it is important to document any and all past illnesses. Details of these conditions must be noted regardless of whether the treatment was successful or resulted in residual dysfunction. Although this section is named "past medical history," it must include surgical, trauma, and behavioral history.

In performing this review, it is essential to obtain accurate data for all conditions, particularly when personal injury, workers' compensation claims, or litigation are involved. Often it becomes necessary to give a patient an extra opportunity to admit to old symptoms in the same body region as a recent compensable injury that is supposedly the sole cause of current suffering. The value of this approach can only be fully appreciated when the content of a record is challenged in deposition or court. The omission of any documentation by health professionals (many must keep separate health records) of prior illness and treatment of a patient seeking compensation or disability status can often reduce the credibility of the patient and the physician. Unfortunately, the beginning physician can only be warned that most patients with compensation claims against a second or third alleged injury have very poor insight regarding the separation of old pain, new pain, and new exacerbations of old pain mechanisms.

Medication history

An individual's history of pharmacologic treatment for the control of pain or unrelated illnesses must be approached with the utmost discretion, tact, and professional confidentiality. Nevertheless, use extreme caution and a healthy, nonparanoid index of clinical suspicion when dealing with a new patient who is more interested in long-term symptom control with a moderate or strong opioid analgesic than in complying with tests to confirm the definitive cause of the pain.

The physician should develop a method for quantifying the amount of analgesics used by the patient to determine if a specific treatment has helped to reduce medication intake. Since new pain patients may be taking large amounts of narcotic, nonnarcotic, and adjunctive medicines, it can be helpful to compare the potency of each daily dosage to the gold standard of 10 mg of morphine sulphate given intramuscularly. The total daily intake of a narcotic analgesic for a large person may not have the same effect on a small individual. By combining the equianalgesic dose calculation method[27] with a weight-related correction factor, a reasonable range of milligrams per kilogram per day may be considered for acute pain control. In patients who request daily oral opioid therapy for an apparently benign chronic pain condition, two principles must be considered: first, ask whether the patient is seeking drugs or seeking relief from pain[28] and secondly, determine the most effective ways to perform objective diagnostic tests that will lead to the specific treatment for the pain etiology.

Allergy history

Without question this portion of a patient's history should be given a significant amount of attention. Adverse side effects or minor or gastrointestinal (GI) upsets should be clearly differentiated from serious allergies with potentially life-threatening cardiovascular and respiratory consequences. Regardless of how inconsistently a patient relates an allergic reaction to a specific agent, the most cautious action is to react as if the patient were markedly sensitive to that agent and to avoid whole families of medicines that have any pharmacologic similarity. Additional monitoring and quantification of medication usage may be necessary in patients who claim allergies to all nonopioid analgesics but who have no known allergies to narcotics.

Family history

The family medical history, when adequately recorded, represents the true biological foundation of the patient's hereditary tendencies toward health and disease. However, the family history should not just list the current health status or cause of death of each family member, but should establish a genetic pedigree for the occurrence of the patient's chief complaint of clinical pain.

Although the global health of the family may not be specifically representative of the patient, any history of disability resulting from chronic pain in one or more members may be a significant determinant of potential tolerance, amplification, or augmentation of symptoms.

Social history

The social history section accounts for the position of the patient within a domestic or other potentially supportive social system. As an extension of the family medical history, it documents the patient's past and present marital status and current social and financial dependents. These data can provide preliminary indicators of stress associated with debilitating pain or illness and the stressful emotional effects this can have on the caregiver, the quality of the care, and the recipient.

A list of the patient's previous social habits and personal or public contacts (shopping, visiting friends, attending church) can be more meaningful if those habits that can no longer be done or enjoyed because of pain, fear of pain, or financial duress caused by lost employment are included. When socially acceptable interactions are disrupted, socially unacceptable actions often fill the void. Therefore this section should include personal habits (alcohol consumption, tobacco use, drug use, gambling) or conflicts with the law. Significant perturbation in the patient's usual social interactions, mood, or affect or new tendencies toward violence or suicidal ideation are sometimes reviewed in this portion of the history.[29]

Occupational history

The first formal work for most North Americans is attending school. Therefore the occupational history should begin with documentation of the highest level of education attained by the patient. Since competitive access to employment may be dependent not only on amount but type of education, it is helpful to list any work-related training in the final determination of equivalency. The patient should list previous jobs and general duties and then describe the specific job-related tasks of the most recent employment. If the patient is currently not working, note if their leave is medically approved in writing or if it occurred only by the patient's own actions. Within this section it may be helpful to note if the patient has undergone any assessment of work-related disability, functional capacities evaluation, or vocational rehabilitation programs before proceeding on to the physical examination.

General physical examination for pain

How to perform the general physical examination and record physical findings is universally available in undergraduate and postgraduate or specialty textbooks in medicine. As a consequence, most physicians assume that their fellow physicians perform complete physical examinations at the initial assessment. However, most anecdotal evidence provided by patients indicates that pain physicians provide more detailed general and specialty examinations than non-algologists. Therefore this section is limited to those specific elements that differentiate the general examination from the physical examination for pain.

Initial examination. First, observe the patient's room for the presence of any acute-care or intermediate-care medical equipment or assistive devices and note the patient's general appearance. Much information can be obtained from critically reviewing the room for any objects within immediate reach, such as tobacco products, food, flowers, and reading materials. The interpretation of these observations and the sequential (rostral/caudal) method using basic principles of inspection, auscultation, palpation, and percussion to conduct the examination have been described in detail elsewhere.[13,14,15] In pain medicine, however, the specific features of three specialty screening examinations should be added: pain behavior, musculoskeletal, and neurologic.

Examination for pain behavior. The patient's face should be examined for expression of pain at the first visual encounter. Before any verbal exchange begins, the physician should inspect the color, muscular contractions, and general animation of the face, and should note any focal or lateralized changes in skin and subcutaneous tissue contour. Emotional changes in facial expression, including grimacing, often may be seen in pain; formal studies of patients with organic and fictitious pain have revealed important differences seen in scoring systems developed for that purpose.[30]

Early in the pain history, the patient may demonstrate speech patterns that indicate abnormalities of articulation or content. Dysarthria resulting from intoxication relating to alcohol or excessive use of prescribed narcotic analgesics must be differentiated from slurred speech patterns caused by cerebral, cerebellar, or bulbar lesions. In general, the content of speech should be relatively consistent with normal mental function. Specifically, the physician should be able to recognize verbal behavior that would indicate delusion, hallucinations, mental retardation, and the classic forms of psychoneurosis because any of these can destroy the validity of the pain assessment. Most pain patients use words that are specific and thereby helpful in the diagnosis of the underlying illness.[27] Others will at least use language that can help determine which component of pain is dominant (affective, sensory). Occasionally patients who lack effective control of chronic organic pain will indicate that suicide would be preferred over suffering.[29] Even the most subtle suggestion that a patient is considering suicide should be taken seriously, with rapid referral for crisis intervention. If the pain has been sufficiently severe and chronic to reduce specificity, the diffusion of pain language can interfere significantly with diagnosis and treatment.[31] Many patients who seek financial compensation for their conditions understand that the examining physicians cannot "see" their pain. Consequently they believe it is necessary to augment their verbal reports of debilitating pain by grunting, breath holding, shaking or tightening trunk and limb muscles, and applying excessive weight on assistive devices. Unfortunately, these activities can change heart and respiratory rate, blood pressure (BP), and perspiration through Valsalva's maneuver, thereby reducing the value of tests for verbal/ autonomic mismatch as a sign of symptom amplification or augmentation.

One study of nonorganic pain behavior that is often cited is the report by Waddell and colleagues,[32] who studied several clinical features of patients with chronic low back pain, regardless of etiology. Waddell et al. found that there were at least five simple test maneuvers (axial loading, skin pinch, hip rotation, differential straight leg raising, and exaggerated behavior) that elicited separate responses in patients whose pain behavior was thought to be based on conditions other than organic back disease. Unfortunately, this method has often been applied to detect malingering, for which this test was not designed to detect or proven truly effective.

Musculoskeletal examination. Many standard reference works on orthopedics, physical medicine, and neurology contain sections dedicated to the integrated clinical examination of bones, muscles, joints, and connective tissue.[33,34] When methods of examining the function of the brain, spinal cord, nerve roots, and peripheral nerves are added, the anatomic and etiologic diagnoses of many painful musculoskeletal conditions can become much more accurate.[35]

Although many patients who have pain in the spine or extremities claim associated weakness, relatively few are able to state definitively whether their reduced power is caused by true paresis, guarding caused by pain upon movement, or that the fear of pain has created a reduction in maximum voluntary effort. Repeated measures of motion through a joint should be recorded objectively; if a unilateral deficit is found, the contralateral limb should be tested for comparison. If there is any obvious anatomic pathology at rest, structural measurements such as true limb length or circumferential measurements of limbs should be taken. Currently, to document upper-extremity and lower-extremity bulk, measure the circumferences above and below the elbows and knees at a constant distance, e.g., 5 in.

For static measurements of regions other than the major limb segments, always use bony landmarks as reference points. Asymmetry can be determined by using homologous sample sites. For dynamic measurements of joint and spi-

nal action, the previously popular goniometer is being replaced by manual or computer-assisted inclinometry for calculation of limb or spinal impairment. Repeated measurements are recommended because each test session should include comparative data and should indicate a consistency of effort.[36,37]

Neurosensory and autonomic examinations. Most standard textbooks of clinical neurology include chapters on how to conduct a complete neurologic examination. Specific aspects of the mental status (behavior and speech), and the motor examination have already been described. Of the many subtests in the physical examination of the nervous system, there are two that are very important to the clinical algologist—the sensory examination and the evaluation of the autonomic nervous system.

In the sensory examination, most pain physicians are already familiar with the structure and function of the pathways for cold, touch, vibration, and each of the subsystems involved in the transmission and central processing of pain.[23] Exposure to a wide range of patients with pain symptoms allows physicians to understand that lesions that are irritative are liable to cause increased sensation to a specific modality, where lesions that are destructive without much irritation tend to cause decreased sensation. By applying various sensory stimuli to the skin, it is possible to map out regions of increased or decreased function and compare this with the standard body schema for cutaneous nerves, roots, or referred zones.[18,19] When the pattern suggests a specific nerve or pathway, then objective tests such as electromyography, nerve conduction studies,[38] and magnetic resonance imaging[39] can be ordered to confirm or refute the clinical impression.

After certain traumas, neural connections between peripheral, central, and automatic centers can become so irregular that severe, paroxysmal pain can follow a relatively mild stimulus (hyperpathia) or even a stimulus that ordinarily would not evoke any pain (allodynia). In most instances, these terrible pain experiences are part of one or more conditions in which nociceptive messages induced by minor injury do not resolve but in fact become part of a "vicious circle" where sympathetic efferent pathways, excited by the afferent signal to the spinal cord, provide positive feedback to the original focus of pain. This condition is variably known as sympathetically mediated pain or reflex sympathetic dystrophy syndrome.[40]

The dystrophic changes are based on abnormalities of growth, health and maintenance of the skin, hair, and cutaneous blood vessels that can occur within the painful territory. The location of such changes reflects the somatotopic distribution of the disrupted or irritated sympathetic efferent paths. The type of change observed in the skin is based upon which fibers are irritated or have been destroyed. For example, if sympathetic sudomotor fibers are irritated, the skin within this territory will be damper than the surrounding tissue because of increased local sweating.[41] If vasomotor fibers are also hyperactive, then their constrictive effects can create cool, pale, or mottled skin on the affected limb. On the other hand, complete destructive lesions of sympathetic outflow paths with little or no irritation will result in warm, dry, and shiny skin on the affected area. In order to improve the evaluation of sympathetically mediated pain and reflex sympathetic dystrophy syndrome, Gibbons and Wilson developed a scoring method[42] that assigns values to clinical signs and symptoms, and the sum of those values determines the likelihood of a correct diagnosis. The clarity and simplicity of this system should result in widespread acceptance in clinical pain practice.

CLINICAL DIAGNOSTIC WORKUP

After the results of the pain history and the general and specialized physical examination have been documented, the medical record should contain enough data so that the physician can begin formulating a differential diagnosis list. Since this list only contains *possible* diagnostic impressions, the next logical step in the process would be to order objective tests that might confirm which of the listed elements represents the true cause of symptoms.

In general the diagnostic procedures used in any workup can be divided into three major categories: tests of structure (radiographic procedures), tests of somatic function (electrodiagnostic tests), and procedures to evaluate internal homeostasis (hematologic/biochemical laboratory tests).

The primary purpose of radiographic investigation for pain is to identify any structural pathology that may be causally related to the patient's symptoms. In current clinical practice, important radiography studies are so important that they are frequently among the first tests to be ordered in any medical workup. However, the number and technical complexity of diagnostic imaging procedures currently applicable to pain evaluation deserve a more detailed discussion than can be presented fairly in this chapter. Therefore the reader is referred to earlier reviews[39,43,44] and subsequent sections within this volume.

In addition to tests of structure, somatic function within the neuromuscular system must be assessed relative to either the cause or effect of any underlying painful condition. Regardless of the neurologic pathophysiologic mechanisms, sensorimotor functions can only be objectively assessed using electrodiagnostic or clinical neurophysiologic tests. For a description of these procedures, refer to later sections of this text and other external reviews.[38,41,45]

Medical laboratory investigation of clinical pain problems serves three purposes: first, the more general tests can be helpful in detecting abnormalities of hematologic, biochemical, and metabolic or endocrine function that are commonly associated with the production of pain. Second, these tests can reveal early or unsuspected dysfunction in a previously asymptomatic system. Since early detection of any disease process may result in more effective treatment, this serendipitous effect is usually beneficial. Third, it is important to establish the functional integrity of hepatic and renal systems, since both systems are essential in the biochemical breakdown and elimination of most pharmacologic agents used for the treatment of pain. Early laboratory detection of compromise within hepatic or renal systems can often prevent potentially hazardous reactions to common pharmacologic agents.

Specific reviews of the medical laboratory assessment of the patient with pain have been reported by Kennedy and Longmire.[46] In addition, most classic textbooks of general or internal medicine, surgery, or pediatrics provide instructions for using laboratory studies to evaluate an immense range of clinical syndromes, where pain is the major symptom.

Nevertheless, there are some basic principles by which laboratory results may be documented specifically as they relate to pain management.

The first request for medical laboratory data, regardless of the putative clinical diagnosis, should be for past laboratory results, particularly those that are most recent. The information gained from this action is invaluable. Obtaining current results of investigations performed elsewhere can often reduce costs associated with repeating tests unnecessarily. Comparing recent results with those obtained at the initial visit can also reflect trends of improvement or worsening of a subclinical state that may require urgent treatment.

If medical laboratory results are urgently needed, there may not be time to wait for earlier records. Nevertheless, ordering new laboratory tests must be performed thoughtfully and cautiously to avoid erroneous assumptions about their validity. For example, the individual values obtained in any biochemical profile are analogous to the elements found in a still photograph of a team sports event. Specifically, the laboratory data provided by a single sample can only reflect individual serum levels present at that particular moment. Even when allowing for normal diurnal variations, the results obtained from a single blood sample cannot adequately represent the dynamic interactions of internal homeostasis.

One common method of laboratory assessment in clinical algology is based on applying standard tests in a manner that will confirm or refute the presence of certain possible etiologic mechanisms that may create pain. When the results support the clinical differential diagnosis, this approach may vindicate the physician's assessment. Although many schools of medical education frown on using abbreviations as learning aids, the "VINDICATE" mnemonic has become popular in pain medicine. Based upon the organization of the first letters of common pain etiologies, this mnemonic reminds the physician of possible pathophysiologic processes for which laboratory or other investigations should be ordered.

1. "V" stands for virus, as an example of infection by any agent, including bacteria or fungus. A complete blood count (CBC) is usually obtained and can emphasize total white cell count and differential analysis. This is especially important when determining whether infective processes are caused by a virus or bacteria. Although any bacterial infection can cause significant pain, one example of a common local virus is associated with herpes zoster and is known for its severe clinical state, known as *postherpetic neuralgia*. Widespread pain caused by viral disease is noted in acquired immunodeficiency syndrome (AIDS). With bacterial involvement, it is not uncommon to have craniofacial pains caused by sinus and other upper respiratory or dental infections, or colicky visceral pain caused by GI infections. In addition to

blood profiles and smears, blood cultures are often required.

2. "I" (inflammation). Although many arthritides degenerate joints and irritate surrounding tissue, most laboratory values associated with such conditions only reflect the primary cause of inflammation (infection, tissue damage). However, there are many vasculopathies, neuropathies, and arthropathies that create changes in the erythrocyte sedimentation rate (ESR) and white blood cell count. Specific tests for connective tissue and rheumatologic disorders and human leukocyte antigen (HLA) profiles are also applicable.

3. "N" (neoplasia). Many diagnostic tests used to confirm the presence of neoplastic disease rely on changes in structure so that a radiologic assessment of pain is necessary. To read about the radiologic procedure for pain and for a more multifaceted approach to the evaluation and treatment of cancer pain, see references on p. 34.[39,43,44,47]

4. "D" (degenerative). Connective tissue profile, ESR, biochemical profile for abnormal release of specific intracellular enzymes into the blood stream, and specific assays can assess hereditary or progressive destruction of neural parenchyma.[48]

5. "I" (ischemia) or hypoxemia. These etiologies are often considered together since both can create neural hyperexcitability and clinical pain when oxygen supply to tissues is inadequate. A CBC with special interest in hemoglobin, red cell count and indices, arterial blood gases, and lipid profile, can provide evidence to indicate ischemia caused by reduced vascular lumen and atherosclerotic disease.

6. "C" (congenital). Chromosome studies, serum and urinary protein abnormalities, and detailed amino-acid profiles may help to determine certain genetic diseases. However, certain inborn errors of metabolism may result in delayed neurologic development with aberrant pain and sensory processing, which, if severe, can be associated with autonomous behavior.[49]

7. "A" (autoimmune). HLA antigen/antibody studies, host-response cellular changes, protein metabolism, and molecular structural properties of those amino-acid sequences that infer antigenic properties are all specialized tests often available only at tertiary centers. The effects of demyelinating phenomena are felt to be the result of these mechanisms and are frequently a collective cause of neuropathic pain or painful paresthesias.[50]

8. "T" (trauma). The admixture of ischemia (from traumatic disruption of circulation) with inflammation, enzyme induction and release, and direct partial injury to exposed nerve endings can accompany the pain of acute somatic insult. Delwaide,[51] Critchley,[52] and Windebank[53] described the painful toxic neuropathies and laboratory investigations for alcohol, drugs, and chemical toxins.

9. "E" (endocrine/metabolic). The relative levels of certain hormones appear to be associated with the general excitability of neural tissue and sensory receptors.[54] Although laboratory values for thyroid function, for example, may be borderline or only minimally abnormal, there is sufficient evidence to suggest that correction of even minor deficiencies can improve pain control.

Ordinarily, painful sensory disorders are associated with abnormalities of glucose metabolism, but abnormally low levels may be implicated as much as the elevated levels seen chronically in diabetes mellitus. In fact, transient hypoglycemia is as important in the provocation of acute recurrent headache and craniofacial pain as the serum hyperglycemia (and tissue hypoglycemia) seen in painful diabetic neuropathy.

Serum electrolyte variations, particularly hypokalemia, are often empirically associated with increased clinical pain that abates with treatment. Similarly, other deficiency syndromes can provide chronic insidious neural changes that do not express themselves severely until the functional reserve for those pathways is exceeded.

As noted previously, some laboratory results can be helpful in confirming the etiologic diagnosis of certain painful disorders. Nevertheless, many pathophysiologic processes can be verified only after obtaining data from many tests (radiologic, neurophysiologic/electrodiagnostic, and laboratory) and adding those results to the pain history and findings from the physical examination.

SUMMARY

In this generation of clinical practice, it is no longer adequate to record the specific elements of the medical history and physical examination that led to the initial differential diagnosis. Today physicians must document in great detail all observations, interpretive mental processes, and physical or treatment interventions that were performed or even considered on behalf of each patient. For many primary care practitioners and specialists, the time required to manually record all essential positive and negative data at each patient encounter is sufficiently prohibitive to reduce the patient access to these physicians. Obviously this effect would negate the efforts of agencies at administrative levels to increase the availability of health care services to the public.

Fortunately, professional societies and collaborative pain management centers currently support the systematic style of collecting health data and performing treatment outcome analysis. Perhaps in the future this style of data collection may serve as a model for the basic medical evaluation of many other nonpainful conditions.

REFERENCES

1. Bonica JJ: History of pain concepts and therapies. In Bonica JJ, editor: *The Management of Pain,* ed 2. Philadelphia, Lea & Febiger, 1990.
2. Chen ACN: Human brain measures of clinical pain: A review. I. Topographic mappings. *Pain* 54:115-132, 1993.
3. Bonica JJ: Multidisciplinary/interdisciplinary pain programs. In Bonica JJ, editor: *The Management of Pain,* ed 2. Philadelphia, Lea & Febiger, 1990.
4. MacBryde CM, Blacklow RS: *Signs and Symptoms,* ed 6. Philadelphia, JB Lippincott, 1983.
5. Judge RD, Zuidema GD, Fitzgerald FT: *Clinical Diagnosis.* Boston, Little, Brown, 1988.

6. Longmire DR: The classification of pain and pain syndromes. *Pain Digest* 2:229-233, 1992.
7. Merskey H: Classification of chronic pain, descriptions of chronic pain syndromes and definitions of pain terms. *Pain Suppl* 3:229-233, 1986.
8. DeGowin EL, DeGowin RL: *Bedside Diagnostic Examination,* ed 5. New York, Macmillan, 1991.
9. Bouchier IAD, Morris JS: *Clinical Skills: A System of Clinical Examination,* ed 2. London, WB Saunders, 1982.
10. Maciewicz R, Martin JB: Pain: Pathophysiology and Management. In Wilson JD, Braunwald E, Isselbacher KJ et al, editors: *Harrison's Principles and Practice of Internal Medicine, vol 1,* ed 12. New York, McGraw-Hill, 1991.
11. Spence AA: Relieving acute pain. *Br J Anaesth* 52:245-246, 1980.
12. Rawal N: Postoperative pain and its management. In Raj PP, editor: *Practical Management of Pain,* ed 2. St. Louis, Mosby, 1992.
13. Raj PP: History and physical examination of the pain patient. In Raj PP, editor: *Practical Management of Pain,* ed 2. St. Louis, Mosby, 1992.
14. Bonica JJ, Loeser JD: Medical evaluation of the patient with pain. In Bonica JJ, editor: *The Management of Pain,* ed 2. Philadelphia, Lea & Febiger, 1991.
15. Longmire DR: The medical pain history. *Pain Digest* 1:29-33, 1991.
16. Longmire DR: The physical examination: Methods and application in the clinical evaluation of pain. *Pain Digest* 1:136-143, 1991.
17. O'Brien JP: Mechanisms of spinal pain. In Wall PD, Melzack R, editors: *Textbook of Pain.* Edinburgh, Churchill Livingstone, 1984.
18. Foerster O: The dermatomes in man. *Brain* 56:1-39, 1933.
19. Head H: On disturbances of sensation with special reference to the pain of visceral disease. *Brain* 16:1-132, 1983.
20. Melzack R: The McGill Pain Questionnaire. Major properties and scoring methods. *Pain* 1:275-299, 1975.
21. Margolis RB, Tait RC, Krause SJ: A rating system for use with patient pain drawings. *Pain* 24:57-65, 1986.
22. Melzack R, Torgerson WS: On the language of pain. *Anesthesiology* 34:50-59, 1971.
23. Fields H: *Pain.* New York, McGraw-Hill, 1987.
24. Gracely RH: Methods of testing pain mechanisms in normal man. In Wall PD, Melzack R, editors: *Textbook of Pain.* Edinburgh, Churchill Livingstone, 1989.
25. Jenson MP, Karoly P: Self-report scales and procedures for assessing pain in adults. In Turk DC, Melzack R, editors: *Handbook of Pain Assessment.* New York, Guilford Press, 1992.
26. Melzack R, Katz J: The McGill Pain Questionnaire: Appraisal and current status. In Turk DC, Melzack R, editors: *Handbook of Pain Assessment.* New York, Guilford Press, 1992.
27. Hill CS Jr: Oral opioid analgesics. In Patt RB, editor: *Cancer Pain.* Philadelphia, JB Lippincott, 1993.
28. Portenoy RK: Inadequate outcome of opioid therapy for cancer pain: Influences on practitioners and patients. In Patt RB, editor: *Cancer Pain.* Philadelphia, JB Lippincott, 1993.
29. Fishbain DA, Goldberg M, Rosomoff RS: Homicide-suicide and chronic pain. *Clin J Pain* 5:275-277, 1989.
30. Craig KD, Prkachkin KM, Grunau KM: The facial expression of pain. In Turk DC, Melzack R, editors: *Handbook of Pain Assessment.* New York, Guilford Press, 1992.
31. Craig KD: Emotional aspects of pain. In Wall PD, Melzack R, editors: *Textbook of Pain.* London, Churchill Livingstone, 1984.
32. Waddell G, McCulloch JA, Kummell E et al: Nonorganic physical signs in low back pain. *Spine* 5:117-125, 1980.
33. Hoppenfeld S: *Physical Examination of the Spine and Extremities.* New York, Appleton Century Crofts, 1976.
34. Travell J, Simons DG: *Myofascial Pain and Dysfunction: The Trigger Point Manual.* Baltimore, Williams & Wilkins, 1983.
35. Hoppenfeld S: *Orthopedic Neurology: A Diagnostic Guide to Neurologic Level.* Philadelphia, JB Lippincott, 1977.
36. Waddell G, Turk DC: Clinical assessment of low back pain. In Turk DC, Melzack R, editors: *Handbook of Pain Assessment.* New York, Guilford Press, 1992.
37. Polatin PB, Mayer TG: Quantification of function in chronic low back pain. In Turk DC, Melzack R, editors: *Handbook of Pain Assessment.* New York, Guilford Press, 1992.
38. Longmire D: Electrodiagnostic studies in the assessment of painful disorders. *Pain Digest* 3:116-120, 1993.
39. Leak WD: Radiologic assessment of chronic pain. *Pain Digest* 2:63-67, 1992.
40. Stanton-Hicks M d'A: Blocks of the sympathetic nervous system. In Stanton-Hicks M d'A, editor: *Pain and the Sympathetic Nervous System. Current Management of Pain.* Boston, Kluwer Academic Publishers, 1990.
41. Longmire DR: Clinical neurophysiology of pain-related sympathetic sudomotor dysfunction. *Pain Digest,* 3:202, 1993.
42. Gibbons JJ, Wilson PR: RSD score: Criteria for the diagnosis of reflex sympathetic dystrophy and causalgia. *Clin J Pain* 8:260-263, 1992.
43. Group M, Stanton-Hicks M: Neuroanatomy and pathophysiology of pain related to spinal disorders. *Radiol Clin North Am* 29:665-673, 1991.
44. Lowry PA: Radiology in the diagnosis and management of pain. In Raj PP, editor: *Practical Management of Pain,* ed 2. St. Louis, Mosby, 1992.
45. Roongta SM: Electromyography. In Raj PP, editor: *Practical Management of Pain,* ed 2. St. Louis, Mosby, 1992.
46. Kennedy LD, Longmire DR: Medical/laboratory evaluation of pain patients. *Pain Digest* 1:306-311, 1992.
47. Patt RB: *Cancer Pain.* Philadelphia, JB Lippincott, 1993.
48. Cherry S, Mayer RF: Hereditary neuropathy and liability to pressure palsies. In Vinken PJ, Bruyn GW, Klawans HL et al, editors: *Neuropathies. Handbook of Clinical Neurology, Rev Series 7.* Amsterdam, Elsevier, 1987.
49. Moffie D: Congenital insensitivity to pain. In Vinken PJ, Bruyn GW, Klawans HL et al, editors: *Neuropathies. Handbook of Clinical Neurology, Rev Series 7.* Amsterdam, Elsevier, 1987.
50. Dyck PJ, Arnason BGW: Chronic inflammatory demyelinating polyradiculoneuropathy. In Dyck PH, Thomas PK, Lambert EH et al, editors: *Peripheral Neuropathy.* Philadelphia, WB Saunders, 1984.
51. Delwaide PJ: Alcoholic neuropathy. In Vinken PJ, Bruyn GW, Klawans HL et al, editors: *Neuropathies. Handbook of Clinical Neurology, Rev Series 7.* Amsterdam, Elsevier, 1987.
52. Critchley EMR: Neuropathies due to drugs. In Vinken PJ, Bruyn GW, Klawans HL et al, editors: *Neuropathies. Handbook of Clinical Neurology, Rev Series 7.* Amsterdam, Elsevier, 1987.
53. Windebank AJ: Peripheral neuropathy due to chemical and industrial exposure. In Vinken PJ, Bruyn GW, Klawans HL et al, editors: *Neuropathies. Handbook of Clinical Neurology, Rev Series 7.* Amsterdam, Elsevier, 1987.
54. Hogenhuis LAH: Endocrine polyneuropathies. In Vinken PJ, Bruyn GW, Klawans HL et al, editors: *Neuropathies. Handbook of Clinical Neurology, Rev Series 7.* Amsterdam, Elsevier, 1987.

QUESTIONS: EVALUATION OF THE PAIN PATIENT

1. Within the medical history, limitations of activity created by painful disorders are often recorded as part of the:
   A. Chief complaint
   B. Systems review
   C. Past medical history
   D. Social occupational history
2. Data that should be collected by inspection early in the physical examination includes:
   A. Observations of facial expression
   B. The patient's comments regarding weakness
   C. Results of upper- and lower-extremity reflexes
   D. Skin texture at sites of sympathetic dystrophy
3. Components for Waddell's signs of nonorganic low back pain behavior include tests of:
   A. Axial loading
   B. Hip rotation
   C. Skin pinch
   D. Heel-shin coordination
4. Which of the following tests of sensory function usually provides the most clinically relevant information regarding radicular pain?
   A. Application of cold and/or warm stimuli
   B. Presence of graphesthesia
   C. Pin and/or point stimulation
   D. Vibration and/or positions assessment
5. A history of being "allergic" to a specific analgesic medication should be checked to determine whether the symptoms that occurred following ingestion represented:
   A. An unexpected bitter taste
   B. A common unpleasant side effect
   C. Reduced efficacy of the medicine
   D. A potentially serious adverse reaction

ANSWERS

1. D
2. A
3. C
4. A
5. B

4 Pain Measurement*

Marc A. Valley

Modern medicine is based upon the treatment of disease processes; treatment is guided by the appropriate interpretation of test results. This is true in the evaluation and treatment of patients with pain syndromes. However, patients with pain also often have concurrent psychologic overlays, either secondary to or in conjunction with the pain syndrome. These psychologic overlays affect both the selection and interpretation of tests used to evaluate pain. The purpose of this chapter is to introduce the reader to a variety of the most commonly used pain assessment tools, describe the mechanics of their administration and interpretation, and critique their advantages and disadvantages. The second part of this chapter presents a model for determining what assessment tool to use and discusses some concerns about specific syndromes and situations.

PATIENT SELF-REPORT USING A SINGLE DIMENSION PAIN SCALE

The most commonly used assessment tools for pain are based upon patient self-reporting and involve only a single dimension (Box 4-1). These single dimension pain scales are easy for the patient to use and understand and are relatively inexpensive. The primary limitations of the single dimension scales are that they risk oversimplifying a patient's pain syndrome and can potentially lose validity with haphazard and careless administration.

Verbal descriptor scales

Verbal descriptor scales use a standard set of five to seven words as pain descriptors. Melzack and Torgerson[1] introduced the following five-word scale that is often used: "Mild, Discomforting, Distressing, Horrible, Excruciating." The major concern with this test was that it was open ended. The problem was remedied when Aitken[2] added defined endpoints, "no pain" and "unendurable." This type of scale allows for standardized descriptors and correlates with the visual analog scale (VAS) in many situations,[3] while potentially being more useful in experimental pain situations than VAS.[4] In addition, more patients may be able to complete the verbal descriptor scale than the VAS or numerical scales.[5]1

The disadvantages of the verbal descriptor scale include: limited number of possible responses and the scale is non-continuous so that the use of nonparametric statistics for analysis is required, which potentially makes this scale weaker than the VAS.[6]

Numerical pain scales

The numerical pain scale is an ordinal method of assessing pain using an 11-point scale where "0" = "no pain" and "10" = "most excruciating pain imaginable." The advantages of this scale are: no special training is required to administer it, it gives consistent and reproducible measurements, it allows for interpatient assessment and the changes within a patient during treatment,[7,8] and this scale may be a better assessment of remembered chronic pain.[9] The numerical pain scale can be used in small children with poker chips representing "pieces of hurt" that are added together to equal the child's pain.[10] A disadvantage of the numerical pain scale is that it can be statistically weak because of the required nonparametric analysis; however, this is probably clinically insignificant.

Visual analog scale

The VAS is a progression of the numerical pain scale that allows for continuous data analysis and uses a 10 cm line with 0 ("no pain") on one end and 10 ("worst pain") on the other end. Patients are asked to place a mark along the line to denote their level of pain. The VAS can be used with a variety of mechanical devices and computer programs to allow for consistent results and to minimize observer bias.[11] The primary advantage of the VAS is that it can give valid data for chronic and experimental pain that can be assessed parametrically.[12-14] However, other studies have questioned its validity when it is used to measure retrospective pain scores[15] or assess treatment efficacy.[16] A second concern is that some patients, especially the elderly, may not be able to complete the scale. Studies have shown that 11% to 26% of patients could not complete the VAS or found it confusing.[5,17] A third concern is that the VAS can be derived from other scores or that the VAS can be modified to a 5 cm scale in order to somehow facilitate its use. Neither derivation or modification has proven reliable.[18,19]

Other single dimension pain scales

Numerous variations of the numeric scale exist: the 11-point box scale (the numbers 0 through 10 are placed in individual boxes and patients are instructed to mark out the box that best corresponds to their pain); the 101-point numerical rating scale (patients are instructed to write the number between 0 and 100 that best describes their pain); and the four-point and five-point verbal rating scale. These methods have similar accuracy and validity to the VAS.[20] A problem com-

*The views expressed in this article are those of the author and do not reflect the official policy of the Department of Defense or other Departments of the United States Government.

Box 4-1 SINGLE DIMENSION PAIN SCALES

---

1. **Verbal descriptor scale:**
   Instructions: From the list below, choose the word that best describes your present pain level.
   (   )Mild
   (   )Discomforting
   (   )Distressing
   (   )Horrible
   (   )Excruciating

2. **Behavioral rating scale (BRS-6):**
   (   )No pain
   (   )Pain present, but can easily be ignored
   (   )Pain present, cannot be ignored but does not interfere with everyday activities
   (   )Pain present, cannot be ignored, interferes with concentration
   (   )Pain present, cannot be ignored, interferes with all tasks except taking care of basic needs such as toileting and eating
   (   )Pain present, cannot be ignored, rest or bedrest required

3. **Simple numerical rating scale:**
   Instructions: Choose a number from 0 to 10 to indicate how strong your pain is right now.
   0 = No pain at all 1 2 3 4 5 6 7 8 9 10 = Worst pain imaginable

4. **Numerical rating scale (NRS-101):**
   Instructions: Indicate on the line below the number between 0 and 100 which indicates how strong your pain is right now. A zero (0) would mean "no pain" and a hundred (100) would mean "Worst Pain imaginable."

   ———————

5. **Point box scale (BS-11):**
   Instructions: Zero (0) means "no pain" and ten (10) means "Worst Pain imaginable" on this scale of 0 to 10. Place an "X" through the number that best represents your pain level.
   0   1   2   3   4   5   6   7   8   9   10

6. **Visual analog scale (VAS):**
   Instructions: Place a mark on the following line to show the intensity of pain that you are feeling.
   No Pain_____Worst Pain

7. **Pain relief scale:**
   Instructions: Make a mark on the line below to indicate the amount of relief you feel from your pain right now as compared to yesterday.
   No Relief_____Complete Relief

---

mon to all numerical and descriptive pain scales is that they rely on the intact language skills of an intelligent patient. Facial drawings (Fig. 4-1) are reliable markers of pain designed specifically for use with children, the mentally handicapped, or patients with poor language skills.[21]

PATIENT SELF-REPORT USING A MULTIDIMENSIONAL PAIN SCALE

Single dimension pain evaluation is probably the most commonly used method of evaluation in the pain clinic. However, if more than one dimension (intensity, duration, therapeutic efficacy, etc.) is desired, patients should be blinded to their previous VAS ratings,[16] or the data obtained is suspect. In addition, pain has a motivational-affective dimension that may not be appropriately measured on a single dimension assessment scale.[22] To overcome this limitation, multidimensional assessment tools were created to simultaneously evaluate multiple pain parameters. The McGill Pain Questionnaire (MPQ) and its derivatives are the major tools within this category.

McGill Pain Questionnaire

The MPQ[23] (Fig. 4-2) was developed in 1975 by Melzack and colleagues at McGill University in an attempt to organize pain descriptors into a comprehensive evaluative tool.[24,25] It consists of three major measures: (1) pain rating index, which is based on the numerical score assigned to the descriptors; (2) total number of words chosen; and (3) the present pain intensity, which is a modification of the single dimension, five-point verbal descriptive scale that is used to evaluate the intensity of pain at the time of completing the questionnaire. The present pain intensity should be considered when evaluating the pain rating index because the present intensity of pain modifies the patient's memory of past pain.[26] The major strength of the MPQ is the pain rating index which is also an area of controversy.

The pain rating index is an organized list of words divided into subcategories of related words, which are rated on a common-intensity scale.[1] By evaluating the patient's responses (the number of words chosen) and the total score based upon each subclass's intensity scale, it is possible to compare diagnosis and treatment in patients with varied pain syndromes. The pain rating index section of the MPQ has been used in a variety of clinical settings including dentistry,[27] postoperative pain and complications,[28] low back pain evaluation,[29] and obstetric pain.[30]

The major sections in the pain rating index are designed to assess the three components of pain postulated by the gate control theory: the sensory, the affective, and the evaluative dimensions. The subclasses of the pain rating index have been found to be reliable and valid measures of pain under diverse conditions.[24,25,31] However, there has been concern that a composite numerical pain rating index (derived from the ten subscale scores) may not adequately discriminate patients[32,33] and whether there is one sensory component[24,34] or two.[32] These considerations are beyond the scope of this chapter.

A major modification of the MPQ occurred when the short form MPQ[35] was introduced by Melzack in 1987 (Fig. 4-3). The major advantage of this questionnaire is in its simplicity and ease of use while it correlates well with the full MPQ. To simplify the administration of the MPQ, give it by interview.[36] The MPQ has been translated into a variety of different languages[37-39] and has been modified to incorporate somatic interventions and changes in patient self-esteem.[40]

Other multidimensional pain scales

Numerous multidimensional inventories have been created to assess general chronic pain patients and specific pain syndromes. These inventories are, in general, modifications of the MPQ or Minnesota Multiphasic Personality Inventory

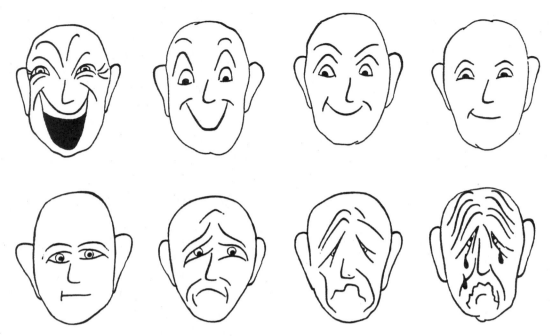

Fig. 4-1 Facial pain expressions. (From Frank AJM, Moll LMH, Hort JF: A comparison of three ways of measuring pain. *Rheumatology and Rehabilitation* 21:211-217, 1982.)

(MMPI), and possess the strengths and weaknesses of those inventories. Table 4-1 lists a representative sample of these inventories and their uses.

PSYCHOLOGIC AND BEHAVIORAL ASSESSMENT TOOLS

A major premise in the evaluation of pain is the assumption that pain can be evaluated using a disease process model. With this model, the patient's cognitive assessment of pain is consistent with physical findings and single dimension or multidimensional self-assessment tools are used for pain measurement. However, this premise may not be valid in all patients. In situations where the physical findings are absent or are insufficient to explain the extent of the patient's pain syndrome, behavioral analysis is indicated.[41] When monitoring pain behavior, the operant conditioning that may have taken place is a major consideration. For example, in patients who benefit from being in pain, physical findings may be exaggerated. Conversely, physical behavior may be blunted in stoic patients. The analysis of pain behavior can be accomplished by observing the patient's physical activity, measuring medication intake, or evaluating the patient's pain diary or pain drawing.

Observation of the pain patient

The most common method of determining the behavioral component of a patient's pain is direct observation. A primary requirement for behavioral observation is a consistent exam that considers the potential psychologic pathology of the patient[41] and potential future therapeutic interventions.[42] Numerous paradigms have been developed for assessment in adults[43,44] and in children.[45] All paradigms rate the occurrence and frequency of response to various activi-

ties such as walking, working, eating, and sex. Particular attention must be given to the affected region. Keefe and co-workers[46] found that patients with head and neck cancer predominantly showed facial motion (e.g., spasms, grimacing, twisting) and not global manifestations of their pain. Keefe and Hill[47] and others combined observation with direct physical measurement of body motion.

The physician will typically assess the history and physical exam and then categorize the patient by using a rank-ordered scheme such as no pain or minimal, mild, or severe pain. Other physicians classify patients using a four-category system,[48] where Class 1 consists of patients with low organic and high behavioral determinants, Class 2 patients have low organic and low behavioral determinants, Class 3 patients have high organic and high behavioral determinants, and Class 4 patients have a predominantly organic component to their pain. However, there are several weaknesses with this classification.[49] First, pain cannot be observed; it can only be inferred from observed actions. Second, rater bias based on the patient's sex, age, weight, or race can affect the rating. Finally, these ratings are judgments, not true pain measurements. The use of multiple raters may partially alleviate these weaknesses.

Pain diary

To assess pain behavior outside the clinical setting, various types of pain diaries have been used. Diaries assess nocturnal variation of the pain, factors that may aggravate or diminish it, and the effect of pain on activity and mobility. Pain diaries may be used independently[50] or in conjunction with other psychologic and self-assessment tools.[51] A potential weakness of the pain diary is that it may not correspond to what the medical staff observes.[52]

McGill-Melzack
PAIN QUESTIONNAIRE

Patient's name _____ Age _____

File No. _____ Date _____

Clinical category (e.g. cardiac, neurological, etc.):

_____

Diagnosis: _____

_____

Analgesic (if already administered):

1. Type _____
2. Dosage _____
3. Time given in relation to this test _____

Patient's intelligence: circle number that represents best estimate

1 (low)   2   3   4   5 (high)

****

This questionnaire has been designed to tell us more about your pain. Four major questions we ask are:

1. Where is your pain?
2. What does it feel like?
3. How does it change with time?
4. How strong is it?

It is important that you tell us how your pain feels now. Please follow the instructions at the beginning of each part.

© R. Melzack, Oct. 1970

Part 1.   Where is your Pain?

Please mark, on the drawings below, the areas where you feel pain. Put E if external, or I if internal, near the areas which you mark. Put EI if both external and internal.

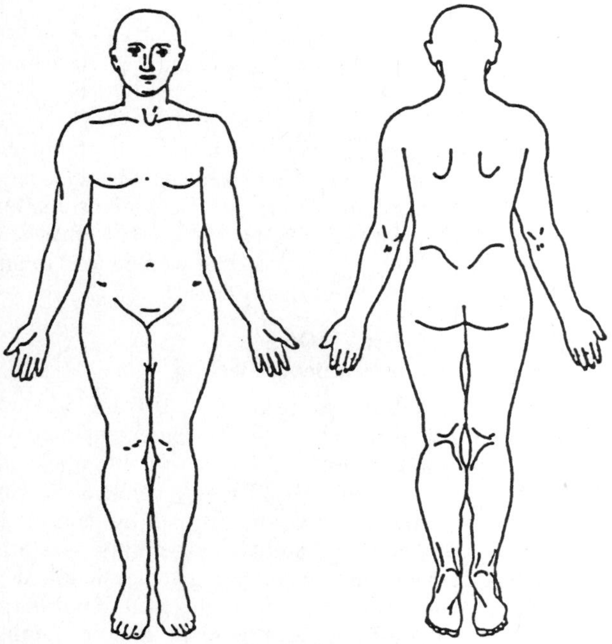

Part 2.   What Does Your Pain Feel Like?

Some of the words below describe your present pain. Circle ONLY those words that best describe it. Leave out any category that is not suitable. Use only a single word in each appropriate category—the one that applies best.

1	2	3	4
Flickering	Jumping	Pricking	Sharp
Quivering	Flashing	Boring	Cutting
Pulsing	Shooting	Drilling	Lacerating
Throbbing		Stabbing	
Beating		Lancinating	
Pounding			

5	6	7	8
Pinching	Tugging	Hot	Tingling
Pressing	Pulling	Burning	Itchy
Gnawing	Wrenching	Scalding	Smarting
Cramping		Searing	Stinging
Crushing			

9	10	11	12
Dull	Tender	Tiring	Sickening
Sore	Taut	Exhausting	Suffocating
Hurting	Rasping		
Aching	Splitting		
Heavy			

13	14	15	16
Fearful	Punishing	Wretched	Annoying
Frightful	Grueling	Blinding	Troublesome
Terrifying	Cruel		Miserable
	Vicious		Intense
	Killing		Unbearable

17	18	19	20
Spreading	Tight	Cool	Nagging
Radiating	Numb	Cold	Nauseating
Penetrating	Drawing	Freezing	Agonizing
Piercing	Squeezing		Dreadful
	Tearing		Torturing

Part 3.   How Does Your Pain Change With Time?

1. Which word or words would you use to describe the pattern of your pain?

1	2	3
Continuous	Rhythmic	Brief
Steady	Periodic	Momentary
Constant	Intermittent	Transient

2. What kind of things relieve your pain?

3. What kind of things increase your pain?

Part 4.   How Strong Is Your Pain?

People agree that the following 5 words represent pain of increasing intensity. They are:

1	2	3	4	5
Mild	Discomforting	Distressing	Horrible	Excruciating

To answer each question below, write the number of the most appropriate word in the space beside the question.

1. Which word describes your pain right now?   _____
2. Which word describes it at its worst?   _____
3. Which word describes it when it is least?   _____
4. Which word describes the worst toothache you ever had?   _____
5. Which word describes the worst headache you ever had?   _____
6. Which word describes the worst stomach-ache you ever had?   _____

Fig. 4-2 The McGill Pain Questionnaire. (From Melzack R: The McGill Pain Questionnaire: Major properties and scoring methods. *Pain* 1:277-299, 1971.)

Short-form McGill pain questionnaire
Ronald Melzack

Patient's name: _____ Date: _____

	None	Mild	Moderate	Severe
Throbbing	0) _____	1) _____	2) _____	3) _____
Shooting	0) _____	1) _____	2) _____	3) _____
Stabbing	0) _____	1) _____	2) _____	3) _____
Sharp	0) _____	1) _____	2) _____	3) _____
Cramping	0) _____	1) _____	2) _____	3) _____
Gnawing	0) _____	1) _____	2) _____	3) _____
Hot-burning	0) _____	1) _____	2) _____	3) _____
Aching	0) _____	1) _____	2) _____	3) _____
Heavy	0) _____	1) _____	2) _____	3) _____
Tender	0) _____	1) _____	2) _____	3) _____
Splitting	0) _____	1) _____	2) _____	3) _____
Tiring-exhausting	0) _____	1) _____	2) _____	3) _____
Sickening	0) _____	1) _____	2) _____	3) _____
Fearful	0) _____	1) _____	2) _____	3) _____
Punishing-cruel	0) _____	1) _____	2) _____	3) _____

PPI

No pain |———————————————| Worst possible pain

0 No pain   _____
1 Mild   _____
2 Discomforting   _____
3 Distressing   _____
4 Horrible   _____
5 Excruciating   _____

© R. Melzack, 1984

Fig. 4-3 The short form McGill Pain Questionnaire. Descriptors *1-11* represent the sensory dimension of pain experience, and *12-15* represent the affective dimension. Each descriptor is ranked on an intensity scale of 0 = none, 1 = mild, 2 = moderate, 3 = severe. The Present Pain Intensity of the standard long form McGill Pain Questionnaire (LF-MPQ) and VAS are also included to provide overall intensity scores. (From Melzack R: The short form McGill Pain Questionnaire. *Pain* 30:191-197, 1987.)

Pain drawing

A major source of information in assessing pain is the patient's graphical depiction of the pain (Fig. 4-4). These drawings help identify the location of the pain and the type of pain perceived at the various locations on the body. Pain drawings have been extensively used in patients with back pain.[53] Organic pain is represented by clearly defined areas that are logical results of potential pathology; for example, the demarcated lancinating pain in the legs that results from a herniated disc compressing a nerve root. Nonorganic pain, however, is characterized by diffuse, global, poorly defined patterns that are not a logical result of physical pathology. In addition to general patient assessment, specific findings are possible when these drawings are evaluated by physicians who routinely use them.[54] Recent developments have used computers in the production and analysis of pain drawings.[55]

Medication use

Another method of monitoring patient behavior is to document medication use either with the aid of the patient, or by enlisting the patient's family or a member of the medical staff. Ready et al.[56] found that chronic pain patients tend to underestimate their drug usage, and this underestimation occurred more often with narcotic analgesics than other pain medications. In addition, they found that women tend to underestimate drug usage more than men.

SPECIAL CONSIDERATIONS
Guidelines for test instrument selection

Before discussing specific pain situations, it is important to have an organized approach to the measurement of pain. Almost all patients can use at least one of the single dimension pain measurement tools. These tools are easily understood by the patient, easily administered by pain clinic staff, display appropriate reliability and validity, and produce results that can be used in assessing analgesic efficacy. Most patients can also understand the multidimensional tests, but their administration can be more time consuming than single dimension tests. Behavioral testing is appropriate in many patients, especially those with a possible functional component to their pain. Perry et al.[57] showed that

Table 4-1 Multidimensional pain assessment inventories

Name	Comments
Pain Disability Index[a]	Modified numeric pain scale which includes categories defining activity. Useful in assessing patient's function.
Neck Disability Index[b]	Modification of the pain disability index.
Dallas Pain Questionnaire[c]	16-item VAS with items describing activity, personal relationships, and emotional status. Used in assessing back pain.
West Haven-Yale Multidimensional Pain Inventory (WHYMPI)[d]	Psychometric inventory including personal assessment, perceptions of significant others' attitudes toward the patient, and responses to defined activities.
Illness Behavior Questionnaire (IBQ)[e]	Similar to MMPI, with seven scales: hypochondriasis, disease conviction, psychologic perception of illness, affective inhibition, affective disturbance, denial, irritability. Useful in assessing functional pain.
Western Ontario and McMaster (WOMAC) Osteoarthritis Index[f]	Specifically designed to assess osteoarthritis patients, this inventory consists of five dimensions: pain, stiffness, physical function, social function, and emotional function.
Descriptor Differential Scale (DDS)[g]	12-descriptor items (faint to extremely intense) for each dimension studied. Subject then marks on a 10-point scale whether perception is greater or less than each of the descriptors. This allows for easier scaling and intersubject evaluation. Usable for any chronic pain syndrome.
Wisconsin Brief Pain Questionnaire (WBPQ)[h]	Modified numeric pain scale measuring pain and therapy efficacy. Specifically designed for cancer pain but usable for any chronic syndrome.
Sickness Impact Profile[i,j]	Assesses functional status and correlates well with MMPI regarding emotional and affective condition of patient.
Abu-Saad Pediatric Pain Assessment Tool[k]	A modified MPQ for children. Written in Dutch.

[a]Tatt RC, Chibnall JT, Krause S: The Pain Disability Index: Psychometric properties. *Pain* 40:171-182, 1980.
[b]Vernon H, Mior S: The neck disability index: A study of reliability and validity. *J Manipulative Physiol Ther* 14:409-415, 1991.
[c]Lawlis GF et al: The development of the Dallas Pain Questionnaire: An assessment of the impact of spinal pain on behavior. *Spine* 14:511-516, 1989.
[d]Kerns RD, Turk DC, Rudy TE: The West Haven-Yale Multidimensional Pain Inventory (WHYMPI). *Pain* 23:345-356, 1985.
[e]Pilowsky I et al: The Illness Behavior Questionnaire as an aid to clinical assessment. *Gen Hosp Psychiatry* 6:123-130, 1984.
[f]Bellamy N: Pain assessment in osteoarthritis: Experience with the WOMAC Osteoarthritis Index. *Semin Arthritis Rheum* 18:14-17, 1989.
[g]Gracely RH, Kwilosz J: The Descriptor Differential Scale: Applying psychophysical principles to clinical pain assessment. *Pain* 35:279-288, 1988.
[h]Daut RL, Cleeland CS, Flanery RC: Development of the Wisconsin Brief Pain Questionnaire to assess pain in cancer and other diseases. *Pain* 17:197-210, 1983.
[i]Bergner M et al: The Sickness Impact Profile: Development and final revision of a health status measure. *Med Care* 19:787-805, 1981.
[j]Follick MJ, Smith TW, Ahern DK: The Sickness Impact Profile: A global measure of disability in chronic low back pain. *Pain* 21:67-76, 1985.
[k]Abu-Saad HH, Kroonen E, Halfens R: On the development of a multidimensional Dutch pain assessment tool for children. *Pain* 43:249-256, 1990.

patients with a poor correlation between the present pain intensity scale of the MPQ and VAS had a larger component of functional pain than patients with a close present pain intensity and VAS correlation. A sample algorithm[58] for pain evaluation is presented in Fig. 4-5.

Laboratory methods of pain management

Quantitative measurement of pain under laboratory conditions began a century ago with the psychometric studies of von Frey. Pain measurement in the laboratory consists of giving a defined, readily controlled stimulus. This stimulus should be conveniently applied, produce minimal tissue damage, closely associate with the changes that cause pain, and reproduce the quantitative measurements of the pain threshold under the same conditions.[59] The stimuli include controlled mechanical stimulation,[60] dolorimeters,[61] the algometer,[62] and CO_2 laser.[63] The major differences between laboratory and clinical pain measurement are as follows: (1) laboratory pain is usually acute, therefore the psychologic overlays present in patients with chronic pain do not play a major role; and (2) the subject understands that the pain will be limited and can be terminated at any time. Furthermore, these differences

make direct comparisons between laboratory data and clinical scenarios difficult.

Cancer pain

The evaluation of cancer pain remains a clinical problem. Cancer pain may have an insidious onset and is often due to many factors. In addition, the characteristics and intensity of the pain are dependent upon the type of pain (bone, musculoskeletal, neuropathic, or visceral). Often the patients are on narcotics and other medications that may affect their ability to communicate. Verbal rating scales, VAS, and the MPQ have been used but each has specific weaknesses.[64] Verbal rating scales and VAS only rate pain intensity and are not affective components; yet the MPQ is often misunderstood by the elderly and debilitated patients who make up this population. Because the VAS is easy to use, there have been attempts to improve it with some success.[65]

A major problem in the treatment of cancer pain remains in the lack of correlation between the patient's self-reporting and the assessment of clinical staff.[66,67] In two studies, the patient's pain was underestimated by nursing staff, physician staff, and family members which often resulted in poor pain control.

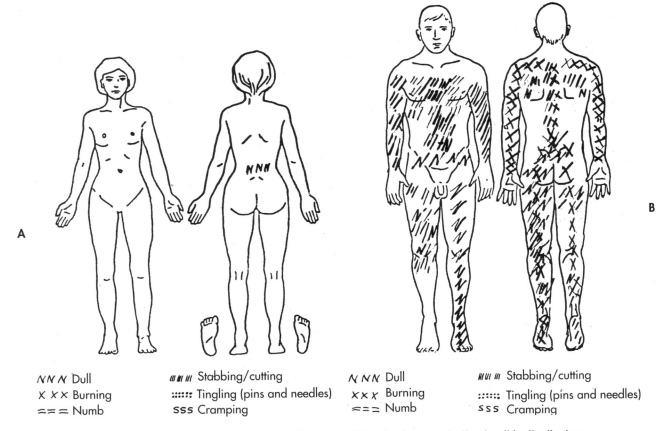

NNN Dull   ⫫⫫⫫ Stabbing/cutting
XXX Burning   :::::: Tingling (pins and needles)
≈≈≈ Numb   sss Cramping

NNN Dull   ⫫⫫⫫ Stabbing/cutting
XXX Burning   :::::: Tingling (pins and needles)
≈≈≈ Numb   sss Cramping

Fig. 4-4 A, An organic pain drawing. Note the well localized, anatomically plausible distribution of pain. **B,** A nonorganic pain drawing. Note the widespread, poorly defined pattern of pain distribution. (From Udén A, Åströmm M, Bergenudd H: Pain drawings in chronic back pain. *Spine* 13:389-392, 1988.)

Psychiatric pain

The psychiatric assessment of pain is an important but complicated part of the evaluation. However, its comprehensive review is beyond the scope of this chapter. As previously discussed, the diagnosis of functional pain should be entertained if there is disparity between the patient's VAS and the present pain intensity section of the MPQ.[57] In addition, certain psychiatric diseases may present with pain: hypochondriasis, depression, and occasionally, psychosis.[68,69] Therefore, in patients with a possibility of psychiatric illness, it is appropriate to obtain psychiatric consultation and to administer the MMPI and other psychiatric assessment tests.

Geriatric pain

A recent study found that approximately 80% of patients in nursing homes complain of pain.[70] The assessment of pain in this population can be complicated by communication difficulties resulting from stroke or dementia and confusion with the instructions for the commonly used assessment tools.[71] These patients often do better with simple tests such as a numerical rating scale, especially when given by interview. In addition, many of these patients are on numerous medications for other medical illnesses, which may cause a change in mental acuity that may also limit the assessment of their pain.

Pediatric pain

Over the last two decades dramatic progress has been made in the assessment of pediatric pain. It is now known that even neonates experience pain.[72] A child's perception of pain is based upon the following factors: sex, age, cognitive level, previous experience of pain, family learning, and culture. Before understanding and completing a VAS, observed behavior (crying, nervousness, grimacing, etc.) is the major assessment tool. Older children can be tested with the modified MPQ and the VAS. For younger children, the faces pain scale is used,[21,73] which is a modification of the numerical rating scale. However, a major limitation in the assessment of pediatric pain, like that of cancer pain, is the poor correlation between patient self-assessment and observer ratings.[74] Manne and colleagues[75] found that nurses' ratings were based upon overt distress, whereas parents' ratings were based upon the parents' subjective perception of the child's pain. The child's ability to rate pain, as mentioned previously, was based upon cognitive level.

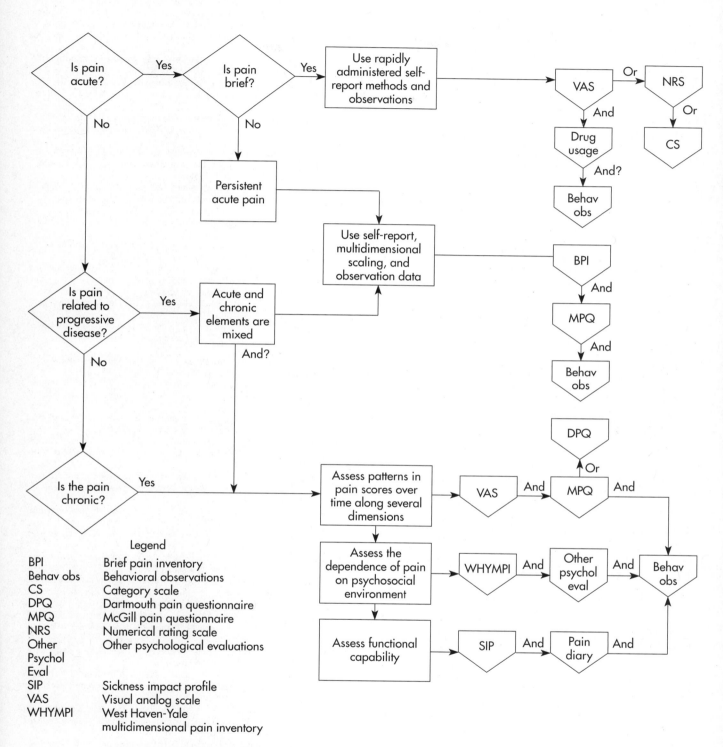

Fig. 4-5 Algorithm for selection of pain measurement instruments. (From Chapman CR, Syrjala KL: Measurement of pain. In Bonica JJ, editor: *The Management of Pain,* ed 2. Philadelphia, 1990, Lea & Febiger.)

SUMMARY

This chapter describes a variety of pain assessment tools and gives an organized approach to determine which test to use in specific situations. However, pain ratings per se cannot be used as an endpoint; clinical correlation and individualized treatment must be used. Remember to *act* on what you learn; this is all that really matters.

REFERENCES

1. Melzack R, Torgerson WS: On the language of pain. *Anesthesiology* 34:50-59, 1971.
2. Aitken RCB: Measurement of feelings using visual analog scales. *Proc Soc Lond [Biol]* 62:17-24, 1969.
3. Woodfore JM, Merskey H: Correlation between verbal scale and visual analogue scale and pressure algometer. *J Psychom Res* 16:173-178, 1971.
4. Duncan GH, Bushnell MC, Lavigne GJ: Comparison of verbal and visual analogue scales for measuring the intensity and unpleasantness of experimental pain. *Pain* 37:295-303, 1989.
5. Kremer E, Atkinson JH, Ignelzi RJ: Measurement of pain: Patient preference does not confound pain measurement. *Pain* 10:241-248, 1981.
6. Ohnhaus EE, Adler R: Methodological problems in the measurement of pain: A comparison between the verbal rating scale and the visual analog scale. *Pain* 1:379-384, 1975.
7. Ferraz MB et al: Reliability of pain scales in the assessment of literate and illiterate patients with rheumatoid arthritis. *J Rheumatol* 17:1022-1024, 1990.
8. Joos E et al: Reliability and reproducibility of visual analog scale and numeric rating scale for therapeutic evaluation of pain in rheumatic patients. *J Rheumatol* 18:1269-1270, 1991 (letter).
9. Linten SJ, Götestam KG: A clinical comparison of two pain scales: Correlation, remembering chronic pain, and a measure of compliance. *Pain* 17:57-65, 1983.
10. Mackey D, Jordan-Marsh M: Pediatric update: Innovative assessment of children's pain. *J Emergency Nursing* 17:250-251, 1991.
11. Spens H, Pugh GC: Measurement of VAS pain scores with a 'magic screen.' *Anaesthesia* 47:359-360, 1992 (letter).
12. Price DD et al: The validation of visual analog scales as ratio scale measures for chronic and experimental pain. *Pain* 17:45-56, 1983.
13. Phillip BK: Parametric statistics for evaluation of the visual analog scale. *Anesth Analg* 71:708-713, 1990 (letter).
14. Flandry F et al: Analysis of subjective knee complaints using visual analog scales. *Am J Sports Med* 19:112-118, 1991.
15. Lui WHD, Aitkenhead AR: Comparison of contemporaneous and retrospective assessment of postoperative pain using the visual analog scale. *Br J Anaesth* 67:768-771, 1991.
16. Carlsson AM: Assessment of chronic pain. I. Aspects of the reliability and validity of the visual analog scale. *Pain* 16:87-101, 1983.
17. Walsh TD: Letter to the editor. *Pain* 19:96, 1984.
18. Revill SI et al: The reliability of a linear analogue for evaluating pain. *Anaesthesia* 31:1191-1198, 1976.
19. Thompson MJ, Hand DJ, Everitt BS: Contradictory correlations between derived scales. *Stat Med* 10:1315-1319, 1991.
20. Jensen MP, Karoly P, Braver S: The measurement of clinical pain intensity: A comparison of six methods. *Pain* 27:117-126, 1986.
21. Frank AJM, Moll LMH, Hort JF: A comparison of three ways of measuring pain. *Rheumatology and Rehabilitation* 1982, 21:211-217.
22. Melzack R: Concepts of pain measurement. In Melzack R, editor: *Pain Measurement and Assessment*. New York, Raven Press, 1983.
23. Melzack R: The McGill Pain Questionnaire: Major properties and scoring methods. *Pain* 1:277-299, 1975.
24. Prieter EJ, Geisinger KF: Factor-analytic studies of the McGill Pain Questionnaire. In Melzack R, editor: *Pain Measurement and Assessment*. New York, Raven Press, 1983.
25. Melzack R: The McGill Pain Questionnaire. In Melzack R, editor: *Pain Measurement and Assessment*. New York, Raven Press, 1983.
26. Eich E, Jaeger B, Graff-Radford SB: Memory for pain: relation between past and present pain intensity. *Pain* 23:375-379, 1985.
27. Van Buren J, Kleinknecht RA: An evaluation of the McGill Pain Questionnaire for use in dental pain assessment. *Pain* 6:23-33, 1979.
28. Cohen MM, Tate RB: Using the McGill Pain Questionnaire to study common postoperative complications. *Pain* 39:275-279, 1989.
29. Haas M, Nyiendo J: Diagnostic utility of the McGill Pain Questionnaire and the Osweatry Disability Questionnaire for classification of low back pain syndromes. *J Manipulative Physiol Ther* 15:90-98, 1992.
30. Melzack R et al: Labour is still painful after prepared childbirth training. *Can Med Assoc J* 125:357-363, 1981.
31. Reading AE: The McGill Pain Questionnaire: An appraisal. In Melzack R, editor: *Pain Measurement and Assessment*. New York, Raven Press, 1983.
32. Holroyd KA et al: A multi-center evaluation of the McGill Pain Questionnaire: Results from more than 1700 chronic pain patients. *Pain* 48:301-311, 1992.
33. Turk DC, Rudy TE, Salovey P: The McGill Pain Questionnaire reconsidered: Confirming the factor structure and examining appropriate uses. *Pain* 21:385-397, 1985.
34. Lowe NK, Walker SN, MacCallum RC: Confirming the theoretical structure of the McGill Pain Questionnaire in acute clinical pain. *Pain* 46:53-60, 1991.
35. Melzack R: The short form McGill Pain Questionnaire. *Pain* 30:191-197, 1987.
36. Klepac RK et al: Interview vs. paper-and-pencil administration of the McGill Pain Questionnaire. *Pain* 11:241-246, 1981.
37. Vanderiet K, Adriensen H, Carton H et al: The McGill questionnaire constructed for the Dutch language (MPQ-DV). Preliminary data concerning reliability and validity. *Pain* 30:395-408, 1987.
38. Strand LI, Wisnes AR: The development of the Norwegian pain questionnaire. *Pain* 46:61-66, 1991.
39. Boureau F, Luu M, Doubrére F: Comparative study of the validity of the four French McGill Pain questionnaire (MPQ) versions. *Pain* 50:59-65, 1992.
40. Corson JA, Schneider MJ: The Dartmouth Pain Questionnaire: An adjunct to the McGill Pain Questionnaire. *Pain* 19:59-69, 1984.
41. Fordyce WE: The behavioral analysis of pain. In Fordyce WE, editor: *Behavioral Methods for Chronic Pain and Illness*. St Louis, Mosby, 1976.
42. Keefe FJ, Gil KM: Behavioral concepts in the analysis of chronic pain syndromes. *J Consult Clin Psychol* 54:776-783, 1986.
43. Vlaeyen JWS et al: Assessment of the components of observed chronic behavior: The Checklist for Interpersonal Pain Behavior (CHIP). *Pain* 43:337-347, 1990.
44. Keefe FJ, Block AR: Development of an observation method for assessing pain behavior in chronic low back pain patients. *Behavior Therapy* 13:363-375, 1982.
45. Broome ME: Measurement of behavioral response to pain. *J Pediatr Oncology Nursing* 8:180-182, 1991.
46. Keefe FJ et al: Behavioral assessment of head and neck cancer pain. *Pain* 23:327-336, 1985.
47. Keefe FJ, Hill RW: An objective approach to qualifying pain behavior and gait patterns in low back pain patients. *Pain* 21:153-161, 1985.
48. Hammonds W, Brenna S: Pain classification and vocational evaluation of chronic pain states. In Melzack R, editor: *Pain Measurement and Assessment*. New York, Raven Press, 1983.
49. Osterweis M et al, editors: *Pain and Disability: Clinical, Behavioral, and Public Policy Perspectives*. National Academy Press, Washington, DC, 1987.
50. Follick MJ, Ahern DK, Laser-Wolston N: Evaluation of a daily activity diary for chronic pain patients. *Pain* 19:373-382, 1984.
51. Tursky B, Jamner LD, Friedman R: The Pain Perception Profile: A psychophysical approach to the assessment of pain report. *Behavior Therapy* 13:376-394, 1982.
52. Kremer EF, Block A, Gaylor MS: Behavior approaches to treatment of chronic pain: The inaccuracy of patient self report measures. *Arch Phys Med Rehabil* 62:188-191, 1981.
53. Udén A, Åströmm M, Bergenudd H: Pain drawings in chronic back pain. *Spine* 13:389-392, 1988.
54. Mann NH III, Brown MD, Enger I: Expert performance in low-back disorder recognition using patient pain drawings. *J Spinal Disord* 5:254-259, 1992.
55. North RB et al: Automated 'pain drawing' analysis by computer-controlled, patient-interactive neurological stimulation system. *Pain* 50:51-57, 1992.

56. Ready LB, Sarkis E, Turner JA: Self-reported vs. actual use of medications in chronic pain patients. *Pain* 12:285-294, 1982.

57. Perry F, Heller PH, Levine JD: A possible indicator of functional pain: Poor pain scale correlation. *Pain* 46:191-193, 1991.

58. Chapman CR, Syrjala KL: Measurement of pain. In Bonica JJ, editor: *The Management of Pain,* ed 2. Philadelphia, Lea & Febiger, 1990.

59. Wolff BB: Laboratory methods of pain measurement. In Melzack R, editor: *Pain Measurement and Assessment.* New York, Raven Press, 1983.

60. Kohllöffel LUE, Koltzenburg M, Handwerker HO: A novel technique for the evaluation of mechanical pain and hyperalgesia. *Pain* 46:81-87, 1991.

61. Smythe HA et al: Control of "fibrocystic" tenderness: Comparison of two dolorimeters. *J Rheumatol* 19:768-771, 1992.

62. Hageweg JA et al: Algometry: Measuring pain threshold, method, and characteristics in healthy subjects. *Scand J Rehabil Med* 24:99-103, 1992.

63. Anton F, Euchner I, Handwerker HO: Psychophysical examination of pain induced by defined CO_2 pulses applied to the nasal mucosa. *Pain* 49:53-60, 1992.

64. Deschamps M, Band P, Coldman AJ: Assessment of adult cancer pain: Shortcomings of current methods. *Pain* 32:133-139, 1988.

65. Grossman SA, Sheidler VR, McGuire DB: A comparison of the Hopkins Pain Rating Instrument with standard visual analog and verbal descriptor scales in patients with cancer pain, *J Pain Symptom Manage* 7:196-203, 1992.

66. Grossman SA, Sheidler VR, Swedeen K: Correlation of patient and caregiver ratings of cancer pain. *J Pain Symptom Manage* 6:53-57, 1991.

67. Cleeland CS: Measurement and prevalence of pain in cancer. *Semin Oncol Nurs* 1:87-92, 1985.

68. Tyrer S: Psychiatric assessment of chronic pain. *Br J Psychiatry* 160:733-741, 1992.

69. Pilowsky I et al: The Illness Behavior Questionnaire as an aid to clinical assessment. *Gen Hosp Psychiatry* 6:123-130, 1984.

70. Roy R, Thomas MR: A survey of chronic pain in an elderly population. *Can Fam Physician Med Fam Can* 32:513-516, 1986.

71. Herr KA, Mobily PR: Complexities of pain assessment in the elderly: Clinical considerations. *J Gerontological Nursing* 17:12-19, 1991.

72. McGrath PA: Evaluating a child's pain. *J Pain Symptom Manage* 4:198-214, 1989.

73. Bieri D et al: The Faces Pain Scale for the self-assessment of the severity of pain experienced by children: Development, initial validation, and preliminary investigation for ratio scale properties. *Pain* 41:139-150, 1990.

74. LeBaron S, Zeltzer L: Assessment of acute pain and anxiety in children and adolescents by self-reports, observer reports, and a behavior checklist. *J Consult Clin Psychol* 52:729-738, 1984.

75. Manne SL, Jacobsen PB, Redd WH: Assessment of acute pediatric pain: Do child self-report, parent ratings, and nurse ratings measure the same phenomenon? *Pain* 48:45-52, 1992.

QUESTIONS: PAIN MEASUREMENT

1. The most commonly used assessment tools for chronic pain are based upon:
   A. Health care staff observations
   B. Patient medication usage
   C. Patient self-reporting
   D. Psychiatric assessment

2. Disadvantages of the Verbal Descriptor Scale include:
   (1) It requires nonparametric statistics to analyze the data.
   (2) It cannot be used in experimental pain situations.
   (3) There is a limitation on the possible number of responses.
   (4) It is difficult to administer.
   A: 1, 2, and 3
   B: 1 and 3
   C: 2 and 4
   D: 4
   E: All of the above

3. A VAS score of 5:
   A. Represents the same level of pain that another patient with a VAS of 5 feels
   B. Is not affected by the patient's cultural upbringing
   C. Can be used as an indicator of the efficacy of a treatment regimen
   D. Represents a measurement of pain behavior

4. Which of the following patient characteristics affect that patient's ability to measure pain?
   A. Age
   B. Gender
   C. Culture
   D. The amount of suffering, as perceived by the patient

5. Which of the following groups of patients are at risk for inadequate measurement?
   A. Elderly
   B. Pediatric
   C. Burn patients
   D. Low back pain patients

ANSWERS

1. C
2. B
3. D
4. E
5. E

5 Laboratory Investigations

L. Douglas Kennedy

There is no laboratory substitute for a careful history and physical examination on the initial consultation and on follow-up visits.[1] This is covered in detail in Chapter 3. Laboratory tests, however, when applied in a logical, systematic method, can enhance the process. This not only improves patient care but also reduces cost. The step after the history and physical examination is development of a laboratory "data base."[2]

History + Physical examination + "Database" = Initial evaluation

After the initial evaluation, a problem list is made, and this results in a differential diagnosis. The differential diagnosis is confirmed or denied based on specific diagnostic tests. In this systematic approach, laboratory and other tests are not used in a random "shotgun" manner. This is discussed later.

Medical laboratory investigations in the clinical pain practice serve three main purposes:

1. They aid in diagnosis of the disease that is responsible for producing the pain.
2. They aid in following the disease course. A progression or regression of the disease with a subsequent response to treatment may be determined. A serum carcinoembryonic antigen (CEA) drawn upon diagnosis of colon cancer can be used to follow the course of the disease. A CEA increase may precede clinical advancement of colon cancer by 2 to 6 months.[3]
3. They help to prevent iatrogenic complication(s). For example, by testing the periodic blood urea nitrogen and creatinine in a geriatric patient, the lab results can determine if nonsteroidal antiinflammatory drugs (NSAIDs) are causing a decrease in renal function. These are discussed in detail.

REVIEW OF PREVIOUS LABORATORY TESTS

By conservative estimate, many patients referred for consultation to the pain medicine physician have already been evaluated and treated by more than five other physicians. Previous reports must be evaluated to prevent unnecessary duplication of testing, which in turn reduces cost and risk to the patient. The trade-off is increased time, cost, and risk to the patient for that test. There is also a trade-off in increased time and cost to physicians and their staff to locate and record those test results. Therefore the physician's staff should be in the habit of requesting patients to obtain their own previous records. Be specific when instructing patients on what to obtain. This not only saves valuable staff time

but allows the patient to become a more active participant in their own care. If the patient is not able to obtain the reports, then the facsimile machine is an excellent option; it can transfer information in a timely manner. The data are transferred while the patient is in the clinic. This cuts down on the number of items the staff must remember to do later and aids in staff efficiency. It also compresses the diagnostic and therapeutic time line significantly, therefore patients receive the correct diagnosis quicker, which results in expeditious treatment. Fewer visits result and cost is reduced.

LABORATORY "DATABASE"

A laboratory "database" for the pain patient generally consists of the following:

1. Complete blood count (CBC)
2. Biochemical profile (renal function, liver function, electrolytes)
3. Urinalysis
4. Sedimentation rate
5. Specific tests as indicated by the results of the history, physical examination, and database.

These laboratory results will not only help in the diagnosis of the underlying illness but also help to estimate the patient's ability to distribute, metabolize, and eliminate a drug (i.e., the patient's pharmacokinetic drug profile). Two excellent references for the practicing algologist are *Interpretation of Diagnostic Tests*[3] and *A Manual of Laboratory Diagnostic Tests*[4], which is extremely useful to the physician and allied health care professional. Normal values, explanation of tests, and clinical application are readily and quickly found. Many of the normal values and explanations of specific laboratory tests were derived from this text. The former reference is a more detailed text and is commonly used by physicians and clinical pathologists. Both are available in softbound editions and are affordable.

Certain facts should be remembered when interpreting laboratory results. For any laboratory result, a "normal value" range will be given based on the assumption that each test will have been derived from a curve containing 95% of the sample/control population. Therefore by definition 5% of the "normal" population will have "abnormal" laboratory values. Does this mean that laboratory test results are of concern or are truly abnormal? No, not necessarily. The selection of these control populations must be assessed within this equation, and features such as age, sex, and ethnicity must be taken into account. False-positive results may occur in some instances in individual patients. If there is a question, the local clinical pathologist can provide helpful insight. Clinical reference manuals are published nationally both on the physician level and for allied health professionals.[3,4] Most hospital and clinical laboratories provide manuals for normative reference ranges, and many of these make age distinction.

Complete blood count hemogram

The complete blood count (CBC) is performed from a peripheral blood sample. It is routinely automated but can be performed manually and is commonly called a *hemogram* when a white blood cell (WBC) differential count is included. Components include WBC, WBC differential (WBC diff), red blood cell count (RBC count), hematocrit (HCT), hemoglobin (HGB), RBC indicae, and platelet count. RBC indexes include the mean red cell volume (MCV), mean red cell hemoglobin concentration (MCHC), and mean red cell hemoglobin (MCH).

White blood cell count. The adult normal range WBC or leukocyte count is 5000 to 10,000 per microliter. The WBCs are integrally involved with the body's immune response; change in absolute number and relative number of types of leukocytes provides important clinical information. An increase in the leukocyte absolute number is termed *leukocytosis* (WBC count greater than 10,000 per microliter). Reasons for leukocytosis include infection, trauma, tissue necrosis, malignancy, toxins, steroid exposure, leukemia, and many others. A decrease in the leukocyte count less than 5000 per microliter is termed *leukopenia*. It is seen in aplastic anemia, chemotherapy, radiation therapy, overwhelming sepsis, anaphylactic shock, collagen vascular disease, and others. Usually one type of leukocyte will be elevated or decreased. Thus the differential leukocyte count is helpful in further limiting the differential diagnosis.

An increase or decrease in the relative type of leukocytes also provides important clinical information. The types of leukocytes and a partial differential of leukocytosis and leukopenia follow.

Neutrophils. Neutrophils (PMNs, polymorphonuclear neutrophils, "segs," "polys") are normally 50% to 60% of the total leukocyte count. They can be further differentiated into "immature" and "mature" neutrophils. The "immature" PMNs (also known as stabs or segs) are elevated with ongoing infection, particularly bacterial. This is also known as a "left shift" (neutrophilia). In elderly and debilitated patients the absolute leukocyte count may not be elevated and the "left shift" may be the only hematologic abnormality. A shift toward the "mature" neutrophils is known as a "right shift." This may be seen with allergies, tissue necrosis or injury, certain drugs, and hemolysis. A neutropenia of less than 500 per cubic millimeter is a medical emergency. The patient is particularly vulnerable to infection, especially bacterial, and should be placed in isolation.

Eosinophils. Eosinophils are normally 1% to 4% of the total leukocyte count. Their number greater than 5% (eosinophilia) may indicate pathology. The mnemonic NAACP can help in remembering the following diseases and syndromes in which eosinophilia can occur:

N = Neoplasm
A = Addison's disease
A = Allergy
C = Collagen vascular disease
P = Parasitic infection

Monocytes. Monocytes are capable of phagocytosis and production of interferon. The normal monocyte range in the WBC differential is 2% to 6%. Monocytosis is seen with tuberculosis, viral infections (e.g., infectious mononucleosis), parasitic infection, lymphoma, multiple myeloma, and others.

Lymphocytes. The normal range is 20% to 40% of the leukocyte count. They are migratory cells and move toward sites of inflammation. Lymphocytes produce serum immunoglobulins and are important in cellular immunity. Lymphocytosis is found in infectious mononucleosis, tuberculosis, syphilis, lead intoxication, viral upper respiratory tract infections and viral infections, in general. A lymphocytopenia of less than 500 per cubic millimeter is a medical emergency. The patient must be isolated and protected against infection, particularly viral.

Hematocrit and hemoglobin (H&H). Hematocrit determines the space occupied by red blood cells in the blood, and hemoglobin determines the content/concentration of the oxygen-carrying molecules within the red blood cell. Normal values for each are age- and sex-dependent. Hematocrit range in the adult man is 40% to 54% and in the adult woman is 37% to 47% of the packed red cell volume. Hemoglobin range in the adult man is 13.5 to 17.5 grams per deciliter and in the adult woman is 12 to 16 grams per deciliter. They are important in determining the amount of oxygen-carrying material in the blood stream but they do not assure the quality of that material. Sickle cell anemia patients have a decrease in the absolute amount and quality of their hemoglobin. Increased hematocrit values may be seen in polycythemia and dehydration (hemoconcentrated state). Decreased hematocrit may be seen in leukemia, blood loss (after intravascular volume has been replaced with non-RBC fluid), collagen vascular disease, hyperthyroidism, and others.

Red blood cell. The red blood count indexes defines the size and hemoglobin content of the red blood cell. They are helpful in differentiating the anemias. It is important to note that these indexes are averaged values and are but one of the assays in the diagnosis of anemia. Examination of the peripheral blood smear and bone marrow aspiration and examination are essential tools to be deferred in the differential diagnosis of anemia; if average values or indices alone are used, diagnoses may be missed. For an example, schistocytes can be present in the peripheral blood smear. Schistocytes are fragmented irregularly shaped RBCs caused by hemolysis, artificial heart values, and disseminated intravascular coagulation. Anisocytosis is the abnormal variation in size of the RBC and may be seen in vitamin B_{12}, folate, and iron deficiency. Microcytic hypochromic anemia presents with a low MCV and MCHC and is often seen with iron deficiency anemia. Macrocytic RBC indexes with anemia are seen with folate and vitamin B_{12} deficiency.

Platelet count. The platelet count is included with the hemogram. Platelets (thrombocytes) are formed in the bone marrow and are fragments of megakaryocytes. Platelet life span is approximately eight days. This becomes important to the algologist when using NSAIDs. Acetylated salicylates (aspirin) inhibit platelet function in an irreversible fashion for the life of the platelet (eight days). Nonacetylated salicylates (most NSAIDs) inhibit platelet function in a reversible fashion. Their platelet inhibition relates to their elimination half-life, which is important when planning procedures with anticipated blood loss and for postoperative and posttraumatic analgesia. Interestingly, one commercially available salicylate, choline magnesium trisalicylate (Trilisate), does not appreciably inhibit platelet function, and it has been useful in treatment for thrombocytopenic cancer pain patients.

One third of the platelets available for immediate clotting are located in the reticuloendothelial system, mainly in the spleen. The rest (two thirds) are found in the circulating blood stream. The normal adult platelet count is 150,000 to 350,000 per cubic millimeter. An increased platelet count (thrombocythemia) may occur with cancer, splenectomy, trauma, and infection. Unexpected thrombocythemia is often found in undiagnosed malignancy. Decreased platelet count (thrombocytopenia) may occur with infection, chemotherapy, drug toxicity, allergic conditions, pulmonary embolism, disseminated intravascular coagulation (DIC), and idiopathic thrombocytopenia purpura. As with the measure of erythrocytes, platelet count does not address the functional state of the platelet. If platelet dysfunction is suspected, then the platelet count and bleeding time should also be checked. Tests of platelet function include the template bleeding time and the ivy bleeding time. An example of a hereditary condition where platelet count is normal but function is abnormal is von Willebrand's disease. It is an autosomal dominant deficiency of a plasma protein (von Willebrand factor) that mediates adherence of platelets.[3]

Biochemical profiles

Automated "biochemical profiles" have become the norm, resulting in a relatively less expensive, reliable, and rapid method of obtaining body chemistry results. Each clinical laboratory is directed by a clinical pathologist who determines what will be included with each standard biochemical profile. Some common acronyms that are often included are Chem 7, Astra 7, and SMA 7. Renal function is determined. This is particularly important with the use of NSAIDs in the geriatric population because nephrotoxicity can occur rapidly in this patient population.

Biochemical profiles can also indicate the homeostasis between the cardiovascular and renal systems. This is especially important to the algologist in determining how a patient will distribute and eliminate a particular drug (pharmacokinetics). A single glucose determination is made but this should be read with caution. If diabetes mellitus is suspected, then fasting glucose and glycosalated hemoglobin (glycohemoglobin) should be checked. These tests contain serum glucose, blood urea nitrogen (BUN), creatinine (Cr), and serum electrolytes (sodium, potassium, chloride, and carbon dioxide).

Other biochemical profiles are more extensive and include the acronyms SMA 24, SMA 18, Chem 18, Chem 24, Chemzyme, and Chemzyme plus. Normative values are derived for the patient population as discussed previously. Besides the above seven tests, hepatic enzymes are determined and commonly include lactate dehydrogenase (LDH), creatinine phosphokinase (CPK), and alkaline phosphatase, to name a few. Baseline liver function and periodic checks should be performed therefore when a patient has been using opioids, anticonvulsants, and acetaminophen. Chronic pain patients commonly ingest large quantities of over-the-counter NSAIDs and acetaminophen, and the database can screen for potential problems of the renal and hepatic systems. Albumin is routinely reported. Because of its ability to variably bind drugs, albumin is important for estimation of a drug's pharmacokinetics, and total protein is helpful in determining the overall nutritional state.

Urinalysis

Urinalysis (U/A) is a relatively inexpensive and low risk method to obtain a great deal of information by using a chemical and microscopic examination. The chemical properties determined are: color, odor, turbidity, specific gravity, pH, glucose, ketones, blood protein, bilirubin, nitrate, and leukocyte esterase. The microscopic properties determined are: presence and type of cells (RBCs, WBCs), casts (WBC, RBC, granular), organisms (bacteria), and crystals (crystine, calcium phosphate, calcium oxalate, uric acid). WBC casts are associated with pyelonephritis, RBC casts with glomerulonephritis, and waxy casts are associated with severe renal damage.

Urinalysis can also be used to determine the presence of a drug or drugs. Most patients who truly seek adequate control of pain do not fear the results of serum or urine drug screening tests. Those who are compliant recognize that the values obtained will compare favorably with the type and amounts of medications prescribed by their treating physicians. These patients generally agree to such testing in order to verify that their medication use does not include excessive illicit drug intake. Documentation of this phenomenon can frequently be used to exonerate the pain patient who has been falsely accused of unauthorized analgesic ingestion. Some patients may fear the erroneous laboratory result that could create social, occupational, or legal problems. Legal issues vary by state, and ethical issues should be addressed. There are procedures for obtaining a witnessed urine sample.[4] Generally, patients should be aware of the purpose of the specimen and give consent. Reasons for obtaining a urine drug screen include to confirm clinical or after-death diagnosis, differentiate drug-induced disease from an intrinsic organ process, and determine adherence to a drug regimen, whether for taking a prescribed drug or abstaining from a banned drug.

Erythrocyte sedimentation rate and C-reactive protein

The erythrocyte sedimentation rate (ESR, "sed rate") is the rate at which red blood cells settle in unclotted blood in 1 hour. Inflammation and tissue necrosis result in a change in serum proteins, causing aggregation of erythrocytes and increasing the rate of fall (increased "sed rate"). The test is therefore inherently nonspecific. The ESR may be helpful in diagnosis of occult disease, in differential diagnosis, and to follow the course of an inflammatory process, for example, how rheumatoid arthritis or a respiratory infection respond to treatment. There may be a short delay time between development of a pathologic state and a change in the ESR. For this reason a C-reactive protein (CRP) may be used. CRP is a specific protein released into the blood with inflammation of any tissue, and it appears to work with the complement system. CRP is an antigen-antibody test and is reported as a titer; any titer, 1:2 or 1:64, is significant. For these reasons, the CRP is a more specific indicator of inflammation and tissue damage, whereas the ESR is a much less specific test. Both of these tests are relatively cost effective when building a database and establishing a working diagnosis.

Vindicate

Vindicate, in *Webster's New Collegiate Dictionary* (1981), is defined as, "to confirm, substantiate; to provide justification or defense for; to set free, deliver; to lay claim to, avenge, exonerate, absolve." These are lofty and worthwhile goals in providing care for the pain patient.

This is especially true because by conservative estimate the chronic pain patient has been seen by an average of five other physicians. The mnemonic VINDICATE PS is a list of etiologies that cause disease that may result in pain. This list of etiologies of disease are cross-indexed with the various organ system(s) suspected as the cause of pain (Box 5-1). Notice that PS has been added to the original mnemonic. This takes into account secondary gain (social, financial, workers compensation, personal injury) and behavioral issues.

After the comprehensive initial evaluation (history, physical examination, and establishing a database), other laboratory tests may be indicated. Once again a systematic rather than a random or "shotgun" approach is utilized. The VINDICATE mnemonic is reviewed and then cross-indexed with the suspected organ system(s) to develop a differential diagnosis. The suspected diagnosis is then confirmed or denied based on selective diagnostic tests. The VINDICATE mnemonic can compress the diagnostic and therapeutic time line to result in correct treatment being rendered faster. It also reduces the possibility of missed diagnoses. Some chronic pain patients will have more than one patho-

logic process present. VINDICATE can also reduce cost and risk to the patient.

In summary, the following sequence is recommended for the evaluation (initial and ongoing) and treatment of patients with pain related disorders:

- Perform thorough initial history and physical examination
- Document prior diagnostic workup and therapy
- Confirm that "routine" health care issues are current
- Obtain routine database
- Develop problem list
- Develop differential diagnosis
- VINDICATE PS the patient's differential diagnosis
- Cross-index with the indicated organ system(s)
- Obtain specific diagnostic tests to limit the differential diagnosis (confirm or deny the diagnosis)
- Develop a working diagnosis
- Develop and institute resultant treatment plan in an expeditious manner

Discussion of specific laboratory tests based on the VINDICATE PS mnemonic is listed in order.

Viral (microbial). This is one example of infection but may encompass other microbes including bacteria and fungi. Viral (microbial) etiologies are "screened" with the CBC in the data base. Emphasis is placed on the WBC and differential (see Laboratory "Database" on p. 47). The WBC differential is often "left shifted" with bacterial infection while a relative increase in lymphocytes or monocytes usually indicates viral infection. The ESR (sed rate) and/or CRP are also discussed on p. 49. They can also be helpful in determining presence of an occult infection and in following the course, treatment, and recovery.

Testing for the antibody to the human T-cell lymphotropic virus (HTLV-III) for acquired immunodeficiency syndrome (AIDS) virus is performed using the enzyme-linked immunoabsorbent assay (ELISA) method. The ELISA method is also used to detect other viruses. It is 93% to 99% sensitive and 99% specific for the anti-HTLV-III antibody. It is a qualitative test, and other confirmatory tests should be performed if it is positive or clinical index is high even with a negative ELISA; then the Western blot technique should be employed, which is more specific but less standardized then the ELISA method. The anti-HTLV-III antibody is used to screen blood bank specimens and is not recommended to diagnose AIDS. Seroconversion (formation of the antibody to the HTLV-III antigen) may not occur until 6 months after a person has contracted the virus.

There are a wide variety of other serologic tests and cultures available to confirm active or previous exposure to viruses that cannot be included in this chapter. For details, see the reference section.

Microscopic examination of tissue samples with and without special staining techniques are available. Gram staining for bacteria and tuberculosis (TB) are commonly used. Skin testing can determine previous exposure to TB. Aerobic and anaerobic cultures are also routinely available.

Inflammatory. Inflammation can be present for a variety of reasons. These reasons can be divided into primary, secondary, or no microbial infection. See the previous section for the discussion about diagnosis of infectious disease.

Box 5-1 EXPLANATION OF VINDICATE PS

V:	Viral/bacterial	Musculoskeletal
I:	Inflammatory	Nervous
N:	Neoplastic	Gastrointestinal
D:	Degenerative	Integumentary
I:	Ischemia	Genitourinary
C:	Congenital/genetic	Reproductive
A:	Autoimmune/collagen vascular disease	Cardiovascular
T:	Traumatic/mechanical	Pulmonary
E:	Endocrine/metabolic	Renal
P:	Psychogenic	Hematologic
S:	Secondary gain	Immune

Secondary microbial infection can be divided into two other groups, those with evidence of autoimmune disorder, including certain neuritides, arthritides, and collagen vascular disease, and those resulting from trauma. There will be obvious overlap between some of these VINDICATE PS groups, which can decrease the chance of a missed diagnosis.

Infectious or noninfectious inflammation can be followed by an ESR (sed rate). If the process is suspected in the very early stages, then the ESR may not yet be elevated. The CRP may be a better test because it becomes positive early in the disease process; see Laboratory "Database" on p. 47. The CRP decrease and normalization of the ESR can provide useful information regarding the patient's successful response to treatment, for example, how a patient's rheumatoid arthritis would react to treatment with salicylates. The ESR combined with clinical examination can provide enough information to decide whether to place the patient on corticosteroids. Specific etiologies resulting in inflammation are discussed later in the chapter.

Neoplastic. Most diagnoses of cancer are based on history and physical examination. It is essential to confirm that the chronic pain patient is current on routine health maintenance, including a chest radiograph for smokers, pelvic and breast examinations for women, and prostate examinations for men. Diagnostic tests to confirm the presence of cancer rely on changes in structure. These imaging studies are discussed in other sections of this text.

Checking for occult blood in stool samples is a cost effective and low risk screening method for occult carcinoma of the colon. It may also be used to diagnose occult gastrointestinal (GI) bleeding induced by NSAIDs. For a thorough discussion, see *A Manual of Laboratory Diagnostic Tests.*[4]

Acid phosphatase is an enzyme found in many tissues and is found in the prostate 100 times greater than in other tissues. It can be used to diagnose metastatic prostate cancer but may be elevated in other disorders such as Paget's disease, multiple myeloma, other cancer that has metastasized to bone, and hepatitis. The prostatic specific antigen (PSA) is more specific and, coupled with a routine prostate examination, is a highly specific and sensitive test for prostate cancer.

Alkaline phosphatase is useful as a potential tumor marker when combined with clinical history and physical examination. It is an enzyme present in liver, kidney, and mainly in the bone, therefore it can indicate disease in those tissues. In the liver, biliary obstruction is the main cause of elevated alkaline phosphatase. Bone diseases such as Paget's disease, osteogenic sarcoma, and metastatic bone cancer lead to elevated alkaline phosphatase. Alkaline phosphatase can be further divided into heat labile and heat stable fractions. The heat labile fraction is predominately from the liver; the heat stable fraction is predominately from bone.

The CBC has been discussed previously. Many neoplasms have an accompanying anemia. Besides the CBC, the peripheral blood smear and bone marrow aspirate are helpful if evaluating suspected neoplasms. A microscopic "smear" evaluation of peripheral blood or of marrow can help diagnose anemia (aplastic, pernicious, or agranulocytosis), leukemia or lymphoma, and purpura.

Tumor-related antigens are widely available cancer markers. It is important to know which antigens are considered early detection tests and which ones can be used to follow the course of the neoplasm after diagnosis. None of them should be used in place of a careful history, follow-up, and regular health care checkups. *Interpretation of Diagnostic Tests* is an excellent reference text for this purpose.[3] Carcinoembryonic antigen (CEA) is a nonspecific cancer test and is not considered an early cancer screening test. There is a wide overlap of values between neoplastic and nonneoplastic disease. Cigarette smokers may have a CEA level greater than 2.5 ng/ml, whereas 97% of nonsmokers have CEA levels less than 2.5 ng/ml. The CEA is useful in following the course of cancer once diagnosed. Rapid elevation of CEA in a patient being treated for colon cancer probably indicates advancement of disease. This often precedes any clinical evidence or deterioration in the patient's condition. Other newer tumor markers include CA 19-9, which may be altered in colon and pancreatic cancer.

Multiple myeloma is a neoplasm that may present with diffuse and varied symptoms. The technetium-99 ("bone scan") will be normal because this is a plasma cell tumor. Plain radiographs and elevated serum calcium and protein are helpful to establish a diagnosis. Different types of myeloma produce various immunoglobulins. The majority have an elevated serum protein. Protein immunoelectrophoresis of the serum and the urine yield a diagnosis in more than 98% of the patients with multiple myeloma.[3]

Degenerative. Degenerative disease is usually crossindexed or checked against the musculoskeletal system and the nervous system. Within the musculoskeletal system a further subdivision is made between the autoimmune/collagen vascular disease disorders and degeneration caused by weight bearing and use. Specifically, this later degenerative condition is due to deterioration in the weight bearing joints (lumbar or cervical spine, knee joints, hip joints). Laboratory values are generally normal in this group. Diagnosis is made with physical examination and imaging studies. Plain radiographs of the affected joint are followed by computer assisted tomography (CT) scan or magnetic resonance imaging (MRI) as needed. The discussion of autoimmune musculoskeletal disease is in the following section.

Nervous system degenerative disease is demonstrated in multiple sclerosis. This progressive demyelinating disease of the nervous system can be difficult to diagnose because it can present with a myriad of signs and symptoms. An MRI of the spinal cord and/or the brain can demonstrate "plaques" within those structures. Analysis of the cerebrospinal fluid (CSF) can be diagnostic for multiple sclerosis. Protein immunoelectrophoresis of albumin and immunoglobulin G (IgG) evaluates the integrity of the blood brain barrier and the production of IgG within the CNS. Multiple sclerosis can be diagnosed by the presense of increased IgG in the cerebrospinal fluid (CSF) with normal serum albumin plus the presence of IgM and oligoclonal bands. Exceptions do exist and are discussed in *A Manual of Laboratory Diagnostic Tests.*[4]

Ischemia. This condition results when tissues receive inadequate oxygen supply, which results in inadequate cellular respiration. Any abnormality in the delivery system (cardiovascular), oxygen-carrying system (hematopoietic), or in the cellular respiratory level can lead to ischemia. Abnormalities in the cardiovascular system are generally defined by electrophysiologic (electrocardiogram, intracardiac conduction) and mechanical flow studies of the coronary arteries, central vessels, and peripheral vessels. Noninvasive flow studies of the larger peripheral vessels are commonly used (Doppler flow). The adequacy of erythrocytes is measured in the CBC. If pathology is suspected, then a peripheral blood smear should be checked. The clinical pathologist can assist with this. Hemolysis of erythrocytes, for example, caused by mechanical heart valves or transition reaction and abnormal erythrocyte morphology can be quickly diagnosed, for example, the sickle cell anemia that occurs during a "sickle cell crisis." Small arteriole disease caused by diabetes mellitus or an arthritides can only be suspected, not diagnosed, with a laboratory test. These are discussed in other parts of this chapter. The end result of significant ischemia can be measured by the development of metabolic acidosis (inadequate cellular respiration). Obtain an arterial blood gas along with a SMA-7 (see Laboratory "Database" on p. 47). This establishes and confirms the ischemic event on a metabolic level. Treatment of the painful condition consists of palliating the pain while identifying the pathology. After determining the underlying cause, treatment can then be curative or at least helpful.

Congenital/genetic. These disorders may result from acquired (prepartum or postpartum) or hereditary etiologies. Laboratory analysis is less important in this category, but certain disorders do merit special mention. Sickle cell disease is one of them.[4] Sickle cell anemia affects millions worldwide. Confirmation of diagnosis is based on the type of hemoglobin found in the erythrocyte. Normal hemoglobin is made up predominantly of hemoglobin A (>95%). Because of a change in one of the terminal amino acids in the hemoglobin molecule, the hemoglobin under lowered oxygen tensions becomes viscous, "sticky," and causes the erythrocytes to clump and "sickle." This is due to the replacement of the normal hemoglobin A with the abnormal hemoglobin S. There are two types of abnormal sickle cell patients. Since it is a hereditary autosomal recessive trait, a patient will have either 0.5 or 1.0 (all) of the gene expressed for the abnormal hemoglobin. The *Sickledex Test* screens for all patients with hemoglobin S. Those testing positive must then submit a blood sample for hemoglobin electrophoresis. Determination of patients with sickle cell trait (partial expression) is made. These patients are not usually symptomatic but can be in extreme situations. Those with full expression of the sickle cell trait have sickle cell disease and often are symptomatic with anemia and suffer frequently from ischemic pain.

Autoimmune and collagen vascular disease. Serologic tests are the mainstay in confirming the presence or the absence of autoimmune and collagen vascular disease, which include systemic lupus erythematosus (SLE), rheumatoid arthritis (RA), polymyositis/dermatomyositis, ankylosing spondylitis, polymyalgia rheumatica, mixed connective tissue disease, temporal arteritis, and scleroderma. Abnormalities in the database and laboratory work are associated with many of these diseases. Anemia, thrombocytopenia, and elevated ESR are common. Specific tests can help make the definitive diagnosis in many cases. Occasionally a definitive diagnosis is not possible with laboratory tests and a tissue biopsy is necessary, for example, with temporal arteritis. If systemic autoimmune/collagen vascular disease is suspected after the initial patient evaluation, screening tests may consist of antinuclear antibody (ANA) with or without an anti-DNA antibody test, rheumatoid factor (RA test), and ESR. The antinuclear antibodies are gamma globulins that react to specific antigens and produce patterns that are relatively specific for certain autoimmune diseases. The ANA test is often combined with the antiDNA antibody test. If these are positive, then other more specific tests are available to differentiate the specific autoimmune disorder. The RA test is useful as a general screening test. Rheumatoid arthritis is mainly a clinical diagnosis. The RA test is positive in only 60% of RA patients. Besides the potential false negative, a number of other disorders cause a positive RA test. These include lupus erythematosus, endocarditis, tuberculosis, syphilis, sarcoidosis, cancer, viral infections, diseases of major organs, and allograft transplant patients. The ESR was discussed in detail in previous sections.

Cryoglobulins (cold agglutinins) are antibodies that cause the agglutination of erythrocytes at 0° to 10° C. Normally, these antibodies are found in serum in small amounts. In certain disease states, they are present in sufficiently high titers to cause agglutination in the acute phase and none in the convalescent phase. They can therefore be used as a general screening test and can help determine disease resolution. Acute increases are found in mycoplasma pneumonia, influenza A and B, infectious mononucleosis, mumps, orchitis, and Raynaud's syndrome. Chronically high titers are seen with hemolytic anemia, cirrhosis, and lymphatic leukemia.[4]

Monoarticular inflammation must be aspirated and examined for bacterial infection (gram stain, cell count, culture) and for presence and type of crystals. Suspected cases of fibrositis/fibromyalgia are diagnosed by exclusion because there are no confirmation laboratory tests; ESR and other indicators of inflammatory reaction are normal. SLE has a positive lupus erythematosus (LE) cell preparation in 60% of cases. Proteinuria, anemia, and thrombocytopenia are common. ANA is the most sensitive laboratory test for SLE and is positive in 95% of cases.

Traumatic/mechanical. Few laboratory studies are helpful here. Diagnosis is made with history, physical examination, and imaging studies (usually plain radiographs). However, the cause of the trauma should be considered and may be diagnosed with a laboratory test. For example, when there is a change in mental status and subsequent trauma caused by metabolic disorder: diabetes mellitus with abnormal blood glucose, electrolyte imbalance with resultant cardiac arrythmia, syncopal episode and drug (prescription and nonprescription) use. This is especially true when dealing with the geriatric population or patients with end stage organ disease (e.g., renal dialysis, cirrhosis, pulmonary). Secondary painful disorders may result from the primary trauma. Posttraumatic infection or inflammation can be diagnosed and followed with CBC by a WBC differential and ESR.

Endocrine/metabolic. Thyroid disease and diabetes mellitus are the most common metabolic endocrine diseases when considering the pain patient. In addition, many pain patients suffer from an affective component such as dysthymia and depression, which can significantly render a pain treatment program ineffective.

A "thyroid profile" and thyroid stimulating hormone (TSH) should be obtained, which may consist of a T3 RIA (T3 by radioimmunoassay) and a total T4. The T3 RIA is the total amount of triiodothyronine concentration in the blood and is the test of choice for the diagnosis of thyrotoxicosis. This test is of limited value in diagnosing hypothyroidism. For general screening purposes of hypothyroidism and hyperthyroidism, the T4 RIA and the T3 uptake ratio (T3UR) are recommended. The T4 RIA is a measure of the total circulating thyroxine. The T3UR is the ratio between the patient specimen and the standard control expressed in a percent, the normal range being 25% to 35%. Increased levels are seen in hyperthyroidism, nephrosis, and neoplasm with metastases. Decreased levels are seen in hypothyroidism, normal pregnancy, and estrogen therapy patients. TSH is used to diagnose primary hypothyroidism. Increased levels are associated with primary hypothyroidism while decreased levels are seen with hyperthyroidism and secondary and tertiary hypothyroidism.

Hypothyroidism is not common but does occur in a significant number of the general population. It can be readily treated and treatment can result in dramatic improvement once it is diagnosed. Diabetes mellitus (DM) is divided into seven categories. The first two are most relevant to the practicing algologist. DM Type I is insulin dependent while DM Type II is insulin independent. The best method to diagnose DM is to obtain a fasting blood sugar (patient must not have caloric intake for 12 hours before drawing blood sample). Blood glucose levels greater than 120 mg/dl are considered abnormal. Some "borderline" patients may have a normal fasting glucose level. A glycosalated hemoglobin (hemoglobin A1c, glycohemoglobin) is determined from a standard venous blood sample. Hemoglobin A1 changes when exposed to glucose. The change is in direct relation to the average amount of glucose present over a set period of time. The erythrocyte life span is 120 days, and during that time glucose becomes bound to the hemoglobin based on the glucose concentration. This is reported as the percent of the total amount of hemoglobin bound to glucose or glycosalated. Normal values are 4% to 7%. These values may be used to diagnose diabetes mellitus or to follow the treatment. Elevated blood glucose and subsequently higher glycohemoglobin levels may cause a more rapid deterioration of the microvascular system and hasten organ compromise and failure. This may be particularly true in diabetic peripheral neuropathy. Optimal control of the blood glucose levels is a cornerstone for reducing further damage to the microvasculature. The pain related to diabetic peripheral neuropathy may then be better controlled.[4]

Hypoglycemia is a relatively rare occurrence. In the practice of algology, the complaint of hypoglycemia should result in a thorough evaluation for psychogenic causes. Pain patients with affective disorders may complain of this malady. A 5-hour glucose tolerance test may be used, but 25% of males may have a fasting blood glucose level less than 50 mg/dl.[3] True pathologic hypoglycemia may rarely be caused by insulinoma.[3]

Osteoporosis is a disorder of low bone mass with a normal ratio of mineral to osteoid (the organic matrix of bone). These patients often develop significant nociceptive pain from compression fractures of the vertebrae. This occurs postmenopausally in the vast majority of cases but can be due to other causes, such as immobilization, hyperthyroidism, primary hyperparathyroidism, renal osteodystrophy, and myeloma. The chemistry profile is commonly comprised of the total calcium levels but should include any serum albumin abnormality and/or the ionized calcium should be checked. If this is present, then metastatic cancer or primary hyperparathyroidism should be ruled out.

Metabolic disease may result in pain for many other reasons. Vitamin B_{12} deficiency can lead to a painful peripheral neuropathy. This can be diagnosed with nerve conduction velocity testing, anemia with megaloblastic erythrocyte indices, and abnormal vitamin B_{12} levels. Heavy metal toxicity can be diagnosed with a "heavy metal screen" obtained from a blood sample.

Psychogenic. Laboratory tests can exclude other significant nociceptive or neuropathic etiologies. They can also confirm compliance with a drug regimen. This is especially important in the dual diagnosis patient—those that have a physical cause of pain but also have psychologic factors that affect their physical condition. Qualitative assays are available for a wide number of substances, and quantitative assays are routinely used for tricyclic antidepressants and anticonvulsants.

These assays become important when determining the adequacy of a drug trial. One of three events must occur for a therapeutic drug to be considered a failure: (1) side effects of the drug are unacceptable, (2) the desired clinical effect has not been achieved (sleep improved, depression treated, pain relief achieved), (3) "therapeutic" blood levels are reached without benefit. The therapeutic blood levels are defined for the tricyclic antidepressant agents as those generally necessary to treat depression. Amitriptyline, nortriptyline, imipramine, desipramine, and doxepin (nordoxepin) blood levels are available including the serotonin specific reuptake inhibitors sertraline, paroxetine, fluoxetine, trazodone, and bupropion. The maximum "therapeutic" levels should not be exceeded because toxicity may result. Blood levels of the anticonvulsants carbamazepine (Tegretol), diphenylhydantoin (Dilantin), and divalproex (Depakote) are also available. The therapeutic range is defined as the usual successful blood level needed to control seizure activity.

Toxicology screening tests of the blood and urine may be used to determine qualitative compliance (i.e., if the patient is taking the drug as prescribed). Issues of informed consent were discussed previously and are especially important when screening for nonprescription and illicit drug use.

Secondary gain. Few laboratory tests exist in this category to assist the algologist. Lack of objective evidence on physical examination, physical pathology on imaging studies, and normal laboratory studies help diagnose by exclusion.

Once the diagnosis is made and a treatment plan instituted, laboratory tests can help to prevent iatrogenic complications. These include stool testing for occult blood and CBC for patients taking NSAIDS for weeks or months to detect early signs of GI bleeding. Renal function should be checked periodically, especially in geriatric patients taking NSAIDS. Drug blood levels, CBC, and liver function studies should be obtained periodically from patients taking long term tricyclic antidepressants or anticonvulsants. Acetaminophen overuse (hepatotoxicity) and overuse of over-the-counter NSAIDs (potential organ damage) can be prevented with a regular, preventive regimen of laboratory tests.

SUMMARY

In this chapter, I have attempted to place laboratory testing in proper perspective. It is not a panacea, nor is it to be used as the sole method of diagnosis. It is not a substitute for a careful history and physical examination. Rather, it is a method by which to include or exclude possible diagnoses. Used logically within this framework, laboratory testing becomes a safe, complementary, and cost effective service that may also prevent iatrogenic complications. Medications can be used safely even in some population groups that may be at risk if preventive testing is performed regularly. Adequate "therapeutic trials" of drugs can be confirmed and inadequate absorption of a drug can be determined with documented blood levels. In addition, patient compliance with prescription, nonprescription, and illicit drugs can be monitored by laboratory testing after obtaining informed consent.

REFERENCES

1. Longmire DR: Tutorial 1: The Medical Pain History. *Pain Digest* 1:29-34, 1991.
2. Kennedy LD, Longmire DR: Tutorial 4: Medical/Laboratory Evaluation of Pain Patients. *Pain Digest* 1:306-312, 1992.
3. Wallach JB: *Interpretation of Diagnostic Tests,* ed 4. Boston, Little, Brown, 1986.
4. Fischbach FF, editor: *A Manual of Laboratory Diagnostic Tests,* ed 3. Philadelphia, JB Lippincott, 1988.

QUESTIONS: LABORATORY INVESTIGATIONS

1. Which of the following is LEAST true of laboratory tests?
   A. They may be used as a confirmation of the working diagnosis.
   B. They may aid in following the course of the disease.
   C. They may help prevent iatrogenic complications.
   D. They should be performed before the development of the initial differential diagnosis.

2. A standard laboratory "Database" includes all of the following EXCEPT:
   A. Urinalysis
   B. Complete blood count
   C. Serum protein electrophoresis
   D. Sedimentation rate

3. All of the following are true of interpretation of laboratory values EXCEPT:
   A. "Normal" values are within one standard deviation of the general population.
   B. False-positive results may occur in some individual patients.
   C. "Normal" values are established within control populations in a given region.
   D. "Normal" values are based on the assumption that 5% of the "normal" control population will fall within the "abnormal" value range.

4. All of the following are true of the WBC EXCEPT:
   A. A WBC greater that 10,000/microliter is defined as a "leukocytosis."
   B. Leukocytosis may result from corticosteroid exposure.
   C. A "left shift" is defined as a shift toward the "mature" white blood cell types.
   D. A "left shift" may be an indication of microbial infection.

5. A WBC "differential" has all of the following components EXCEPT:
   A. Basophils
   B. Neutrophils
   C. Eosinophils
   D. Microphils

ANSWERS

1. D
2. C
3. A
4. C
5. D

6 Radiography and Neuroimaging

Christopher M. Loar and P. Prithvi Raj

The role of radiology in pain management is primarily diagnostic. In patients with pain symptoms, the goal is to establish the specific etiology of the pain in order to prescribe appropriate proper therapeutic measures.

A proper radiologic workup should provide a thorough, diagnostically accurate evaluation of the specific disorder. Cost, availability, risks or side effects, and acceptability to the patient should be considered. A radiographic test should be obtained only when the results may alter the patient's subsequent management.

With the advent of multiple new radiographic modalities, thoughtful selection and planning of radiologic evaluation is crucial to efficiently derive the diagnostic benefits while controlling the substantial costs (and sometimes risk or discomfort) involved.

More than ever, it is important to consult with a radiologist when any doubt exists regarding the efficacy or appropriateness of a planned radiologic workup for a patient in order to avoid unnecessary studies. Furthermore, radiologic examinations are often tailored to fit the individual patient in order to best answer the diagnostic question. Therefore communication between clinician and radiologist thus directly results in more accurate diagnosis and ultimately benefits the patient.

CONVENTIONAL RADIOGRAPHY

Conventional radiographs are often used as an initial evaluation, especially in patients with musculoskeletal pain. Radiographs are readily available in nearly all medical facilities; they may be obtained and interpreted quickly, and cost is substantially less than other special modalities. Their noninvasive nature and short exposure times (a fraction of a second) make plain radiographs acceptable to most patients. Patients with moderate discomfort may be able to cooperate with radiographic positioning for a short duration, whereas the necessity of longer immobilization for magnetic resonance imaging, computed tomography, or nuclear scanning may not be feasible.

Radiographs are indicated for evaluation of a number of skeletal abnormalities. Their obvious primary utility is for diagnosis of fracture (including documentation of healing or complications), arthritis, and primary bone tumors. The fine anatomic resolution is not equaled by any other modality and maximizes precision of diagnosis in these types of disorders.

Trauma

Fractures are usually easily detected provided that there is sufficient disruption of bony architecture to alter the contour or cortical margin. If fracture is highly suspected but not visible by plain radiography, several options for further evaluation exist. Tomography can demonstrate thin sections of the area in question by x-ray tube motion that blurs the planes above and below the area of interest; superimposing structures may then be excluded, thus delineating the area in focus. Follow-up radiographs may reveal healing changes such as callus formation even if the fracture was not promptly detected, thus providing retrospective diagnosis. Radionuclide bone scan is the most sensitive means to detect subtle bone alterations, but it lacks good anatomical resolution. Bone scanning is discussed in a later section.

After documented skeletal trauma, radiographs evaluate fracture unions and bone alignments. Complications such as osteomyelitis (appearing as lytic bone destruction), and osteoporosis caused by disuse or reflex sympathetic dystrophy may be detected as well.

Pathologic fractures may occur following minimal trauma, evidenced by radiographs that demonstrate a fracture superimposed on a destructive bone lesion (metastases, multiple myeloma) or on a generalized skeletal disorder such as osteoporosis.

Bone tumors

Radiographs are fundamental in the evaluation of primary bone tumors. They detail the morphologic characteristics of a lesion, which may allow a limited differential diagnosis to be formulated with accuracy when combined with clinical information and anatomic sites.[1]

Tomography may delineate the margins of the lesion and tumor matrix without spurious shadows of overlying structures.[2] The nidus of osteoid osteoma may be better delineated by tomography than by conventional radiography.

Metastatic disease is usually better detected by radionuclide bone scanning than by the radiographic skeletal survey. As many as 66% of metastatic lesions may not be seen radiographically despite visualization on bone scan.[3] Multiple myeloma, however, is a notable exception: radiography is more sensitive in this disease and more accurately estimates the extent of skeletal involvement.[4]

Arthritis

The fine anatomic detail provided by radiographs enables precision in the diagnosis of arthritic disorders. The morphology of articular lesions and the distribution within the body are important in establishing a diagnosis.[5] In the hands, for example, osteoarthritis often involves the distal and proximal interphalangeal joints and the first carpometacarpal joint; osteophytes and sclerosis are typical. Conversely, predominant involvement of the metacarpophalangeal joints is typical of rheumatoid arthritis, and findings usually include joint space narrowing and marginal erosions.

Low back pain

The role of radiography in evaluation of low back pain has been controversial. The relatively low diagnostic yield and the relatively high radiation dose to skin, marrow, and gonads weigh against the indiscriminate use of lumbosacral spine series, particularly in young persons with acute or subacute onset.[6] These patients usually have muscular strain that resolves with conservative therapy; radiographs may be performed later in those few patients in whom symptoms persist.

Radiographic findings that are likely to be associated with low back pain include: spondylolisthesis, marked narrowing of disk spaces, congenital kyphosis, scoliosis, osteoporosis, ankylosing spondylitis, and Scheuermann's disease. In patients without a clinically evident cause of pain, only the radiologic diagnoses of ankylosing spondylitis, trauma, infection, or neoplasm are likely to alter treatment.[7] However, even normal radiographs may provide some therapeutic value by excluding major pathology, reassuring the patient, and ensuring medicolegal coverage.[6]

Oblique views of the lumbar spine have traditionally been used to evaluate apophyseal joint abnormalities and pars interarticularis defects (spondylolysis). However, the diagnostic benefit of oblique views has been questioned, since apophyseal degenerative changes are usually accompanied by narrowed disk spaces and hypertrophic spurring easily demonstrated on routine anteroposterior and lateral views.[8]

Evaluation of a suspected herniated disk requires using a modality to image soft tissue structures. This may be done by directly imaging the spine and disk material by computed tomography or magnetic resonance imaging or indirectly visualizing the herniated disk by taking an impression of the thecal sac and nerve roots (myelography).

MAGNETIC RESONANCE IMAGING

Magnetic resonance imaging (MRI) evaluates the CNS and its surrounding structures by using strong magnetic fields and electromagnetic radiation in the radiowave frequency spectrum to create two-dimensional images.

Components of the imaging system

There are several important components of the system that create the image: the magnet, coils, and computer[9] (Fig. 6-1). To understand MRI, an explanation of the system components is important.

Magnet system. The several different types of magnets used in clinical imaging include the fixed, resistive, superconducting, and gradient magnets.

Fixed magnets. Fixed magnets are permanent magnets that always maintain their magnetic properties. These magnets may weigh several tons and are usually in the low to mid field strength range (up to 0.3 tesla). These magnets are very cost efficient to operate; however, at the lower field strength the images are not as sharp and crisp. These magnets cannot be built in the high field strength range because of the sheer size and weight of the apparatus.[9,10]

Resistive magnets. The resistive magnet is actually an electromagnet. This magnet is created by a current-carrying wire that is wrapped around a cylinder. A simple analogy is the elementary-school experiment that consists of wrapping a copper wire around a nail. The copper wire is then connected to a battery, and when current flows in the wire, the nail becomes electromagnetic and is capable of lifting iron

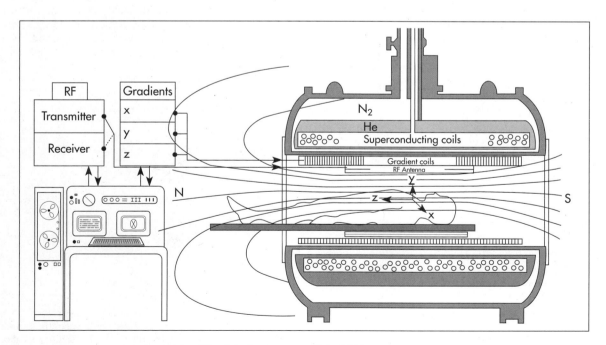

Fig. 6-1 Components of the MRI system.

filings or other ferromagnetic materials. Imagine that this theoretic magnet is attached to a stronger current source with more circular wrappings made of copper wire. If the nail is removed from the coil, then the magnet would function like resistive magnets. Resistive magnets can generate a magnetic field by turning on the electrical current and allowing it to flow into the circular wires.

A related principle of electricity and magnetism is that an oscillating electrical current in a wire will produce a fluctuating magnetic field termed *electromagnetic radiation.* Conversely, an oscillating magnetic field that occurs inside a closed circuit will cause an oscillating electrical current to flow.

Superconducting magnets. The most common magnet used in clinical neuroimaging is the superconducting magnet, a variation of the traditional resistive magnet. In the superconducting magnet, there are multiple coils of current-carrying wire made of a metal alloy that becomes superconducting at temperatures near 0 K. When superconductivity occurs, there is no resistance to electrical flow and an electrical current will flow in a closed circuit perpetually. The continually flowing electrical current will therefore generate a continuous magnetic field. This, however, requires that the current-carrying wires be kept at temperatures near 0 K. In order to achieve superconducting conditions, the coils are bathed in liquid helium with a temperature near 0 K. The inner jacket of helium and coils are kept cool by an outer jacket of less expensive liquid nitrogen. The outer jacket is then surrounded by an insulating casing much like a thermos bottle that prevents the cryogens (liquid helium and nitrogen) from boiling off. The conditions of superconductivity cannot be easily created, but once created, conditions can be maintained if cryogens are replaced as needed. For these reasons it is not practical to turn the magnetic field on and off. Persons working in the area of the scanner should be aware that the large magnetic fields are always present and should beware of metallic objects on their and the patients' clothing that may be pulled into the scanner at high speed and potentially cause harm.

Gradient magnets. Gradient magnets are another part of the MRI system. These are primarily resistive magnets that may be less than one tenth as strong as the primary magnet. These magnets are arranged in any of three directions to create gradient magnetic fields superimposed on the main magnetic field and are termed the *x, y,* and *z axes* (see Fig. 6-1). The z axis is usually parallel to the lines of flux of the main magnetic field. These gradient fields function in the creation of the three-dimensional imaging process.

Coils. The *body coil* is sometimes called the "stimulating coil" or "gradient coil" and may function as the stimulator and receiver. This coil is different from the coil of wires that creates the magnetic field; it acts as a stimulator when an electric current oscillates in the wires, thereby generating electromagnetic radiation. A specific frequency in the radio-wave portion of the electromagnetic spectrum will stimulate the subject.

When the current is turned off, the coil can function as a receiver. The coil detects the electromagnetic radiation signals that come from the subject. These signals create the image. Specially designed receivers called *surface coils* are being used in place of the body coil to detect the electromagnetic signal from the subject and to improve image quality. These surface coils are placed on the surface of the subject in the area of interest. The body coil then functions as the stimulator and a separate surface coil functions as the receiver.[9,10]

Computer. All MRI systems have a computer. The computer translates the received signals into images. The signals are received in a coded format that determines their three-dimensional location. The amount of signal coming from each area is mapped on a gray scale; a high signal appears white and a low signal appears dark or black. It is the overall collection of these spatially located signals of different intensity that ultimately creates the image.

The principle of magnetic resonance

Magnetic resonance occurs primarily in nuclei with unpaired protons. Hydrogen, with its one proton and no neutrons, has the property of net spin. When the nucleus spins, it creates a magnetic dipole with a positive and a negative direction[11] (Fig. 6-2). In any substance with hydrogen, e.g., a glass of water, the nuclei are spinning randomly, and this causes many small magnetic dipoles to cancel each other out. Thus the glass of water does not demonstrate net magnetic properties.

Substances that demonstrate magnetic resonance can be affected by an external magnetic field. In the presence of a strong magnetic field, a fraction of the nuclei will align themselves with the lines of flux in the magnetic field. This gives the object a net magnetic field. The direction with the field is a low-energy position.[11,12]

The small magnetic dipoles can be induced to a higher energy position by using the energy of a specific wavelength. The magnetic dipoles that align opposite the direction of the outside magnetic field are in a high-energy position, which requires the absorption of energy[3] (Fig. 6-3). Only a certain type of energy will be absorbed by the nuclei to cause them to move to the high-energy state. The

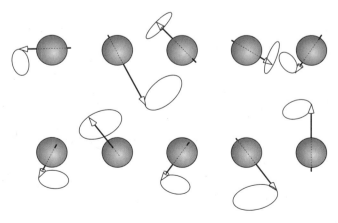

Fig. 6-2 In the absence of an external magnetic field, individual hydrogen nuclei are oriented randomly. Their dipoles cancel each other out producing no net magnetization.

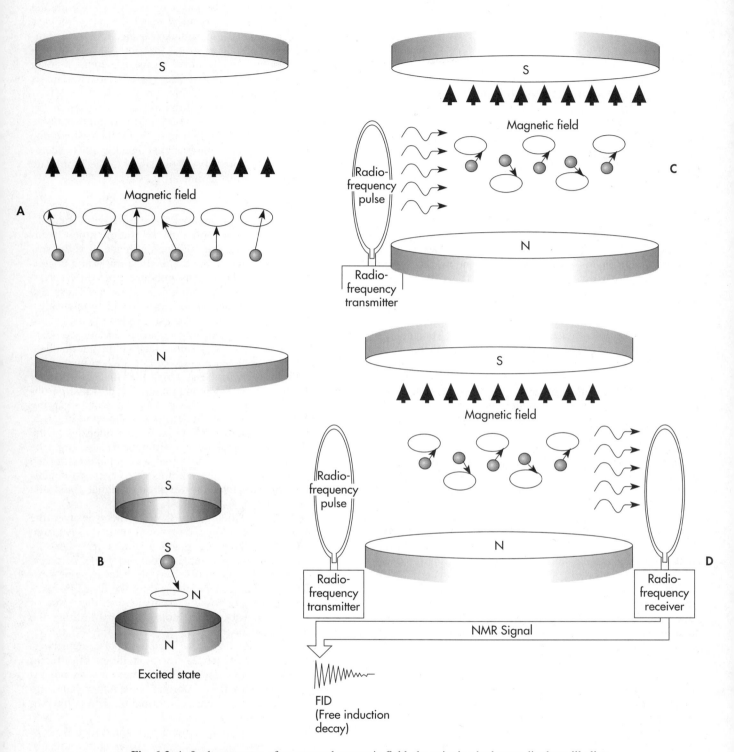

Fig. 6-3 A, In the presence of an external magnetic field, the spinning hydrogen dipoles will align with the magnetic field in a low-energy state. **B,** An excited state can be induced by the absorption of energy where the magnetic dipole is oriented opposite the external magnetic field. **C,** After the MRI system is stimulated, some of the spinning nuclei occupy a high-energy state. **D,** When these spinning nuclei relax back to the low-energy state, they create a signal that can be detected by the receiver coil.

wavelength of the energy required is described by the Larmour equation[11,12]

$$w = y*B_o$$

where

w = wavelength of electromagnetic radiation required

y = the gyromagnetic constant, specific for the type of nucleus

B_o = the magnetic field strength

The energy that is required to stimulate these spinning nuclei can then be described by the equation

$$E = h\nu$$

where

E = the energy of the electromagnetic radiation

h = Planck's constant

v = the wavelength of the electromagnetic radiation

Different wavelengths will not be able to induce the nuclei into the higher energy state.[11,12]

T_1 and T_2 relaxation

The high-energy magnetic dipoles give off energy in a process called *relaxation*. Once the stimulating electromagnetic radiation or the "pulse" is turned off, the high-energy system will begin to decay. This decay process is a relaxation back to a lower energy state, where the magnetic dipoles are aligned with the main magnetic field. As the system relaxes back to a lower energy state, electromagnetic radiation is given off and this is then detected and used to create the image[13] (Fig. 6-4).

T_1 and T_2 are the two types of relaxation.* T_1 and T_2 relaxation times can be compared to the half-life of radioactive substances, where one half of a radioactive substance will decay to its components in a specified time. This process can theoretically continue indefinitely. A similar process occurs with T_2 relaxation time, where two thirds of the signal will decay after a specified time (see Fig. 6-4, *A*). Of the remaining one third of the original signal, two thirds of that will decay after another T_2 relaxation time, and so on.

The T_1 relaxation time is similar; however, the signal returns from a negative direction toward its baseline amplitude. The signal grows by two thirds of the baseline amplitude for every T_1 time period (see Fig. 6-4, *B*). After one T_1 time period, the remaining one third (approximately) of the total missing signal will be two-thirds replaced after another T_1 time period. This can conceivably continue indefinitely before the system is completely relaxed back to baseline amplitude. However, after five T_1 time periods, the system has essentially relaxed back to baseline.

The rate of relaxation is an exponential process related to the T_1 and T_2 relaxation time. The slope of the graph describing this changing signal relates indirectly to the T_2 relaxation time (see Fig. 6-4).

---

*An in-depth description of T_1 and T_2 relaxation times is beyond the scope of this chapter. For more information, refer to other sources listed in the reference section.

Various mechanisms have been employed to measure the T_2 relaxation time. One of these mechanisms employs a varying pulse sequence of stimulating electromagnetic radiation. A signal is then recorded from the sample at alternating times, and the amplitudes are used to create a graph that describes an exponential decay of the signal. This is then used to calculate the T_2 relaxation time.

The rate of relaxation of different tissues varies. If the rate of relaxation of one tissue is rapid and another tissue relaxation rate is slow, a point may be reached where one tissue may produce much more signal than the other. Therefore, based on the intensity of the signals, one tissue can be discriminated from the other (Fig. 6-5).

Image construction

Although individual tissues may have different T_1 and T_2 relaxation times, these individual relaxation times themselves are not important in creating an image. It is the amplitude of the detected signal that is most important in constructing the image. Signals are obtained from different areas at a particular time in the relaxation process. These signals create a two-dimensional map of signal intensities, which becomes the image. When the signal intensities are translated into a gray scale, high signals are assigned a white color; low signals are assigned a black color. Intermediate signals are then assigned a shade of gray. When images are obtained this way, the time at which the signal is obtained in the relaxation process is important; the information obtained at different times in this process may show varying distribution of T_1, T_2, or spin density. As shown in Fig. 6-5, if the signal was obtained at point X, the intensity of the amplitude of this signal in two different tissues might be very similar. However, if the signal was obtained from the two tissues at point Y, the amplitudes of the two signals might be very different. This variation in signal could discriminate one tissue from another.

Theoretically, it would seem that the more decayed the tissue the easier it would be to discriminate that tissue from others. However, there are practical limits on when the "echo" or signal can be sampled from the tissue. At a certain point the background noise may have the same or similar amplitude as the signal coming from the tissue of interest. It may then be impossible to distinguish the tissue of interest from the background noise, thereby limiting the usefulness of the image.

MRIs are obtained in three different pulse sequences. Each of these pulse sequences creates an image of different T_1, T_2, or spin density distribution. One pulse sequence increases the amount of T_1 information, another pulse sequence maximizes spin density information, and a third sequence maximizes T_2 information.

Of all the types of images, the T_2 weighted scan is probably the most important because on T_2 weighted images, pathologic variations are most easily seen. The T_2 weighted scan may best demonstrate the difference between a tumor and surrounding normal brain tissue, but it does not display good anatomic detail. Tissue resolution is best seen on T_1 or spin density weighted images.[9,10]

During the imaging process one portion of a slice is imaged at a time. When an MRI image is created, a section of

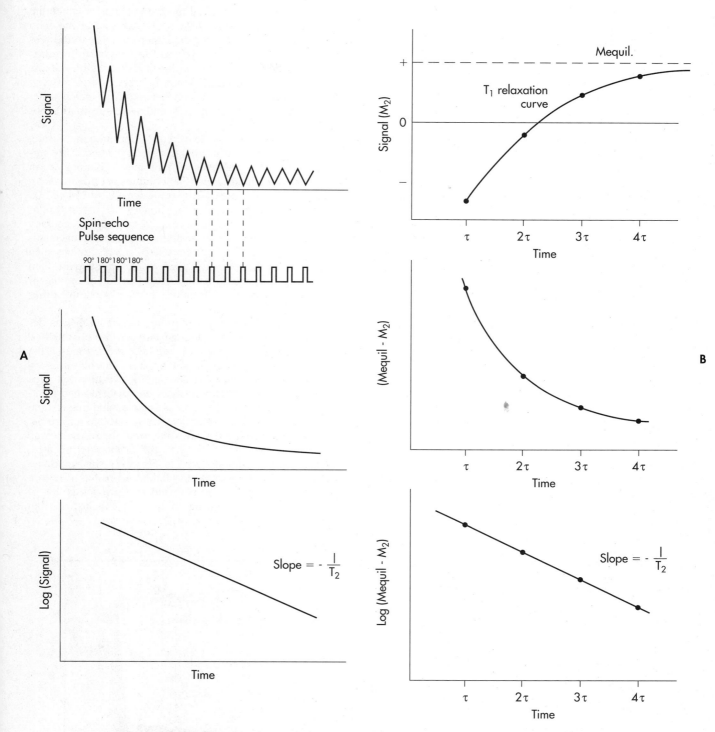

Fig. 6-4 A, The T_2 relaxation curve is constructed by a spin-echo pulse sequence composed of alternating radio frequency stimulations. The amplitude of the received signal is plotted against time. If this graph is then plotted as the logarithm of the signal against time, the slope will be a straight line and is equal to $-1/T_2$. **B,** The T_1 relaxation curve is similar to the T_2 relaxation curve but uses a different pulse sequence. The amplitude appears to grow with progressive time from the stimulus. When the recorded signal amplitude is subtracted from the initial steady state amplitude and this product is plotted against time, an exponential decay curve is produced. If the logarithm of this product is plotted against time the slope of that straight line will be equal to $-1/T_1$.

tissues is selected, then one particular thin column is selected, and signals are obtained. No other signals are obtained from the rest of the tissue in that slice (Fig. 6-6). The tissue in the slice is allowed to relax back to steady state. Another column immediately adjacent to the previously selected column is then stimulated and signals are recorded from that area. The signals are recorded in such a way that it is possible to tell what intensity was obtained from what segment of the column of tissue. Then numerous columns of the image are collected and put together to produce a two-dimensional image. More detailed descriptions of the process of image construction can be found in other references.

The imaging process may require a considerable amount of time. After a section of tissue is selected for stimulation, the tissue is pulsed several times with electromagnetic radiation in the radiowave spectrum. The tissue is allowed to relax for a short period of time (generally between 30 to 120 msec) and then a signal or "echo" is recorded and used

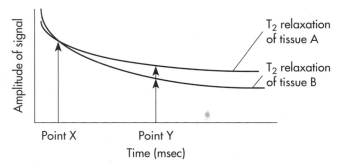

Fig. 6-5 The T_2 relaxation curves of two different tissues are plotted superimposed. At Point X the amplitude of the recorded signal is essentially the same for the two tissues. At Point Y the amplitudes of the two tissues vary considerably.

to create the two-dimensional image. The time at which the echo is recorded is called *TE* or *echo time*. After the echo is recorded, it takes time for the system to relax to the prestimulation state. This time period for the system to relax, from the time of stimulation back to prestimulation state, is called *TR;* repetition time or time to relaxation is between 0.5 and 2.0 sec. Once the system has relaxed to steady state, the tissue can be stimulated again and more information obtained.

Imaging one slice can take a considerable amount of time. The length of time that it takes to collect the necessary signals from one slice depends on how many columns are in the image. Many imagers use 254 columns per picture. With a TR or repetition time of 2.0 sec, at least 2×254 or 508 secs, must be used to create one image. Even with a relatively long imaging time like this, resolution or accuracy must often be improved by obtaining the signal in each column more than one time. If two sets of signals are obtained to create an average of each pixel or picture element, then the imaging time would double. One can easily see that if one slice were to be collected at a time, scanning times would be extremely long.

In order to reduce imaging times, *interleaving* was developed. With this technique many images are obtained simultaneously. The imaging procedure is essentially the same: One slice is selected, then a particular column is selected and pulsed, and the echo obtained. While that slice is allowed to relax to steady state, an adjacent slice is selected; a column from that slice is selected and pulsed, and an echo obtained. Then the next slice is selected and so on. The process is continued until the first slice has relaxed back to its steady state and then the process is repeated. This principle is demonstrated in Fig. 6-7. This interleaving of images allows multiple planes or images to be obtained simultaneously. The unfortunate drawback is that, if the patient is moving during stimulation, not just one but

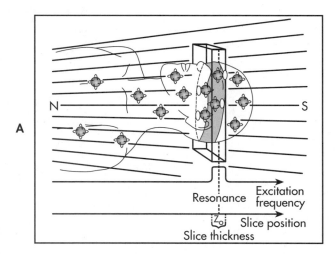

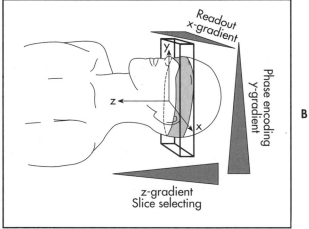

Fig. 6-6 A, In a magnetic gradient, a defined radiofrequency pulse will only stimulate a slice of this sample. By changing gradients, individual slices of the sample can be selected for imaging. **B,** After the slice is selected, other gradients are applied to the sample in order to select and encode a single column of the slice. Thus one acquisition provides all the information needed for a complete image line.

essentially all of the images may be affected by motion artifact. It is therefore imperative that the patient remain still during the imaging process.

Image contrast

The T_1, T_2, and spin density images can be easily distinguished and provide important clinical information. Fig. 6-8 summarizes T_1, spin density, and T_2-weighted images and their relative appearance on film. The T_2-weighted images are easily identified because the cerebrospinal fluid (CSF) appears white. The resolution of detail on T_2 images is not as precise as other images. The T_2-weighted scans will have a long TR time, around 2 secs; and the TE time is also relatively long at about 80 to 120 msec.[14]

The T_1-weighted image is also easily discerned by visual inspection. The spinal fluid appears black or dark and the resolution of the anatomical structures is clear, thus supporting the theory that T_1-weighted images give the sharpest pictures. T_1-weighted images can also be verified by inspecting the TR and TE times. Although the TR and TE

times will change depending on the field strength of the magnet, the TR is generally short, approximately 0.5 sec. The TE time is also short and may be less than 30 msec. Because T_1-weighted images have short TR times, they can be performed relatively quickly, thereby allowing for multiple imaging planes.[14]

Spin density scans are also good for anatomical detail. They can be recognized by the long TR like the T_2-weighted scans, but they have a much shorter TE of 20 to 30 msec.

Some physicians use the T_2-weighted scans to locate the approximate area of suspected pathology because pathologic features stand out on this scan. The T_1-weighted or spin-density images are then used to define the anatomic region of suspected pathology.

Gadolinium contrast enhancement may be given to alter the signal characteristics of some abnormal tissues. Gadolinium primarily affects those structures within a disrupted blood-brain barrier and penetrates into the surrounding tissues by passive diffusion. The paramagnetic properties of gadolinium decrease the T_1 relaxation time of nearby hydrogen atoms. Abnormal tissues will have a relatively high signal on T_1-weighted images. Gadolinium is often used to differentiate edema from tumor. On T_2-weighted scans, edema and tumor appear bright with a high signal detected (see Fig. 6-8). On T_1-weighted scans without gadolinium, both tissues may appear alike and may differ only slightly from the surrounding normal tissue. Since the blood-brain barrier is intact in edematous tissue but disrupted in tumor, gadolinium will penetrate the tumor tissue but not the edema. On T_1-weighted gadolinium-enhanced scans, the tumor will appear white and the surrounding edema will stay dark or gray.[14]

Indications

MRI may help evaluate the central nervous system (CNS) in the pain patient. MRI provides different types of information when performed on the head and spine. In general, MRI is good for soft tissue structures, and CT is good for bone.

In the head, MRI is superior for evaluating many disorders of the brain. In comparative studies of CNS lesions evaluated by CT or MRI, MRI was found to be superior in the evaluation of most disease states.[14-16] MRI is more sensitive than CT, particularly in the evaluation of demyelinating disease, neoplastic disease of the brain, degenerative disease, and cerebral infarction. Chronic hemorrhage is better defined on MRI, but acute hemorrhage, including subarachnoid hemorrhage and disorders of the skull, are seen better on CT.[17,18]

Spinal MRI is especially important in the pain patient because it can demonstrate high sensitivity for soft tissue structures (Fig 6-9). Surface-coil MRI of the spine is an excellent investigation for possible spinal canal stenosis or herniated disk.[19] This is also true in the cervical and lumbosacral areas. MRI can be too sensitive in some instances. In 20% of asymptomatic individuals, MRI has shown herniated disks. It is therefore important to correlate the patient's history and physical exam with the MRI findings.

There are other advantages of MRI besides the information that can be obtained. MRI has no ionizing radiation, is

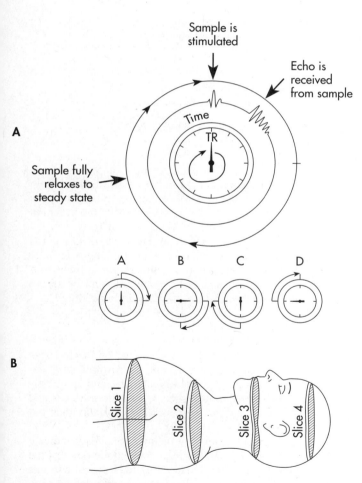

Fig. 6-7 A, During a TR time cycle, most of the time is spent waiting for the system to fully relax to the prestimulation steady state. **B,** The technique of interleaving allows imaging data to be obtained during most of the TR time. During **A,** data is obtained for slice #1. During **B,** data is obtained for slice #2, etc. At the end of time *D,* the cycle is repeated.

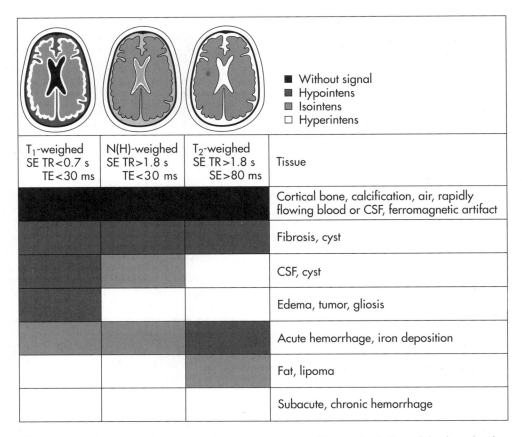

T$_1$-weighed SE TR<0.7 s TE<30 ms	N(H)-weighed SE TR>1.8 s TE<30 ms	T$_2$-weighed SE TR>1.8 s SE>80 ms	Tissue
			Cortical bone, calcification, air, rapidly flowing blood or CSF, ferromagnetic artifact
			Fibrosis, cyst
			CSF, cyst
			Edema, tumor, gliosis
			Acute hemorrhage, iron deposition
			Fat, lipoma
			Subacute, chronic hemorrhage

■ Without signal
■ Hypointens
■ Isointens
□ Hyperintens

Fig. 6-8 Relative signal intensities of various tissues on T$_1$-weighted, T$_2$-weighted, and spin density-weighted scans.

not as invasive as myelography, and has the ability to easily construct multiple imaging planes. One major disadvantage of MRI is its increased cost, which is approximately twice the cost of a CT scan.[10,17]

MRI is not the best study for evaluating bony structures because it detects very little signal from bone; therefore anatomic detail of the bony structures is absent. It is for this reason that suspected spinal facet disease or radiculopathy from osteophyte encroachment at the neural foramen is not well defined on MRI.[10,12,18]

Monitoring and anesthetic factors

During the MRI procedure, traditional cardiorespiratory monitoring procedures are usually restricted. In particular, monitoring with electronic instruments is limited because some equipment may not be compatible with the MRI scanners; their use may interfere with signal acquisition and patient safety. One central rule is that if monitors are used, they should be positioned outside the shielded area. Traditional cathode ray tubes do not make the best monitoring screens because their image may be severely distorted by the magnetic fields. Liquid crystal displays are preferred and digital liquid emitting diode readouts may also be reliable.[14]

Cardiovascular or respiratory monitoring equipment must often use nonmetallic instruments such as the precordial esophageal stethoscope for auscultating heartbeat, but in this situation, long sections of connective tubing may be necessary unless the anesthesiologist is inside the scanning area. An electrocardiogram (ECG) can usually be recorded on the subject during an MRI scan. However ECG records are subject to alteration by the surrounding magnetic field. A peripheral pulse recording or pulse oximetry may provide good monitoring results of respiration and pulse but can in some instances disturb the imaging procedure.[14]

Contraindications

There are several devices that, if present inside the subject's body, will contraindicate the performance of MRI. These devices include: cardiac pacemakers, neurostimulators, cerebral aneurysm clips, recent surgical clips, and some aortic valve prostheses. The presence of metallic implants and prosthetic devices may be permissible on an individual basis.[10,14]

Cardiac pacemakers and neurostimulators contraindicate MRI scanning because the fluctuating magnetic fields of the imaging process may cause inappropriate electrical currents to flow into the wires of the device, possibly delivering a relatively large electrical current to the heart or other neurologic structure. These devices also could malfunction in the presence of a high magnetic field. Cerebral aneurysm clips and surgical clips can also contraindicate an MRI ex-

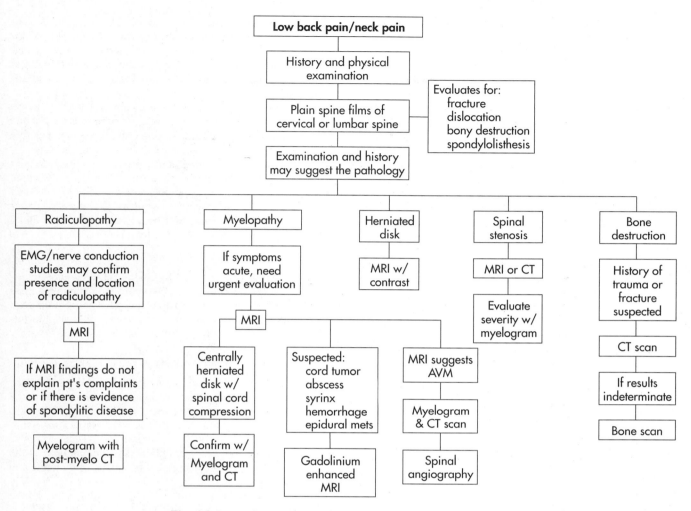

Fig. 6-9 Evaluation decision tree for back and neck pain complaints.

amination because the fluctuating magnetic fields may cause movement of the clip off of important vascular structures.[10,14]

Relative contraindications for performing MRI evaluations include claustrophobia and the inability to remain immobile during the imaging process. The MRI scanner often will appear as a threatening structure and may increase patients' anxiety levels to such an extent that they are not capable of completing the procedure. If these individuals cannot be sedated so that their anxiety is relieved yet are still able to follow directions, then alternative methods of neuroimaging must be found.

Individuals in constant discomfort or with alterations in alertness levels may not be good candidates for MRI. In addition, individuals who are unable to follow directions because of pain or as a result of confusional states may not be able to remain immobile for the scanning time of 30 to 60 minutes. Anesthesia can be given so that the patient can tolerate the scanning procedure; however, the risks of this level of anesthesia and the potential benefits must be weighed carefully.[10,14]

COMPUTED TOMOGRAPHY

CT is a well-known diagnostic study. The technique uses ionizing x-radiation to create two-dimensional images of the body.

Indications

CT scanning can be performed on the skull and spine. In both areas, CT is the preferred technique in patients with suspected trauma. Trauma patients often must be evaluated rapidly with monitoring of vital signs, and sedation may not be possible to allow for MRI scanning. The trauma patient may also be combative or unable to follow directions. Rapid CT evaluation is possible by using a scanning time of less than 5 seconds per slice.

CT of the brain and skull is also important in the patient with suspected acute intracranial hemorrhage. Acute subarachnoid, intraparenchymal, and epidural hemorrhage are visualized best by CT. The patient with subarachnoid hemorrhage may come to a pain specialist with complaints of acute severe headache. This relatively uncommon headache presentation is potentially life-threatening if there is associated aneurysmal rupture. CT scan is the study of choice in this setting.

CT scanning can detect lesions where increased calcification is a prominent feature or bony destruction is present. Calcified lesions that may be seen on CT include meningioma or craniopharyngioma. These are often poorly seen on MRI because of the low signal detected from calcified lesions. Lesions of the skull caused by bony destruction for neoplastic, inflammatory, or traumatic injuries are also evaluated best with CT.[17]

Spinal CT with myelogram in the lumbar or cervical spine is beneficial for the evaluation of suspected radiculopathy (see Fig. 6-9). In settings where radiculopathy may be from disk herniation, neural foramen encroachment, or spinal canal stenosis, CT or a myelogram will be helpful.[17]

MYELOGRAPHY

Myelography is often performed in combination with CT scan in individuals who do not tolerate MRI or as an emergent procedure in patients with acute myelopathy.

Indications

Myelography, when compared with spinal CT, may be superior in evaluating the conus. On myelogram, the conus and upper lumbar disk segments are routinely visualized and only the portion of the spinal canal and thecal sac that are reasonably distended are seen. At L_5-S_1 there is an increased epidural fat layer that essentially hides the disk herniation.[17,18]

In the clinical setting, myelography is especially good for evaluating the nerve roots of cervical radiculopathy with osteophyte encroachment of the neural foramen. Myelogram may detect the abnormality better than CT or MRI alone.[17,18]

BONE SCANNING

Radionuclide bone scanning has long been known for its high degree of sensitivity in detecting a variety of bone lesions. In recent years, applications of bone scanning to various orthopedic, traumatic, neoplastic, and infectious processes have proven the usefulness of this modality in detecting clinically significant but often radiographically elusive problems.

The value of bone scanning, as in many nuclear imaging studies, lies in its ability to reflect physiologic changes rather than anatomic detail. While other radiographic modalities excel in providing defined, precise anatomic information, nuclear scans by their inherent nature are not able to define small structures or provide high resolution images. In fact, radiographs and bone scanning often provide complementary information in evaluation of skeletal pain. The greatest value of bone scanning is its high level of sensitivity for detection of early or subtle bone abnormalities. For this purpose, the bone scanning technique is not likely to become obsolete in the face of new, anatomically-oriented modalities.

Physiologic basis for bone scanning

Technetium labeled bone-seeking radiopharmaceuticals localize in bone by exchanging or adsorbing the hydroxyapatite component of bone. The amount of deposition of technetium tracer is affected by two factors: (1) the rate of local repair and remodeling of bone,[21] and (2) local skeletal blood flow, which delivers the tracer to the extracellular space, thus making it available for local exchange and adsorption.[20,22]

Any active process in bone that causes a local increase in bone turnover will result in a larger surface area of bone available for tracer accumulation. Thus a region of active bone turnover such as a normal growth plate, fracture, tumor, infection, or any other active process results in locally increased tracer deposition or a "hot spot." At the same time, any process that results in increased blood flow, such as cellulitis or sympathectomy, will locally increase tracer deposition based on increased tracer delivery to the site.[23] This will also result in a "hot" area on bone scan.

Technique

Bone scanning is performed following intravenous (IV) injection of Technetium TC-99M methylene diphosphonate (99mTc-MDP) or a similar diphosphonate compound. Approximately 2 to 3 hours after injection, scintigraphic images are obtained with a gamma camera of specific areas of interest or the entire skeleton.

In some cases, a "three-phase bone scan" may be used:

1. A radionuclide angiogram or flow study of the area of interest is obtained during the IV injection of the tracer. As the tracer passes through the arterial circulation, rapid-sequence images are obtained to evaluate the vascularity of the region being scanned.
2. A "blood pool" image, obtained immediately after the flow study, displays regional perfusion of the bone and soft tissues.
3. Routine, delayed "static" images taken after 2 to 3 hours demonstrate active bony abnormality, which is reflected by locally increased deposition of tracer in the skeleton.

Comparison of early phases (flow and blood pool) to the delayed phase (static) may yield useful information about inflammatory processes and other vascular changes such as those found in reflex sympathetic dystrophy.

The radiation dose to the patient is relatively low; a whole body dose is approximately 0.02 rad per administered mCi.[24] For the usual adult dose of 20 mCi, a total body dose of 0.4 rad per examination is obtained, which is less than the radiation dose from a lumbar spine series.[25] Since iodinated contrast material is not used, side effects and allergic contrast reactions are uncommon.

Common clinical indications for bone scanning

Whereas a substantial loss of bone must occur before a destructive lesion or demineralization becomes radiographically visible, bone scanning does not rely on the actual amount of bone loss to demonstrate pathology. Consequently, destruction caused by metastases and osteomyelitis may be detected much earlier on bone scans than on radiographs. Similarly, subtle trauma sufficient to incite a local repair process, such as a stress fracture, may also be obvious on bone scans but radiographically invisible.

The phrase "sensitive but nonspecific" is commonly applied to bone scanning. Although many different bone abnormalities result in "hot spots," careful attention to characteristics of the lesions will usually reveal a specific diagnosis when juxtaposed with the appropriate clinical information. The number, location, and distribution of lesions, as well as the clinical history (such as trauma or known primary malignancy) are important. When radiographic correlation is obtained, an even more precise and specific diagnosis is possible.

Since the advantage of bone scanning is high sensitivity, certain painful conditions are more appropriately detected by bone scanning than by radiographs, where findings may be subtle or even undetectable.

Metastatic tumor. Bone scanning is the primary modality for detection and follow-up of skeletal metastases. Metastases often appear on bone scans long before they become evident radiographically. The bone scan is a convenient way to evaluate the entire skeleton in a single examination and provides an accurate means for follow-up. The usual pattern is to scan multiple areas with increased uptake, predominately involving the axial skeleton. However, a single focus may represent metastasis in a high percentage of cases, especially in a patient with a known primary tumor.[26]

Infection. Acute osteomyelitis may not be detectable radiographically for at least 7 to 10 days after onset, since radiographs reflect the amount of bone destruction present. However, because of the very active nature of the process, osteomyelitis can usually be detected by bone scan at the onset. Three-phase bone scanning demonstrates markedly increased vascularity and focally intense tracer uptake at the site of infection. The appearance is easily differentiated from cellulitis where there may be hyperemia in the soft tissues but absence of focal tracer deposition in the bone.

Trauma. Occult fractures may be too subtle to be visible radiographically because of very subtle alterations of the bony architecture. However, bone scans will become positive in most patients within a short period of time; approximately 95% of patients under age 65 demonstrate abnormal bone scans within 24 hours after fracture, and 100% of the same age group demonstrate abnormal scans within 3 days.[27] The sensitivity of bone scanning may detect fractures that may not be detectable even with CT.

Stress fractures are a common cause of pain in athletes, military recruits, and in other persons who abnormally stress an otherwise normal bone. Radiographically, the fractures may not be visible in the early stages, and may or may not develop periosteal reaction and cortical thickening in the healing stage. However, they are usually readily detectable by bone scanning despite normal radiographs.

A focal area of intensity representing the stress fracture may be graded according to its extension through the diameter of the bone, thus the approximate duration of rest required for healing can be predicted.[28] "Shin splints" may be demonstrated by diffusely increased cortical uptake along the tibias without the focal appearance typical of stress fractures.

Arthritis. Inflammatory joint disorders are best characterized by conventional radiographs but may also be easily detected by bone scan. Active inflammation, such as rheumatoid or septic arthritis, will show increased flow on the three-phase bone scan and increased periarticular uptake on delayed views. Osteoarthritis, on the other hand, rarely appears hypervascular on early images. As in conventional radiography, distribution of involved joints is a primary means of differentiating the various forms of arthritis. Occasionally, acute inflammation in a joint may cause severe pain and swelling mimicking osteomyelitis, but bone scanning can usually differentiate the two conditions easily. In arthritis, the increased tracer uptake is symmetrical around the joint; in osteomyelitis, there is focal activity localized to the involved bone on one side of the joint.

Osteonecrosis. Avascular necrosis of the bone may be associated with trauma, hemoglobinopathies, infiltrative processes or steroid administration, or it may be idiopathic.[29] Bone scan evaluation has historically been performed with either radiocolloid bone marrow scans, which demonstrate absent marrow activity at the involved site, or conventional bone scintigraphy, which usually demonstrates increased uptake reflecting the active repair process. In very early stages, the infarcted bone will appear as a "cold" spot of absent radioactivity; however, scans are rarely obtained in the early stages because most patients are asymptomatic.[30] In later stages, radiographic changes become characteristic, including flattening of the femoral head, subchondral lucency, and sclerotic changes. Once these changes occur, the bone scan adds no information. Recently MRI has been studied as a more sensitive means to detect avascular necrosis of the femoral head, and it may demonstrate marrow abnormality when radiographs and bone scans are normal.[31]

Paget's disease. The increased vascularity and active bone turnover in Paget's disease yield a fairly characteristic bone scan appearance. Typically, there is intense tracer uptake in the involved bones and the bones often show visible enlargement. Bone scanning may suggest the diagnosis and delineate additional sites of involvement; however, radiographs are usually necessary to confirm Paget's disease because the scan appearance might be mimicked by osteomyelitis or metastasis.

ULTRASOUND

Ultrasound is one of the most important and rapidly progressive imaging modalities. By using an ultrasound beam that is transmitted and reflected from tissues, images are obtained without patient discomfort and without using ionizing radiation.

Ultrasound excels in characterizing tissues based on their *echogenicity,* or reflective characteristics. Fluid can easily be distinguished from solid tissue, allowing for differentiation of cysts from solid masses in the kidney, liver, or thyroid. Fluid-containing structures, such as the common bile duct and renal collection systems, are likewise well delineated. Gallstones are identified clearly; ultrasound has replaced the oral cholecystogram in the evaluation of suspected gallbladder disease. Using the fluid-filled bladder as a "window," the uterus and adnexae are easily visualized. The lack of ionizing radiation makes ultrasound examination ideal for women of child-bearing age and children, since no adverse effects have been demonstrated.

Masses or abscesses may be visualized if they are located in the pelvis or upper abdomen where bowel gas cannot interfere with transmission of the sound beam. Bone and air do not adequately transmit sound, which precludes evaluation of the chest, middle of the abdomen, and musculoskeletal system.

Doppler flow scanning in conjunction with ultrasound imaging of the vascular system has become popular for the detection of arterial occlusions and venous thrombosis. New transcranial Doppler is being applied to cerebrovascular disease. Ultrasound has gained wide popularity with patients and physicians and will certainly remain one of the most versatile and informative modalities in the future.

REFERENCES

1. Resnick D, Niwayama G: *Diagnosis of Bone and Joint Disorders,* ed 3. Philadelphia, WB Saunders, 1988.
2. DeSantos LA: The radiology of bone tumors: Old and new modalities. *CA Cancer J Clin* 30:66-89, 1980.
3. Brady LW, Croll HN: The role of bone scanning in the cancer patient. *Skeletal Radiol* 3:217, 1979.
4. Woolfenden JM et al: Comparison of bone scintigraphy and radiology in multiple myeloma. *Radiology* 134:723-728, 1980.
5. Resnick D: The target area approach to articular disorders: A synopsis. In Resnick D, Niwayama G, editors: *Diagnosis of Bone and Joint Disorders,* ed 2. Philadelphia, WB Saunders, 1988.
6. Gehweiler JA, Daffner RH: Low back pain: The controversy of radiologic evaluation. *AJR* 140:109-112, 1983.
7. Hall FM: Back pain and the radiologist. *Radiology* 137:861-863, 1980.
8. Eisenberg RL et al: Optimum radiographic examination for consideration of compensation awards. II. Cervical and lumbar spines. *AJR* 135:1071-1074, 1980.
9. Gademann G: Physical principles and techniques of MR imaging. In Huk WJ, Gademann G, Friedmann G, editors: *Magnetic Resonance Imaging of Central Nervous System Disease.* Berlin, Springer-Verlag, 1992.
10. Lufkin RB: Magnetic resonance imaging. In Mazziotta JC, Gilman S, editors: *Clinical Brain Imaging: Principles and Applications.* Philadelphia, FA Davis, 1991.
11. Harms SE et al: Principles of nuclear magnetic resonance imaging. *Radiographics* 4:26, 1984.
12. Maudsley AA: Principles of nuclear magnetic resonance. In Budinger TF, Margulis AR, editors: *Medical Magnetic Resonance Imaging and Spectroscopy.* Berkeley, CA, Society of Magnetic Resonance in Medicine, 1986.
13. Loar CM: T_1 and T_2 measurements on the IBM PC-10 spectrometer. From syllabus for postgraduate course in magnetic resonance imaging, Baylor University College of Medicine, Houston, 1986.
14. Huk WJ, Gademann G, Friedmann G: Practical aspects of the MR examination. In Huk WJ, Gademann G, Friedmann G, editors: *Magnetic Resonance Imaging of Central Nervous System Disease.* Berlin, Springer-Verlag, 1992.
15. Bradley WG et al: Comparison of CT and MRI in 400 patients with suspected disease of the brain and cervical spinal cord. *Radiology* 152:695, 1984.
16. Haughton VM et al: A blinded clinical comparison of MR imaging and CT in neuroradiology. *Radiology* 160:751, 1986.
17. Gibby WA, Zimmerman RA: X-ray computed tomography. In Mazziotta JC, Gilman S, editors: *Clinical Brain Imaging: Principles and Applications.* Philadelphia, FA Davis, 1991.
18. Kirkwood RJ: *Essentials of Neuroimaging.* New York, Churchill Livingstone, 1990.
19. Modic MT et al: Imaging of degenerative disk disease. *Radiology* 168:177, 1988.
20. Jones AG, Francis MD, Davis MA: Bone scanning: Radionuclide reaction mechanisms. *Semin Nucl Med* 6:3-18, 1976.
21. Mitchell MD et al: Avascular necrosis of the hip: Comparison of MR, CT, and scintigraphy. *AJR* 147:67-71, 1986.
22. Dalinka MK et al: Modern diagnostic imaging in joint disease. *AJR* 152:229-240, 1989.
23. Charkes ND: Skeletal blood flow: Implications for bone-scan interpretation. *J Nucl Med* 21:91-98, 1980.
24. Graham LS, Krishnamurthy GT, Blahd BH: Dosimetry of skeletal-seeking radiopharmaceuticals. *J Nucl Med* 15:496, 1974.
25. Scleien B, Tucker TT, Johnson DW: The mean active bone marrow dose to the adult population of the United States from diagnostic radiology. Dept of Health, Educ, and Welfare Pub No 77-8013. Washington, DC, 1977, US Government Printing Office.
26. McNeil BJ: Value of bone scanning in neoplastic disease. *Semin Nucl Med* 14:277-286, 1984.
27. Matin P: Bone scintigraphy in the diagnosis and management of traumatic injury. *Semin Nucl Med* 13:104-122, 1983.
28. Zwas ST, Elkanovitch R, Frank G: Interpretation and classification of bone scintigraphic findings in stress fractures. *J Nucl Med* 28:452-457, 1987.
29. Solomon L: Mechanisms of idiopathic osteonecrosis. *Orthop Clin North Am* 16:655-667, 1985.
30. Bonnarens F, Hernandez A, D'Ambrosia R: Bone scintigraphic changes in osteonecrosis of the femoral head. *Orthop Clin North Am* 16:697-703, 1985.
31. Jergeson HE, Heller M, Genant HK: Magnetic resonance imaging in osteonecrosis of the femoral head. *Orthop Clin North Am* 16:705-716, 1985.

QUESTIONS: RADIOGRAPHY AND NEUROIMAGING

1. T_2-weighted scans can be distinguished by their TR and TE times. Which of the following could produce a T_2-weighted scan?
   A. The TR is short (0.5 sec), and the TE is short (25.0 msec)
   B. The TR is short (0.5 sec), and the TE is long (80.0 msec)
   C. The TR is long (2.0 sec), and the TE is short (25.0 msec)
   D. The TR is long (2.0 sec), and the TE is long (80.0 msec)

2. T_1-weighted scans can be distinguished by their TR and TE times. Which of the following could produce a T_1-weighted scan?
   A. The TR is short (0.5 sec), and the TE is short (25.0 msec)
   B. The TR is short (0.5 sec), and the TE is long (80.0 msec)
   C. The TR is long (2.0 sec), and the TE is short (25.0 msec)
   D. The TR is long (2.0 sec), and the TE is long (80.0 msec)

3. On T_1-weighted scans the CSF appears:
   A. Black
   B. Gray
   C. White

4. Magnetic resonance imaging is not the study of choice in which disease state of the brain?
   A. Neoplasm
   B. Inflammation
   C. Acute hemorrhage
   D. Demyelinating disease

5. Myelography is the most useful method to evaluate which suspected disease state of the spine?
   A. Herniated nucleus pulposus with radiculopathy
   B. Osteophyte encroachment of neural foramen
   C. Vertebral body metastatic disease
   D. Spinal trauma with fracture of the posterior elements

ANSWERS

1. D
2. A
3. A
4. D
5. B

PART TWO

Special Examinations

7 Neurophysiologic Studies

David R. Longmire

One of the many diagnostic responsibilities of the practicing algologist is to confirm the presence of any organic condition that can reasonably produce clinical pain. Failure to complete this task often results in reduced symptom control and inadequate treatment of the causative dysfunction or anatomic lesion. Unfortunately, despite the current technical sophistication of imaging procedures,[1-3] there are many organic pain syndromes in which no structural abnormalities can be demonstrated radiologically. When patients are told that their radiographic findings are normal, they often interpret this information to mean that there is no proof that their pain is physical. Furthermore, many patients become concerned that family, friends, or employers who learn of the negative results will believe that the patient's pain is only psychogenic in origin. If anxiety and depression develop in response to this situation, there is a greater chance that the physician may be further misled by the clinical stigmata of these behavioral reactions at subsequent clinical visits.

In order to avoid this problem, the physician must improve accuracy in objectively assessing pain by considering etiologies other than just structural pathology. Since the transmission and translation of pain responses in animals and humans occur in conjunction with electrical impulses in nerve cells and fibers,[4,5] it would seem appropriate to include measurements of such neurophysiologic activity in the assessment of pain-related somatic dysfunction.

Unfortunately, the art and science of clinical neurophysiology have not been developed as fully for the objective evaluation of clinical pain as they have for the diagnostic assessment of neuromuscular diseases or nonpainful sensory or cerebral disturbances. Algologists are therefore left with two personal educational tasks:

1. To acquire a basic understanding of any tests which are commonly used for electrodiagnosis of nervous system disorders, regardless of whether such conditions are painful or not
2. To attain facility with the successful theories and methods previously used in pain research and those methods that are used currently in clinical pain evaluation[6-12]

Completion of these tasks may broaden pain assessment skills.

The purpose of this chapter will be to review those methods used to measure certain electrical functions of the central and peripheral nervous systems relative to pain.

HISTORICAL PERSPECTIVES

The early histories of scientific disciplines such as electrophysiology, electrodiagnosis, and clinical neurophysiology are often dated by the work of Galvani in the late eighteenth century.[13-15] His observations of the electrical induction of muscular contraction in the legs of the frog have become classic material for biology students in most developed nations. In reality, there are many earlier natural[16] and scientific[17-22] publications that confirm the relationship between electricity and neurological function. Although the reasons for reduced interest in these prior observations are not completely known, there has been much speculation that many other scientific discoveries of that period were also overshadowed by the heated debate between Galvani and Volta regarding the true mechanism of electrical activation of muscular contraction.[23,24]

Gradually, however, the introduction of electrical stimulators and measuring instruments for the assessment of somatic functions in the human body grew within circles of European medicine and science. By the middle of the nineteenth century, these methods became recognized as a specialty[25,26]; textbooks on electrophysiology appeared shortly thereafter.[27]

With rapidly growing interest, nineteenth century physicians debated whether the value of this science was greater for treatment of diseases (many of which were painful), or for the diagnosis of disordered nervous function. These differences were never really settled, but the competitive nature of medical practice eventually resulted in physicians who separately promoted themselves as specialists in electrotherapy, electrodiagnosis, or electromedicine.[28-31]

The electrotherapists developed skills sufficiently effective to be used as cornerstones of physical medicine and rehabilitation. For specialists in electrodiagnosis, they had to first establish that potential electrical changes in nerve and muscle function could be quantified.[32,33] These early observations were subsequently validated in states of normal function and disease, and gradually the idea that specific abnormalities could occur in patients with neuromuscular illness was accepted.[34]

Nevertheless, around the turn of the century, the great mysteries of the human nervous system continued to be unsolved. As a result, much of the research effort in the field of electrodiagnosis was directed by neurologists, neuropsychiatrists, and neurosurgeons.[31] Consequently there was a period during which the term *electrodiagnosis* was so often used to indicate exploration of the nervous system that the field became known by a second name, "clinical neurophysiology."

However, this restrictive view did not prevent the development of other tests of electrical function generated outside the nervous system. Most of the new methods were named by adding the prefix *electro-* and the suffix *-graphy* to the root name of the organ being studied. Following the introduction of *electrocardiography* as the name for the electrical recording of the heart,[35,36] studies of the brain and muscle became known as *electroencephalography,*[37,38] and *electromyography,*[39] respectively.

CLASSIFICATION OF ELECTROPHYSIOLOGIC ACTIVITY

Gradually, electrophysiologic methods became so specialized that multiple fields of study were developed around individual organs or tissue types. Despite this tendency toward a narrower field of electrodiagnosis for each body system, the limited access to electronic equipment for research that was created by the advent of World War II forced physiologists to use available equipment for as many different applications as possible. This led to the realization that, if the same instrument could be used effectively to monitor different body systems, then perhaps the ways in which physiologic phenomena could be expressed electrically were limited. This position was summarized by Walter in 1950[40] and restated in 1963 as a framework of principles for which any electrophysiologic or electrodiagnostic procedure could be developed. Simply stated, Walter directed the organization of all electrophysiology to be based on the type of electrical phenomenon to be measured, not on the region of the body where the pain originated. In today's application of electrodiagnosis to pain medicine, Walter's approach can be divided into the passive and active electrical characteristics of tissue.

Passive electrophysiologic phenomena includes how body tissues respond to externally applied current as an electrical load. For pain medicine, the ability to resist, impede, or conduct electricity has become an important new field for objective measurement; these changes are among the few that are currently applicable to painful disorders of the sympathetic nervous system.[7,41]

Active bioelectric changes may fall into one of three distinct types:

1. Bioelectric changes generated by dissimilar levels of chemical ionic concentration, which create electrical potential differences between the inside and outside of cell membranes; in the Walter schema, these phenomena are considered to be steady states; the absolute levels change with metabolic shifts within tissue
2. Bioelectric changes that are noted when voltage levels fluctuate rapidly or when bioelectric currents flow as an expression of living activity
3. Bioelectric changes that occur when the system has been manipulated or stimulated externally in order to elicit a response

The test stimulus usually consists of a measurable form of physical energy that can be adjusted through a sufficient range to evoke different reactions. These responses can be analyzed differentially to provide a better understanding of the dynamic functional capabilities of the tissues being studied.

A review of the essential features of electronic devices is provided in the following section. Since the equipment used for the evaluation of active phenomena has been in existence longer, this will be considered first, followed by a review of more modern methods of assessing passive electrical characteristics.

INSTRUMENTATION SYSTEMS FOR ELECTRODIAGNOSIS

Over the past 30 years, engineers and clinical scientists have modified and improved instrumentation used in clinical electrodiagnosis. Despite advances in new equipment (e.g., for data analysis and topographic display), any electrodiagnostic system must still include five structural elements.

Electrodes

The first interface between the human subject and the equipment designed to record or measure bioelectric activity is the electrodes. Most of these contacts consist of small disks of semiprecious metal used for surface recording, or fine disposable needles for recording from deeper tissues such as muscle.

Amplifiers

Since the purpose of the system is to record any changes detected at the electrodes, one might expect the next component in the sequence to be a monitoring device or an oscillograph. However, the level of power required to drive a display monitor or electrical recorder is generally much greater than the potential differences created within biologic tissue. Therefore most electronic instruments of this type must include amplifying circuits that can increase the effective strength of weak signals by several hundred thousand times. This means that electrical changes occuring between two electrodes connected to the input of an amplifier not only increase the power of the signals of interest but would also equally increase any electrical noise. The quality of an amplifier is often judged by how well it can reject interference while amplifying true signals.

Monitors and recording devices

After amplification, monitoring and recording devices such as oscilloscopic displays or oscillographic ink- or heat-writing instruments can be driven readily. A limited system of this type can record slow, average volume changes that occur spontaneously and are ordinarily measured during rest or activity.

Stimulators

Although there should be detectable differences between painful and pain-free states, it is also important to study specific responses evoked in sensory pathways. Therefore complete systems must include an additional device to stimulate receptors or neural fibers. In human neurophysiology, electrical stimulation of nerves and muscles is most common, but flash, visual pattern reversal, audible clicks, and tones are also used for specific tests. Since many of the expected responses in nerve or brain are particularly weak and often masked by stronger spontaneous activity, it is usually necessary to analyze only the most pertinent period of wave fluctuation after each stimulus. Therefore all stimulators are equipped with synchronous pulses that act as temporal reference points.

Computer-assisted analysis components

After the early recommendations of Dawson,[42] superimposition of poststimulus potentials made researchers realize that a great deal of important information was being lost or at least masked by unwanted bioelectric noise. The advent of special-purpose averaging computers helped remove unwanted signals electronically. Soon afterward, an entire range of test procedures known as *evoked potential studies*[43,44] was developed.

In early neurophysiology, electrical pulses were the most common form of stimulation. Flash, visual pattern reversal, clicks, tones, and the laser were also being used to elicit changes in specific sensory systems.

Resistance and selective tissue conductance devices

In order to provide adequate electrodiagnostic services for clinical pain facilities, the active test elements described previously must be supplemented by apparatus and technology that permit the measurement of body tissue as a passive electrical load. Early studies showed that destructive but painless nerve lesions were associated with increased skin resistance.[45] In conditions functionally anesthetized by sympathetic blockade, the regional skin conductance also drops.[7,46] In painful conditions, however, the increase in sympathetic outflow to the skin causes a regional increase in conductivity.[7,47,48] The most current devices avoid artifactual phenomena by combining bipolar surface recording, subsensory test currents, and short sample times to measure selective tissue conductance and not simply resistance.

CLINICAL APPLICATION TO REGIONAL PAIN SYNDROMES

In order to better understand how these instruments and methods can be applied in clinical pain practice, the following sections attempt to consider symptoms that are ordinarily associated with certain sections of the body. By following a standard sequence of physical examination as a guideline,[49] various electrodiagnostic techniques can be potentially applied to the diagnosis of regional pain syndromes.

Headache

Headache and craniofacial pain syndromes are common disorders to which objective neurophysiologic testing can be applied. In a superb review, Chen summarized 28 studies regarding the relationships between electrophysiologic data and various headache syndromes.[10] While some reports were based on the identification of abnormal waveforms in the electroencephalograms (EEGs) of patients with progressive or recurrent headaches, it became evident that many of these abnormalities were not induced by clinical pain, but by the pathologic processes in the brain causing the headaches. Previously there had been hope that specific EEG patterns would be found in various headache types in the same way that they were found for seizure disorders. When abnormalities of resting brain activity were not found to be pathognomonic for any of the classic headache syndromes, methods were introduced to activate latent, but important, etiologic dysfunction.

The first of these activation methods is voluntary hyperventilation, which the patient performs for 2 to 3 minutes in the supine or seated position.[50] As carbon dioxide is exhaled in excessive amounts, respiratory alkalosis and arteriolar constriction occur, the latter creating irritation of central neurons through relative ischemia. If local areas of the cortex have been made more susceptible to hyperventilation by previous headaches with regional vasospasm, the EEG can reveal intermittent slow, sharp or, occasionally, spike activity in the appropriate distribution. In waveform classification, these patterns would be more often expected in the EEG of any individual with active seizures or an epileptiform diathesis, instead of headaches. The cumulative research on both these conditions confirms a potential, if not complete, relationship between migraine and seizures. Headache patients whose symptoms increase after long periods of dietary indiscretion, specifically those with reactive hypoglycemia, show a different pattern. During overbreathing, the frontal regions show a very high-amplitude delta EEG pattern bilaterally synchronous at approximately 2.5 Hz. Following the cessation of hyperventilation, the pattern generally disappears in less than 90 seconds.

Intermittent rhythmic photic stimulation by a stroboscopic lamp at rates of 1 to 30 flashes per second can evoke certain specific epileptiform abnormalities.[51,52] In patients with headache, irritative responses may be induced by this method, but they are generally less specific in morphology. Flash rate-dependent myoclonus and subjective complaints of photosensitivity or photophobia are the most common behavioral responses with this EEG activation.

Patterns of respiratory change during spontaneous sleep are generally documented by polysomnography, which uses a synchronous recording of EEG and other physiologic variables.[53] The headaches created by recurrent reductions of serum p_{O2} or frequent desaturation phases caused by obstructive sleep apnea, resemble headaches of individuals affected by acute mountain sickness.[54] EEGs performed at sea level in healthy civilian volunteers and military personnel revealed two distinct and unexpected patterns during hyperventilation. Those who had little or no slowing of background rhythms and no anterior slow response during overbreathing suffered the greatest headaches. Conversely, those who had the most dramatic slow-wave response to hyperventilation were spared the excruciating pain. Although the specific mechanisms underlying this EEG/clinicopathologic interaction are not completely understood, this study emphasizes that hypoxemia, not just ischemia or anemia,[55] may play a role in pain modulation.

In North America, the applications of computers or other special devices to the automatic analysis of EEG frequencies, amplitudes, power, and topography are almost as old as clinical EEG.[37,38] *Quantitative EEG* uses Fourier analysis, integration, and diagnostic algorithms and provides more than just a numeric expression or topographic display of brain/scalp activity.[56] Instead, it compares the digitized EEG activity from an individual with similar data obtained from large populations who have no similar symptoms or illness.

Eye and periorbital pain

Persistent pain, in or around the orbit or within the globe, requires ophthalmologic attention regardless of severity. Any acute onset of ocular pain also associated with a sudden reduction in vision must be considered an emergency. This often means that electrophysiologic testing of the eye, optic nerve, tracts, and thalamocortical pathways must be temporarily deferred in favor of angiographic, tonometric, or imaging techniques.

On an elective basis, the assessment of subacute or chronic eye pain can be supplemented using one or more of the following techniques.

Surface electrodes placed in horizontal or vertical pairs around the orbits can detect those fluctuations in electrical potential that accompany eye movement. Such changes can be better understood if the eye is considered a cylindric electrical dipole that has been inflated into a generally spherical shape. The direct current (DC) potential difference of the eye is created by a net electrical charge that is negative at the retina and relatively positive at the cornea. If the front of the eye moves closer toward one of the periorbital electrodes, this corneofundal potential field shift will make that electrode relatively positive by volume conduction. If the direction of the eye changes, then the polarity of the detected periorbital signal will reverse. This standard method of recording such change is known as electrooculography.[57,58] When this recording method is applied to studies of nystagmus and vestibular dysfunction, it is called electronystagmography.[59] Electrooculography can assess certain forms of painful or nonpainful ocular disease. One valuable application is in the detection of dysfunctional disease near or in the retina, particularly involving the pigment epithelium. The electrooculography levels are measured during alternate fixation between two flashing calibration lights for a few seconds, approximately once every minute for 30 minutes, during which time ambient light is eliminated (dark adaptation) then replaced (light adaptation). In normal subjects, the amplitude of the electrooculography created during alternate fixation increases twofold after the light has been replaced, but in patients with painful diseases of the pigment retina, this response is absent. The presence of ocular pain, as is described by those individuals, occurs immediately after the reintroduction of ambient light but not during the dark phase.

If the electrooculographic activity for a single eye is measured with two electrode pairs (one horizontal and one vertical) and each channel is plotted against the other in a Lissajou figure, the resulting vector electrooculogram may be used to monitor the dynamic path of the optic axis. Although this method has been used to assess neuromuscular deficits during circular-pursuit eye movements,[60] it can be modified to localize specific zones of transient pain, often in the frontal or temporal regions of headache patients, during specific directions of gaze when the orbicularis oculi is also active.[61]

Further tests of ocular disorders heralded by pain include direct or indirect electroretinography.[62,63] Direct electroretinography measures the electrical potential changes evoked in retinal receptors and their associated neuronal layers through a fine wire imbedded in a glass or plastic contact lens. The expected waveform created by exposing the eye to a brief, intense flash consists of a biphasic or triphasic wave, and the components are designated "a," "b," and "c" in order of their poststimulus latencies. Indirect electroretinography recording only differs from the direct technique in that the potential changes created in each of the retinal or neuronal layers which generate electroretinography waves are measured without using a corneal contact lens. Instead, the electroretinography responses are detected indirectly by volume conduction, using electrodes placed on or near the sclera or on the skin around the orbit. Electroretinography measures electrical function at a retinal/neural level and, although it may be abnormal in some conditions in which eye pain is a feature, it does not measure the pain of ocular or periorbital disease.

Ear, periaural, and temporal pain

The most common pains of the ear involve inflammatory mechanisms. The associated hyperemia and edema with the related distortion of anatomy and hyperexcitability of sensory nerve fibers can occur at many craniofacial sites and yet can still be felt as ear pain. A detailed review of this effect has been provided by Lynn and Mazzocco.[64] Whereas disorders of the temporomandibular joints and related craniocervical musculature are often implicated, seeking objective diagnoses through needle electromyographic (EMG) recordings has actually been more painful than productive. Instead, computer analysis of multiple muscle fields measured by surface EMG is a more acceptable and accurate method and continues to grow in popularity.[65] When combined with biomechanical data measured via transducers or clinical examination, the diagnostic value of this noninvasive technique is increased significantly.

For assessing those individuals whose symptoms suggest sympathetic mediation or maintenance of temporomandibular disorder pain, selective tissue conductance measurements of the fields surrounding the joint may be helpful. The results of an earlier, double-blind pilot study[66] suggested that consistent patterns of selective tissue conductance abnormality could be measured during type-B (unstaged) testing.[7] The most common type is when the basal selective tissue conductance level is significantly higher ($>3:1$ ratio) on one side than the other when the mouth is closed but the jaws are not clenched. When the mouth is opened, the basal level at the hyperhidrotic side falls rapidly, whereas the basal level on the hypohidrotic side rises almost instantaneously. When the jaw is returned to a closed but unclenched position, the resting level returns to or near the original values.

Although many other conditions that affect the ear are painless and therefore not referred to pain physicians, additional testing of sensorineural function using a brainstem or middle-latency auditory response recording may be of diagnostic value.[43,44]

Nasal and paranasal sinus pain

Pain in the nose resulting from trauma or local infection usually shows little or no abnormality in tests that record active bioelectric phenomena. One of the first studies to relate sinus pain and electrophysiologic abnormalities incorporated the passive measurement of skin resistance. More than 50 years ago, van Metre[47] first reported a spatial relationship between reduced skin resistance (increased skin conductance) of the frontal and facial skin over regions of painful sinusitis compared with nonpainful regions. Open label studies of patients with similar symptoms confirmed this report, particularly when a type C, stage I, linear gradient Selective Tissue Conductance test procedure was used.[7]

Dental and orofacial pain

One of the most pivotal studies in the neurophysiology of pain was performed by recording the cerebral responses evoked by dental stimulation using electrical pulses applied through wire electrodes implanted in the tooth pulp.[67] For the first time an objective relationship between the intensity of a physical stimulus, the severity of the pain it induced, and the amplitude of the brain it evoked was demonstrated. This work also confirmed that certain components of the evoked response were more directly related to the stimulus properties than the subjective report of pain intensity, since the amplitudes of both stimulus and early-response components were generally proportional. On the other hand, the amplitude of later components related more to the subject's report. Although the invasive nature of this evoked potential method could not be generalized to clinical practice, it stimulated further study regarding the pathophysiology of dental and trigeminal nerve pain.[68-70] Before this, most diagnostic tests of the trigeminal nerve were limited to electrical stimulation of the supraorbital limb of the blink reflex, and the results only determined relative patency of fibers, not pain responses. When it became evident that evoked response recording could assess physiologic phenomena to painful stimulation, new interest in electrodiagnostic procedures extended into algology and clinical neurosciences to the benefit of both fields.

Cardiac pain

The medical workup for any recurrent or persistent chest pain invariably includes electrodiagnostic studies of the heart: 12-lead electrocardiography, Holter monitoring, or continuous bedside monitoring of a prolonged rhythm strip usually precedes invasive cardiac stimulation or intravascular pharmacologic challenge. These tests are important in determining the presence of electrophysiologic changes created by acute myocardial ischemia and are therefore most often performed on an emergency basis.

The acute pains of angina pectoris and myocardial infarction are frequently accompanied by diffuse, transient elevation in sympathetic efferent activity. Increased vasoconstrictor tone to the skin and diffuse sweating with associated upward shifts in Selective Tissue Conductance level are common general responses to the acute pain experience. Between attacks, Selective Tissue Conductance levels are reduced to normal except in the skin over the chest, where occasional minor pains occur. Although there is some potential benefit in using local changes in skin conductivity over precordial or reference regions as a method to detect early referred sympathetic responses to focal cardiac ischemia, this type of testing is not applied clinically.

Chest pain of noncardiac origin

Electromyography of the chest wall has been helpful in monitoring disorders of intercostal muscle or paralysis of one half of the diaphragm. It is also useful to determine the electrical patency of nerve fibers and the mechanical neuromuscular response to phrenic nerve stimulation. When disease or trauma to the ribs, postsurgical recovery, or inflammation of the pleura creates pain and reactive splinting of the chest wall, such features are usually so evident clinically that they do not require diagnostic EMG testing. Chronic pain syndromes or conditions where there is active guarding against mechanical exacerbation of intensity may be studied electively using multisite surface EMG recordings.[71]

Surface pain of the type found in postherpetic neuralgia is commonly assessed by Selective Tissue Conductance, since these meters are fitted with sterilizable surface electrodes that can be changed to prevent spread of any remaining virus. In active or early postinfective stages, the most common findings include extremely high selective-tissue-conductance levels that occur in a bandlike distribution usually over one hemithorax. Late changes may show low selective-tissue-conductance levels, since scar tissue formed at the sites of previous lesions is generally anhidrotic. This is the exception rather than the rule, however, since patients who continue to have pain of postherpetic neuralgia usually demonstrate healed lesions with border zones that are both hyperesthetic and moderately hyperhidrotic (high Selective Tissue Conductance levels) when compared to the surrounding skin.

Abdominal and gastrointestinal pain

Electrodiagnostic tests using the three phenomena of Walter's classification do not appear to have been applied often or successfully in the objective assessment of abdominal or visceral pain. Instead, electrophysiologic changes associated with gastrointestinal (GI) pain are measured as variations in the cutaneous expression of increased sympathetic efferent function. Such reflex phenomena are often more sudomotor than vasomotor, but both functions may become abnormal during pain induced by intraluminal irritants or peristaltic contraction against an obstruction. This differs from somatic excitation of the spinal sympathetic efferent reflexes only in that the transmission of nociceptive impulses is along visceral afferent pathways.

Studies of the upper intestinal tract in patients with painful chronic esophagitis associated with hiatal hernia revealed increased levels of selective-tissue-conductance, the superior margin of which approximates the levels of inflammation created by reflux. This phenomenon was noted by Bonica[72] who translated the original report by Teodori and Galletti[73] that indicated a close relationship between passive electrical changes in the skin and local pain induced by stretching the esophagus. Using an intraluminal balloon stimulation technique, those authors noted that the electrical resistance of the skin over the sternum and upper abdomen decreased markedly whenever the balloon was dilated. As the level of the balloon tip was changed by retracting or introducing the catheter further, the regions of electrodermal abnormality shifted appropriately.

These local changes in the ability of the skin to conduct electricity appear to be directly proportional to sympathetic sudomotor efferent activity. At the present time, increased Selective Tissue Conductance tends to be found over symptomatic regions only if the referred visceral pain is accompanied by local sympathetic hyperactivity. This effect was noted as early as 1982 in a patient with severe pain of recurrent pancreatitis and was reported by Longmire and Parris.[41] Longmire and Woodley[7] presented a separate case report in which local and referred pain caused by acute cholecystitis were also associated with regional elevations in Selective Tissue Conductance. Since that time, other patients with similar electroclinical correlations have been studied. Each of these patients revealed a similar pattern, although not always identical, to zones described by Head[74] for visceral pain referral to the abdominal wall.

Spine and extremity pain

Application of radiologic studies to the evaluation of pain in the spine and extremities has been described in most textbooks of pain management and in reviews by Leak[1] and Group and Stanton-Hicks.[2] Those radiologic procedures are often ordered urgently to identify any pathologic lesion requiring rapid surgical removal. Acute surgical intervention reduces the possibility of progressive motor deficits that can result from prolonged nerve, root, or spinal cord compression.

Regardless of the value of structural tests, if the spatial distribution of spinal pain extends from the midline to involve one or both of the upper or lower extremities, it would become necessary to provide diagnostic procedures to confirm the presence of a lesion or dysfunction involving the spinal nerve roots or the spinal cord. The test procedure that has been most widely accepted for achieving this goal is electromyography.[8,11,75-78] By recording the electrical patterns that occur at rest or during activity in specific muscles,[79] the integrity of motor innervation can be obtained.

The electromyographic recording consists of introducing a presterilized fine wire or needle electrode through the skin so that the tip first rests in close proximity to the motor endplate zone or another selected territory of the muscle surface. The individual bursts of electricity which can be detected at that site are very low in voltage and are called miniature endplate potentials. As with other bioelectric phenomena, these weak signals must be amplified to increase their effective power sufficiently to be displayed or recorded. In addition to visual display methods, electromyographic activity is simultaneously connected to an internal loudspeaker, through which audible changes in frequency or duration of motor potentials may aid in diagnostic interpretation.

In the classical form of electromyography, the needle electrode is pushed deeper into the muscle tissue, which creates bursts of rapid, fairly short-duration potentials, known as *insertional activity.* When the muscle is allowed to rest between changes in electrode position, it becomes relatively silent from an electrical point of view. Persistence of insertion-like potentials, or spontaneous firing of motor units in small populations (fibrillations) or in large groups (fasciculations), can constitute evidence for hyperexcitability caused by partial denervation or irritative lesions, which are often associated with neuropathic or radiculopathic pain.

Individual electromyographic potentials can be created when neural messages generated by a single anterior horn cell travel along their respective axons and excite the several muscle cells on which their terminals rest. Since this relationship between nerve cell, axon, and muscle cell act with a single purpose in creating movement, the combination thereof is considered to be a functional entity known as the *motor unit.*[80] Naturally, the specialized purposes for which most muscles have been developed are intimately related to the number of motor units that control their contraction. Muscles that are anatomically small but have daily functions involving a significant requirement for fine control may have many more motor units than large muscles that are involved in more powerful but coarse activities.

In addition to histopathologic data to confirm this difference, noninvasive electrophysiologic methods have also been used to estimate the number of functional motor units in selected muscles in health and disease.[81,82] Recordings of individual motor unit potentials have been made using very small-diameter wire electrodes introduced percutaneously into the muscles of the hand.[83,84] Detailed voluntary control of these signals has been demonstrated through single motor unit training using both visual and auditory feedback methods.[39] In the past decade, studies of the temporal variability of motor unit potential intervals, or *jitter,* have been found to be clinically useful in the assessment of neuromuscular illnesses such as various types of muscular dystrophy and a wide range of myopathies.[85,86]

Ordinarily, the most common electromyographic patterns used in clinical diagnosis of painful and nonpainful disorders are those occurring when motor unit potentials are recruited so rapidly that their individual waveforms run together to form a pattern of interference. The relative density or frequency of this interference pattern is dependent upon the number of motor units recruited during voluntary contraction. Less than maximum voluntary effort will create interruptions in the interference pattern and reduced density of motor unit potentials. Unfortunately, people who wish to create an apparent deficit within their test results in order to obtain secondary gain may only offer a weak effort. This results in reduced electromyographic activity but cannot create potentials with pathologic configuration.

One waveform particularly important to electromyographers and pain physicians is the positive sharp wave. This is a pattern of electrical discharge which is as morphologically different from its surrounding (normal) motor unit potentials as a single rose in a garden of vidalia onions. By convention, the visual display of most electrophysiologic phenomena has been oriented with a polarity in which important negative phenomena are directed upward. This is quite the opposite from the expected direction of graphs using Cartesian coordinates, but the inversion has been accepted in neurophysiology for nearly a century. Therefore, monophasic electrical transients that are positive are displayed or recorded so that their peaks are directed downward. Waveforms that have this characteristic shape and have a longer duration than normal motor unit potentials are known as positive sharp waves. They can be found in a wide range of neuropathic pain syndromes and, when recorded from multiple muscles that are innervated by the same root level, can provide valuable objective evidence to support a clinical diagnosis of radiculitis or radiculopathy. It is also important to note that these waveforms cannot be produced voluntarily or fictitiously by patients who claim compensable injury and who wish to create the impression of debilitating motor deficits. Specifically, the interference pattern of motor unit potentials created during voluntary contraction can be reduced in patients who cannot or will not provide maximum effort. This effect, based upon decreased cooperation during test performance, must not be considered as objective as positive sharp waves occurring involuntarily at a regional level of tissue irritation or damage.

In addition to this clear morphologic difference, the relative frequency of sharp waves recorded from muscles driven by dysfunctional nerve roots may be used as a semiquantitative guideline to the amount of irritation, but not to the anatomic severity of, for example, bulging or herniation of intervertebral disks.

This lack of electroclinical or clinicopathologic correlation is based on the fact that dysfunction is not just caused by pressure on the nerve fibers, but also by the ischemia created by compression of the vasa nervorum and associated metabolic changes accompanying local edema and inflammation. Techniques performed as part of the usual electromyographic examination are known as nerve conduction velocity or sensory nerve action potential studies. Motor fibers of mixed nerves in the extremities can be evaluated by applying electrical stimuli along the path of the nerve through the intact skin. When the polarity and intensity of the stimuli excite orthodromic nerve action potentials, observable and recordable motor responses can be found at muscles which are supplied by that nerve. When measuring the latencies of these responses following stimulation at proximal and distal sites and at multiple points along the nerve, comparison of the distances traveled can mathematically determine the velocity of conduction, which relates to the health of nerve function.

When sensory nerve trunks are stimulated, responses may be recorded proximally or distally, but access to effective conduction velocity recording is reduced because the potential levels created in sensory nerves are lower than those noted in muscles used for motor nerve conduction velocity testing.

For this reason, local compressive changes in nerve or plexus tend to be assessed using motor conduction velocity measurement. As the stimulating electrode is moved along the axis of peripheral nerves in the extremities, a sudden reduction in the ability of a particular nerve segment can be compared to signs or symptoms of local entrapment. The most classic examples of this effect include compression of nerve, trunk, or cord by neoplastic bone or muscule at the brachial plexus and beyond (thoracic outlet syndrome); of the median nerve at the wrist (carpal tunnel syndrome); or of the ulnar nerve as it passes across the ulnar groove at the elbow.

Other methods of testing patency in afferent pathways from the extremities all the way to the spinal nerve roots, spinal cord, brainstem, and the thalamocortical projections usually involve somatosensory (computer-averaged) evoked potentials.[9,43,44]

Integument and sympathetically related pain

Studies of the electrical properties of the human skin have been applied to the assessment of painful nerve injuries for over 100 years.[45] The early establishment of the electrodiagnostic service at La Salpêtrière Hospital, Paris, was funded to complement the world famous neurology department, directed at that time by Charcot. Electrical resistance had been important before the turn of the century, but the inverse relationship between this resistance and sympathetic efferent supply to the skin was not confirmed for several decades. Currently reciprocal phenomenon (i.e., skin conductance) is more applicable in the assessment of sympathetic dysfunction since its basal, tonic shifts are analogous to sudomotor function.

Phasic changes in palmar skin potential, or skin conductance, have been recorded as a method by which anesthesiologists can determine the relative success of sympathetic blockade.[87] The theoretical basis for this is that successful stellate ganglion block could reduce efferent control of sudomotor function in the skin. However, selective tissue conductance studies by Parris and colleagues[46] not only revealed a significant reduction of selective tissue conductance on the side of blockade but a marked elevation contralaterally, possibly as an escape phenomenon.

Unfortunately for the field of pain medicine, recognition of the clinical value of the passive electrical characteristics of tissue was delayed for decades. The main reasons for this appear to have been technical. The test currents, which were often painful, generally flowed through sensitive body tissues including the heart, and true values were often distorted by the iontophoretic effect. In the early 1960s research efforts were directed at correcting these deficiencies and resulted in the final development of Selective Tissue Conductance instrumentation and technology. In this method, a very weak, subsensory level of DC current was applied through a bipolar concentric surface electrode for very brief periods of time. Early open-label and double-blind single- and multicentered trials indicated potential benefits of this method to quantify sudomotor changes created by sympathetic blocks[7,46] and for comparative topographic analysis of regional hyperhidrosis and local clinical pain.[88] After the registration of an operational definition for classification of Selective Tissue Conductance devices by the Food and Drug Administration (FDA)[89] and publication of practice guidelines,[7] use of this technology has become more widespread among anesthesiologists and algologists in North America.

REFERENCES

1. Leak WD: Tutorial 5, Radiologic assessment of chronic pain. *Pain Digest* 2:63-68, 1992.
2. Group M, Stanton-Hicks M: Neuroanatomy and pathophysiology of pain related to spinal disorders. *Radiol Clin North Am* 29:665-673, 1991.
3. Lowry PA: Radiology in the diagnosis and management of pain. In Raj PP, editor: *Practical Management of Pain*, ed 2. St Louis, Mosby, 1992.
4. Bonica JJ: Anatomic and physiologic basis of nociception and pain. In Bonica JJ, editor: *The Management of Pain*, ed 2. Philadelphia, Lea & Febiger, 1990.
5. Balter K: Tutorial 8: A review of pain anatomy and physiology. *Pain Digest* 2:306-330, 1992.
6. Longmire DR: Tutorial 10: Electrodiagnostic studies in the assessment of painful disorders. *Pain Digest* 3:116-122, 1993.
7. Longmire DR, Woodley WE: Tutorial 11: Clinical neurophysiology of pain-related sympathetic sudomotor dysfunction. *Pain Digest* 3:202-209, 1993.
8. Roongta SM: Electromyography. In Raj PP, editor: *Practical Management of Pain*, ed 2. St Louis, Mosby, 1992.
9. Waldman HJ: Evoked potentials. In Raj PP, editor: *Practical Management of Pain*, ed 2. St Louis, Mosby, 1992.
10. Chen ACN: Human brain measures of clinical pain: A review. I. Topographic mapping. *Pain* 4:115-132, 1993.
11. Spindler HA: Medical electrodiagnostics. In Tollison CD, editor: *Handbook of Chronic Pain Management*. Baltimore, Williams & Wilkins, 1989.
12. Stolov WC: Electrodiagnostic evaluation of acute and chronic pain syndromes. In Bonica JJ, editor: *The Management of Pain*, ed 2. Philadelphia, Lea & Febiger, 1990.
13. Galvani L: *De Viribus Electricitatis in Motu Musculari: Commentarius*, 1791.
14. Capelli L: *Memorie ed Esperimenti Inediti di Luigi Galvani*, Bologna, 1937.
15. Brazier MAB: *A History of Neurophysiology in the 17th and 18th Centuries: From Concept to Experiment*. New York, Raven Press, 1984.
16. Kellaway P: The part played by electric fish in the early history of bioelectricity and electrotherapy. *Bull Hist Med* 20:112-137, 1946.
17. Gray S: A letter to Cromwell Mortimer MD, Sec. RS, containing several experiments concerning electricity. *Phil Trans Roy Soc* 37:18-44, 1731.
18. Hales S: *Statickal Essays: Containing Haemastaticks*. London, Manby & Woodward, 1733.
19. Newton I: General scholium. *Principia mathematica, vol 2*. London, 1713.
20. Von Haller A: Observatio de schirro cerebelli. *Phil Trans Roy Soc* 43:100-101, 1744.
21. Beccaria G: *Dell' electricismo artificale e naturalae, vol 1*. Turin, Campana, 1753.
22. Von Haller A: *Memoires sur la nature sensible et irritable des parties du corps animal, vol 1*. Lausanne, 1756.
23. Volta A: Memoria prima sull'elettricita animale. *Giornale fisico-medico* 2:146-187, 1792.
24. Volta A: Account of some discoveries made by Mr. Galvani of Bologna. *Phil Trans Roy Soc* 83:10-44, 1793.
25. DuBois-Reymond E: *Untersuchungen uber thierische Electricitat, vol 1*. Berlin, Reimer, 1848.
26. DuBois-Reymond E: *Untersuchungen uber thierische Electricitat, vol 2*. Berlin, Reimer, 1849.
27. Biedermann W: *Electro-physiology*. London, Macmillan, 1898.
28. Duchenne Du Boulogne M: Memoire sur la galvanisation localisee. *Arch Gen de Medecine* 257-420, 1850.
29. Dunglison R: *New Remedies with Formulae for Their Administration*. Philadelphia, Blanchard and Lea, 1851.
30. Beard GM, Rockwell AD: A practical treatise on the medical and surgical uses of electricity, including localized and general electrization. New York, William Wood, 1871.
31. Mills CK: Electrodiagnosis and electroprognosis. In Mills CK, editor: *The Nervous System and Its Diseases*. Philadelphia, JB Lippincott, 1898.
32. Lucas K: *The Conduction of the Nervous Impulse* (revised by ED Adrian). London, Longmans, Green, 1917.
33. Adrian ED, Lucas K: On the summation of propagated disturbances in nerve muscle. *J Physiol (Lond)* 44:68-124, 1912.
34. Buchtal F: The electromyogram: Its value in the diagnosis of neuromuscular disorders. *World Neurol* 3:15, 1962.
35. Hoffman BF, Cranefield PF: *Electrophysiology of the Heart*. New York, McGraw-Hill, 1960.
36. Hurst JW, Myerburg RJ: *Introduction to Electrocardiography*, ed 2. New York, McGraw-Hill, 1973.
37. Berger H: Uber das elektrenkephalogramm des menschen. *Arch Psych Nervenkr* 87:527-570, 1929.
38. Gloor P: Hans Berger on the electroencephalogram of man. *Electroencephalogr Clin Neurophysiol Suppl* 28, 1969.
39. Basmajian JV: *Muscles Alive: Their Functions Revealed by Electromyography*, ed 2. Baltimore, Williams & Wilkins, 1967.
40. Walter WG: Introduction. In Hill D, Parr G, editors: *Electroencephalography: A Symposium on its Various Aspects*. London, Macdonald, 1950.
41. Longmire DR, Parris WCV: Selective tissue conductance in the assessment of sympathetically mediated pain. In Parris WCV, editor: *Contemporary Issues in Chronic Pain Management*. New York, Kluwer Academic Publishers, 1991.
42. Dawson G: A summation technique for the detection of small evoked potentials. *Electroencephalogr Clin Neurophysiol* 6:153-154, 1954.
43. Chiappa KH: *Evoked Potentials in Clinical Medicine*. New York, Raven Press, 1983.
44. Spehlmann R: *Evoked Potential Primer: Visual, Auditory, and Somatosensory Evoked Potentials in Clinical Diagnosis*. Boston, Butterworth Publishers, 1985.
45. Vigouroux R: Sur le role de la resistance electrique des tissue dans l'electrodiagnostic. *C R Seances Soc Biol Fil* 31:336-339, 1879.
46. Parris WCV et al: The effect of stellate ganglion block on skin conductance using Epi-Scan 5000. Paper presented at the annual meeting of the American Pain Society, Phoenix, 1989.
47. Van Metre TH Jr: Electrical skin resistance studies of the region of pain in painful acute sinusitis. *Bull Johns Hopkins Hosp* 85:409, 1949.
48. Riley LH, Richter CP: Uses of the electrical skin resistance method in patients with neck and upper extremity pain. *Johns Hopkins Med J* 137:69-74, 1975.
49. Longmire DR: Tutorial 2. The physical examination: Methods and application in the clinical evaluation of pain. *Pain Digest* 1:136-143, 1991.
50. Billinger TW, Frank GS: Effects of posture on EEG slowing during hyperventilation. *Amer J EEG Technol* 9:22-27, 1969.
51. Takahashi T: Activation methods. In Niedermeyer E, Lopes da Silva F, editors: *Electroencephalography: Basic Principles, Clinical Applications and Related Fields*, ed 2. Baltimore, Urban and Schwarzenberg, 1987.
52. Jeavons PN, Harding GFA: *Photosensitive Epilepsy: A Review of the Literature and a Study of 460 Patients*. London, Heinemann, 1975.
53. Broughton RJ: Polysomnography: Principles and applications in sleep and arousal disorders. In Niedermeyer E, Lopes da Silva F, editors: *Electroencephalography: Basic Principles, Clinical Applications and Related Fields*, ed 2. Baltimore, Urban and Schwarzenberg, 1987.
54. Powles ACP et al: Electroencephalogram in acute mountain sickness. *Clin Res* 23:642, 1975.
55. Kennedy LD, Longmire DR: Tutorial 4: Medical/laboratory evaluation of pain patients. *Pain Digest* 1:306-312, 1992.
56. Lopes da Silva F: EEG analysis. Theory and practice. In Niedermeyer E, Lopes da Silva F, editors: *Electroencephalography: Basic Principles, Clinical Applications and Related Fields*, ed 2. Baltimore, Urban and Schwarzenberg, 1987.
57. Venables PH, Christie MJ: Mechanisms, instrumentation, recording techniques and quantification of responses. In Prokasy WF, Roskin DC, editors: *Electrodermal Activity in Psychological Research*. New York, Academic Press, 1973.
58. Papakostopolous D, Winter A, Newton P: New techniques for the control of eye potential artifacts in multichannel CNV recordings. *Electroenceph Clin Neurophysiol* 34:651-653, 1973.
59. Barber HO, Stockwell CW: *Manual of Electronystagmography*. St Louis, Mosby, 1976.
60. Zahoruk R, Longmire DR: Recent modifications in the vector electro-oculographic (VEOG) assessment of oculomotor dysfunction. Pro-

ceedings of the Association for Research in Vision and Ophthalmology, Miami, 1975.

61. Travell J, Simons D: *Myofascial Pain and Dysfunction: The Trigger Point Manual, vol 1*. Baltimore, Williams & Wilkins, 1983.

62. Gouras P: Electroretinography: Some basic principles. *Invest Ophthalmol* 9:557-569, 1970.

63. Armington JC: Electroretinography. In Aminoff MJ, editor: *Electrodiagnosis in Clinical Neurology*. Edinburgh, Churchill Livingstone, 1980.

64. Lynn JM, Mazzocco ME: Neuromuscular differentiation of craniocervical pain: Is it headache or TMD? *AJPM* 3:181-190, 1993.

65. Cram JR, Engstrom D: Patterns of neuromuscular activity in pain and nonpain patients. *Clinical Biofeedback and Health* 9:106-115, 1986.

66. Jones ED, Longmire DR, Leak WD: Selective tissue conductance changes over the cranial, facial and cervical regions. Paper presented at the Annual Meeting of the American Pain Society, New Orleans, 1991.

67. Chatrian GE et al: Cerebral responses to electrical tooth pulp stimulation in man. An objective correlate of acute experimental pain. *Neurology (Minn)* 25:745-757, 1975.

68. Chen ACN, Chapman CR, Harkins SW: Brain evoked potentials are functional correlates of induced pain in man. *Pain* 6:305-314, 1979.

69. Chapman CR, Chen ACN, Harkins SW: Brain evoked potentials as correlates of laboratory pain: A review and perspective. In Bonica JJ, Liebeskind JC, Albe-Fessard D, editors: *Advances in Pain Research and Therapy, vol 3*. New York, Raven Press, 1979.

70. Bromm B: Evoked cerebral potentials and pain. In Fields HL, editor: *Advances in Pain Research and Therapy, vol 9*. New York, Raven Press, 1985.

71. Cram JR: *Clinical EMG for Surface Recordings, vol 2*. Nevada City, Clinical Resources, 1990.

72. Bonica JJ: Applied anatomy relevant to pain. In Bonica JJ, editor: *The Management of Pain*, ed 2. New York, Lea & Febiger, 1990.

73. Teodori U, Galletti R: *Il Dolore Nelle Affezioni Defli Organi Interni del Torace*. Roma, L Pozzi, 1962.

74. Head H: On disturbance of sensation with special reference to the pain of visceral disease. *Brain* 16:1, 1893.

75. Johnson EW: *Practical Electromyography*, ed 2. Baltimore, Williams & Wilkins, 1988.

76. Kimura J: *Electrodiagnosis in Diseases of Nerve Muscle: Principles and Practice*. Philadelphia, FA Davis, 1989.

77. Ludin H: *Electromyography in Practice*. New York, Georg Thieme Verlag, 1980.

78. Liveson JA, Spielholz NI: *Peripheral Neurology: Case Studies in Electrodiagnosis*. Philadelphia, FA Davis, 1979.

79. Delagi EF et al: *Anatomic Guide for the Electromyographer*, ed 2. Springfield, Charles C Thomas, 1980.

80. Sherrington CS: *The Integrative Action of the Nervous System*. New York, Charles Scribners Sons, 1906.

81. McComas AJ et al: Physiological estimates of the numbers and sizes of motor units in man. In Stein R, editor: *Control of Posture and Locomotion*. New York, Plenum Press, 1973.

82. Sica REP et al: Motor unit estimations in small muscles of the hand. *J Neurol Neurosurg Psychiatry* 37:55-67, 1974.

83. Basmajian JV, Stecko G: A new bipolar indwelling electrode for electromyography. *J Appl Physiol* 17:849, 1962.

84. Basmajian JV, Forrest WJ, Shine G: A simple connector for fine-wire electrodes. *J Appl Physiol* 21:1680, 1966.

85. Stalberg E, Trontelj J: *Single Fibre Electromyography*. Old Woking, Surrey, Mirville Press, 1979.

86. Stalberg E, Trontelj J: Clinical neurophysiology: The motor unit in myopathy. In Rowland LP, DiMauro S, editors: *Handbook of Clinical Neurology*. Amsterdam, Elsevier, 1992.

87. Lofstrom JB, Lloyd JW, Cousins MJ: Sympathetic neural blockade of upper and lower extremity. In Cousins MJ, editor: *Neural Blockade in Clinical Anesthesia and Management of Pain*. Philadelphia, JB Lippincott, 1980.

88. Longmire DR et al: Computerized contour mapping of selective tissue conductance in sympathetically mediated craniofacial pain. Proceedings of the VIth World Congress of the International Association for the Study of Pain (Suppl 5). Amsterdam, Elsevier, 1990.

89. Longmire DR, Woodley WE: 1988 Selective tissue conductance meter, K874850A. Office of Device Evaluation, Food and Drug Administration, US Dept of Health and Human Services, Washington, DC, 1988.

QUESTIONS: NEUROPHYSIOLOGIC STUDIES

1. Single-fiber electromyographic recordings are helpful in assessing:
   A. Sensory nerve fibers affected by ABC syndrome
   B. Jitter that occurs in some myopathies
   C. Postherpetic neuralgia
   D. Trigeminal neuralgia
2. The most significant difference between the active and passive phenomena measured during electrodiagnostic testing is that:
   A. The former are associated with spontaneous or evoked changes in electrical potential difference
   B. The latter are only created by passive stretching of nerve roots
   C. The former may be used to diagnose severe active joint disease
   D. Measurements of the latter may be made on neural, but not nonneural, tissue
3. Frontal headaches that are present early on awakening in patients who do not drink alcohol may be related to:
   A. Occult trauma
   B. Obstructive sleep apnea
   C. Migraine with aura
   D. Lumbar pain
4. Changes in sudomotor function over the frontal and molar regions can be assessed using:
   A. Skin resistance or conductance
   B. Somatosensory evoked potentials
   C. Dental stimulation
   D. Electromyography of the frontal scalp muscles
5. Painful paresthesias of the hands occurring at night may be associated with:
   A. Slow nerve conductors across the ulnar grove
   B. Prolonged distal latencies at the wrist
   C. Reduced electromyographic amplitude
   D. Reduced somatosensory evoked response amplitude

ANSWERS

1. B
2. A
3. B
4. A
5. B

8 Diagnostic Nerve Block

P. Prithvi Raj

Differential neural blockade provides an objective means of establishing a diagnosis to pain mechanism that far exceeds the efficacy of clinical judgment, even in the seemingly "clear-cut case." But the greatest usefulness of differential neural block is in that group of patients who exhibit no demonstrable organic cause for that pain.

It is important to emphasize that differential neural blockade is not intended to replace a careful history, physical examination, and, particularly, a thorough neurologic examination; nor to minimize the value of appropriate laboratory or psychologic studies. However, it is equally important to appreciate that all of these diagnostic efforts may fail to yield an identifiable cause of the patient's pain or to indicate an appropriate form of therapy. In these patients, differential neural blockade can provide an accurate diagnosis of the mechanism underlying the patient's pain; and the results of these diagnostic maneuvers may indicate a different mechanism from that indicated by the results of the usual diagnostic workup. Such results will explain the failure of previous therapeutic efforts to relieve the patient's pain and indicate the therapy that is appropriate for that particular syndrome.

Before performing a diagnostic differential nerve block, the following questions should be considered:

1. Is there a reversible nociceptive process present?
2. Which anatomic structures are involved?
3. Which peripheral nerves carry the sensations?
4. Is there an autonomic component?
5. Is there referred pain?
6. Which central pathways are involved?
7. Are nonnociceptive processes involved (e.g., contractures)?
8. Is there central (neuropathic) pain?
9. Is there psychogenic pain?
10. Are neurolytic blocks indicated?

LIMITATIONS OF DIAGNOSTIC DIFFERENTIAL BLOCK

Peripheral nerves contain fibers of all diameters and functions. It is not possible with local anesthetics to block selective fibers of a specific function (Table 8-1). In general, the fine unmyelinated fibers tend to be blocked before the larger myelinated fibers. However, several factors are involved: the length of the fiber exposed to the local anesthetic, the frequency of fiber firing, and the duration of exposure. There are probably other factors as well. It is a common clinical observation that 0.125% bupivacaine can produce a profound motor block in some patients by both peripheral and epidural administration, whereas in others, 0.5% bupivacaine might only produce minimal blockade. The same concentration of local anesthetic administered epidurally to different individuals produces threefold to fivefold differences in several neurophysiologic variables.[1]

It is therefore impossible to make any valid physiologic inference from the outcome of a diagnostic block based on the concentration of the injected local anesthetic. This renders the interpretation of differential peripheral nerve, epidural, and subarachnoid blocks misleading at best and counterproductive at worst, because such blocks are not able to answer any of the fundamental questions listed previously.

Overlapping

There may be overlap of nerves at the peripheral level, and there is variation from one individual to the next in the peripheral distribution of a particular nerve. When the nerve enters the spinal cord, its terminals spread over several spinal segments. A joint tends to be innervated by the spinal segments and peripheral nerves of the muscles that move it. For example, joint nociceptors in the facet joints are highly unlikely to be blocked by disrupting a single nerve to the joint (as in facet *rhizotomy*). Similarly, a femoral nerve block is unlikely to denervate the knee joint and render it anesthetic. On the other hand, intraarticular local anesthetic is likely to be effective for its particular duration because all intraarticular nerve endings, nociceptive and nonnociceptive, will be blocked.

Sympathetic/somatic interaction

Any sympathetic block interrupts both afferent and efferent activity; indeed, the measure of successful sympathetic blockade is a rise in temperature (indicating blockade of efferent vasoconstrictor fibers). It is theoretically possible that pain relief might be secondary to the increased blood flow and not indicative of sympathetically maintained pain. Conversely, a somatic nerve block also interrupts the sympathetic fibers traveling in that nerve.

TECHNIQUES OF DIFFERENTIAL NEURAL BLOCKADE

There are basically two approaches to the performance of differential neural blockade—a pharmacologic approach and an anatomic approach.

Pharmacologic approach

A differential spinal block provides the simplest pharmacologic approach with the most discrete endpoints. The basis for the pharmacologic approach is the fundamental physi-

Table 8-1 General classification of mixed peripheral nerve fibers

Fiber	Diameter (μ)	Conduction velocity (m/sec)	Function Sensory	Motor
A fibers	2-20	6-120	Muscle tendon and spindle	Skeletal muscle and spindle control
Alpha	10-20	60-120	Vibration	
Beta	5-15	30-80	Deep pressure touch	
Gamma	3-7	10-50		
Delta	2-5	6-30	Pricking pain, cold, warmth	
C fibers	0.5-2	0.5-2	Crude touch, pressure, tickle, aching pain, cold, warmth	Sympathetic

From Raj PP, editor: *Practical Management of Pain,* ed 1. St Louis, Mosby, 1986.

ologic research performed years ago by Gasser and Erlanger, who showed that different sizes of nerve fibers are blocked by different concentrations of local anesthetics.[2] They demonstrated in a very simple but elegant experiment that the size of a nerve fiber is probably the most important single factor that determines virtually all of the functional characteristics of a nerve. These researchers showed that when one stimulates a nerve and then records the response only a few millimeters away, the record shows a compound action potential. However, as the recording electrode is moved further away from the stimulating electrode, the compound action potential can consist of several smaller spikes, each representing an impulse that is travelling at a different rate along the different sized nerve fibers. The action potentials might be compared to runners in a race who become separated along the course as the faster contestants outstrip the slower; thus in a record at 82 mm from the point of stimulation, three waves are shown, whereas at 12 mm, the potentials are fused and only one large wave appears. The delta wave is not shown in the record (Fig. 8-1).

Thus the smallest fibers require the least concentration of local anesthetic to be blocked, and the largest fibers require the highest concentration. Recent studies[3-6] have indicated that the situation is not quite as "simplistic" as the studies of Gasser and Erlanger would indicate: in addition to fiber size and concentration of local anesthetic applied, differential neural blockade is also a function of the length of the nerve exposed to the local anesthetic and the frequency of incoming impulses. However, *functionally,* the Gasser and Erlanger concept is valid and for our purposes provides us with a sound and useful clinical tool.

Conventional "sequential" differential spinal.[7,8] In carrying out a differential spinal, four solutions should be prepared in four separate syringes as indicated in Box 8-1: normal saline, 0.25% procaine, 0.5% procaine, and 1% procaine, all in normal saline.

After preparation of the solutions, the patient is told that a single needle will be placed in the back, after which each of the solutions will be injected sequentially. The patient is instructed to tell the physician which solution, if any, relieves the pain. The solutions are referred to as Solution A, Solution B, Solution C, and Solution D so that the physicians can discuss the solutions freely in front of the patient. Solution A is normal saline, which serves as a placebo. So

---

Box 8-1 PREPARATION OF SOLUTION: CONVENTIONAL "SEQUENTIAL" DIFFERENTIAL SPINAL

Solution A: Draw 10 ml of normal saline to equal 10 ml of 0% procaine (placebo)

Solution B: To 5 ml of 0.5% procaine, add 5 ml normal saline to equal 10 ml of 0.25% procaine (sympathetic blockade)

Solution C: To 5 ml of 1% procaine, add 5 ml normal saline to equal 10 ml of 0.5% procaine (sensory blockade)

Solution D: To 1 ml of 10% procaine, add 9 ml of normal saline to equal 10 ml of 1% procaine (motor blockade)

From Winnie AP, Collins VJ: The Pain Clinic I: Differential neural blockade in pain syndromes of questionable etiology. *Med Clin North Amer* 52:123-129, 1968.

---

lution B, 0.25% procaine, is the mean sympatholytic concentration of procaine, i.e., the concentration that is sufficient to block B fibers but insufficient to block A-delta and C fibers. Solution C, 0.5% procaine, is the mean sensory blocking concentration of procaine, i.e., the concentration that is sufficient to block B fibers, A-delta, and C fibers but insufficient to block A-alpha, beta, and gamma fibers. Finally, Solution D, 1% procaine, provides complete blockade of all fibers. If this concentration is insufficient to produce complete motor, sensory, and sympathetic block, the concentration should be increased to 5%.

It is extremely important that each of the injections be carried out in a manner that is identical to and indistinguishable from the rest. In addition, it is equally important that the observations that the physician makes after each injection (Box 8-2) be carried out in an identical manner. Thus after each injection the physician must question the patient about subjective changes in the level of pain at rest and during attempts to mechanically reproduce the pain, and carry out appropriate tests to determine the presence or absence of sympathetic, sensory, and/or motor blockade (see Box 8-2).

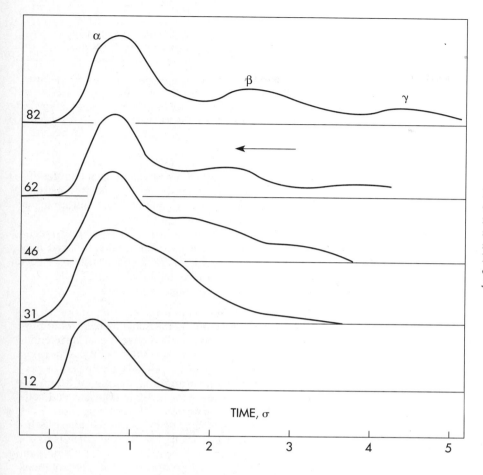

Fig. 8-1 Cathode ray oscillograph records of the action current in a bullfrog's sciatic nerve after conduction from the point of stimulation through the distances (mm) shown at the left. (From Gasser HS, Erlanger J: Role of fiber size in establishment of nerve block by pressure or cocaine, *Am J Physiol* 88:581-591, 1929.)

Box 8-2 OBSERVATIONS AFTER EACH INJECTION

1. Blood pressure
2. Pulse rate
3. Patient's subjective evaluation of pain at rest
4. Mechanical reproduction of pain
5. Signs of sympathetic block (temperature change, psychogalvanic reflex)
6. Signs of sensory block (response to pinprick)
7. Signs of motor block (ability to move toes, feet)

Results of differential spinal. If the patient's pain is relieved after the first injection, the mechanism underlying the patient's pain is classified as *psychogenic.* It is well established that 30% to 35% of all patients who have true organic pain will obtain relief from an inactive agent, so relief after the injection of the normal saline may simply represent a placebo reaction (technically, a psychogenic response). However, this can usually be differentiated clinically from true psychogenic pain, since the placebo reaction is usually of rather short duration and is self-limiting, whereas pain relief provided by a placebo in a patient suffering from true psychogenic pain is usually extremely long lasting, if not permanent. The possibility that the pain is entirely psychogenic will be substantiated or refuted by the findings of the psychologic evaluation.

If the patient does not obtain relief from the placebo injection and relief is obtained after the injection of 0.25% procaine, a sympathetic mechanism is indicated provided that there are signs of sympathetic blockade and not signs of sensory blockade concomitant with the onset of pain relief. Although 0.25% procaine is the mean or usual sympatholytic concentration, there will be a few patients who may have a decreased critical sensory blocking threshold; they will get relief from this concentration of procaine, but only because it is actually producing analgesia, i.e., sensory block. However, that is the exception and not the rule.

If the 0.25% procaine solution does not provide pain relief but 0.5% does, the pain relief is provided by means of a sensory block, i.e. blockade of the A-delta and/or C fibers. This blockade indicates a somatic or organic basis for the patient's pain, provided the patient exhibited signs of sympathetic blockade after the injection of 0.25% procaine and showed signs of sensory blockade after the 0.5% procaine.

If the patient does not obtain relief with 0.25% or 0.5% procaine, 1% procaine (or if necessary, 5% procaine) is injected to produce blockade of all modalities. If this increase in concentration relieves the pain, the mechanism is still considered to be somatic, presuming that the patient has an elevated critical sensory blocking threshold. If the patient fails to obtain relief in spite of complete sympathetic, sensory, and motor blockade, a *central mechanism* is indicated. Possible central mechanisms include: (a) a lesion higher in the central nervous system (CNS) than the level of spinal anesthesia; (b) encephalization*; (c) psychogenic pain; (d) malingering.

If the patient is anticipating financial benefit from pending litigation, it would be a disadvantage for the patient to state that anything removed the pain. For this reason many pain control centers refuse to accept patients involved in litigation. Although it is difficult to rule out malingering, in several patients with pending litigation, a differential spinal produced useful information in two patients who exhibited placebo reactions. It is our contention that a placebo reaction, because it depends on a positive motivation to obtain relief, is impossible in a malingerer. Clearly, there is no way to prove or disprove this thesis.

Whereas this conventional ("sequential") technique of differential spinal blockade has been extremely effective, it does have several drawbacks:

1. This technique is time-consuming. The physician must wait a sufficient time after each injection to allow the various responses to become evident, and in cases where the 1% concentration of procaine does not provide complete blockade of all modalities, an additional injection of 5% procaine is necessary.
2. Each injection deposits increasing amounts of procaine in the subarachnoid space, so after blockade of all modalities, a considerable period of time is necessary for full recovery. This is essential because the vast majority of the patients in our pain control center are outpatients and must be fully able to ambulate before discharge.
3. This technique requires the needle to remain in place throughout the procedure, which requires the patient to remain in the lateral position throughout. This poses a problem when a patient only experiences pain in a particular position and the needle in situ disallows that position.

Modified differential spinal.[9,10]   In an effort to streamline the conventional technique and therefore increase its utility, the conventional technique has recently been modified. In preparation for the modified technique, only two solutions need be prepared as indicated in Box 8-3, normal saline (Solution A), and 5% procaine in cerebrospinal fluid (CSF) (Solution D).

After lumbar puncture has been accomplished, 2 ml of normal saline are injected, and the same observations are made as in the conventional technique (see Box 8-2). If the patient obtains no relief (or only partial relief) from the placebo injection, then 2 ml of 5% procaine in CSF is injected, the needle is removed, and the patient is returned to the supine position. Since 5% procaine in CSF is hyperbaric, the

---

*Encephalization is the phenomenon whereby severe agonizing pain, originally peripheral in origin, moves centrally after being endured for a prolonged period of time. After time even removal (or blockade) of the peripheral mechanism that originally produced the pain fails to provide relief and the pain becomes self-sustaining at a central level.

Box 8-3 PREPARATION OF SOLUTIONS: MODIFIED DIFFERENTIAL SPINAL

1. Solution A: Draw 2 ml of normal saline to equal 2 ml of 0% procaine
2. Solution D: To 1 ml of 10% procaine, add 1 ml of CSF to equal 2 ml of 5% procaine (hyperbaric)

---

position of the table may be manipulated to obtain the desired level of anesthesia. After the development of anesthesia to an appropriate level, the same observations are made as with the conventional technique.

In interpreting the modified differential spinal, this technique correlates the recovery of the various blocked modalities with the return of the patient's pain instead of correlating the onset of blockade with the relief of pain.

Modified differential spinal interpretation

1. If the pain is relieved after the injection of normal saline, the interpretation is the same as pain relief provided by the placebo in the conventional differential spinal, i.e., the pain is considered to be of *psychogenic origin*. Again, if the pain relief is prolonged or permanent, then the pain origin is considered truly psychogenic, but if the pain relief is transient and self-limiting, this is considered a placebo response.
2. If the patient does not obtain pain relief after the injection of the 5% procaine in CSF, then the diagnosis is the same as when the patient does not obtain pain relief following the injection of all of the solutions with the conventional technique, i.e., the mechanism is considered to be "central." Again, this diagnosis is intended to include four possibilities: the patient may have a true organic lesion above the level of the spinal block; the pain may have become *encephalized* because of its long duration; the pain may be truly psychogenic in origin; and the patient could be malingering.
3. If the patient does develop complete pain relief after the injection of the 5% procaine solution, the mechanism is considered to be somatic (to be subserved by A-delta and C fiber pathways) if the pain returns concomitant with the return of the appreciation of pinprick (recovery from analgesia).
4. The mechanism is considered to be sympathetic (to be subserved by B fiber pathways) if the pain relief persists for a considerable period of time after recovery from analgesia.

The primary advantage of the modified differential spinal block over the conventional technique is time; the modified technique has consistently provided identical diagnostic information in approximately half the time. The modified technique allows a better evaluation of the patient's subjective pain, because without the need to keep the needle in the back throughout the procedure, the patient can lie in the supine position and change positions or passively move the legs if required to produce the pain.

Another advantage of this technique is the simplicity with which sympathetic and somatic mechanisms can be differentiated from each other.

Differential epidural block

I advocate the use of a differential diagnostic epidural block instead of a differential spinal.[11] With this proposed technique, Solution A is still a placebo but Solution B is 0.5% lidocaine or mepivacaine, which is presumed to be the mean sympatholytic concentration of these agents in the epidural space. According to this proposal, Solution C is 1% lidocaine or mepivacaine, which is presumed to be the mean sensory blocking concentration of these agents in the epidural space; and Solution D is 2% lidocaine or mepivacaine, a concentration sufficient to block all modalities. In short, the technique to perform a differential epidural block is virtually identical to the technique used in a conventional differential spinal, except that the local anesthetic is injected sequentially into the epidural space and the concentrations have been modified accordingly.

There are two problems with this technique. First of all, because of the slower onset of blockade of each modality after injection of local anesthetics into the epidural space, a longer period of time must be allowed between injections before the usual observations can be made. However, an even more serious drawback with this approach is that the variations in the critical sympathetic, sensory, and motor blocking concentrations of local anesthetics frequently fail to give discrete endpoints when injected into the epidural space.

Nonetheless, a differential epidural approach is inherently appealing, since it avoids lumbar puncture and the possibility of postlumbar puncture headache in a predominantly outpatient population. We now carry out a differential epidural as follows.[10] After placing a needle in the epidural space at an appropriate level, we sequentially inject normal saline and either 3% chloroprocaine, 2% lidocaine, or 2% mepivacaine. The interpretation is virtually identical to the interpretation of a modified differential spinal: (1) if the patient experiences pain relief after the injection of saline, the presumptive diagnosis is psychogenic pain and that diagnosis includes a placebo reaction and true psychogenic pain; (2) if the patient does not experience pain relief after the injection of 3% chloroprocaine, 2% lidocaine, or 2% mepivacaine into the epidural space (in spite of complete anesthesia of the painful area), then the diagnosis is considered to be "central." That diagnosis includes four possibilities: true organic pain caused by a lesion above the level of the epidural block, encephalization, psychogenic pain, or malingering.

This approach to differential epidural blockade has been used extensively now and has provided the same valuable information as that obtained from the modified differential spinal technique without the possibility of postspinal headache. In addition, it is a useful alternative to differential spinal when the patient refuses spinal anesthesia or when spinal anesthesia is contraindicated, although these two indications are rare. For examples of cases with antegrade differential epidural block and their interpretation, see Tables 8-2 to 8-4.

Anatomic approach

Differential brachial plexus block. In a manner similar to a differential epidural block, a differential brachial plexus block can be extremely useful as a diagnostic technique in the patient with upper extremity pain.

To obviate the problems related to high spinal (or epidural) anesthesia, particularly in an outpatient, and when the location of a patient's pain is in the upper part of the body, it is perhaps safer and certainly more appropriate to use an anatomic approach. After the injection of a placebo and the sympathetic and sensory and/or motor fibers are sequentially blocked, inject the local anesthetic at points where one modality can be interrupted without blocking another. Table

Table 8-2 Retrograde differential epidural block*

| Time (min) | BP (mm Hg) | Pulse (beats/min) | Subjective feelings | Objective findings | | | | Temp (° F) | |
| | | | | Motor power | | | Sensation on pinprick | | |
				Leg	Knee bend	Toes		Right leg	Left leg
Control	134/84	60	Burning pain in left foot	—	—	—	—	91	86
0	148/80	64	Burning pain in left foot	X	X	X	X	90	86
10	120/80	88	75% pain relief	25%	X	X	T_{10}	95	90
20	114/82	76	Total pain relief	—	—	—	T_8	95	92
60	140/96	64	Total pain relief	X	X	X	T_{12}	95	92
70	140/96	64	Total pain relief	X	X	X	X	94	92
80	138/94	64	Total pain relief	X	X	X	X	92	90

*The results of a differential epidural block (20 ml of 3% 2-chloroprocaine) in a 22-year-old man with pain in the left foot. At first evaluation at the pain control center patient gave the history of motor vehicle accident 6 months previously. He sustained a medical malleolar fracture at the ankle which was surgically corrected and put in a cast. The fracture healed normally, but the patient complained of burning pain in his left foot, especially after weight-bearing. A diagnosis of reflex sympathetic dystrophy of the left leg was made and retrograde differential epidural block was done to confirm the diagnosis. The findings above show that total relief of pain was obtained by blocking the C fibers only. A-delta and A-alpha nerve fibers did not transmit the nociceptive impulses. A series of six lumbar sympathetic blocks (left) were done at 2-week intervals with adjuvant physical therapy. The patient recovered completely.
From Raj PP, editor: *Practical Management of Pain,* ed 1. St Louis, Mosby, 1986.

Table 8-3 Retrograde differential epidural block*

| Time (min) | BP (mm Hg) | Pulse (beats/min) | Subjective feelings | Objective findings | | | | Temp (° F) | |
| | | | | Motor power | | | Sensation on pinprick | Right leg | Left leg |
				Leg	Knee bend	Toes			
Control	116/65	72	Pain and discomfort in back, left hip, and left thigh	X	X	X	X	86	88
0	120/76	76	Same as above	X	X	X	X	86	88
10	112/70	72	Feeling of warmth, some pain	—	—	—	to T_9	89	93
20	120/60	72	No pain	—	—	—	to T_6	92	94
60	120/60	72	No pain	X	X	X	to T_9	96	96
70	120/60	72	Some return of pain	X	X	X	X	90	92
80	120/60	72	Return of pain to pre-block level	X	X	X	X	88	89

*The results of differential epidural block (20 ml of 3% 2-chloroprocaine injected into epidural space at zero minute) in a 45-year-old man with pain in the low back, left hip, and left thigh and a history of four surgical procedures in the lumbar area. Findings showed that the pain was transmitted via A-delta and C fibers. Following the investigative differential blocking, the relief obtained by a series of sympathetic blocks was not enough. Stimulation by percutaneously inserted epidural electrodes gave the patient 70% pain relief. Note that blood pressure and pulse were stable during the differential study. Hypotension may make the test unreliable.
From Raj PP, editor: *Practical Management of Pain,* ed 1. St Louis, Mosby, 1986.

Table 8-4 Retrograde differential epidural block*

| Time (min) | BP (mm Hg) | Pulse (beats/min) | Subjective feelings | Objective findings | | | | Temp (° F) | |
| | | | | Motor Power | | | Sensation on pinprick | Right leg | Left leg |
				Leg	Knee bend	Toes			
Control	106/88	100	Severe pain in abdominal region	X	X	X	X	88	91
0	110/70	128	Pain in same abdominal region	X	X	X	X	88	91
10	110/70	100	Pain—same	25%	X	X	T_{10}	86	90
20	106/88	92	Pain—same	—	—	75%	T_4	94	92
60	118/70	92	Pain—same	X	X	X	T_{10}	90	91
70	120/70	92	Pain—same	X	X	X	X	89.5	90
80	120/70	92	Pain—same	X	X	X	X	88.5	90

*The results of a differential epidural block (20 ml of 3% 2-chloroprocaine injected into epidural L_2-L_3 space at time zero) in a 24-year-old woman with chronic abdominal pain. Before admission to the pain control center the patient had a diagnosis of chronic pancreatitis for 12 months. During her previous workup and treatment, she had cholecystectomy and multiple ERCP. She became dependent on narcotics and in the interim found it difficult to wean herself off the drugs. At initial pain evaluation, it was unclear whether her pain was visceral, somatic, or central. First, a celiac plexus block was carried out which intensified her pain. Second, a retrograde differential epidural block was done to diagnose peripheral versus central pain. The findings given in the table show clearly that the pain was central in origin since total motor, sensory, and sympathetic nerve fiber loss of function did not change her perception of pain. Her subsequent treatment consisted of behavioral therapy and a drug withdrawal program, with moderate success.
From Raj PP, editor: *Practical Management of Pain,* ed 1. St Louis, Mosby, 1986.

8-5 summarizes the procedural sequences for the differential nerve blocks administered for pain in different parts of the body.

Techniques utilized in the different regions of the body.
If a placebo injection does not produce relief for pain in the head, neck, and arm, then a stellate ganglion block is administered with any short-acting local anesthetic agent. If the sympathetic block cannot be administered without spill-over onto somatic nerves innervating the painful area, then the sequential blocks should be carried out on two separate occasions, thereby allowing the sympathetic block to wear off before proceeding with the somatic block. In any case, if the patient does not obtain relief after the stellate ganglion block, then a block of the somatic nerves to the painful area should be administered.

For pain in the thorax, the safest procedure is to administer a differential segmental epidural. Relief after an extensive sympathetic block indicates a possible sympathetic mechanism and may indicate visceral (rather than somatic) pain because visceral pain is mediated by sympathetic fibers. If this is the case, the patient's pain can usually be relieved (on a different occasion) by a stellate ganglion

Table 8-5 Anatomical approach: procedural sequence in differential diagnostic nerve blocks

Site of pain	Solutions to be injected and sites of injection		
	First injection (saline)	Second injection (local anesthetic)	Third injection (local anesthetic)
Head	Placebo block	Stellate block	Block of C_2
			Block of Trigeminal I, II, III (or branches)
Neck	Placebo block	Stellate block	Cervical plexus block (or individual nerve)
Arm	Placebo block	Stellate block	Brachial plexus block (or individual nerve)
Thorax*	Placebo block	Paravertebral somatic block	Paravertebral sympathetic block
Abdomen†	Placebo block	Paravertebral somatic or intercostal block	Celiac plexus block
Leg	Placebo block	Lumbar paravertebral sympathetic block	Lumbar paravertebral somatic block

From Winnie AP, Collins VJ: The Pain Clinic I: Differential neural blockade in pain syndromes of questionable etiology. *Med Clin North Amer* 52:123-129, 1968.

*In the opinion of A. Winnie, thoracic paravertebral sympathetic blocks carry such a high risk of pneumothorax that a pharmacologic approach should be utilized.

†Because of the simplicity of intercostal blocks compared to celiac plexus blocks, the procedural sequence is altered for abdominal pain.

block. If it is unwise to perform a differential thoracic epidural because of possible cachexia, hypovolemia, etc., an alternative procedure is to perform paravertebral or intercostal blocks of the appropriate dermatomes with these possible results: failure to provide relief indicates a visceral origin of the patient's pain; complete relief of the pain with return following the recovery from anesthesia indicates a peripheral, somatic mechanism; and complete relief, which persists long after recovery of sensation, indicates a peripheral but reflex sympathetic mechanism.

If a placebo injection fails to provide relief for abdominal pain, before attempting a celiac plexus block, a paravertebral or intercostal block of the appropriate dermatomes should be performed to be sure that the origin of pain is not somatic (body wall). Patients have difficulty localizing "abdominal pain" and therefore cannot differentiate pain caused by a body wall extension of a lesion from that caused by true visceral involvement. However, if the paravertebral or intercostal blocks fail to provide relief, then a celiac plexus block should be administered to establish that the pain is truly visceral in origin.

For pain in the leg, a differential spinal or epidural is preferable, but differential nerve blocks can be used when the pharmacologic approach is contraindicated or undesirable. After a placebo block, lumbar paravertebral sympathetic blocks are administered at the level of L_2, L_3, and L_4. If these fail to provide relief, then lumbar paravertebral somatic block of the appropriate dermatomes or any appropriate peripheral nerve block is administered.

Relief after a placebo injection indicates a "psychogenic mechanism," which can represent a placebo reaction or true psychogenic pain. Relief after sympathetic blocks indicates a sympathetic mechanism, usually a sympathetic dystrophy; and relief after the blockade of the somatic nerves indicates an organic somatic mechanism. Failure to obtain relief in spite of the establishment of complete anesthesia in any of these areas would indicate a "central mechanism," which could represent any of the four possibilities mentioned earlier. Interpretation of the results of differential blocks for thoracic and abdominal pain have already been discussed.

Placebo effect

The placebo effect occurs when an intervention that is not expected to have an effect produces one.[12] The effect can be in any realm of biologic function (e.g., sporting performance, learning, anxiety control, wound healing, weight loss, or analgesia). In analgesia, "sugar pills" produce significant reductions in reported pain intensity in about 30% of the population. Pain cannot be measured directly; likewise, the placebo effect cannot be measured accurately. The existence of this effect has made the *double-blind crossover* design mandatory. Exhaustive statistics and large numbers of subjects are essential to evaluate any intervention. The intervention in analgesia research can be physical (TENS), psychologic (biofeedback), or pharmacologic (narcotic). As this placebo effect appears to be present in so many areas of human function, the presence of placebo analgesia implies that some individuals may be more able than others to modulate processing of nociceptive information. There is no psychologic or other test than can predict the existence of the placebo effect or of its "potency" in a given individual. Similarly, there is no information on the presence of the placebo effects in multiple areas of function. Therefore, the presence of placebo analgesia cannot be used to infer the absence of a nociceptive process. This critical point is often ignored by those who claim to be able to interpret differential spinal, epidural, or peripheral nerve blocks. It is also often ignored by the proponents of novel therapies that produce 30% to 40% "success" attributed to a "real" effect. To illustrate this point, consider the successes claimed for some 50 different therapies for reflex sympathetic dystrophy.[13] The hypothesis that the placebo analgesic effect is endorphin-mediated has neither been confirmed nor refuted.[12]

Nocebo effect

Just as interventions that are theoretically ineffective may produce beneficial effects, so may ineffective interventions produce adverse effects. Such "negative placebo" effects may also be known as "nocebo" effects. All placebo-controlled studies produce a significant incidence of adverse effects produced by the placebo itself, which cannot be explained in conventional terms. These adverse effects are often the same as those expected from the active agent, especially when the subject has been fully informed of the potential adverse effects of the active agent. Again, the occurrence of the nocebo effect during diagnostic or therapeutic maneuvers during pain management does not imply either presence or absence of nociceptive processes or of psychogenic pain. There are no confirmed hypotheses for the mechanisms of the nocebo effect and no psychologic tests to predict its occurrence.

However, diagnostic nerve blocks are particularly important in determining the relative contributions of putative somatic and visceral nociception. For example, low back pain could arise from any structure in the lumbar spine and could also be referred from intraabdominal pathology. Injections of local anesthetics into specific structures, such as a facet joint, intervertebral disc, ligament or muscle attachment, sacroiliac joint, a specific nerve root, or even the epidural space, might define the structures involved in generation of the pain.

Diagnostic nerve blocks are of limited value in predicting the extent, intensity, and duration of "permanent" nerve blocks. In a negative prediction, it can be assumed that if the diagnostic block did not produce significant relief, then neither will the neurolytic block.

REFERENCES

1. Wilson PR, Wedel DJ, Daube JR: Evoked potentials during epidural anesthesia. *Anesthesiology* 69:A390, 1988.
2. Gasser HS, Erlanger J: Role of fiber size in establishment of nerve block by pressure or cocaine. *Am J Physiol* 88:581-591, 1929.
3. Gissen AJ, Covino BG, Gregus J: Differential sensitivities of mammalian nerve fibers to local anesthetics. *Anesthesiology* 53:467-474, 1980.
4. Strichartz GR, Ritchie JM: The action of local anesthetics on ion channels of excitable tissue. In Strichartz GR, editor: *Local Anesthetics, Handbook of Experimental Pharmacology, vol 81*. New York, Springer-Verlag, 1987.
5. Fink BR: Mechanism of differential axial blockade in epidural and subarachnoid anesthesia. *Anesthesiology* 70:851-858, 1989.
6. Raymond SA et al: The role of length of nerve exposed to local anesthetics in impulse blocking action. *Anesth Analg* 68:563-570, 1989.
7. McCollum DE, Stephen CR: Use of graduated spinal anesthesia in the differential diagnosis of pain of the back and lower extremities. *South Med J* 57:410, 1964.
8. Winnie AP, Collins VJ: The Pain Clinic I: Differential neural blockade in pain syndromes of questionable etiology. *Med Clin North Amer* 52:123-129, 1968.
9. Akkineni SR, Ramamurthy S: Simplified differential spinal block. Abstracts of scientific papers, Annual Meeting of the American Society of Anesthesiologists, 1977.
10. Winnie AP: Differential diagnosis of pain mechanism. *ASA Refresher Courses in Anesthesiology* 6:171-186, 1978.
11. Raj PP: Sympathetic pain mechanisms and management. Paper presented at the second annual meeting of the American Society of Anesthesiologists. Hollywood, Fla, Mar 10-11, 1977.
12. Grevert P, Albert LH, Goldstein A: Partial antagonism of placebo analgesia by naloxone. *Pain* 16:129-143, 1983.
13. Wilson PR: Sympathetically-maintained pain. In Stanton-Hicks M, editor: *Pain and the Sympathetic Nervous System*. Boston, Kluwer Academic Publishers, 1990.

QUESTIONS: DIAGNOSTIC NERVE BLOCK

1. The basis for differential nerve block is the study by Gasser and Erlanger. They showed that as the recording electrode is moved away from the nerve, the compound action potential shows several smaller spikes traveling at different rates. These data are interpreted as due to:
   A. Different-sized nerve fibers
   B. Same-sized nerve fibers
   C. Topographic arrangement of nerve fibers
   D. Stimulation of spinal neurons

2. Differential spinal block requires preparation of four solutions containing normal saline or different procaine concentrations. Which of the solutions should contain normal saline?
   A. Solution A
   B. Solution B
   C. Solution C
   D. Solution D

3. During the performance of a differential spinal block the patient does not obtain pain relief from normal saline but does obtain relief after the injection of 0.25% procaine. This is commonly interpreted as due to:
   A. Somatic mechanism
   B. Sympathetic mechanism
   C. Neurogenic mechanism
   D. Psychogenic mechanism

4. The principle of modified differential spinal block is to observe changes in the patient's pain:
   A. At the onset of the block
   B. During the effect of the block
   C. At the recovery of the block
   D. After the recovery of the block

5. Differential epidural block is inherently appealing because it:
   A. Avoids lumbar puncture headache
   B. Takes longer time than differential spinal block
   C. Can be done by a small-gauge needle
   D. Needs to be done as an outpatient

ANSWERS

1. A
2. A
3. B
4. C
5. A

9 Thermography

Gabor B. Racz and Donald L. Kramer

Medical thermography is based on the fact that central homeostatic controls result in reliable symmetry of cutaneous blood flow. As thermal asymmetry is the hallmark of abnormality in thermography, the patients serve as their own control. Fluctuation from this symmetry occurs as a result of a disruption in the homeostasis. Uematsu and colleagues[1] carefully mapped the temperature symmetry of 90 healthy volunteers in 40 body regions. Asymmetry of fingers was 0.43° C ± 0.26 and toes 0.59° C ± 0.27. The remaining areas of the body showed thermal asymmetry of less than 0.40° C. In the extremities, thermal gradients progress from proximal to distal. The fingers and toes are cooler than the arms and legs, yet the symmetry remains.[2] Thermography does not picture pain itself but reveals pathophysiologic conditions associated with pain syndromes from characteristic thermal dysfunction.[3]

Skin temperature below 20.0° C is almost entirely controlled by skin blood flow, which, in turn, is controlled by the sympathetic nervous system. Active impulses of the sympathetic nerves cause the walls of the blood vessels to constrict; as they subside the walls dilate passively.

Skin temperature is continually fluctuating in response to internal physiologic and external environmental conditions.[4] The hands and feet respond rapidly because of a large blood volume in relation to the small skin surface. The arms and legs are slower to respond because of a less favorable relationship between the heat content and the skin surfaces.[5] The skin has a heat transfer coefficient of 0.98; therefore, it is essentially transparent to heat and acts as a window to the vasculature beneath it. Thermography may reveal the existence of pathophysiologic states that alter the cutaneous blood flow and result in thermal dysfunction.[3]

Two distinctly different techniques to measure skin temperature are commonly used: contact thermography and infrared telethermography. Contact thermography uses plates of cholesterol esters embedded in flexible body contouring sheets that are applied directly to the back, neck, and extremities. They are extremely sensitive to temperature change and have specific color responses, with blue representing the warmer and brown the cooler end of physiologic temperature. They can distinguish differences of 0.30° C.[6]

In contrast, infrared telethermography is a noncontact method of determining skin temperature. The infrared scanning device converts radiated thermal energy into electronic signals that are amplified and transmitted to a video monitor.[7] The images of infrared thermography can be displayed in color or black and white. In black and white one sees a continuous gray scale. This scale represents qualitative temperature gradients and is difficult to interpret. Electronic

pseudocolor can be added. This is a digital technique and is set up to produce stepwise color changes at certain preset temperature increments. The assignment of a color to a specific temperature is arbitrary, and colors are used only to aid in interpretation.[2] Infrared thermography has now achieved a high level of technical performance. With current technology, videothermograms can distinguish temperatures with as little as a 0.15° C difference and can visualize areas ranging from 1 cm^2 to the entire body at once.[8] At a camera-to-object distance of 50 cm, precise measurements can be made of skin surface areas as small as 1 mm.^{2}[2,9] Scanning speeds range from 1 to 60 frames per second.[4] Laser Doppler flowmeter, with its rapid response time, provides an even more sensitive index of local vasoconstriction than that recorded thermally. However, this test is not widely available.[10]

With the advances in infrared thermography, contact thermography can be considered a less valuable tool clinically. Its major advantage is its inexpensive cost. The liquid crystal technique has been criticized for a number of reasons. First, the technique is especially dependent on the training and the expertise of the person performing the study. Precise technique is needed for an adequate study. Second, the difficulty of contouring flexible sheets to the round and bony areas of the trunk and extremities leads to uneven pressure and unequal temperature mapping. Third, the crystals have a "heat sink" effect, which can produce unreliable data when both sides of the body are not imaged in the same picture.[7] Finally, the application of mylar sheets reduces evaporative heat loss from the skin and produces a warming of the surfaces beneath.

The thermographer must follow a standard patient preparation protocol if there is to be any hope of obtaining reproducible data. The American Academy of Thermology published standards in 1986[9] (Box 9-1), which are scheduled to be updated. The thermographer must understand that there are a number of exogenous and endogenous artifacts that can affect the study. Exogenous artifacts can be due to lotions, creams, jewelry, physical therapy, sunburn, recent injections, or tatoos that cause an inflammatory response. Endogenous artifacts include obesity, hyperhidrosis, or acute dermatologic lesion.[3] Thermography is also sensitive to smoking, medications, eating, and ambient temperatures that have a large influence on skin blood flow.[11] Any technique that attempts to monitor skin temperature must therefore standardize environmental factors.

Room temperature is critically important to control. In a warm room patients will sweat. The primary source of heat loss from the skin will be evaporative rather than the radi-

Box 9-1 PREPARATION FOR THERMOGRAPHY

Prior to the thermographic examination visit, each patient should be instructed on the following points:

a. The patient should not smoke for four (4) hours prior to the examination.

b. It is recommended that the patient shower or bathe on the morning of the visit. No powders, cosmetics, lotions, or ointments should be applied to the body on the day of the examination.

c. There should have been no physiotherapy treatment earlier on the day of the examination.

d. The patient should not use a TENS unit nor have an EMG/nerve conduction evaluation or acupuncture treatment within 24 hours prior to the examination.

e. No brace, splint, or supportive collar should be worn for at least 6 hours prior to the visit unless absolutely essential for some other condition and then should be noted by the technician.

f. Sunburn or other excessive exposure to the sun should be avoided for ten (10) days prior to the examination.

TENS, Transcutaneous electrical nerve stimulation; EMG, electromyogram.
From Roberts WJ, Foglesong ME: A neuronal biasis for sympathetically maintained pain. *Thermology* 2:2-6, 1986.

ant energy that is measured by the thermograph. Generally, room temperatures are kept at 20.0 to 24.0° C, and the patient must be allowed 20 minutes for equilibration. A cooler temperature of 20.0° C is preferred to allow for maximal sympathetic stimulation.[12] Failure to allow for adequate temperature equilibration will result in false-negative results. Application of ice to either a proximal limb or to the trunk may accentuate the sympathetic tone differences.[11] In studies of the upper body, the patient should be disrobed to the waist. In studies of the lower body, nothing but a paper drape should be worn.

Understanding the role of the sympathetic nervous system is critical, since thermography is rooted in the principle that nerve impingement alters sympathetic outflow. In traditional neuroanatomic teachings, sympathetic preganglionic cell bodies are confined to the thoracic and upper lumbar area.[7] This may not be true. Mitchell[13] found preganglionic cell bodies at all levels of the spinal cord. This work received direct support from Randall and co-workers,[14] who found anatomic and physiologic evidence for the entry of preganglionic fibers at all lumbar levels of the sympathetic trunk. Anatomically, postganglionic sympathetic cell bodies involved in the control of cutaneous vessels lie largely in the sympathetic chain ganglia, located just outside the intervertebral canal. These ganglia are connected by rami with the spinal nerves distal to the dorsal root ganglia. Some postganglionic cell bodies have also been noted within spinal nerves and the brachial and lumbosacral plexuses. These unmyelinated postganglionic fibers accompany the various peripheral nerves into the extremities, where some ultimately project to the blood vessels, sweat glands, and erector pili muscles. The sympathetic fibers to the blood vessels form a terminal reticulum or sympathetic ground plexus in the myoadventitial junction. Vasoconstriction and sweating are normal responses to sympathetic stimulation.[15]

Although thermography is somewhat analogous to nerve conduction studies, it reflects dysfunction of the small, sympathetic nerve fibers, whereas nerve conduction studies demonstrate the activity of large, myelinated A fibers.[9] Recognition of thermal patterns and their asymmetrical disorders requires expert medical interpretation.

The clinician is interested in detecting aberrations in skin temperature over a small area and in relating it to pathology.[5] Thermography has been used as a diagnostic aid in the evaluation of radiculopathy, reflex sympathetic dystrophy, nerve entrapment syndromes, and a variety of neuropathic and nociceptive pain states. The literature is polarized in its view toward using thermography in the nonresearch setting of clinical practice. The number of well-controlled, blind studies without significant methodologic error are few, and anecdotal and case reports are many. The emotional pitch in the literature has been fed by a perception that some clinicians have used this test primarily for financial gain. We have summarized the current literature concerning the utility of thermography.

RADICULOPATHY

The definition of a control population is a significant problem to overcome. It is known that 80% of the population has, or is, experiencing low back pain; and that 24% to 50% of asymptomatic individuals have abnormalities on myelography, discography, and computed tomography (CT) scan. Thus in a study of thermography, it would be impossible to use the general population of low back sufferers because no independent measure of disease is available for comparison.[16]

The criterion of abnormality—a 0.8° to 1.0° C difference affecting 25% of the surface area of a dermatome compared to its contralateral dermatome—seems to have been adopted uncritically by many advocates of thermography. Using strict environmental controls, So and coworkers analyzed thermographic findings in patients with clinically unequivocal cervical radiculopathy. Using three standard deviations from the normal mean as criteria for abnormality, thermography was abnormal in only 43% of patients.[17]

In a separate report, So and colleagues[18] studied 21 patients with symptoms and clinical signs of radiculopathy, and 17 of the 21 (81%) had abnormal thermographic studies. However, thermography determined the correct level of the lesion, as judged clinically, in only three of these patients. It was impossible to identify definitely the symptomatic side on thermographic grounds.

Many investigators have had difficulty explaining thermographic abnormalities in lumbosacral radiculopathy, since it has been traditionally accepted that preganglionic sympathetic fibers do not exit through the neural foramina below the level of L_2. Sympathetic fibers are, therefore, not directly compressed in most patients with lumbosacral radiculopathy. A number of investigators have proposed possible mechanisms, but none have been clearly demonstrated.[19,20]

Some thermographers report a well-defined dermatomal distribution in radiculopathy, but these results are suspect because dermatomal distribution cannot be expected unless peripheral nerves are directly involved, and this is not the case in radiculopathy. A more likely explanation of the increased heat pattern of radiculopathy is as follows. The sinovertebral nerve is a recurrent branch of the spinal nerve that originates just distal to the dorsal root ganglia. It frequently unites with the autonomic nerves, giving it a dual spinal and autonomic composition, and supplies the spinal elements, vascular structures, longitudinal ligaments, the periosteum of the vertebrae, the synovial capsules of the apophyseal joints, and the articular surfaces. It may also reunite or communicate with the spinal nerves to contribute fibers to the skin and the muscles of the back. Another possible explanation for the increased heat is that substance P is produced by the affected sensory nerve and antidromically travels toward the skin, where it produces vasodilation.[5]

Failing to understand the complexity of sympathetic neuroanatomy and clinical correlations obscures interpretation of thermographic data in radiculopathy and back pain.[12]

Thermographic study of patients with spinal root compression nearly always reveals thermal asymmetry, with decreased temperatures in the involved dermatome.[9] Thomas et al.[21] reported that lumbar sympathetic thermatomes follow a cutaneous dermatomal distribution that is sclerotomal-myotomal, i.e. not dermatomal. For example, an L_5 unilateral nerve root impingement produces thermographic changes beyond the L_5 dermatome. This concept is necessary in the clinical interpretation of thermographic data in patients with back pain. In addition, thermatomes may overlap.

In a separate study, Thomas and co-workers[21,22] found the anterior leg region particularly reliable in thermographic diagnosis of L_5 and S_1 radiculopathy. They cited excellent correlation between infrared thermography and myocardial infarction (94%), thermography and CT scan (87%), and thermography and myelography (80%) in 57 patients with chronic low back pain and radiation in the distribution of a unilateral radiculopathy.

Literature regarding thermography for diagnosing lumbar radiculopathy was evaluated in 1991 by Hoffman and colleagues.[23] From 81 relevant citations, only 28 could be analyzed for diagnostic-accuracy data (sensitivity and specificity). The remainder had significant methodologic flaws that overestimated test performance. Of the remaining 28 reports, the data varied so widely that no meaningful meta-analysis could be performed; hence pooled summary statistics could not be reported. Yet certain conclusions could be drawn. Thermographic literature preferentially used anatomic imaging as a reference standard despite the fact that thermography is not truly an anatomic study. The thermographic literature for radiculopathy has focused almost exclusively on diagnostic accuracy and technical ability. No study offered data evaluating thermography's diagnostic impact, i.e. the relationship between thermographic results and the need for further testing. Thermography is relatively nonspecific, yet there were no discussions of diagnostic algorithms or clinical outcomes for the false-positive subjects. They concluded that the current literature does not support using thermography to diagnose lumbar radiculopathy and that its role remains in research protocols.

Harper and co-workers[24] looked at using thermography in the diagnosis of lumbosacral radiculopathy. Thermograms from 37 patients with healthy backs and 55 patients with clinical evidence of lumbosacral radiculopathy were presented in a blind fashion to three experienced readers. The results showed only a moderate degree of agreement in thermographic diagnosis in the tests of intraobserver and interobserver variabilities. They concluded that thermography compared well with the sensitivity of CT scans, electromyography, and myelography. However, thermography was less reliable than either electromyography or myelography in predicting the level of radiculopathy as found clinically or at the time of operation, and was therefore not specific.

Thermography has been suggested as a screening modality.[25] Low specificity means that if thermography was employed as a routine screening test a large number of patients would incorrectly carry the diagnosis of radiculopathy.

Advocates of thermography claim that such a finding may indicate subclinical conditions in which pain is not currently felt, and therefore false-positive results are rare. This hypothesis is unsupported.

Ochoa[26] discussed the mechanical hyperalgesia seen with light touch in patients with known radiculopathy. These burning sensations, which may be mediated by C fibers, are often relieved by decompression of the affected nerve root. Antidromic vasodilation caused by these fibers may be consistent with the changes seen in thermography of radiculopathy. This theory is supported by Kajander and Bennett,[27] who showed that in a distal to snug ligation of the sciatic nerve in rats, the nerve became depopulated to an almost pure C fiber preparation (presumed to contain a mixture of afferent and sympathetic efferents). The hyperalgesic neuropathic pain that resulted and the fluctuations in temperature were probably due to an interplay of orthodromic and antidromic impulses within these C fibers.

The Therapeutics and Technology Subcommittee of the American Academy of Neurology (AAN) in 1990[28] concluded that thermography is probably not indicated for patients who have mild or short-lived neck or back pain with neurologic findings, for those who will not be considered for surgical treatment, or for those patients who have an obvious clinical radiculopathy that would require the more definitive studies of CT, magnetic resonance imaging, or myelography. In addition, they opposed the use of thermography as a screening test for patients with neck or back pain.

The AAN report was followed by a dissenting commentary[29] signed by 39 neurologists who emphasized that the AAN report did not emphasize the value of thermography as a test of autonomic nerve physiology.

In valuing thermography over electromyography for specificity in the diagnosis of radiculopathy, weigh the fact that of the 43 muscles in the lower extremity 37 have at least three different nerve roots innervating them and 6 have only dual innervation. In addition, innervation of these muscles can vary significantly. Needle electromyography conceptually cannot be any more specific for nerve root level than a dermatomal sensory map with its areas of overlap, or a thermogram.[12] Electromyography evaluates the alpha (motor) fibers, and thermography evaluates the sensory/autonomic, or C fibers.[30]

NERVE ENTRAPMENT SYNDROMES

Tchou and co-workers[32] assessed the sensitivity and specificity of thermography in 61 patients with electromyographic diagnosis of unilateral carpal tunnel syndrome and 40 volunteers entirely negative for carpal tunnel. Using a thermal asymmetry of 1.0° C, they found sensitivities of 79% in the dorsum of hands, 89% in combined dorsal and palmar areas, and 90% in combined dorsal and thenar areas. The specificities were all greater than 95%.

The Therapeutics and Technology Subcommittee of the AAN in 1990[28] found that the use of thermography in evaluating trapped nerves was not promising.

MYOFASCIAL PAIN

Thermographers have evaluated the muscles of patients with suspected trigger points using the reasoning that thermography is well suited to assess problematic symptomatology.[6]

Sherman and colleagues[33] presented a series of 125 thermograms to a blind panel of trained evaluators. The raters were not able to efficiently differentiate between the subgroups of healthy patients and those reporting current pain in the shoulder and neck caused by muscle tension. When raters were asked to sort through a group of thermograms, they frequently guessed where the pain was because they were usually given thermographs of only one part of the body. However, when they were presented with thermographs of the entire body, they were unsuccessful in defining the painful area.

Palpation of areas with suspected trigger points can induce local changes that may obviate thermographic results. Kruse and Christiansen[34] found that after compression of trigger points, there was a drop in temperature of 0.4° to 0.8° C. They found no change in areas that were devoid of trigger points and in patients whose trigger points were secondary to a more diffuse myofascial pain syndrome.

Swerdlow and Dieter[35] studied 165 randomly selected subjects from their headache clinic population and found that 97 had "hot spots" of greater than 1.0° C in the upper back and neck. Of the subjects, 50% *with* trigger points exhibited hot spots, but 60% of the patients *without* trigger points also exhibited hot spots. In addition, there was no difference in the kilogram pressure that was comfortably sustained by hot spot and nonhot spot areas. The authors concluded that thermographic hot spots observed on the upper back are not associated with active trigger points.

Since thermogram patterns can be nonspecific in nonradicular muscle pain, the thermogram must be correlated clinically; it simply serves to objectively augment that impression.[7]

POSTHERPETIC NEURALGIA

Rowbotham and Fields[36] looked at 12 patients (who were otherwise healthy) with longstanding postherpetic neuralgia before and after skin infiltration with subcutaneous lidocaine. Treatment was not blind and no placebos were used. The site of pain was trigeminal in seven cases and thoracic in five. Thermographic findings were abnormal in 6 of the 11 patients with interpretable thermograms; average skin temperature was warmer in 6 and cooler in 2. Areas of warmth correlated well with reported areas of maximal pain, sensory loss, and allodynia. Cool areas were extensively scarred, with mild sensory loss and no allodynia. The local anesthetic that was infiltrated into the warmer areas provided a more profound relief, with longer duration than the local anesthetic that was infiltrated into the cooler areas. Rowbatham and Fields concluded that excessive sympathetic nervous system activity is a major contributor to postherpetic neuralgia. Thermography may indicate areas that may be best treated with local anesthetics.

REFLEX SYMPATHETIC DYSTROPHY

Medical thermography may have its greatest use in the evaluation of patients with reflex sympathetic dystrophy because of alterations in autonomic activity. Unfortunately, the literature does not cover any long-term series that relate clinical progress to progress seen on thermograms of a subject with reflex sympathetic dystrophy.[8] Advocates of thermography claim that this procedure can objectively quantify thermal dysfunction associated with regional pain syndromes[3] and can monitor the effects of sympathetic blockade.[7] However, central neural processes, rather than peripheral interactions, between sympathetic neurons and specific sensory receptors may contribute to the pain of reflex sympathetic dystrophy.[37] In any case, the clinician is usually interested in monitoring the pain levels of reflex sympathetic dystrophy, not in ongoing temperature changes.

Thermographic findings in reflex sympathetic dystrophy are hypothermic in the majority of patients, although areas of hyperthermia may also be seen. Both hypothermic and hyperthermic reactions are abnormal and may represent different stages of the disease because there should be no significant temperature differential between normal extremities.[38] Over time a cooling in the distal limb that gradually progresses throughout can be observed.[8]

Cooke and co-workers[39] studied temperature changes after a mild cold stress in the hands of 20 patients with reflex sympathetic dystrophy involving the hands. They were compared against 10 patients with chronic upper-extremity pain of uncertain etiology. No significant difference in thermographic results was found.

Strong and colleagues[40] used thermography and pinprick to evaluate the duration of sympathetic and sensory block in the lumbar roots following infusion of epidural 2% lidocaine with epinephrine. They found an unpredictable duration of sympathetic block compared with sensory block and cautioned against using differential epidural blockade to diagnose sympathetically-mediated pain.

SUMMARY

The literature is replete with references to the unique role of thermography in the diagnosis of painful syndromes, such as whiplash, sprains, and strains that do not show up on other imaging studies. Furthermore, thermography is often claimed as the only method available to document sensory nerve involvement. If thermography has any clinical merit, it is to assess the functional integrity of the autonomic component of a mixed nerve root and not sensory nerve involvement.[41]

In the legal courtroom, thermographic pictures with their striking colors are presented as evidence of pain. Visceral pain, breast cancer risk evaluation, thrombophlebitis, and temporomandibular joint dysfunction are but a few of the many conditions for which thermography has been employed in the uncontrolled clinical setting.

Many investigators have thought of thermography as an indirect indicator of pain, which it is not.[15] Thermography may be measuring something completely different than electromyography. Whatever thermography is measuring, it lacks the specificity of other imaging studies.[12] In the absence of standardized laboratory temperatures, standardized equipment, and clinically appropriate circumstances, the technique may produce results capable of overinterpretation or misreading.[7]

We were unable to find reports of blind, controlled studies where variables such as intrasubject change with time and pain intensity were considered.

In some minds, thermography is a diagnostic aid like the CT scan and myelogram and must be interpreted and evaluated as part of the entire diagnostic picture, which includes patient history and physical examination.[3]

A diagnostic test is most useful in clinical situations where the diagnosis is uncertain. Thermography in its current form is nonspecific[17] and, to some, of limited value.[29]

REFERENCES

1. Uematsu S et al: Quantification of thermal asymmetry. *J Neurosurg* 69:552-555, 1988.
2. Spence VA et al: Precision thermal imaging of the extremities. *Orthopedics* 9:379-382, 1986.
3. Thermography as a diagnostic aid in the management of chronic pain: An update. From Aronoff G, editor: *Evaluation and Treatment of Chronic Pain.* 1985.
4. Will RK et al: Infrared thermography: What is its place in rheumatology in the 1990s? *Br J Rheumatol* 31:337-344, 1992.
5. Edeiken J, Shaber G: Thermography: A reevaluation. *Skeletal Radiol* 15:545-548, 1986.
6. Feldman F: Thermography of the hand and wrist: Practical applications. *Hand Clin* 7:99-112, 1991.
7. Schwartz R: Neuromuscular thermography. In: *American Academy of Physical Medicine & Rehabilitation Handbook.* Chicago, American Academy of Physical Medicine and Rehabilitation, 1955.
8. Karstetter KW, Sherman RA: Use of thermography for initial detection of early reflex sympathetic dystrophy. *J Am Podiatr Med Assoc* 81:198-205, 1991.
9. American Medical Association Scientific Council: Thermography in neurological and musculoskeletal conditions. *Thermology* 2:600-607, 1987.
10. Hardy PA: Quantification of sympathetic blockade by thermography. *Br J Anaesth* 59:664-665, 1987.
11. Spence VA et al: Quantification of sympathetic blockade by thermography. *Br J Anaesth* 59:665, 1987.
12. Hubbard JE: Thermography. *Neurology* 42:701-703, 1992.
13. Mitchell GG: Anatomy of the autonomic nervous system. In: *American Academy of Physical Medicine & Rehabilitation Handbook.* Chicago, American Academy of Physical Medicine and Rehabilitation, 1955.
14. Randall WC et al: Direct examination of sympathetic outflow in man. *J Appl Physiol* 7:688-698, 1955.
15. Perelman RB, Adler D, Humphreys M: Reflex sympathetic dystrophy: Electronic thermography as an aid in diagnosis. *Orthop Rev* 16:561-566, 1987.
16. Frymoyer JW, Haugh LD: Thermography: A call for scientific studies to establish its diagnostic efficacy. *Orthopedics* 9:699-700, 1986.
17. So YT, Olney RK, Aminoff MJ: A comparison of thermography and electromyography in the diagnosis of cervical radiculopathy. *Muscle Nerve* 13:1032-1036, 1990.
18. So YT, Aminoff MJ, Olney RK: The role of thermography in the evaluation of lumbosacral radiculopathy. *Neurology* 39:1154-1158, 1989.
19. The newly recognized painful ABC syndrome: Thermographic aspects. *Thermology* 2:65-107, 1986.
20. Sato A, Schmidt RF: Somatosympathetic reflexes: Afferent fibers, central pathways, discharge characteristics. *Physiol Rev* 53:916-947, 1973.
21. Thomas D et al: Infrared thermographic imaging, magnetic resonance imaging, CT scan and myelography in low back pain. *Br J Rheumatol* 29:268-273, 1991.
22. Thomas D et al: Infrared thermographic imaging, magnetic resonance imaging, CT scan and myelography in low back pain. *Br J Rheumatol* 29:268-273, 1991.
23. Hoffman M, Kent DL, Deyo RA: Diagnostic accuracy and clinical utility of thermography for lumbar radiculopathy. *Spine* 16:623-628, 1991.
24. Harper CM et al: Utility of thermography in the diagnosis of lumbosacral radiculopathy. *Neurology* 41:1010-1014, 1991.
25. Chafetz N, Wexler CE, Kaiser JA: Neuromuscular thermography of the lumbar spine with CT correlation. *Spine* 13:922-925, 1988.
26. Ochoa JL: Neuropathic pains, from within: Personal experiences, experiments, and reflections on mythology. In Dimitrijevibe MR, Wall PD, Lindblom, V, editors: *Recent Achievements in Restorative Neurology 3: Altered Sensation and Pain.* Basel, Switzerland, Karger, 1990.
27. Sugimoto T, Bennett GJ, Kajander KC: Strychnine-enhanced transsynaptic degeneration of dorsal horn neurons in rats with an experimental painful peripheral neuropathy. *Neurosci Lett* 98(2):139-143, 1989.
28. Van den Noort S et al: Assessment: Thermography in neurologic practice. *Neurology* 40:523-525, 1990.
29. Harden N et al: Commentary on the AAN thermography report. *Neurology* 40:728, 1990.
30. So YT, Olney RK, Aminoff MJ: Comparison of thermography and electromyography. *Muscle Nerve* 14:785-787, 1991.
31. So YT et al: Evaluation of thermography in the diagnosis of selected entrapment neuropathies. *Neurology* 39:1-5, 1989.
32. Tchou S et al: Thermographic observations in unilateral carpal tunnel syndrome: Report of 61 cases. *J Hand Surg [Am]* 17:631-637, 1992.
33. Sherman RA, Barja RH, Bruno GM: Thermographic correlates of chronic pain: Analysis of 125 patients incorporating evaluations by a blind panel. *Arch Phys Med Rehabil* 68:273-279, 1987.
34. Kruse RA, Christiansen JA: Thermographic imaging of myofascial trigger points: A follow-up study. *Arch Phys Med Rehabil* 73:819-823, 1992.
35. Swerdlow B, Dieter JN: An evaluation of the sensitivity and specificity of medical thermography for the documentation of myofascial trigger points. *Pain* 48:205-213, 1992.
36. Rowbotham MC, Fields HL: Post-herpetic neuralgia: The relation of pain complaint, sensory disturbance, and skin temperature. *Pain* 39:129-144, 1989.
37. Sato J, Perl ER: Adrenergic excitation of cutaneous pain receptors induced by peripheral nerve injury. *Science* 251:1608-1610, 1991.
38. Lightman H, Pochaczeysky R, Aprin H: Thermography in childhood reflex sympathetic dystrophy. *J Pediatr* 111:551-555, 1987.
39. Cooke ED et al: Reflex sympathetic dystrophy: Temperature studies in the upper limb. *Br J Rheumatol* 28:399-403, 1989.
40. Strong WE et al: Does the sympathetic block outlast sensory block: A thermographic evaluation. *Pain* 46:173-176, 1991.
41. Newman DL et al: Cervical radiculopathy revisited. *Orthop Rev* 17:199, 1988.

QUESTIONS: THERMOGRAPHY

For questions 1-4, choose from the following:
  A. 1, 2, and 3
  B. 1 and 3
  C. 2 and 4
  D. 4
  E. All of the above

1. Which of the following statements about medical thermography is (are) true?
  1. It may be used as a graphic representation of a patient's pain.
  2. Thermal asymmetry of more than 0.6° C is typically abnormal.
  3. Proximal changes occur before distal changes.
  4. Skin temperature continually fluctuates in response to physiologic and environmental conditions.

2. Contact thermography:
  1. Is more reliable than infrared thermography
  2. Is best performed at normal room temperatures
  3. Can picture the entire body
  4. Is less expensive than infrared thermography

3. Thermography is best performed:
  1. With room temperature at 20° to 24° C
  2. With the examined body part exposed
  3. Without any skin lotions or creams
  4. After a challenge with intravenous caffeine

4. In evaluating a patient with back pain:
  1. Thermography provides a radicular picture
  2. Thermography correlates well with other imaging studies to define the level of pathology
  3. Thermography is a reliable screening test of the general population
  4. Infrared thermography is more reliable than contact thermography

ANSWERS:

1. B
2. D
3. A
4. C

10 Psychologic Evaluation and Treatment

Jennifer F. Kelly

PSYCHOLOGIC EVALUATION

The evaluation of psychosocial factors is an important part of the initial assessment of the pain patient. The goal of the psychologic evaluation is to determine the contribution of affective, cognitive, and behavioral factors to the pain experience.[1] This will assist the treatment team in formulating reasonable treatment goals.

Different clinical psychologic pictures are observed in patients experiencing acute and chronic pain.[2] Acute pain, or pain of relatively short duration, is usually accompanied by anxiety. As the patient's pain becomes more chronic, habitual autonomic responses occur. The clinical picture includes sleep disturbance, increased somatic focus, decreased libido, and appetite changes. These symptoms are characterized as depressive symptomatology.[3]

Some of the psychologic symptoms observed are secondary to the pain complaint, whereas others may have been in existence before the pain occurred. Regardless of the chronologic order, an adverse effect on a patient's response to treatment is likely to occur if the psychologic factors are not identified and treated.

The psychologic evaluation should assess the following dimensions: (a) the current status of pain sensations, cognitions, pain behaviors, and mood; (2) premorbid personality functioning; and (3) environmental factors that can influence pain.[4] Although various assessment methods exist, they all should focus on assessing the psychosocial factors that can influence a patient's response to treatment. Most treatment facilities have a standard battery for assessing pain patients. These include the clinical interview, a structured pain inventory, and psychometric testing. Box 10-1 outlines the evaluation method.

Clinical interview

Information about the individual's premorbid level of functioning should be obtained during the clinical interview. Educational background, social functioning, psychosocial stressors, and vocational history can all influence success in a pain rehabilitation program. Patients with good premorbid level of functioning are believed to have a more positive response to treatment.[4] Interviewing the spouse or other close relatives can also provide background information to assist in diagnosing and treating the patient.

Structured pain inventories

There are numerous structured pain inventories available, including the Psychosocial Pain Inventory,[5] the McGill Comprehensive Pain Questionnaire,[6] the West Haven-Yale Multidimensional Pain Inventory,[1] and the Pain Profile.[7]

The structured interviews are designed to obtain information about the pain complaint, medical history, reinforcers of pain behaviors, and other psychosocial influences such as financial status and litigation. The pain inventories are usually easy to administer and score and can provide objective data to use when developing an appropriate treatment plan.

Many of the areas assessed in the pain inventory may appear redundant with the clinical interview. However, the clinical interview focuses more on the premorbid level of functioning, whereas the structured pain inventories emphasize the psychosocial correlates of the pain experience. Additionally, because the clinical interview is unstructured, the psychologist can focus on the patient's affective responses and interaction with the interviewer.

Psychometric testing

Various objective psychologic test measures are used to evaluate pain patients. Among them are the McGill Pain Questionnaire (MPQ),[8] Minnesota Multiphasic Personality Inventory (MMPI),[9] the Symptom Checklist-90 (SCL-90),[10] and the Millon Behavioral Health Inventory.[11] Brief inventories are also available for use in assessing this population. They include, but are not limited to, the Beck Depression Scale[12] and the State-Trait Anxiety Inventory.[13]

The MPQ and MMPI are widely used by psychologists working with the pain population. The revised version of the MMPI, the MMPI-2, is now being used more frequently. The MMPI has been useful in assessing emotional disorders that occur secondary to the pain experience or preexistent personality factors that could potentially adversely affect a patient's response to treatment. Neither the MMPI nor any other structured psychologic test has been useful in determining the difference between "psychogenic" and "organic" pain in patients.[14]

It is common for chronic pain patients to have a profile configuration on the MMPI known as *conversion V*. This profile is characterized by high elevations on the hypochondriasis and hysteria scales and a relatively lower score on the depression scale. Research with this configuration rendered its original interpretation of conversion symptoms as being unsupported by pain populations, since studies have shown that pain patients with these profiles usually have an organic basis for the pain experienced and they are not experiencing their pain as a conversion reaction.

Studies have been conducted that evaluate the usefulness of the MMPI in predicting treatment outcome. They have yielded inconsistent findings regarding its predictive validity. This may be related to the fact that studies often used subjective and poorly defined indexes of success. Additionally, differences in the patient population examined could account for the inconsistent results.[15]

A disadvantage of the MMPI is the length of the test, which consists of 566 items. Additionally, many patients become defensive when responding to the test because they tend to feel that the questions are implying that there is no physiologic basis for the pain.

The MPQ contains adjectives that patients can select to characterize their pain experience. The questionnaire assesses affective, sensory, and evaluative dimensions of pain. Information on the relative intensity of each aspect and the patient's evaluation of the overall intensity of pain is also provided.[16] Research indicates that the MPQ is a valid and reliable instrument that can fairly and quickly assess a patient's subjective pain experience.[17]

The SCL-90 is a checklist that allows the patient to rate symptoms of physical and emotional distress on a five-point scale. Because it consists of only 90 items, it is viewed as a viable alternative to the MMPI. The main disadvantage of this instrument is that its standardization sample consisted of psychiatric and not pain patients. This renders its generalization to the pain population questionable.

The Millon Behavioral Health Inventory[11] is another alternative to the MMPI. This self-report inventory consists of 150 true-false items that measure personality styles and attitudes relevant to specific illnesses. Additionally, it contains a prognostic index that can predict response to treatment. Although there is no conclusive evidence to validate this instrument with pain patients, it is an instrument that deserves further investigation.

There are numerous brief psychometric measures to use with the pain population that can quickly assess negative affective states such as anxiety and depression. These negative states can adversely affect the patient's response to treatment. Advantages of these instruments are their relatively brief time to administer, score, and interpret. However, they generally only measure the presence or absence of specific symptoms instead of providing a more global assessment of the patient's psychologic adjustment.

In assessing pain patients, it is important to integrate all data instead of relying exclusively on information from only one source. Only then can one have a comprehensive psychologic assessment of the patient.

PSYCHOLOGIC APPROACHES TO MANAGEMENT OF CHRONIC PAIN

Studies have shown that psychologic techniques such as contingency management and cognitive-behavioral strategies are associated with improved functioning in chronic pain patients. Observed improvements include the use of more appropriate coping strategies, decreased pain perception, improved psychologic functioning, and the appropriate use of the health care system. One of the main goals of the psychologic approaches is to teach patients techniques so that they can manage their condition appropriately. The psychologic interventions have been categorized by the pain experience component that they are to target: physiologic, subjective, or behavioral (Fig. 10-1). Biofeedback and relaxation training are used to treat the physiologic compo-

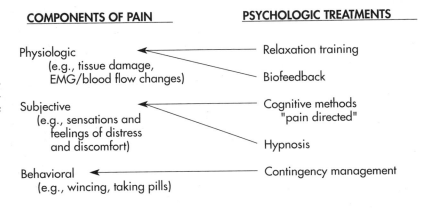

Fig. 10-1 Psychologic approaches to pain management. (From Pearce S: A review of cognitive-behavioural methods for the treatment of chronic pain. *J Psychosom Res* 27:431-440, 1983.)

nent of the pain experience. For example, electromyographic biofeedback is used to treat muscle contraction headache. Cognitive approaches and hypnosis focus on sensations and feelings of distress and discomfort. The operant approaches, or contingency management, target the behavioral component of the pain experience, such as pill-taking behavior. A patient may be treated with all of the various methods because the treatments are not mutually exclusive.[18]

Biofeedback

Biofeedback is a noninvasive procedure that has become a widely accepted treatment of chronic pain. The effectiveness of biofeedback relies on the patient's participation. Biofeedback involves the use of electronic equipment to reveal involuntary physiologic events. With this information, patients can learn to bring the involuntary responses under voluntary control.[19] Biofeedback is used to treat a variety of pain syndromes: muscle contraction and migraine headache, low back pain, and arthritis.[20]

There are several rationales for using biofeedback to treat chronic pain, and they are:

1. Modification of the specific physiologic process that underlies the pain disorder. For example, electromyographic biofeedback is used to treat muscle contraction headache. It is believed that the reduction in muscle tension achieved through biofeedback training will result in a corresponding decrease in muscle contraction headache. This rationale is not supported in the treatment of syndromes for which the etiology is unclear.[21,22]

2. Facilitation of the relaxation response. A reduction in autonomic arousal can lead to a corresponding reduction in pain. If stress and tension exacerbate pain, then relaxation should be associated with its relief.

3. Self-regulation. Through biofeedback training, patients become more aware of their own contribution to the pain experience and their ability to influence the pain. In order for biofeedback to be effective, patients must take responsibility for management of their pain.[21] Patients learn that their pain can be internally, as opposed to externally, controlled.[23] The patients' view of the pain may change, which could result in greater acceptance of personal responsibility for the

pain behavior. The internal focus can also facilitate the patients developing a more optimistic outlook for the future. The patients' affective states may improve, and participation in the treatment process can increase.

The most common forms of biofeedback used with the chronic pain population are electromyographic biofeedback and skin temperature or thermal biofeedback. Alpha biofeedback has been investigated as a treatment for chronic pain, but this form of biofeedback is not regularly used at pain management centers.

Electromyographic biofeedback provides a measure of the electrical discharge in the muscle fibers, indicating relaxation or contraction of the muscles. The effective use of electromyographic biofeedback should result in reduction in muscle tension, which in turn decreases the pain experienced.[21] The pain syndromes that electromyographic biofeedback has been used to treat include muscle contraction headache, temporomandibular joint pain, and myofascial pain.

A potential problem with electromyographic feedback is that the electromyographic readout may not be an accurate representation of the muscle tension level. The pain could be the result of deep muscle tension that is not easily measured by electromyographic surface electrodes, or the pain may originate at a site different from where it is experienced.[21,24] Some studies have failed to consistently show a positive correlation between reported pain relief and reduction in electromyography. It is possible for a patient to be successfully trained in electromyographic biofeedback yet not have a reduction in pain.[25] One possible explanation for this occurrence is that there may be a delay between reduction of electromyography and the corresponding reduction of pain.[26]

The basis for using skin temperature or thermal biofeedback in treating chronic pain is that activity in the sympathetic nervous system may result in vasoconstriction of peripheral arterioles, and that reduced sympathetic nervous system activity is associated with vasodilation. The goal of skin temperature biofeedback is to teach patients to increase the skin temperature in their extremity, usually their finger, thereby increasing vasodilation and reducing sympathetic nervous system activity. Additionally, an increase in skin temperature is associated with a full relaxation response.[21,27] The pain syndrome that skin temperature biofeedback is most commonly used to treat is migraine headaches. However, the exact physiologic mechanism by which this form of biofeedback works with migraine headache remains unclear.[22,28]

Studies evaluating the effectiveness of skin temperature biofeedback in treating migraine headache have yielded mixed results.[27,29,30] The analysis of studies evaluating its effectiveness is frequently complicated by the use of additional techniques, such as autogenic relaxation training. It seems that the use of skin temperature biofeedback is effective in treating selected cases of migraine. Its usefulness may be related to the nonspecific factors in biofeedback therapy, such as relaxation and the patients' perceived control over the pain.[31]

Electroencephalogram biofeedback assists patients in producing alpha brain activity (8 to 13 Hz). This is a relaxed state incompatible with pain.[32] Early studies examining the use of this form of biofeedback in reducing pain yielded positive findings; however, they were not well controlled.[33,34] These studies did prompt further investigation of the procedure in the management of pain, but they have not provided sufficient support for the use of this form of biofeedback for pain control.

Relaxation training

The main purpose for using the various relaxation techniques in pain management is to elicit the relaxation response. Studies have shown that physiologic changes consistent with decreased sympathetic nervous system activity often accompany the relaxation response.[35-37] The changes observed include decreases in oxygen consumption, reduction in heart rate, and a marked decrease in arterial blood lactate concentration. Relaxation is believed to reduce pain by reducing arousal. Additionally, it facilitates a patient's ability to use suggestion and imagination to provide relief of pain.[21] The process of focused concentration helps the patients learn to disrupt preoccupying thoughts, especially those related to pain.[38]

Relaxation has also been used to teach chronic pain patients body awareness. Patients experiencing pain, especially myofascial pain, frequently tense their muscles in response to pain or in anticipation of pain. By becoming more aware of the physical sensations in their bodies, patients can learn to reliably decrease the muscle tension and thereby cope with the pain more effectively.

Numerous relaxation approaches are used with chronic pain patients. Progressive muscle relaxation is the most common approach. This technique involves tensing and relaxing the major muscle groups. The purpose is for the patients to learn to relax the tense muscles that contribute to pain. When the patients have consistently achieved success with progressive muscle relaxation, a shorter version of the technique is usually substituted. The eventual goal is to reduce tension by recall, thus eliminating the need to actively tense muscle groups. As patients become more advanced using the technique, they can incorporate visual imagery and autogenic phrases to elicit relaxation.[22]

Relaxation training has been successfully used to treat a wide variety of pain disorders, including muscle contraction headache,[39,40] migraine headaches,[41-43] temporomandibular joint pain,[44,45] chronic back pain,[46,47] and myofascial pain syndrome.[48,49]

Comparison between biofeedback and relaxation training

Numerous studies have compared the relative effectiveness of biofeedback and relaxation training in treating chronic pain. The majority of the studies indicate that relaxation and biofeedback training are equally effective in the management of pain.[50] However, the two approaches can be useful to the patients in different ways. Biofeedback provides patients with an overt indicator of the relationship between behaviors and cognitions and changes in physiologic processes. When provided with this feedback, patients can develop control over the specific physiologic mechanism that contributes to pain.[51] With biofeedback, patients can be provided with objective data on the progress made during the treatment sessions. Additionally, patients tend to favor the instrumentation and technology associated with feedback. The main advantage of relaxation training is that it is more practical and cost effective.[52]

Biofeedback and relaxation are generally used as conjunctive treatments. The relaxation training can alter physiologic processes, and the biofeedback can shape the patient's relaxation response. The biofeedback can pinpoint the training problems and open up new intervention tactics. By providing objective data to the patients, the instrumentation and measurement techniques can place the techniques in a "scientific" explanatory framework.[53] In the treatment sessions, the patients should verbalize the control strategies, attend to sensations experienced during the training sessions, and use conditioned verbal cues to generalize learned techniques to daily life. The patient should not develop excessive reliance on the machine.[54]

Hypnosis

The dramatic pain relief that patients have achieved with hypnosis is not well understood. Studies have indicated that the hypnotic analgesia is not mediated by the endorphin system.[55-58] Research supports the theory that cognitions play an important role in hypnosis and hypnotic analgesia.[59] In managing chronic pain, hypnosis focuses on the subjective component of the pain experience, such as feelings of distress and discomfort.

Hypnosis can provide an analgesic experience for many patients, but the technique itself is not expected to cure chronic pain. It provides a sensation of peacefulness and comfort, and short-term relief of pain can be experienced. In order for lasting benefit to occur, it should be part of a broader psychotherapeutic regime.[60] It is more effective in managing pain of organic etiology than with psychogenic, or functional, pain. This is because persistent psychogenic pain often has complicating factors that need to be addressed, such as secondary gain.[61] Using hypnosis to treat disorders with secondary gain may result in symptom substitution.[62]

Generally, the effectiveness of hypnosis depends on two factors: the patient's imagination and the clinician's ability to capitalize on that imagination. Hypnotic responsiveness varies considerably among individuals, and hypnotizability can be modified by various means, such as operant training and biofeedback.[63,64]

Various hypnotic methods can achieve hypnotic pain control, and they include[60,65]:

1. Altering the perception of the pain. Analgesia or anesthesia is obtained by suggesting that the pain is diminishing, changing, or that the area is becoming numb.
2. Substituting the painful sensation with a different or less painful sensation. Some patients can use this technique more effectively if the substituted feeling is not totally pleasant; for example, substituting stabbing pain with a pinching sensation.
3. Moving the pain to another area of the body. The new location of the pain should be an area of lesser psychologic vulnerability. For example, a writer who has pain in the dominant hand can be given a hypnotic suggestion that the pain is moving to the tip of the small finger. The eventual goal is for the pain to be moved to another part of the body.
4. Dissociating awareness of the pain. The technique is useful when patients do not need to be functional, such as when they are undergoing medical or dental procedures or in the latter stages of a terminal illness. The patient is taught to experience another state, place, or time, such as in a vivid daydream.
5. Altering the meaning of the pain for the patient. With this technique the pain becomes less meaningful and less debilitating to the patient.
6. Distorting time. Patients are taught ways to distort time so that the amount of time experiencing a pain sensation is altered. The patient can be taught to perceive that a painful sensation is rapidly passing.

An important component of using hypnosis with pain patients is to teach them self-hypnosis. In this way, they can use the hypnotic techniques themselves to self-regulate the pain.

Cognitive approaches

Expectations, attitudes, and beliefs affect the way in which patients cope with pain. The premise of the cognitive approach is that change in negative cognitions can result in better pain control.[66] Inadequate coping mechanisms in chronic pain patients are related to errors in cognitions. Patients who misinterpret their experience of pain are more severely disabled.[67,68] The goal of intervention is to correct faulty thought processes that contribute to prolonged suffering and disability, and maladaptive beliefs are replaced with more adaptive ones.[69] Studies conducted support using cognitive approaches in treating chronic pain.[70,71] The cognitive approaches have been associated with the following benefits:

1. Patients will have the necessary coping skills to deal with the pain more effectively.
2. Patients learn to live more satisfying lives despite the presence of physical discomfort.
3. There is decreased reliance on the health care system and a reduction in dependence on analgesic medications,

which is a message emphasized to patients that they are not helpless in dealing with their pain and that it should not control their lives.[72]

There are a wide variety of therapeutic techniques under the cognitive model but they have common elements. The interventions are structured, action oriented, and usually limited to a certain period of time. The approaches can be taught in individual or group sessions.[73]

Turk and associates[73] describe three phases of the intervention of the cognitive approaches:

1. Patients are taught how thoughts and feelings influence pain.
2. Patients are taught a specific method for coping with pain that includes:
   · Preparing for minor painful sensations
   · Confronting more severe pain
   · Coping with feelings that exacerbate pain, such as anxiety or frustration
   · Learning to reinforce self for successfully coping with the episode of pain
   The pain methods are: relabeling painful sensations, attention diversion, reinterpreting pain sensations, relaxation, and imagery.
3. Patients are taught to generalize the skills to use in situations outside the clinical setting by practicing in the office setting and then using the techniques in outside situations, such as the work or home environment.

Operant approaches

The operant approach to the management of chronic pain is based on the assumption that patients' behaviors are governed by consequences, and that the environmental consequences of a behavior determine whether or not the behaviors will return. If the reinforcers are positive, then there is an increased likelihood that the behavior will recur, whereas negative reinforcement decreases the likelihood. The goal of operant approaches, or contingency management, is to replace learned maladaptive behaviors with behaviors incompatible with the sick role.[74] Environmental contingencies are changed so that appropriate "healthy" behaviors are reinforced and pain behaviors are not rewarded. For this to occur, the targeted behaviors and possible reinforcers need to be identified and the reinforcers should be manipulated. Family members and health care providers are instructed to reinforce appropriate behaviors and to ignore pain behaviors such as complaints of pain, use of narcotics, and inactivity. Other forms of intervention, such as marital counseling, family therapy, and vocational planning, can be incorporated in the treatment.[75,76]

SUMMARY

There is support in the literature for the use of these treatments in managing chronic pain patients. In order for the approaches to be successful, the patients must accept responsibility for successful management of the pain. To be the most beneficial, the treatments should be incorporated into a comprehensive pain management program.

REFERENCES

1. Turk DC, Rudy TE: Toward an empirically derived taxonomy of chronic pain patients: Integration of psychological assessment data. *J Consult Clin Psychol* 56:233-238, 1988.
2. Sternbach RA: *Pain Patients: Traits and Treatment.* New York, Academic Press, 1974.
3. Sternbach RA: The psychologist's role in the diagnosis and treatment of pain patients. In Barber J, Adrian C, editors: *Psychological Approaches to the Management of Pain.* New York, Brunner/Mazel, 1982.
4. Degood DD: A rationale and format for psychosocial evaluation. In Lynch NT, Vasudevan SV, editors: *Persistent Pain: Psychosocial Assessment and Intervention.* Boston, Kluwer Academic Publishers, 1988.
5. Getto CJ, Heaton RK: *Psychosocial Pain Inventory Manual.* Odessa, Fla, Psychological Assessment Resources, 1985.
6. Monks R, Taenzer P: A comprehensive pain questionnaire. In Melzack R, editor: *Pain Measurement and Assessment.* New York, Raven Press, 1983.
7. Duncan GH, Gregg JM, Ghia JN: The Pain Profile: A computerized system for the assessment of chronic pain. *Pain* 5:275-284, 1978.
8. Melzack R: The McGill Pain Questionnaire: Major properties and scoring methods. *Pain* 1:277-299, 1975.
9. Hathaway SR, McKinley JC: *Minnesota Multiphasic Personality Inventory: Manual for Administration and Scoring.* Minneapolis, University of Minnesota Press, 1983.
10. DeRogatis L: SCL-90. *Administration, Scoring, and Procedure Manual - I, Revised Version.* Baltimore, L DeRogatis, 1977.
11. Millon T, Green C, Meagher R: The MBHI: A new inventory for the psychodiagnostician in medical settings. *Professional Psychology* 10:529-539, 1979.
12. Beck AT et al: An inventory for measuring depression. *Arch Gen Psychiatry* 4:561-571, 1961.
13. Spielberger CD, Gorsuch RL, Lushene RE: Manual for the State-Trait Anxiety Inventory. Palo Alto, CA, Consulting Psychologists Press, 1970.
14. Elkins GR, Barrett ET: The MMPI in evaluation of functional versus organic low back pain. *J Pers Assess* 48:259-264, 1984.
15. Trief PM, Yuan HA: The use of the MMPI in a chronic back pain rehabilitation program. *J Clin Psychol* 39:46-53, 1983.
16. Melzack R: The McGill Pain Questionnaire. In Melzack R, editor: *Pain Measurement and Assessment.* New York, Raven Press, 1983.
17. Melzack R: Concepts of pain management. In Melzack R, editor: *Pain Measurement and Assessment.* New York, Raven Press, 1983.
18. Pearce S: A review of cognitive-behavioural methods for the treatment of chronic pain. *J Psychosom Res* 27:431-440, 1983.
19. Basmajian JV: Introduction: Principles and background. In Basmajian JV, editor: *Biofeedback: Principles and Practice for Clinicians.* Baltimore, Williams & Wilkins, 1983.
20. Jessup BA: Biofeedback. In Wall PD, Melzack R, editors: *Textbook of Pain.* New York, Churchill Livingstone, 1984.
21. Schuman M: Biofeedback in the management of chronic pain. In Barber J, Adrian C, editors: *Psychological Approaches to the Management of Pain.* New York, Brunner/Mazel, 1982.
22. Grzesiak RC, Ciccone DS: Relaxation, biofeedback, and hypnosis in the management of pain. In Lynch NT, Vasudevan SV, editors: *Persistent Pain: Psychosocial Assessment and Intervention.* Boston, Kluwer Academic Publishers, 1988.
23. Ciccone DS, Grzesiak RC: Cognitive dimensions of chronic pain. *Soc Sci Med* 19:1339-1345, 1984.
24. Linton SJ: Behavioral remediation of chronic pain: A status report. *Pain* 24:125-141, 1986.
25. Peck CL, Kraft GH: Electromyographic feedback for pain related to muscle tension. *Arch Surg* 112:889-895, 1977.
26. Philips C: The modification of tension headache pain utilizing EMG feedback. *Behav Res Ther* 15:119-129, 1977.
27. Chapman SL: A review and clinical perspective on the use of EMG and thermal biofeedback for chronic headaches. *Pain* 27:1-43, 1986.
28. Nigl AJ: *Biofeedback and Behavioral Strategies in Pain Treatment.* New York, SP Medical and Scientific Books, 1984.
29. Sargent JD, Green EE, Walters DE: Psychosomatic self-regulation of migraine and tension headaches. *Sem Psychiat* 5:415-428, 1973.
30. Turin A, Johnson WG: Biofeedback therapy for migraine headaches. *Arch Gen Psychiatry* 33:577-579, 1976.
31. Turk DC, Meichenbaum DH, Berman WH: Application of biofeedback for the regulation of pain: A critical review. *Psychol Bull* 86:1322-1338, 1979.
32. Pelletier KR, Peper E: Developing a biofeedback model: Alpha EEG feedback as a means for pain control. *Int J Clin Exp Hypn* 25:361-371, 1977.
33. Coger R, Werbach M: Attention, anxiety, and the effects of learned enhancement of EEG in chronic pain: A pilot study in biofeedback. In Crue B, editor: *Pain: Research and Treatment.* New York, Academic Press, 1975.
34. Gannon L, Sternbach RA: Alpha enhancement as a treatment for pain: A case study. *J Behav Ther Exp Psychiatry* 2:209-213, 1971.
35. Benson H, Pomeranz B, Kutz I: The relaxation response and pain. In Wall PD, Melzack R, editors: *Textbook of Pain.* New York, Churchill Livingstone, 1984.
36. Levander VL et al: Increased forearm blood flow during a wakeful hypometabolic state. *Federation Proceedings* 31:405, 1972.
37. Wallace RK, Benson H: The physiology of meditation. *Sci Am* 226:84-90, 1972.
38. Sachs LB: Teaching hypnosis for the self-control of pain. In Barber J, Adrian C, editors: *Psychological Approaches to the Management of Pain.* New York, Brunner/Mazel, 1982.
39. Fichtler H, Zimmerman RR: Changes in reported pain from tension headaches. *Percept Mot Skills* 36:712, 1973.
40. Tasto DL, Hinkle JE: Muscle relaxation treatment for tension headaches. *Behav Res Ther* 11:347-349, 1973.
41. Andreychuk T, Skriver C: Hypnosis and biofeedback in the treatment of migraine headache. *Int J Clin Exp Hypn* 23:172-183, 1977.
42. Hay KM, Madders J: Migraine treated by relaxation therapy. *J R Coll Gen Pract* [Occas Pap] 21:664-669, 1971.
43. Warner G, Lance J: Relaxation therapy in migraine and chronic tension headache. *Med J Aust* 1:298-301, 1975.
44. Funch DP, Gale EN: Biofeedback and relaxation therapy for chronic temporomandibular joint pain: Predicting successful outcomes. *J Consult Clin Psychol* 52:982-989, 1984.
45. Gessel AH, Alderman MM: Management of myofascial pain dysfunction syndrome of the temporomandibular joint by tension control training. *Psychosomatics* 12:302-309, 1971.
46. Sanders SH: Component analysis of a behavioral treatment program for chronic low-back pain. *Behavior Therapy* 14:697-705, 1983.
47. Turner JA: Comparison of group progressive-relaxation training and cognitive-behavioral group therapy for chronic low back pain. *J Consult Clin Psychol* 50:757-765, 1982.
48. Crockett DJ et al: A comparison of treatment modes in the management of myofascial pain dysfunction syndrome. *Biofeedback Self Regul* 11:279-291, 1986.
49. Stenn PG, Mothersill KJ, Brooke RI: Biofeedback and a cognitive behavioral approach to treatment of myofascial pain dysfunction syndrome. *Behavior Therapy* 10:29-36, 1979.
50. Blanchard EB et al: Migraine and tension headache: A meta-analytic review. *Behavior Therapy* 11:613-631, 1980.
51. Cott A et al: Long-term efficacy of combined relaxation: Biofeedback treatments for chronic headache. *Pain* 51:49-56, 1992.
52. Schneider CJ: Cost effectiveness of biofeedback and behavioral medicine treatments: A review of the literature. *Biofeedback Self Regul* 12:71-91, 1987.
53. Stoyva J: Guidelines in cultivating general relaxation: Biofeedback and autogenic training combined. In Basmajian JV, editor: *Biofeedback: Principles and Practice for Clinicians.* Baltimore, Williams & Wilkins, 1983.
54. Budzynski TH: Biofeedback procedures in the clinic. *Sem Psychiat* 5:537-548, 1973.
55. Hilgard ER, Hilgard JR: Hypnosis in the relief of pain. Los Altos, CA, William Kaufmann, 1975.
56. Goldstein A, Hilgard E: Lack of influence of the morphine antagonist naloxone on hypnotic analgesia. *Proc Nat Acad Sci USA* 72:2041-2043, 1975.
57. Finer B, Terenius L: Endorphin involvements during hypnotic analgesia in chronic pain patients. Paper presented at the Third World Congress on Pain of the International Association for the Study of Pain. Edinburgh, Scotland, September, 1981.

58. Barber J, Mayer D: Evaluation of the efficacy and neural mechanism of a hypnotic analgesia procedure in experimental and clinical dental pain. *Pain* 4:41-48, 1977.
59. Hilgard ER: The alleviation of pain by hypnosis. *Pain* 1:213-231, 1975.
60. Barber J: Incorporating hypnosis in the management of chronic pain. In Barber J, Adrian C, editors: *Psychological Approaches to the Management of Pain.* New York, Brunner/Mazel, 1982.
61. Orne MT: Hypnotic methods for managing pain. In Bonica JJ, Albe-Fessard GG, editors: *Advances in Pain Research and Therapy.* New York, Raven Press, 1983.
62. Orne MT, Dinges DF: Hypnosis. In Wall PD, Melzack R, editors: *Textbook of Pain.* New York, Churchill Livingstone, 1984.
63. Sachs L: Construing hypnosis as modifiable behavior. In Jacobs AB, Sachs LB, editors: *Psychology of Private Events.* New York, Academic Press, 1971.
64. London P, Cooper LM, Engstrom DR: Increasing hypnotic susceptibility by brain wave feedback. *J Abnorm Psychol* 83:554-560, 1974.
65. Barber J, Gitelson J: Cancer pain: Psychological management using hypnosis. *Cancer* 30:130-136, 1980.
66. Brownell KD: Behavioral medicine. *Ann Rev Behav Ther* 9:180-210, 1984.
67. Lefebvre MF: Cognitive distortion and cognitive errors in depressed psychiatric and low back pain patients. *J Consult Clin Psychol* 54:222-226, 1986.
68. Smith TW et al: Cognitive distortion and disability in chronic low back pain. *Cog Ther Res* 10:201-210, 1986.
69. Ciccone DS, Grzesiak RC: Cognitive therapy: An overview of theory and practice. In Lynch N, Vasudevan S, editors: *Persistent Pain: Psychosocial Assessment and Intervention.* Boston, Kluwer Academic Publishers, 1988.
70. Nicholas MK, Wilson PH, Goyen J: Comparison of cognitive-behavioral group treatment and an alternative non-psychological treatment for chronic low back pain. *Pain* 48:339-347, 1992.
71. Manne SL, Zautra AJ: Coping with arthritis: Current status and critique. *Arthritis Rheum* 35:1273-1619, 1992.
72. Turk DC, Meichenbaum D: A cognitive-behavioral approach to pain management. In Wall PD, Melzack R, editors: *Textbook of Pain.* New York, Churchill Livingstone, 1984.
73. Turk DC, Meichenbaum D, Genest M: *Pain and Behavioral Medicine: A Cognitive-Behavioral Perspective.* New York, Guilford Press, 1983.
74. Sternbach RA: Behaviour therapy. In Wall PD, Melzack R, editors: *Textbook of Pain.* New York, Churchill Livingstone, 1984.
75. Fordyce WE et al: Some implications of learning in problems of chronic pain. *J Chronic Diseases* 21:179-190, 1968.
76. Turner JA, Chapman CR: Psychological interventions for chronic pain: A critical review. II. Operant conditioning, hypnosis, and cognitive-behavioral therapy. *Pain* 12:23-46, 1982.

QUESTIONS: PSYCHOLOGIC EVALUATION AND TREATMENT

For questions 1-5, choose from the following:
- A. 1, 2, and 3
- B. 1 and 3
- C. 2 and 4
- D. 4
- E. All of the above

1. The purpose of the psychologic evaluation is:
   1. To determine the current status of pain sensations, cognitions, pain behaviors, and mood
   2. To assess environmental factors that influence pain
   3. To assess the premorbid personality function
   4. To determine if the pain is psychogenic or organic
2. The following symptoms of depression are observed in chronic pain patients:
   1. Sleep disturbance
   2. Appetite disturbance
   3. Suicidal ideation
   4. Poor concentration and memory disturbance
3. Common forms of biofeedback used to manage chronic pain include:
   1. Electromyographic biofeedback
   2. Thermal or skin temperature biofeedback
   3. Alpha biofeedback
   4. Pulse wave velocity biofeedback

4. The following therapeutic approaches are useful in treating chronic pain patients:
   1. Cognitive-behavioral
   2. Contingency management or operant approaches
   3. Hypnosis
   4. Psychoanalytic therapy
5. The following are methods of achieving hypnotic pain control:
   1. After the perception of pain
   2. Substitute the painful sensation with a different or less painful sensation
   3. Move the pain to another area of the body
   4. Distortion of time

ANSWERS

1. A
2. E
3. B
4. A
5. E

11 Functional Evaluation

Elise A. Trumble and *Margaret P. Krengel*

The role of physical therapy in the management of patients with pain is to evaluate the involved tissue for stage of healing and possible biomechanical causative factors that contribute to the pathology. Treatment includes evaluation, tissue preparation and pain-relieving modalities, soft tissue mobilization, joint mobilization, therapeutic exercise, postural education, and injury prevention.

INITIAL EVALUATION
History

A complete history should be compiled including the current condition and any previous similar conditions. If a previous similar condition existed, detail the frequency, severity, and character of the previous episodes.

The area and behavior of the pain are charted by the therapist, who should carefully question whether the pain is constant or intermittent. Note any irritating movements or behaviors and the length of time that the activity can be tolerated.[1] This information is important for future treatments to evaluate the effectiveness of treatment and the progress. This form of questioning also starts the educational process, helping patients to understand the control they have over their pain.

Other facts included in a complete history are previous surgeries; treatments, especially physical therapy or another manual approach; and the actual treatments tried and whether they were effective. Medications, diagnostic tests and results, the primary treating physician, and any other physicians involved in the patient's management are also noted.

Visual inspection

The visual inspection directs the examiner's attention to a particular area or areas of the system that might be dysfunctional. A thorough visual inspection requires that the involved body part and the joints above and below are completely exposed to the examiner in adequate lighting. This point is obvious for spinal problems, but it is also important that the body from the waist up be visible for evaluation of any upper-extremity problem and, conversely, that the entire body from the waist down be exposed for a lower-extremity problem.

Note any abnormalities of symmetry, muscle tone, atrophy, alignment, skin, body type, and condition. A patient with pain will posture himself or herself to relieve painful structures and change position depending on the irritability of the problem.[2]

Active movements

Active movements should be tested before passive movements because the patient will perform these within his or her own limits of pain, and therefore in safety. Assessments of these movements will indicate the severity of the disability and guide the examiner in determining how much passive handling the joint or limb will tolerate.[1] Note the rhythm, range, feel, arc, pattern, and pain behavior.[3]

Objective baseline measurement of range of motion is obtained by the use of a goniometer. Several studies have tested the reliability of various measurement techniques and have found that the goniometer produces high reliability within and between testers.[4,5] A specific instrument* was designed to measure the cervical range of motion. A recent study by Garrett and co-workers found this cervical range of motion instrument to be reliable in the measurement of forward head posture.[6]

Palpation

On palpation examination, note skin temperature and sweating, and soft-tissue changes.

Skin temperature elevation and sweating could indicate an inflammatory condition such as rheumatoid arthritis that would be treated differently and possibly require medical direction and communication.

Soft-tissue evaluation and treatment have been developed significantly in the past 10 years. The extensibility and integrity of the superficial to deep myofascial structures are evaluated in a layer method. The superficial palpatory exam includes tissue temperature, moisture, and light touch to determine the extensibility of the superficial connective tissues. Tissue rolling is one technique that is particularly useful. The deep palpatory examination includes compression, which is palpation through layers of tissue perpendicular to the tissue, and shear. Palpable structures are muscle bellies, muscle sheaths, tendons, myotendinous junctions, tenoperiostial junctions, joint capsules, and the deep periosteal layers of tissue. Note any tissue texture abnormalities and restrictions.[7]

Joint mobility

Testing joint mobility by palpation involves techniques that are used for evaluation and treatment. The test seeks not only range of motion but "end feel" of the range, the behavior of the pain throughout the range, and the quality of any resistance or muscle spasm that may be present.[1]

---

*Obtained from Performance Attainment Associates, Roseville, Minn.

Table 11-1 Stages, signs, symptoms, and suggested appropriate rehabilitation treatments

Phase	Times	Signs	Symptoms	Treatments
Inflammatory Acute	0-48 hrs	Swelling Redness Muscle spasm	Constant, severe pain Guarding No movement Protective posture	Education Inflammation-reducing modalities, postures Protective splints/braces Activities of daily living
Cellular Subacute	2 days-2 wks	Decreased edema Localized pain Pain-free at rest Limited movement	Variable pain	Irritation control Pain-free range of motion Isometrics Stretching Gentle soft tissue mobilization Light functional activities
Proliferative Settled	2 wks-6 wks	Movement patterns Muscle shortening Scar formation	Stiffness	Educational Weaning from splints, supporters Modified work simulation Reconditioning Lumbar stabilization Soft tissue mobilization
Maturation Progressive	6 wks-3 mos 3-6 mos	Weakness Fatigue Increased functional ability Limited end range movement		Work simulation Adaptive equipment Reconditioning Job analysis Physical capacity evaluation Med-Ex
	6 mos	Phase 1, 2, and 3 signs and symptoms		Pain treatment center

Functional tolerances

More and more physical therapists are including functional tolerances in their initial assessments. Pressure to address these tolerances has increased in past years because employers and insurance companies are more interested in what patients can do compared to how they feel. The examiner who asks the right functional tolerance questions can obtain many benefits and information, and they are:

1. A functional baseline that is meaningful to both the therapist and the patient can be established.
2. Irritability of the affected tissue can be indirectly assessed.
3. A life-style pattern can be noted and sleep disturbances identified.
4. Patients will be active participants in their programs by being able to note increases or decreases in tolerances.
5. An exercise program can be prescribed for reconditioning or work.

Occupational therapists have assessed functional skills for many years and are still using the information in a therapeutic manner more than physical therapists. However, the physical therapist involved in pain rehabilitation must be able to integrate functional tolerances so that the entire rehabilitation team has similar goals and can communicate more easily.

TREATMENTS
Heat and cold

Stages, signs, symptoms, and suggested appropriate rehabilitation treatments are shown in Table 11-1. An exhaustive review of the thermal modalities was performed by Vasudevan and colleagues in 1992.[8] Generally the modalities are used more during the acute stage when reduction of inflammation and pain and increased circulation are important.

Electrical modalities

A transcutaneous electrical nerve stimulator (TENS) is a very effective modality in the relief of pain.[9-11] The TENS unit works through neuronal stimulation and peripheral nerve stimulation. The pain signal from the injured tissue is masked by the TENS stimulation, which is less noxious, allowing the patient to carry on with his or her normal daily activities more comfortably.

Muscle stimulators have become more useful for preventing or retarding disuse atrophy, increasing of local blood supply, maintaining or increasing range of motion, relaxing muscle spasms, and reeducating muscle.[12-15] Muscle stimulators are different from TENS units in that a muscle contraction is achieved by the muscle stimulators. Advances have been made in modifying the waveform characteristics, such as focusing on pulse width and strength-duration curves, instead of on voltage and resistance. These advances have enabled clinicians to choose a device for a specific goal, and because of advances in portability, most devices can be used by the patient at home. This is important during the acute stages when more frequent or continual stimulation is desired.

Soft-tissue mobilization

Soft-tissue mobilization is a primary treatment that can be used in the acute through the chronic stages. It is most important for a patient with pain in a structure for 3 to 6 months to be treated by a therapist with strong soft-tissue mobilization skills because layers of soft-tissue restrictions develop over time.

Soft tissue is generally considered to be everything but the joint. The soft tissue has all the histologic features that tissues have and responds to trauma in very predictable ways. The trained physical therapist knows what to do to allow the tissue to heal itself as quickly as possible and to restore that tissue to its preinjury length, tension, and action.

Soft-tissue mobilization techniques can be direct or indirect. The treatment is based on localizing the restriction and moving in the direction of the restriction, which, in the superficial fascia for example, may be in many different directions.[7]

Joint mobilization

Joint mobilization is a primary technique that can be applied to the acute through the chronic stages. The techniques are gentle, and rhythmic oscillations are performed within or at the limit of the range. There are four grades of movements:[16]

1. Grade I is a small amplitude movement near the starting position of the range.
2. Grade II is a large amplitude movement that carries well into the range and can occupy any part of the range that is free of stiffness or muscle spasm.
3. Grade III is also a large amplitude movement but does move into stiffness or muscle spasm.
4. Grade IV is a small amplitude movement stretching into stiffness or muscle spasm.

Select grades of mobilization by the feel at the end range of the joint. The techniques are not used in any set, rigid pattern, but they should be varied, modified, reversed, and used again until the intention is achieved.

Therapeutic exercise

The benefits of exercise are not generally disputed in the overall well-being of an individual. Recent studies have found that general fitness plays a role in the prevention of and recovery from injuries.[17]

Consequently, the focus of the exercise therapist is not only on the strength and endurance of the injured area but also on the general condition of the individual. Rainville and co-workers found that chronic pain patients do not consistently report changes in pain measures with increased physical performances. Medical recommendations for subjects' involvement should not be based solely on the reported association of pain with those activities.[18]

Initial evaluation. The exercise therapist questions patients on their previous perceived physical condition to establish interests so that the exercises can be enjoyable and transferable to their previous life-style.

Address any limitations to exercise such as cardiac or pulmonary limitations, incontinence, or discomfort of the individual.

Stretching and strengthening exercises. Stretching and strengthening techniques are essential components of an exercise program. Myofascial pain problems require stretching but are best applied in specific ways.[19] A recent multimodal study found that systematic stretching enhanced the functional gains of chronic low back pain patients compared to a control group.[20]

Whereas stretching and strengthening techniques are most commonly associated with exercises, the concept of stabilization has been developed in recent years. The lumbar stabilization program has filled a void in the rehabilitation of low back pain. The basic theory is that there is one position in which the spine will function optimally.[21] This position will vary with different body positions and is therefore called the *functional position* of the spine. This is the position of the spine in which the patient experiences the least amount of pain. Stabilization exercises should be included in the rehabilitation exercise program and instituted during the acute stages. Higher level stabilization classes can be taught in groups that provide a more relaxed, enjoyable, and varied experience for the patients.

Specialty equipment. Dynamic testing devices have been developed in the past 25 years. Early devices used isokinetics that measured the amount of torque generated around the axis of the involved joint at various speeds. Examiners made assumptions about performance expectations based on the data. The data could be useful for extremities, because there was usually a normal or uninvolved limb to compare the data to, but this was not true with the spinal population. Data banks have been created, but published results are population specific to the studies' criteria and should not be applied to individuals generally. The tests do have value in establishing a baseline, which can be used as exercise devices when postexercise testing is performed.[22-24]

A new generation of testing devices has addressed the limitations of early devices, i.e. isolation of the joint being tested and control of the effects of impact and friction. This has been accomplished with the use of a static, isometric testing procedure that is currently ongoing around the country.[24,25]

OCCUPATIONAL THERAPY AND MANAGEMENT OF PAIN PATIENTS

Occupational therapy services rendered when pain causes an inability to carry out life tasks include: work simplification with emphasis on proper methods of body mechanics, activity assimilation, work simulation, psychologic support, behavior modification, job analysis, and functional capacity assessments.[26]

Evaluation

A thorough history of the patient's work and leisure activities is collected and should include medical history, past surgeries, and therapeutic intervention. Patients are asked to fill out a personal inventory questionnaire describing their level of independence in activities of daily living. When reviewed by the therapist, this information reveals the patients' perceptions of how limited they are by the pain or injury.

To determine if the reported pain is consistent with the experienced pain, tests can be given that confuse the patient into responding with signs that are contradictory to usual clinical examination.[27]

An assessment of activities of daily living and body mechanics is given to the patient and examined by the therapist. This part of the evaluation allows the therapist to match function with perceived limitations. Also, the body mechanic evaluation can be videotaped and used as part of treatment to educate the patient in correct posture while performing activities of daily living.

Behavior is also observed to determine how a patient expresses pain. Nonverbal pain behavior adds dimensions to be assessed such as facial expressions, contortions, moaning, and also excessive rubbing of a body part that is painful.[28,29]

Impaired function is further assessed by measuring range of motion and decreased mobility, avoidance of occupation, and impaired personal relationships.[28,29]

Another method for gathering information on meaningful human behaviors is to have patients keep an activity diary of their "up" time versus "down" time, sleep patterns, and specific task performance.[30] Close observation and review are needed with this method because self-reported behaviors often do not match the observed behaviors, causing some unreliability.[31]

When asking a patient to describe pain, there are several methods available.

1. Body diagrams. Have the patient color in the areas that are painful on an anatomic figure. Kellegren was the first to identify and diagram specific pain-referral patterns arising from muscles.[32] Clinicians use a grid to determine the percentage of the body affected, which relates directly to a patient's pain perception.[33]
2. McGill Pain Questionnaire.[34] This is a descriptive word list for patients to choose from to describe the quality and intensity of their pain. A written questionnaire with specific forms is used to gather more comprehensive and descriptive information about a patient's problem and can include the following parts: word descriptor subcategory lists to assess sensory, effective, and evaluative components of pain; body diagrams marked by the patient for external pain and internal pain; specific questions concerning the duration and activities affecting pain intensity. Pain intensity is determined at the time of the test by asking the patient to describe pain using a range of adjectives for worst to least pain.[35]
3. Visual Analogue Scale (VAS).[36-38] The method of administering the VAS is simple. The patient is given a piece of paper with a 10 cm line drawn horizontally or vertically. The ends of the line are marked with the labels "no pain" and "pain as bad as it could be." The

scale is then divided into 20 portions to measure the distance from "0" (no pain) to the patient's mark. This test is performed initially and throughout treatment with reevaluations. Though this test shows good construct validity, there are no norms. The advantages of this test are: it has a greater sensitivity than other pain rating scales because of the infinite number of points between two extremes, it is quick and easy to use, it has vertical and horizontal scales to check consistency of rating in the same session, and it can be used as a quick check of the effectiveness of treatment. The disadvantages are that it is subjective, there is a higher failure rate because of confusion and lack of structure for some patients who therefore may not be able to complete the test, supervision is recommended while the patient is taking the test, and repeated trials may show increased errors of pain estimation.

Objective evaluation

Patients who complain of pain frequently have limited range of motion; therefore it is important for the occupational therapist to take accurate measurements.[39] The objective of measuring range of motion is to provide data regarding the quality of available active range of motion, passive range of motion, or total range of motion at a specific joint.[39] The initial evaluation is used to establish a baseline for comparison when changes occur over time. Standard methods used can be found in an occupational therapy text such as *Occupational Therapy for Physical Dysfunction.*[40]

Davidoff suggested a specific method of measuring joint pain by palpation using a four-point scale.[41]

0 = No pain

1 = Mild pain to deep palpation

2 = Severe pain to deep palpation

3 = Severe pain to mild palpation

4 = Hyperesthesia

This scale provides an objective means of measuring joint pain; however, the reliability and validity may be reduced because of varying pain thresholds and anticipated pain among patients.

Manual muscle testing is performed on general muscle groups. The therapist looks for functional movement patterns and muscles working in synergistic balance. It is a way to establish gross muscle function. It should not be used as a sole means of evaluation, but should be used in conjunction with other extremity evaluation tools and techniques.[42]

Strength can be compared between left and right hands using the Jamar dynamometer*, and this comparison can determine maximal effort exerted and consistency. Using the Jamar dynamometer, Bechtol noted that variations occurred in submaximal efforts compared to previous grip values.[43] The Jamar dynamometer, when calibrated according to specific standards, has been shown to be an extremely accu-

---

*Available from Preston, Inc., Clifton, NJ.

rate and reliable instrument with a minimum selection criterion of +0.994 correlation coefficient.[44]

In a study by Bechtol, when normal subjects were tested, scores from the five handles produced a slightly skewed bell-shaped curve, with the highest strengths occurring in the second or third handle positions.[43] The bell-shaped curve is the expected result when the patient is giving a consistent effort. A less sincere effort can produce a flat curve according to Stokes[45] (Fig. 11-1).

When the evaluation process is completed, the occupational therapist should be able to identify specific areas in which therapeutic intervention can restore or improve independence in activities of daily living, mobility, communication, and pain management skills.

Treatment

Body mechanics and activities of daily living. When training the patient in body mechanics, educating how the body works and how gravity acts upon the body is essential. Gravity acts upon a mass as if all of the mass were concentrated at one point, the center of gravity.[46] The center of gravity has been determined to be just anterior to sa-

---

NAME ___Joe Smith___   Date ___6/14/93___

Hand Tested ___Both___

Dx. CTS right hand. patient has c/o inability to hold things in right hand. Patient did not form a bell shape curve in the right hand, indicating inconsistent effort.

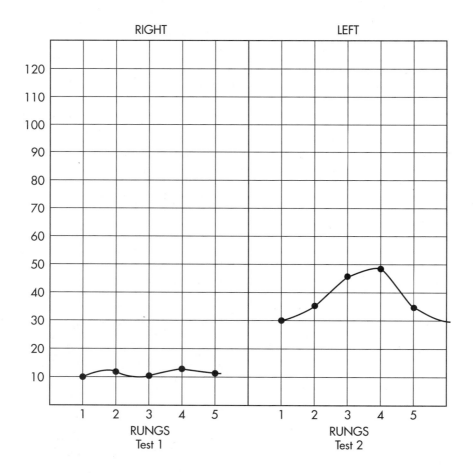

Inconsistent effort: Flat curve
Consistent effort: Bell shaped curve

Fig. 11-1 Jamar Dynamometer five handle grip test.

cral vertebra 2 if the subject is in the anatomic position.[46] As soon as the individual changes position, the center of gravity also changes its location. This principle is applicable in all activities of work or daily living. When lifting and carrying objects, keeping the object close to the center of gravity is the most relevant factor.

Stages of healing. The following stages categorize the healing process of an injury according to the stages of recovery.

Stage I. The occupational therapist can treat an injury by understanding its cause. In the case of cumulative trauma, during the first 48 hours after tendinitis, sprains, or strains, it is recommended to avoid movement and try to rest the affected body part.[47] Custom splints or manufactured braces can be applied to immobilize the injured body part. Also, the application of inflammation-reducing modalities such as ice or electrical stimulation is used. The patient should be educated on how postures and work habits can aggravate the condition. If, for instance, a back injury is sustained, the occupational therapist will instruct the patient how to modify activities of daily living to reduce the strain on affected muscle or joints.

Stage II. At this stage the pain has somewhat subsided, and movement through range of motion can be attempted. Early movement is important to reduce scar tissue, muscular and soft-tissue shortening, and in increasing circulation. In a 1981 study, Gelberman and associates demonstrated biochemical and microangiographic evidence that early controlled passive motion improved the quality of the healing response by stimulation of maturation and remodeling of scar in dogs' tendons.[48]

The patient then progresses to light functional activities with application of body mechanics. This early intervention restores confidence in patients and allows them to gain some control of self-care without increased pain. Work restrictions are also entailed and recommended by the treating physician. A temporary transfer to a different job may need to be considered.[47]

Therapeutic modalities such as heat are applied at this stage to relieve pain and relax muscle before or after activity.

External supports are worn to restrict or avoid activities that cause pain or stress to the injured body area.[47] Splints or braces immobilize movement of the joints or muscles to reduce pain or inflammation by supporting the body part in a position of low stress.[47] Three problem areas need to be considered when using external supports:

1. Inactivity can weaken muscle.
2. Long periods of inactivity can cause loss of normal range of motion in the supported joints.
3. If the worker with a splint or brace is assigned jobs that require major movements of the supported area, these motions may be even more stressed with the splint than without it.[47]

Stage III. In this stage of recovery the occupational therapist focuses on increasing activity level by increasing range of motion and strength. The weaning of supportive devices is initiated to prevent physical and psychologic dependency. Work transition is initiated by gradually preparing patients to return to their previous occupation. Education in body

mechanics is reinforced and practiced with modified simulated work activities. Pacing and work simplification techniques are discussed so patients can accomplish more during the day with less strain and fatigue. Therapeutic modalities are continued to control pain from flare-ups, but they are used less frequently.

Stage IV. At 6 weeks the patient should be experiencing less pain, increased range of motion, increased strength, and ability to sustain activity. There may be residual weakness and fatigue from prolonged inactivity. Reconditioning of endurance and muscle strengthening will be performed in physical therapy or by the exercise physiologist.

The occupational therapist at this time will assist the patient in returning to the full duty of occupational demands. A job analysis is performed to identify sources of cumulative trauma so recurrence of an injury is prevented. Ideally, a job analysis should include a method for measuring the worker's exposure to each of the major biomechanic risk factors: force, posture, and repetition.[49] The information from a job analysis is useful when setting up a work-simulation program or performing a physical capacity evaluation. The essential functions of a job can be identified so the return-to-work process is compliant with the Americans with Disabilities Act. At this stage of recovery, it is critical that the patient resume normal physical activity. According to Chapman, the transition period is when the injury heals, the person goes on to a "good recovery" and resumes a role in society, or the residual disabilities closely correlate with the residual impairments.[50]

Individuals lost in the rehabilitation process and destined not to return to their former jobs may benefit from a work or physical capacity evaluation.[51]

As defined by Matheson and Niemayer, a work capacity evaluation is a systematic process of measuring and developing an individual's capacity to dependably sustain performance in response to broadly defined work demands.[52] The actual evaluation process can be combined with rehabilitation in a work hardening program as described below. As subjects participate in work capacity evaluation programs, they are evaluated in terms of current work tolerances and inferences are made about their potential work capacity.[52]

Matheson defined a work tolerance screening as an intensive short-term (usually 1 day) evaluation that focuses on major physical tolerance abilities related to musculoskeletal strength, endurance, speed, and flexibility. The information from this type of evaluation is usually marketed to the vocational rehabilitation community, and data are used to determine employability.[52]

Components of a physical capacity evaluation include:[28]

1. Lifting and carrying
2. Pushing and pulling
3. Reaching
4. Grasping and handling
5. Manipulation
6. Standing, sitting, and walking
7. Kneeling, crouching, crawling, and stooping
8. Endurance
9. Sequential testing for consistency and maximum effort

Work hardening/transition. Matheson[52] defines work hardening as:

1. A prescriptive productivity development program
2. A highly structured productivity-oriented treatment program that uses the injured worker's involvement in real or simulated work activities as its principal means of treatment
3. An individualized, work-oriented treatment process involving the client in simulated or actual work tasks that are structured and graded to progressively increase physical tolerances, stamina, endurance, and productivity[53]

Work hardening is especially useful with patients who are primarily limited by their pain. They can be taught to control their symptoms while performing a job. Patients may continue to report no change in pain level, while at the same time they demonstrate and experience a major improvement in functional capacity.[52] The primary goal of the occupational therapist when treating a patient with pain is to teach the patient how to function in everyday life in spite of pain.

Specialty equipment. The work simulator* has been refined over the last few years and can be found in many clinics.[52] This device can be used for evaluation and exercise. It has numerous attachments that may be applied in various positions to simulate almost any type of work. The computerized printout gives information on force, distance, and work produced. With the Quest component, coefficient of variation is determined and information can be stored for comparison of tests at later dates. It can be used in an isometric mode or dynamic isotonic mode.

REFERENCES

1. Maitland GD: *Vertebral Manipulation,* ed 5. Boston, Butterworth, 1986.
2. Charnley J: Orthopedic signs in the diagnosis of the disc protrusion. *Lancet* 1:186, 1951.
3. Cyriax J: *Textbook of Orthopedic Medicine, vol 2,* ed 8. London, Baltimore, Balliere Tindall, 1982.
4. Riddle DL, Rothstein JM, Lamb RL: Goniometric reliability in a clinical setting: Elbow and knee measurements. *Phys Ther* 63:1611-1655, 1983.
5. Youdas JW, Carey JR, Garrett TR: Reliability of measurements of cervical spine range of motion: Comparison of three methods. *Phys Ther* 71:98-104, 1991.
6. Garrett TR, Youdas JW, Madson TJ: Reliability of measuring forward head posture in a clinical setting. *J Sports Physical Ther* 17:155-160, 1993.
7. Cantu RI, Grodin AJ: Myofascial manipulation, theory and clinical application. Aspen, CO, Aspen Publications, 1992.
8. Vasudevan S et al: Physical methods of pain management. In Raj PP, editor: *Practical Management of Pain,* ed 2. St Louis, Mosby, 1992.
9. Barr JO, Nielsen DH, Soderberg GL: Transcutaneous electrical nerve stimulation characteristics for altering pain perception. *Phys Ther* 66:1515-1521, 1986.
10. Bending G: TENS in a pain clinic. *Physiotherapy* 75:292-294, 1989.
11. Paris PM: No more pain: Transcutaneous nerve stimulation. *Emerg Med* 18:57-60, 1986.
12. Currier DP, Mann R: Muscular strength development by electrical stimulation in healthy individuals. *Phys Ther* 66:937-943, 1986.
13. Fulbright JS: Electrical stimulation to reduce chronic toe-flexor hypertonicity. A case report. *Phys Ther* 64:515-523, 1984.
14. Gould N et al: Transcutaneous muscle stimulation to retard disuse atrophy after open meniscectomy. *Clin Orthop* 178:190-197, 1983.
15. Liu HI, Currier DP, Threlkeld AJ: Circulatory response of digital arteries associated with electrical stimulation of calf muscles in healthy subjects. *Phys Ther* 47:340-345, 1987.
16. Grieve GP: *Common Vertebral Joint Problems.* Edinburgh, Churchill Livingstone, 1980.
17. Nachemson AL: Exercise, fitness, and back pain. In Pavi Nurmi, editor: *Congress Book—Advanced European Course on Sports Medicine,* Abo, Finland, The Finnish Society of Sports Medicine, 1989.
18. Rainville J et al: The association of pain with physical activities in chronic low back pain. *Spine* 17:1060-1064, 1992.
19. Travell J, Simons D: Myofascial Pain and Dysfunction. In *The Trigger Point Manual.* Baltimore, Williams & Wilkins, 1983.
20. Khalil TM et al: Stretching in the rehabilitation of low back pain patients. *Spine* 17:311-317, 1992.
21. Morgan D: Concepts on functional training and postural stabilization for the low back injuries. *Top Acute Care Trauma Rehab* 2:8-17, 1988.
22. Berger RA: Comparison of static and dynamic strength increases. *Res Q Exerc Sport* 33:329-333, 1962.
23. Langrana NA, Lee CK: Isokinetic evaluation of trunk muscles. *Spine* 9:171-175, 1984.
24. Graves JE et al: Quantitative assessment of range of motion isometric lumbar extension strength training frequency and specificity on isometric lumbar extension strength. *Spine* 15:289-293, 1990.
25. Grave JE et al: Effect of training frequency and specificity on isometric lumbar extension strength. *Spine* 15:504-509, 1990.
26. Hopkins HL, Smith HD: *Willard and Spackman's Occupational Therapy,* ed 5. Philadelphia, JB Lippincott, 1978.
27. Omer GE Jr: Management of pain syndromes in the upper extremity. In Hunter JM et al, editors: *Rehabilitation of the Hand,* ed 3. St Louis, Mosby, 1990.
28. Fredrickson LW, Lynd RS, Ross J: Methodology in the measurement of pain. *Behav Ther* 9:486-488, 1978.
29. Keeke FJ: Behavioral assessment and treatment of chronic pain: Current status and future directions. *J Consult Clin Psychol* 50:896-911, 1982.
30. Craig KD, Prkachin KM: Nonverbal measure of pain. In Melzack R, editor: *The Measurement and Assessment of Pain.* New York, Raven Press, 1983.
31. Ready LB: Self reported vs actual use of medication in chronic pain. *Pain* 12:285-295, 1982.
32. Kellegren JM: Observation on referred pain arising from muscles. *Clin Sci* 3:175-190, 1938.
33. Toomey TC et al: Stability of self report methods of improvement in chronic pain. *Pain* 12:273-283, 1982.
34. Melzack R: The McGill Pain Questionnaire: Major properties and scoring method. *Pain* 1:227, 1975.
35. Melzack R: The Short-form McGill Pain Questionnaire. *Pain* 30:191-197, 1987.
36. Downie WW et al: Studies with pain rating scale. *Ann Rheum Dis* 37:378-381, 1978.
37. Jenson MP, Karoly P, Brover S: The measurement of clinical pain intensity: A comparison of six methods. *Pain* 27:117-126, 1986.
38. Michlovitz S: *Thermal Agents in Rehabilitation,* ed 2. Philadelphia, FA Davis, 1990.
39. Adams LS, Greene LW, Topoozian E: *Clinical Assessment Recommendations,* ed 2. Chicago, The American Society of Hand Therapists, 1992.
40. Trombly CA, Scott AD: *Occupational Therapy for Physical Dysfunction,* ed 3. Baltimore, Williams & Wilkins, 1989.
41. Davidoff G et al: Pain measurement in reflex sympathetic dystrophy syndrome. *Pain* 32:27, 1988.
42. Kienan LS: *Clinical Assessment Recommendations,* ed 2. Chicago, The American Society of Hand Therapists, 1992.
43. Bechtol CD: Grip test: Use of a dynamometer with adjustable handle spacing. *J Bone Joint Surg Am* 36A:820-824, 1954.
44. Fess EE: A method for checking Jamar dynamometer calibration. *J Hand Ther* 1:28-32, 1987.
45. Stokes HM: The seriously uninjured hand: Weakness of grip. *J Occup Med* 25:683-684, 1983.

---

*Available from Baltimore Therapeutic Equipment, Balitmore, Md.

46. Schenek JM, Cordova DF: *Introduction to Biomechanics,* ed 2. Philadelphia, FA Davis, 1980.

47. Fine L: Medical diagnosis and treatment. In Anderson V-P, editor: *Cumulative Trauma Disorders. A Manual for Musculoskeletal Diseases of the Upper Limbs.* Bristol, PA, Taylor & Francis, 1992.

48. Gelberman RH et al: The influence of protected passive mobilization on the healing of flexor tendons: A biochemical and microangiographic study. *Hand* 13:120-128, 1981.

49. Anderson V-P, editor: *Cumulative Trauma Disorders. A Manual for Musculoskeletal Diseases of the Upper Limbs.* Bristol, PA, Taylor & Francis, 1992.

50. Berna SF, Chapman SL: Pain and litigation. In Wall PD, Melzack R, editors: *Textbook of Pain.* New York, Churchill Livingstone, 1984.

51. Kadsan ML: *Hand Therapy of Occupational and Upper Extremity Injuries and Diseases.* Philadelphia, Hanley & Belfus, 1991.

52. Matheson LW, Niemayer LO: *The Work Capacity Evaluation Manual,* 1-3–1-7. Anaheim, CA, Employment and Rehabilitation Institute of California, 1988.

53. Vocational Evaluation and Work Adjustment Association and American Occupational Therapy Association: *Work Hardening Guidelines.* The Associations, 1986.

PART THREE

Modalities of Pain Management

12   Pharmacokinetics and Pharmacodynamics of Analgesic Agents

Laurence E. Mather, Donald D. Denson, and P. Prithvi Raj

GENERAL PRINCIPLES

This chapter describes fundamental pharmacokinetic concepts and modeling methods as applied to analgesic agents used in pain therapy.

Clearance and volume of distribution

Two primary terms are commonly encountered in pharmacokinetics: *clearance* (the efficiency of the body in eliminating drug) and *volume of distribution* (the degree of dilution of the drug within the body). From these, the more familiar secondary term *half-life* (the time required for drug blood concentrations to be altered by a factor of two) may be derived.

In physiologic terms, clearance (Cl) by any organ or tissue is equal to the product of blood flow to that organ and the extraction ratio by that organ; thus it has the dimensions of flow. In this context, extraction ratio is the difference in drug concentrations entering and leaving an organ, divided by the entering concentration. The mean total body clearance (ClT) (usually and imprecisely referred to as *clearance*) is the time-averaged pharmacokinetic property measured experimentally from serial blood drug concentration-time data and is the sum of all organ or regional clearances. Renal clearance (ClR) is equal to the total body clearance multiplied by the fraction of the dose eliminated via the kidneys, and so on for other organs. Clearance is related to time, so it can be thought of as the functional mean drug "output." If drug "input" is made over a period of time (e.g., by multiple doses or continuous infusion), the ratio of the mean rate of input to the mean output gives the mean steady-state drug blood concentration, which is an important index of drug exposure.

The volume of distribution is more complicated because there are several varieties. Any volume may be thought of as a precise proportionality constant between an amount and a concentration. Pharmacokinetic volumes are "apparent" volumes because they are not (generally) homogenous anatomic or physiologic spaces but are the average of heterogeneous partitioning of drug into different organs and tissues. The volume of distribution thus expresses the proportionality between the amount of drug in the body and the concentration of drug in the fluid sampled (traditionally blood, plasma, or serum). Its value increases to a limiting value with time after drug administration because equilibra-

tion is governed by the differing rates of delivery to, and uptake by, different organs and tissues.[1] Therefore there are two principal volumes of distribution: an initial dilution volume, sometimes called a central compartment volume, which reflects drug dilution and distribution within tissues that rapidly equilibrate with the blood, and a total volume of distribution, which measures overall drug equilibration with all tissues (Fig. 12-1).

The volume of distribution at steady state equilibrium defines the extent of dilution of drug at the time of peak distribution. The volume of distribution during pseudoequilibrium defines the extent of drug dilution during the so-called elimination phase when blood and tissues are giving up drug at the same proportional rates, and its value is referenced to this rate. It is sometimes called volume of distribution (area) or volume of distribution (β) since it relates the dose, area under the blood (or plasma, etc.), drug concentration time curve, and the rate of decay of concentrations (often called the β phase in the traditional "two-compartmental model" of drug disposition).

Half-life

The term half-life (sometimes referred to as half-time) defines the time required for the blood concentration to change by a factor of two from an original condition (Table 12-1). This may be an increase if the drug is given by infusion, but most commonly it is a decrease after drug administration. The half-life is a measure of how fast concentrations change and is related to both the clearance (inversely) and the volume of distribution (directly) of the drug. Drugs may appear to have several half-lives, depending on the time after administration as the result of the tissue uptake gradually becoming completed during redistribution. According to most traditional pharmacokinetic models, the concentrations in blood and tissues decay in parallel (pseudoequilibrium), and the half-life is described by a single terminal half-life only when tissue equilibration is complete. This is the commonly referenced value of half-life of the drug and provides useful information on when the drug dose may need repeating, not on how much drug may need to be given.

Because most body processes concerning drug absorption, distribution, and elimination occur by first-order rate processes (i.e., their rates are proportional to how much drug there is at that time), there are finite limits on the blood

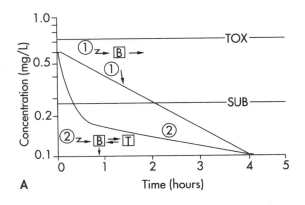

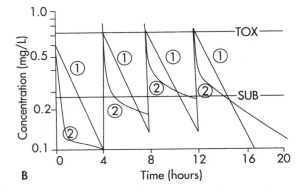

Fig. 12-1 Fundamental pharmacokinetic properties of drugs. Simulated time courses of drug "blood concentrations" for two hypothetical drugs 1 and 2 in relation to their subeffective *(SUB)* and threshold-toxic *(TOX)* concentrations. Drug 1 distributes essentially instantaneously in the body so that its blood *(B)* and tissue concentrations cannot be differentiated. Its half-life is 1.5 hours. The rate of distribution of Drug 2 is slower than its rate of elimination; therefore a biphasic curve is evident with a fast (loosely called the *distribution*) half-life and a slow half-life (loosely called the *elimination*) half-life. The slow half-life is 5.0 hours. The (total) apparent volume of distribution of Drug 1 (40 liters) is equal to the initial dilution volume of Drug 2 so that their initial concentrations are equal. Drugs similar to Drug 1 are sometimes said to be represented by a "one compartment model," those similar to Drug 2 are sometimes said to be represented by a "two compartment model." Real drug examples of the former are rare; the now obsolete analgesic antipyrine is one known example. Most "real drugs" behave like Drug 2, at least with respect to blood drug concentrations in the arm vein, but even this is an oversimplification; Drug 2 represents the behavior of meperidine. **A,** Equal single dose comparison shows that compared with Drug 1, Drug 2 becomes subeffective quite quickly because of tissue distribution *(T)*. **B,** Multiple equal 4 hourly dose comparison shows that compared to Drug 1, accumulation in blood of Drug 2 occurs so that the duration of action becomes longer with each dose until a steady state occurs with dosing for at least 5 times the slow half-life of the drug. (From Raj PP, editor: *Practical Management of Pain,* ed 2. St Louis, Mosby, 1992.)

Table 12-1 Change in concentration as a function of terminal half-life

Cumulative half-life (multiples)	Approach to final steady state* (% completed)
0	0
1	50
2	75
3	87.7
4	93.8
5†	96.9
6†	98.4

*Accumulation to or removal from an original steady state.
†Considered to be the completed steady state for clinical purposes.

zero at the same rate, theoretically in proportion to the existing concentration.

Therefore in one half-life, concentrations will change by 50% from the original steady state, and in two half-lives, concentrations will change again by 50% from the newly reached steady state (i.e., to 75% of the original) and so on (Figs. 12-1 and 12-2).

Redistribution

Drug redistribution is very important during drug treatment. In acute care, pseudoequilibrium or steady state conditions generally do not occur. Many drugs are used routinely so that their duration of action is terminated by their redistribution into nonresponsive tissue mass; therefore the time (half-life) for distribution is important information for acute care. For example, it is well known that patients awaken from thiopental anesthesia as the thiopental redistributes progressively from responsive brain tissue into muscle mass and fat. Fentanyl analgesia dissipates for the same reason. However, reported values from the literature of fast half-lives (or redistribution phase) should be interpreted with caution. Because the rate of redistribution decreases with time after drug administration, the redistribution half-lives are sensitive to the times when the blood samples are taken for measurement and to the region from which the blood samples are taken.

If blood sampling in a pharmacokinetic experiment is stopped too soon, the measured half-life will be smaller than the true value of the terminal half-life because some blood-tissue redistribution will also be occurring simultaneously. The body responds to the arterial drug concentrations as the tissues take up the drug. Therefore arterial drug concentrations generally provide a more valid correlate of the pharmacologic effect. However, the duration of response depends on the tissue concentration, and this is better reflected by the venous concentration draining the responsive tissue. Clinical pharmacokinetic studies usually rely on drug concentrations in blood samples drawn from a vein in the arm. These reflect the rate of drug equilibration in the arm tissue and may bear no relation whatsoever to that in the responsive tissue. Therefore arterial concentrations provide a better guide as to the rate of drug redistribution because venous concentrations are damped locally.

concentrations attained. This means that a drug given at a constant rate will not accumulate on continuous dosing but will approach a steady state (plateau) concentration equal to the quotient of rate of administration and clearance. Conversely, after administration, concentration will approach

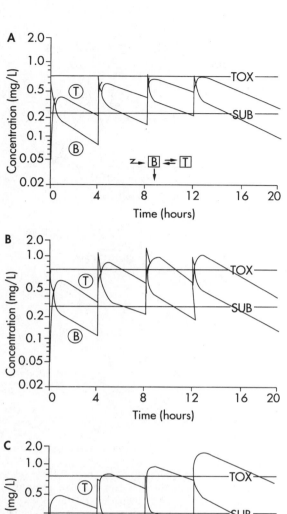

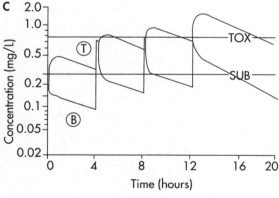

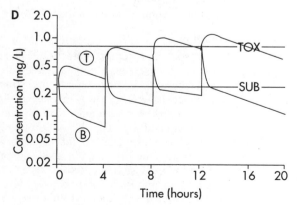

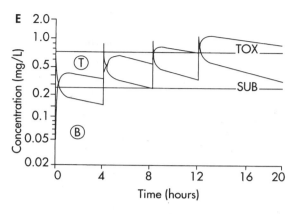

Fig. 12-2 Alterations to the fundamental pharmacokinetic properties of hypothetical Drug 2 of Fig. 12-1 are shown in blood and tissue concentration simulations in the different panels for multiple equal (50 mg) doses. These alterations could represent the values for the same drug in different subjects, the effects of physiopathologic changes, or different drugs. **A,** The original properties (as in Fig. 12-1) resemble those of meperidine. The mean total body clearance is 36 L/hr, the initial dilution volume is 80 L, and the slow half-life is 5.0 hours. **B,** The mean total body clearance is still 36 L/hr but the initial dilution volume is halved to 40 L. This might occur with a redistribution of cardiac output from peripheral to central perfusion as, for example, in circulatory shock. As a result, the fractional elimination rate is doubled and the slow half-life is now 2.7 hours and the drug comes to a steady state in the body more rapidly. **C,** The properties as in *A* but the rate of transfer from blood to tissues is now doubled. This might occur with a redistribution of cardiac output from central to peripheral perfusion as, for example, with peripheral vasodilatory drug treatment. A greater amount of drug is now transferred to tissues from which it takes longer to wash out. As a result, the slow half-life is now 8.2 hours. **D,** The properties are the same as in *A* but the rate of transfer from tissues to blood is now halved. This might occur, for example, with gross obesity. A greater amount of drug now remains in the tissues from which it takes longer to wash out. As a result, the blood concentrations are lower but the slow half-life is now increased to 8.6 hours. **E,** The properties are the same as in *A* but the fractional rate of elimination is halved as might occur, for example, with liver dysfunction. The mean total body clearance is also halved. As a result, the slow half-life is now 9.7 hours. (From Raj PP, editor: *Practical Management of Pain,* ed 2. St. Louis, Mosby, 1992.)

Steady state

Steady state refers to the constancy in time of blood drug concentrations and requires that blood-tissue drug equilition exists. Blood-tissue drug equilibration is difficult to ascertain in practice because it requires knowledge of the constancy (and usually equality) of arterial and relevant venous blood to drug concentrations. In practical terms, steady state occurs when the average sampled blood to drug concentrations do not increase or decrease systematically over time with continuous or repeated dosing.

A steady state of blood to drug concentrations is achieved only after approximately five to six times the terminal half-life. However, the rate of approach to the steady state concentration depends on the relative contribution of the fast phase in filling the tissues. Steady state can be achieved with anesthetic agents; for example, in a patient within the normal time frame of exposure during surgery for drugs with low tissue solubility (e.g., nitrous oxide) but not with drugs of high tissue solubility (e.g., halothane). Under these circumstances, an alternative is to give a loading dose to fill the tissues plus a maintenance dose so that a steady state can be achieved within the given time frame (Fig. 12-3).

These principles apply to treatment with analgesic agents. Short-term control of acute pain can be obtained with agents having low tissue solubility or rapid removal from the blood either by redistribution or by clearance. Alfentanil provides the closest representation of an agent having these properties. The difference becomes apparent when prolonged control of pain is required. Repeated doses of an agent with a redistribution-limited duration of action leads to cumulation after the redistribution phase has dominated. For such agents (e.g., fentanyl), potentially late-onset prolonged respiratory depression may ensue. In principle, repeated doses of an agent with a predominantly clearance-limited duration of action would not lead to cumulation at the same rate, but it is difficult to find relevant examples of drugs with a clearance-limited duration of action. Succinylcholine is an example that is familiar to anesthesiologists. For the majority of analgesic agents, redistribution and clearance are important determinants of duration of action and therefore of dosing frequency.

For acute pain therapy, there are two fundamental choices in the selection of analgesic agents: repeated doses of an agent with a higher clearance or fewer repeated doses of an agent with a lower clearance. The repeated use of a high-clearance agent may mean periods of fluctuating analgesia and an injection whenever analgesia is required. The alternative use of a low-clearance (long-acting) agent may avoid fluctuating analgesia and frequent injections, but if complications occur, then the complications are also long lasting. Repeated doses with higher clearance agents can be replaced by continuous IV infusions. Then, should adverse effects occur, cessation of infusion will mean that no more drug will be admitted to the circulation, and blood concentrations will start to decrease immediately. This contrasts with drug administration by an absorption route, where absorption will continue relentlessly, irrespective of adverse effects. For routine chronic therapy, the IV route provides little use, except perhaps as part of a diagnostic workup of the patient. During chronic therapy, absorption routes re-

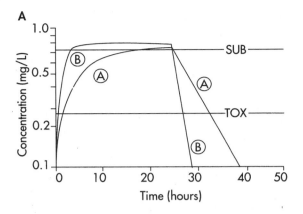

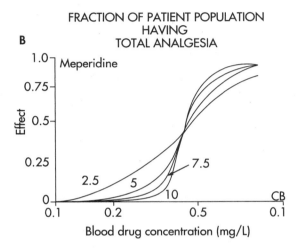

Fig. 12-3 The tissue solubilities of hypothetical Drug A is greater than Drug B. As a result, the slow half-lives are, respectively, 4.8 and 1 hour. Drug A resembles meperidine. Drug B resembles alfentanil. **A,** It takes much longer for Drug A to equilibrate during washing, say during infusion, and to washout after cessation of infusion. **B,** The "effect" curves derived from these blood drug concentrations also reflect the rates of washing and washout equilibration. The numbers 2.5, 5, 7.5, and 10 represent the "steepness factors" of the sigmoidal equation described by the Hill equation. (From Raj PP, editor: *Practical Management of Pain,* ed 2. St Louis, Mosby, 1992.)

quire knowledge of absorption rates and bioavailability in addition to the fundamental pharmacokinetic properties.

Protein drug binding

Most drugs act by a specific receptor interaction. The reaction leading to drug response stems from the free (or unbound) drug concentration in the blood, and this is measured by the concentrations of drug in plasma water. The remaining part, which is presumed to be pharmacologically inert, is regulated by the plasma protein and blood cell binding. This is estimated in the laboratory by the nondialyzable fraction or the fraction that cannot be ultrafiltrated from blood, plasma, or serum. The bound fraction is considered an important pharmacokinetic characteristic of the drug or of the recipient of the drug, but its importance is sometimes misunderstood or overemphasized. A greater correlation between plasma unbound drugconcentrations and response would be expected than between drug dose or plasma total drug concentrations and response, but more often this has been assumed rather than verified experimentally.

Proteins that bind drugs

Endobiotic substances such as hormones bind specifically to carrier proteins; acidic drugs such as salicylates usually bind nonspecifically to albumin; and several plasma proteins bind to weak organic bases, including opioid analgesic drugs and local anesthetics. Endobiotic substances compete for the drug in proportion to the relative abundance of, and the affinity constants for, each protein. In particular, α-acid glycoprotein (AAG) has a high affinity for basic drugs but has a low capacity, albumin has a low affinity but has a high capacity, and lipoproteins also may play a role. Because AAG is an acute-phase reactant protein, its abundance in plasma depends on the state of health, recent trauma, and concurrent drug therapy. Thus disease states and other factors that influence the concentrations of protein or the affinity of drugs for the binding sites have the ability to alter the drug fraction that is bound. Similarly, a greater extent of binding occurs in maternal plasma compared to fetal plasma and is believed to be the reason that transplacental gradients of many drugs such as fentanyl and bupivacaine still exist at delivery. This is believed to be due in part to a relatively lower concentration of binding proteins in fetal blood.

The plasma protein binding of the clinically important alkaloidal opioid analgesics and amide-type local anesthetics has been reported extensively. Broadly, the more lipophilic the agent, the higher the fractional binding, which suggests that hydrophobic interactions between drug and protein are more important than ionic attractions. At therapeutic plasma concentrations found after analgesic procedures in adult patients, fentanyl and meperidine are approximately 85% and 50%, respectively, bound in adult human plasma.

Although minimum effective analgesic concentrations are useful guidelines for the design and interpretation of analgesic dosage regimens, interpatient variation of the drug to blood concentration-response relationship thwarts the blind application of pharmacokinetically-derived dosage regimens. It has been calculated that for an optimum postoperative analgesic response, patients require a dosage rate of opioid analgesics to average, not the product of the minimum effective analgesic concentration and clearance, but approximately 1.6 times this value.

The therapeutic window should be taken into account when designing dosage regimens, but data relating to toxic effects are sparse. For the most part, deciding on acceptable steady state concentrations is far more difficult for drugs used for regional nerve block than for opioid analgesics. There is little relationship between their plasma concentrations and the actual effect of the drug on the nerve. For long-term continuous epidural infusions of bupivacaine, there is a good correlation between the plasma concentration and the type of nerve fibers blocked in normal patients. This reemphasizes the need for more interactive pharmacokinetic and pharmacodynamic data. In cases of prolonged perineural block, either by multiple injection or by continu-

ous infusion, knowledge of plasma concentrations can prevent untoward effects. In multiple dosing circumstances such as these, an understanding of the principles of absorption and bioavailability is imperative.

Drug absorption and systemic bioavailability of analgesic agents

In addition to the global pharmacokinetic parameters, the rate of drug absorption and extent of drug availability to the systemic circulation need to be considered. These factors markedly influence the magnitude and the time course of blood to drug concentrations and therefore the pharmacodynamic response.

Drugs for the relief of pain may be administered by a variety of routes: intravenously (IV), intramuscularly (IM), subcutaneously, orally, epidurally, or intrathecally. These can be divided into routes where the drug is administered to have direct access to receptors by diffusion or bulk flow (principally epidural, intrathecal, and intracerebroventricular), and those routes where the drug is administered to be carried in the blood to the receptors (IV, IM, subcutaneous, and oral), thereby having indirect access. The direct routes of administration of opioid analgesics offer the possibility of regionally selective effects and allow minimal doses to be used because the dose is placed close to the site of action in the required region. In contrast, the indirect routes lead to drugs being dispersed in the general circulation. Therefore regional selectivity is highly improbable, and all regions of the body receive distribution of the drug in proportion to their share of the cardiac output.

In contrast to the indirect routes, the direct routes necessitate a greater invasion of the body and require a greater expertise by the pain therapist. Therefore the benefit to risk and cost ratios becomes a relevant consideration.

Oral administration. Oral administration is the most frequently used route of administration of medication. The most significant barrier to admission of drug to the systemic circulation comes from oral enteral administration, where absorption locally results in collection by the portal venous system and presentation to the liver en route to the systemic circulation. Drugs that are removed from the body by enzymatic biotransformation in the liver may be rendered totally useless if given orally, while they are perfectly useful if given parenterally. This effect can usually be predicted from knowledge of the drug clearance.

The drug's total body clearance is made up of the sums of clearances by individual organs and tissues. The hepatosplanchnic clearance, which can usually be estimated from the difference between total body and renal clearances, can be used to predict the oral bioavailability. The regional clearance (the product of the regional blood flow and extraction ratio) and the transmission fraction (1 − extraction ratio) can be used to estimate the amount of drug escaping extraction (i.e., the regional bioavailability).

The transmission fraction equals 1 − hepatosplanchnic clearance/hepatosplanchnic blood flow. The value for clearance should be based on blood drug concentrations to relate to the hepatosplanchnic blood flow. Plasma or serum concentrations are not believed to be as reliable because of uncertain drug uptake into blood cells. Although individual values of organ blood flow may show time-related and patient-related variability, the use of an average value (e.g., adult human hepatosplanchnic blood flow, 1.5 L/min) gives a reasonable estimate for purposes of estimating the probable drug bioavailability after oral administration. For example, meperidine total body clearance is approximately 0.7 L/min with negligible renal clearance; thus the hepatosplanchnic transmission fraction equals $1 - 0.7/1.5$ or 0.53; the average measured oral bioavailability = 0.59.

Drugs are cleared by tissues such as the liver in a series of events resulting in their chemical transformation to metabolites. As a general rule, metabolites are more polar (i.e., less lipophilic) than their parent drugs and, as a consequence, have less propensity for penetrating the central nervous system (CNS) and greater propensity for excretion by the kidney. Compared to the parent drug, the pharmacologic activity of metabolites may range from being totally inactive to being the active product for which the drug is given. Metabolites may have similar or totally different pharmacokinetic properties than the parent drug. Although an oral regimen can be scaled for dose to account for drug lost by first-pass hepatic clearance, it is important to remember that the resultant drug metabolites should not produce adverse effects, especially on accumulation.

Intravenous administration. The most important aspects of IV drug administration are that it avoids the uncertainties of drug absorption and that it allows innovative and complete control over the rate of drug delivery. Virtually all opioids can be given IV if appropriate pharmaceutical preparations are available, and the method is suitable for almost all patients in whom venous access can be obtained.[2-4] Cautions against this route pertain more to the rate of drug administration than to any intrinsic unsuitability of particular agents. The most important disadvantages of this route are that aseptic techniques are critical and that some skill of the therapist is necessary in instituting and maintaining venous access.

It is relatively easy to design an infusion regimen to produce a target blood to drug concentration (Css) from a set of pharmacokinetic parameters.[5-9] The regimen, in its simplest form, should consist of a loading dose equal to Css $\times$ V to increase the blood concentration to account for dilution, followed immediately by an infusion equal to Css $\times$ Cl to account for elimination. However, drug concentrations produced by such a regimen will "sag" below the "target value" soon after injection of the loading dose until steady state is ultimately achieved. This is because equilibration between blood and tissues of most drugs takes hours, and additional drug has to be added to the body to provide for the amount distributing into tissues from blood at a concentration equal to that determined by the initial dilution volume (Vc) and that determined by the total distribution volume (Vss).

Perhaps the most suitable method for the infusion is the three stage method described previously. This is usually referred to as the BET method, where B is bolus for loading; E is elimination to be matched by constant infusion; and T is the transfer between blood and tissues to be matched by exponentially decreasing infusion. Although it is ideally delivered by a computer-controlled infusion pump, it may be

approximated manually or by dilution flask. Those agents having the shortest half-life or highest Cl present the greatest ease of alteration of blood concentrations by rapid elimination. However, the design of safe and satisfactory infusions depends on better understanding of pharmacodynamic aspects.

Intramuscular administration. Intramuscular injections represent the most frequently used method of administration of opioids for acute pain management. As stated previously, they are subject to vagaries because of the uncertain perfusion of the region into which the drug is deposited.

Consequently, blood drug concentrations can vary widely between patients intended to be dosed in the same way and even from successive doses in the same patient. To help overcome this problem, the use of an indwelling soft catheter may be possible, but the clinical value of this approach has not yet been evaluated.

Intramuscular injections may be frightening to some patients, especially children, so that they may prefer their pain to that caused by the injection. It is surprising that this route of administration has become the standard in most hospitals. Its only commendable features are its relative simplicity and cheapness.

Subcutaneous administration. Subcutaneous injection was the standard form of administration of opioids until the 1950s, when IM injection became more widespread. Like IM administration, it is believed to generate unpredictable drug absorption rates but, as its use predates contemporary pharmacokinetics methodology, few data exist to substantiate this opinion. It is now clear that continuous subcutaneous infusion does not cause problems from poor drug absorption and has been used to advantage in the treatment of both acute and chronic pain using a simple Butterfly needle and a reliable infusion device. Prolonged subcutaneous infusions require that the infusion site be changed every 4 to 7 days.

Sublingual and buccal routes. In recent tests with sublingual formulations, the lipophilic opioids buprenorphine (55% absorption), fentanyl (51%), and methadone (34%) were all absorbed more efficiently than morphine (18%); levorphanol, hydromorphone, oxycodone, and heroin were all absorbed to a lesser extent than morphine.[10] Although buprenorphine has been used by this route for many years, there appears to be scope for further exploration of other agents. Studies with buprenorphine indicate successful pain management is possible in patients with acute[11,12] and chronic pain,[13] although it is generally agreed that it is helpful to use a parenteral loading dose to provide analgesia during the long and variable period of absorption. Although early reports suggested great promise for the buccal administration of morphine,[14] slow absorption and variability like those from sublingual administration have been noted in more recent reports of buccal tablet preparations.[15] The drug bioavailability from sublingual and buccal preparations depends on the relative amounts of the dose absorbed through the oral mucosa and swallowed.

Rectal route. The rectal route is underutilized in contemporary practice, but it has been used for the administration of opioid analgesics in patients for whom the oral or parenteral routes may be unsuitable, notably children or debilitated patients.[16] Drug bioavailability is especially sensitive to the position of the preparation in the rectum.[17] Correct placement in the rectum leads to absorption principally via the inferior and middle rectal veins into the systemic system and thereby largely avoids the hepatic first-pass effect.[18,19] Placement too high in the rectum results in greater absorption via the superior rectal veins into the portal system; placement too low (in the anus) may result in the preparation's expulsion before sufficient absorption has taken place. Undoubtedly, variability of placement is a major cause of intersubject variability of bioavailability commonly reported in studies.

The rectal route is sensitive to formulation of the drug, with hydroalcoholic formulations resulting in much more efficient and rapid absorption than fatty suppositories. With morphine, rectal hydrogel bioavailabilities of around 50% compare favorably with oral bioavailabilities of around 25%. Some work has been reported for other analgesics.[20-27] With codeine, similar oral and rectal bioavailabilities have been reported. With methadone, hydromorphone, and oxycodone, the rectal bioavailability has been reported as inferior to oral bioavailability, but the reasons (placement or formulation) have not been established. With meperidine, rectal bioavailability of around 80% compared favorably with 50% oral bioavailability. Except for hydrogel preparations, slower absorption from rectal suppositories than from oral tablets usually occurs, but this may be useful to provide sustained nighttime analgesia in patients with chronic pain.

Transdermal route. An extensive trial of transdermal preparation of fentanyl has been carried out in patients with postoperative pain.[28-33] Self-adhesive skin patches of 10, 20, 30, and 40 cm^2 deliver fentanyl transdermally at rates equivalent to IV infusions of 25, 50, 75, and 100 μg/hr, respectively. The delivery rate is regulated by a rate-controlling membrane in the preparation so that the doses are determined by the area of product applied. When applied to a nonhairy region of the body (e.g., the anterior chest wall), this preparation has been shown to be efficacious in delivering fentanyl and providing pain relief. Dosage regimens have been studied that reliably deliver fentanyl at rates equivalent to 50 to 125 μg/hr. Pharmacokinetic studies have shown that the skin provides a depot for fentanyl; consequently, there is a lag of some 6 to 12 hours before steady state blood fentanyl concentrations are obtained, and there is a corresponding lag before they decay to below effective concentrations when the preparation is removed. This preparation holds particular promise for patients who are unable to receive analgesic agents by mouth or injection where sustained blood fentanyl concentrations are required. Other opioid analgesic agents such as meperidine[34] and hydromorphone[35] also have suitable pharmacokinetic properties for transdermal drug delivery, but the larger masses of drug required for clinical analgesia may limit their feasibility in practice.

Therapeutic monitoring. The success of dosing regimens devised as described in the previous section is limited by the potentially large variability between patients in volume of distribution, clearance, absorption, and bioavailability. Therapeutic monitoring seems an ideal solution to these problems.

Richens and Warrington[36] suggested seven major reasons for monitoring plasma drug concentrations:

1. When there is a wide variation between individuals in the metabolism
2. When saturation kinetics occur
3. When the therapeutic ratio of a drug is low
4. When signs of toxicity are difficult to recognize clinically
5. When gastrointestinal, hepatic, or renal disease is present
6. When drug interactions are suspected
7. When patient noncompliance is suspected

Clinical judgment, in association with blood concentration data, is required to determine treatment efficacy. This can be illustrated by the examination of a patient being treated with epidural bupivacaine for terminal cancer pain. Clinical experience suggests that a rate of 25 mg/hr of bupivacaine would provide adequate analgesia. Blood concentrations monitored daily revealed that the bupivacaine concentration continued to accumulate, reaching a mean steady state value of 6.5 mg/L in this patient. However, this patient had an AAG level of 260 mg/dL and a free fraction concentration of 0.12 mg/L of bupivacaine. The increased plasma concentration of AAG caused an increase in the binding level accompanied by a decreased bupivacaine clearance. The free concentration of 0.12 mg/L was well below that usually associated with bupivacaine-induced CNS toxicity. However, it would be considered a normal practice to reduce the rate of bupivacaine infusion if blood bupivacaine concentrations of greater than 2.0 to 2.5 mg/L were measured, unless all aspects of the blood concentration data were understood. The result of such a reduction in infusion rate would be unsatisfactory analgesia.

Accurate and prudent monitoring of selected patients also allows the physician to separate the psychologic contributions to pain from the nonefficacy of the selected dosing regimen. No matter what, it cannot replace careful observation and adjustment of dose.

REFERENCES

1. Niazi S: Volume of distribution and tissue level errors in instantaneous intravenous input assumption. *J Pharm Sci* 65:750-752, 1976.
2. Millar AJ, Rode H, Cywes S: Continuous morphine infusion for postoperative pain in children. *S Afr Med J* 72:396-398, 1987.
3. Olkkola KT et al: Kinetics and dynamics of postoperative intravenous morphine in children. *Clin Pharmacol Ther* 44:128-136, 1988.
4. Tanguy M et al: Prolonged intravenous infusion of morphine: Pharmacokinetic study. *Ann Fr Anesth Reanim* 6:22-28, 1987.
5. Sitar DS et al: Kinetic disposition of morphine in young males after intravenous loading and maintenance infusion. *Can Anaesth Soc J* 33:145-149, 1986.
6. Alvis JM et al: Computer-assisted continuous infusions of fentanyl during cardiac anesthesia: Comparison with a manual method. *Anesthesiology* 63:41-49, 1985.
7. McMurray TJ et al: A method for producing constant plasma concentrations of drugs. *Br J Anaesth* 58:1085-1090, 1986.
8. Sear J: General kinetic and dynamic principles and their application to continuous intravenous anaesthesia. *Anaesthesia* 38(Suppl):10-15, 1983.
9. Schwilden H, Schüttler J, Stockel H: Pharmacokinetics as applied to total intravenous anaesthesia. *Anaesthesia* 38(Suppl):51-56, 1983.

10. Weinberg DS et al: Sublingual absorption of selected opioid analgesics. *Clin Pharmacol Ther* 44:335-342, 1988.
11. Tolksdorf W et al: Sublingual buprenorphine in the therapy of postoperative pain. *Anaesth Intensivmed Notfallmed Schmerzther* 19:117-123, 1984.
12. Cuschieri RJ, Morran CG, McArdle CS: Comparison of morphine and sublingual buprenorphine following abdominal surgery. *Br J Anaesth* 56:855-895, 1984.
13. Adriaensen H, Mattelaer B, Vanmeenen H: A long-term open, clinical and pharmacokinetic assessment of sublingual buprenorphine in patients suffering from chronic pain. *Acta Anaesthesiol Belg* 36:33-40, 1985.
14. Bell MD et al: Buccal morphine—a new route for analgesia? *Lancet* 1:71-73, 1985.
15. Fisher AP, Fung C, Hanna M: Serum morphine concentrations after buccal and intramuscular morphine administration. *Br J Clin Pharmacol* 24:685-687, 1987.
16. Jacobsen J et al: Comparative plasma concentration profiles after I.V., I.M. and rectal administration of pethidine in children. *Br J Anaesth* 60:623, 626, 1988.
17. Katagiri Y et al: Enhanced bioavailability of morphine after rectal administration in rats. *J Pharm Pharmacol* 40:879-881, 1988.
18. Aungst BJ, Lam G, Shefter E: Oral and rectal nalbuphine bioavailability: First-pass metabolism in rats and dogs. *Biopharm Drug Dispos* 6:413-421, 1985.
19. DeBoer AG, DeLeede LG, Breimer DD: Drug absorption by sublingual and rectal routes. *Br J Anaesth* 56:69-82, 1984.
20. Burgess HA et al: The relative bioavailability of paracetamol after rectal administration of suppositories containing a mixture of paracetamol, codeine phosphate and buclizine hydrochloride in healthy volunteers. *Curr Med Res Opin* 9:634-641, 1985.
21. Spahn H et al: The bioavailability of combination preparations of acetylsalicylic acid and codeine phosphate. *Arzneimittelforschung* 35:973-976, 1985.
22. Moolenaar F et al: Preliminary study on the absorption profile after rectal and oral administration of methadone in human volunteers. *Pharm Weekbl Sci* 6:237-240, 1984.
23. Ellison NM, Lewis GO: Plasma concentrations following single doses of morphine sulfate in oral solution and rectal suppository. *Clin Pharm* 3:614-617, 1984.
24. Westerling D, Andersson KE: Rectal administration of morphine hydrogel: Absorption and bioavailability in women. *Acta Anaesthesiol Scand* 28:540-543, 1984.
25. Lipman AG, Anderson BD: Bioavailability of morphine from rectal suppositories. *Am J Hosp Pharm* 41:636-638, 1984.
26. Kummer M, Mehlhaus N: Bioavailability of codeine and paracetamol in a combination preparation following oral and rectal administration. *Fortschr Med* 102:173-178, 1984.
27. Moolenaar F et al: Rectal versus oral absorption of codeine phosphate in man. *Biopharm Drug Dispos* 4:195-199, 1983.
28. Duthie DJ et al: Plasma fentanyl concentrations during transdermal delivery of fentanyl to surgical patients. *Br J Anaesth* 60:614-618, 1988.
29. Holley FO, van Steennis C: Postoperative analgesia with fentanyl: Pharmacokinetics and pharmacodynamics of constant-rate I.V. and transdermal delivery. *Br J Anaesth* 60:608-613, 1988.
30. Von Bormann B et al: Postoperative pain therapy by transdermal fentanyl. *Anasthesiol Intensivmed Notfallmed Schmerzther* 23:3-8, 1988.
31. Gourlay GK et al: The transdermal administration of fentanyl in the treatment of postoperative pain, pharmacokinetics and pharmacodynamic effects. *Pain* 37:193-202, 1989.
32. Varvel JR et al: Absorption characteristics of transdermally administered fentanyl. *Anesthesiology* 70:928-934, 1989.
33. Plezia PM et al: Transdermal fentanyl: pharmacokinetics and preliminary clinical evaluation. *Pharmacotherapy* 9:2-9, 1989.
34. Ritschel WA, Sathyan G, Denson DD: Transdermal drug delivery of meperidine. *Methods Find Exp Clin Pharmacol* 11:165-172, 1989.
35. Chang SF, Moore L, Chien YW: Pharmacokinetics and bioavailability of hydromorphone: effect of various routes of administration. *Pharm Res* 5:718-721, 1988.
36. Richens A, Warrington S: When should plasma drug levels be monitored? *Drugs* 17:488-500, 1979.

QUESTIONS: PHARMACOKINETICS AND PHARMACODYNAMICS OF ANALGESIC AGENTS

1. The time required for drug to blood concentration to be alleved by a factor of two is called in pharmacokinetic terms:
   A. Clearance
   B. Volume of distribution
   C. Half-life
   D. Redistribution
2. In acute pain therapy when one selects an analgesic agent, the choice is:
   A. Fewer repeated doses of high-clearance drug
   B. Fewer repeated doses of low-clearance drug
   C. Frequent repeated doses of low-clearance drug
   D. Oral administration
3. In chronic pain therapy the best route of drug administration is:
   A. Intraspinal
   B. Intravenous
   C. Oral
   D. Transdermal
4. Which of the following routes allow analgesic drugs to have direct access at the target receptor by diffusion?
   A. Rectal
   B. Epidural
   C. Subcutaneous
   D. Intravenous

5. When prescribing sublingual or buccal route of administration, the best drug (55%) for absorption is:
   A. Methadone
   B. Fentanyl
   C. Morphine
   D. Buprenorphine

ANSWERS

1. C
2. B
3. C
4. B
5. D

13 Opioids and Nonsteroidal Antiinflammatory Analgesics

Jeffrey A. Katz

OPIOID ANALGESICS

Research in the area of opiate receptors and opiate receptor agonists and antagonists is an ongoing process, with new information being developed on what seems like a daily basis. However, specialty examinations in pain will attempt to emphasize information that is clinically relevant, not esoteric, and relatively noncontroversial. As a result this chapter emphasizes information that adheres to those standards. Research compounds that are not in clinical use are not mentioned in an effort to simplify the material presented. Likewise, data that only relate to animals is also kept to a minimum, and discussion of theories that have no scientific data to support them is minimized. Generic drug names only are used.

Chemistry

There are three classification schemes generally used when describing opioids. One classification characterizes the drug as either weak or strong; this is the simplest because only codeine and propoxyphene are considered weak, whereas the rest are considered strong (although some references include oxycodone and hydrocodone as weak opioids). Another classification scheme divides the opioids into four categories: agonists (which include all of the drugs not in the other categories), partial agonists (only buprenorphine), agonist/antagonists (butorphanol, nalbuphine, pentazocine, and dezocine), and antagonists (naloxone, naltrexone, and cholecystokinin). The final categorization method is based on the chemical derivation of the drugs and divides them into naturally occurring, semisynthetic, and synthetic compounds, with each group having subgroups (Box 13-1).

Opioids are morphine-like substances. The term *opioids* is derived from opium (from the Greek term for juice), which is an extract from the poppy plant. Opium contains 20 different alkaloids that have been isolated; among them are morphine, codeine, and papaverine.

Opium contains two alkaloid types, the phenanthrene series (from which morphine and codeine are derived) and the benzylisoquinoline series (from which papaverine, a completely nonanalgesic drug, is derived). Modification of the morphine molecule while retaining the basic five ring structure results in the semisynthetic agents heroin and hydromorphone (Fig. 13-1). When the furan ring is removed from morphine, the resulting four ring synthetic opioid levorphanol is formed. The phenylpiperidines, e.g., meperidine, fentanyl, and the phenylheptylamines (metha-

done and propoxyphene all have only two of the original five rings of the basic morphine molecular structure. All the opioids, despite the diverse molecular structures, share an N-methylpiperidine moiety that seems to confer analgesic activity.[1]

After the discovery of opioid receptors in the early 1970s, the search began for endogenous substances that were the agonists for the opioid receptors. In 1975 these agonists were identified: enkephalins, endorphins, and dynorphins. By the early 1980s three precursor molecules to these agonists were identified and named after the active fragments: proenkephalin, proadrenocorticotropic hormone (pro-ACTH) ACTH endorphin (also called proopiomelanocortin), and prodynorphin (Fig. 13-2).[2]

Mechanism of action

In 1973 three separate research groups identified the opioid receptor system through which opioids exert their clinical effects. There are at least three opioid receptors known to mediate analgesia. The μ *receptor* was named after its first known agonist, morphine; and was found to produce analgesia, miosis, and respiratory depression. The κ *receptor* was named after an early known agonist, ketocyclazocine, which also produced analgesia but with less respiratory depression than morphine. The proprietary compound SKF 10,047 was the source for naming the opioid ς *receptor,* which produced excitation and dysphoria but little analgesia. As a result, some do not even consider the ς receptor to be in the opioid receptor class.[2] Another receptor similar in action to the μ receptor but distinct was identified in studies of mouse vas deferens, hence the name δ *receptor.*[3]

The proposed receptor system has recently undergone some modifications. The identification of μ receptor subclasses revealed that a μ_1 receptor subtype may mediate opioid analgesia, whereas a μ_2 receptor subtype may mediate respiratory depression. In addition, subtypes of the κ and δ receptors have recently been examined.[4] The actions of many of these discovered receptors, however, remains to be identified. The μ_1, δ, and κ receptors comprise about 40%, 10%, and 50%, respectively, of *opioid spinal receptors.*[5]

It has been demonstrated that different opioids have different affinities. These are: morphine—$\mu_1 > \mu_2 > \kappa_3 > \kappa_1 > \delta$; codeine— $\kappa_3 > \mu$; nalorphine— $\mu_1 > \mu_2 > \kappa_1 > \kappa_3 > \delta$; levorphanol—$\kappa_3 > \kappa_1$; pentazocine— $\kappa_1 > \kappa_3$; nalbuphine—$\kappa_1 > \delta > \mu_1 > \kappa_3 > \mu_2$.[4] Note that, despite co-

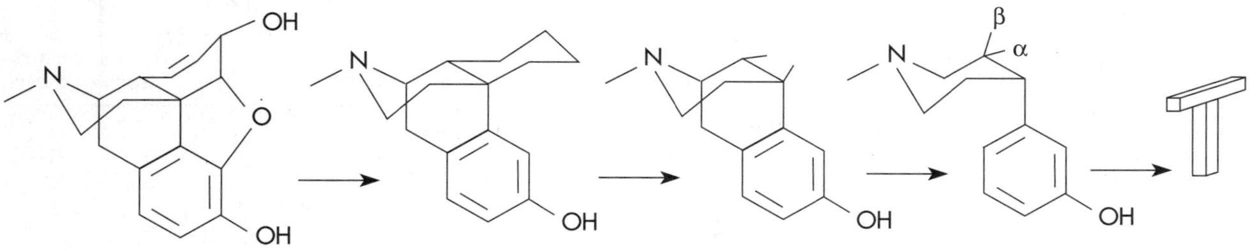

Fig. 13-1 Synthetic opioids are produced by successive removal of ring structures from the five-ring phananthrene structure of morphine. However, a common core, envisaged as a T, is shared by all opioids. A piperidine ring (which is believed to confer "opioid-like" properties to a compound) forms the crossbar, and a hydroxylated phenyl group forms the vertical axis. (From Ferrante FM, Vadeboncouer TR, editors: *Postoperative Pain Management.* New York, Churchill Livingstone, 1993.)

BOX 13-1 CLASSIFICATION SCHEME OF OPIOIDS BASED ON DERIVATION OF DRUG

Naturally occurring opium alkaloids

Phenanthrene derivatives
  Morphine
  Codeine
Benzylisoquinoline derivatives
  Papaverine

Semisynthetic derivatives of opium alkaloids

Morphine derivatives
  Oxymorphone (dihydrohydroxymorphinone)
  Hydromorphone (dihydromorphinone)
  Heroin (diacetylmorphine)
Thebaine derivatives
  Buprenorphine
  Oxycodone

Synthetic opioids

Morphinans
  Levorphanol
  Nalbuphine
  Naloxone
  Naltrexone
Phenylheptylamines
  Methadone
  Propoxyphene
Phenylpiperidine
  Alfentanil
  Fentanyl
  Meperidine
  Sufentanil

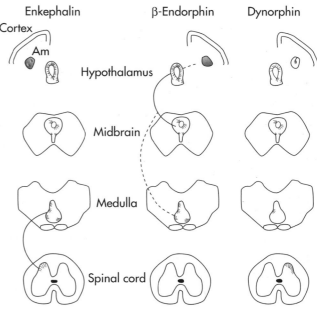

Fig. 13-2 Distribution of endogenous opioid peptides in CNS. Left, proenkephalin-derived peptides have the most extensive distribution. They are present in cells and terminals in the amygdala *(AM),* the hypothalamus, the midbrain periaqueductal gray matter, the rostroventral medulla, and the dorsal horn of the spinal cord and lamina X. Middle, β-endorphin in CNS. β-endorphin is largely derived from cells in the arcuate nucleus of the hypothalamus. There is a significant amount of β-endorphin in the periaqueductal gray matter and much less in the medulla and spinal cord. Right, dynorphin-related peptides roughly parallel the distribution of enkephalins, but there is much less dynorphin in the hypothalamus and the rostroventral medullas. (From Fields HL: Central nervous system mechanism for control of pain transmission. In Fields HL, editor: *Pain.* New York, McGraw-Hill, 1987.)

---

deine's stronger κ affinity, it is considered mostly a μ agonist, whereas nalorphine is considered a κ agonist despite its stronger μ affinity.

The site of action of the opioids is at the supraspinal and spinal levels, although recent research has questioned whether there are mechanisms of opioid analgesia outside the central nervous system (CNS).[6,7] Furthermore, basic science research has confirmed what has often been observed clinically: Supraspinal and spinal opioid analgesic mechanisms are synergistic.[8] This could explain why medications such as fentanyl and sufentanil produce more profound analgesia when delivered epidurally than when delivered systemically, despite the similar blood concentrations observed with both routes of administration.

Table 13-1 Pharmacokinetic and physicochemical variables for opioid analgesics

Drug	Vc (L/kg)	Vd (L/kg)	Cl (mL/min/kg)	T1/2β (min)	Partition coefficient (octanol/water)
Morphine	0.23	2.8	15.5	134	1
Hydromorphone	0.34	4.1	22.7	15	1
Meperidine	0.6	2.6	12	180	21
Methadone	0.15	3.4	1.6	23hr	115
Levorphanol		10	10.5	11hr	
Alfentanil	0.12	0.9	7.6	94	130
Fentanyl	0.85	4.6	21	186	820
Sufentanil	0.1	2.5	11.3	149	1750
Buprenorphine	0.2	2.8	17.2	184	10,000
Nalbuphine	0.45	4.8	23.1	222	
Butorphanol		5	38.6	159	
Dezocine		12	52	156	

Vc, central volume of distribution; Vd, volume of distribution; Cl, clearance, T1/2β, elimination half-life.
From Hill H, Mather L: Patient-controlled analgesic, pharmacokinetic and therapeutic considerations. *Clin Phamacokinet* 24: 124-140, 1993 and O'Brien J, Benfield P: Dezocine: A preliminary review of its pharmacodynamic and pharmacokinetic properties, and therapeutic efficacy. *Drugs* 38: 226-248, 1989.

Pharmacokinetics

The pharmacokinetic variables and partition coefficients (in octanol/water) for several of the opioid analgesics are summarized in Table 13-1. When reviewing the table, it is more critical to note how the parameters of the drugs relate to each other rather than the numbers themselves. For example, fentanyl and morphine have similar elimination half-lives, which can explain how the drugs develop similar durations of action when high doses of fentanyl are used.

Pharmacodynamics

The potency, speed of onset, and duration of action of the opioid analgesics are perhaps the most clinically relevant pharmacodynamic measures. The relative potencies are listed in Table 13-2. Apparent potencies, however, can change over time and can be a function of the route of administration. For example, morphine administered over a long period of time may seem to become more potent; this may be a result of gradual accumulation of active metabolites from the previously administered doses. The potencies listed are based on acute administration only. The potency of a drug used intravenously (IV) will differ from its potency when used by extravascular routes (e.g., oral, rectal), and this is a function of the drug's bioavailability. To convert from a parenteral dosage of a drug to its oral form, divide the parenteral dose by the bioavailability. So a 10 mg IV dose of morphine is approximately equivalent to a 30 mg oral dose based on a bioavailability of 0.3.

Probably of greatest importance in determining the speed of onset of analgesia of systemically administered analgesics is the gradient between blood and brain tissue. Although other factors such as percentage of free, unionized drug in blood and lipid solubility would appear to play a significant role in the rate of drug entry into the CNS, empirically these factors do not correlate to drug onset. For example, alfentanil is known to have a shorter time to onset of drug effect than either fentanyl or morphine. However, fentanyl is over 7 times more lipid soluble than alfentanil, and morphine has 16 times more unionized free drug avail-

Table 13-2 Relative potencies of opioid analgesics

Drug	Relative potency IM	Relative potency oral
Morphine	10	30
Hydromorphone	1.5	7.5
Meperidine	75	300
Methadone	10	12.5
Codeine	120	200
Levorphanol	2	4
Nalbuphine	10	
Oxycodone		30
Pentazocine	60	180

able to enter the CNS for any given dose. Alfentanil's rapid onset is likely due to its small volume of distribution, which allows a greater blood to brain gradient to persist than either morphine or fentanyl.[9]

All of the opioid agonists have similar clinical effects that vary in degree from one drug to another. In addition to analgesia, sedation, respiratory depression, nausea, constipation, cough suppression, euphoria, dysphoria, and miosis are also known dose-dependent effects of the opioid agonists. The respiratory depression is likely the result of activation of μ_2 receptors located in the brainstem.[10]

The gastrointestinal (GI) effects include constipation, nausea, and vomiting. Constipation is likely the result of decreased GI transit via action on μ_2 receptors within the brain and in the peripheral nerve plexus.[11,12] The nausea and vomiting are likely the result of stimulation of the chemoreceptor trigger zone in the medulla, but it is unclear whether it involves opioid receptors specifically.[4]

Increased tone of smooth muscle sphincters can also occur with opioid use. This has been reported in the sphincter of Oddi but study results conflict. One study demonstrated that morphine produces greater biliary sphincter spasm than meperidine, whereas another demonstrated no significant differences between morphine and meperidine; but fentanyl produced even larger increases in intrabiliary pressure.[13,14]

Both studies demonstrated that pentazocine clearly produced less biliary sphincter spasm than any of the other opioids studied. The increase in smooth muscle tone can also result in urinary retention via action on the vesical sphincter. However, the tone of the detrusor muscle is enhanced, possibly leading to a sensation of urgency. The effect of opioids on the ureters in humans is variable.[15]

Typically, opioid agonists have few cardiovascular effects at the therapeutic doses in supine patients. At high doses, however, most opioids produce significant bradycardia, probably via medullary vagal stimulation.[16] An exception is meperidine, which can often cause tachycardia, either as a result of its similarity in structure to atropine or via a reflex response to hypotension.[17,18] Morphine may cause tachycardia as a reflex to the hypotension resulting from histamine release.[19,20] Histamine release is less with meperidine, sufentanil, and fentanyl.[20]

Endocrinologic effects of opioids include release of vasopressin and inhibition of the stress-induced release of corticotropin and the gonadotropins from the pituitary. Thyrotropin release from the adenohypophysis is also inhibited. Basal metabolic rate and temperature may also be decreased in patients receiving chronic opioids, although animal data indicate that acute administration systemically or intrathecally can increase temperature.[21,22]

Intraspinal delivery

Opioids delivered via the epidural or subarachnoid routes behave very differently in onset, duration, and side effects than the same drugs given systemically. Pain unresponsive to systemic opioids may respond to the same opioids given centrally, reducing some side effects while increasing the incidence of others.[23]

Drugs with higher lipid solubilities (see Table 13-1) tend to be rapidly absorbed into the spinal tissues after central administration, which results in a faster onset of action. However, higher lipid solubility is also associated with a small area of distribution of the drug along the length of the spinal cord and therefore a more limited area of analgesia. Higher lipid solubility is also associated with faster clearance of the drug out of the epidural and intrathecal space, possibly resulting in a shorter duration of action and higher blood concentrations of the opioid (with subsequent systemic side effects).[23,24]

INDIVIDUAL AGENTS
Agonists

Naturally occurring opioids: phenanthrene derivatives

Morphine. The pharmacodynamics of morphine have been well described (Fig. 13-3). However, newer, slow-release formulations of the drug have become popular in the treatment of cancer pain and many benign pain states, since regular morphine taken orally requires dosing intervals every 4 hours. These slow-release formulations use either hydrophilic or hydrophobic matrices in pill form to allow a gradual release of morphine as the pill passes through the GI tract at dosing intervals of 6 to 12 hours. Thus the duration of action of morphine is prolonged by virtue of a sustained, controlled release while the elimination of the drug is unchanged. The pills cannot be crushed; doing so results in im-

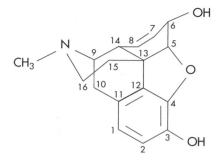

Fig. 13-3 Morphine. (From Ferrante FM, Vadeboncouer TR, editors: *Postoperative Pain Management.* New York, Churchill Livingstone, 1993.)

mediate release of all the morphine. These slow-release medications take about 2.5 hours to reach peak plasma concentrations of morphine after oral administration, versus about 1 hour for regular morphine preparations.[25]

In patients with renal failure, morphine produces a more prolonged effect and often excessive sedation. It is currently believed to be a result of an active metabolite, morphine-6-glucuronide (M6G) (Fig. 13-4). Morphine is glucuronidated at both the "3" (producing morphine-3-glucuronide, M3G) and "6" positions (producing M6G) in a 2:1 ratio.[15] Once inside the CNS, the M6G metabolite is 100 times more potent than the parent morphine drug, while the M3G metabolite is inactive.[26] However, the greater hydrophilicity of M6G normally impedes its passage into the CNS. However, after chronic dosing, and in patients unable to renally excrete the M6G metabolite, concentrations of M6G can exceed the collected morphine in the blood; and M6G may be able to enter the CNS by mass action.

Codeine. Codeine is considered a weak opioid and is generally not used for severe pain. It is also considered to have less tendency toward developing addiction, but this is likely a dose-related effect. It has good antitussive activity, but on a weight basis it is a less potent antitussive than morphine (Fig. 13-5). Codeine's analgesia and addiction potential may stem from its biotransformation to morphine.[27]

Semisynthetic opioids

Hydromorphone. Derived from morphine in the 1920s, hydromorphone has a global pharmacokinetic profile similar to morphine (Fig. 13-6).[25] It is well absorbed from oral, rectal, or parenteral sites. Because of its lipid solubility, it is often used instead of morphine for central administration when a wide area of analgesia is needed. Few studies have been performed on hydromorphone relative to morphine; but, because of the lack of any identified significantly active metabolites, it is sometimes recommended for patients with renal failure.[4]

Diacetylmorphine. Diacetylmorphine is also known as heroin, and is metabolized to morphine during first pass through the liver and before reaching the CNS target site. It has little advantage over morphine in clinical practice (Fig. 13-7).[28]

Oxycodone. Since oxycodone has only relatively recently been approved for use in the United States as a sole agent (previously sold only in combination with aspirin or acet-

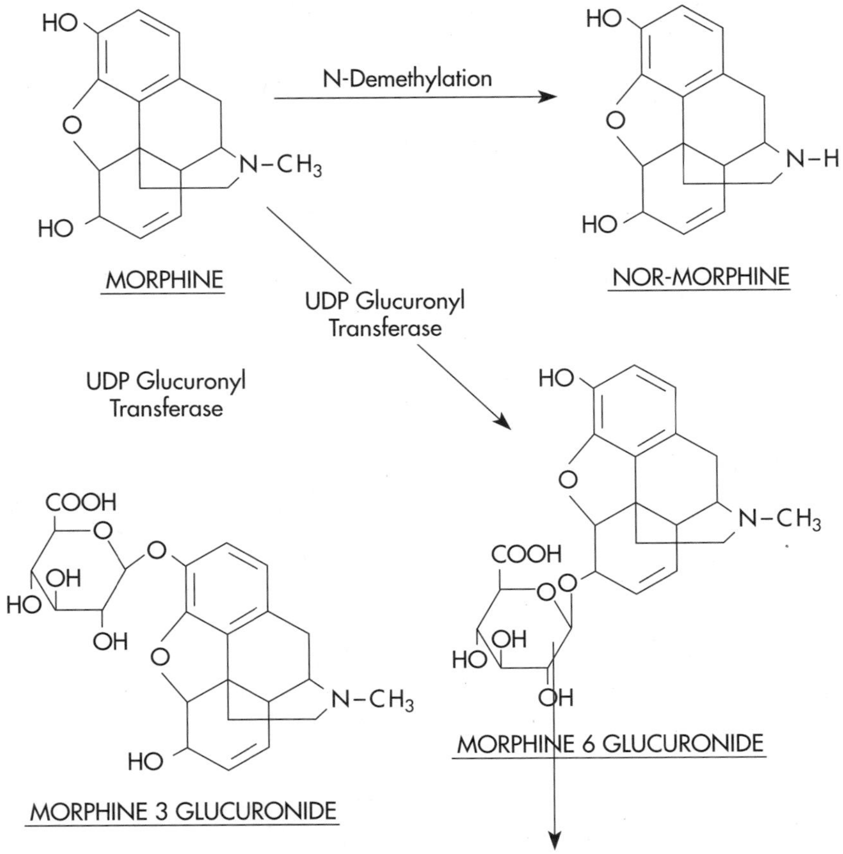

Fig. 13-4 Metabolism of morphine. Morphine-3-glucuronide and morphine-6-glucuronide are major metabolites. Morphine-6-glucuronide possesses significant analgesic activity and may substantially contribute to morphine's analgesic effects. Both metabolites are excreted in the urine, and accumulation may occur after repetitive dosing in patients with renal failure. Demethylation is a minor pathway for morphine metabolism. (From Ferrante FM, Vadeboncouer TR, editors: *Postoperative Pain Management.* New York, Churchill Livingstone, 1993.)

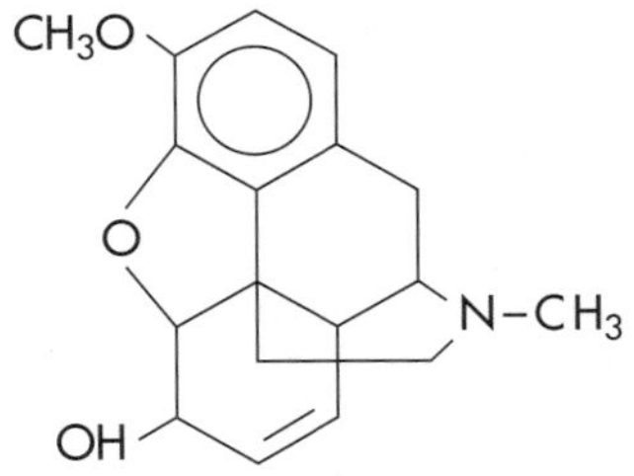

Fig. 13-5 Codeine is the result of substitution of a methyl group on carbon 3 of morphine. Codeine is a naturally occurring alkaloid that has significant efficacy after oral administration because of limitation of first-pass metabolism. (From Ferrante FM, Vadeboncouer TR, editors: *Postoperative Pain Management.* New York, Churchill Livingstone, 1993.)

aminophen), little has been published regarding its use alone. Its relative potency compared to codeine is estimated at 7.7 times that of codeine.[29]

Synthetic opioids

Methadone. Supplied as a racemic mixture of two optical isomers, most of methadone's activity comes from the L-isomer (Fig. 13-8). Unlike most opioids, methadone has a very long half-life, which allows less frequent dosing. Since its prolonged effect is the result of extensive protein binding with slow release and the result of a lower intrinsic ability of the liver to metabolize it, methadone does not require a special formulation and can be administered as a liquid, unlike sustained-release morphine. It also has the advantages of a high bioavailability and no active metabolites. However, drawbacks of methadone include accumulation (which results when a drug is administered more frequently than the half-life) and a longer time to reach steady state than other opioids (on the order of days for methadone versus hours for morphine).[30]

Propoxyphene. Although structurally related to methadone, propoxyphene was considered a nonopioid when introduced; but its frequent use, combined with clinical observations regarding tolerance and psychologic dependence and addiction, indicated it was indeed an opioid (Fig. 13-9).[25] Its analgesic efficacy has been claimed to be even less than that of aspirin.[31] Unlike other opioids, it causes depression of the cardiac conduction systems similar to that produced by lidocaine, which constitutes a significant risk

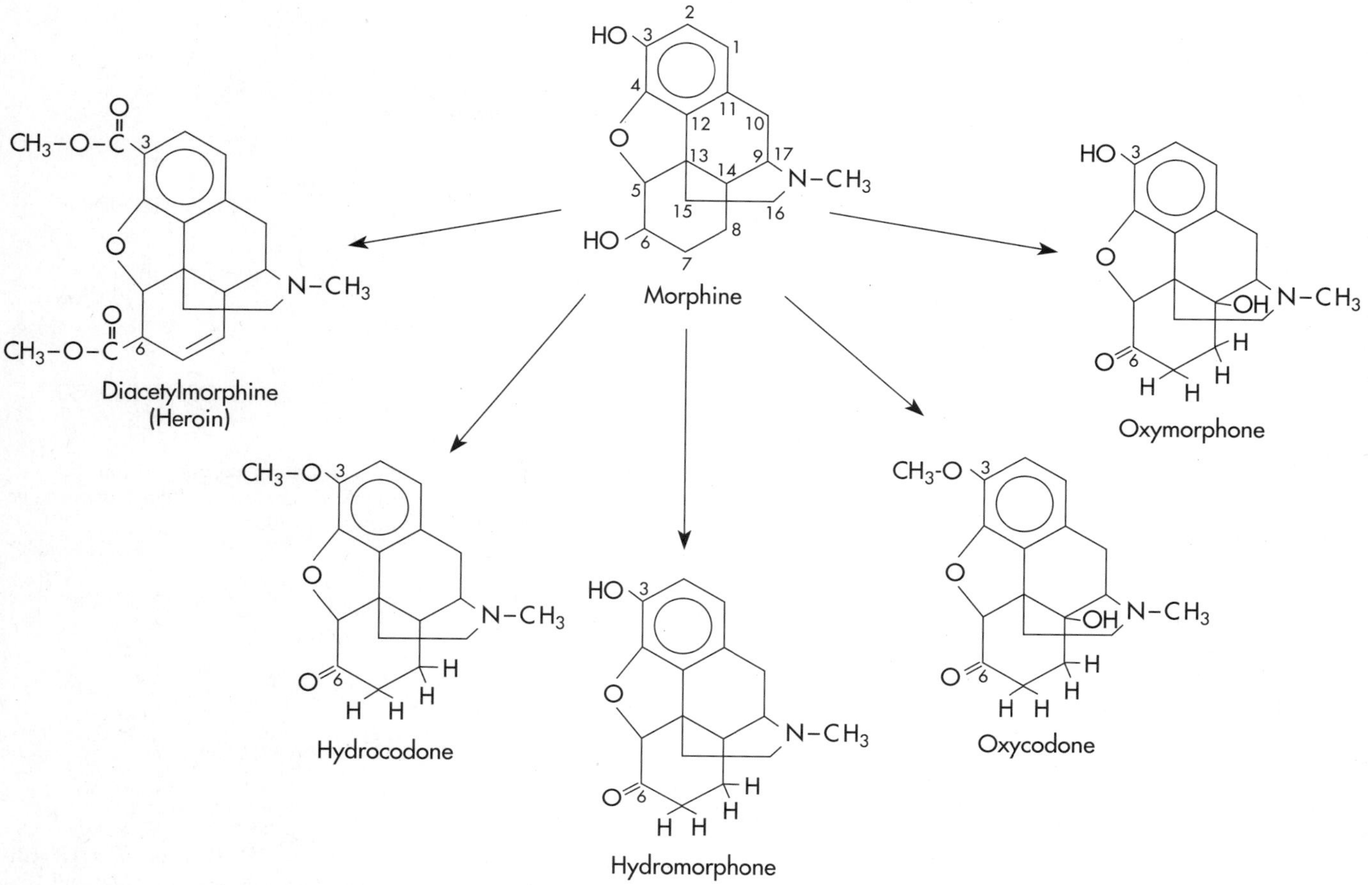

Fig. 13-6 Semisynthetic opioids are created by modification of functional groups on the morphine molecular skeleton. (From Ferrante FM, Vadeboncouer TR, editors: *Postoperative Pain Management*. New York, Churchill Livingstone, 1993.)

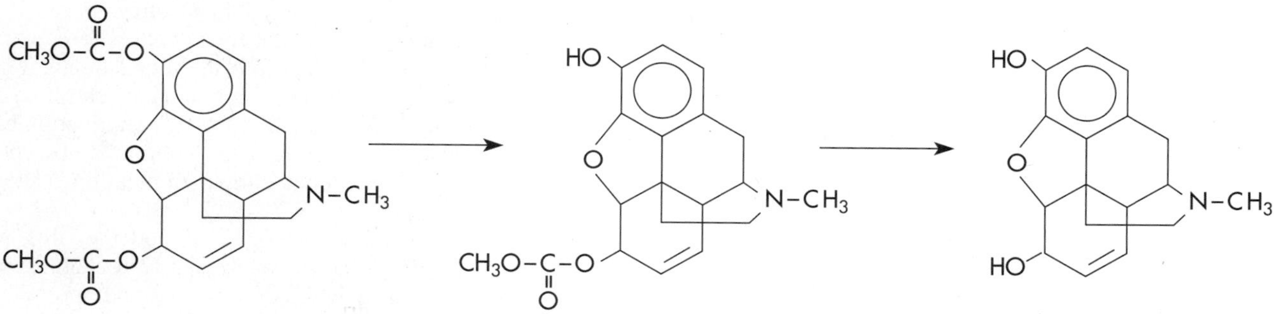

Fig. 13-7 Diacetylmorphine is a prodrug that is rapidly hydrolyzed in the plasma to monoacetyl-morphine (analgesically active) and morphine. (From Ferrante FM, Vadeboncouer TR, editors: *Postoperative Pain Management*. New York, Churchill Livingstone, 1993.)

in cases of overdose.[32] In fact, animal data demonstrate that it is a potent local anesthetic.[33]

Patients with hepatic disease are at particular risk for propoxyphene toxicity, since there is significant first-pass metabolism to norpropoxyphene.[34] Also, patients with renal failure develop very high blood concentrations of both propoxyphene and norpropoxyphene; and because of their high protein binding, neither is removed well by hemodi-

alysis.[25] Finally, exercise caution when giving propoxyphene to patients taking carbamazepine, since propoxyphene inhibits carbamazepine metabolism to the point of inducing toxicity.[35]

Meperidine. Meperidine is noteworthy because of a metabolite, normeperidine, which is about half as analgesic as meperidine but lowers the seizure threshold and induces CNS excitability (Figs. 13-10 and 13-11). Normeperidine's

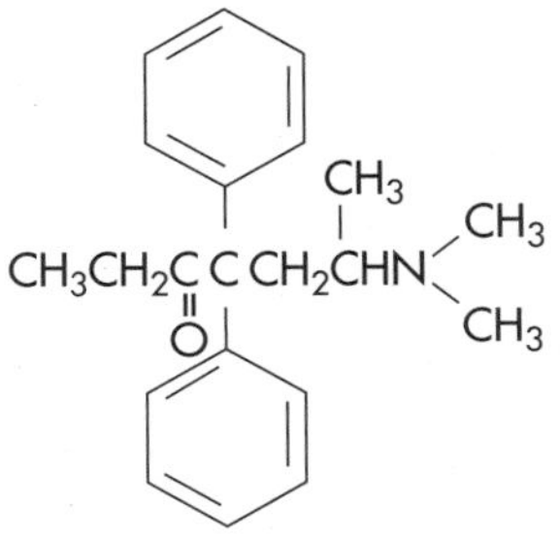

Fig. 13-8 Methadone. (From Ferrante FM, Vadeboncouer TR, editors: *Postoperative Pain Management.* New York, Churchill Livingstone, 1993.)

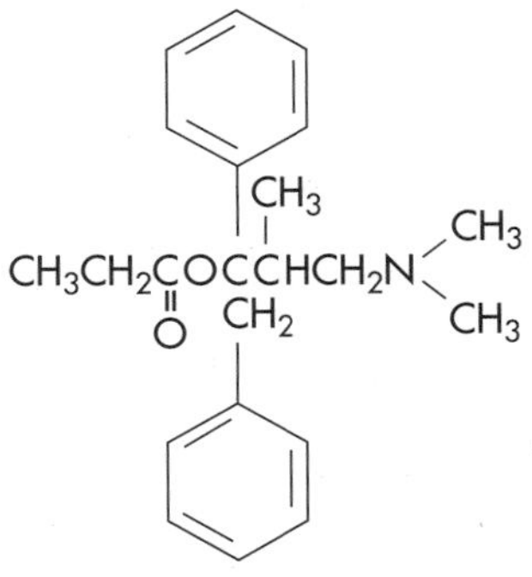

Fig. 13-9 Propoxyphene. (From Ferrante FM, Vadeboncouer TR, editors: *Postoperative Pain Management.* New York, Churchill Livingstone, 1993.)

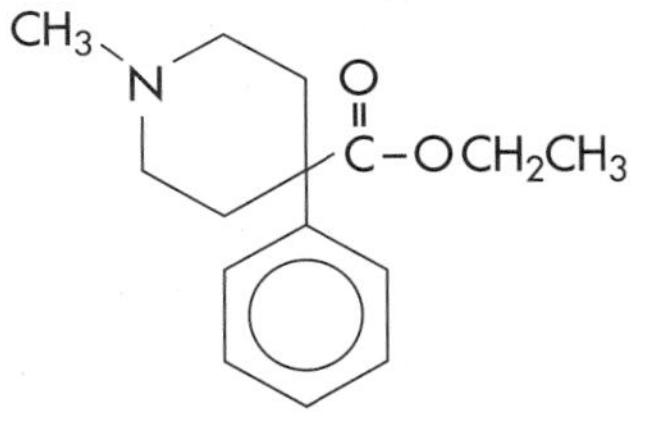

Fig. 13-10 Meperidine. (From Ferrante FM, Vadeboncouer TR, editors: *Postoperative Pain Management.* New York, Churchill Livingstone, 1993.)

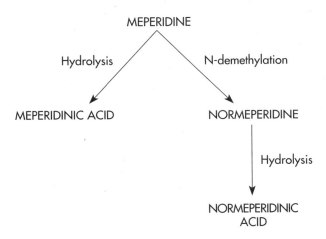

Fig. 13-11 Hepatic metabolism of normeperidine. (From Ferrante FM, Vadeboncouer TR, editors: *Postoperative Pain Management.* New York, Churchill Livingstone, 1993.)

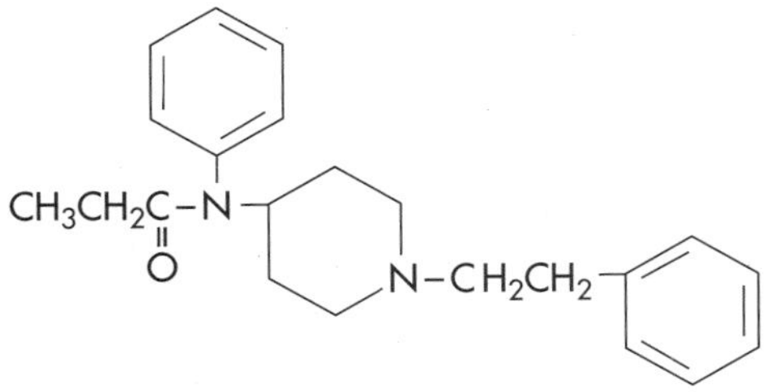

Fig. 13-12 Fentanyl. (From Ferrante FM, Vadeboncouer TR, editors: *Postoperative Pain Management.* New York, Churchill Livingstone, 1993.)

elimination half-life is significantly longer than that of meperidine (8 to 21 hours). Patients with renal failure or cancer patients receiving very high doses of meperidine can significantly accumulate this metabolite; the use of meperidine in those clinical settings should be limited.[36] Meperidine administered systemically has been reported to cause corneal anesthesia, thus blunting the corneal reflex. It also produces local anesthesia when applied locally, but it can also cause significant local tissue irritation.[21]

Fentanyl. Although initially used for intraoperative IV anesthesia, fentanyl later became used IV for postoperative patient-controlled analgesia (Fig. 13-12). However, recent introduction of the transdermal delivery system for fentanyl has provided an alternative method of analgesia with a longer duration for a given dose. The amount of fentanyl released from the transdermal patches is proportional to the surface area, with 25 μg/hr released per 10 cm^2 of patch. It takes up to 24 hours after the application of a patch for blood concentrations of fentanyl to stabilize because the drug must saturate the a subcutaneous depot before the fentanyl is consistently absorbed into the bloodstream. When the patch is removed, the decline in blood concentration follows an apparent 17 hour half-life; the true elimination half-life of fentanyl is about 3 hours, but continued absorption from the subcutaneous depot during elimination makes it appear longer.[21]

Tramadol. A synthetic analogue of codeine, this new agent produces analgesia via weak μ receptor agonism in addition to blocking reuptake of serotonin and norepinephrine. Developed for oral or IV use, its T½β is 5 hours, but the T½β of its primary active M1 metabolife is 9 hours. Oral doses peak at about 2 hours, and oral bioavailability is approximately 0.68.[37]

Partial agonists and agonists/antagonists

Pentazocine. This drug has analgesic and very weak antagonistic effects, but its mechanisms of action are not well characterized (Fig. 13-13). It is thought to be a competitive antagonist at the μ receptors and an agonist at κ and ς receptors. Although it does not reverse morphine-induced respiratory depression, it can precipitate withdrawal in morphine-dependent patients. It was originally intended to

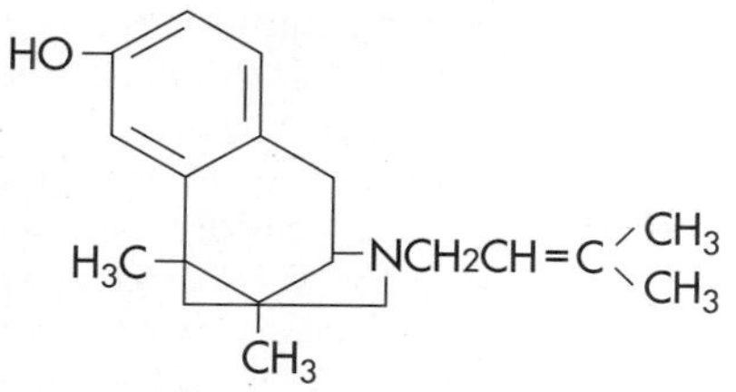

PENTAZOCINE

Fig. 13-13 Pentazocine. (From Ferrante FM, Vadeboncouer TR, editors: *Postoperative Pain Management*. New York, Churchill Livingstone, 1993.)

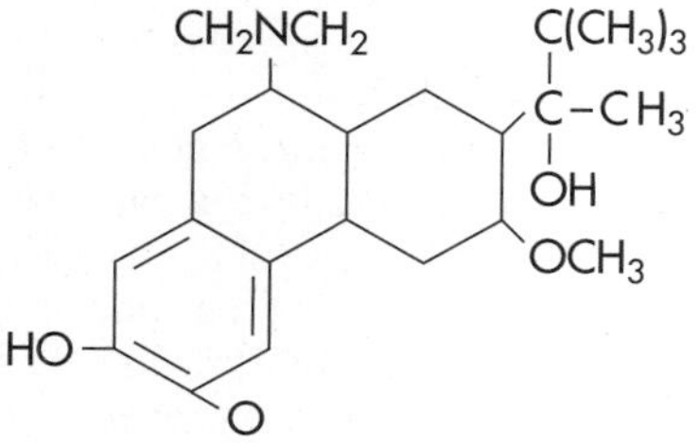

Fig. 13-14 Buprenorphine. (From Ferrante FM, Vadeboncouer TR, editors: *Postoperative Pain Management*. New York, Churchill Livingstone, 1993.)

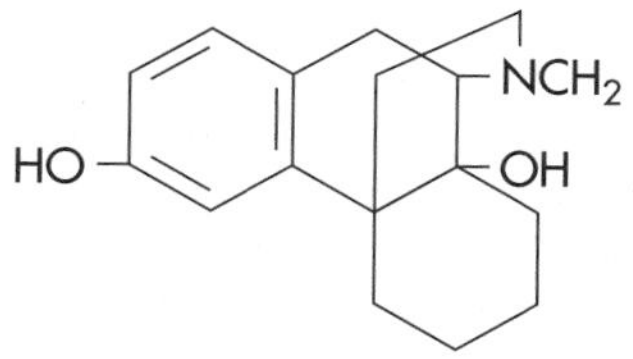

BUTORPHANOL

Fig. 13-15 Butorphanol. (From Ferrante FM, Vadeboncouer TR, editors: *Postoperative Pain Management*. New York, Churchill Livingstone, 1993.)

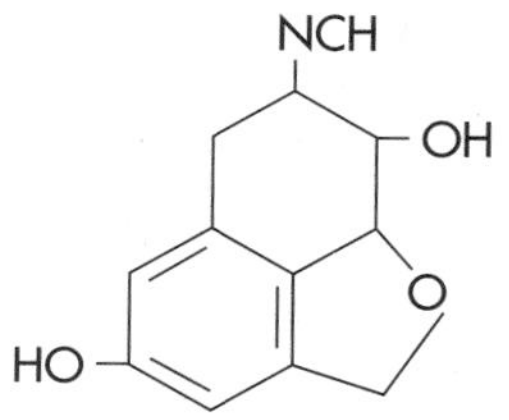

Fig. 13-16 Nalbuphine. (From Ferrante FM, Vadeboncouer TR, editors: *Postoperative Pain Management*. New York, Churchill Livingstone, 1993.)

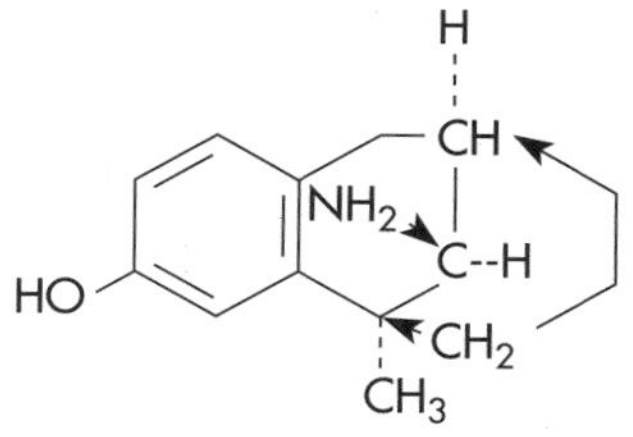

Fig. 13-17 Dezocine. (From Ferrante FM, Vadeboncouer TR, editors: *Postoperative Pain Management*. New York, Churchill Livingstone, 1993.)

serve as a nonaddicting opioid, but its abuse liability became apparent with clinical use.[21,25]

Buprenorphine. This semisynthetic derivative is the only partial agonist opioid, binding mostly to the μ receptor (Fig. 13-14). Its slow dissociation from the receptor is thought to contribute to its long duration of action (as long as 8 hours). This high affinity for the μ receptor may also account for naloxone's reduced ability to reverse the effects of buprenorphine relative to other opioids. Although clinically significant respiratory depression can occur with therapeutic doses of buprenorphine, it demonstrates a ceiling effect where increasing the dose does not increase the respiratory depression; this is believed to be the result of the antagonistic effects of the drug becoming more apparent at higher dosages.[21] Like the agonists/antagonists, buprenorphine can precipitate withdrawal in patients addicted to opioid agonists and has minimal effect on GI motility and smooth-muscle sphincter tone.

Butorphanol and nalbuphine. Although mechanisms are not well characterized for butorphanol or nalbuphine, it is thought that both of these IV agents exert their effects mostly through κ and ς receptor agonism and μ receptor antagonism (Figs. 13-15 and 13-16). A ceiling effect similar to buprenorphine and difficulty reversing the effect with naloxone have also been demonstrated for these drugs.[21,25] Overall, they have clinical effects similar to buprenorphine. Butorphanol has recently been approved as a nasal spray formulation without the controlled substance restriction; however, it may have an abuse liability similar to other opioids (Personal communication, Sgt. J.J. Burke, Cincinnati Police Department, Pharmaceutical Diversion Unit, 8/93).

Dezocine. Dezocine is the newest of the opioid agonist/antagonist drugs (Fig. 13-17). It has characteristics similar to the older agonist/antagonist drugs but demonstrates greater anesthetic sparing effect. It appears to have much less affinity for sigma receptors than the older agonists/antagonists, but it does have significant activity at the κ receptor and may be a partial μ agonist.[38] It is currently not considered a controlled substance and is available for IV use only.

NONSTEROIDAL ANTIINFLAMMATORY ANALGESICS

The nonopioid analgesics most often used are the nonsteroidal antiinflammatory drugs. In 1984, it was estimated that one in seven Americans was treated with a nonsteroidal antiinflammatory drug.[39] The class of nonsteroidal antiinflammatory drugs contains compounds that are often chemically unrelated, and they are grouped together based only on their therapeutic actions.[40] Unlike the opioids, the nonsteroidal antiinflammatory drugs do not demonstrate tolerance and are often more effective at controlling certain pain conditions with fewer side effects than the opioids.[41]

One must be cautious when reviewing the literature on nonsteroidal antiinflammatory drugs, since the vast majority of studies involve responsiveness of patients treated for rheumatic or other arthritic conditions. In those studies, inflammation of the joints rather than analgesia is often emphasized as the measured variable. Although such data are useful in predicting the ability of a nonsteroidal antiinflammatory drug to prevent inflammatory damage to joint structures, they have little bearing on nonsteroidal antiinflammatory drug efficacy for analgesic purposes, since there is clearly a documented lack of association between analgesia and the antiinflammatory effect of these drugs.[42] Similarly, most toxicity studies of nonsteroidal antiinflammatory drugs have been performed in elderly patients with concomitant medical conditions. Subsequently, there are not much toxicity data specifically in healthier patients using the nonsteroidal antiinflammatory drugs solely for pain.

Mechanism of action

All nonsteroidal antiinflammatory drugs have analgesic properties. Traditional teaching indicates that the nonsteroidal antiinflammatory drugs provide analgesia primarily through actions outside the CNS by inhibiting the formation of prostaglandins. When cell membranes are damaged, a class of substances called the *eicosanoids* (which includes arachidonic acid) is released. Arachidonic acid is then broken down by the lipooxygenase system or the cyclooxygenase (also called the prostaglandin synthetase) enzyme system.

tem. Although all nonsteroidal antiinflammatory drugs inhibit cyclooxygenase, several also inhibit lipooxygenase (Fig. 13-18).

The metabolites of the lipooxygenase system are the leukotrienes. Some of the leukotrienes are involved in affecting pain transmission: leukotriene B4 produces thermal hyperalgesia in humans. The cyclooxygenase system produces prostaglandins, which can sensitize nociceptors to respond to what are normally nonnoxious stimuli, possibly by altering sodium channel permeability. Prostacyclin (PGI$_2$), prostaglandin (PGE$_1$), and PGE$_2$ are most likely involved in inflammatory pain via promotion of the response of nociceptors to other inflammatory mediators.

However, more research has been indicating that the nonsteroidal antiinflammatory drugs may produce analgesia at least partially through a mechanism in the CNS.[43-47] Nonsteroidal antiinflammatory drugs cross the blood-brain barrier to enter the CNS, sometimes in proportion to plasma concentrations.[48] The central mechanisms of nonsteroidal antiinflammatory drugs to produce analgesia may involve facilitation of the descending pathways involved in pain inhibition or possible inhibition of peripheral inflammation through nonprostaglandin mechanisms in the CNS.[46,49] Furthermore, there is evidence that nonsteroidal antiinflammatory drugs have cellular effects unrelated to the synthesis of prostaglandins, such as inhibiting the release of inflammatory mediators from neutrophils and macrophages.[50]

Evidence has indicated that the analgesic response to a particular nonsteroidal antiinflammatory drug will vary depending on the individual. The mean response of a popula-

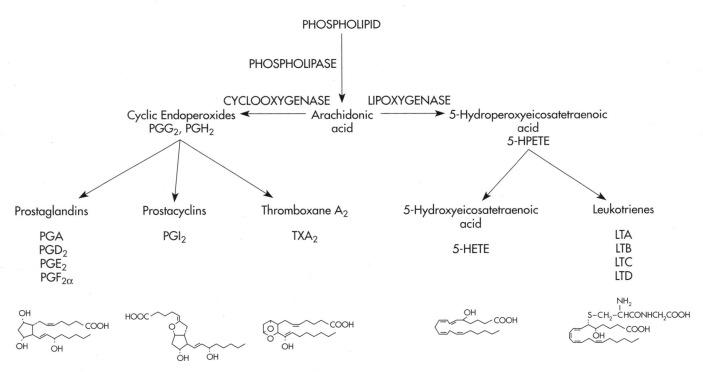

Fig. 13-18 Arachidonic acid metabolism. Five major groups of metabolites are formed: prostaglandins, prostacylclins, thromboxanes, 5-HETE, and leukotrienes. (From Ferrante FM, Vadeboncouer TR, editors: *Postoperative Pain Management*. New York, Churchill Livingstone, 1993.)

tion is the same for all nonsteroidal antiinflammatory drugs, but the individual response can be highly variable. This is reflected in clinical situations where patients respond well to some nonsteroidal antiinflammatory drugs and do not respond to others.[51,52] Some studies have stated that, because of the interpatient variability in side effects, efficacy, and pharmacokinetics, 10 to 15 nonsteroidal antiinflammatory drugs are necessary to provide a reasonable range of alternative therapy.[53]

Pharmacokinetics

Basic pharmacokinetic data of most nonsteroidal antiinflammatory drugs are summarized in Table 13-3. Reviews of the clinical pharmacokinetics of nonsteroidal antiinflammatory drugs have been previously published.[54] Overall, the nonsteroidal antiinflammatory drugs have similar pharmacokinetic characteristics: They are rapidly and extensively absorbed after oral administration, tissue distribution is very limited (because of high protein binding), they are metabolized extensively in the liver with little dependence on renal elimination, and they have low clearances.[55] Of particular clinical relevance is the observation that toxicity of many nonsteroidal antiinflammatory drugs may be related to their plasma half-lives—the longer the elimination half-life, the greater the risk of toxicity.[56]

Despite the overall similarity between nonsteroidal antiinflammatory drugs in their pharmacokinetic profiles, there are subclasses of the drugs with unique features. The most studied nonsteroidal antiinflammatory drugs are the salicylates, which demonstrate increasing half-life with increasing dose (Michaelis-Menten kinetics). It takes about 2 days to achieve steady-state blood concentrations when 1.5 g/day of aspirin is given to adults, while more than 1 week may be needed to achieve steady-state concentrations when the

dose is 3 g/day.[57] Salicylates also displace other nonsteroidal antiinflammatory drugs such as naproxen and phenylbutazone from plasma binding sites, increasing the free concentrations of those drugs and increasing the risk of toxicity.[58] Other clinically relevant pharmacokinetic characteristics are described in the sections describing the individual agents.

Differences in efficacy between nonsteroidal antiinflammatory drugs may be more related to the relative doses of the drugs being compared than to the properties of the medications. For example, one paper compared diclofenac, indocin, and piroxicam and noted wide differences in bioavailability and elimination between patients. This study suggested that these pharmacokinetic differences contributed to the phenomena of interpatient differences in drug responsiveness.[59] Such data must be interpreted relative to the data mentioned previously regarding individual variability in pharmacodynamic response to nonsteroidal antiinflammatory drugs.

Toxicity

Although they do not demonstrate tolerance or physical dependence like the opioids, nonsteroidal antiinflammatory drugs present a toxicity profile that is very significant. The use of nonsteroidal antiinflammatory drugs increased more than 100% between 1973 and 1983. More recently, the prescription rate has been stable, most likely because of physician awareness of the significance of the complications of nonsteroidal antiinflammatory drugs.[60] Nonetheless, recent studies regarding informed consent before institution of nonsteroidal antiinflammatory drug therapy revealed that, whereas epigastric discomfort was discussed 72% of the time, other side effects were mentioned less than 15% of the time.[61] Such statistics are disconcerting, given the

Table 13-3 Pharmacokinetic data of nonsteroidal antiinflammatory drugs

Drug (generic)	Drug (brand)	T1/2β (hr)	Vd (L/kg)	Cl (L/kg/hr)
Acetaminophen		2.8	1.0	0.25
Aspirin		0.25	0.2	.55
Diclofenac	Voltaren	1-2	0.12	0.04-0.08
Diflunisal	Dolobid	5-20	0.1	0.007
Etodolac	Lodine	7.3	0.362	0.047
Fenoprofen	Nalfon	2-3	0.1	0.02-0.04
Flurbiprofen	Ansaid	3-4	0.1	0.03-0.04
Ibuprofen	Motrin, Nuprin	2-2.5	0.14	0.04-0.05
Indomethacin	Indocin	6	0.12	0.014
Ketoprofen	Orudis	1.5	0.11	0.07
Ketorolac	Toradol	5.5	0.28	0.035
CMT	Trilisate	7	0.11	0.07
Nabumetone	Relafen	26	0.68	0.018
Naproxen	Naprosyn, Anaprox	12-15	0.10	0.005-0.006
Oxaprozin	Daypro	40-60	0.15	0.002
Piroxicam	Feldene	48.5	0.1	0.002
Salsalate	Mono-Gesic	3.8		0.21
Sulindac	Clinoril	1.5	0.52	0.21
Tolmetin	Tolectin	1	0.09	0.07

T1/2β, elimination half-life; Vd, volume of distribution; Cl, clearance.
*Choline magnesium trisalicylate.
From Denson D, Katz J: Nonsteroidal anti-inflammatory agents. In Raj PP: *Practical Management of Pain,* ed 2. St Louis, Mosby, 1992.

rather severe reactions to nonsteroidal antiinflammatory drugs possible in significant numbers of patients. Several reviews documented that complications from nonsteroidal antiinflammatory drugs resulted in an increased mortality in elderly arthritic patients who used nonsteroidal antiinflammatory drugs versus those who did not.[62,63] Also, the risk of toxicity from nonsteroidal antiinflammatory drugs for any organ system is greater with increasing age.[64] The three most common adverse drug reactions to nonsteroidal antiinflammatory drugs are GI, dermatologic, and neuropsychiatric, the last one (oddly) not being age related.[65] However, most clinically significant complications involve the GI, renal, hematologic, and hepatic organ systems.

One question repeatedly asked, particularly by pharmaceutical manufacturers, is whether one nonsteroidal antiinflammatory drug is more toxic than another. One review of 2747 rheumatoid arthritis patients, even controlling for patient factors, found more problems with indomethacin, tolmetin, and meclofenamate. The least toxic were coated or buffered aspirin, salsalate, and ibuprofen. The most toxic drugs were those usually taken in the lowest doses.[66]

GI toxicity

GI bleeding and perforation are the most frequently reported significant complications of nonsteroidal antiinflammatory drug use. One review estimated 7000 deaths and 70,000 hospitalizations per year in the United States among nonsteroidal antiinflammatory drug users.[67] Nonsteroidal antiinflammatory drug injury to the GI system usually involves antral and prepyloric gastric lesions. However, although 50% to 60% of patients taking nonsteroidal antiinflammatory drugs experience dyspepsia, silent ulcerations are still common, which necessitates vigilance by the prescribing physician.[68,69] Recent studies have implicated the bacteria *Helicobacter pylori* in the pathogenesis of peptic ulcer disease; however, prevalence of the bacteria is not affected by nonsteroidal antiinflammatory drug use.[70] The risk factors for nonsteroidal antiinflammatory drug gastropathy include age over 60 years, prior history of peptic ulcer disease, steroid use, alcohol use, multiple nonsteroidal antiinflammatory drug use, and possibly the first 3 months of nonsteroidal anti-inflammatory drug treatment.[71]

To prevent nonsteroidal antiinflammatory drug gastropathy, antacids and enteric coating have been added to some nonsteroidal antiinflammatory drugs and have had limited success. One study found that the use of magnesium hydroxide (Maalox) instead of placebo in combination with naproxen resulted in an increased incidence of gastric lesions.[72] Cimetidine and ranitidine are effective in treating gastric ulcers caused by nonsteroidal antiinflammatory drug use; but most data indicate they are not effective in preventing such ulcers, although some studies claim otherwise.[73-76]

Another drug used to prevent nonsteroidal antiinflammatory drug gastropathy is sucralfate. Sucralfate is a basic aluminum salt of sucrose octasulfate that aids the healing of gastric and duodenal ulcers by: (1) forming a complex with proteins at an ulcer base, thereby protecting it from further erosion; (2) stimulating prostaglandin synthesis in gastric mucosa; and (3) promoting gastric mucus secretion by a prostaglandin-independent mechanism. Its major advantage is a low side-effect profile, but it has not been demonstrated to be very effective in preventing nonsteroidal antiinflammatory drug gastropathy.[77]

The most successful drug available to prevent nonsteroidal antiinflammatory drug gastropathy is misoprostol. It is a synthetic analog of prostaglandin E_1. In a study comparing it to placebo and sucralfate, misoprostol 200 µg taken four times a day resulted in far fewer gastric lesions in patients taking nonsteroidal antiinflammatory drugs.[77] However, diarrhea can occur in up to 50% of patients using 200 µg four times daily, and in 25% of patients using 100 µg four times a day. It is also relatively expensive, so it is probably best to restrict use of the drug to those patients at increased risk of nonsteroidal antiinflammatory drug gastropathy who require nonsteroidal antiinflammatory drug use. There are data to support that the newer $H+/K+$ ATPase inhibitors that reduce acid secretion, e.g., omeprazole, may also be effective in preventing nonsteroidal antiinflammatory drug gastropathy.[78]

Renal toxicity

Prostaglandin regulation of renal blood flow is clinically significant in patients with heart failure, renal insufficiency, or liver disease, but not in normal patients.[79] Hence reduced renal blood flow with subsequent medullary ischemia may result from nonsteroidal antiinflammatory drug use in susceptible individuals.[80] Sulindac has theoretical advantages in the patient at risk for nonsteroidal antiinflammatory drug renal toxicity: It does not block PGE_2 or prostacycline in the kidney and thus should not impair renal blood flow.[81]

The resulting decline in glomerular filtration rate from nonsteroidal antiinflammatory drug use in susceptible individuals can lead to increased water and electrolyte reabsorption in the proximal tubule.[82] This in turn can antagonize antihypertensive therapies and even exacerbate congestive heart failure.[80,83] Nonsteroidal antiinflammatory drugs vary markedly in their effect on blood pressure. One review cited that naproxen and indomethacin produced significant rises in BP, and another study demonstrated that naproxen had a minimal effect on antihypertensive drug therapy.[84,85]

Acute renal injury from nonsteroidal antiinflammatory drug use has been reported. For example, it is possible in acute overdose of ibuprofen to induce acute renal failure with tubular necrosis.[86] Allergic nephritis to nonsteroidal antiinflammatory drugs can occur within 2 to 13 days of use and is accompanied by fever, skin eruptions, and serum IgE elevations. Tubulointerstitial nephritis occurs, and treatment consists of steroids and dialysis. However, not all cases will recover; and since all nonsteroidal antiinflammatory drugs are protein bound, they are not easily dialyzed.[87]

Hematologic toxicity

Nonsteroidal antiinflammatory drugs decrease platelet function with the exception of the nonacetylated salicylates, salsalate, and choline magnesium trisalicylate. Aspirin affects platelet function for the life of the platelet, and therefore can prolong bleeding time for 4 to 7 days after a single 650 mg dose. The other nonsteroidal antiinflammatory drugs induce a reversible platelet inhibition that resolves when the drug is mostly eliminated (in hours).[88] The clinical significance of these effects can be seen in studies of patients undergoing total hip replacement surgery: 140 patients had more intraoperative and postoperative blood loss when using nonsteroidal antiinflammatory drugs than those who did not.[89] Other studies confirmed that finding and noted more complications in patients using nonsteroidal antiinflammatory drugs with half-lives longer than 6 hours.[90]

Hepatic toxicity

Hepatic side effects of nonsteroidal antiinflammatory drugs have been reported to occur in 3% of patients receiving the drugs.[91,92] Reports associating the use of diclofenac with fulminant hepatitis have appeared in American and European literature, but it is not clear whether the incidence of diclofenac-induced hepatitis is higher than the incidence for other nonsteroidal antiinflammatory drugs.[93,94] The mechanism of such hepatotoxicity is not well defined, but it seems advisable to follow liver function tests in patients on long-term nonsteroidal antiinflammatory drug therapy.[95]

Specific drugs

Salicylates

Aspirin. Aspirin is the most studied and commonly used nonsteroidal antiinflammatory drug. Aspirin has an elimination half-life that changes from 2.5 hours at low doses to 19 hours at high doses. It is well absorbed in the stomach and small intestine, with peak blood levels 1 hour after an oral dose. There is then rapid conversion of aspirin to salicylates from high first-pass effect, which occurs in both the wall of the small intestine and the liver.

Diflunisal. Diflunisal is possibly better tolerated in the GI system because it is not metabolized to salicylic acid in plasma. It has a short half-life relative to aspirin.

Choline magnesium trisalicylate and salsalate. Both are nonacetylated salicylates that have minimal effect on platelet function and less effect on GI mucosa than their acetylated counterparts. They produce similar analgesia and blood levels of salicylate to those of the acetylated class.

Acetaminophen. Acetaminophen is a paraaminophenol derivative with analgesic and antipyretic properties similar to those of aspirin. Antipyresis is likely from direct action on the hypothalamic heat-regulating centers via inhibiting action of endogenous pyrogen. Although equipotent to aspirin in inhibiting central prostaglandin synthesis, acetaminophen has no significant peripheral prostaglandin synthetase inhibition. Doses of 650 mg have been shown to be more effective than doses of 300 mg; but little additional benefit is seen at doses above 650 mg, indicating a possible ceiling effect. It has few side effects in the usual dosage range; no significant GI toxicity or platelet functional changes occur with acetaminophen use. It is almost entirely metabolized in the liver, and the minor metabolites are responsible for the hepatotoxicity seen in overdose. Inducers of the P-450 enzyme system in the liver (such as alcohol) increase the formation of metabolites and therefore increase hepatotoxicity.

Acetic acid derivatives. This group of nonsteroidal antiinflammatory drugs contains two subclasses: pyrroleacetic

acids and phenylacetic acids (of which only diclofenac is approved for use in the United States so far).

Indomethacin. Indomethacin has good oral and rectal absorption although the extent of absorption varies widely between patients. There is also a large interpatient variability in elimination half-life, caused by extensive enterohepatic recirculation of the drug. Its clinical use is somewhat limited by a relatively high incidence of side effects.

Sulindac. Sulindac was the result of a search for a drug similar to indomethacin but with less toxicity. The lower GI toxicity with sulindac may be because sulindac is an inactive prodrug that is converted after absorption by liver microsomal enzymes to sulindac disulfide, which appears to be the active metabolite. However, one study demonstrated a relatively high rate of GI hemorrhage with sulindac.[96] As mentioned previously, sulindac was considered in previous studies to be the least nephrotoxic of the nonsteroidal antiinflammatory drugs, but more recent studies have failed to support that contention.[97,98]

Tolmetin and etodolac. Both of these drugs claim fewer side effects than other nonsteroidal antiinflammatory drugs.

Ketorolac. Ketorolac is currently the only parenteral nonsteroidal antiinflammatory drug for clinical analgesic use in the United States. Although indomethacin has been available as an injectable form for years, it was pursued only in low dose as a treatment for patent ductus arteriosus. Ketorolac demonstrates analgesia well beyond antiinflammatory properties that are between those of indomethacin and naproxen; but ketorolac can provide analgesia 50 times that of naproxen. It has antipyretic effects 20 times that of aspirin and thus can mask temperatures when given routinely to patients postoperatively. Several studies have demonstrated efficacy comparable to or exceeding that of morphine for moderate postoperative pain treatment but with fewer side effects.[99,100] Although ketorolac prolongs bleeding time, it does not do so excessively; however, case reports of postoperative bleeding associated with intraoperative ketorolac use have been reported.[101,102] Oral ketorolac was approved for use in the United States approximately 3 years after the parenteral form and has an efficacy similar to that of naproxen and ibuprofen.[103] However, the parenteral form is given in a loading dose of 60 mg followed by 30 mg IM every 6 hours, whereas the oral dose is limited to 10 to 20 mg because of GI toxicity.

Diclofenac. Diclofenac differs from the other nonsteroidal antiinflammatory drugs by having a high first-pass effect and hence a lower oral bioavailability. As mentioned previously, it may also have a significantly higher incidence of hepatotoxicity than the other nonsteroidal antiinflammatory drugs. A parenteral form has been used in Europe, and one study showed it effective in reducing opioid requirements and pain after thoracotomies.[104]

Propionic acid derivatives. This class contains ibuprofen, fenoprofen, ketoprofen, flurbiprofen, and naproxen. A newer drug in this class is oxaprozin, which has received attention because it has a once-daily dosing; but it has no other distinct advantage over other nonsteroidal antiinflammatory drugs.[105]

Oxicam derivatives. The only nonsteroidal antiinflammatory drug in this class in clinical use is piroxicam. Unlike other nonsteroidal antiinflammatory drugs, it has a slow time to peak serum concentration following oral dosing of 5.5 hours. It is also notable for its long elimination half-life of 48.5 hours, so it may take up to one week to achieve steady state blood concentrations, although it does also allow for once-daily dosing.

Pyrazolone derivatives. The only drug in clinical use in this class is phenylbutazone. Although phenylbutazone is a very effective antiinflammatory and analgesic, it has been associated with aplastic anemias and agranulocytosis; therefore it cannot be recommended for long-term use. It is thus not often clinically used.

Anthranilic acid derivatives. These nonsteroidal antiinflammatory drugs are unique because they block prostaglandin synthesis and the tissue response to prostaglandins. Mefenamic acid has been associated with severe pancytopenia and many other side effects. Therefore therapy cannot to be used longer than 1 week.[106] Meclofenamate has a high incidence of GI toxicity and is also not a first-line drug.

Naphthyl-alkanones. This new class of nonsteroidal antiinflammatory drug is most noted for being a nonacidic chemical structure unlike other clinically used nonsteroidal antiinflammatory drugs. Some describe the structure as similar to naproxen. The only clinically available nonsteroidal antiinflammatory drug in this class is nabumetone. Studies have shown that its use results in fewer gastric lesions than aspirin, naproxen, or ibuprofen. Also, doses of 1 g/day for 7 days in volunteers resulted in no change in bleeding time. Only 35% of the drug is converted to its active form after oral administration. None of the parent drug can be measured in plasma after oral administration because of the rapid biotransformation that occurs during first- pass, which makes nabumetone a prodrug.[107]

REFERENCES

1. Colasanti B: Narcotic analgesics and antagonists. In Craig C, Stitzel R, editors: *Modern Pharmacology,* ed 3. Boston, Little, Brown, 1990.
2. Anand KJ, Carr DB: The neuroanatomy, neurophysiology, and neurochemistry of pain, stress, and analgesia in newborns and children. *Pediatr Clin North Am* 36:795-822, 1989.
3. Lord J et al: Endogenous opioid peptides: Multiple agonists and receptors. *Nature* 267:495, 1977.
4. Pasternak G: Multiple morphine and enkephalin receptors and the relief of pain. *JAMA* 259:1362-1367, 1988.
5. Czlonkowski A et al: Opiate receptor binding sites in human spinal cord. *Brain Res* 267:392-394, 1983.
6. Stein C: Peripheral mechanisms of opioid analgesia. *Anesth Analg* 76:182-191, 1993.
7. Junien J, Wettstein J: Role of opioids in peripheral analgesia. *Life Sci* 51:2009-2018, 1992.
8. Bodnar R, Paul D, Pasternak G: Synergistic interactions between the periaqueductal gray and the locus coeruleus. *Brain Res* 558:224-230, 1991.
9. Hill H, Mather L: Patient-controlled analgesia, pharmacokinetic and therapeutic considerations. *Clin Pharmacokinet* 24:124-140, 1993.
10. Ling G et al: Dissociation of morphine's analgesic and respiratory depressant actions. *Eur J Pharmacol* 86:487-488, 1983.
11. Gintzler A, Pasternak G: Multiple mu receptors: Evidence for mu$_2$ sites in the guinea pig ilium. *Neurosci Lett* 39:51-56, 1983.
12. Heyman J et al: Dissociation of opioid antinociception and central gastrointestinal propulsion in the mouse: Studies with naloxonazine. *J Pharmacol Exp Ther* 245:238-243, 1988.
13. Economou G, Ward-McQuaid W: A cross-over comparison of the effect of morphine, pethidine, pentazocine, and phenazocine in biliary pressure. *Gut* 12:218-221, 1971.
14. Radnay P et al: The effect of equi-analgesic doses of fentanyl, morphine, meperidine and pentazocine on common bile duct pressure. *Anaesthetist* 29:26-29, 1980.
15. Jaffe J, Marin W: Opioid analgesics and antagonists. In Gilman A et al, editors: *Goodman and Gilman's The Pharmacological Basis of Therapeutics.* New York, Pergamon Press, 1990.
16. Reitan J et al: Central vagal control of fentanyl induced bradycardia during halothane anesthesia. *Anesth Analg* 57:31-36, 1978.
17. Stanley T et al: Cardiovascular effects of nitrous oxide during meperidine infusion in the dog. *Anesth Analg* 56:836-841, 1977.
18. Freye E: Cardiovascular effects of high dosages of fentanyl, meperidine and naloxone in dogs. *Anesth Analg* 53:40-47, 1974.
19. Rosow C et al: Histamine release during morphine and fentanyl anesthesia. *Anesthesiology* 56:93-96, 1982.
20. Bovill J, Sebel P, Stanley T: Opioid analgesics in anesthesia: With special reference to their use in cardiovascular anesthesia. *Anesthesiology* 61:731-755, 1984.
21. McEvoy G, editor: *American Hospital Formulary Service, 1993.* American Society of Hospital Pharmacists, Bethesda, Md, 1993.
22. Rudy T, Yaksh T: Hyperthermic effects of morphine: Set point manipulation by a direct spinal action. *Br J Pharmacol* 61:91-96, 1977.
23. Cousins M, Mather L: Intrathecal and epidural administration of opioids. *Anesthesiology* 1:276-310, 1984.
24. Bullingham R, McQuay J, Moore R: Unexpectedly high plasma fentanyl levels after epidural use. *Lancet* 1:1361-1362, 1980.
25. Mather L: Clinical pharmacokinetics of analgesic drugs. In Raj PP, editor: *Practical Management of Pain,* ed 2. St Louis, Mosby, 1992.
26. Paul D et al: Pharmacological characterization of morphine 6β-glucuronide, a very potent morphine metabolite. *J Pharmacol Exp Ther* 251:477-483, 1989.
27. Dayer P et al: Bioactivation of the narcotic drug codeine is mediated by the polymorphic monooxygenase catalyzing debrisoquine 4-hydroxylation. *Biochem Biophys Res Commun* 152:411-416, 1988.
28. Inturrisi C et al: Heroin: Disposition in cancer patients. *Clin Pharmacol Ther* 31:235, 1982.
29. Sunshine A, Laska E, Olson N: Analgesic effects of oral oxycodone and codeine in the treatment of patients with postoperative, postfracture, or somatic pain. In Foley K, Inturrisi C, editors: *Advances in Pain Research and Therapy, vol 8.* New York, Macmillan, 1985.
30. Fainsinger R, Schoeller T, Bruera E: Methadone in the management of cancer pain: A review. *Pain* 52:137-147, 1993.
31. Smith R: Federal government faces painful decision on Darvon. *Science* 203:857-858, 1971.
32. Holland D, Steinberg M: Electrophysiological properties of propoxyphene or norpropoxyphene in canine cardiac conducting tissues in vitro and in vivo. *Toxicol Appl Pharmacol* 47:123-133, 1979.
33. Nicklander R, Smits S, Steinberg M: Propoxyphene and norpropoxyphene: Pharmacology and toxic effects in animals. *J Pharmacol Exp Ther* 200:245-253, 1977.
34. Giacomini K et al: Propoxyphene and norpropoxyphene plasma concentrations after oral propoxyphene in cirrhotic patients with and without surgically constructed portacaval shunt. *Clin Pharmacol Ther* 28:417-424, 1980.
35. Hansen B et al: Influence of dextropropoxyphene on steady state serum levels and protein binding of three antiepileptic drugs in man. *Acta Neurol Scand* 61:357-367, 1980.
36. Austin K, Stapleton J, Mather L: Rate of formation of norpethidine from pethidine. *Br J Anaesth* 53:255-258, 1981.
37. Dayer P, Collart L, Desmeules J: The pharmacology of tramadol. *Drugs* 47(S1):3-7, 1994.
38. O'Brien J, Benfield P: Dezocine: A preliminary review of its pharmacodynamic and pharmacokinetic properties, and therapeutic efficacy. *Drugs* 38:226-248, 1989.
39. Clive D, Stoff J: Renal syndromes associated with nonsteroidal antiinflammatory drugs. *N Engl J Med* 310:563-572, 1984.
40. Flower R, Moncada S, Vane J: Analgesic-antipyretics and antiinflammatory agents; drugs employed in the treatment of gout. In Gilman A et al, editors: *The Pharmacological Basis of Therapeutics,* ed 7. New York, Macmillan, 1985.
41. Parr G et al: Joint pain and quality of life: Results of a randomised trial. *Br J Clin Pharmacol* 27:235-242, 1989.
42. McCormack K, Brune K: Dissociation between the antinociceptive and anti-inflammatory effects of the nonsteroidal anti-inflammatory

drugs. A survey of their analgesic efficacy. *Drugs* 41:533-547, 1991.

43. Ferreira S: Prostaglandins: Peripheral and central analgesia. In Bonica JJ, Lindblom U, Iggo A, editors: *Advances in Pain Research and Therapy, vol 5.* New York, Raven Press, 1983.

44. Willer J, De Broucker T, Bussel B: Central analgesic effects of ketoprofen in humans: Electrophysiological evidence for a supraspinal mechanism in a double-blind and cross-over study. *Pain* 38:1-7, 1989.

45. Carlsson K, Monzel W, Jurna I: Depression by morphine and the nonopioid analgesic agents metamizol, lysine acetylate and paracetamol, of activity in rat thalamus neurons evoked by electrical stimulation of nociceptive afferents. *Pain* 32:313-326, 1988.

46. Taiwo Y, Levine J: Prostaglandins inhibit endogenous pain control mechanisms by blocking transmission at spinal noradrenergic synapses. *J Neurosci* 8:1346-1349, 1988.

47. Fabbri A et al: Piroxicam-induced analgesia: Evidence for a central component which is not opioid mediated. *Experientia* 48:1139-1142, 1992.

48. Bannwarth B et al: Clinical pharmacokinetics of nonsteroidal antiinflammatory drugs in the cerebrospinal fluid. *Biomed Pharmacother* 43:121-126, 1989.

49. Catania A et al: Inhibition of acute inflammation in the periphery by central action of salicylates. *Proc Natl Acad Sci USA* 88:8544-8547, 1991.

50. Abramson S: Therapy with and mechanisms of nonsteroidal antiinflammatory drugs. *Curr Opin Rheumatol* 3:336-340, 1991.

51. Day R et al: Variability in response to NSAIDs—fact or fiction? *Drugs* 36:643-651, 1988.

52. Day R et al: Clinical pharmacology of nonsteroidal anti-inflammatory drugs. *Pharmacol Ther* 33:384-433, 1987.

53. Dukes M, Lunde I: The regulatory control of nonsteroidal antiinflammatory drug preparations within individual rheumatology private practices. *J Rheumatol* 16:1253-1258, 1989.

54. Verbeeck R, Blackburn J, Lowewen G: Clinical pharmacokinetics of nonsteroidal anti-inflammatory drugs. *Clin Pharmacokinet* 8:297-331, 1983.

55. Denson D, Katz J: Nonsteroidal anti-inflammatory agents. In Raj PP, editor: *Practical Management of Pain,* ed 2. St Louis, Mosby, 1992.

56. Adams S: Non-steroidal, anti-inflammatory drugs, plasma half-lives, and adverse reactions. *Lancet* 2:1204-1205, 1987.

57. Levy G, Tsuchiya T: Salicylate accumulation kinetics in man. *N Engl J Med* 287:430-432, 1972.

58. Hayes A: Therapeutic implications of drug interactions with acetaminophen and aspirin. *Arch Intern Med* 141:301-304, 1981.

59. Brune K: Clinical relevance of nonsteroidal anti-inflammatory drug pharmacokinetics. *Eur J Rheumatol Inflamm* 8:18-23, 1987.

60. Gabriel S, Fehring R: Trends in the utilization of non-steroidal antiinflammatory drugs in the United States, 1986-1990. *J Clin Epidemiol* 45:1041-1044, 1992.

61. Katz J et al: Informed consent and the prescription of nonsteroidal anti-inflammatory drugs. *Arthritis Rheum* 35:1257-1263, 1992.

62. Griffin M, Ray W, Schaffner W: Non-steroidal anti-inflammatory drug use and death from peptic ulcer in elderly persons. *Ann Intern Med* 109:359-363, 1988.

63. Nuki G: Pain control and the use of non-steroidal analgesic antiinflammatory drugs. *Br Med Bull* 46:262-278, 1990.

64. Weinblatt M: Nonsteroidal anti-inflammatory drug toxicity: Increased risk in the elderly. *Scand J Rheumatol Suppl* 91:9-17, 1991.

65. Clark D, Ghose K: Neuropsychiatric reactions to nonsteroidal antiinflammatory drugs. The New Zealand experience. *Drug Saf* 7:460-465, 1992.

66. Fries J, Williams C, Bloch D: The relative toxicity of nonsteroidal anti-inflammatory drugs. *Arthritis Rheum* 34:1353-1360, 1991.

67. Fries J: NSAID gastropathy: The second most deadly rheumatic disease? *J Rheumatol Suppl* 28:6-10, 1991.

68. Roth S: Non-steroidal anti-inflammatory drugs: Gastropathy, deaths and medical practice. *Ann Intern Med* 109:353-354, 1988.

69. Caruso I, Bianchi Porro G: Gastroscopic evaluation of antiinflammatory agents. *BMJ* 1:75-78, 1980.

70. Laine L: *Helicobacter pylori,* gastric ulcer, and agents noxious to the gastric mucosa. *Gastroenterol Clin North Am* 22:117-125, 1993.

71. Gabriel S, Jaakkimainen L, Bombardier C: Risk for serious gastrointestinal complications related to use of nonsteroidal antiinflammatory drugs. A meta-analysis. *Ann Intern Med* 115:787-796, 1991.

72. Sievert W et al: Low dose antacids and nonsteroidal antiinflammatory drug-induced gastropathy in humans. *J Clin Gastroenterol* 13 (Suppl 1):S145-S148, 1991.

73. Roth S et al: Cimetidine therapy in non-steroidal anti-inflammatory drug gastropathy. *Arch Int Med* 147:1799-1801, 1987.

74. Ehsanullah R et al: Prevention of gastro-duodenal damage induced by non-steroidal anti-inflammatory drugs: Controlled trial of ranitidine. *BMJ* 297:1017-1021, 1988.

75. Rachmilewitz D: The role of H2-receptor antagonists in the prevention of NSAID-induced gastrointestinal damage. *Aliment Pharmacol Ther* 2(S):65-73, 1988.

76. Robinson M, Mills R, Euler A: Ranitidine prevents duodenal ulcers associated with non-steroidal anti-inflammatory drug therapy. *Aliment Pharmacol Ther* 5:143-150, 1991.

77. Agrawal N et al: Misoprostol compared with sucralfate in the prevention of nonsteroidal anti-inflammatory drug induced gastric ulcer. *Ann Intern Med* 115:195-200, 1991.

78. Agrawal N, Dajani E: Prevention and treatment of ulcers induced by nonsteroidal anti-inflammatory drugs. *J Assoc Acad Minor Phys* 3:142-148, 1992.

79. Dunn M et al: Non-steroidal anti-inflammatory drugs and renal function. *J Clin Pharmacol* 28:524-529, 1988.

80. Carmichael, Shankel S: Renal effects of nonsteroidal antiinflammatory drugs. *Am J Med* 78:992-1000, 1985.

81. Clabattoni G et al: Renal effects of anti-inflammatory drugs. *Eur J Rheumatol* 3:210-221, 1980.

82. Donker A et al: Effect of indomethacin on kidney function and plasma renin activity in man. *Nephron* 16:288-296, 1976.

83. Davis A, Day R, Begg B: Interactions between non-steroidal antiinflammatory drugs and anti-hypertensive diuretics. *Aust NZ J Med* 16:537-546, 1986.

84. Weiss Y et al: Maintenance of blood pressure control in elderly hypertensives on ketoprofen. *Scand J Rheumatol Suppl* 91:37-44, 1991.

85. Pope J, Anderson J, Felson D: A meta-analysis of the effects of nonsteroidal anti-inflammatory drugs on blood pressure. *Arch Intern Med* 153:477-484, 1993.

86. Perazella M, Buller G: Can ibuprofen cause acute renal failure in a normal individual? *Am J Kidney Dis* 18:600-602, 1991.

87. Shibasaki T et al: Clinical characterization of drug-induced allergic nephritis. *Am J Nephrol* 11:174-180, 1991.

88. Kantor T: Peripherally-acting analgesics. In Kuhar M, Pasternak G, editors: *Analgesics, Neurochemical, Behavioral, and Clinical Perspectives.* New York, Raven Press, 1984.

89. An HS et al: Effects of hypotensive anesthesia, nonsteroidal antiinflammatory drugs, and polymethylmethacrylate on bleeding in total hip arthroplasty patients. *J Arthroplasty* 6:245-250, 1991.

90. Connelly C, Panush R: Should nonsteroidal anti-inflammatory drugs be stopped before elective surgery? *Arch Intern Med* 151:1963-1966, 1991.

91. Kromaann-Anderson H, Pedersen A: Reported adverse reactions to and consumption of nonsteroidal anti-inflammatory drugs in Denmark over a 17-year period. *Dan Med Bull* 35:187-192, 1988.

92. Rabinovitz M, Van Thiel D: Hepatotoxicity of nonsteroidal antiinflammatory drugs. *Am J Gastroenterol* 87:1696-1704, 1992.

93. Helfgott S et al: Diclofenac associated hepatotoxicity. *JAMA* 264:2660-2662, 1990.

94. Babany G et al: Fulminating hepatitis in a woman taking glafenine and diclofenac. *Gastroenterol Clin Biol* 9:185, 1985.

95. Gay G: Another side effect of NSAIDs. *JAMA* 264:2677-2678, 1990.

96. Carson J et al: The relative gastrointestinal toxicity of the nonsteroidal anti-inflammatory drugs. *Arch Intern Med* 147:1054-1059, 1987.

97. Roberts D et al: Sulindac is not renal sparing in man. *Clin Pharmacol Ther* 38:258-265, 1985.

98. Quintero E et al: Sulindac reduces the urinary excretion of prostaglandins and impairs renal function in cirrhosis with ascites. *Nephron* 42:298-303, 1986.

99. Stouten E et al: Comparison of ketorolac and morphine for postoperative pain after major surgery. *Acta Anaesthesiol Scand* 36:716-721, 1992.

100. Brown C et al: Comparison of repeat doses of intramuscular ketoro-

lac tromethamine and morphine sulfate for analgesia after major surgery. *Pharmacotherapy* 10:45S-50S, 1990.
101. Greer I: Effects of ketorolac tromethamine on hemostasis. *Pharmacotherapy* 10:71S-76S, 1990.
102. Garcha I, Bostwick J: Postoperative hematomas associated with Toradol [letter]. *Plast Reconstr Surg* 88:919-920, 1991.
103. Forbes JA et al: Evaluation of ketorolac, ibuprofen, acetaminophen, and an acetaminophen-codeine combination in postoperative oral surgery pain. *Pharmacotherapy* 10:94S-105S, 1990.
104. Rhodes M: Nonsteroidal anti-inflammatory drugs for postthoracotomy pain. *J Thorac Cardiovasc Surg* 103:17-20, 1992.
105. Miller L: Oxaprozin: A once-daily nonsteroidal anti-inflammatory drug. *Clin Pharm* 11:591-603, 1992.
106. *Medical Letter* 14:31, 1972.
107. Dahl S: Nabumetone: A "nonacidic" nonsteroidal anti-inflammatory drug. *Ann Pharmacother* 27:456-463, 1993.

QUESTIONS: OPIOIDS AND NONSTEROIDAL ANTIINFLAMMATORY DRUGS

For questions 1-4, choose from the following:
A. 1,2, and 3
B. 1 and 3
C. 2 and 4
D. 4
E. All of the above

1. Which of the following opioids are naturally occurring?
   1. Morphine
   2. Hydromorphone
   3. Codeine
   4. Methadone

2. Which of the following statements is (are) true regarding classes of opioid drugs and their analgesic effects?
   1. κ receptor agonists can provide good analgesia.
   2. A potent ς opioid receptor agonist will likely have significant excitatory effects relative to its analgesic properties.
   3. δ receptor agonists will likely produce similar analgesic effects to those of μ agonists.
   4. Agonists of μ_1 and μ_2 receptors produce both analgesia and respiratory depression.

3. Which of the following factors explains the relatively rapid onset of alfentanil as compared with other opioids?
   1. Alfentanil is far more lipid-soluble than most opioids, including fentanyl and morphine.
   2. Alfentanil has a far greater unionized fraction than morphine in plasma.
   3. Alfentanil has a long elimination half-life relative to other opioids such as sufentanil or fentanyl, allowing it to quickly accumulate high blood concentrations.
   4. Alfentanil has a very small volume of distribution compared with most of the other opioids.

4. The following is (are) true regarding nonsteroidal antiinflammatory drug renal toxicity:
   1. The risk of renal toxicity is not related to patient intravascular volume status.
   2. Tubulointerstitial nephritis from nonsteroidal antiinflammatory drugs is a form of allergic reaction.
   3. Even normal patients are highly dependent on prostaglandins for regulation of renal blood flow.
   4. Renal effects of nonsteroidal antiinflammatory drugs can antagonize the effects of antihypertensive drugs and worsen preexisting heart failure.

5. Oral morphine sustained-release formulations and oral methadone are both used to provide prolonged analgesia in patients with cancer pain. Which of the following comparisons between the two drugs is true?
   A. Sustained-release formulations provide longer effect than regular morphine preparations by prolonging the elimination half-life of morphine.
   B. Methadone is far more likely to accumulate in the bloodstream than morphine because of its much longer half-life.
   C. Like methadone, slow-release morphine preparations can be prepared in elixir form.
   D. Slow-release morphine preparations are *less* dependent upon variations in GI transit than methadone.

ANSWERS

1. B
2. E
3. D
4. C
5. B

14 Coanalgesic Agents*

J. David Haddox

The objective of this chapter is to review a practical guide for using adjunctive agents in pain management.

ANTIDEPRESSANTS

Since being introduced about three decades ago, antidepressants have become the mainstay of the pharmacologic treatment of depression. Clinical use has gradually increased, usually by serendipity, to include the treatment of several nonaffective conditions, such as generalized anxiety disorders, phobias, panic disorder, enuresis, eating disorders, peptic ulcer disease, and pain syndromes.[1] Their use for pain has evolved from anecdotal reports and observations that many depressed patients complain of pain problems that seem to resolve when their depression lifts.[2] There are similarities between patients with chronic pain and depression: sleep disturbance, somatic focus, fatigue, hopelessness, etc.[3-15] Some authors have suggested that patients whose pain complaints responded to antidepressant medication were in fact exhibiting a somatic delusion or another manifestation of an otherwise "masked" depression. The relationship between depression and pain has recently been explored by Turk and Rudy in a series of articles that comprehensively analyzes the extant literature.[16]

The first drugs to be marketed as *antidepressants* are generally referred to as the *tricyclic* antidepressants because they all are three ringed with more or less substitution on the middle ring. The tricyclics are further subclassified as secondary or tertiary amines based on the terminal substitution of the side chain. Secondary amines can be derived in the body from tertiary amines (with the exception of amoxapine) and tend to have less side effects than the parent tertiary compound.

With the introduction of maprotiline, the term *tetracyclic* has been used to describe this drug. Currently, there are several other drugs available (trazodone, bupropion) that make a general classification system cumbersome. The term *heterocyclics* has been used, but there is no agreement as to precisely what this denotes. For these reasons the term *antidepressants* will be used in this chapter.

Pharmacology

The antidepressants are generally well absorbed after oral administration,[1] although this may be decreased by the anticholinergic activity of these drugs.[1,17-19] They undergo extensive first-pass hepatic metabolism[20] and are highly bound to serum proteins, especially alpha$_1$ acid glycoprotein. Since this is an acute-phase reactant that increases in response to acute myocardial infarction, burns, and infections, it can increase binding and total serum levels with no change in clinical effect.[20] These drugs are highly lipophilic and have correspondingly large apparent volumes of distribution, on the order of 10 to 50 L/kg.[1,21] Their elimination half-lives are long (1 to 4 days), and they frequently have active metabolites, some of which are synthesized and marketed: desipramine from imipramine, nortryptiline from amitriptyline.[1,17,21] The drugs are generally oxidized by the hepatic microsomal system and conjugated with glucuronic acid.[1] Elimination occurs via urine and feces.[22]

There is wide variability among individuals in serum levels from these drugs, due most likely to variation in clearance.[18,20,23] Addition or reduction of other drugs can also affect levels within a patient.[23-27] Serum levels are available for all antidepressants and should report not only the concentration of the drug being given, but also the level of any active metabolites because these may account for different effects than the parent drug.[1,20,21] Interpretation of serum levels can be influenced by a number of factors,[20] and sampling time for a given patient should be the same time before the next dosing interval or after the patient is thought to have reached a steady state concentration.[1,20,21,28] Therapeutic ranges have been established for most of these drugs, and their effectiveness for affective disorders and toxicity appears to correlate with the ranges.[1,29] Therapeutic serum levels for use in pain management independent of depression have not been determined.[30]

Antidepressants exert their actions on affect by altering monamine neurotransmitter activity at the level of the synapse.[1,17,31] Specifically, they block the presynaptic reuptake of serotonin and norepinephrine by the amine pump. This is an almost immediate effect, yet it is well-accepted clinically that there is a typical lag of 1 to 4 weeks between initiation of therapy and onset of effect when the drugs are used for the treatment of depression. A similar latency to maximum benefit when used for pain has been demonstrated in some studies[6,32,33,34] and not in others.[35-37] Antidepressants also cause sedation, but this has not been felt to be the primary therapeutic effect.[34] Problems not frequently mentioned in ascertaining the mechanism of action of these drugs in pain treatment are the difference between older and newer uptake-blockade-assay methodologies[17] and the differences between acute and chronic administration of antidepressants.[17,21,31] It appears that neurotransmitter modulation is the probable mechanism.

*Text derived from Haddox JD: Neurophyschiatric drug use in management. In Raj PP, editor: *Practical Management of Pain*, ed 2. St Louis, Mosby, 1992.

The anticholinergic effects of antidepressants are generally confined to muscarinic receptors and may contribute to xerostomia, visual accommodation difficulties, constipation, tachycardia, urinary retention, reduced gastric motility and delayed emptying, reduced secretion of gastric acid, and worsening of narrow-angle glaucoma.[1,17,38] The cholinomimetic bethanechol has been used to overcome antimuscarinic effects,[39] but with the wide variation in antimuscarinic profiles found today, it is probably more prudent to change drugs than to add a new one in most instances.[17]

Many of the currently available antidepressants are potent antihistaminics as well.[17] These drugs may block both the H_1 and the H_2 receptors. Imipramine was synthesized in a search for potential antihistaminic and sedative drugs, and its antidepressant efficacy was discovered incidentally.[1] Cell culture studies have shown that doxepin is one of the most potent histamine receptor blockers known.[17] The brain contains H_1 receptors, and the antihistaminic potency of the antidepressants correlates fairly closely to the sedation experienced by many patients.

Blockade of the H_2 receptors associated with gastric acid secretion may be a desirable effect in many patients who have a past or current problem with reflux, ulcers, or are at risk for these diseases. Some receptor affinity assay studies have shown that certain antidepressants are more potent at blocking the H_2 receptor than cimetidine. Although extrapolating directly from receptor studies in animal tissues to intact humans is not always reliable, there have been some studies that show that trimipramine[38] and doxepin[40] hasten healing of gastric ulcers in humans.

Perhaps one of the most potentially dangerous side effects of antidepressants is the occurrence of orthostatic hypotension. This effect is generally thought to be mediated by α_1-adrenergic blockade. There are also data that suggest that the orthostatic hypotension may be due to serotonin reuptake blockade.[17] Radioligand studies show the antidepressants to be relatively weak antagonists of the central presynaptic α_2-adrenergic receptor.[17]

Antidepressants do not appear, based on current information, to have any antagonistic effects on benzodiazepine, γ-aminobutyric acid, and β-adrenergic or opiate receptors.[17]

Antidepressants are not considered to have an addiction liability in the true sense; that is, their use is not associated with a drive to obtain and use the drug. They may, however, be associated with withdrawal syndromes.[41] These are generally precipitated by abrupt discontinuation of substantial doses of the drugs. The symptoms most likely to occur in the pain population, who generally benefit from dosages smaller than those employed in the treatment of affective diseases, are associated with the effects of these drugs on sleep structure. Abrupt stopping of antidepressants can lead to sleep disruption characterized by the perception of nearly constant, extremely vivid and colorful dreams that are usually not dysphoric, but stand out because of their intensity. Patients will often report that they feel as though they have "been at the movies all night." This will generally resolve in a few days. Other phenomena include gastrointestinal distress, restlessness, and occasional psychic activation. Some authors have noted that these symptoms are suggestive of cholinergic rebound and have recommended treatment with anticholinergic drugs.[41] In practice, these problems can virtually always be prevented by gradually discontinuing these drugs over 5 to 10 days. Emergence of any symptoms can be managed by reducing the rate of the withdrawal schedule or reinstituting the drug.

The presenting signs of an antidepressant overdose are related to extreme manifestations of their sedative effects, anticholinergic actions, and their influence on the cardiac conduction system, which is similar to that of quinidine. The most common presentation of substantial overdose is coma.[1,18,42,43] This is frequently accompanied by significant hypotension,[1,18,43,44] which may be unresponsive to fluids and dopamine but may respond to norepinephrine.[45] An anticholinergic syndrome consisting of mydriasis, dry skin and mucosae, flushed appearance, warm skin, decreased bowel function, urinary retention, tachycardia and, if conscious, delirium is usually a predominant feature.[1,18,43] Disturbances of cardiac conduction manifest as a prolonged QT interval and superventricular dysrythmias.[1,18,42,43] Adult respiratory distress syndrome[46] and respiratory depression may also complicate the postoverdose course.[1,18,43] Seizures may be present in about 10% of overdose cases.[43] A particularly dangerous aspect of overdose with these drugs is the potential to develop late (after 72 hours) complications, which may be fatal.[1,18,43] A recent review of the management of this type of overdose stated that patients should be aggressively managed until they have been symptom free for 24 hours.[18]

Initial treatment of overdoses requires the immediate institution of airway management, ventilatory and cardiovascular support, gastric lavage, and control of seizures. Physostigmine was once recommended as the "antidote" for antidepressant toxicity because of its ability to cross the blood-brain barrier and reverse the antimuscarinic features by inhibiting acetylcholine esterase. It has little effect on the cardiac manifestations of overdose and may cause other serious complications, such as bradycardia.[18] Dialysis does not seem to significantly alter the course of treatment.[1,18] A more detailed discussion of the problem is found in the review by Frommer et al.[18]

Antidepressants can cause a number of other side effects ranging from skin rashes, which may be photosensitive,[47,48] to jaundice.[1] Fluctuation in weight can be a problem. The earlier drugs tend to cause weight gain,[1] and some of the newer drugs are associated with little change or weight loss.[49-51] The occasional patient will complain of sexual difficulties while taking antidepressants.[1] With the notable exception of lithium, clinical experience has shown little teratogenic potential of the antidepressants, even when taken early in gestation.[52,53] It is, of course, advisable to avoid the use of any nonessential medication during pregnancy and lactation.

Efficacy in pain management

Most review articles conclude that either the use of antidepressants for various pain states is widespread but not well-supported[31,54,55] or that they have special utility in treating chronic pain.[9,56] All reviewers mention the relationship between the monoamine hypothesis of affective disorders and the role these compounds are thought to have in the descending pain inhibitory pathways.[9,31,54-58] In a review attempting to explain the mechanism of action of the antidepressants in pain relief, Feinmann[57] postulated three possibilities: alleviation of overlying depression, which intensified the suffering of the individual; a common underlying biochemical substrate integral to the experience of pain and depression; and neuromodulatory effects of these drugs on the endogenous opioid systems. Despite much research, all three of these explanations have some merit, and the definitive answer awaits discovery.

Max and colleagues[59] published an important article that employed an "active" placebo, that is, a formulation (anticholinergic, with sedative added in early part of study) that mimicked the side effects of amitriptyline. The two compounds were given to patients with diabetic neuropathy over a six-week period. They found that amitriptyline was associated with significant improvement in pain of neuropathy, regardless of the affective state of the patient. The analgesia from amitriptyline was not associated with altered mood. A similar finding was obtained using low (30 mg) and high (150 mg) dose amitriptyline versus placebo in chronic facial pain.[33] This study found analgesia independent of mood effects. These studies would argue for a mechanism independent of depression alleviation.

Davis and colleagues[36] published one of the first reports citing that amitriptyline or fluphenazine, alone or in combination, provided a significant reduction in pain. This series of eight cases showed that pain relief ensued within days (five or less). The pain relief occurred much sooner than the usual lag time between instituting an antidepressant and the depression response, which is generally 1 to 2 weeks.

This brief overview of a few of the many studies that have been done would indicate that the antidepressants, alone or in combination with other drugs such as neuroleptics, can be beneficial to the patient suffering from a variety of painful conditions.

Individual drugs

Amitriptyline. Amitriptyline is one of the drugs that is often written about in articles dealing with pain. It has a tertiary amine tricyclic structure and blocks the reuptake of norepinephrine somewhat better than it blocks serotonin. It is a potent antimuscarinic and should not be used in patients with narrow-angle glaucoma. Amitriptyline is sedating and blocks α_1-adrenergic receptors. It is available as a parenteral preparation for intramuscular (IM) injection in a concentration of 10 mg/ml.

Doxepin. Doxepin is also a tertiary amine tricyclic antidepressant and is equipotent to amitriptyline. It is sedating, has a high degree of norepinephrine reuptake blockade, and has less antimuscarinic activity than amitriptyline. It is a potent blocker of H_1 and H_2 receptors. It can cause orthostatic hypotension because of its adrenergic blockade. Doxepin is available as an oral concentrate of 10 mg/ml that contains no alcohol.

Imipramine. Imipramine has a tertiary amine tricyclic structure that inhibits reuptake of norepinephrine and serotonin, with norepinephrine reuptake being affected most. Its antimuscarinic activity is similar to doxepin. It may cause

less orthostatic hypotension than doxepin or amitriptyline and may also be less sedating. It is also available in an IM preparation in a concentration of 12.5 mg/ml.

Trimipramine. Also a tertiary amine tricyclic, trimipramine inhibits norepinephrine reuptake somewhat better than it does serotonin reuptake. It is a potent H_2 receptor antagonist and also blocks H_1 receptors. It has significant antimuscarinic activity, is sedating, and is associated with orthostatic hypotension.

Desipramine. The active metabolite of imipramine, desipramine is a secondary amine tricyclic and can be considered a relatively pure norepinephrine reuptake blocker. It is not generally sedating, has little antihistaminic activity, and does not demonstrate much antimuscarinic effect. It has less propensity to cause changes in upright blood pressure than the tertiary amines and may be given in the morning.

Nortriptyline. A tricyclic with a secondary amine side chain, nortriptyline is the active metabolite of amitriptyline. It is associated with less cardiovascular problems[60] and is the only antidepressant for which a therapeutic window in serum levels has been demonstrated.[30] It is primarily a norepinephrine reuptake blocker with some mild sedative and antihistaminic effects. It is generally given in a dose equivalent to about half of the usual amitriptyline daily dose (75 mg as opposed to 150 mg) when treating depression. Because it is well-tolerated with regard to cardiovascular effects and its low antimuscarinic profile, it is often recommended for use in elderly patients. It is available as a liquid containing 2 mg/ml in an alcohol base.

Protriptyline. This secondary amine tricyclic is a relatively selective inhibitor of norepinephrine reuptake, with moderate antihistaminic and sedative properties and significant antimuscarinic activity.

Amoxapine. Structurally related to the neuroleptic loxapine, this drug somewhat selectively interferes with norepinephrine reuptake. It has little antimuscarinic action, is moderately sedating, and blocks dopamine receptors to a clinically significant degree. Because of its dopamine receptor antagonism, it is capable of causing acute extrapyramidal side effects, such as akathisia and drug-induced parkinsonian features.[61] It could cause tardive dyskinesia. It has been associated with the development of neuroleptic malignant syndrome. Amoxapine is particularly prone to causing seizures in overdosage in the absence of much cardiovascular effect. Rhabdomyolysis from repetitive seizures is felt to be the genesis of renal failure secondary to acute tubular necrosis that may occur as a late consequence of overdosage.

Maprotiline. Maprotiline is the only tetracyclic on the U.S. market and is a selective norepinephrine reuptake inhibitor. It has little antimuscarinic activity and is touted as having fewer cardiac side effects. Maprotiline is moderately sedating and may cause seizures in a small portion of the population who do not have a preexisting seizure diathesis.

Trazodone. Trazodone ia a triazolopyridine derivative that is marketed for its relative lack of side effects. It is about one half as potent as amitriptyline. It is a serotonergic reuptake blocker, although binding studies indicate that its inhibition constant is small (0.53 versus 2.4 for impramine).[62] It should be taken with food because bioavailability will be enhanced. Trazodone has been associated with priapism at an incidence of about 1:10,000. Any alteration of erectile function should prompt discontinuation. It is mildly sedating and generally well tolerated.

Fluoxetine. Fluoxetine is a benzenepropanamine compound that has recently been released on the U.S. market. It is a selective serotonin reuptake blocker and has minimal antimuscarinic effects. There have been some incidences of nausea, nervousness, and insomnia.[51] A dose of 20 mg should be taken each morning for the treatment of depression and advanced to 20 mg morning and noon if necessary. The maximum recommended dose is 80 mg per day. Anorexia has been reported in some studies,[51] and the ensuing weight loss may actually benefit some patients. Preliminary reports indicate that fluoxetine may inhibit the metabolism of tricyclic antidepressants and may cause dramatic increases in serum concentration of these drugs. Because of the long half-life of fluoxetine, there may be a delay of weeks between its institution and its effect on concurrent administration of another antidepressant.[63] There have been no studies of its use in pain patients to date.

Bupropion. Bupropion is the newest antidepressant available. It is a propiophenone derivative and is unusual in that some patients will respond to this drug for depression treatment when they have been resistant to others.[49] The mechanism of action is unknown, and it has little effect on the reuptake of norepinephrine or serotonin.[49,62] Minimal orthostatic hypotension has been associated with its use, it has little effect on cardiac conduction,[64] and it may cause weight loss.[49] It has been associated with seizure activity[50] and may be somewhat stimulating.[49] It is recommended that initial doses be 100 mg in the morning and evening.

Guidelines for using antidepressants

The monamine oxidase inhibitors, although useful in some types of chronic pain, should not be recommended to patients by the nonpsychiatric physician because of their pharmacologic side effects and medicolegal ramifications. Concomitant use of these drugs with other antidepressants has been associated with a syndrome of rigidity, hyperthermia, and seizures.[65]

When selecting an antidepressant for use in pain management, the problems experienced by the patient should be matched with the drug most likely to have an effect on that problem. Most pain patients will, for example, have poor sleep patterns. This would lead one to select a tertiary amine tricyclic or trazodone. As many chronic pain patients are very somatically focused, it is important to start the medications slowly and to inform the patient of what the side effects will likely be ahead of time. It is also helpful to inform patients that, in general, antidepressants are associated with "nuisance" side effects as opposed to serious effects. Fortunately, most patients will develop rapid tolerance to the daytime sedation that is commonly experienced when starting a sedating antidepressant. Sleep effects are frequently noted on the first dose.

Antimuscarinic tolerance typically takes weeks and can

be a reason for stopping the drugs. Tolerance to the analgesic effects has not been reported. Long-term use of these drugs is generally safe, but withdrawal must be gradual to avoid insomnia and abdominal discomfort. Gradually decreasing the dosage for 1 to 2 weeks is usually sufficient to obviate any significant withdrawal phenomena.

To institute antidepressants for pain treatment, start with 25 mg of amitriptyline or an equivalent dosage of another compound, to be taken about 1 to 2 hours before sleep. If the individual is frail, elderly, or predisposed to untoward side effects, a starting dose of 10 mg would be appropriate. This should be monitored and increased every few days by 25 mg (or 10 mg if that was the starting dose), using sleep as the initial target symptom. If unacceptable side effects ensue, maintain or decrease the current dose, depending on the nature and severity of the problem. Any signs of toxicity should prompt a serum level determination. It must be stressed to pain patients that these drugs have some potential to reduce pain but are not typical analgesics, and must therefore be taken on a fixed schedule to have a predictable effect.

To summarize, antidepressants are used as one part of a comprehensive approach to the management of pain and its associated problems. They have analgesic activity, are nonaddicting hypnotics and anxiolytics, and may enhance ulcer healing. They have a myriad of pharmacologic actions, and this must be recognized by the prescribing physician. Serum levels are useful in determining compliance or toxicity but have not yet been correlated to efficacy in pain treatment. These drugs are highly protein bound. Therefore the potential for pharmacokinetic alterations by disease states and coadministration of other drugs must be considered.

NEUROLEPTICS

The terminology of neuroleptics has been confusing in the past. Because a phenothiazine nucleus was originally employed in the development of this line of drugs, it was traditional to call all antipsychotics "phenothiazines." This terminology is no longer acceptable, since antipsychotics now include several chemical classes. The term *neuroleptic* was originally used to describe these drugs based on the regularity with which antipsychotic efficacy was associated with extrapyramidal side effects in animal assays, and its meaning implies the ability to produce a neurologic disorder.[22] Although this association between side effects and efficacy generally still exists, there are exceptions and a great incentive to develop new drugs that lack side effects. This makes the name neuroleptic somewhat less than precise, but tradition has established its use.

Within the major classes of neuroleptics, there are several distinct subclasses

1. Phenothiazines—aliphatic (chlorpromazine), piperidines (thioridazine), and piperazines (fluphenazine)
2. thioxanthenes—aliphatic (chlorprothixene) and piperazine (thiothixene)
3. butyrophenones—haloperidol and droperidol
4. dibenzazepines—dibenzoxapines (loxapine) and dibenzodiazepines (clozapine)

The literature discussing the use of these drugs in chronic pain tends to be more anecdotal than that concerning the antidepressants.[34,37,55,66]

Pharmacology

A major problem in the psychiatric use of neuroleptics is the unreliability of gastric absorption after oral administration. Baldessarini states that IM administration can increase the availability of the active drug by four to ten times.[1] The drugs are highly lipophilic and are largely bound to proteins and membranes. They cross the placenta easily and are not dialyzable.[1] They do accumulate in the brain tissue in disproportionate amounts relative to their plasma concentrations.

The half-lives of all the neuroleptics tend to exceed 24 hours, with some as long as 40 hours.[1] This feature makes once-a-day dosing feasible, which will increase compliance. The drugs may be taken at night so that any sedative effects will have their greatest impact when the patient is likely to be sleeping.

Depot-injectable forms exist for fluphenazine and haloperidol. These are created by esterifying the parent compound to a long-chain fatty acid and result in a decanoate preparation that, when injected IM, can exert pharmacologic effects for weeks.

The primary metabolism of these drugs is by hepatic microsomal oxidation.[1] There exists a significant first-pass effect.[20] Conjugation also occurs. The metabolites are excreted in the urine and, via bile, the feces. Cimetidine has been reported to increase serum levels of chlorpromazine, presumably by competing with the cytochrome P450 oxidase system.[67] Perphenazine has been reported to increase amitriptyline levels, and haloperidol may inhibit metabolism of nortriptyline.[25,68]

The mechanism of antipsychotic action of the neuroleptics is presumed to be dopamine receptor blockade. Excess levels of brain dopamine are associated with psychosis, and dopaminergic activity blockade is associated with resolution or control of psychotic processes. These associations have led to a "dopamine hypothesis" of schizophrenia. The neuroleptics are potent blockers of dopamine receptors but are relatively nonspecific.[69] Although there is no clearcut explanation for the possible benefit of these drugs for patients with pain syndromes, there has been some study of the interaction of various drugs and opiate receptors.[21] This is not entirely surprising when one realizes that the butyrophenones were developed by Janssen by altering derivatives of meperidine.[1]

The side effects of the neuroleptics have some commonalities with those of the antidepressants. Side effects that are unique to dopamine-blocking drugs include extrapyramidal reactions such as acute dystonias, akathisia syndrome, drug-induced parkinsonism, and tardive dyskinesia. These reactions are thought to be due to the blockade of dopamine receptors in the caudate nucleus or its related pathways.[22]

Akathisia (Greek for not *[-a]* sit still *[- kathisis]*) is a syndrome caused by dopamine blockade, which is frequently misdiagnosed. The condition is characterized by an intensely uncomfortable desire on the part of the patient to move about. Agitation (excess purposeless motor activity) is frequently observed, and may include foot tapping, pac-

ing, and rocking.[70] Patients may describe this as "wanting to jump out of my skin" or as a profound sense that something is wrong; they may be unable to elaborate with specific concerns.

Drug-induced parkinsonism is a later complication of using these drugs and is characterized by the classic signs of Parkinson's disease: shuffling gait, bradykinesia, akinesia, mask facies, and cogwheel rigidity.[22] It can be very subtle in its onset; the patient may not be aware of the early symptoms until they are pointed out. Treatment involves an antimuscarinic or amantadine. It is less common with lower-potency drugs, since their inherent antimuscarinic activity may counteract the dopaminergic blockade in the caudate nucleus.

The most significant adverse effect of dopamine blockade is tardive (late-onset) dyskinesia. The syndrome consists of involuntary choreiform movements that affect the orolinguobuccal musculature classically, but can also involve the trunk or respiratory or extremity muscles.[70] The cause of tardive dyskinesia has not been delineated.[70] Tardive dyskinesia can be permanent, tends to increase initially after reduction or withdrawal of medication, and can be masked, but is probably worsened, by increased doses of neuroleptics.[22,71] From a medicolegal perspective, informed consent should be obtained before instituting a neuroleptic, and frequent assessment of side effects and continued efficacy are prudent.[71]

Neuroleptic malignant syndrome is a rare but serious condition that can occur after the use of these drugs. It presents in fashion reminiscent of malignant hyperthermia and is characterized by skeletal muscle hypertonicity, hyperthermia, delirium, and autonomic instability.[72-74] Temperatures may exceed 41° C. Laboratory abnormalities include elevated liver enzymes, very high creatine kinase levels, and leucocytosis.[73] Rhabdomyolysis and renal failure may occur. Although dehydration, concurrent brain diseases, and exhaustion may predispose to the development of this syndrome, duration of exposure to the drug does not correlate with incidence of neuroleptic malignant syndrome.[73] Dantrolene, pancuronium amantadine, and bromocriptine have all been used as specific therapy with variable results.[73,75]

Dopaminergic blockade interferes with prolactin regulation; dopamine is now known to be a prolactin-inhibiting factor. Thus when dopamine activity is decreased by these drugs, prolactin levels may increase, which leads to gynecomastia in men and galactorrhea in both sexes.[22] This is usually seen only in long-term therapy.

Neuroleptics have other side effects that are apparently unrelated to their dopaminergic blockade. These include agranulocytosis, jaundice, photosensitivity, retrograde ejaculation, and pigmented retinopathy.[1,22,48] The latter two conditions have especially been related to use of thioridazine.

Dependence and withdrawal symptoms do not occur with these drugs.[55,76,77] In overdose, these drugs have a remarkably low lethal potential.[22]

Efficacy in pain management

Few publications have speculated on the precise mechanism of action in regard to analgesia. Most studies that have shown some efficacy have been difficult to interpret, due to small numbers, mixed diagnoses, or a variety of drugs and dosing schedules. There is a trend, however, to suggest that these drugs may have some usefulness in diabetic neuropathy[36,66] and postherpetic neuralgia,[34,55,66] specifically. Many studies employed a combination of an antidepressant and a neuroleptic, making the therapeutic agent difficult to specify,[34,36,66,78] and it is possible that the neuroleptic exerted an effect by increasing serum levels of the antidepressants.[68]

Clarke reviewed his experiences with the combination of amitriptyline and perphenazine in 120 patients with various diagnoses.[79,98] The daily dose was 25 mg of the antidepressant and 2 mg of perphenazine each morning, and double doses of each at night. Ten patients were withdrawn because of unacceptable side effects (dry mouth, urinary retention, drowsiness, and dissociation). The remainder completed the 2-month study period. Of 13 patients, 7 had postherpetic neuralgia, and 10 of 19 patients with postsurgical scar pain were "improved." Results were not as good with failed laminectomies and other diagnoses. Overall, 33.6% of the patients improved to such a degree that no other treatment was deemed necessary.

Methotrimeprazine has been studied by numerous French investigators and has been felt to have analgesic properties. Montilla et al., in one of the earliest U.S. studies, compared methotrimeprazine to morphine in 105 patients with a variety of diagnoses, from postherpetic neuralgia to cancer to coronary occlusion.[76] They used a double-blind design, and all assessments of pain in a given patient were done by the same investigator. Morphine 10 mg or methotrimeprazine 15 mg was administered subcutaneously. In addition, 44 received the opiate and 61 received the neuroleptic during the study period. The methotrimeprazine group had a greater average pain score initially (3.18 versus 2.09 on a 0 to 4 scale) but had similar postdrug scores throughout the 4-hour observation period (approximately 1.5).

Individual drugs

Fluphenazine. Fluphenazine is a very potent drug that has been used in treating several pain disorders. It is relatively nonsedating but has a significant incidence of dopaminergic, blockade-mediated side effects. It is usually given in 1 mg doses starting at night and advancing up to 4 mg in 1 mg increments with several days at each dose.

Perphenazine. Perphenazine is somewhat less potent than fluphenazine and has less propensity to cause extrapyramidal side effects. It is available as a tablet and in combination with amitriptyline in various dosages. It is usually given in 4 to 12 mg doses for analgesia.

Haloperidol. Haloperidol is also a potent drug, and doses of 0.5 to 10.0 mg in divided doses can be useful in pain management. It is generally well tolerated in terms of cardiovascular side effects, even in the debilitated patient. It is available as a tablet, an injection, and a decanoate preparation.

Chlorprothixine. Chlorprothixine is less potent and therefore more sedating than the drugs listed previously. It is usually given in doses of 25 to 50 mg orally, which is increased gradually to several doses a day. It has been used in pain associated with zoster.

Thioridazine. Thioridazine is a less potent neuroleptic that may show some preference for blockade of limbic dopamine receptors over nigrostriatal receptors. It is associated with a lower incidence of extrapyramidal reactions and possibly a lower risk of tardive dyskinesia. Thioridazine is associated with ejaculatory difficulties and retinitis pigmentosa, especially in doses exceeding 900 mg per day. It can be used in similar doses to chlorpromazine.

Chlorpromazine. Chlorpromazine is also a low-potency sedating neuroleptic with a low incidence of extrapyramidal side effects. It has a significant antimuscarinic profile. Chlorpromazine has been associated with reversible agranulocytopenia, jaundice, and photosensitivity. Doses range from 25 to 100 mg once a day to several times a day.

Guidelines for using neuroleptics

When choosing a neuroleptic for use in pain management, weigh the risk of side effects against possible benefit. Although this is sound policy for any medical decision, it is especially important here because tardive dyskinesia can be permanent. Prudence would dictate starting an antidepressant first and adding a neuroleptic only if there was no change in pain after the patient's sleep pattern had normalized. At that point, there is no clear indication of which drug to add. Higher-potency drugs offer the advantage of little daytime sedation but have higher risks of side effects mediated through dopaminergic blockade. Low-potency drugs may enhance sleep but have high antimuscarinic and alpha$_1$ adrenergic blockade. Perphenazine can be coadministered with amitriptyline in one formulation, which may enhance compliance but decreases dosing flexibility. Methotrimeprazine can cause sedation and hypotension, but in a nonambulatory terminal cancer patient, this may not be an issue. All of the neuroleptics can raise prolactin levels over time.

Neuroleptics should be instituted gradually, starting at night and increasing the dose to include daytime doses only if nocturnal administration is inadequate for symptom control. Monitor frequently for the development of akathisia, cogwheel rigidity, and orthostatic hypotension. A family history of Parkinson's disease may indicate a greater propensity for these adverse reactions from these drugs.

To summarize, the neuroleptic drugs may have some benefit in pain management, especially in regard to neuropathic pain syndromes. Presently, there are no reasons to choose one particular drug; physician experience and side-effect profile appear to be the deciding factors.

ANTICONVULSANTS

The anticonvulsants are a heterogenous group of drugs including four which have been used in pain management. Phenytoin (originally called diphenylhydantoin), valproic acid, carbamazepine, and clonazepam have been used primarily in neuralgic syndromes, but like most of the drugs in this chapter, have been tried in a variety of painful states, occasionally with some success.[80,81]

Pharmacology

Phenytoin has a variable absorption when given orally.[82] Its peak serum level can occur anywhere from 3 to 12 hours after a dose, with peaks likely to occur in the 4 to 8 hour range.[82,83] It is extensively bound to proteins, primarily albumin, but also α_1 acid glycoprotein; and in the normal situation it has a free fraction of 10%.[31,82,84] In reduced protein-binding situations such as hypoalbuminemia or uremia, the free fraction can be as high as 30%, leading to toxicity at what would normally be a therapeutic dose.[20,84] Conversely, when acute-phase reactants are elevated, increased serum total drug levels can be seen without any increase in clinical effect.[20] Metabolism occurs primarily by hepatic microsomal enzymes.[82] The serum half-life is about 22 hours but can be increased in higher doses.[82,83]

Valproic acid is rapidly absorbed, reaching a peak serum level within 1 to 4 hours.[85] It is highly bound (90% to 95%) to albumin. Valproic acid undergoes glucuronidation in the liver and is primarily excreted in the urine.[85] Its half-life is about 10 hours but can be increased in higher dose ranges.[83,85]

Carbamazepine, which is structurally similar to imipramine, is slowly and unpredictably absorbed after oral dosing.[81,82] Peak concentrations are generally reached between 2 and 8 hours but can be delayed longer.[82,83] Carbamazepine is 75% protein bound to albumin and α_1 acid glycoprotein. It is metabolized to the 10, 11 epoxide form, and this species has substantial anticonvulsant activity of its own. Subsequently, it undergoes glucuronidation and urinary excretion.[82] The serum half-life with chronic administration averages 14 hours, with a range of 10 to 20 hours.[82,83] Acute half-lives are longer, owing to enzyme induction with continued use.

Clonazepam is well-absorbed after oral administration and reaches a peak concentration in serum about 1 to 4 hours after it is taken.[82] It is 85% protein bound and is metabolized by the liver to an inactive form.[82] The serum half-life averages about a day.[82,83]

Serum levels are routinely measured in the treatment of epilepsy, but the usefulness of doing this in pain management has not been clearly established. Valproic acid, because of its short half-life, should be sampled at the same time interval after a dose to decrease variability.[85] Optimal levels are between 50 to 100 μg/ml.[83] Phenytoin shows a fairly good correlation between serum level and efficacy for epilepsy and toxicity.[82] The therapeutic range for epilepsy is 10 to 20 μg/ml.[82,83] Carbamazepine, in a range of 4 to 10 μg/ml is felt to be best for epilepsy, and some scientific evidence suggested that this should be an effective range for use in pain management.[83,86] Clonazepam concentrations range from 5 to 70 ng/ml for treatment of epilepsy, but these are not felt to be tightly correlated with effect or toxicity.[82]

The mechanisms of action of all four of these drugs are not well understood, but are probably unique to each drug. Phenytoin has a stabilizing effect on all neuronal membranes and alters sodium, calcium, and potassium flux which is associated with an action potential.[82] Valproic acid increases γ-aminobutyric acid (GABA) activity by interfering with GABA transaminase.[82,85] Carbamazepine reduces sodium and potassium conductance and decreases the amount of spontaneous activity in experimental neuromas in rats.[86] Clonazepam is a benzodiazepine and most likely acts through the benzodiazepine receptor-linked chloride channel to enhance the efficiency of GABA binding or activity.[82,87]

Phenytoin is associated with hirsutism, ataxia, diplopia, confusion, epigastric pain, nausea, and vomiting.[82] Gingival hyperplasia is a side effect peculiar to phenytoin and may be related to stimulation of a particular type of fibrocyte.

Valproic acid is associated primarily with GI symptoms that tend to ameliorate with time.[82,85] Nausea, vomiting, anorexia, and diarrhea can all occur and may be less frequently seen with the use of the enteric coated preparations.[81,82,85] Central nervous system (CNS) effects include sedation, tremor, and ataxia.[82,85] Rashes, transient alopecia, and altered liver function tests have been reported.[82,85] Weight gain has also been reported.[81]

Carbamazepine is known for its propensity to cause hematologic abnormalities.[82] Thrombocytopenia, agranulocytosis, anemia, and pancytopenia have occurred with its use. Ataxia, diplopia, and sedation can also occur,[82] and nausea is sometimes seen.[81]

Clonazepam may cause transient drowsiness, ataxia, and some signs of disinhibition, such as hostility, emotional lability, and agitation.[81] Lethargy and fatigue may occur early in a course of use but tend to subside with chronic administration.[82] A withdrawal syndrome was demonstrated in dogs and, given the potential of the benzodiazepines for dependence, it is reasonable to assume that this could be seen in humans after prolonged use.[88]

Overdosage with any of these drugs may be fatal except with clonazepam, which seems to share the customary wide therapeutic index of the other benzodiazepines.[82]

Anticonvulsants should be avoided during pregnancy and in females not using contraceptives. Phenytoin may interfere with the efficiency of oral contraceptives.[82] Calabrese and Gulledge state that carbamazepine and clonazepam have the least teratogenic potential.[89]

The levels of these drugs can be changed by the coadministration of other drugs, including other anticonvulsants. Phenytoin binding can be decreased by salicylates, diazepam, valproic acid, and phenylbutazone.[82,84] Clonazepam levels can be decreased by the coadministration of carbamazepine, whereas high concentrations of valproic acid, phenytoin, and aspirin can increase the free fraction of clonazepam.[90,91] Clonazepam can reduce the serum level of desipramine.[24] The metabolism of carbamazepine may be inhibited by propoxyphene, while phenobarbital and phenytoin may increase it.[82] Diltiazem and verapamil can interact with carbamazepine, causing an acute rise in serum levels resulting from inhibition of liver metabolism.

All of the anticonvulsants can cause cognitive and behavioral effects[92,93]: alterations in memory, mental processing, and motor response time in tests.[94]

Efficacy in pain management

Swerdlow has compiled the most extensive review of efficacy in pain management to date.[81] Hatangdi and co-workers reported on the treatment of 34 patients with postherpetic neuralgia who had been symptomatic for months to years and half experiencing symptoms for more than a decade.[95] Many of these patients had received neuroleptics without benefit. They used carbamazepine in therapeutic blood levels supplemented with nortriptyline 50 to 100 mg per day in divided doses. Of the 34 subjects, 18 (53%) had complete relief on this regimen, 9 had "good" relief, 3 had "partial" relief, and 4 discontinued the drugs because of side effects from either agent.

Young and Clarke used an algorithmic approach to the treatment of diabetic neuropathy, where clonazepam was the only anticonvulsant and the last drug employed and was used only after failure of simple analgesics, two different antidepressants, and one of two neuroleptics.[96] They studied 80 patients, and three progressed through the protocol to enter the clonazepam phase of the study. Two of the patients obtained relief and commented that clonazepam was useful in treating the syndrome of restless legs.

Bouckoms and Litman treated 21 patients who had symptoms suggestive of deafferentation pain, with clonazepam in a range of 1 to 4 mg per night.[97] Six of the study group responded with "marked or complete" relief. Of the 12 who met several of their criteria for deafferentation pain, the 6 who responded to treatment had allodynia as a presenting finding, while 5 of the 6 who were nonresponders to clonazepam did not have allodynia. Based on these results, Bouckoms and Litman suggested that allodynia may be predictive of clonazepam responsiveness.

Individual drugs

Phenytoin. Phenytoin is available in capsules, extended-release capsules, suspension, and a parenteral form. The average adult starting dose is 100 mg two to three times a day. Vitamin supplementation should be considered. If a patient is to be on this medication for an extended period, a dental consultation aimed at maximizing oral hygiene should be obtained.

Valproic acid. Valproic acid is available as a capsule, a syrup, and an enteric-coated tablet. The usual adult starting dose is 15 mg/kg per day in divided doses. This can be increased by 5 to 10 mg/kg per day every week until adequate response is obtained or a maximum dose of 60 mg/kg per day is reached. Baseline and periodic liver function tests are recommended. Hepatic failure resulting in death has been rarely reported with this agent.

Carbamazepine. Carbamazepine is available in tablets and chewable tablets. The usual range to achieve therapeutic serum levels in adults is 800 to 1200 mg per day in divided doses. This range is reached with doses of 200 mg twice daily and then gradually increasing the drug. Obtain baseline hematologic studies including reticulocyte, leukocyte, and platelet counts, along with hematocrit and hemoglobin. These should be repeated biweekly early in therapy, and the frequency can be decreased later.

Clonazepam. Clonazepam is available in strengths of 0.5, 1, and 2 mg tablets. The usual doses reported in the pain literature range from 1 to 4 mg per day. Most authors recommend giving the drug at night to minimize sedative effects during the day. The sedative effects of this drug can be potentiated by other drugs with sedation profiles. Ataxia and dizziness can be especially bothersome early in the course of therapy but tend to ameliorate with time. A withdrawal syndrome similar to that seen with any other benzodiazepine can occur upon abrupt cessation of this group.

When discontinuing any anticonvulsant, a schedule of tapering decreases in dose should be employed to reduce the possibility of seizures. These may occur even in the patient without a preexisting seizure diathesis.

Summary

Even though anticonvulsants have significant potential side-effects, they can be useful in the management of pain that has been refractory to other therapy. They appear to be particularly useful in the treatment of neuropathic pain states. Anticonvulsants are considered the treatment of choice in trigeminal neuralgia and are gaining status in the management of other neuralgias. Serum levels have generally not been correlated with pain response, but toxicity concerns mandate using established ranges as target levels.

SEDATIVE-HYPNOTICS AND ANXIOLYTICS

Drugs to alleviate anxiety and promote sleep are some of the most widely prescribed agents. Although there are several types of drugs that may be used to treat insomnia and anxiety disorders, such as the antidepressants discussed previously, in terms of numbers the benzodiazepines are clearly prescribed most often. Chronic pain patients frequently take benzodiazepines for a myriad of perceived reasons, such as pain, muscle spasm, and anxiety.[98] Most authors recognize the usefulness of these drugs for short-term indications but feel there is little benefit from using benzodiazepines in the management of chronic pain.[55,56,99,100]

Pharmacology

The pharmacokinetics of benzodiazepines are quite variable among drugs and among routes of administration of the same drug. Diazepam, the most used drug of this class, is well-absorbed after being taken orally but erratically absorbed after IM administration.[101] It is highly lipid soluble and enters the brain rapidly. This lipid solubility may offset its effects via peripheral redistribution.[102] Other drugs in this class, such as lorazepam and chlordiazepoxide, are less lipophilic and have a relatively slower onset but tend to have a longer residence in the brain.[102]

Metabolism of this class occurs by hepatic oxidation and conjugation. Some drugs undergo both processes (diazepam, chlordiazepoxide, and flurazepam), whereas others undergo conjugation alone (lorazepam, oxazepam, and temazepam).[101] Since oxidation is more easily influenced by pathologic processes and other concurrent drug administration, the half-lives of drugs metabolized by these pathways tend to be more variable.[101,102] Without extraneous factors, the benzodiazepines have a wide range of half-lives from 3 to 200 hours.[103,104] The half-lives are further influenced by the clearance of the drug, route of administration, and occurrence of multiple dosing, which allows accumulation of active metabolites.[101-103]

The mechanism of benzodiazepine action is through binding with a specific receptor that is complexed to a $GABA_A$ receptor.[87] When the drug binds to its receptor, it causes the action of GABA to be enhanced.[102,105] This, in turn, mediates the opening of chloride channels, which lowers the transmembrane potential and decreases the ability of the neuron to conduct an action potential.[105,106] Thus benzodiazepines facilitate the inhibitory actions of GABA.[102,105,106] Exactly how this receptor interaction gives rise to the various actions of these drugs is not completely understood, but it would seem that more inhibitory activity of the nervous system would be associated with sedation and sleep. There is some evidence that diazepam, in particular, exerts an additional direct effect on muscle contraction via alteration in calcium flux.[107]

The side effects of the different benzodiazepines are similar with a few exceptions, although some drugs in this class may have a higher or lower incidence of a particular effect. Sedation substantial enough to impair psychomotor performance is more likely to occur with the long half-life drugs. It is somewhat offset by tolerance with chronic administration.[108] Amnesia can occur and may be especially a problem with triazolam and lorazepam,[98,108] and disinhibition that results in agitation, hostility, and anger has been described.[109] Cognitive and intellectual dysfunction can be troublesome, especially in the elderly or with chronic usage.[90,100,108] Chlordiazepoxide has been associated with extrapyramidal symptoms on rare occasions.[110] Although this class can induce sleep, it typically alters sleep architecture by suppressing rapid eye movement and Stage 3 and 4 sleep. It is recommended that it be used for the shortest time necessary and in the lowest effective dose.[103,104]

When withdrawal occurs, it may include sweating, tremors, sensitivity to light and sound, tachycardia, dysphoria, headache, hostility, muscle twitching or weakness, delirium, or psychosis.[98,100,109] Seizures can occur in some patients.[98,108] The manifestations of acute withdrawal may vary considerably from patient to patient.[111] The drugs with longer half-lives tend to show a somewhat lower incidence and severity of withdrawal symptoms because of their gradual disappearance from the body after cessation.[108]

Fatalities resulting solely from benzodiazepine overdose are extremely rare.[98] Their use in pregnancy has been associated with a higher incidence of oral clefts in some studies and not in others.[53]

Buspirone is a new nonbenzodiazepine anxiolytic that is said to be relatively free of sedation.[112] It is rapidly absorbed when given orally and undergoes extensive first-pass metabolism.[113] It is highly protein bound, and its half-life is about 3 hours.[113] It appears to interact with a serotonin receptor subtype and blocks dopamine receptors to some degree.[113,114] Buspirone is useful in treating anxiety but has a lag time of 1 to 2 weeks and may not be as effective in patients who have used benzodiazepines on a chronic basis.[113] Nausea, initial anxiety, diarrhea, and tingling in the extremities can occur.[112] It does not appear to cause dependence or withdrawal and does not potentiate the CNS depressive effects of alcohol.[112,113] It can interact with monamine oxidase inhibitors, causing severe hypertension.[112]

Efficacy in pain management

Few studies focus on the use of benzodiazepines in pain management. Diazepam is commonly used to treat the muscle spasm and pain presumed to arise from pain problems.[98,115]

Singh et al. studied the effects of acute postoperative administration of diazepam in a group of 35 patients who underwent upper abdominal surgery.[116] After fully recovering from a standardized anesthetic technique, baseline pain ratings were obtained. They were randomized into groups receiving either morphine 10 mg, diazepam 10 mg, or a mixture of 5 mg of each IM. They found indistinguishable relief at 30 minutes postinjection, but thereafter diazepam alone was not as effective and caused more pain at the injection site than either of the other two treatment options.

Hollister and colleagues studied 108 neurosurgical clinic patients who had been taking diazepam in doses of 5 to 40 mg per day for up to 16 years.[115] The drug was being taken for muscle spasm in 36% of the cases, as an analgesic in 30%, and for "nerves" and to aid sleep in 34% of patients with pain and spasm.

Alprazolam appears to be unique among this class in that it seems to have particular efficacy in the treatment of panic disorder and has demonstrated an antidepressant efficacy in several placebo-controlled, double-blind, multicenter studies.[103,117,118] The mean doses for antidepressant action were 2.87 and 3.0 mg per day in two studies by Feighner and Rickels.[117,118] With the exception of drowsiness occurring in some patients, alprazolam was associated with fewer side effects than the tricyclic antidepressants used in the studies.

Summary

The anxiolytics are commonly used by patients suffering from chronic pain, despite little evidence to substantiate that use. The benzodiazepines are useful when given for a limited time for acute anxiety and insomnia. The risk of dependence and withdrawal may be greater in the chronic-pain population. Alprazolam appears to have some unique assets, but also has all of the drawbacks of this class, including the particular difficulty in discontinuing.[108] Buspirone lacks many of the disadvantages of the other drugs in this section but has not demonstrated any efficacy as an analgesic to date.

ANTIHISTAMINES AND MUSCLE RELAXANTS

This section discusses hydroxyzine and the muscle relaxants, a group of drugs with diverse pharmacologic actions that are used to treat pain ostensibly arising from muscle spasm.[56,99]

Pharmacology

Hydroxyzine is a diphenylmethane antihistamine like diphenhydramine and has antiemetic and anxiolytic effects.[110,119] It is extensively metabolized in the liver.[120] Like diphenhydramine, it has significant antimuscarinic properties. It is sedating and may cause ataxia and disinhibition[110] but has rarely been associated with convulsions in high doses.[110]

The skeletal muscle relaxants have pharmacologic profiles that are basically similar despite their different structures.[121,122] They act by depressing polysynaptic reflexes, but this property is not unique to these drugs. They do not interfere with neuromuscular transmission as do curare and related neuromuscular blockers.[121] All of the agents undergo hepatic metabolism, and the half-lives vary from about 1 hour (chlorzoxazone) to 3 days (cyclobenzaprine). Some are marketed in combination with analgesics. Cyclobenzaprine has a structure that is quite similar to that of the tricyclic antidepressants, while the others in this group have varied structures. Several of them can cross the placenta. Drowsiness is the most frequently reported side effect, and headache, dizziness, blurred vision, nausea, and vomiting have also been reported.[121,122] Predictably, cyclobenzaprine can cause antimuscarinic symptoms. Chlorzoxazone has been reported to cause jaundice.[122] Central nervous system depression characterizes overdose, and an anticholinergic syndrome may result from large doses of orphenadrine. Orphenadrine overdose can be fatal.[121]

Baclofen, which has antispasticity properties and acts on the $GABA_B$ receptor, has been used in some painful conditions where its efficacy seems to stem from its ability to decrease muscle spasm.[56,99,105] It may also reduce substance P release.[56] Dantrolene acts by direct peripheral action on the muscle and can reduce muscle tone.[56]

Efficacy in pain management

Hydroxyzine has been studied for a potent analgesic that lacks respiratory depression. At the First World Congress on Pain, Beaver and Feise reported their results of a study involving 96 postoperative patients who received placebo, 8 mg of morphine, 100 mg of hydroxyzine or the same doses of both active drugs simultaneously. All drugs were given IM on one occasion in the early postoperative period, and the patients were questioned hourly for pain ratings for 6 hours after the injection. Using change in pain intensity versus time, the results showed that morphine alone was superior to placebo, but there was no significant difference between the response curves of morphine and hydroxyzine. Furthermore the combination had an additive rather than synergistic effect. This relationship also held when the patients were stratified by the severity of their baseline pain.[118]

Hydroxyzine 100 mg combined with morphine 10 mg provided superior analgesia over morphine alone in 82 postoperative patients who were enrolled in a double-blind, single-dose study.[123] The combination also provided better pain relief than morphine 5 mg by itself or combined with 100 mg of hydroxyzine. Larger doses of morphine and hydroxyzine in combination produced more drowsiness than any of the other treatments.

Studies of efficacy of the skeletal muscle relaxants generally showed some improvement in acute muscle problems versus placebo.[121] Evidence of effect in chronic cases is less convincing; only cyclobenzaprine showed possible benefit.[121] Elenbaas concluded that there was no evidence to suggest superiority of any particular drug, or to suggest superiority of these drugs over sedatives or analgesics.

Hydroxyzine has inherent analgesic properties that may be clinically relevant but has a ceiling effect that does not warrant the use of the drug in doses beyond 150 mg. The skeletal muscle relaxants have been inadequately studied,

given their frequency of use. They are probably effective for acute muscle problems but do not appear to have utility in chronic pain syndromes. Care must be used in prescribing cyclobenzaprine because of its long half-life and its antimuscarinic effects.

REFERENCES

1. Baldessarini RJ: Drugs and the treatment of psychiatric disorders. In Gilman AG et al, editors: *The Pharmacological Basis of Therapeutics.* New York, Macmillan, 1985.
2. Paoli F, Darcourt G, Corsa P: Note preliminaire sur l'action de l'imipramine don les etats douloureaux. *Rev Neurol* 102:503-504, 1960.
3. Krishnan KRR, France RD, Houpt JL: Chronic low back pain and depression. *Psychosomatics* 26:299-302, 1985.
4. Lindsay PG, Wyckoff M: The depression-pain syndrome and its response to antidepressants. *Psychosomatics* 22:571-577, 1981.
5. Ward N et al: Antidepressants in concomitant chronic low back pain and depression: Doxepin and desipramine compared. *J Clin Psychiatry* 45:54-59, 1984.
6. Hameroff SR et al: Doxepin's effect on chronic pain and depression: A controlled study. *J Clin Psychiatry* 45:47-52, 1984.
7. Romano JM, Turner JA: Chronic pain and depression: Does the evidence support a relationship? *Psychol Bull* 97:18-34, 1985.
8. Hendler N: Depression caused by chronic pain. *J Clin Psychiatry* 45:30-36, 1984.
9. Rosenblatt RM, Reich J, Dehring D: Tricyclic antidepressants in the treatment of depression and chronic pain: Analysis of the supporting evidence. *Anesth Analg* 63:1025-1032, 1984.
10. Lindsay PG, Olsen RB: Maprotiline in pain-depression. *J Clin Psychiatry* 46:226-228, 1985.
11. France RD et al: Differentiation of depression from chronic pain with the dexamethasone suppression test and DSM-III. *Am J Psychiatry* 141:1577-1579, 1984.
12. Von Knorring L et al: Pain as a symptom in depressive disorders. I. Relationship to diagnostic subgroup and depressive symptomatology. *Pain* 15:19-26, 1983.
13. Lopez Ibor JJ: Masked depressions. *Br J Psychiatry* 120:245-258, 1972.
14. Lesse S: Masked depression—A diagnostic and therapeutic problem. *Diseases of the Nervous System* 29:169-173, 1968.
15. Ward NG, Bloom VL, Friedel RO: The effectiveness of tricyclic antidepressants in the treatment of coexisting pain and depression. *Pain* 7:331-341, 1979.
16. Turk DC, Rudy TE, Stieg RL: Chronic pain and depression. *Pain Management* 1:17-25, 1987.
17. Richelson E: Pharmacology of antidepressants in use in the United States. *J Clin Psychiatry* 43:4-11, 1982.
18. Frommer DA et al: Tricyclic antidepressant overdose. *JAMA* 257:521-526, 1987.
19. Ancill RJ, Kennedy JS: Variability of plasma levels of antidepressants in the elderly: A possible mechanism. Proceedings of the American Psychiatry Association's 140th Annual Meeting. Washington, DC, 1987.
20. Friedman H, Greenblatt DJ: Rational therapeutic drug monitoring. *JAMA* 256:2227-2233, 1986.
21. Oxman T, Denson DD: Antidepressants and adjunctive psychotropic drugs. In Raj PP editor: *Practical Management of Pain.* St. Louis, Mosby, 1986.
22. Baldessarini RJ: *Chemotherapy in Psychiatry.* Cambridge, Harvard University Press, 1977.
23. Van Brunt N: The clinical utility of tricyclic antidepressant blood levels: A review of the literature. *Ther Drug Monit* 5:1-10, 1983.
24. Deicken RF: Clonazepam-induced reduction in serum desipramine concentration. *J Clin Psychopharmacol* 8:71-72, 1988, (letter).
25. Gram LF, Overo KF, Kirk L: Influence of neuroleptics and benzodiazepines on metabolism of tricyclic antidepressants in man. *Am J Psychiatry* 131:863-866, 1974.
26. Maany I et al: Increase in desipramine serum levels associated with methadone treatment. *Am J Psychiatry* 146:1611-1613, 1989.
27. Abernethy DR, Todd EL: Doxepin-cimetidine interaction: Increased

doxepin bioavailability during cimetidine treatment. *J Clin Psychopharmacol* 6:8-12, 1986.

28. Goodkin K, Gullion CM: Antidepressants for the relief of chronic pain: Do they work? *Annals of Behavioural Medicine* 11:83-101, 1989.

29. Preskorn SH, Simpson S: Tricyclic-antidepressant-induced delirium and plasma drug concentration. *Am J Psychiatry* 139:822-823, 1982.

30. Rubin EH, Biggs JT, Preskorn SH: Nortriptyline pharmacokinetics and plasma levels: Implications for clinical practice. *J Clin Psychiatry* 46:418-424, 1985.

31. Walsh TD: Antidepressants in chronic pain. *Clin Neuropharmacol* 6:271-295, 1983.

32. Woodforde JM et al: Treatment of post-herpetic neuralgia. *Med J Aust* 2:869-872, 1965.

33. Sharav Y et al: The analgesic effect of amitriptyline on chronic facial pain. *Pain* 31:199-209, 1987.

34. Taub A, Collins WF: Observations on the treatment of denervation dysesthesia with psychotropic drugs: Postherpetic neuralgia, anesthesia dolorosa, peripheral neuropathy. In Bonica JJ, editor: *Advances in Neurology, vol 4*. New York, Raven Press, 1974.

35. Kvinesdal B et al: Imipramine treatment of painful diabetic neuropathy. *JAMA* 251:1727-1730, 1984.

36. Davis JL et al: Peripheral diabetic neuropathy treated with amitriptyline and fluphenazine. *JAMA* 238:2291-2292, 1977.

37. Merskey H, Hester RA: The treatment of chronic pain with psychotropic drugs. *Postgrad Med J* 48:594-598, 1972.

38. Wetterus S et al: The effect of trimipramine on symptoms and healing of peptic ulcer: A double blind study. *Scand J Gastroenterol* 12:33-38, 1977.

39. Everett HC: The use of bethanechol chloride with tricyclic antidepressants. *Am J Psychiatry* 132:1202-1204, 1975.

40. Mangla JC, Pereira M: Tricyclic antidepressants in the treatment of peptic ulcer disease. *Arch Intern Med* 142:273-275, 1982.

41. Dilsaver SC, Greden JF: Antidepressant withdrawal phenomena. *Biol Psychiatry* 19:237-256, 1984.

42. Beaumont G: The toxicity of antidepressants. *Br J Psychiatry* 154:454-458, 1989.

43. Callaham M, Kassel D: Epidemiology of fatal tricyclic antidepressant ingestion: Implications for management. *Ann Emerg Med* 14:1-9, 1985.

44. Shannon M, Merola J, Lovejoy FH: Hypotension in severe tricyclic antidepressant overdose. *Am J Emerg Med* 6:439-442, 1988.

45. Teba L et al: Beneficial effect of norepinephrine in the treatment of circulatory shock caused by tricyclic antidepressant overdose. *Am J Emerg Med* 6:566-568, 1988.

46. Varnell RM et al: Adult respiratory distress syndrome from overdose of tricyclic antidepressants. *Radiology* 170:677-680, 1989.

47. Walter-Ryan WG et al: Persistent photoaggravated cutaneous eruption induced by imipramine *JAMA* 254:357-358, 1985, (letter).

48. Litvak R, Kaelbling R: Dermatological side effects with psychotropics. *Diseases of the Nervous System* 33:309-311, 1972.

49. Weintraub M, Evans P: Bupropion: A chemically and pharmacologically unique antidepressant. *Hosp Forum* 24:254-259, 1989.

50. Davidson J: Seizures and bupropion: A review. *J Clin Psychiatry* 50:256-261, 1989.

51. Wernicke JF: The side effect profile and safety of fluoxetine. *J Clin Psychiatry* 46:59-67, 1985.

52. Calabrese JR, Gulledge AD: Psychotropics during pregnancy and lactation: A review. *Psychosomatics* 26:413-425, 1985.

53. Cohen LS, Heller VL, Rosenbaum JF: Treatment guidelines for psychotropic drug use in pregnancy. *Psychosomatics* 30:25-33, 1989.

54. France RD, Houpt JL, Ellinwood EH: Therapeutic effects of antidepressants in chronic pain. *Gen Hosp Psychiatry* 6:55-63, 1984.

55. Atkinson JH, Kremer EF, Garfin SR: Psychopharmacological agents in the treatment of pain. *J Bone Joint Surg Am* 67-A:337-342, 1985.

56. Aronoff GM, Wagner JM, Spangler AS: Chemical interventions for pain. *J Consult Clin Psychol* 54:769-775, 1986.

57. Feinmann C: Pain relief by antidepressants: Possible modes of action. *Pain* 23:1-8, 1985.

58. Melzack R, Wall PD: Pain mechanisms: A new theory. *Science* 150:971-979, 1965.

59. Max MB et al: Amitriptyline relieves diabetic neuropathy pain in patients with normal or depressed mood. *Neurology* 37:589-596, 1987.

60. Thayssen P et al: Cardiovascular effects of imipramine and nortriptyline in elderly patients. *Psychopharmacology* 74:360-364, 1981.

61. Price WA, Giannini AJ: Amoxapine-induced extrapyramidal effects. *Psychosomatics* 27:464-465, 1986, (letter).

62. Richelson E: Antidepressants: Pharmacology and clinical use. In Karasu TB editor: *Treatments of Psychiatric Disorders*. Washington, DC, American Psychiatric Association, 1989.

63. Goodnick PJ: Influence of fluoxetine on plasma levels of desipramine. *Am J Psychiatry* 146:552, 1989, (letter).

64. Roose SP et al: Cardiovascular effects of imipramine and bupropion in depressed patients with congestive heart failure. *J Clin Psychopharmacol* 7:247-251, 1987.

65. Richards GA et al: Unusual drug interactions between monoamine oxidase inhibitors and tricyclic antidepressants. *J Neurol Neurosurg Psychiatry* 50:1240-1241, 1987, (letter).

66. Kocher R: Use of psychotropic drugs for the treatment of chronic severe pain. In Bonica JJ, Albe-Fessard D, editors: *Advances in Pain Research and Therapy, vol 1*. New York, Raven Press, 1976.

67. Byrne A, O'Shea B: Adverse interaction between cimetidine and chlorpromazine in two cases of chronic schizophrenia. *Br J Psychiatry* 155:413-415, 1989.

68. Linnoila M, George L, Guthrie S: Interaction between antidepressants and perphenazine in psychiatric inpatients. *Am J Psychiatry* 139:1329-1331, 1982.

69. Borison RJ: Pharmacology of antipsychotic drugs. *J Clin Psychiatry* 46(4, sec 2):25-28, 1985.

70. Baldessarini RJ: Clinical and epidemiologic aspects of tardive dyskinesia. *J Clin Psychiatry* 46(4, sec 2):8-13, 1985.

71. Jeste DV, Wyatt RJ: Prevention and management of tardive dyskinesia. *J Clin Psychiatry* 46(4, sec 2):14-18, 1985.

72. Liskow BI: Relationship between neuroleptic malignant syndrome and malignant hyperthermia. *Am J Psychiatry* 142:390, 1985, (letter).

73. Guze BH, Baxter LR: Neuroleptic malignant syndrome. *N Engl J Med* 313:163-166, 1985.

74. Caroff SN et al: Malignant hyperthermia susceptibility in neuroleptic malignant syndrome. *Anesthesiology* 67:20-25, 1987.

75. Sangal R, Dimitrijevic R: Neuroleptic malignant syndrome: Successful treatment with pancuronium. *JAMA* 254:2795-2796, 1985.

76. Montilla E, Frederick WS, Cass LJ: Analgesic effect of methotrimeprazine and morphine. *Arch Intern Med* 111:91-94, 1963.

77. McGee JL, Alexander MR: Phenothiazine analgesia—fact or fantasy? *Am J Hosp Pharm* 36:633-640, 1979.

78. Mendel CM et al: A trial of amitriptyline and fluphenazine in the treatment of painful diabetic neuropathy. *JAMA* 255:637-639, 1986.

79. Clarke IMC: Amitriptyline and perphenazine (Triptafen DA) in chronic pain. *Anaesthesia* 36:210-211, 1981.

80. Maciewicz R, Bouckboms A, Martin JB: Drug therapy of neuropathic pain. *Clin J Pain* 1:39-49, 1985.

81. Swerdlow M: Anticonvulsant drugs and chronic pain. *Clin Neuropharmacol* 7:51-82, 1984.

82. Rall TW, Schleifer LS: Drugs effective in the therapy of the epilepsies. In Gilman AG et al editors: *The Pharmacological Basis of Therapeutics*. New York, Macmillan, 1985.

83. Morley GK, Erickson DL, Morley JE: The neurology of pain. In Joynt RJ, editor: *Clinical Neurology*. Philadelphia, JB Lippincott, 1989.

84. Fitzsimmons WE: The role of metabolites and protein binding in antiepileptic monitoring. *Resident Staff Physician* 33:151-159, 1987.

85. Bruni J, Wilder BJ: Valproic acid: Review of a new drug. *Arch Neurol* 36:393-398, 1979.

86. Burchiel KJ: Carbamazepine inhibits spontaneous activity in experimental neuromas. *Exp Neurol* 102:249-253, 1988.

87. Snyder SH: Drug and neurotransmitter receptors. *JAMA* 261:3126-3129, 1989.

88. Scherkl R, Frey H: Physical dependence on clonazepam in dogs. *Pharmacology* 32:18-24, 1986.

89. Calabrese JR, Gulledge AD: Carbamazepine, clonazepam use during pregnancy. *Psychosomatics* 27:464, 1986, (letter).

90. Kimura S et al: Plasma protein binding of clonazepam in vitro: Interaction with other drugs in the effect of pH and plasma dilution. *Jpn J Psychiatry Neurol* 41:527-530, 1987.

91. Sunaoshi W, Miura H, Shirai H: Influence of concurrent administra-

tion of carbamazepine on the plasma concentrations of clonazepam. *Jpn J Psychiatry Neurol* 42:589-591, 1988.

92. Whyte J, Wroblewski B: Effects of phenytoin on cognitive function. *N Engl J Med* 321:53, 1989 (letter).

93. Dodrill CB: Effects of phenytoin on cognitive function. *N Engl J Med* 321:53, 1989.

94. Reynolds EH, Trimble MR: Adverse neuropsychiatric effects of anticonvulsant drugs. *Drugs* 29:570-581, 1985.

95. Hatangdi VS, Boas RA, Richards EG: Postherpetic neuralgia: Management with antiepileptic and tricyclic drugs. In Bonica JJ, Albe-Fessard D, editors: *Advances in Pain Research and Therapy.* New York, Raven Press, 1976.

96. Young RJ, Clarke BF: Pain relief in diabetic neuropathy: The effectiveness of imipramine and related drugs. *Diabet Med* 2:363-366, 1985.

97. Bouckoms AJ, Litman RE: Clonazepam in the treatment of neuralgic pain syndrome. *Psychosomatics* 26:933-936, 1985.

98. Greenblatt DJ, Shader RI, Abernethy DR: Current status of the benzodiazepines (1). *N Engl J Med* 309:410-416, 1983.

99. Digregorio GJ, Kozin SH: Adjuvant drug therapy for pain. *Am Fam Physician* 33:227-232, 1986.

100. Hendler N et al: A comparison of cognitive impairment due to benzodiazepines and to narcotics. *Am J Psychiatry* 137:828-830, 1980.

101. Lader M: Clinical pharmacology of benzodiazepines. *Annu Rev Medicine* 38:19-28, 1987.

102. Greenblatt DJ, Shader RI, Abernethy DR: Current status of the benzodiazepines (2). *N Engl J Med* 309:354-358, 1983.

103. Drugs and Insomnia: The use of medications to promote sleep. *JAMA* 251:2410-2414, 1984.

104. Hollister LE: A look at the issues. *Psychosomatics* 21(suppl):4-8, 1980.

105. Oreland L: The benzodiazepines: A pharmacologic overview. *Acta Anaesthesiol Scand* 32(88 suppl):13-16, 1987.

106. Gottlieb DI: GABAergic neurons. *Sci Am* 258:82-89, 1988.

107. Bianchi CP: Basic mechanisms of action and therapeutic applications of the benzodiazepines. *Postgrad Med* June: 10-18, 1983.

108. Choice of benzodiazepines. *Med Lett Drugs Ther* 30:26-28, 1988.

109. Drugs that cause psychiatric symptoms. *Med Lett Drugs Ther* 28:81-86, 1986.

110. Drugs for psychiatric disorders. *Med Lett Drugs Ther* 25:45-52, 1983.

111. Ayd FJ: Benzodiazepine dependency and withdrawal. In Usdin E et al editors: *Pharmacology of Benzodiazepines.* Weinheim, Verlag Chemie, 1984.

112. Schatzberg AF: New treatment for anxiety: Update on buspirone. *Harvard Medical School Mental Health Letters* 4:8, 1988.

113. Buspirone: A non-benzodiazepine for anxiety. *Med Lett Drugs Ther* 28:117-119, 1986.

114. Straughan JL, Conradie EA: Buspirone—frontrunner of a new genre of anxiolytics. *S Afr Med J* 74:441-444, 1988.

115. Hollister LH et al: Long-term use of diazepam. *JAMA* 246:1568-1570, 1981.

116. Singh PN et al: Clinical evaluation of diazepam for relief of postoperative pain. *Br J Anaesth* 53:831-835, 1981.

117. Feighner JP et al: Comparison of alprazolam, imipramine and placebo in the treatment of depression. *JAMA* 249:3057-3064, 1983.

118. Rickels K, Feighner JP, Smith WT: Alprazolam, amitriptyline, doxepin, and placebo in the treatment of depression. *Arch Gen Psychiatry* 42:134-141, 1985.

119. Beaver WT, Feise G: Comparison of the analgesic effects of morphine, hydroxyzine, and their combination in patients with postoperative pain. In Bonica JJ, Albe-Fessard D, editors: *Advances in Pain Research and Therapy, vol 1.* New York, Raven Press, 1976.

120. Kantor TG, Steinberg FP: Studies of tranquilizing agents and meperidine in clinical pain. Hydroxyzine and meprobamate. In Bonica JJ, Albe-Fessard D, editors: *Advances in Pain Research and Therapy, vol 1.* New York, Raven Press, 1976.

121. Elenbaas JK: Centrally acting oral skeletal muscle relaxants. *Am J Hosp Pharm* 37:1313-1323, 1980.

122. Franz DN: Drugs for Parkinson's disease. In Goodman LS, Gilman AG editors: *The Pharmacological Basis of Therapeutics.* New York, Macmillan, 1975.

123. Hupert C, Yacoub M, Turgeon LR: Effect of hydroxyzine on morphine for the treatment of postoperative pain. *Anesth Analg* 59:690-696, 1980.

QUESTIONS: COANALGESIC AGENTS

1. The anticholinergic effects of antidepressants (e.g., xerostomia, poor visual accommodation, tachycardia, urinary retention) are due to their:
   A. Nicotinic action
   B. Muscarinic action
   C. Histaminic action
   D. α_1 adrenergic action

2. When selecting an antidepressant for use in pain management, one should consider all of the following EXCEPT:
   A. Match the patient's pain syndrome with the drug that most likely will effect it.
   B. Consider a tricyclic or trazadone for patients with poor sleep.
   C. Start with a high dose and decrease gradually.
   D. Inform the patient about the drug's side effects ahead of time.

3. Side effects of neuroleptics include all of the following EXCEPT:
   A. Dystonia
   B. Akathisia
   C. Drug-induced parkinsonism
   D. Muscular flaccidity

4. When choosing a neuroleptic for use in pain management, one should consider all of the following EXCEPT:
   A. Start the antidepressant first.
   B. Use of antidepressant is ineffective even with improved sleep.
   C. The liver function test is normal.
   D. The institution of neuroleptic should be done fast.

5. The mechanism of benzodiazepine is through binding with a specific receptor that is complexed to:
   A. Dopamine receptor
   B. GABA$_A$ receptor
   C. Opiate receptor
   D. α adrenergic receptor

ANSWERS

1. B
2. C
3. D
4. D
5. B

15 Organization and Function of Nerve Block Facility

P. Prithvi Raj

Nerve blocks useful for chronic pain include somatic peripheral nerve blocks, intravertebral central neural blocks, and sympathetic blocks. They can be spectacularly effective in acute pain relief; they are used daily in medical and dental operative procedures to interrupt the transmission of nociceptive stimuli from the peripheral to the central nervous system. Because the mechanisms of chronic pain are frequently different from those of acute pain, nerve blocks may be less effective in chronic pain states. Nevertheless, they still have an important part to play in the diagnosis, prognosis, and sometimes therapy of chronic pain.

FACILITIES

A pain control center should provide a comfortable and relaxing area for its patients who are having such invasive procedures as nerve blocks. Adequate space and equipment are imperative to ensure proper preparation and care of the patient undergoing such procedures.

To perform the more invasive procedures (e.g., epidural blocks, celiac plexus blocks, lumbar sympathetic blocks, and stellate ganglion blocks), large, major treatment rooms are necessary. They should be equipped to accommodate emergencies that may arise. A list of essential equipment for such invasive procedures follows.

· Locking stretcher or surgical table that can be easily and quickly placed into many different positions
· Anesthesia machine ready for emergency situations
· Oxygen tank with Ambu bag, oxygen mask, and nasal cannula available for emergencies
· Suction machine and catheter
· Cardiac monitor with defibrillator
· Emergency crash cart with medication and intubation equipment
· Intravenous (IV) tray that can be easily carried into an examination room should the need arise
· IV pole
· Two Mayo stands
· Large supply cabinets and counters to store medication, procedure trays, gloves, extra supplies, etc.
· X-ray view box

ROLE OF THE NURSE

The nurse plays an extremely important role in patient preparation and education before a procedure; the nurse helps allay the patient's fears and apprehension.

It is the responsibility of both the physician and the nurse to inform the patient of the purpose of the procedure, how it is done, the expected outcome, and the side effects and risks. Unless the procedure is urgent, this explanation is given on the visit before the procedure. To reinforce the verbal explanation, the patient receives a simple, written explanation of the procedure. Patients are told to bring an escort to accompany them home after the procedure. Written consent is obtained; although this is the responsibility of the physician, the nurse verifies that this was done.

When first seen at the pain control center, the chronic pain patient has already been examined by many professionals in various hospitals and has undergone various tests and procedures. This experience makes the patient fearful and apprehensive of seeing another new set of medical professionals. Nerve blocks are often foreign to patients and can be a source of apprehension. The patient must be reassured that nerve blocks are a standard form of therapy and are performed by experts at the pain control center.

During the procedure, the nurse not only sets up equipment, positions the patient, monitors vital signs, and assists as required during the procedure but also helps the patient relax and anticipates the patient's needs and any problems that may arise.

The nurse helps the patient relax by employing techniques of relaxation, distraction, or guided imagery. It is important that the patient knows what to expect at each step of the procedure so that the patient is less likely to make sudden, unexpected movements. The nurse offers comfort as needed, including proper positioning of extremities with pillows and premedication if necessary.

The nurse is knowledgeable about the anatomy and physiology of the region to be blocked and the pharmacology of the drugs to be used. Knowing drug complications and side effects is imperative in anticipating problems and dealing with emergencies.

After the procedure, patients are closely monitored as long as necessary, usually 30 minutes to 1 hour, to evaluate the success of the block and its sequelae.

Verbal and written instructions are given to the patient before discharge. This includes a list of side effects that commonly occur with the block and the length of time they should last. Patients are also informed how and when to call the personnel in the pain control center should problems arise.

ADJUVANT TECHNIQUES FOR SUCCESSFUL NERVE BLOCK

Many procedures that involve placement of a catheter for continuous infusion or a neurolytic block are done under fluoroscopy. Because of the nature of the block and the potential risks involved, it is imperative that a nurse accompany the physician. Essentially, the nurse provides the same assistance during this type of procedure as during any other nerve block.

A mobile cart is essential and should be stocked with supplies necessary for the procedure: IV supplies, procedure trays, appropriate needles and catheters, temperature probes, syringes, medication, emergency drugs, and intubation equipment.

Before the procedure, a thorough explanation is given to the patient and written consent obtained. An IV line is started in all patients.

The nurse's role during the procedure in the x-ray unit is critical. The nature of these blocks and the presence of large pieces of x-ray apparatus increase patient's apprehension. The nurse provides relaxation techniques and medications to lessen this apprehension. Diazepam, although often used, may cause generalized peripheral vasodilation that may make evaluation of the degree of sympathetic block more difficult.

After the procedure, the patient is monitored as necessary and reminded of what to expect. A post-block pain assessment is done to evaluate the success of the block, and arrangements are made for the safe transfer of the patient to a hospital bed or to the pain control center before the patient is discharged home.

Radiologic localization is indicated when difficulty is anticipated because of poor landmarks or anatomic anomalies, when deep nerves or plexuses are to be blocked, and when neurolytic procedures are planned.

Contrast materials should not be injected if the patient has a history of allergy to iodine-containing solutions. Metrizamide may inadvertently be injected into the subarachnoid space during the procedure. Even though this is usually innocuous, generalized muscle twitching may occur because of the action of metrizamide on the spinal cord. Repeated doses of diazepam (0.1 mg/kg IV) may be needed for 24 hours before the muscle twitching subsides. However, in general, intravascular injection of any contrast material has not been deleterious.

MONITORING

Preparation of the patient for regional anesthesia should include a complete explanation of the procedure to be performed and informed consent before or while the patient is brought to the area where the block will occur. This room should be quiet, undisturbed, of adequate size, and have good lighting. The characteristics and design of an ideal regional anesthesia block room have been described by Rosenblatt and Shal.[1] Complete resuscitation facilities must be available and should include equipment to provide positive-pressure oxygen and suction, intubation equipment with appropriate laryngoscope blades and handles already tested for working order, appropriate-sized endotracheal tubes and oral airways, and emergency drugs. Essential emergency drugs that should be available include succinylcholine, atropine, thiopental or diazepam, ephedrine, and lidocaine (Table 15-1). A functioning IV catheter is essential for all regional anesthesia procedures, except for small (2 to 3 ml) injections of local anesthetics into muscle trigger points or single peripheral nerve blocks. Minimal monitoring should include continuous electrocardiographic (ECG) monitoring, heart rate, blood pressure, respiratory rate, oxygen saturation if sedative or narcotic analgesic medications will be given before or during the block, and level of consciousness.[2]

Central neural blockade

Spinal anesthesia. Once the patient is taken to the facility where the block will occur, a functioning IV catheter should be started, and blood pressure and heart rate should be measured before administration of the block. These measurements must be continued throughout the procedure with continuous ECG monitoring, because the most important physiologic response to spinal anesthesia involves the cardiovascular system. This response is mediated primarily by the combined effects of sympathetic denervation and, with higher block (T_1-T_4), unopposed vagal nerve dominance. Sympathetic denervation produces arterial, and more importantly, arteriolar vasodilation. This vasodilation is not complete, however, because the vascular smooth muscle on the arterial side maintains a significant degree of autonomous tone. The venous system has little smooth muscle present within its walls, and maintains no residual tone with complete sympathectomy. Venodilatation and reduced preload result in a reduction in cardiac output and can cause hypotension after spinal anesthesia, which needs clinical management.[3] Bradycardia can occur after spinal anesthesia and may be due to blockade of the cardioaccelerator fibers (arising from T_1 to T_4) or decreased venous return activation of the great vein and right atrial cardiac receptors, which reflexively slow the heart rate.[4]

Respiratory rate must be determined before the block and adequacy of ventilation monitored throughout the procedure. It is important to monitor closely the level of consciousness throughout the period of spinal anesthesia to detect any change before it becomes a problem.[5] The level of spinal anesthesia should be followed in anticipation of an untoward event, such as blockage of the cardioaccelerator fibers with a high thoracic block (T_1-T_4).

When spinal narcotics are administered, monitor for delayed respiratory depression and assess for sedation and excessive somnolence, which usually occurs before overt respiratory depression. The respiratory rate and depth of respiration must be followed closely. Pulse oximetry can help detect inadequate arterial oxygenation. Monitor patients for at least 12 hours after administering the last dose of intrathecal opioids.[6]

Epidural blockade. Whenever epidural anesthesia is attempted, there is a potential for local anesthetic toxicity because significantly higher volumes of local anesthetic will be used to achieve anesthesia.

Before initiation of an epidural block, determine baseline blood pressure, heart rate, and level of consciousness. The anesthesiologist must continuously monitor blood pressure

Table 15-1 Routine emergency drugs required during regional anesthesia procedures

Drug	Suggested dosage (70 kg adult)	Indication
Atropine	0.2-0.4 mg IV increments	Bradycardia from vagal dominance
Diazepam	2.5-5 mg IV increments	Local anesthetic; seizure activity
Ephedrine	5-10 mg IV increments	Hypotension from sympathetic block
Lidocaine	50-100 mg IV bolus	Ventricular arrhythmias
Thiopental	50-100 mg IV increments	Local anesthetic; seizure activity
Succinylcholine	100 mg IV bolus	Muscle relaxation airway control

and the ECG. If sedative or narcotic analgesic medication is given during the block, continuous pulse oximetry is mandatory. Before giving a full dose of local anesthetic, verify that the needle is in the epidural space by administering a test dose of 3 ml of local anesthetic with 15 μg of epinephrine, and constantly observing the patient.[7] In the event of intravascular injection, this dose of epinephrine should elevate heart rate greater than 30 (beats per minute) bpm within 25 seconds of injection. If the subarachnoid space has inadvertently been entered and the test dose has been administered, the patient will have an identifiable level of anesthesia; thus it is critical to monitor the patient for any signs of nerve block. There is a continuing controversy over the validity of epidural test doses in obstetrics.[8] Once it has been determined that the epidural space has been reached, the volume of local anesthetic to achieve the desired level may be administered in divided doses of 5 ml each. Continue monitoring the patient's level of consciousness, respiratory rate, blood pressure, ECG, heart rate, and the extent of neural blockade.

Sympathetic ganglion blocks

Stellate ganglion blocks. Functioning IV access must be available before the block in the event of an intravascular injection and the occurrence of seizure activity.[9] A system for positive-pressure oxygen delivery and suction should be available nearby. Before the block, determine resting blood pressure, heart rate, and level of consciousness. If the patient is to receive sedative or narcotic medications, a pulse oximeter is necessary during the block and throughout the recovery period. Monitor temperature probes on a fingertip of each hand before the block to get a baseline temperature, and after the block to objectively assess the effectiveness; an elevation of temperature on the blocked side will indicate blocked sympathetic fibers.[10] The patient must fast at least 8 hours before the block to prevent intraoperative aspiration.

Because of the proximity of the ganglion to critical vascular structures, a test dose is mandatory. Administer 0.25 ml of the local anesthetic and constantly monitor the patient for any type of toxic reaction.[11] After repeat aspiration, inject the local anesthetic in divided doses. The patient must be continuously monitored for any change in the level of consciousness or for toxic reaction. Adequate placement of the local anesthetic after the block is complete can be confirmed by elevated temperature on the blocked side and evidence of Bernard-Horner syndrome (myosis, ptosis, and enophthalmos).[10]

Lumbar sympathetic ganglion blocks. A functioning IV catheter must be present in the event of an accidental intraspinal injection, and if sedatives or narcotic analgesics are needed during the procedure. Obtain baseline blood pressure, heart rate, level of consciousness, and lower-extremity temperatures before performing the block. Continuously monitor these parameters during the block and recovery period. Inadvertent intravascular injection can cause seizure activity, and subarachnoid placement of local anesthetic will cause complete spinal anesthesia; thus the anesthesiologist must be prepared for this rare outcome. The patient should fast at least 8 hours before the block. If the patient receives sedative or narcotic analgesic medications, use a pulse oximeter to monitor arterial oxygenation. It is also important to assess the patient's level of consciousness during the injection of local anesthesia and to maintain verbal contact after the block is complete. Monitor the patient for lower extremity motor strength and sensation because a somatic nerve block is possible, and continue monitoring after the block is complete.

Use fluoroscopic assistance to confirm proper needle placement especially when neurolytic agents are used. If fluoroscopy is not available, take baseline foot temperatures as another monitor of correct needle placement. After needle placement is complete, inject a small amount of 3% chloroprocaine and wait for a temperature elevation of at least 1.5° C before injecting a larger volume of a longer-acting local anesthetic.[10]

Celiac plexus blocks. Before proceeding with the block, establish an adequate intravenous access and determine baseline blood pressure, heart rate, respiratory rate, and level of consciousness. Resuscitation facilities should be available in the event of an inadvertent intravascular injection during the block. During the performance of the block and in the recovery period, continuously monitor the patient's blood pressure and ECG. Because the sympathetic nervous system supply to the abdominal viscera is interrupted with this block, hypotension is common and must be anticipated.[12] If sedative or analgesic drugs are used during the block, continuous pulse oximetry must be available. Use fluoroscopy to monitor correct needle placement and adequate spread of contrast dye before performing the block.

Somatic nerve blocks

With a somatic nerve block, confirm accurate placement of the needle with a nerve stimulator. Paresthesia can also be used to monitor proximity to the brachial plexus, but the incidence of peripheral nerve injury is higher when this technique is used to localize the nerve.[13]

Intercostal nerve blocks

The patient should have continuous monitoring of blood pressure, ECG, respiratory rate, and level of consciousness. Frequently these patients receive intravenous sedation, and therefore pulse oximetry should be used. After the patient has received the block, monitoring should be continued in the recovery period with special attention to respiratory and hemodynamic status. The incidence of pneumothorax following intercostal nerve block has been reported to be between 0.0083% and 19%.[14] Any patient complaining of dyspnea and chest pain accentuated by deep breathing and coughing should be suspected of having a pneumothorax and should have a chest x-ray for evaluation.

Lumbosacral plexus and its branches

Sciatic nerve blocks. Minimal monitoring should include continuous regulating blood pressure, ECG, and level of consciousness. If the patient receives any sedative or narcotic medications during the block, use a pulse oximeter. A peripheral nerve stimulator can greatly enhance the success rate of a sciatic nerve block by helping to avoid significant patient discomfort. Assess the extent of the block by examining motor function, which is primarily a somatic nerve.

Head and neck blocks. Insert a functioning IV catheter before performing the block, and resuscitation facilities must be available if a seizure should occur.[11] Continuously monitor blood pressure, ECG, respiratory rate, and level of consciousness throughout the block and during the recovery period. If IV sedatives or narcotics are used, use pulse oximetry.

EQUIPMENT

To perform successful regional anesthesia, the correct equipment should be available, including needles, syringes, and ancillary equipment necessary for the block. If continuous infusions are planned, adequate tubing and pumps must be available.

A nerve block tray, whether commercially or hospital prepared, should contain sufficient equipment to perform the intended regional anesthesia procedure (Box 15-1). Basic items on each nerve block tray should include items for sterile skin preparation and draping; containers for sterile antiseptic solution and local anesthetic; syringes for skin infiltration anesthesia and performance of the block; and an assortment of needles for skin infiltration and drawing up local anesthetic solutions, preparing the skin, and performing the block. Injection tubing should be available, and if continuous infusions are planned, appropriate catheters should also be available. If drugs are to be added to regional block trays, consult with the hospital pharmacy to ensure stability and potency of the drug and so that sterility can be maintained during the sterilization process.

Using reusable regional anesthesia trays or commercially available trays is a personal preference, ultimate cost and arguments can be made in favor of either choice. McMahon recently discussed the merits of reusable trays versus disposable trays.[15]

Box 15-1 CONTENTS OF MULTIPURPOSE REGIONAL ANESTHESIA BLOCK TRAY

Routine items

Prep tray
Container for antiseptic solution (50 ml)
Antiseptic solution
Prep sponges (3)
4 × 4 gauze sponges
Ruler (15 cm)
Sterility indicator
Sterile drapes (4)
IV extension tubing
Container for local anesthetic (2, 50 ml each)
Local anesthetic solution for infiltration (1.5% lidocaine, 10 ml)
Epinephrine (1 mg/ml)
Syringes
    1 ml to dispense epinephrine
    3 ml for skin infiltration
    5 ml glass to identify the epidural space
    10 ml to inject local anesthetic
Needles
    25 x 2.5 cm (1 inch) for skin infiltration of local anesthetic
    22 x 7.5 cm (3 inch) for deeper skin infiltration
    22 x 11.8 cm (4.5 inch) for deep skin infiltration
    18 x 3.8 cm (1.5 inch) to pierce skin and draw up solutions

Contents specific for procedure

Block needles
    Spinal
    Spinal introducer needle
    Epidural
    Blunt bevel needles, appropriate size
Catheter for continuous infusions; spinal, epidural, peripheral nerve
Local anesthetic for nerve block
Contrast agent and container
Neurolytic solution and container

Needles

Nerve injury can occur after injection of local anesthetic for regional anesthesia and involves one of three mechanisms:

1. Direct injury may occur to the nerve from the cutting edge of the needle.
2. Local anesthetic injection into the nerve sheath under high pressure can cause direct neural damage or ischemia of the nerve.
3. A toxic effect of the local anesthetic or its preservative may be responsible for neural toxicity.

During peripheral or plexus nerve block procedures, a needle with a short, blunt bevel has produced less nerve trauma than the conventional hypodermic needle, which has a long or cutting bevel.[16] It is important to use the smallest diameter needle possible to avoid tissue trauma and undue discomfort. However, it is essential that the needle be large enough to inject local anesthetics and aspirate blood easily should an accidental intravascular injection occur; therefore a 22-gauge needle is recommended for most nerve blocks.

For procedures that require deep penetration, such as a celiac plexus or hypogastric plexus block, an 18- or 20-gauge needle is preferred for better control in guiding the needle and for ease of aspiration. A 25- or 27-gauge needle should be used to infiltrate the skin and subcutaneous tissue before proceeding with a larger needle for the nerve block. If a catheter is to be used for a continuous infusion technique, prepare the skin first by making a nick with a larger (18-gauge) needle to avoid disrupting the catheter tip as it is inserted into the skin. If a styletted needle is used, the stylet nust fit flush with the bevel of the needle to avoid coring the tissue and possible obstruction of the needle tip during insertion. Extension tubing can be beneficial when directly attached to the needle because the syringe can then be changed when multiple injections are to be used, such as with confirmation of needle placement using contrast agents under fluoroscopy.

The incidence of spinal headaches appears to be directly related to the size of needle used and the orientation of the needle in performing spinal anesthesia.[17] Mihic established the important relationship between postspinal headaches and the orientation of the needle bevel to the longitudinal dural fibers.[18] It is thought that the spinal needle oriented parallel to the dura separates the fibers rather than cuts them, as a spinal needle oriented perpendicular to the dural fibers does, and produces a smaller defect in the dura mater.

Catheters

There are a wide variety of catheters available for insertion through both spinal and epidural needles and for placement on peripheral nerves and plexuses for continuous infusion techniques. The primary difference between these catheters is the material from which they are made and their physical properties. The ideal material for catheter construction should have the properties described by Bromage[19] (Box 15-2). The material should be inert, nonirritating, and supple enough to avoid cracking during placement. It should possess tensile strength to prevent breakage caused by traction and during insertion, and should allow rigid maneuvers. The length of the catheter should be long enough to reach up over the shoulder from the lumbar region and still have sufficient length to enter the epidural space. The external diameter should be small enough to allow it to easily pass through an epidural needle, and the internal diameter lumen must be large enough to inject fluids and to aspirate blood and cerebrospinal fluid (CSF). The wall of the catheter must be thick enough to avoid kinking and obstruction. The catheter tip should be smooth, dull, and flexible to prevent perforation of veins or dura. Radiopaque catheters can allow verification of correct placement with radiographic guidance, and graduated markings facilitate control of the depth of catheter insertion into the epidural space.

Recently subarachnoid catheters have been introduced for continuous spinal infusions.[20] Continuous spinal catheter infusion is not a new technique of regional anesthesia; it was described by Tuohy in 1944.[21] An epidural catheter can be used for continuous subarachnoid infusion, however, the incidence of spinal headache with an 18- to 20-gauge catheter would be too high in younger patients. The present sub-

---

Box 15-2 IDEAL CHARACTERISTICS OF AN EPIDURAL CATHETER*

Biochemically inert and nonirritating
High tensile strength
Low coefficient of friction
Resistant to kinking and obstruction
Maneuverable rigidity
Smooth and nontraumatic tip
Indicator of catheter length
Radioopacity

---

*From Hurley RJ, Lambert DH: Continuous spinal anesthesia with microcatheter techniques: The experience in obstetrics and general surgery. *Reg Anesth* 14:S3, 1989.

---

arachnoid catheter is small enough to be used clinically without an unacceptably high incidence of spinal headache.[22] These catheters are 27-, 28-, or 32-gauge, and have internal diameters large enough to inject medications. One of the problems associated with such a small catheter is the force that must be generated to overcome the resistance of the catheter. However, a recent study confirmed that infusion pumps can accurately deliver a continuous infusion into the 32-gauge catheter.[23]

Catheters are available for continuous peripheral nerve, plexus, and sympathetic ganglion infusions. They should have most of the properties of an ideal epidural catheter (see Box 15-2), but they should be sufficiently rigid to maintain their initial placement and avoid migration away from the area to be blocked. The 18-gauge Longdwel thin-wall Teflon catheter* has been used for prolonged infusions of sympathetic ganglia, peripheral nerves, and plexi.[24] It is available in 4, 6, and 8 inches.

Tubing and pumps

Continuous infusions of local anesthetics or anesthetic-narcotic combinations are commonly used to provide anesthesia, prolong analgesia postoperatively, and relieve chronic pain conditions.

Adequate tubing must be available and should be a caliber small enough to reduce dead space, and ideally should be a color different from regular IV tubing to clearly identify that it is carrying a potentially toxic substance. It must not have injection ports and should be clearly labeled that it is not an IV line to prevent accidental injection or infusion of another drug.

Several commercial pumps are available that are capable of providing continuous infusions: IV infusion pumps, patient-controlled analgesia pumps with basal rate capability, and syringe pumps. The pump must generate enough force to infuse the medication through the resistance of the narrow tubing without exceeding its limits and causing frequent high pressure alarms. The pump should be easy to operate and should be able to set the rate delivered per hour, maximum volume over a certain time period, and volume

---

*Available from Becton Dickinson & Co., Franklin Lakes, NJ.

Box 15-3 MANAGEMENT OF ANAPHYLAXIS*

Initial therapy

1. Stop administration of antigen (contrast agent)
2. Maintain airway with 100% oxygen
3. Start IV volume expansion (2 to 4 L crystalloid with hypotension)
4. Discontinue any supplemental analgesic or sedative agents
5. Give epinephrine (4 to 8 μg IV bolus with hypotension, titrate as needed; 0.1 to 0.5 mg IV bolus with cardiovascular collapse)

Secondary treatment

1. Antihistamines (diphenhydramine 0.5 to 1 mg/kg)
2. Catecholamine infusions (starting doses: epinephrine 2 to 4 μg/min, norepinephrine 2 to 4 μg/min, or isoproterenol 0.5 to 1 μg/min as a drip, and titrated to desired effects)
3. Aminophylline (5 to 6 mg/kg over 20 min with persistent bronchospasm)
4. Corticosteroids (hydrocortisone 0.25 to 1 g; alternately methylprednisolone 1 to 2 g)†
5. Sodium bicarbonate (0.5 to 1 mEq/kg with persistent hypotension or acidosis)
6. Airway evaluation (before extubation)

*Doses are representative for a 70 kg adult.
†Methylprednisolone may be the drug of choice if the reaction is suspected to be mediated by complement.

Table 15-2 Radiologic contrast agents

Agent	Type	Use
Diatrizoate (Renografin, Hypaque)	Ionic	Nerve plexus blocks
Iothalamate (Conray)	Ionic	Nerve plexus blocks
Metrizamide (Amipaque)	Nonionic	Central neural blockade
Iopamidol (Isovue)	Nonionic	Central neural blockade
Iohexol (Omnipaque)	Nonionic	Central neural blockade

infused, and should have a locking system to prevent tampering with the preset rate. Because these infusion volumes are frequently small, the pump must be capable of infusing small volumes (to 1 ml/hour with subarachnoid infusions). Alarm capabilities are important; and the unit should signal low infusion volumes, obstruction to flow, increased pressure, and tampering.

Fluoroscopy

Fluoroscopy is an invaluable adjunct in the performance of difficult regional anesthetic procedures in morbidly obese patients with poor anatomic landmarks or during celiac or hypogastric plexus blocks. Fluoroscopy is essential to verify accurate needle placement and spread of opaque contrast material before injecting neurolytic agents.

The ideal contrast material should provide opacification of blood vessels and tissue during fluoroscopy without any accompanying toxicity or alteration in physiologic function. These agents are commonly used to delineate different tissue planes and spread of the injected solution before introduction of local anesthetic or neurolytic substances. They can be used to confirm epidural placement of permanent catheters and to detect subdural or subarachnoid catheter placement or intravascular location.[25] Since these substances may be injected into the central nervous system (CNS) or intravascularly, the potential toxicity of the different agents must be considered.

The amount of contrast agents used during regional anesthesia procedures is usually small, therefore the clinical effects described with larger volumes during radiographic procedures are usually not produced.[26] The possibility of a true anaphylactic reaction to contrast agents is extremely rare but can occur; therefore a treatment plan must be prepared in anticipation of such an event. Carefully take the history of any patient scheduled to receive contrast agents to identify any previous adverse reaction to x-ray procedures or contrast material. It is essential to be able to provide airway support and intravascular volume expansion, and to be able to deliver 100% oxygen and epinephrine to treat any hypotension and hypoxia that could occur from vasodilation, increased capillary permeability, and bronchospasm in an anaphylactic reaction. Levy has provided an excellent review of anaphylactic reaction management. Box 15-3 provides a protocol for managing anaphylaxis that may occur after the injection of contrast material.[27] Emergency drugs and fluids should be readily available.

The contrast agents that are commonly used have a fully substituted, triiodinated benzene ring structure and may have an ionic or nonionic formulation (Table 15-2). The nonionic contrast agents provide opacification of the CNS and reduce CNS toxicity after subarachnoid injection. Metrizamide was the first nonionic formulation to be clinically used and has been used for years to provide state-of-the-art imaging during myelography. However, it comes in a powder that must be prepared before use, and the frequency of seizures with its use is unacceptably high relative to the newer agents available.[28] When contrast agents are used near the central axis and the potential for subarachnoid injection exists, use iopamidol or iohexol because they have a lower potential for CNS toxicity, are water soluble, and are provided in a liquid form that is easy to use.[29] In other regions of the body, the ionic contrast agents diatrizoate or iothalamate can be used without any significant clinical effects or adverse sequelae if the volume is limited to 10 to 15 ml.

REFERENCES

1. Rosenblatt RM, Shal R: The design and function of a regional anesthesia block room. *Reg Anesth* 9:12, 1984.
2. Smith DC, Crul JF: Oxygen desaturation following sedation for regional anesthesia. *Br J Anaesth* 62:206, 1989.
3. Ward RJ et al: Epidural and subarachnoid anesthesia: Cardiovascular and respiratory effects. *JAMA* 191:275, 1965.
4. Mackey DC et al: Bradycardia and asystole during spinal anesthesia: A report of three cases without morbidity. *Anesthesiology* 70:866, 1989.

5. Caplan RA et al: Unexpected cardiac arrest during spinal anesthesia: A closed claim analysis of predisposing factors. *Anesthesiology* 68:5, 1988.
6. Rawal N et al: Present state of extradural and intradural opioid analgesia in Sweden. A nationwide follow-up survey. *Br J Anaesth* 59:791, 1987.
7. Moore DC, Batra MS: The components of an effective test dose prior to epidural block. *Anesthesiology* 55:693, 1981.
8. Dain SL, Rolbin SH, Hew EM: The epidural test dose in obstetrics: Is it necessary? *Can J Anaesth* 6:601, 1987.
9. Korevaar W, Burney RG, Moore PA: Convulsions during stellate ganglion block: A case report. *Anesth Analg* 58:329, 1979.
10. Benzon HT, Avram MJ: Temperature increases after complete sympathetic blockade. *Reg Anesth* 11:27, 1986.
11. Kozody R et al: Dose requirement of local anesthetic to produce grand mal seizure during stellate ganglion block. *Can Anaesth Soc J* 29:489, 1982.
12. Thompson GE, Moore DC: Celiac plexus, intercostal and minor peripheral blockade. In Cousins MJ, Bridenbaugh PO editors: *Neural Blockade in Clinical Anesthesia and Management of Pain.* Philadelphia, JB Lippincott, 1988.
13. Ellis JC, Ramamurthy S: More problems with the Arrow-Racz epidural catheter. *Anesthesiology* 65:124, 1985.
14. Bridenbaugh LD: Should regional anesthesia be used during upper abdominal surgery? *Problems in Anesthesia* 1:567, 1987.
15. McMahon D: Managing regional anesthesia equipment. *Problems in Anesthesia* 1:592, 1987.
16. Selander D, Dhuner KG, Lundberg G: Peripheral nerve injury due to injection needles used for regional anesthesia. *Acta Anaesthesiol Scand* 21:182, 1977.
17. Eckstein KL et al: Prospective comparative study of postspinal headaches in young patients (less than 51 years). *Reg Anesth* 5:57, 1982.
18. Mihic DN: Postspinal headache and relationship of needle bevel to longitudinal dural fibers. *Reg Anesth* 10:76, 1985.
19. Bromage BR: *Epidural Analgesia.* Philadelphia, WB Saunders, 1978.
20. Hurley RJ, Lambert DH: Continuous spinal anesthesia with microcatheter techniques: The experience in obstetrics and general surgery. *Reg Anesth* 14:S3, 1989.
21. Tuohy EB: Continuous spinal anesthesia: Its usefulness and technic involved. *Anesthesiology* 5:142, 1944.
22. Moote CA, Varkey GP, Komar WE: The incidence of headache is similar after both continuous spinal anaesthesia and conventional spinal anaesthesia. *Reg Anesth* 15(Suppl 1):59, 1990.
23. Flanagan J et al: Evaluation of four infusion pumps with a 32-gauge microspinal catheter for continuous infusion. *Reg Anesth* 15(Suppl 1):67, 1990.
24. Brown RE et al: Continuous peripheral nerve of local anesthetic for management of pain due to reflex sympathetic dystrophy. *Reg Anesth* 15 (Suppl 1):88, 1990.
25. Mehta M, Maher R: Injection into the extra-arachnoid subdural space. *Anaesthesia* 32:761, 1977.
26. Bettmann MA, Morris TW: Recent advances in contrast agents. *Radiol Clin North Am* 24:347, 1986.
27. Levy J: *Anaphylactic Reactions in Anesthesia and Intensive Care.* Boston, Butterworth, 1986.
28. Kieffer SA et al: Lumbar myelography with iohexol and metrizamide: A comparative multicenter prospective study. *Radiology* 151:665, 1984.
29. Lamb JT: Iohexol vs. iopamidol for myelography. *Invest Radiol* 20:537, 1985.

16 Local Anesthetics

Mark J. Williams

The placement of local anesthetics at various sites along the neural axis to produce anesthesia or analgesia is classified as *regional anesthesia*. These techniques are used for surgical anesthesia, postoperative analgesia, and acute or chronic pain management modalities.

Local anesthetics can be combined or used with other adjuvant medications to potentiate speed of onset and duration of action or to increase the intensity of anesthesia or analgesia. It is important to know the pharmacology of these medications to select the appropriate drug for a specific therapeutic task.

The chemical structure determines metabolism and elimination of these drugs from the body. Local anesthetics exist in two chemical forms, amino esters and amino amides (see Fig. 16-1). Amino esters are ester derivatives of paraaminobenzoic acid and are metabolized by plasma cholinesterase. The metabolic byproduct is paraaminobenzoic acid, which is a known allergen, and allergic reactions are therefore common. On the other hand, amino amides are compounds with amide linkages and are metabolized for the most part by the liver. The potentials for allergic reactions are extremely rare.

Local anesthetics can also be classified on the basis of their clinical properties[1] into three basic categories:

1. Low potency/short duration—procaine, 2-chloroprocaine
2. Intermediate potency/intermediate duration—lidocaine, mepivacaine, prilocaine
3. High potency/long duration—bupivacaine, tetracaine, etidocaine

The difference in clinical activities among the local anesthetics can be explained by their inherent physicochemical properties.

PHYSICAL AND CHEMICAL PROPERTIES

Lipid solubility, protein binding, and pKa of the local anesthetic agents are important factors that directly influence potency, onset of action, and duration of action (Table 16-1). In addition, some local anesthetics exist as chemical isomers (chiral forms), which may further create differences in their inherent activity and toxicity.

Lipid solubility

The potency of a local anesthetic is influenced in a nonlinear manner by its lipid solubility.[2] The more lipid soluble a local anesthetic is, the more potent the local anesthetic effect. The major determinant of the lipid solubility is the aromatic group (benzene ring) found on the local anesthetic molecule. The measurement of solubil-

ity is performed by studying the base form's solubility in organic solvents. However, experimental evaluations of solubility differ from clinical effect in that local anesthetics' clinical potency increases to a point and then levels off. This leveling off occurs at a lipid partition coefficient of about four. The plateauing of clinical potency is related to the surrounding fat and blood vessel adjacent to the nerve. These may act as a depot and pull the local anesthetic away, thereby decreasing the total amount of drug available to the nerve.

Protein binding

Local anesthetics bind to plasma and tissue proteins. A local anesthetic with a high protein-binding capacity will stay on the protein receptor for a longer time, thereby producing an increased duration of effect. Also, when these molecules are bound to the plasma proteins, they are not pharmacologically active; this has implications on their activity, toxicity, and metabolism. The two main binding plasma proteins are albumin and α_1-acid glycoprotein. α_1-acid glycoprotein has a high affinity and low capacity for binding with the local anesthetics, whereas albumin has a lower affinity and higher capacity. In other words, albumin has less affinity but will bind larger amounts of local anesthetics long after the α_1-acid glycoprotein binding capacity has been maximized. This capacity for binding local anesthetics is concentration dependent and decreases in a curvilinear manner as concentration increases. The clinical importance of this is that the potential for toxicity increases disproportionately with increased plasma concentrations.

Protein binding is also influenced by the pH of the plasma. The percentage of the bound drug decreases as the pH decreases. Therefore in acidotic states, for a given total concentration, there is an increased fraction of free active drug in the circulation; this potentiates toxicity. This also occurs at the receptor proteins in the sodium channels and may decrease duration of the local anesthetic effect.

Ionization

The amino acid group on the local anesthetic molecule determines the ionization of the molecule and thus the hydrophilic activity. This amino group is capable of accepting a hydrogen ion (H+) and then converting the unionized base form into the cationic form of the drug. The proportions of these forms present in solution are determined by the pKa of the drug and the pH of the solution. The pKa is defined as: the pH where 50% of the local anesthetic remains in the uncharged (basic) form, and 50% exists in the charged (cationic) form. This relationship between the pH and the

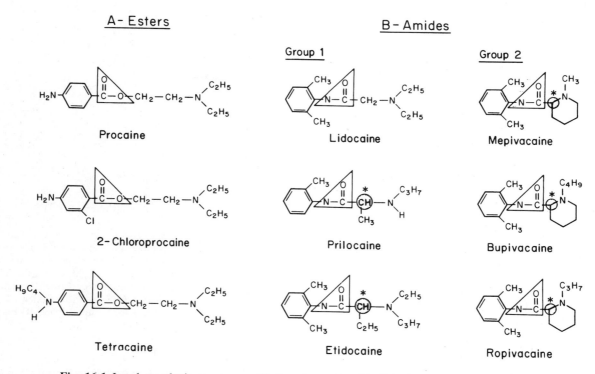

Fig. 16-1 Local anesthetic structures with the ester and amide link shown within the superimposed triangle. When present, the asymmetric carbon is circled, shaded, and marked with an asterisk (*). (From DiFazio CA, Woods AM: Pharmacology of local anesthetics. In Raj PP, editor: *Practical Management of Pain,* ed 2. St Louis, Mosby, 1992.)

Table 16-1 Physical properties and equipotent concentrations of local anesthetics

	Procaine	Lidocaine	Mepivacaine	Bupivacaine	Etidocaine	Ropivacaine
Molecular weight	236	234	246	288	276	274
pK$_a$	8.9	7.7	7.6	8.1	7.7	8.0
Lipid solubility	1	4	1	30	140	2.8
Partition coefficient	0.02	2.9	0.8	28	141	9
Protein binding	5	65	75	95	95	90-95
Equipotent conc ck	—	2.0	1.5	0.5	1.0	0.75

From DiFazio CA, Woods AM: Pharmacology of local anesthetics. In Raj PP, editor: *Practical Management of Pain,* ed 2. St Louis, Mosby, 1992.

pKa and the concentrations of the cation and the base forms is described by the Henderson-Hasselbalch equation:

$$pKa = pH + log(cation/base)$$

The pKa is important in determining the speed of onset of the local anesthetic. It is believed that the unionized form is responsible for diffusion across the nerve membrane and the ionized form produces blockade of the sodium ion movement through the sodium channel by binding to the receptor proteins. Hence both uncharged and charged forms are important for local anesthetic neural blockade. For local anesthetics, the pKa falls within a range of 7.6 to 8.9; thus these drugs at equilibrium exist predominantly in the cationic form at normal pH. Still agents with a pKa closest to the body's pH will have the fastest onset of action because a major portion will exist in the uncharged forms.

Chiral forms

The identification of stereo isomers for some local anesthetics like bupivacaine, mepivacaine, etidocaine, prilocaine, and ropivacaine has led to further evaluations of potential differences in potency, toxicity, and duration between these drugs. For stereo isomers to exist, an asymmetric carbon atom must be present in the molecule. The nomenclature to describe these isomers has changed in recent years; terms like *D* and *L* have been replaced by *R* and *S* respectively. The details of these differences are presented in Table 16-2. As a rule, the *S* form is less toxic and has a longer duration of anesthesia than the *R* form.

MECHANISMS OF LOCAL ANESTHETIC FUNCTION

A good way to explain the mechanism of local anesthetic action is to relate anesthetic activity to the transmission of

Table 16-2 Anesthetic duration and toxicity of local anesthetic isomers

Drug	Duration	Toxicity
Etidocaine	S = R	S = R
Mepivacaine	S > R	S = R
Bupivacaine	S > R	S < R
Ropivacaine	S > R	S < R

From DiFazio CA, Woods AM: Pharmacology of local anesthetics. In Raj PP, editor: *Practical Management of Pain,* ed 2. St Louis, Mosby, 1992.

the nerve impulse. Stimulation of the nerve results in a propagated impulse that passes along the course of the nerve. This electrical signal results from a propagation of ionic currents. These currents are created by a transient fluctuation in the ion concentrations across a lipoprotein membrane. The main ionic species are Na+, which is mostly concentrated extracellularly; and K+, which is primarily concentrated intracellularly. These gradients are maintained by an ion-translocating Na+K+ adenosine triphosphate (ATP) pump mechanism within the nerve cell. The resulting resting electrical potential across the membrane is about −90 mV, with a positive exterior. For the most part, this is due to a difference in the membrane's permeability for K+ over Na+. In otherwords, the ionic leakage down the concentration gradient occurs more for the K+ than for the Na+ ions at the resting potential.

As the nerve impulse spreads, partial depolarization exceeds the threshold potential and triggers depolarization via a major increase in the permeability to Na+. With the influx of Na+, the membrane potential transiently becomes negative relative to the inside, and depolarization is electrically conducted to the adjacent areas of the membrane. At the same time, K+ ion outflow commences. This occurs at a slower rate and later than for Na+ and peaks after the Na+ influx has subsided. In the late phase of depolarization, the membrane again becomes less permeable to Na+; and as the ATP ion pump exchanges ions, the membrane returns to its resting potential. This sequence of events occurs successively as the impulse spreads down the nerve. At present, investigators postulate that the action potential causes conformational changes in the nerve membrane lipoproteins, and this change results in the actual opening of the Na+ channel gates, which consist of two proteins designated as *m* and *h* gate proteins. These channels, because of their size and charges, are specific for the Na+ ion.

Local anesthetics act on the membrane by interfering with its ability to undergo the specific changes that result in the altered permeability to Na+. Thus local anesthetics increase the threshold for electrical excitation in the nerve, slow the propagation of the impulse, reduce the rate of rise of the action potential, and eventually block the conduction. Several theories have been postulated over the years as to the exact mechanism of local anesthetics.

Presently, the most popular theories are a combination of the receptor[3] and membrane expansion theories[4] (Fig. 16-2). The membrane expansion theory states that the local anesthetic, in its uncharged base form, dissolves in the nerve

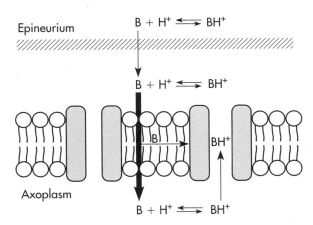

Fig. 16-2 Local anesthetic access to the sodium channel. The uncharged molecule diffuses most easily across lipid barriers and interacts with the channel through the axolemma interior. The charged species formed in the axoplasm gains access to a specific receptor via the sodium channel pore. (From Carpenter RL, Mackey DC: Local anesthetics. In Barash PG, Cullen BF, Stoelting RK, editors: *Clinical Anesthesia.* Philadelphia, JB Lippincott, 1989.)

membrane and causes an expansion of the membrane. This changes the conformation between proteins and their association with membrane lipids and results in a partial collapse of these ionic channels, which impedes the passage of Na+ ions.

The receptor theories basically state that local anesthetics bind to receptors at the cell membrane and prevent the opening of channels or pores for the passage of ions.

The local anesthetics diffuse through the lipid bilayer structure of the cell membrane in a lipid-soluble, uncharged base form. They then equilibrate in the axoplasm of the nerve into charged cationic and uncharged forms in accordance with the drug's pKa and the pH of the axoplasm. It is the cationic form that enters the Na+ channel from the intracellular side, binds to the anionic site within the Na+ channel, and physically or ionically blocks the movement of the Na+ ions. Therefore the local anesthetic prevents the action potential from developing in the nerve by inhibiting the movement of Na+ into the cell, which results in a nondepolarization block similar to the action of curare at the neuromuscular junction.

NERVE FIBER SIZE

The varying effect on nerve conduction is termed *differential blockade.* Although each local anesthetic has its own inherent hydrophilic or hydrophobic properties that produce this effect, there are also other factors to explain this phenomenon. Nerve-fiber diameter and myelinization play an important role in the physical function and modality of the nerve. They also affect the sensitivity of the nerve fiber to local anesthetic blockade. Nerve fibers are categorized into three major anatomical classes (Table 16-3). Myelinated somatic nerves are called *A fibers,* myelinated preganglionic autonomic nerves are called *B-fibers,* and nonmyelinated axons are called *C fibers.* The A fibers are further divided

Table 16-3 Classification of nerve fibers

Conduction/biophysical classification	Anatomic location	Myelin	Diameter (μ)	Rate (ms⁻¹)	Function
A fibers					
Alpha	Afferent to and efferent from muscles and joints	Yes	6-22	30-85	Motor and proprioception
Beta					
Gamma	Efferent to muscle spindles	Yes	3-6	15-35	Muscle tone
Delta	Sensory roots and afferent peripheral nerves	Yes	1-4	5-25	Pain, temperature, touch
B fibers	Preganglionic sympathetic	Yes	<3	3-15	Vasomotor, visceromotor, sudomotor, pilomotor
C fibers					
sC	Postganglionic sympathetic	No	0.3-1.3	0.7-1.3	Vasomotor, visceromotor, sudomotor, pilomotor
drC	Sensory roots and afferent peripheral nerves	No	0.4-1.2	0.1-2.0	Pain, temperature, touch

From Carpenter RL, Mackey DC: Local anesthetics. In Barash PG, Cullen BF, Stoelting RK, editors: *Clinical Anesthesia.* Philadelphia, JB Lippincott, 1989.

into four groups according to decreasing size: alpha, beta, gamma, and delta.

In general, the thicker the nerve, the greater the amount of local anesthetic required to block the conduction.[5] B fibers (preganglionic autonomic fibers) are an exception to the rule because although they are myelinated, they are more easily blocked than other fiber groups. This explains why the sympathetic blockade with epidural or subarachnoid blocks extends several segments beyond the cutaneous block.

The geographical arrangement of the nerve fibers within a peripheral nerve is another factor[6] (Fig. 16-3). Simply stated, the nerve fibers that are located in the outer layers of the nerve bundles will be exposed to and blocked by the effects of the local anesthetic before more internal ones.

Next there is the concept of conduction safety.[7] The distance between the nodes of Ranvier increases as the size of the myelinated nerve fibers increases. Conduction safety requires that at least three nodes of Ranvier must be exposed to local anesthetic before conduction can be halted. Therefore the variation in the distances between the nodes of Ranvier plays a major role in the variability of blockade (Fig. 16-4).

In addition, the degree of impulse activity, effects of CO_2 tension, pH, local ion gradients, degree of myelination on the nerve, and the concentration of the local anesthetic all contribute to this known clinical phenomena. The importance of the differential block of nerve conduction plays a major role in the proper utility of these medications and adds to the armamentarium of those proficient in regional anesthesia.

EXTERNAL FACTORS THAT AFFECT BLOCKADE
Volume and concentration

The total amount of the agents will dictate the onset, quality, and duration of the block. For example, increasing the dose of a local anesthetic can make the onset faster and the

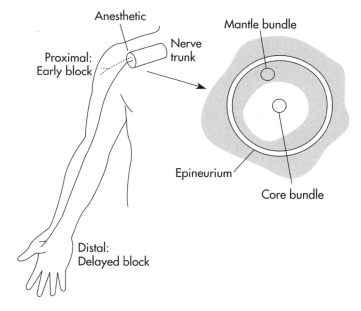

Fig. 16-3 Representation of the somatotopic arrangement of fibers in the trunks of the brachial plexus. Nerve fibers in the mantle (or peripheral) bundles innervate the proximal arm, and fibers in the core (or central) bundles innervate the distal arm. The concentration gradient that develops during initial diffusion of local anesthetic into the nerve trunk causes onset of anesthesia to proceed from proximal to distal. (From Carpenter RL, Mackey DC: Local anestetics. In Barash PG, Cullen BF, Stoelting RK, editors: *Clinical Anesthesia.* Philadelphia, JB Lippincott, 1989.)

duration longer (Table 16-4). Using the same volume, rapid onset, better quality, and duration of the block can be observed with varying concentrations of local anesthetics.[8,9] On the other hand, in epidural administration when the concentration is varied and the volume is adjusted to maintain

Table 16-4 Effects of dose and epinephrine on local anesthetic properties

	Increased dose (concentration or volume)	Addition of epinephrine
Onset time	↓	↓ (Minimal effect for etidocaine)
Degree of motor blockade	↑	↑
Degree of sensory blockade	↑	↑
Duration of blockade	↑	↑
Area of blockade	↑	↑
Peak plasma concentration	↑	↓

From Covino BG: Clinical pharmacology of local anesthetic agents. In Cousins MJ, Bridenbaugh PO, editors: *Clinical Anesthesia and Management of Pain.* Philadelphia, JB Lippincott, 1988.

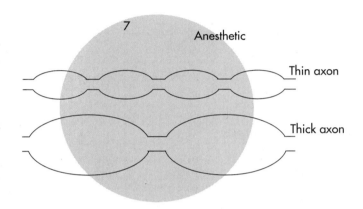

Fig. 16-4 Differential blockade of myelinated nerve fibers of differing diameters. Intermodal distance is proportional to axon diameter, and conduction blockade occurs when at least three adjacent nodes of a nerve fiber are exposed to blocking concentrations of the local anesthetic agent. Thus equivalent spread of local anesthetic may produce conduction blockade of a *thin axon,* but not the adjacent *thick axon.* (Modified from Franz DN, Perry RS: Mechanisms of differential block among single myelinated and non-myelinated axons by procaine, *J Physiol (Lond)* 236:193, 1974.)

the same milligram dosage, there is no difference noted in the onset, duration, and quality of the block. However, the spread of the block may be higher when using a larger volume. There is also a potential for increased serum levels and toxicity with increased dosages.

Addition of vasoconstrictor agents

Epinephrine, norepinephrine, and phenylephrine are often used with different local anesthetics to hasten onset and improve the quality and duration of the analgesia[10] (Table 16-5). These drugs reverse the known intrinsic vasodilatation effects found in most local anesthetics. Vasoconstriction caused by these chemicals will reduce the absorption of the local anesthetics; hence more agent is available for the neural blockade.

Site of injection

The proximity of the site of injection to nervous tissues and anatomic structures can influence onset, duration, and peak

serum levels. For example, the subarachnoid route of administration has a faster onset than an epidural placement.

Decreased duration of effect and increased serum levels of local anesthetics are related to the amount of blood flow at the site of injection. The potential for these effects is listed in decreasing order: intercostal, caudal, epidural, brachial plexus, and then sciatic or femoral nerves.[11]

Bicarbonation and carbonation of local anesthetics

The addition of bicarbonate to local anesthetics is associated with faster onset and spread of the block. Local anesthetics are often supplied at low pH to prolong the shelf life. The addition of bicarbonate will increase the pH of these solutions and ultimately the percentage of the uncharged form, which is important for diffusion through the nerve membrane.

The mixing of CO_2 (700 mm Hg) with a local anesthetic will also shorten the onset time but by a different mechanism. The CO_2 diffuses rapidly across the axonal membrane and thus decreases the intracellular pH.[12] This will increase the concentration of the charged form of the local anesthetic, which is important for receptor binding and neural blockade.

Temperature

Warming the local anesthetic reduces the onset of epidural blockade because the temperature elevation decreases the pKa of the drug.[13]

Pregnancy

The requirements for local anesthetic in parturients are decreased compared to their nonpregnant counterparts.[14] Onset has been faster with epidural and spinal anesthesia and peripheral nerve blocks; progesterone is suspected to be a factor.[15]

Combination of local anesthetics

Local anesthetics have been combined to hasten the onset of action and to improve the quality of the block. However, this may not always be the case. For example, the combination of 2-chloroprocaine with bupivacaine improved the onset and quality of the sensory block but shortened the duration of bupivacaine. The cause may be related to the possible interference by 2-chloroprocaine or its metabolites with the binding of bupivacaine to the receptors.[16]

Table 16-5 Comparative onset times and analgesic durations of various local anesthetic agents and effects of epinephrine on duration and peak plasma levels

Anesthetic technique	Anesthetic agent	Usual concentration (%)	Average onset time (min ± SE)	Average analgesic duration (min ± SE)	Addition of EPI* % change	
					Duration	C_{max}
Brachial plexus block (40-50 ml)	Lidocaine	1.0	14 ± 4	195 ± 26	+ 50	− 20-30
	Mepivacaine	1.0	15 ± 6	245 ± 27	—	− 20-30
	Bupivacaine	0.25-0.5	10-25	572	—	− 10-20
	Etidocaine	0.5	9	572	—	− 10-20
Epidural anesthesia (20-30 ml)	Lidocaine	2.0	15	100 ± 20	+ 50	− 20-30
	Mepivacaine	2.0	15	115 ± 15	+ 50	− 20-30
	Bupivacaine	0.5	17	195 ± 30	+ 0-30	− 10-20
	Etidocaine	1.0	11	170 ± 57	+ 0-30	− 10-20
Local infiltration	Lidocaine	0.5	—	75 (35-340)	+ 200	− 50
	Mepivacaine	0.5	—	108 (15-240)	+ 120	—
	Bupivacaine	0.25	—	200 ± 33	+ 115	—

*5µg/ml.
From Carpenter RL, Mackey DC: Local anesthetics. In Barash PG, Cullen BF, Stoelting RK, editors: *Clinical Anesthesia*. Philadelphia, JB Lippincott, 1989.
C_{max}, peak plasma levels; SE, standard error.

LOCAL ANESTHETICS
Esters

Cocaine. Cocaine is a rather complex alkaloid originally obtained from the Peruvian coca plant and used solely for topical anesthesia. Because of its unique vasoconstrictive action, which is related to its abilities to inhibit the reuptake of norepinephrine, it is especially useful during procedures on the oral and nasal cavities. Addiction and high toxicity are the main drawbacks to its use. The metabolism is by two pathways of hydrolysis, but 20% is still excreted in the urine unchanged.

Procaine. Procaine (Novocain) was one of the first synthetic paraaminobenzoic acid esters. Its use declined because of low potency, slow onset, short duration of action, and the advent of the more lipid-soluble amide-linked anesthetics. Although the potential for systemic side effects is low, procaine can cause allergic reactions. Currently it is mainly used for local infiltration anesthesia and in differential spinal blocks to evaluate chronic pain patients.

2-Chloroprocaine. Chloroprocaine (Nesacaine) is an analogue of procaine but is hydrolyzed four times faster than procaine in human plasma; thus it is less toxic. It has a rapid onset, brief duration, and low systemic toxicity, which has made it popular, especially in obstetrics, because it can be metabolized by the fetal enzyme system. It is not used intrathecally secondary to reports of neurotoxicity. However, this has been associated with the low pH and buffers used in the solution mixture. It is also proven to be valuable for peripheral nerve blocks.

Tetracaine. Tetracaine (Pontocaine, Amethocaine, Pantocaine) is also an analogue of procaine with radically different local anesthetic properties. It is ten times more potent and toxic but about four times slower to hydrolyze than procaine. Tetracaine's main benefit is its long duration of action, which can be further potentiated by the use of vasoconstrictors. Because of its poor diffusion qualities, it is not a good agent for peripheral nerve blockade except when combined with other fast onset local anesthetics. Also, its potential for systemic side effects is increased with the larger dosages required for these types of nerve blocks. Tetracaine does possess excellent topical anesthetic properties. Previously it was used to topically anesthetize the oral mucosa; however, rapid absorption with aerosol mixtures led to some reports of fatalities. It is eliminated excretion by the biliary tree.

Benzocaine. Benzocaine is an ethyl ester of paraaminobenzoic acid that lacks the hydrophilic amine tail. In addition, the pKa of benzocaine is well below physiologic range, which means it exists almost entirely as the unionized base form. These differences make it nearly insoluble in water and limit its sole use to topical application because it causes irritation on injection.

Amino amides

Lidocaine. Lidocaine (Xylocaine, Lignocaine) remains the most versatile and commonly used local anesthetic because of its inherent potency, rapid onset, and moderate duration of action. It is used in infiltration, peripheral nerve block, and epidural, spinal, and topical anesthesia. Given intravenously (IV), it acts as a systemic analgesic by blunting the response to intubation in the operating room and in the treatment of certain chronic pain syndromes secondary to its direct effects on the CNS. Generally, the duration of lidocaine is 1 to 3 hours for various regional anesthetic procedures; however, the addition of epinephrine to the dosage will increase onset, extend duration, and simultaneously decrease toxicity by limiting peak levels in the serum. Lidocaine is metabolized in the liver and, although the metabolites are excreted by the biliary tree, they are reabsorbed by the circulation only to be excreted in the urine. Only a small portion of lidocaine is excreted in the urine unchanged.

Bupivacaine. Bupivacaine (Marcaine, Sensorcaine) is a butyl derivative of a ringed piperidine carboxylic acid amide. It is used in infiltration, peripheral nerve block, and epidural and spinal anesthesia. It is not used for topical anesthesia. Bupivacaine has a duration that is two to three times longer then lidocaine but it has a severe toxic profile that prevents its use as an IV regional or systemic anesthesia. Because it offers excellent differential blockade between different nerve fibers, it has gained popularity for use in obstetric, acute postoperative, and chronic pain anesthetic techniques. Its longest duration of action occurs when it is used for peripheral nerve blockade and then it has been reported to last hours or longer. The addition of epinephrine does influence its vascular absorption and effect on target sites. As an intrathecal agent, it has a better anesthetic effect than tetracaine and reportedly has less potential for hypotensive side effects. Also, the degree of motor blockade is greater when isobaric solutions of bupivacaine are used as opposed to hyperbaric formulations.

Etidocaine. Etidocaine (Duranest) is a longer-acting derivative of lidocaine that is four times more potent and toxic than lidocaine. It is characterized by a very rapid onset, prolonged duration, and profound sensory and motor blockade. It is formulated for infiltration, peripheral nerve block, and epidural uses. It differs from bupivacaine in that it produces a more profound motor block than sensory block, which makes it primarily used for surgical procedures that require muscle relaxation, but limits its use for obstetric and postoperative analgesia.

Mepivacaine. Mepivacaine (Carbocaine) is a methyl derivative of a ringed piperidine rather than an alkl-amino compound. Its duration is slightly longer than lidocaine. It has some vasoconstrictive activity, but the addition of epinephrine affects the duration, onset, and potential for toxicity just as it does for lidocaine. It is used in infiltration, peripheral nerve, and epidural anesthesia in the United States, but it is not effective as a topical agent. Also, the metabolism is markedly decreased in the fetus and the newborn, so it is infrequently used in obstetric anesthesia.[17] Although it is eliminated by the same mechanism as lidocaine, the metabolites are also excreted by the salivary glands and gastric mucosa.

Prilocaine. Prilocaine (Citanest, Propitocaine) is a secondary amine analogue of lidocaine. It is as potent as lidocaine, but it is the least toxic of all the amino amide local anesthetics. This is due to the fact that levels in the blood are cleared quickly secondary to rapid uptake by the tissues. It has a rapid onset, a moderate duration, and profound depth of conduction blockade. Prilocaine is used in infiltration, peripheral nerve blocks, and epidural anesthesia. No specific formulas for topical or spinal use are available because of its short duration of action. During metabolism it is biotransformed to an amino phenol end product. This compound can oxidize hemoglobin to methemoglobin that can result in cyanosis; thus, the total dose needs to be limited to 600 mg. Also, its use in obstetric anesthesia and IV analgesic techniques has been abandoned. The metabolism of prilocaine is via the lung, liver, and kidney.

Ropivacaine. Ropivacaine is a propyl derivative of an n-alkyl piperidine amide. Ropivacaine is a chiral drug, but in its production the racemic mixture exists almost as a pure solution of one isomer. It is believed that this isomer possesses the most therapeutic qualities and the safest cardiac profile.[18] In fact, one of the main advantages of ropivacaine over bupivacaine is its reduced cardiotoxic potential. The physicochemical properties of ropivacaine are similar to those of bupivacaine, except for the fact that it is less lipid soluble (see Table 16-5). This may explain why, although ropivacaine and bupivacaine have equipotent effects on C-fiber action potentials, ropivacaine is less potent in blocking A-fiber activity. In other words, when compared with bupivacaine, the sensory anesthetic profiles of the two drugs were similar in onset, depth, and duration; but the depth and duration of the motor block were less with ropivacaine.[19] Ropivacaine may possess an even greater potential for a differential sensory motor blockade compared to bupivacaine. However, this differential blocking effect has been overcome by increasing the concentration of the ropivacaine. This would make ropivacaine superior to bupivacaine and an extremely useful agent for obstetric anesthesia and postoperative epidural analgesia. Ropivacaine has been an effective local anesthetic agent for infiltration, epidural, spinal, and brachial plexus anesthesia. Also, the addition of epinephrine has not altered the onset or duration of its action significantly because of its own inherent vasoconstrictive activity.[20] A clinical profile of local anesthetics is presented in Table 16-6.

TOXICITY OF LOCAL ANESTHETICS

Allergic reactions to local anesthetics occur mainly with the amino ester-linkage local anesthetics. This has been especially documented for procaine, but crossover hypersensitivity has also been seen with the other ester amide-linkage drugs. This is thought to occur because of a cross sensitivity with paraaminobenzoic acid.[21] True allergic reactions to amino amide local anesthetics are extremely rare and are usually related to the preservative methylparaben and not to the drug.[22] Paraben esters have excellent bacteriostatic and fungistatic properties and are widely used in multidose vials. In the past, those suspected of possible allergic reactions to local anesthetics were skin tested to identify those patients. However, this may not be scientifically reliable because only a small amount of drug is used, and there may need to be a conjugation of the drug with a carrier molecule before allergic reactions can occur. Also, the possibility of a severe anaphylactic reaction could put the patient's life at risk.

Local tissue toxicity

Tissue toxicity is rare when proper technique and concentrations of local anesthetics are used. However, serious neurotoxicity may result from intraneural injections, needle trauma, injections of large concentrations or volumes, chemical contamination, and neural ischemia produced by local neural compression or systemic hypotension.[23] The neurologic deficits reported with the use of

2-chloroprocaine in epidural anesthesia are an example. Although 2-chloroprocaine did not appear to have neurotoxic effects at the clinical level, the preservative sodium bisulfite[24] and the low pH[25] of the solution were felt to be the culprits. This resulted in the reformulation of this local anesthetic.

There are recent reports of neurotoxicity with the administration of local anesthetics through small gauge subarachnoid catheters.[26] At present, the proposed theory is that the use of these catheters results in a maldistribution of local anesthetic. This, in turn, leads to localized areas of the cauda equina being continuously exposed to high concentrations of local anesthetics, which results in direct local anesthetic neurotoxicity. Therefore there is a ban on the use of these smaller catheters until further investigation.

Systemic toxicity

The systemic effects of local anesthetic, which ranges from therapeutic to toxic, can best be described as a continuum that is dependent on blood level concentrations. Systemic toxicity most frequently arises from one of two causes: accidental vascular injections, or administration of an excessive dose (Table 16-7). The main toxic effects occur in the CNS and cardiovascular systems, but the cardiovascular system is four to seven times more resistant to these effects, i.e., seizures will occur with lower concentrations than those required to produce cardiovascular collapse.

CNS toxicity

The continuum of symptoms related to CNS toxicity appears to be not only related to concentration but also to the rate at which the concentration presented is to the nervous system.

For example, small amounts of local anesthetic can induce side effects, including seizures, if their application to the CNS is instantaneous, as with inadvertent intraarterial injections. On the other hand, high blood concentrations can be tolerated without signs of systemic toxicity if they are applied over long periods of time with continuous perineural and epidural infusions. The progression of CNS toxic symptoms results from selective depression of inhibitory fibers or centers in the CNS that results in excessive excitatory input. Early signs of toxicity differ between the ester and amide-linkage local anesthetics. Ester-linked anesthetics generally produce stimulant and euphoric symptoms, whereas amide-linked anesthetics tend to produce sedation and amnesia. Beyond this, all local anesthetics produce similar toxic symptoms. Commonly reported symptoms associated with rising blood levels are headache, lightheadedness, numbness and tingling of the perioral area or distal extremities, tinnitus, drowsiness, a flushed or chilled sensation, and blurred vision or difficulty focusing the eyes. Objectively, signs of obtundation, confusion, slurred speech, nystagmus, and muscle tremors or twitches can be observed. It is important to recognize these signs because they can foreshadow an impending seizure. The seizures appear to arise from subcortical levels in the brain, mainly the amygdala and the hippocampus. They subse-

quently spread, producing a generalized grand mal seizure.[27]

There are other factors that affect the CNS toxicity of local anesthetics. Increases in P_{CO_2} may have an effect by increasing cerebral blood flow and therefore increasing delivery to the CNS, as well as enhancing excitatory effects on the brain tissue.[28] Similarly, a decrease in pH may increase the concentration of the active cationic form in the brain cells. Cimetidine can also increase the toxicity of local anesthetics by slowing their elimination.[29]

Likewise, the toxic effects of local anesthetics can be decreased by the effects of barbiturates, benzodiazepines, and inhalation anesthetics by raising the seizure threshold of the CNS.

Cardiovascular system toxicity

Although the cardiovascular system (CVS) is more resistant to the toxic effects of local anesthetics, CVS toxicity can be severe and difficult, if not impossible, to treat. Decreases in myocardial contractility, rates of cardiac electrical impulse conduction, and effects on smooth muscle contractual functions are dose dependent. Cardiac arrhythmias and hypertension develop as dosages increase. At one time the potency of the local anesthetics was thought to be directly related to their cardiac toxicity. However, now it is known that bupivacaine and etidocaine have a more profound effect on the electrophysiology of the heart. Bupivacaine is approximately 70 times more potent than lidocaine in blocking cardiac conduction, yet it is only four times more potent in blocking the conduction of nerves.[30] This is due to the slower dissociation of bupivacaine from the cardiac Na+ channels than that of lidocaine. This lack of complete dissociation leads to a progressive number of blocked Na+ channels during diastole, which leads to subsequent cardiac depression and failure. Also, there is an indirect contribution to the cardiac toxicity by the local anesthetic's suppressive effects on the CNS. In addition, local anesthetics have a direct and an indirect (via the autonomic system) effect on the vascular smooth muscle tone, which results in either vasoconstriction and/or vasodilatation in different vascular beds, and is related to different levels of dosages. Cardiovascular toxicity is increased by hypoxia, acidosis, pregnancy, and hyperkalemia.[31]

PROCEDURAL USE OF LOCAL ANESTHETICS

Before the application of neural blockade, assess the patient's present physical condition and take a complete history to assure appropriateness of the procedure. It is important to ascertain if the patient has had any past reactions to local anesthetics. Patients scheduled for nerve blocks should refrain from eating 4 hours before the procedure because vomiting may occur either as a psychogenic response or secondary to a systemic reaction. Ambulatory patients need to be transported home; they should not be permitted to drive. Obtain consent only after full disclosure as to the purposes of the blockade, the procedural steps, effect and duration of the medications, and possible side effects and complications. Assure IV access and monitor vital signs. Sedation with a benzodiazepine will allay apprehension and pro-

Table 16-6 Clinical profile of local anesthetic agents

Agent	Concentration (%)	Clinical use	Onset	Usual duration (hours)	Recommended maximum single dose (mg)	Comments	pH of pain solutions
Amides							
Lidocaine	0.5-1.0	Infiltration	Fast	1.0-2.0	300	Most versatile agents	6.5
	0.25-0.5	IV regional		1.0-3.0	500 + epinephrine		
	1.0-1.5	Peripheral nerve blocks	Fast		500 + epinephrine		
	1.5-2.0	Epidural	Fast	1.0-2.0	500 + epinephrine		
	4	Topical	Moderate	0.5-1.0	500 + epinephrine		
	5	Spinal	Fast	0.5-1.5	100		
Prilocaine	0.5-1.0	Infiltration	Fast	1.0-2.0	600	Least toxic agents	4.5
	0.25-0.5	IV regional	Fast	1.5-3.0	600	Methemoglobinemia occurs usually above 600 mg	
	1.5-2.0	Peripheral nerve blocks			600		
Mepivacaine	2.0-3.0	Epidural	Fast	1.0-3.0	400	Longer duration of plain solutions than lidocaine without epinephrine	4.5
	0.5-1.0	Infiltration	Fast	1.5-3.0	500 + epinephrine		
	1.0-1.5	Peripheral nerve blocks	Fast	2.0-3.0	100	Useful when epinephrine is contraindicated	
	1.5-2.0	Epidural	Fast	1.5-3.0	175		
	4.0	Spinal	Fast	1.0-1.5	225 + epinephrine		
Bupivacaine	0.25	Infiltration	Fast	2.0-4.0	225 + epinephrine	Lower concentrations provide differential sensory/motor block; ventricular arrhythmias and sudden cardiovascular collapse reported following rapid IV injection	4.5-6
	0.25-0.5	Peripheral nerve blocks	Slow	4.0-12.0	225 + epinephrine		
	0.25-0.5	Obstetric epidural	Moderate	2.0-4.0	225 + epinephrine		
	0.5-0.75	Surgical epidural	Moderate	2.0-5.0	20		
	0.5-0.75	Spinal	Fast	2.0-4.0	300		
Etidocaine	0.5	Infiltration	Fast	2.0-4.0	400 + epinephrine	Profound motor block used for surgical anesthesia but not for obstetrical analgesia	4.5
	0.5-1.0	Peripheral	Fast	3.0-12.0	400 + epinephrine		
	1.0-1.5	Surgical epidural	Fast	2.0-4.0	400 + epinephrine		

Drug	Concentration (%)	Clinical use	Onset	Duration (min)	Maximum dose (mg)	Comments	pH
Dibucaine	0.25–0.5 hyperbaric	Spinal	Fast	2.0–4.0	10	Only recommended for spinal and topical use	
	0.00067 hypobaric	Spinal	Fast	2.0–4.0	10		
	1.0	Topical	Slow	30–60	50		
Esters							
Procaine	1.0	Infiltration	Fast	30–60	1000	Used mainly for infiltration and differential spinal blocks; allergic potential after repeated use	5–6.5
	1.0–2.0	Peripheral nerve blocks	Slow	30–60	1000		
	2.0	Epidural	Slow	30–60	1000		
	10.0	Spinal	Moderate	30–60	200		
Chloropro- caine	1.0	Infiltration	Fast	30–60	800		
	2.0	Peripheral nerve block	Fast	30–60	1000 + epinephrine		
	2.0–3.0	Epidural	Fast	30–60	1000 + epinephrine 1000 +		
Tetracaine	0.5	Spinal	Fast	2.0–4.0	20	Lowest systemic toxicity of all local anesthetics. Intrathecal injection may be associated with sensory/motor deficits. Use is primarily limited to spinal and topical anesthesia	2.7–4
	2.0	Topical	Slow	30–60	20		
Cocaine	4.0–10.0	Topical	Slow	30–60	150	Topical use only; addictive, causes vasoconstriction; CNS toxicity, marked excitation ("Fight and Flight" response); may cause cardiac arrhythmias owing to sympathetic stimulation	
Benzocaine	Up to 20	Topical	Slow	30–60	200	Useful only for topical anesthesia	4.5–6.5

From Covino BG: Clinical pharmacology of local anesthetic agents. In Cousins MJ, Bridenbaugh PO, editors: *Clinical Anesthesia and Management of Pain.* Philadelphia, JB Lippincott, 1988.

tect the patient from possible systemic reaction by increasing the level for CNS seizure threshold. Calculate in advance the appropriate amount of the drug needed to avoid toxic dose potentials by understanding the anatomic considerations and knowing the optimal site for injection to attain the desired effects with the least amount of local anesthetic solution.

Injection should be unhurried with frequent aspirations for blood or cerebrospinal fluid (CSF), and multiple test doses are encouraged. Continuous conversation with the patient assures the patient and it also alerts the physician to possible adverse reactions secondary to the drug misplacement. Monitor for adverse reactions or delayed complications; Table 16-8 lists possible reactions. Record complete summary of the procedure, drug dosages, effects, and adverse reactions. At the end of the procedure debrief the patient about the experience and inform the patient what to do if an untoward reaction occurs.

Table 16-7 Comparable safe doses of local anesthetics (mg/kg)*

| | | Areas injected | | |
| | | Central blocks† | | |
Drugs	Peripheral blocks†	Plain	With Epinephrine 1:200,000	Intercostal blocks‡ with Epinephrine 1:200,000
2-Chloroprocaine	—	20	25	—
Procaine	—	14	18	—
Lidocaine	20	7	9	6
Mepivacaine	20	7	9	6
Bupivacaine	5	2	2	2
Tetracaine	—	2	2	—

* Estimated to produce peak plasma levels that are less than half the plasma levels at which seizures could occur.
†Areas of low vascularity, i.e., axillary blocks using local anesthetic solutions containing 1:200,000 epinephrine.
‡Areas of high vascularity, i.e., intercostal blocks using local anesthetic solutions containing 1:200,000 epinephrine.
From DiFazio CA, Woods AM: Pharmacology of local anesthetics. In Raj PP, editor: *Practical Management of Pain.* ed 2. St Louis, Mosby, 1992.

Table 16-8 Differential diagnosis of local anesthetic reactions

Etiology	Major clinical features	Comments
Local anesthetic toxicity		
Intravascular injection	Immediate convulsion and/or cardiac toxicity	Injection into vertebral or a carotid artery
Relative overdose	Onset in 5 to 15 min of irritability, progressing to convulsions	may cause convulsion after administration of small dose
Reaction to vasoconstrictor	Tachycardia, hypertension, headache, apprehension	May vary with vasopressor used

Vasovagal reaction	Rapid onset
	  Bradycardia
	  Hypotension
	  Pallor, faintness
		Rapidly reversible with elevation of legs

Allergy		
Immediate	Anaphylaxis ($\downarrow$ BP, bronchospasm, edema)	Allergy to amides extremely rare
Delayed	Urticaria	Cross-allergy possible, for example, with preservatives in local anesthetics and food

High spinal or epidural block	Gradual onset
	  Bradycardia*
	  Hypotension
	  Possible respiratory arrest
		May lose consciousness with total spinal block and onset of cardiorespiratory effects more rapid than with high epidural or with subdural block

Concurrent medical episode†	May mimic local anesthetic reaction	Medical history important

* Sympathetic block above T_4 adds cardioaccelerator nerve blockade to the vasodilatation seen with blockade below T_4, total spinal block may have rapid onset.
† Asthma attack, myocardial infarction.
From Covino BG: Clinical pharmocology of local anesthetic agents. In Cousins MJ, Bridenbaugh PO, editors: *Clinical Anesthesia and Management of Pain.* Philadelphia, JB Lippincott, 1988.

APPENDIX

Eutectic mixture of local anesthetic

Lidocaine (Xylocaine, Astra) and prilocaine (Citanest, Astra) are the two active ingredients of eutectic mixture of local anesthetic (EMLA).[32] They are mixed together in a 1:1 ratio, which not only increases the efficacy of the local anesthetics but forms a mixture with a melting point that is lower than that of either local anesthetic alone. Specifically, lidocaine has a melting point of 67° C, prilocaine has a melting point of 37° C, and EMLA has a melting point of 18° C.[33] Therefore the 1:1 mixture of lidocaine and prilocaine forms an oil at room temperature. This property of depressing of melting point when two substances are combined is called a *eutectic mixture.*

To make the 1:1 eutectic mixture of lidocaine and prilocaine into a clinically useful formulation, the local anesthetics are compounded into an emulsion with Arlatone 289, a caster oil derivative, which functions as a nonionic surfactant. The compound is then thickened to form a cream to keep it from running off the skin with the neutralized carbomer Carbopol 934. The pH of the compound is then adjusted to 9.4, with sodium hydroxide to maximize the amount of local anesthetic that is in base form (Box 16-1). The local anesthetics in EMLA exist in three separate forms:

1. A freely dissolved fraction
2. An emulsified fraction
3. Surfactant-solubilized fraction[34]

The emulsified and surfactant-soluble substances serve as a reservoir that replenishes the freely dissolved fraction as it is absorbed into the skin.[35] This results in a relatively constant release of dissolvable local anesthetics that can diffuse more rapidly through the tissue, relative to a local anesthetic used alone or in a nonemulsified formulation.

Pharmacokinetics. As a rule, plasma concentrations of both lidocaine and prilocaine are well below toxic levels.[36-38] Very low levels are detectable in the general circulation after application of 5% EMLA cream, although they can be detected in the veins draining the treated area.[39]

Factors affecting absorption. Factors affecting the absorption of EMLA include the site of application and the condition of skin on which it is applied. In general the more vascular the area, the more rapid the absorption.

Time-response studies. The minimum application time required when using EMLA to obtain reliable dermal analgesia is 40 to 60 minutes.[40-43] An increase in analgesia will generally continue for an additional 60 minutes, even if the cream is removed, as the local anesthetics that accumulated in the stratum corneum of the skin during the application period continue to diffuse into the deeper layers of the skin.[44-46]

Duration of analgesia. A 1-hour application of EMLA will provide 1 to 5 hours of dermal analgesia.[47] It has been further demonstrated that EMLA can be left on the skin for several hours without any decrease in analgesic efficacy. This has important clinical implications when applied at home by the patient before outpatient procedures.

Pharmacokinetics of EMLA when applied to mucous membranes. EMLA has been applied on the oral and genital mucosa. It provides effective analgesia of the buccal and palatal mucosa after a 2 to 5 minute application time, respectively.[48] Maximal analgesic efficacy for the gingival mucosa was achieved after an application time of 10 to 20 minutes.[49]

Effective analgesia of the genital mucosa sufficient to allow cautery of genital warts occurred after a 10 minute application of EMLA.[50] Analgesic efficacy appears to decrease gradually with applications of 15 minutes or longer, presumably secondary to the more rapid absorption and diffusion, because of the lack of stratum corneum in mucosal structures.[51] The lack of stratum corneum also accounts for the faster onset of analgesia relative to that required for intact skin.

Side effects of EMLA

Local circulatory effects. After a 30 to 60 minute application of EMLA, a pallor or blanching of the skin may occur.[52] This effect, which lasts for 1 to 2 hours, is due to the vasoconstriction of underlying capillary loops.[53] Interestingly, after longer application times of 2 to 4 hours, erythema of the skin caused by vasodilatation may be observed.[54] Both of these reactions may be related to the di-

---

Box 16-1 CHEMICAL FORMULATION OF EMLA

Lidocaine	25 mg
Prilocaine	25 mg
Arlatone	19 mg
Carbopol	10 mg
Sodium hydroxide to pH	9.6
Purified water sufficient to produce 1 g	

Box 16-2 HOW TO APPLY EMLA CREAM

1. Apply 5 g of cream (one half the 5 g tube) over a 2″ x 2″ area in a thick layer at the site of the procedure
2. Take the occlusive dressing and remove the center outer piece
3. Peel the paper from the paper frame dressing
4. Cover the EMLA cream so there is a thick layer underneath; do not spread the cream
5. Smooth down the dressing edges carefully to ensure adequate contact
6. Remove the paper frame from the top of the dressing
7. Mark the time of application directly on the occlusive dressing
8. After appropriate application time, remove the occlusive dressing
9. Wipe off the EMLA cream and clean the entire area with antiseptic solution

rect effect of the local anesthetic on vascular smooth muscle, with resultant vasoconstriction at low concentrations and vasodilatation occurring when higher concentrations are achieved.[48] Localized edema in the area of EMLA application has also been observed.[54,55] It will generally disappear within 2 to 3 hours after removal of the cream.[56-58] Although the clinical observations of pallor, erythema, and/or edema are not harmful, to avoid undue concern and anxiety, the patient should be warned that such side effects may occur. These side effects may have a quicker onset and greater intensity when EMLA is used in patients with diseased skin.[52]

Methemoglobinemia. High plasma concentrations of prilocaine can cause an increase in the formation of methemoglobin.[59] High levels of methemoglobin can result in tissue hypoxia. With normal doses of EMLA, plasma levels of prilocaine are well below levels that would cause significant methemoglobinemia in adults or infants above 3 months of age.[60]

Clinical Considerations. EMLA is supplied as a 5% cream/5 g tube. Two transparent occlusive dressings are also supplied. Box 16-2 provides step-by-step instructions on the use of EMLA. A thick layer of cream should be used at the procedure site to increase efficacy. Application of 1 hour for procedures involving needle puncture and 2 hours for split-thickness skin grafts is recommended. The application time should be decreased to 15 minutes when used on mucosal surfaces. As mentioned previously, prolonged mucosal application times may decrease the efficacy of EMLA cream.

Box 16-3 PROCEDURES INVOLVING NEEDLE PAIN

Venipuncture
Arterial cannulation
Hemodialysis
Allergy testing
Immunocompetence testing
Lumbar puncture
Subcutaneous drug reservoir puncture
Vaccination

Box 16-4 SUPERFICIAL SURGICAL PROCEDURES WHERE EMLA IS EFFECTIVE

Collagen implants
Dermabrasion
Pruritis
Curettage of minor skin lesions
Harvesting of split-thickness skin grafts
Port wine removal

Clinical indications for EMLA cream.

1. Procedures involving needle pain
2. Minor dermatologic procedures
   (See Boxes 16-3 and 16-4)

FUTURE USES OF EMLA

Clinical studies are currently underway to assess the efficacy of EMLA in the treatment of postherpetic neuralgia, ischemic neuropathy, and a variety of deafferentation pain states.[61,62] EMLA cream may also have a place in treating the pain of recurrent herpes Type I and Type II infections.[63] Clinical trials to assess the efficacy of EMLA in providing analgesia for circumcision in older children are also underway.

REFERENCES

1. Covino BG, Vassello HG: *Local Anesthetics, Mechanism of Action and Clinical Use.* New York, Grune & Stratton, 1976.
2. Covino BG: Pharmacology of local anesthetic agents. *Br J Anaesth* 5:701-706, 1986.
3. Hille B: Local anesthetics: Hydrophilic and hydrophobic pathways for the drug-receptor reaction. *J Gen Physiol* 69:497-575, 1977.
4. Seeman P: The membrane expansion theory of anaesthesia. In Fink BR, editor: *Molecular Mechanisms of Anesthesia. Progress in Anesthesiology, vol 1.* New York, Raven Press, 1975.
5. Raymond SA, Gissen AJ: Mechanisms of differential nerve block. In Strichartz GR, editor: *Local Anesthetics.* Berlin, Springer-Verlag, 1987.
6. Winnie AP et al: Clinical pharmacokinetics of local anaesthetics. *Can Anaesth Soc J* 24:252, 1977.
7. Franz DN, Perry RS: Mechanisms of differential block among single myelinated and non-myelinated axons by procaine. *J Physiol (Lond)* 236:193, 1974.
8. Littlewood DG et al: Comparative study of various local anesthetic solutions in extradural block in labour. *Br J Anaesth* 51:47, 1979.
9. Scott BD et al: Effects of concentration of local anaesthetic drugs in extradural block. *Br J Anaesth* 52:1033, 1980.
10. Covino BG: Clinical pharmacology of local anesthetic agents. In Cousins MJ, Bridenbaugh PO, editors: *Clinical Anesthesia and Management of Pain.* Philadelphia, JB Lippincott, 1988.
11. Tucker GT, Mather LE: Clinical pharmacokinetics of local anaesthetic. *Clin Pharmacokinet* 4:241, 1979.
12. Catchlove RFH: The influence of CO_2 and pH on local anesthetic action. *J Pharmacol Exp Ther* 181:291, 1972.
13. Metha PM, Theriot E, Mehrotra D: A simple technique to make bupivacaine a rapid-acting epidural anesthetic. *Reg Anesth* 123:135, 1987.
14. Fagraeus L, Urban BJ, Bromage PR: Spread of epidural analgesia in early pregnancy. *Anesthesiology* 58:184, 1983.
15. Datta S et al: Differential sensitivities of mammalian nerve fibers during pregnancy. *Anesth Analg* 62:1070, 1983.
16. Corke BC, Carlson CG, Dettbarn WD: The influence of 2-chloroprocaine on the subsequent analgesic potency of bupivacaine. *Anesthesiology* 60:25, 1984.
17. DiFazio CA, Woods AM: Pharmacology of local anesthetics. In Raj PP, editor: *Practical Management of Pain,* ed 2. St Louis, Mosby, 1992.
18. Arthur GR, Feldman HS, Covino BG: Acute IV toxicity of LEA-103, a new local anesthetic, compared to lidocaine and bupivacaine in the awake dog. *Anesthesiology* 65:724, 1986.
19. Bader AM, Datta S, Flanagan H: Comparison of bupivacaine and ropivacaine induced conduction blockade in the isolated rabbit vagus nerve. *Anesth Analg* 68:724, 1989.
20. Kopacz DJ, Carpenter RL, Mackey DC: Effects of ropivacaine on uterine blood flow in pregnant sheep. *Anesthesiology* 71:69, 1989.
21. Fisher MM, Pennington JC: Allergy to local anesthesia. *Br J Anaesth* 54:893-894, 1982.
22. Aldrete AJ, Johnson DA: Allergy to local anesthetic. *JAMA* 207:356, 1969.

23. Kane RE: Neurologic deficits following epidural or spinal anesthesia. *Anesth Analg* 60:150, 1981.
24. Wang BC et al: Chronic neurological deficits and nesacaine-CE—An effect of the anesthetic, 2-chloroprocaine, or the antioxidant, sodium bisulfite? *Anesth Analg* 63:445, 1984.
25. Ravindran RS, Turner MS, Muller J: Neurologic effects of subarachnoid administration of 2-chloroprocaine-CE, bupivacaine, and low pH normal saline in dogs. *Anesth Analg* 61:279, 1982.
26. Rigler M et al: Cauda equina syndrome after continuous spinal anesthesia. *Anesth Analg* 72:275-281, 1991.
27. Wagman IH, DeJong RH, Prince DA: Effects of lidocaine on the central nervous system. *Anesthesiology* 28:155, 1967.
28. Englesson S: The influence of acid-base changes on central nervous system toxicity of local anesthetic agents. *Acta Anaesthesiol Scand* 18:79, 1974.
29. Kim KC, Tasch MD: Effects of cimetidine and ranitidine on local anesthetic central nervous system toxicity in mice. *Anesth Analg* 65:840, 1986.
30. Clarkson CW, Hondeghem LM: Mechanism for bupivacaine depression of cardiac conduction: Fast block of sodium channels during action potential with slow recovery from block during diastole. *Anesthesiology* 62:396, 1985.
31. Carpenter RL, Mackey DC: Local anesthetics. In Barash PG, Cullen BF, Stoelting RK, editors: *Clinical Anesthesia.* Philadelphia, JB Lippincott, 1989.
32. Reference deleted in proofs.
33. Brodin A et al: Phase diagram and aqueous solubility of the lidocaine-prilocaine binary system. *J Pharm Sci* 73:481-484, 1984.
34. Nyqvist-Mayer AA, Brodin AF, Frank SG: Phase distribution studies on an oil-water emulsion based on a eutectic mixture of lidocaine and prilocaine as the dispersed phase. *J Pharm Sci* 74:1192-1195, 1985.
35. Nyqvist-Mayer AA, Brodin AF, Frank SG: Drug release studies on an oil-water emulsion based on a eutectic mixture of lidocaine and prilocaine as the dispersed phase. *J Pharm Sci* 75:365-373, 1986.
36. Evers H et al: Dermal effects of compositions based on the eutectic mixture of lignocaine and prilocaine (EMLA). *Br J Anaesth* 57:997-1005, 1985.
37. Manner T et al: Reduction of pain at venous cannulation in children with a eutectic mixture of lidocaine and prilocaine (EMLA Cream): Comparison with placebo cream and no local premedication. *Acta Anaesthesiol Scand* 31:735-739, 1987.
38. Scott DB et al: Factors affecting plasma levels of lignocaine. *Br J Anaesth* 44:1040, 1972.
39. Juhlin L, Hagglund G, Evers H: Absorption of lidocaine and prilocaine after application of a eutectic mixture of local anesthetics (EMLA) on normal and diseased skin. *Acta Derm Venereol (Stockh)* 69:18-22, 1989.
40. Arendt-Nielsen L, Bjerring P: Laser-induced pain for evaluation of local analgesia: A comparison of topical application (EMLA) and local injection (lidocaine). *Anesth Analg* 67:115-123, 1988.
41. Ehrenstrotm-Reiz G, Reiz S, Stockman O: Topical anaesthesia with EMLA, a new lidocaine-prilocaine cream and the Cusum technique for detection of minimal application time. *Acta Anaesthesiol Scand* 27:510-512, 1983.
42. Maddi R et al: Evaluation of EMLA as a topical anesthetic. *Reg Anesth* 10:39 (Abstr 27), 1985.
43. Arendt-Nielsen L, Bjerring P: The effect of topically applied anaesthetics (EMLA cream) on thresholds to thermode and argon laser stimulation. *Acta Anaesthesiol Scand* 33:469-473, 1989.
44. Hallen B, Olsson GL, Uppfeldt A: Pain-free venipuncture. Effect of timing of application of local anaesthetic cream. *Anaesthesia* 39:969-972, 1984.
45. Bjerring P, Arendt-Nielsen L: Depth and duration of skin analgesia to needle insertion after topical application of EMLA cream. *Br J Anaesth* 64:173-177, 1990.
46. Lahteenmaki T et al: Topical analgesia for the cutting of split-skin grafts; a multicenter comparison of two doses of a lidocaine/prilocaine cream. *Plast Reconstr Surg* 82:458-462, 1988.
47. Juhlin L, Evers H: EMLA: A new topical anaesthetic. *Adv Dermatol* 5:75-92, 1990.
48. Holst A, Evers H: Experimental studies of new topical anaesthetics on the oral mucosa. *Swed Dent J* 9:185-191, 1985.
49. Haasio J et al: Topical anesthesia of gingival mucosa by 5% eutectic mixture of lidocaine and prilocaine or by 10% lidocaine spray. Twentieth Congress of the Scandinavian Society of Anaesthesiologists, Copenhagen, Denmark, June 26-30, 1989.
50. Ljunghall K, Lillieborg S: Local anaesthesia with lidocaine/prilocaine cream (EMLA) for cautery of condylomata acuminata on the vulval mucosa. The effect of timing of application of the cream. *Acta Derm Venereol (Stockh)* 69:362-365, 1989.
51. Rylander E et al: Local anesthesia of the genital mucosa with a lidocaine/prilocaine cream (EMLA) for laser treatment of condylomata acuminata. A placebo-controlled study. *Obstet Gynecol* 75:302-306, 1990.
52. Juhlin L, Rollman O: Vascular effects of a local anesthetic mixture in atopic dermatitis. *Acta Derm Venereol (Stockh)* 64:439-440, 1984.
53. Bjerring P, Andersen PH, Arendt-Nielsen L: Vascular response of human skin after analgesia with EMLA cream. *Br J Anaesth* 63:655-660, 1989.
54. Uppfeldt A, Hallen B, Carlsson P: A new topical preparation reduces pain from venepuncture. *Acta Anaesthesiol Scand Suppl* 27 (78):Abstr 97, 1983.
55. Hallen B, Carlsson P, Uppfeldt A: Clinical study of lignocaine-prilocaine cream to relieve the pain of venepuncture. *Br J Anaesth* 57:326-328, 1985.
56. Ohlsen L, Englesson S, Evers H: An anaesthetic lidocaine/prilocaine cream (EMLA) for epicutaneous application tested for cutting split skin grafts. *Scand J Reconstr Surg* 19:201-209, 1985.
57. Bucyk B et al: Evaluation of EMLA in providing split thickness skin graft donor site analgesia. *Can J Anaesth* suppl 35, 1988.
58. Andersen C, Danielson K, Ladefoged J: EMLA cream for pain prevention in hemodialysis patients. *Dial Transplantation* 18:684-685, 1989.
59. Frayling IM et al: Methaemoglobinaemia in children treated with prilocaine-lignocaine cream. *BMJ* 301:153-154, 1990.
60. Radford M, Pinder A-M: Methaemoglobinaemia in children treated with prilocaine-lignocaine cream. *BMJ* 301:495, 1990.
61. Milligan KA, Atkinson RE, Schofield PA: Lignocaine-prilocaine cream in postherpetic neuralgia. *BMJ* 298:253, 1989.
62. Stow PJ, Glynn CJ, Minor B: EMLA cream in the treatment of postherpetic neuralgia. Efficacy and pharmacokinetic profile. *Pain* 39:301-305, 1989.
63. Cassuto J: Topical local anaesthetics and herpes simplex. *Lancet* i:100-101, 1989.

QUESTIONS: LOCAL ANESTHETICS

For questions 1-4, choose from the following:

A. 1 and 3
B. 2 and 4
C. 1, 2, and 3
D. 4
E. All of the above

1. Name the local anesthetic(s) most likely to produce an allergic reaction.
   1. Prilocaine
   2. Ropivacaine
   3. Etidocaine
   4. Benzocaine

2. Which of the following statements regarding bupivalaine is (are) true?
   1. The degree of motor blockade is greatest when isobaric solutions of bupivacaine are used as opposed to hyperbaric formulations.
   2. One of the disadvantages with the use of bupivacaine is that it does not produce a good enough differential blockade when used for postoperative pain management.
   3. Bupivacaine has produced neural blockade for longer than 10 hours.
   4. In the United States the use of bupivacaine for IV analgesic techniques has been banned secondary to its metabolites' ability to oxidize hemoglobin to methemoglobin.

3. Which of the following local anesthetics exist as chiral forms?
   1. Bupivacaine
   2. Mepivacaine
   3. Etidocaine
   4. Prilocaine

4. Which of the following statements is (are) true about local anesthetic physicochemical properties?
   1. Lipid solubility influences the duration of the neural blockade.
   2. The protein binding has significant effect on the potency of the local anesthetic.
   3. The nonionic form of the local anesthetic molecule has been postulated to have no direct effect on the conduction of ions through the $Na+$ channels.
   4. It is believed that the stereoisomers known to exist for some of the local anesthetics may have inherent differences in potency, toxicity, and duration.

5. The addition of epinephrine has the following effects on local anesthetic properties EXCEPT:
   A. Increases the degree of motor blockade
   B. Increases the area of the blockade
   C. Increases the time of onset
   D. Decreases the peak plasma concentration

ANSWERS

1. D
2. A
3. E
4. D
5. C

17 Techniques

P. Prithvi Raj

A. TOPOGRAPHIC INDICATIONS

Box 17-1 lists various topographic indications for nerve blocks.

Box 17-1 TOPOGRAPHIC INDICATIONS FOR NERVE BLOCK

Area of pain	Appropriate nerve block
Head	
Face	Trigeminal nerve blocks
Orbit and contents, ethmoidal cells, sphenoid sinus, eyelids, forehead, anterior two thirds of scalp, root of nose	Ophthalmic nerve block
Forehead	Supraorbital and supratrochlear nerve block
Upper jaw, maxillary antrum, distribution of infraorbital nerve	Maxillary nerve block
Lower eyelid, cheek, lateral aspect of nose, upper lip, temple	Infraorbital nerve block
Lower jaw, lower lip, anterior two thirds of tongue, teeth, floor of mouth, distribution of mental nerve	Mandibular nerve block
Lower jaw and lower lip	Mental nerve block
Nose, palate	Sphenopalatine (pterygopalatine) block
Posterior one third of tongue, parotid gland, soft palate to larynx	Glossopharyngeal nerve block
Scalp, back of neck	Greater occipital nerve block
Neck	
Shoulder and upper neck	Cervical plexus block
	Cervical paravertebral block (C_1-C_4)
Larynx, trachea	Laryngeal nerve block
	Deep cervical plexus block
Structures superficial to deep fascia in neck	Superficial cervical plexus block
Back of neck	Greater occipital nerve block
	Spinal accessory nerve block
Upper extremity	
Entire extremity including shoulder	Brachial plexus block
	Interscalene approach
	Supraclavicular approach
	Subclavian perivascular approach
	Supracapsular nerve block
Shoulder and scapular region	Brachial plexus block
	Supracapsular nerve block
Mid-upper arm to hand	Brachial plexus block, all approaches
Elbow, forearm	Brachial plexus block, all approaches
	Intravenous regional anesthesia
Lower forearm, wrist, hand	Brachial plexus block, all approaches
	Elbow block
	Intravenous regional anesthesia

Continued.

Box 17-1 TOPOGRAPHIC INDICATIONS FOR NERVE BLOCK—cont'd.

Hand, metacarpus	Brachial plexus block, all approaches
	Elbow block
	Wrist block
Digits	Wrist block
	Hand and digital block
Thorax	
Chest, parietal and visceral pleura	Intercostal nerve block (ribs I-VIII)
	Thoracic epidural block
	Thoracic paravertebral block
Integumentary structures superficial to deep fascia	Field block for mammoplasty
Cavity (chest wall and viscera of thorax)	High thoracic epidural block (T_1-T_5) in combination with vagal nerve block and thoracic sympathetic nerve block
Abdomen	
Abdominal wall and abdominal and pelvic viscera	Lumbar epidural block
	Subarachnoid block
	Lumbar paravertebral block
	Intercostal nerve block (ribs VI-XII)
	Field block for upper and lower abdomen in combination with splanchnic nerve and celiac plexus block
All structures of inguinal region	Field block for inguinal region
Greater pelvis (including hips, pelvic, viscera, perineal floor)	Subarachnoid block
	Lumbar epidural block
Hip joint	Lumbar paravertebral block (T_{12}-L_3)
Lesser pelvis (pelvic, viscera, renal tract, genital structures, overlying dermatomes)	Subarachnoid block
	Lumbar epidural block
	Caudal epidural block
Perineum and urinary tract	Transsacral nerve block (as supplement to caudal epidural block)
Perineum and genital structures	Pudendal nerve block
Os cervix	Paracervical nerve block
	Field block for lower abdomen
Penis	Penile block
Anus	Anal block
Pelvic viscera, perineal floor	Caudal epidural block
Rectum, bladder, genital tract	Transsacral nerve block
	Sacrococcygeal plexus block
Lower extremity	
Entire extremity including hip	Subarachnoid block
	Lumbar epidural block
	Lumbosacral plexus block (unilateral block of lower extremity) in combination with femoral nerve (3-in-1) block
	Caudal epidural block
	Sciatic nerve block in combination with psoas compartment block
Hip, anterolateral thigh	Femoral nerve (3-in-1) block
	Obturator nerve block
	Lateral femoral cutaneous nerve block
Knee and leg	Sciatic nerve block in combination with femoral nerve block and obturator nerve block
Knee	Sciatic, femoral, and obturator nerve block
Leg	Common peroneal and tibial nerve block at knee
Medial aspect of leg	Saphenous nerve block at knee
Ankle, foot	Common peroneal and tibial nerve block
	Saphenous nerve block at knee
	Ankle block (anterior and posterior ankle block)
	Intravenous regional anesthesia
Distal one third of foot and toes	Metatarsal block
	Intravenous regional anesthesia

Continued.

TOPOGRAPHIC INDICATIONS FOR NERVE BLOCK—cont'd.

Obstetrics

Vaginal delivery (labor and delivery)	Lumbar epidural block
	Caudal epidural block
	Subarachnoid block (emergency)
	Pudendal nerve block in combination with paracervical nerve block
Stage I labor	Paracervical block
Stage II labor	Pudendal nerve block
Abdominal delivery	Lumbar epidural block
	Subarachnoid block (emergency)
Cerclage	Subarachnoid block (saddle block)
	Caudal epidural block

B. CRANIAL NERVES

Indications for somatic nerve blocks of the head fall into two primary categories: (1) the diagnosis and treatment of pain syndromes secondary to cancer and the therapies used to treat cancer (e.g., radiation osteitis), and (2) the management of tic douloureaux. Rarer problems include trauma causing a neuropathy of any particular nerve branch, temporomandibular joint dysfunction, postherpetic neuralgia, and, in some instances, atypical facial neuralgia.

TRIGEMINAL (GASSERIAN) GANGLION BLOCK

Anatomy

The gasserian ganglion is formed by the fusion of a series of rootlets starting along the ventral surface of the brain stem at the midpontine level. These rootlets pass forward within the posterior cranial fossa and across the superior border of the petrous temporal bone to enter a recess called Meckel's cave (trigeminal cave). The posterior two thirds of the ganglion are surrounded by an invagination of the dura, which in turn is in direct continuity with the cerebrospinal fluid (CSF) within the brain. From the anterior convex border of the crescent-shaped ganglion, the three major divisions—ophthalmic, maxillary, and mandibular nerves—leave the skull to innervate the head (Fig. 17-1).

Technique

Block of the gasserian ganglion is a technically difficult procedure for the uninitiated. It should be done with x-ray guidance to confirm needle position. The patient lies in the neutral position with the head slightly extended. External landmarks include the midpoint of the zygomatic arch, which should be marked. Insert the needle approximately 1 inch lateral to the corner of the mouth, which should be slightly superior to the upper second molar; after local anesthetic infiltration, advance the 4-inch, 22-gauge block needle through the substance of the cheek. With a finger intraorally guiding the needle, move it just medial to the ramus of the mandible in a cephalad and medial direction. The needle should be going in the general direction of the pupil of the eye. When viewed from the side, the needle should also be noted to pass just deep to the mark on the midpoint of the zygomatic arch. The needle when further advanced will contact the base of the skull, usually slightly anterior to the foramen ovale. After x-ray verification, redirect the needle until it enters the foramen. Paresthesia of the mandibular nerve at this time is occasionally encountered. Withdraw the needle slightly and attempt to have it enter the foramen without eliciting significant paresthesias (Fig. 17-2).

If a diagnostic block is required, inject 1 to 3 ml of local anesthetic slowly after carefully aspirating for both blood and CSF. If a permanent block of the ganglion is required, then inject absolute alcohol, approximately 1 ml in divided doses.

Thermocoagulation, radiofrequency, and retrogasserian phenol installation into Meckel's cave all have been used successfully to manage pain syndromes. The current use of alcohol, therefore, is extremely limited because of the diffuse effect on the ganglion and the resultant complications, including anesthesia dolorosa, painful paresthesias, and keratitis. Similarly, older methods of ganglion destruction, such as the injection of hot water, cold water, or yttrium, are extremely rare procedures.

Problems

The major problem with trigeminal ganglion block has to do with the placement of the needle, which can be painful and technically difficult to achieve. Therefore most patients require a heavy sedation or, in some cases, even a general anesthetic. Once the needle has been placed, aspirate carefully. Small amounts of local anesthetic, if injected directly into the CSF via the dural invagination, can cause rapid loss of consciousness and even cardiac arrest. Therefore full resuscitative means should be available when this block is carried out. In addition, when alcohol is used, the numbness that the patient feels over the entire face may become intolerable, suggesting that before any destructive procedure is done a local block should be carried out first. In addition, the corneal anesthesia that results from permanent block may encourage inflammatory diseases of the involved eye to go undetected for a period of time.

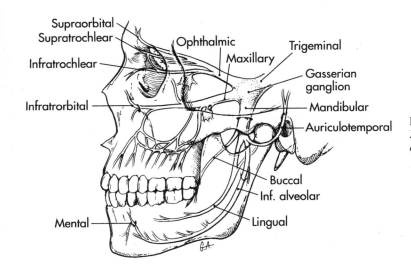

Fig. 17-1 Anatomy of gasserian ganglion block (From Katz J: Somatic nerve blocks. In Raj PP, editor: *Practical Management of Pain,* ed 2. St Louis Mosby, 1992.)

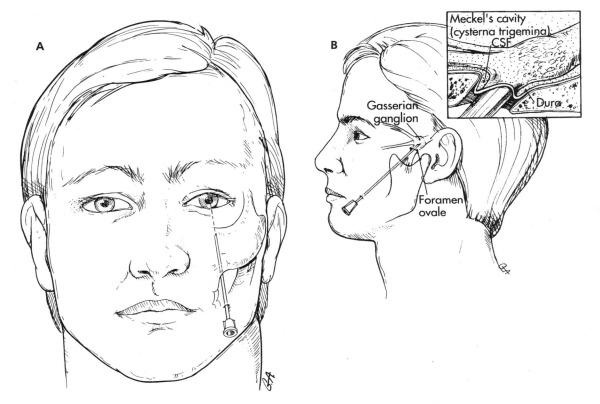

Fig. 17-2 A, Line for directing needle in anteroposterior view. **B,** Line for directing needle in lateral view. Inset shows details of Meckel's cavity. (From Katz J: Somatic nerve blocks. In Raj PP, editor: *Practical Management of Pain,* ed 2. St Louis, Mosby, 1992.)

OPHTHALMIC DIVISION AND ITS BRANCHES
Anatomy

The ophthalmic branch of the trigeminal nerve has three major branches: the *lacrimal, nasocilliary,* and *frontal* nerves. The frontal nerve runs forward beneath the periosteum of the orbital roof, dividing into the larger lateral supraorbital nerve and the smaller medial supratrochlear nerve. The supraorbital nerve leaves the orbit via the supraorbital notch (occasionally through the foramen). The su-

pratrochlear nerve exits over the rim of the orbit in the area where the nasal bone joins the bone of the orbit itself.

Technique

Block of the ophthalmic division per se is not indicated because of factors mentioned above (i.e., keratitis). However, block of the supraorbital nerve could be indicated for the management of tic and occasionally postherpetic neuralgia. Nerve block with local anesthetic is easy to perform (Fig.

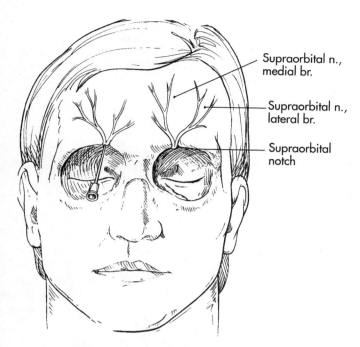

Fig. 17-3 Anatomy of supaorbital nerve and technique of nerve blocking. (From Katz J: Somatic nerve blocks. In Raj PP, editor: *Practical Management of Pain,* ed 2. St Louis, Mosby, 1992.)

17-3). With the palpating finger, the depression on the supraorbital ridge is located usually directly above the pupil of the eye when the patient is looking straight ahead. Insert a short 25-gauge needle to the bone, and inject 2 ml of local anesthetic just above the periosteum to block the nerve. For permanent block inject 1 ml of alcohol in the same area. However, surgical excision of the nerve produces longer satisfactory results. The result of either alcohol or surgical ablation of the nerve produces an area of anesthesia over the entire forehead on the involved side up to the vertex of the skull.

MAXILLARY NERVE AND ITS BRANCHES

The maxillary division of the trigeminal nerve proceeds horizontally forward from the ganglion exiting from the middle cranial fossa through the foramen rotundum to enter the pterygopalatine fossa, where its major branches arise. The major reason for blocking the maxillary nerve itself is for denervation of the areas listed in Box 17-2 and for inflammatory diseases of the nerve itself, such as tic douloureux.

Technique

The patient lies supine with the head turned slightly away from the side to be blocked. Identify the zygomatic arch and the notch of the mandible (Fig. 17-4). After asking the patient to open his mouth slightly, thus giving more room between the notch of the mandible and the zygomatic arch, generously infiltrate the area with local anesthetic. Insert a 3-inch block needle parallel to the base of the skull to come in contact with the lateral pterygoid plate. Once the lateral pterygoid plate is contacted, usually about 1 to 1½ inches below the skin, redirect the needle superiorly and anteri-

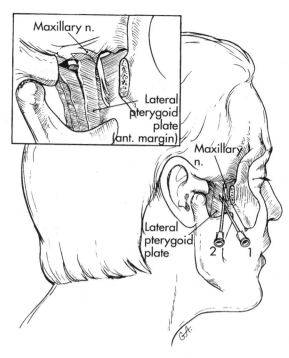

Fig. 17-4 Anatomy of maxillary nerve with two-step technique of blocking. Inset shows details of anatomy of lateral pterygoid plate and relationship of maxillary nerve as it runs anterior to it. (From Katz J: Somatic nerve blocks. In Raj PP, editor: *Practical Management of Pain,* ed 2. St Louis, Mosby, 1992.)

Box 17-2 AREAS INNERVATED BY MAXILLARY NERVE

Maxilla
Maxillary antrum
Teeth of upper jaw
Roof of mouth
Lower part of nose
Nasopharynx
Tonsillar fossa
Skin over middle third of face

---

orly (in the general direction of the orbit of the eye) so that the needle tip passes the anterior border of the lateral pterygoid plate. Advance the needle an additional half inch into the pterygopalatine fossa until a paresthesia to the upper jaw is elicited. At this point, inject 5 to 8 ml of local anesthetic. Use 2 to 3 ml of absolute alcohol for more permanent blocks.

Problems with this block are caused by the difficulties differentiating the lateral pterygoid from other bony aspects of the base of the skull. Another problem is that the lower portion of the pterygoid plate is attached to the bony skull a variable amount, so the space available for the needle to enter into the pterygopalatine fossa may be limited. In addition, the block can be quite painful to perform, and use of local anesthetic and/or sedation should be generous.

The terminal division of the maxillary nerve, the infraorbital nerve, can be blocked by remembering that the nerve courses along the floor of the orbit in the infraorbital groove and then emerges just beneath the bony orbit via the infraorbital foramen. The major indication for blocking this nerve is usually second division tic; occasionally a neuropathy secondary to trauma or infection is indicated. The technique is relatively simple, since the infraorbital foramen lies directly below the pupil when the patient is looking forward. Approach the foramen laterally with a small needle, 22- to 25-gauge (Fig. 17-5), when attempting a diagnostic block, or medially to enter the foramen and canal when attempting a neurolytic block. For diagnosis, once the lip of the foramen is met, 2 to 3 ml of local anesthetic will produce surface anesthesia. If the nerve is to be destroyed, enter the needle into the foramen and the canal for a short distance (2 to 3 mm) and inject ½ ml of absolute alcohol.

MANDIBULAR NERVE AND ITS BRANCHES
Anatomy

The mandibular nerve is the third and largest of the three branches of the gasserian ganglion. It is formed by the fusion of a single motor root with the larger inferior sensory branch from the ganglion and exits the skull via the foramen ovale. At about ½ to 1 inch below the foramen, the nerve divides into its lingual and inferior alveolar branches. Indications for block of this nerve are to denervate structures listed in Box 17-3, as well as tic and peripheral neuropathies.

Techniques

The landmarks are the same as noted earlier for the maxillary nerve. This time, however, when the needle strikes the lateral pterygoid plate, redirect it so that it just goes off its posterior edge, in the general direction of the ear (Fig. 17-6). About ½ inch or less beyond the pterygoid plate a paresthesia to the lower jaw or tongue is elicited. At this point, if the block is diagnostic, inject 5 to 8 ml of local anesthetic after careful aspiration; if the block is to be permanent, inject about 2 to 3 ml of alcohol on a paresthesia.

The difficulties are similar to those mentioned for the maxillary nerve; however, the posterior edge of the lateral pterygoid plate is not attached to any bony structure, and hence the space limitations are not as severe as with the maxillary nerve.

Block of the terminal division of the inferior alveolar branch of the mandibular nerve, the mental nerve, is often

---

Box 17-3 AREAS INNERVATED BY THE MANDIBULAR NERVE

Mandible
Anterior two thirds of tongue
Teeth of lower jaw
External auditory meatus
Temporal region
Anterior part of ear
Temporomandibular joint
Skin over lower third of face

---

useful for diagnosis and treatment. The mental foramen usually can be located in the midmandible, appearing slightly higher in edentulous patients, almost directly inferior to the corner of the mouth. It can be approached from the anterior for diagnostic blocks so that the needle does not enter

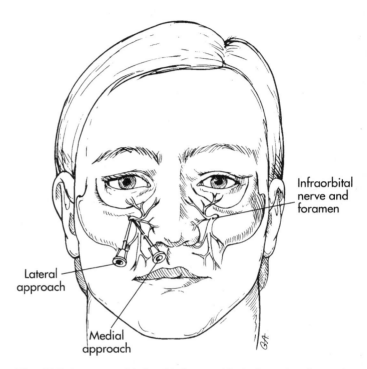

Fig. 17-5 Anatomy of infraorbital nerve block. Lateral and medial approach. (From Katz J: Somatic nerve blocks. In Raj PP, editor: *Practical Management of Pain,* ed 2. St Louis, Mosby, 1992.)

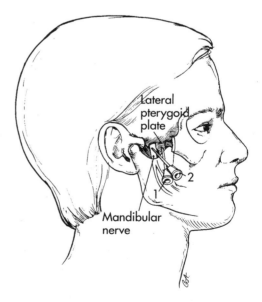

Fig. 17-6 Anatomy of mandibular nerve block. (From Katz J: Somatic nerve blocks. In Raj PP, editor: *Practical Management of Pain,* ed 2. St Louis, Mosby, 1992.)

the mental canal competing for space with the nerve and injuring it, or the canal can be entered from a more posterior approach if neurolysis is required (Fig. 17-7). In the first situation, inject 2 to 3 ml of local anesthetic at the mental foramen. In the latter case, ½ to 1 ml of absolute alcohol when the needle is in the mental canal will produce the desired results.

GLOSSOPHARYNGEAL AND VAGUS NERVES
Anatomy

The rootlets of the glossopharyngeal nerve originate in a groove on the lateral aspect of the medulla. They then fuse to form a single nerve that exits the skull via the jugular foramen. The nerve goes just medial to the styloid process and immediately lateral to the vagus and spinal accessory nerves. It is also just superficial to the internal carotid artery and jugular vein.

The vagus nerve runs in close contact with the spinal accessory nerve as it exits the skull via the jugular foramen, and it begins its descent to the lower portions of the body running in the sheath between the internal jugular vein and internal carotid artery.

Indications for block of the glossopharyngeal and vagus nerves are usually secondary to tumor involvement or mucocitis secondary to treatment in the areas innervated by the terminal divisions of these nerves (see Box 17-4). In particular, pain in the pharyngeal and tonsillar branches of the glossopharyngeal nerve, which innervate the pharyngeal mucosa, tonsillar areas, and posterior third of the tongue, are the major block indications.

Technique

Since both nerves lie near each other, attempted block of one usually results in block of both in addition to the spinal accessory and hypoglossal nerves. Make a skin wheal immediately below the external auditory meatus and just anterior to the border of the mastoid process (Fig. 17-8). Insert a 2-inch block needle perpendicular to the skin; at a depth of about ½ to 1 inch, it contacts the styloid process. At this point withdraw the needle into the subcutaneous tissue, direct it slightly posterior to the styloid process, and advance it an additional ½ to 1 inch. After careful aspiration, inject 3 to 5 ml of local anesthetic.

The block is technically easy to do. However, extreme care is necessary before injecting any local anesthetic, since the needle tip is immediately adjacent to the major vascular structures mentioned earlier.

Box 17-4 AREAS INNERVATED BY GLOSSOPHARYNGEAL AND VAGUS NERVES

IX

Palatine tonsils
Pharyngeal wall
Posterior one third of tongue

X

Base of tongue
Epiglottis
Larynx above cords and adjacent pharynx

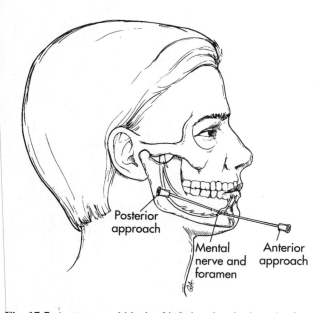

Fig. 17-7 Anatomy and block of inferior alveolar branch of mandibular nerve (mental nerve). (From Katz J: Somatic nerve blocks. In Raj PP, editor: *Practical Management of Pain,* ed 2. St Louis, Mosby, 1992.)

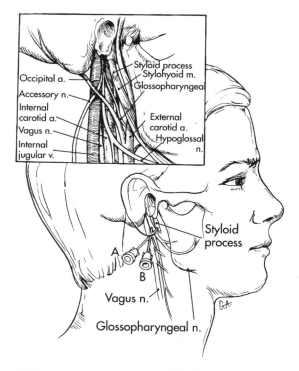

Fig. 17-8 Anatomy and technique of blocking glossopharyngeal and vagus nerves at styloid process. Inset shows details of anatomy of structures coursing through from base of skull in posterior cranial fossa. (From Katz J: Somatic nerve blocks. In Raj PP, editor: *Practical Management of Pain,* ed 2. St Louis, Mosby, 1992.)

QUESTIONS: TECHNIQUES

1. The ganglion that lies in the recess of the petrous portion of the temporal bone on its superior aspect and is surrounded by the invagination of the dura is known as:
   A. Geniculate ganglion
   B. Otic ganglion
   C. Trigeminal ganglion
   D. Sphenopalatine ganglion

2. The landmark commonly used for gangliolysis of trigeminal ganglion is all of the following EXCEPT:
   A. Midpoint of the zygomatic arch
   B. Needle entry point 1 cm lateral to the angle of the mouth
   C. At the level of upper second molar
   D. Root of the nose

3. The rootlets of the glossopharyngeal nerve originate in a groove on the lateral aspect of the medulla. It exits the skull via the:
   A. Foramen lacerum
   B. Foramen ovale
   C. Foramen rotundum
   D. Jugular foramen

4. Areas innervated by the mandibular nerve are all of the following EXCEPT:
   A. Teeth of the lower jaw
   B. Anterior two thirds of the tongue
   C. Temporomandibular joint
   D. Skin over the middle third of the face

5. Areas innervated by glossopharyngeal nerve are all of the following EXCEPT:
   A. Palatine tonsils
   B. Posterior one third of the tongue
   C. Pharyngeal wall
   D. Epiglottis

ANSWERS

1. C
2. D
3. D
4. D
5. D

18 Central Nerve Blocks

P. Prithvi Raj, Hans Nolte, and Michael Stanton-Hicks

A. INTRATHECAL BLOCK

ANATOMY
Spinal column

The spinal column consists of vertebral bodies that together form 7 cervical, 12 thoracic, 5 lumbar, 5 sacral, and 4 coccygeal vertebrae. A typical vertebra consists of two basic parts: the ventral vertebral body and the dorsal vertebral arch. Between the vertebral bodies are the intervertebral disks, which give the spinal column its flexibility. Together, the vertebral bodies and the intervertebral disks form a strong column supporting the head and trunk, and the vertebral arch protects the spinal cord. When the spinal column is viewed from the side, four flexures are visible: The thoracic and the sacrococcygeal flexures are concave ventrally, whereas the cervical and lumbar flexures are convex ventrally. In a supine position, L_3 is the highest point and L_5 the lowest point of the lumbar flexure.

Vertebral canal

The vertebral canal contains the epidural and the subdural/subarachnoid spaces. The shape of the vertebral canal is influenced by the different curves of the columns. It is triangular in regions where there is greater flexibility (cervical and lumbar regions) and round in the thoracic region, where there is less flexibility. The vertebral bodies and the intervertebral disks are the ventral boundaries of the vertebral canal. The dorsal boundaries are comprised of the laminae, the ligamentum flavum, and the vertebral arches. The vertebral arches carry the spinous processes, to which the interspinous ligaments are attached. The lateral boundary of the spinal canal is formed by the pedicles and the laminae. The principal intervertebral ligaments (Fig. 18-1) are (a) the supraspinous ligament, which runs longitudinally over the tips of the spinous processes from C_7 to the sacrum; (b) the interspinous ligaments, which attach to the spinous processes; (c) the ligamentum flavum, which is attached to the vertebral arches and is comprised of yellow, elastic fibers, becoming thicker toward its caudal end; (d) the posterior longitudinal ligament, which runs within the spinal canal on the dorsal surface of the vertebral bodies; and (e) the anterior longitudinal ligament, which runs ventrally along the vertebral bodies. In the median approach for subarachnoid or epidural anesthesia, insert the needle through the supraspinous and interspinous ligaments and the ligamentum flavum (Fig. 18-2); in the lateral approach, penetrate only the ligamentum flavum.

Subdural space. The subdural space, which is very small, is situated between the dura mater and the arachnoid mater. Small amounts of fluid in this space moisten these two membranes, which lie very close to each other. The subdural space is thus of no importance for central nerve blocks.

Subarachnoid space. The contents of the subarachnoid space include the spinal cord and its endings, which are covered by the pia mater; the cerebrospinal fluid (CSF), which is contained by the arachnoid mater; and the blood vessels supplying the spinal cord. The dura and arachnoid mater comprise a double layer that constitutes the dural sac and thus forms the outer boundary surrounding the CSF. Cranially, the spinal dura mater is attached to the circumference of the foramen magnum and to the dorsal surfaces of the bodies of C_2 and C_3.

In 43% of adults the dural sac ends at the transition from S_1 to S_2, in 32% at the middle of S_2, and in 23% at the transition from S_2 to S_3.[1] In some cases it may extend as far as the transition from S_3 to S_4.

Spinal cord. The spinal cord (Figs. 18-3 and 18-4), with an average length of 42 to 54 cm, is the axial part of the central nervous system (CNS), running from the cranial border of the atlas to the superior border of the second lumbar vertebral body. The spinal cord consists of 30 spinal segments: 8 cervical, 12 thoracic, 5 lumbar, and 5 sacral. Except for the sacral segments, all others branch from the subarachnoid space with their meningeal projections through the epidural space. The anterior and posterior communicating roots of the spinal nerves leave the spinal column through the intervertebral foramina and are part of the paravertebral ganglia. The caudal end of the spinal cord forms the conus medullaris (Fig. 18-5), from the tip of which the filum terminale extends to the sacrum. The filum terminale pierces the dura mater and is attached to the periosteum on the dorsal coccyx.

In the fetus the spinal cord occupies the entire spinal canal. As the spinal canal grows very rapidly, the spinal cord becomes proportionately shorter. The nerve roots that run horizontally during the fetal stage become more caudal as the fetus grows. In adults the spinal nerves from the midthoracic region downward have an almost vertical course as they reach their respective foramina. The lumbosacral nerves constitute the cauda equina. The dermatomal distribution of the spinal nerves is shown in Fig. 18-6.

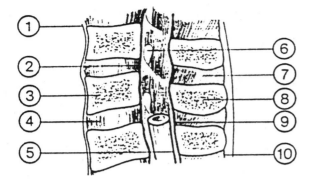

Fig. 18-1 Sagittal section of the spinal column in the lumbar region. *1,* Anterior longitudinal ligament: *2,* posterior longitudinal ligament; *3,* vertebral body; *4,* intervertebral disk; *5,* dura and arachnoid mater; *6,* intervertebral foramen; *7,* interspinous ligament; *8,* spinous process; *9,* ligamentum flavum; *10,* supraspinous ligament. (From Central neural blocks. In Raj PP, Nolte H, Stanton-Hicks M, editors: *Illustrated Manual of Regional Anesthesia.* Heidelberg, Germany, Springer-Verlag, 1988.)

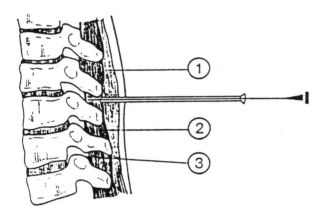

Fig. 18-2 In the median approach for subarachnoid or epidural block, the needle pierces the supraspinous and intraspinous ligaments and the ligamentum flavum. *1,* Supraspinous ligament; *2,* interspinous ligament; *3,* ligamentum flavum. (From Central neural blocks. In Raj PP, Nolte H, Stanton-Hicks M, editors: *Illustrated Manual of Regional Anesthesia.* Heidelberg, Germany, Springer-Verlag, 1988.)

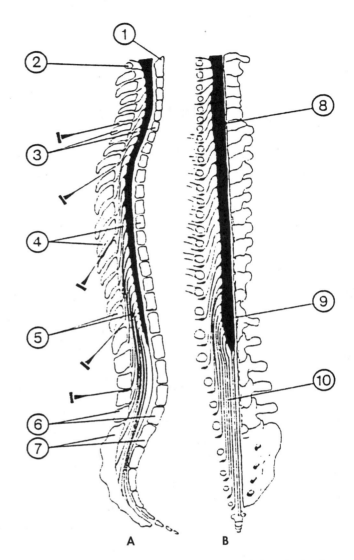

Fig. 18-3 A, Sagittal and **B,** dorsal views of the spinal column with the spinal cord and spinal nerves, showing the angle the needle takes between the spinous processes at each level and the relation of the nerve roots as they exit from the intervertebral foramina. *1,* Body of C_2; *2,* posterior arch; *3,* C_7; *4,* T_7; *5,* T_{12}; *6,* L_5; *7,* S_1; *8,* cervical widening and *9,* lumbar widening of the spinal cord; *10,* cauda equina. (From Central neural blocks. In Raj PP, Nolte H, Stanton-Hicks M, editors: *Illustrated Manual of Regional Anesthesia.* Heidelberg, Germany, Springer-Verlag, 1988.)

The spinal cord widens at two points: in the cervical and lumbar regions. The cervical widening of the spinal cord extends from C_3 to T_2. Its maximum circumference, approximately 38 mm, is at C_6. Similarly, at T_{12}, the circumference of the lumbar spinal enlargement is approximately 35 mm (see Fig. 18-3).

In 44% of adult Europeans the caudal end of the spinal cord extends to the middle of the first lumbar vertebral body. In 20% of cases it is at the level of the intervertebral disk L_1-L_2, in 16% at the intervertebral disk T_{12}-L_1, and in another 16% at the middle of L_2.[1] In very rare cases the spinal cord can extend as far as the middle of the vertebral body of L_4 or even more caudally.

The spinal cord is supplied by two posterior spinal arteries and by one anterior spinal artery. The posterior spinal arteries are most frequently derived from the posterior inferior cerebral or vertebral arteries, and the anterior spinal artery is derived from the vertebral artery at the level of the foramen magnum. The posterior spinal arteries pass caudad as paired or unpaired vessels one in front of and the other behind the dorsal roots of the spinal nerves; they supply the posterior columns of the spinal cord. They are reinforced by communicating branches of spinal vessels from intercostal and lumbar arteries (Fig. 18-7). This additional supply is greatest at the level of T_1 and T_{12}. The anterior median artery descends along the front of the spinal

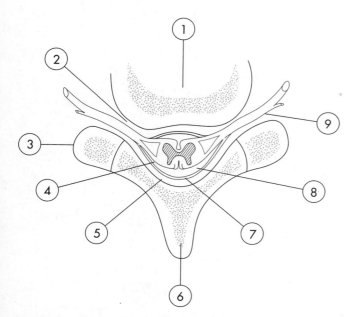

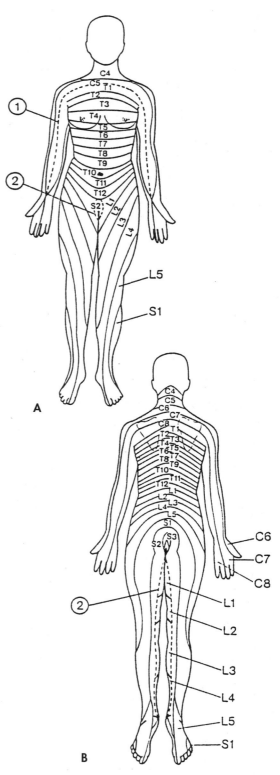

Fig. 18-4 Transverse section of vertebra showing the relation of spinal canal and its contents. *1,* Vertebral body; *2,* intervertebral foramen; *3,* transverse process; *4,* pia mater; *5,* epidural space; *6,* spinous process; *7,* subdural space; *8,* subarachnoid space; *9,* spinal nerve. (From Central neural blocks. In Raj PP, Nolte H, Stanton-Hicks M, editors: *Illustrated Manual of Regional Anesthesia.* Heidelberg, Germany, Springer-Verlag, 1988.)

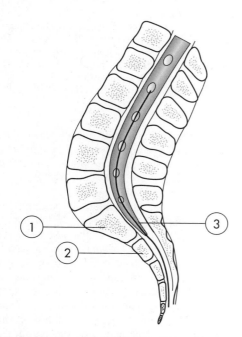

Fig. 18-5 Sagittal section of spinal column in lumbar and sacral regions. *1,* S$_1$; *2,* S$_2$; *3,* end of dural sac. (From Central neural blocks. In Raj PP, Nolte H, Stanton-Hicks M, editors: *Illustrated Manual of Regional Anesthesia.* Heidelberg, Germany, Springer-Verlag, 1988.)

Fig. 18-6 Dermatomal distribution of spinal segments; **A,** anterior and **B,** posterior views. *1,* Ventral axial line of arm; *2,* ventral axial line of leg. (From Central neural blocks. In Raj PP, Nolte H, Stanton-Hicks M, editors: *Illustrated Manual of Regional Anesthesia.* Heidelberg, Germany, Springer-Verlag, 1988.)

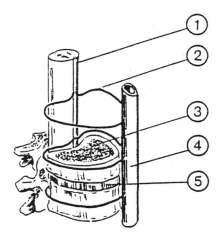

Fig. 18-7 Local blood supply of spinal cord showing distribution of radicular arteries in relation to aorta. *1,* Anterior spinal artery; *2,* radicular artery; *3,* vertebral body; *4,* aorta; *5,* intervertebral disk. (From Central neural blocks. In Raj PP, Nolte H, Stanton-Hicks M, editors: *Illustrated Manual of Regional Anesthesia.* Heidelberg, Germany, Springer-Verlag, 1988.)

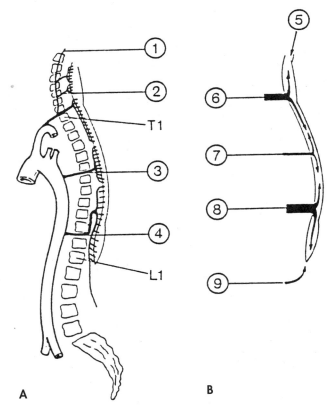

Fig. 18-8 Blood supply of the spinal cord showing **A,** vertical distribution and **B,** direction and proportion of flow. *1,* Vertebral artery; *2,* cervical radicular artery; *3,* thoracic radicular artery; *4,* artery of Adamkiewicz (radicularis magna); *5,* vertebral artery; *6,* cervical region; *7,* upper thoracic region; *8,* thoracolumbar region; *9,* iliac artery. (From Central neural blocks. In Raj PP, Nolte H, Stanton-Hicks M, editors: *Illustrated Manual of Regional Anesthesia.* Heidelberg, Germany, Springer-Verlag, 1988.)

cord and is also reinforced by small segmental arteries. At the conus medullaris the anterior median artery divides into two branches, which pass upward to anastomose with the terminal branches of the posterior spinal arteries. A slender twig continues onto the filum terminale. The largest communicating branch is the arteria radicularis magna, or artery of Adamkiewicz. It enters through the intervertebral foramen, most often on the left side between T_8 and L_3. In rare cases the entrance of the artery of Adamkiewicz can also be at T_5. If the point of entry is high, the caudal end of the spinal cord is supplied by a branch of the iliac artery, which runs cranially from the lower lumbar region (Fig. 18-8).

The veins of the spinal cord are composed of an anterior and a posterior plexus. They drain longitudinally along the nerve roots through the intervertebral foramina into the vertebral veins, the azygos vein, and the lumbar veins.

Cerebrospinal fluid. The CSF plays an important role in spinal anesthesia. It is a clear, colorless, slightly alkaline fluid enclosing the entire CNS and is found in both the spinal and cerebral regions, including the ventricles and cisterns. The volume of the CSF ranges from 100 to 150 ml in an adult. The volume of spinal CSF of relevance to subarachnoid anesthesia as measured from the foramen magnum is about 25 to 35 ml, whereas from T_5 downward it is about 15 to 18 ml. The CSF contains small amounts of protein and glucose and nearly isotonic amounts of sodium and chloride. Bicarbonate is also present. The pH of the CSF is 7.4 to 7.6, and its specific gravity is 1.004 ± 0.004 g/ml at 25° C and 1.0010 ± 0.0003 g/ml at 37° C.

Epidural space. The epidural space is a tissue plane between the spinal dura mater and the periosteum and ligaments within the vertebral canal. Superiorly the epidural space is limited by the foramen magnum, interiorly by the sacrococcygeal membrane, anteriorly by the posterior longitudinal ligament and the vertebral bodies and disks, posteriorly by the laminae and ligamentum flavum,

and laterally by the pedicles and intervertebral foramina. The volume of the epidural space from the foramen magnum to the sacrococcygeal membrane varies from 130 to 150 ml.

The epidural space contains the spinal nerve roots and their dural projections, the internal vertebral venous plexus, loose areolar tissue, segmental blood supply, and lymphatics. An important aspect of the veins found in this space is that they form an arcuate pattern, tending to aggregate at the level of each vertebral body, where they are disposed laterally. The latter fact is important for the technique of epidural block because if the needle always enters the epidural space in the midline, the chance of accidental venous puncture is greatly diminished. Another important aspect is that the veins of the epidural space, being valveless, provide an alternate route of venous return from the body cavities through their segmental connections. This is of great importance for epidural anesthesia: since these veins are also distensible, any increase in their size will encroach on the volume of the epidural space, thereby affecting the spread of solutions within the space. The ligamentum flavum, composed of elastic fibers, is the tough ligament that connects adjacent-laminae and serves as a landmark for epidural puncture. It is thinnest in the cervical region, becoming progressively thicker as the lumbar region is reached. Access to the ligamentum flavum is easiest in the lumbar region, where the interspinous interval is greatest. A midline approach to the thoracic region is also relatively simple between the lower and upper four thoracic spines. Because the laminae and spines overlap each other in the midthoracic region, a midline approach may be all but impossible, in which case a paramedian position of the needle should be adopted. It should be kept in mind that the distance between the ligamentum flavum and the dura mater is about 2 mm in the upper thoracic region and increases to about 5 to 6 mm in the lumbar region.

Surface markings serving as landmarks in epidural anes-thesia include the vertebra prominens (seventh cervical spine) at the base of the neck in the nuchal furrow; the tip of the seventh thoracic spine, which is opposite the inferior scapular angle when the arms are adducted; and the inter-cristal line crossing the spinous process of L_4 or the L_3-L_4 interspace.

REFERENCE

1. Central neural blocks. In Raj PP, Nolte H, Stanton-Hicks M, editors: *Illustrated Manual of Regional Anesthesia.* Heidelberg, Germany, Springer-Verlag, 1988.

SUGGESTED READING

Crock HV, Yoshizawa H: *The Blood Supply of the Vertebral Column and Spinal Cord in Man.* New York, Springer, 1977.

B. SUBARACHNOID BLOCK

HISTORY

In 1764 Cotugno first described the presence of CSF. In 1825 Magendie described its circulation. In 1885 Corning, a neurologist from New York, inadvertently performed the first subarachnoid block with cocaine by puncturing the dura mater of a dog. Lumbar puncture was described in 1891 by Quincke. The first intentional subarachnoid block for surgery on humans was carried out in Kiel, Germany, in 1898 by Bier with a 0.5% cocaine solution.[1]

INDICATIONS

Generally, all operations on the lower half of the body can be carried out with subarachnoid block. The usual indica-tions are operations on the lower extremities and pelvis, uro-logic and genital surgery, and surgery of the perineal re-gions. Unlike epidural block, subarachnoid block is particu-larly suited for (a) geriatric patients, (b) cases where sur-gery must be performed within 20 to 30 minutes, (c) trauma patients who are in severe pain, and (d) emergency obstet-ric procedures (e.g., cesarean section).

TYPES AND METHODS OF SUBARACHNOID BLOCK

Subarachnoid block can be divided into three categories:
   1. High subarachnoid block, where sensory block ex-tends as far as T_4
   2. Midsubarachnoid block, where there is sensory block to T_7
   3. Low subarachnoid block, where sensory block extends below T_{12}
   Saddle block is a special form of subarachnoid block that can be achieved only with hyperbaric agents and in which, depending on the volume injected (0.5 to 1 ml), sensory block extends cranially to S_1-S_2.
   The various forms of subarachnoid block can be per-formed easily by using hyperbaric local anesthetic agents and appropriate positioning of the patient. With isobaric agents a corresponding increase or decrease in the volume of drug is necessary. Thus when isobaric local anesthetic agents are employed, high subarachnoid block requires 4 ml, midsubarachnoid block 3 ml, and low subarachnoid block 2 ml of local anesthetic solution.

Block intended to extend above T_3 may result in total subarachnoid block.

PATIENT PREPARATION

Routine procedure includes the following steps:
   1. Insert a 16- to 18-gauge venous cannula.
   2. Infuse a volume of 500 to 1000 ml lactated Ringer's solution to compensate for vasodilatation.
   3. Monitor blood pressure and pulse before and during the procedure.
   4. Monitor the patient's electrocardiogram (ECG).

PATIENT POSITION

Subarachnoid block can be carried out with the patient in either a sitting or a lateral decubitus position. With the sit-ting position the patient sits on the operating table or bed with the legs hanging down comfortably and the feet sup-ported by a stool. The knees and hips should be flexed at about a 90° angle. The patient bends over slightly so that the lower arms rest on the thighs. For the lateral decubitus position the patient lies with the knees and hips flexed as far as possible and the chin lowered to the chest. The pa-tient's back should be as close as possible to the edge of the table.

TECHNIQUE
Midline approach

Cleanse the skin around the lumbar region with an appro-priate antiseptic solution or spray. To ensure aseptic condi-tions, place a windowed sheet over the area. All equipment must be sterile, and the anesthesiologist must wear sterile gloves.

Subarachnoid block should be performed preferably at the interspaces of L_3-L_4 or L_2-L_3. The intercristal line join-ing the two iliac crests identifies the spinous process of L_4, where it intersects the spinal column. The interspace felt above this point is the interval between L_3 and L_4. At the selected interspace make an intradermal skin wheal in the midline with 1 ml local anesthetic. Insert a 22-gauge needle 2 to 3 cm long perpendicularly through the skin wheal into the interspinous ligament, and inject another 2 ml of local anesthetic to anesthetize the needle path. Through this anesthetized region insert an introducer to a depth of about 3 to 4 cm. Advance a 25-gauge or 26-gauge needle through the introducer (Fig. 18-2). The first clearly felt resistance is usually at the ligamentum flavum. Then advance the needle another 0.8 to 1.2 cm on average to reach the dura mater. With the stylet removed, advance the needle slowly until CSF drips out of the end of the needle, thus indicating that the arachnoid mater has been perforated. Note that since the CSF flows very slowly through a thin needle, it should not be advanced more than 1 to 2 mm at a time. After CSF drips from the needle, attach the syringe with the measured amount of local anesthetic to the needle. This amount varies, depending on whether the technique is high, low, or midsubarachnoid. Inject the local anesthetic appropriately according to the chosen technique, remove the spinal needle and introducer, and cover the puncture site with adhesive dressing. Place the patient in the appropriate position, usually supine, and monitor for the onset of anesthesia. Although only a few minutes are necessary for a subarachnoid block to take effect, the patient's vital parameters must be checked every few minutes and appropriate therapeutic measures taken (e.g., increase of intravenous (IV) fluids or use of vasopressors to treat hypotension or to counteract physiologic changes). In most cases complete onset of subarachnoid block is usually reached in about 10 to 15 minutes, at which time surgery may begin.

Lateral approach

In addition to the midline approach, the lateral approach is also a technique frequently used. In this case make a skin wheal 1.5 to 2 cm lateral to the midline in the middle of the selected lumbar vertebral interspace. After patient preparation as described for the midline approach, insert the needle through the wheal at a 25° angle to the midline until reaching the subarachnoid space. This technique is advisable for obese patients or those with anatomic anomalies such as scars or arthritic changes.

Taylor approach

Another technique for lumbar subarachnoid block is the Taylor approach. Place the patient in a sitting, prone, or lateral decubitus position. Make a skin wheal approximately 1 cm medial and 1 cm cephalad to the posterior superior iliac spine. Insert a spinal needle through the wheal in a medial and cephalad direction at a 55° angle from the midline. If the needle touches the surface of the sacrum, it must be withdrawn slightly and redirected. When correctly positioned, the needle enters the lumbosacral foramen between L_5 and S_1. Since the lumbosacral foramen constitutes the widest opening of the entire vertebral column, the Taylor technique is particularly advantageous for patients who have advanced arthritis or a calcified ligamentum flavum.

TECHNIQUES USING LOCAL ANESTHETIC AGENTS OF VARYING SPECIFIC GRAVITY
Hyperbaric technique

With this technique local anesthetics with a specific gravity significantly higher than that of the CSF (1.003 to 1.006) are used. The extent of the block can be increased or decreased, depending on the patient's position. Thus as much

as 20 or even 30 minutes after initiating the block, repositioning the patient can change the level of anesthesia. The disadvantage of this technique is that when significant hypotension occurs, it is necessary to place the patient in the Trendelenburg position. In such cases the anesthesiologist must take into account that in the first half-hour after injection of the local anesthetic, the block will spread further cephalad. Sympathetic block will also spread further, thus aggravating hypotension. Hyperbaric subarachnoid block can also be used for unilateral techniques if the patient is positioned on the side to be operated on for at least 30 minutes.

Drugs commonly used with the hyperbaric technique include lidocaine 5%, mepivacaine 4%, tetracaine 0.5%, and bupivacaine 0.5%. Hyperbaricity is obtained by adding dextrose 10% to the local anesthetic to obtain a final dextrose concentration of 5% or 8%. The specific gravity thus achieved ranges from 1.018 to 1.035.

Isobaric technique

This technique employs local anesthetic agents of which the specific gravity is the same as that of the CSF. The advantage is that after complete onset is obtained at about 10 to 15 minutes, the level of anesthesia remains relatively constant in any position.

With a maximal dose of 3 ml, cephalad spread is within safe limits. Other advantages of this technique are that (a) conventional local anesthetic solutions can be injected, thus making special preparations unnecessary; and (b) positioning the patient, particularly during the first half hour, can be carried out without sequelae.

The preferred anesthetic is presently bupivacaine 0.5% with epinephrine (1:200,000). The main features of this agent are its long-lasting action and its ability to produce adequate motor block.

Hypobaric technique

With this technique local anesthetics with a lower specific gravity than the CSF are used. It is indicated for procedures in which the surgical site can be positioned higher than the head. This technique has proven popular for pelvic and perineal procedures with the patient in the Trendelenburg position. The hypobaric solution is prepared by mixing a local anesthetic solution with sterile water in a 1:2 weight-by-volume proportion (e.g., 5 mg tetracaine in 10 ml sterile water). A 1:1 weight-by-volume ratio is also used.

CONTRAINDICATIONS

Subarachnoid block is contraindicated with (a) hypovolemia (hemorrhagic shock etc.) and unstable vital functions, (b) infection in the area of the spinal puncture, (c) spina bifida or similar pathologic conditions, (d) coagulopathy, and (e) infectious diseases of the CNS.

COMPLICATIONS

No serious sequelae occur if the technique is performed correctly. However, headache requiring intensive treatment occurs after subarachnoid block in 1% to 3% of all cases. The incidence of spinal headache increases with increasing needle gauge size (22-gauge) and a number of spinal punctures. The incidence decreases in older patients. In combination with postspinal headache, cranial nerve palsy, which is mainly caused by loss of CSF through the puncture hole, may occur. Because of its proximity to the tentorium, the sixth cranial nerve may be affected; it is stretched owing to CSF drainage.

Neurologic sequelae are uncommon and mostly occur as a result of damage to the nerve roots from the spinal needle or intraneural injection of local anesthetic.

C. EPIDURAL BLOCK

HISTORY

Sicard[1] and Cathelin[2] independently published their experience with epidural anesthesia in 1901. For ease of entry into the epidural space they used the caudal route. Only a few proponents advocated the spinal approach, described by Sicard and Forrestier 20 years later, until Dogliotti introduced his *loss of resistance* technique in 1933. This technique provided a reproducible means of identifying the epidural space that could be acquired through a knowledge of anatomy and the possession of normal manual dexterity. Another established means of identifying the epidural space, called the *hanging drop sign,* was described by Gutiérrez (1933) at the same time. Its success depends not so much on manual dexterity as on the fact that a subatmospheric pressure exists in the epidural space.

The introduction of the Huber-tipped Tuohy needle in 1945, originally intended for continuous subarachnoid anesthesia, was adopted for epidural anesthesia by Curbelo in 1949 and provided a simple means of placing an epidural catheter in situ. Other modifications of this needle and equipment designed to facilitate identification of the epidural space have been described, but this discussion is limited to the use of the Tuohy needle in a midline approach and the Crawford needle in a paramedian approach.

CERVICAL APPROACH
Indications

Cervical epidural anesthesia is indicated for surgery on the neck, such as carotid endarterectomy; procedures on the upper limbs; and operations on the chest wall, such as mammoplasty.

Acute pain states such as herpes zoster, Raynaud's disease of the upper extremities, and chronic neurogenic pain or causalgia are all amenable to single-injection or continuous cervical epidural anesthetic techniques.

Practical aspects

Entry into the cervical region is comparatively simple because of good landmarks offered by the sixth and seventh spinous processes and the wide posterior foramina.

Acute flexion of the neck increases the distance between the ligamentum flavum and the dura mater from 1.5-2 mm to 4-5 mm, thereby markedly increasing the safety of the technique. Place the patient either in a sitting position, in which case a midline entry using the hanging drop sign is recommended for identification of the epidural space, or in

a lateral decubitus position, in which case a paramedian approach can be used.

Technique

Midline approach. Entry into the cervical canal is facilitated by using the interspace C_7-T_1 because of the landmarks and size of the posterior foramen. However, the C_6-C_7 interspace can also be used.

Place the patient in a sitting position with the head well anteroflexed and supported by an assistant. Using an aseptic technique, inject the skin and subcutaneous tissue with local anesthetic. With the hands holding the Huber-tipped Tuohy needle, introduce the needle through the spine in a strict midsagittal plane with the tip directed cephalad. At a depth of approximately 2 cm, withdraw the stylet and place a drop of anesthetic solution in its hub (Fig. 18-9). This maneuver increases the subatmospheric pressure in the epidural space, thereby facilitating its identification.

Entry into the epidural space is heralded by a sensation of "release" as the ligamentum flavum is pierced and the immediate disappearance of the drop of fluid from the needle hub, at which point further movement of the needle is arrested. Confirm correct needle placement by injecting into the needle hub a jet of local anesthetic that will vanish inside the epidural space.

Other short, bevelled epidural needles such as the Crawford, Bromage, and Weiss needles may also be used. In addition, where there is considerable familiarity with the loss

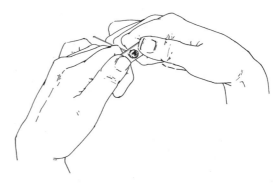

Fig. 18-9 Position of hands and grip used when advancing the winged epidural needle for the midline approach in epidural block. (From Raj PP, editor: *Practical Management of Pain,* ed 2. St Louis, Mosby, 1992.)

Some patients complain of backache lasting from several days to three weeks after a subarachnoid block. This can be caused by repeated spinal punctures or a small hematoma.

REFERENCE

1. Central neural blocks. In Raj PP, Nolte H, Stanton-Hicks M, editors: *Illustrated Manual of Regional Anesthesia.* Heidelberg, Germany, Springer-Verlag, 1988.

of resistance technique, a midline approach can be employed as an alternative to the one just described.

Paramedian approach. This approach, essentially designed to avoid both the spinous processes and their intervening ligaments, facilitates introduction of the epidural catheter and can be adopted for epidural puncture at any vertebral level.

After appropriate skin preparation, make a skin wheal 1.5 cm lateral to the spinous process of C_7 or C_6. Direct a 22-gauge needle (60 to 80 mm) at right angles to the skin down to the lamina, thereby enabling its depth to be determined. Then redirect the same needle while infiltrating the tissues with local anesthetic to assume a parasagittal angle of about 15°, and advance it to contact either the lamina or the ligamentum flavum. The direction taken by the needle is shown in Fig. 18-10. Then replace this needle by a Crawford or Tuohy needle. The bevel of the Crawford needle should face

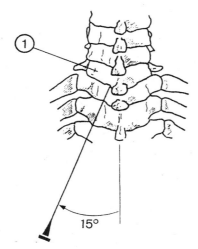

Fig. 18-10 Angle taken by needle for the paramedian approach to the cervical region. *1,* C_7. (From Central neural blocks. In Raj PP, Nolte H, Stanton-Hicks M, editors: *Illustrated Manual of Regional Anesthesia.* Heidelberg, Germany, Springer-Verlag, 1988.)

caudad, whereas that of the Tuohy should face cephalad to minimize the chance of accidental dural puncture. Introduce the epidural needle in the direction taken by the 22-gauge needle, and carefully advance it until it contacts the lamina or ligamentum flavum. Remove the stylet; attach a syringe containing saline; and while applying constant pressure to the plunger, advance the complete unit as shown in Fig. 18-11 until a loss of resistance to the plunger signals entry into the epidural space.

Choice and dosage of agents

The selection of a local anesthetic depends on the purpose and the required duration of anesthesia. In the cervical and thoracic regions the duration of epidural anesthesia is about 15% less than that obtained by an equivalent dose in the lumbar region.

An initial dose of 8 ml, including the test dose, of either a short- or a long-acting local anesthetic is suggested. Place the patient in the Trendelenburg position before injection of the local anesthetic because it is generally difficult to block the upper two cervical segments. This dose should provide anesthesia for all of the cervical and the upper three to four thoracic segments. If after 30 minutes the anesthetic spread is inadequate, an additional 12 ml of local anesthetic can be given. Choose the usual concentrations required to block sympathetic, sensory, or motor elements. Even when using a motor-blocking concentration, it is very difficult to block the phrenic nerves with any of the agents except etidocaine.

Complications

Possible complications of cervical epidural anesthesia include dural puncture, intravenous injection, neural injury, hematoma, and abscess.

THORACIC APPROACH
Indications

Thoracic epidural block is suited for surgery on the chest wall, such as mammoplasty or radical mastectomy. Mediastinal and intrathoracic surgery are well managed by high

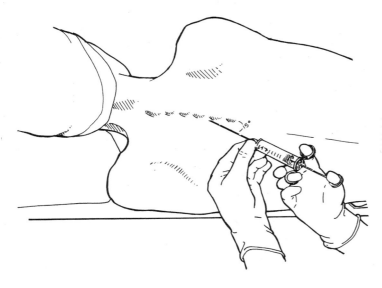

Fig. 18-11 Position of hands and grip used with the loss of resistance method of entry to the epidural space. (From Raj PP, editor: *Practical Management of Pain,* ed 2. St Louis, Mosby, 1992.)

thoracic epidural anesthesia combined with endotracheal intubation and a light general anesthetic. Low thoracic epidural puncture is ideally suited for upper abdominal surgery and for pheochromocytoma in particular as an adjunct to general anesthesia.

Acute pain states induced by, for example, herpes zoster, fractured ribs, and pancreatitis respond well to thoracic epidural block, which can be limited to the affected spinal segments and used as a sequel to general or regional anesthesia for postoperative pain.

Chronic pain such as that stemming from neuropathic and malignant disease is also an indication for epidural block in this region.

Practical aspects

Because of the anatomic disposition of the spinous processes in the thoracic region, it is difficult to attempt a midline entry into the epidural space in the center of the thoracic spine. Midline entry should therefore be restricted to the upper or lower four thoracic interspaces. Paramedian puncture, however, can be performed at any level. Because the zygapophyseal joints in the thoracic regions allow a primary rotational movement around the spinal axis, only a marginal increase in the intervertebral space is achieved by flexion of the spine. However, even this small increase may facilitate entry of the thick epidural needle.

When using the hanging drop sign of Gutiérrez for identification of the epidural space, the patient should assume the sitting position. With the loss of resistance technique from either the midline or paramedian approaches, the lateral decubitus position should be used.

Technique

Midline approach. Palpate the spinous processes defining the desired interspace. If the particular vertebral level is not critical, also palpate adjacent spaces and choose the space with the best definition. As shown in Fig. 18-12, make a wheal exactly midway between the two spinous processes (T_{10}-T_{11}). Infiltrate the deeper tissues with a 22-gauge needle and the epidural needle; then carefully introduce the latter (Weiss, Bromage, or Tuohy needle) to a depth of about 2 cm with the bevel facing cephalad in a strict sagittal plane.

The direction taken by the needle is shown in Fig. 18-13. Remove the stylet and place a drop of local anesthetic in the open hub (see Fig. 18-9). With the hands braced against the back and the thumbs and adjacent fingers holding the needle, as shown in Fig. 18-9, firmly and slowly advance the needle in concert with the patient's inspiration, since during this phase of respiration the subatmospheric pressure within the epidural space is most marked. Pay complete attention to the drop, which should exhibit a good light reflex. Precisely as the bevel of the needle enters the epidural space, the drop of local anesthetic will disappear, at which time a sense of "give" will be transmitted to the hand holding the needle. Then arrest movement of the needle and confirm the needle's position by observing the disappearance of a stream of fluid that is squirted into the hub. Although it is remote, always be alert to the possibility that the needle point may have entered an epidural vein. Therefore do not delay either introducing the catheter or injecting the test dose and capping the needle hub with a syringe to prevent the possibility of air entertainment.

Paramedian approach. This approach is very similar to that in the cervical region, the only difference being the obliquity with which the needle enters the interspace. This angle is determined by the indication of the thoracic lamina. As shown in Figs. 18-13 and 18-14, the point of entry into the T_3-T_4 interspace is 1.5 cm lateral and on a line just caudal to the tip of the third thoracic spinous process. Make a wheal at this point, and then use a 22-gauge needle to infiltrate the subcutaneous and deeper tissues with local anesthetic. At the same time, determine the depth and site of the ligamentum flavum. At this stage the needle forms an

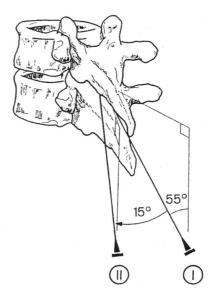

Fig. 18-13 Position of the needle (at a 55° angle from the plane of the back) relative to the spinous processes of the chosen interspace (T_3-T_4) for the midline approach *(I)* and the paramedian approach *(II)* (15° lateral to the midline) for thoracic epidural block. (From Central neural blocks. In Raj PP, Nolte H, Stanton-Hicks M, editors: *Illustrated Manual of Regional Anesthesia.* Heidelberg, Germany, Springer-Verlag, 1988.)

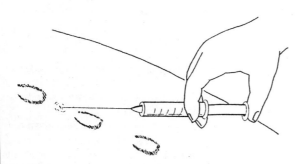

Fig. 18-12 Raising a skin wheal midway between the spinous processes of the selected interspace. (From Central neural blocks. In Raj PP, Nolte H, Stanton-Hicks M, editors: *Illustrated Manual of Regional Anesthesia.* Heidelberg, Germany, Springer-Verlag, 1988.)

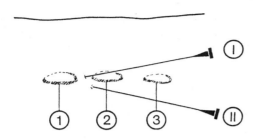

Fig. 18-14 Position of Crawford needle for the paramedian approach in thoracic epidural block, caudad and 1.5 cm lateral to T_3 spinous process. Needle in midline shown for comparison. *I*, Midline approach; *II*, paramedian approach; *1*, T_3; *2*, T_4; *3*, T_5. (From *Central neural blocks*. In Raj PP, Nolte H, Stanton-Hicks M, editors: *Illustrated Manual of Regional Anesthesia*. Heidelberg, Germany, Springer-Verlag, 1988.)

angle of 15° to the sagittal plane and about 55° to the plane of the back. The short-bevelled Crawford needle designed for the paramedian approach should be used, although a Tuohy type of needle may be substituted. If the latter is used, the bevel must face cephalad, whereas the bevel of the Crawford needle is always turned to face caudad to minimize the risk of dural puncture. The needle should assume the same direction as that taken by the 22-gauge needle. Advance it carefully down to the superomedial border of the lamina. Then "walk" the tip of the needle superiorly until it contacts the ligamentum flavum, and at this point attach a 5- or 10-ml freely moving glass or plastic syringe containing saline. With the hands holding the syringe as shown in Fig. 18-11, advance the entire unit through the ligamentum flavum while maintaining constant unremitting pressure on the plunger of the syringe. At the precise moment the needle enters the epidural space, a feeling of "release" is transmitted to the hands holding the needle, and a loss of resistance to injection is immediately sensed. Halt further movement and verify the needle's position by injecting 3 to 4 ml air, which will disappear without any resistance.

Choice and dosage of agents

Similar to the dosage requirements in the cervical region, thoracic epidural doses are approximately 15% less than those needed for segmental anesthesia in the lumbar spine. Whether a short- or long-acting agent is used, the volume of local anesthetic is identical, although it is the dose of drug per unit volume that determines the quality of anesthesia. Therefore for surgical procedures involving the thoracic wall or viscera, muscle relaxation is not as important as it would be for intraabdominal operations.

For acute pain states such as those induced by rib fractures, herpes zoster, and pancreatitis, where the primary objective is to block small pain fibers and sympathetic nerves, bupivacaine 0.25% to 0.37% is the most suitable drug and concentration and is generally administered by intermittent injection. When continuous infusion techniques are employed, even more dilute solutions can be used. The duration of analgesia in the thoracic region tends to be somewhat shorter than that obtained when the same drug is used for similar purposes in the lumbar region.

Complications

Thoracic epidural anesthesia carries with it the risk of complications such as dural puncture, intravenous injection, neural injury, hematoma, and abscess.

LUMBAR APPROACH
Indications

Surgery of the abdomen, particularly when it involves bowel and retroperitoneal structures as in major vascular surgery, is ideally suited for lumbar epidural block. Pelvic surgery and surgery of the extremities are also indications for epidural block in this region. Epidural anesthesia is also used as an adjunct to general anesthetic techniques to provide muscle relaxation, analgesia, and sympathetic block. Lumbar epidural anesthesia is the technique of choice for normal parturition and operative obstetrics. The technique is also valuable for hyperactive uterine contractions and preeclampsia. Acute pain states such as postoperative pain and ischemic pain from vascular occlusion or frostbite in the lower extremities are specific indications. Incidental to the relief of acute disk prolapse is the therapeutic use of epidural steroid injection.

Chronic neurogenic back pain is sometimes treated with a continuous lumbar epidural block, thereby allowing for other treatment modalities without the limitations imposed by the patient's pain.

Practical aspects

As with cervical or thoracic epidural puncture, the patient may adopt a sitting or lateral decubitus position. The hanging drop sign, when used in conjunction with a midline approach to the epidural space in the lumbar region, is subject to a higher failure rate than when it is employed in the cervicothoracic spine. It is important to achieve the greatest amount of spinal flexion when performing lumbar epidural puncture because the plane of the facet joints in the lumbar spine allow for considerable anteroposterior rotation. For a patient with severe degenerative disease of the spine this may make the difference between success and failure in entering the posterior spinal foramen. In such cases a paramedian rather than a median approach greatly increases the chances of successful puncture.

The midline approach can be performed in a sitting or decubitus position, but it is more comfortable for the operator to use the paramedian approach with the patient lying on his or her side.

Technique

Midline approach. The spinous processes are palpated transversely, as shown in Fig. 18-15. Make a skin wheal of local anesthetic with a 25-gauge needle exactly midway between the spinous processes selected. Then use the 22-gauge needle to infiltrate and explore the deeper tissues in preparation for insertion of the Tuohy needle. With a quick twisting motion, introduce the Tuohy needle through the needle site, and firmly but carefully direct it down to the ligamentum flavum. The needle should be almost perpendicular to the skin, as shown (see Fig. 18-15). The increased resistance of the ligamentum flavum must be recognized, and at this point halt further advance of the needle and re-

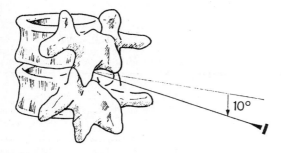

Fig. 18-15 Needle position relative to spinous processes for midline approach to the lumbar epidural space. (From Central neural blocks. In Raj PP, Nolte H, Stanton-Hicks M, editors: *Illustrated Manual of Regional Anesthesia*. Heidelberg, Germany, Springer-Verlag, 1988.)

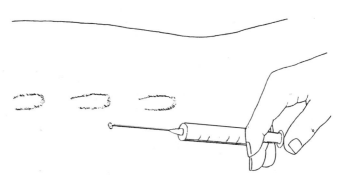

Fig. 18-17 Raising a skin wheal 1.5 cm lateral to caudal tip of spinous process below the chosen interspace. (From Central neural blocks. In Raj PP, Nolte H, Stanton-Hicks M, editors: *Illustrated Manual of Regional Anesthesia*. Heidelberg, Germany, Springer-Verlag, 1988.)

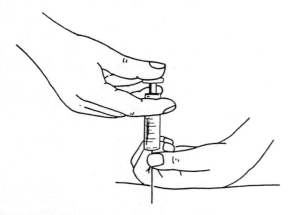

Fig. 18-16 Side view of hand positions used when performing the loss of resistance technique in the lumbar region. (From Central neural blocks. In Raj PP, Nolte H, Stanton-Hicks M, editors: *Illustrated Manual of Regional Anesthesia*. Heidelberg, Germany, Springer-Verlag, 1988.)

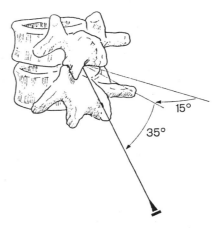

Fig. 18-18 Position of epidural needle alongside the spinous process for the paramedian (paraspinous) approach to the lumbar region. (From Central neural blocks. In Raj PP, Nolte H, Stanton-Hicks M, editors: *Illustrated Manual of Regional Anesthesia*. Heidelberg, Germany, Springer-Verlag, 1988.)

move the stylet. The orifice of the Tuohy needle should always point cephalad. Attach a freely moving 5- or 10-ml glass or plastic syringe filled with saline or air to the needle, and, maintaining constant pressure in the case of fluid or continual tremolo percussion if air is being used, advance the syringe by rocking the holding hand on the back (Fig. 18-16). Precisely as the needle point escapes from the ligamentum flavum and enters the epidural space, cease resistance to the plunger, allowing it to advance suddenly. This movement confirms identification of the epidural space by the so-called loss of resistance method. The hand that controls the advance of both needle and syringe should stop immediately, thereby preventing accidental dural puncture. Then remove the syringe, and in the case of a single-shot injection, slowly administer the therapeutic dose of local anesthetic. Alternatively, if the dose is large (e.g., 20 ml), it can be given in two or three aliquots over a 10-minute interval. This obviates the need for a specific test dose.

Paramedian approach. Raise a skin wheal 1.5 cm lateral to the caudal edge of the spinous process immediately below the chosen interspace (Fig. 18-17). Introduce a

22-gauge needle at right angles to the skin, and while infiltrating ahead of the needle point, carefully but positively advance the needle until contact with the lamina is made. This indicates the depth at which the ligamentum flavum can be expected. Then withdraw the needle to the epidermis, and redirect it, at the same time infiltrating with local anesthetic so as to pass alongside the spinous process until the needle contacts the ligamentum flavum in the midline (Fig. 18-18). The angle of the needle to the sagittal plane is 15° and to the plane of the back approximately 55°, although the latter relation will vary with the depth of tissue in different individuals. Then replace this needle by an 18-gauge Crawford needle, again directing it toward the superomedial aspect of the ipsilateral lamina or ligamentum flavum, whichever is contacted first. In the former case walk the needle superiorly until it engages the ligamentum flavum. Remove the stylet, rotate the needle so that the bevel faces caudad, and attach a syringe containing saline or air. With the hands in the same position as for the paramedian approach in the cervical region (Fig. 18-11), advance the sy-

Table 18-1 Agents of choice for lumbar epidural block

Drug	Sympathetic block		Analgesia		Motor block	
	Concentration (%)	Duration (min)	Concentration (%)	Duration (min)	Concentration (%)	Duration (min)
2-Chloroprocaine	1.0	—	2.0	40-60	3.0	30-50
Lidocaine	0.5	0-100	1.0	60-75	2.0	75-90
Bupivacaine	0.25	180-360	0.5	220-380	0.75	210-300
Etidocaine	0.5	180-360	1.0	240-400	1.5	230-360

ringe andneedle together until the loss of resistance toinjection signals entry of the needle tip into the epidural space.

Choice and dosage of agents

The choice of local anesthetic will depend on the required duration of anesthesia. Most uses of lumbar epidural anesthesia for surgery necessitate a motor-blocking concentration, whereas for acute pain control such as with postoperative pain, a weak concentration of bupivacaine would be the most appropriate anesthetic solution.

Table 18-1 lists the agents of choice with their indications. The required volume of local anesthetic can be roughly calculated from the dosage range, a rectilinear relationship related to the age of the patient and varying between 0.4 and 1.6 ml per spinal segment.

Complications

Lumbar epidural block can give rise to the following complications: dural puncture, intravenous injection, neural injury, hematoma, and abscess.

REFERENCES

1. Sicard JA: Les injections médicamenteuses extra-durales par voie sacro-coccygiene. *CR Soc Biol (Paris)*53:396, 1901.
2. Cathelin MF: Une nouvelle voie d'injection radichienne: méthode des injections épidurales par le procédé du canal sacré (applications àl'homme). *CR Soc Biol (Paris)* 53:452, 1901.

D. CAUDAL BLOCK

HISTORY

Cathelin[2] and Sicard[1] first described the technique of caudal (sacral epidural) block in 1901. Stoeckel[3] introduced the technique in Germany in 1909, and Meeker and Bonar reported its use for obstetrics in the United States in 1923. Edwards and Hingson[4] developed the continuous caudal technique in 1942, which represented the most significant advance in obstetric pain management to that date.

INDICATIONS

The principal surgical uses for caudal anesthesia involve perineal and anal surgery, circumcision, and orthopedic procedures on the feet.

Depending on the dose employed, this route can be varied to provide total pelvic or lower extremity anesthesia. The block can extend from T_{10} to S_5 or, through the so-called *single-shot* technique or low caudal block, provide anesthesia in only the sacral segments when perineal anesthesia is indicated.

Pediatric cases lend themselves especially well to caudal anesthesia, particularly those involving children under 1 year in whom major abdominal conditions such as exomphalos can be repaired under caudal block with supplemental, light, general anesthesia. Outpatient surgery is also a specific indication, where in association with a light general anesthetic, caudal block provides for benign emergence and prolonged postoperative analgesia.

Although caudal analgesia is still occasionally employed for normal parturition, its principal use is now restricted to instrumental delivery and repair during the late second and third stages of labor.

There are few indications for the use of caudal block in pain states. However, patients suffering from spastic paraplegia can often benefit from caudal administration of a dilute neurolytic substance. In addition, patients in whom severe degenerative disease or surgery of the lumbar spine may preclude access for therapeutic injections often respond successfully with a caudal route of administration.

PRACTICAL ASPECTS

Because of the significant variations in the anatomic form of the sacrum, particularly in the adult, landmarks may be indistinct or misleading. Usually the posterior superior iliac spines can be felt, and lines drawn from those points to the tip of the coccyx will pass just medially to the sacral cornua. When the cornua can be readily felt, the inferior base of the triangular sacral hiatus can be easily defined (Fig. 18-19). In the adult the needle should not be advanced more than 1.5 cm superiorly through the sacrococcygeal membrane. In children and infants the needle should only pierce the membrane.

TECHNIQUE

The patient is preferably positioned prone as shown in Fig. 18-19, although if this is impracticable for clinical reasons (e.g., obstetrics), puncture can also be performed in the lateral decubitus position with the hips fully flexed.

As surface landmarks, the posterior superior iliac spines should be identified and marked. The tip of the coccyx is palpated, and the sacral cornua should be sought. At the apex of lines drawn from the posterior inferior iliac crests to the coccyx, the sacral hiatus can be identified.

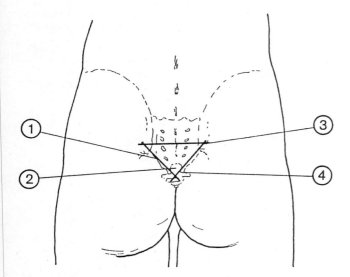

Fig. 18-19 Landmarks for caudal block. *1*, Sacral triangle; *2*, sacral hiatus; *3*, posterior superior iliac spine; *4*, sacral cornu. (From Central neural blocks. In Raj PP, Nolte H, Stanton-Hicks M, editors: *Illustrated Manual of Regional Anesthesia*. Heidelberg, Germany, Springer-Verlag, 1988.)

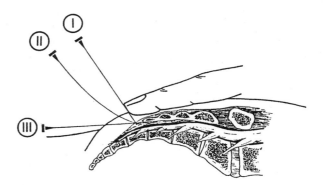

Fig. 18-20 The needle is directed initially at 120° to sacral canal through the sacrococcygeal membrane *(I)*. Then it is moved through an arc of 60° as shown with needles *(II and III)*. When the tip of the coccyx is palpated with the forefinger lying in the natal cleft, the second knuckle lies over the sacral hiatus. The pressure exerted by the finger helps to prevent dislodgement of the needle from the sacral canal during insertion. (From Central neural blocks. In Raj PP, Nolte H, Stanton-Hicks M, editors: *Illustrated Manual of Regional Anesthesia*. Heidelberg, Germany, Springer-Verlag, 1988.)

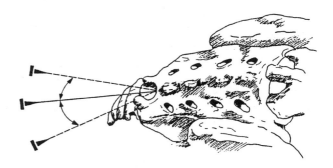

Fig. 18-21 Side-to-side movement of the needle confirms its correct position in the caudal canal. (From Central neural blocks. In Raj PP, Nolte H, Stanton-Hicks M, editors: *Illustrated Manual of Regional Anesthesia*. Heidelberg, Germany, Spinger-Verlag, 1988.) (From Central neural blocks. In Raj PP, Nolte H, Stanton-Hicks M, editors: *Illustrated Manual of Regional Anesthesia*. Heidelberg, Germany, Springer-Verlag, 1988.)

As another guide to the sacral hiatus, when the forefinger is placed on the tip of the coccyx, the middle metacarpophalangeal joint lies over the sacrococcygeal membrane. Before preparing the skin, push a swab into the natal cleft to prevent the antiseptic solution from burning the sensitive perineal skin.

Make a wheal with a 25-gauge needle, and infiltrate the subcutaneous tissues down to the sacrococcygeal membrane with a small amount of local anesthetic. After this procedure it is helpful to use the forefinger to depress the tissues to disperse both the local anesthetic and any edema present. This facilitates recognition of the anatomic features.

For a single injection a 22-gauge needle can be used in adults, but only a 25-gauge 1.5-cm needle should be used in infants or small children. When a continuous technique is desired, an 18-gauge caudal needle should be employed. A 20-gauge 7-cm intravenous cannula can also be employed for continuous techniques in children.

Direct the needle through the sacral hiatus at an angle of 120°, as shown in Fig. 18-20. The tip pierces the sacrococcygeal membrane with a snap. Then rotate it through about 60°, while at the same time maintaining pressure with a finger over the needle point (see Fig. 18-20). Then advance the needle about 1.5 cm into the sacral canal. A confirmatory sign of correct placement is the side-to-side movement of the hub indicating the free movement of the needle tip within the sacral canal (Fig. 18-21). A further confirmatory test is the injection of 5 to 10 ml of air, which will be identified as crepitus or a tumescence dorsal to the sacrum when the needle is not within the sacral canal.

CHOICE AND DOSAGE OF AGENTS

Either a short- or a long-acting local anesthetic can be used, depending on the duration required, although there are few indications for needing a motor-blocking concentration. The volumes used are very unpredictable in the adult because of the loss of local anesthetic from the anterior foramina and the relatively large volume of the sacral canal. Generally, twice as much drug will be needed as would be required for lumbar epidural block.

In children, however, the dose requirements are much more predictable. A useful formula is that developed by Schulte-Steinberg and Rahlfs:[5] 0.1 ml × segment × age in years, with maximum dosages of 10 mg/kg lidocaine 1% or 2.5 mg/kg bupivacaine 0.25%.

COMPLICATIONS

Caudal block is subject to complications such as subarachnoid injection, intravenous injection, abscess, hematoma, and broken epidural catheters. Subarachnoid injection should be preventable by carefully noting the distance to which the needle has been advanced and applying gentle aspiration with a syringe. Administration of the test dose will permit additional recognition of incorrect needle placement in either the subarachnoid or intravascular compartments.

REFERENCES

1. Sicard JA: Les injections médicamenteuses extra-durales par voie sacro-coccy giene. *CR Soc Biol (Paris)* 53:396, 1901.
2. Cathelin MF: Une nouvelle voie d'injection radichienne: méthode des injections épidurales par le procédé du canal sacré (applications à l'homme). *CR Soc Biol (Paris)* 53:452, 1901
3. Stoeckel W: Uber sakrale anästhesie. *Zentralbl Gynaekol* 33:1, 1909.
4. Edwards WB, Hingson RA: Continuous caudal anesthesia in obstetrics. *Am J Surg* 57:459, 1942.
5. Schulte-Steinberg O, Rahlfs VW: Caudal anaesthesia in children and spread of 1% Lignocaine: a statistical study. *Br J Anaesth* 42:1093, 1970.

QUESTIONS: CENTRAL NERVE BLOCKS

1. The epidural space contains the following EXCEPT:
   A. Spinal nerve roots
   B. Vertebral venous plexus
   C. Areolar tissue
   D. Lymphatic duct
2. Cervical epidural anesthesia is indicated for pain relief and surgery for:
   A. Carotid endarterectomy
   B. Cholecystitis
   C. Hysterectomy
   D. Knee replacement
3. In the paramedian approach for cervical epidural block the angle taken by the needle at the skin entry is:
   A. 10°
   B. 15°
   C. 20°
   D. 30°
4. In the lumbar region the position of the epidural needle from the spinous process in the paramedian approach should be:
   A. 15°
   B. 25°
   C. 35°
   D. 45°

5. Landmarks for caudal block are all of the following EXCEPT:
   A. posterior superior iliac spine
   B. anterior superior iliac spine
   C. sacral cornu
   D. sacral hiatus

ANSWERS

1. D
2. A
3. B
4. C
5. B

19 Peripheral Nerve Blocks

P. Prithvi Raj

A. COMMON SOMATIC NERVE BLOCKS
Neck

CERVICAL PLEXUS
Anatomy

The cervical plexus is formed by the ventral primary rami of the upper four cervical nerves, which, via ascending and descending branches, interconnect with each other. Although block of the cervical plexus is a useful anesthetic technique for surgical anesthesia and may be of some benefit in the diagnosis of vague neck discomforts, more definitive diagnostic or therapeutic procedures are usually done on its peripheral extensions, in particular, block of the occipital nerves for the diagnosis and treatment of headaches and occipital neuralgia and block of the suprascapular nerve for the management of shoulder pain, including bursitis, capsulitis, etc. The major motor branch of the cervical plexus, the phrenic nerve, is often blocked as a diagnostic and occasionally therapeutic measure to relieve hiccups. Painful, cancerous invasions of structures of the neck are best treated by subarachnoid dorsal root rhizotomy of the appropriate cervical nerves, usually C_3 and C_4, rather than a block of the cervical plexus itself.

The greater occipital nerve arises from the dorsal primary ramus of the second cervical nerve together with a smaller branch coming from the third cervical nerve. As mentioned above, the indications for this block are primary in the diagnosis and treatment of occipital headaches and neuralgia.

OCCIPITAL NERVE BLOCK
Technique

The technique for block of the greater occipital nerve is as follows (Fig. 19-1). With the patient in the sitting position and the head bent slightly forward, identify the nuchal ridge. With the palpating finger just lateral to the nuchal ligament on the involved side, the occipital artery can occasionally be felt. The nerve runs with the occipital artery innervating the posterior portion of the skull. While identifying the artery or ligamentous structure, which covers both the artery and nerve, insert a 1-inch block needle perpendicular to the superior nuchal line. Before reaching the bone of the skull, paresthesia of the occipital nerve may be elicited. If not, the skull is reached, and withdraw the needle slightly. Inject 5 ml of local anesthetic.

PHRENIC NERVE BLOCK
Technique

The phrenic nerve arises from the anterior primary division of C_4, primarily with contributions from C_3 and C_5. The nerve passes downward in the neck along the anterior surface of the anterior scalene muscle and between it and the sternocleidomastoid muscle. Prime indication for the block is the diagnosis and treatment of hiccups.

The patient lies supine, head turned opposite to the side to be blocked (Fig. 19-2). Identify the sternocleidomastoid muscle, and at the C_6 level insert a needle between the sternocleidomastoid and anterior scalene muscles. Use a 2- to 3-inch, 22-gauge block needle and, at about midpoint of the sternocleidomastoid muscle, inject local anesthetic as the needle is moved back and forth. Approximately 10 ml of a concentrated local anesthetic (e.g., 2% lidocaine or its equivalent) is required. To ascertain the efficacy of the block, it should be done under radiologic controls, the endpoint being disappearance of diaphragmatic activity on the involved side.

Block of the phrenic nerve is aided by use of a nerve stimulator. Using this technique, insert a coated needle electrode in the same anatomic position as described above. When the phrenic nerve is stimulated, the observer will note a diaphragmatic twitch. The use of radiologic control and stimulator for this particular nerve blocking procedure are recommended.

Trunk

THORACIC NERVE ROOT BLOCK

The 12 pairs of thoracic nerve roots can be blocked as they emerge from the thoracic intervertebral foramina. The spine of the thoracic vertebrae inclines downward, especially in the midthoracic area; therefore the tip of the vertebral spine in the thoracic region could be opposite the intervertebral foramen, two levels below. However, from T_1-T_3 and from T_9-T_{12} this overlap does not exceed one level below.

Indications

A thoracic nerve root block is useful for diagnostic, prognostic, and therapeutic purposes and for pain secondary to nerve root irritation or compression at the foramina level or distally. It can be used for treatment of intercostal neuralgia secondary to herpes zoster, fractured ribs, tumors, or metastasis.

Technique

A thoracic nerve root block can be done with the patient prone or in the lateral position with the affected side up.

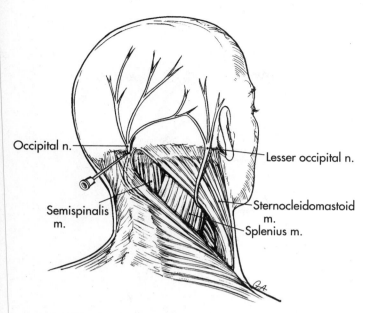

Fig. 19-1 Anatomy and site of nerve blocking for occipital nerve. (From Katz J: Somatic nerve blocks A. In Raj PP, editor: *Practical Management of Pain,* ed 2. St Louis, Mosby, 1992.)

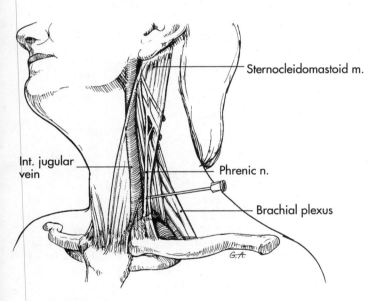

Fig. 19-2 Anatomy and technique of blocking phrenic nerve in lower third of neck anterior to the anterior scalene muscle. (From Katz J: Somatic nerve blocks A. In Raj PP, editor: *Practical Management of Pain,* ed 2. St Louis, Mosby, 1992.)

Vertebrae can be counted from C_7 down and checked again by counting from L_4 up. Fluoroscopy is essential.

Advance a 22-gauge, 8-cm needle perpendicularly through a skin wheal 3 cm lateral to the level of the cephalad edge of the vertebrae to contact the transverse process. Then withdraw the needle and advance it slightly medially (25°) and caudally (20°). If paresthesias are obtained, inject 5 ml of a local anesthetic. If paresthesias are not obtained, advance the needle 2.5 cm deeper than the transverse pro-

cess or until it contacts the posterolateral aspect of the vertebra and inject the local anesthetic there.

The development of cutaneous analgesia in the appropriate dermatome indicates a successful block. It is hard to confirm analgesia of one dermatome because of the overlap of dermatomes. Three roots may have to be blocked to provide good analgesia in one dermatome.

Complications

Pneumothorax is possible but unlikely. If the patient has a coughing spasm or if air is aspirated, the pleura may have been punctured. Observe the patient for the development of a pneumothorax.

Epidural or subarachnoid spread of the injection solution can occur, especially if there is a long dural sleeve. Segmental sympathetic block can result from the block of the sympathetic fibers that accompany the root.

If the volume is increased, solution can spread paravertebrally or epidurally up and down and more roots may be anesthetized. It is important to use small volumes (1 to 3 ml) of local anesthetic when performing a neurolytic block. In addition, use of a small volume defines the contribution of the individual nerve root to the patient's pain.

INTERCOSTAL NERVE BLOCK

The thoracic spinal nerves in the paravertebral region divide into a dorsal branch, which innervates the muscle and skin of the posterior third of the back, and a ventral branch, which forms intercostal nerves for the 11 intercostal spaces and the subcostal nerve below the twelfth rib (Fig. 19-3).

The thoracic ventral branches of T_1 and T_2 also contribute to the formation of the lower trunk of the brachial plexus. Only a small part of T_2 continues first as the intercostal nerve. The second intercostal nerve gives rise to the lateral cutaneous branch, called the intercostobrachial nerve, which innervates the medial side of the upper arm. Each of the other intercostal nerves gives rise to a lateral branch that innervates the skin of the lateral body wall and an anterior cutaneous branch that innervates the anterior body wall; the upper six intercostal nerves innervate up to the xiphisternum, whereas the lower six intercostal nerves innervate from the xiphisternum to the umbilicus.

The upper six intercostal nerves innervate the muscle in the intercostal space. The lower five intercostal nerves and the subcostal nerves innervate the abdominal muscles, in addition to the intercostal muscles. The nerve runs in the neurovascular plane between internal intercostal muscle, and the innermost layer (subcostal, sternocostal, innermost intercostal) is protected by the costal groove in the intermediate part of the rib where the innermost layer of muscle is deficient.

Indications

An intercostal nerve root block is indicated for patients undergoing surgery of the upper abdominal region (in conjunction with a celiac plexus block) and for patients with pain after thoracoabdominal surgery. It is also useful for patients who have incurred trauma to the chest wall, especially fracture of the ribs, and for neurolytic blocks for cancer.

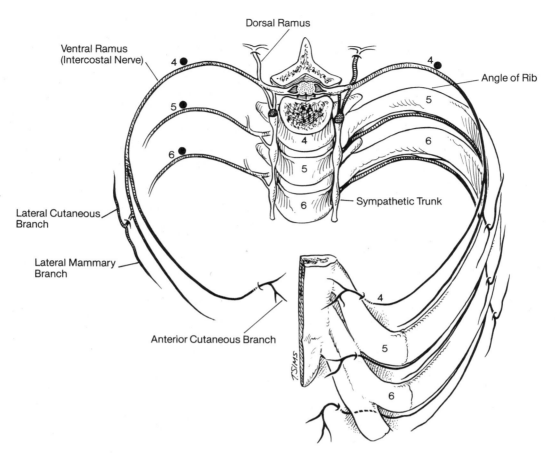

Fig. 19-3 Anatomy of intercostal nerves. (From Raj PP, Pai U, Rawal N: Techniques of regional anesthesia in adults. In Raj PP, editor: *Clinical Practice of Regional Anesthesia.* New York, Churchill Livingstone, 1991.)

Equipment/Drugs

The intercostal nerve root block is performed with a 22-gauge, 1½-inch needle; a 23-gauge, ½-inch needle; 10-ml syringes; and the usual preparation tray.

The volume of injectate is 3 to 5 ml per intercostal nerve. For a short-duration block 1% to 1.5% lidocaine is used; for a long-duration block 0.5% bupivacaine or 1% etidocaine is used. For a neurolytic block 6% to 8% phenol in diatrizoate is used.

Technique

For bilateral intercostal blocks position the patient prone with the arms hanging or elevated above the head. For a unilateral block at the posterior or midaxillary line the patient lies in a lateral position with an arm over the head. For an anterior block to cover the parasternal region the patient lies supine.

The intercostal block can be done (1) at the angle of the rib posteriorly, (2) at the posterior axillary line or midaxillary line laterally, and (3) at the anterior axillary line anteriorly. The patient usually lies prone for bilateral intercostal blocks.

After the skin is prepared, insert the needle over the rib selected for the block. It should touch the lower half of the rib subcutaneously. At this point the operator holds the needle and syringe with one hand (Fig. 19-4) and with the other hand moves the skin caudally over the rib so that the needle point slips off the rib. Push the needle about 3 mm deeper until a click is felt. Then turn the hub downward, and direct the needle tip under the lower edge of the rib cephalad about 2 to 3 mm. Aspiration is done for air or blood. If the aspiration test is negative, inject 3 ml of a local anesthetic. For one intercostal space to be blocked, three intercostal nerves, one above and one below the nerve selected, must be injected. A single-catheter technique can be used for postoperative and trauma pain relief.

An intercostal nerve block provides analgesia in the intercostal region. Respiratory excursion is usually improved because of pain relief. There may be hypotension, nausea, and fainting because of fast systemic absorption of the drug injected.

Precautions

Large volumes of local anesthetics should not be used for intercostal blocks, since they are more readily absorbed at this site than at other sites. The risks associated with this block are intravascular injection and pneumothorax. Pneumothorax can be prevented if the operator is careful, is slow,

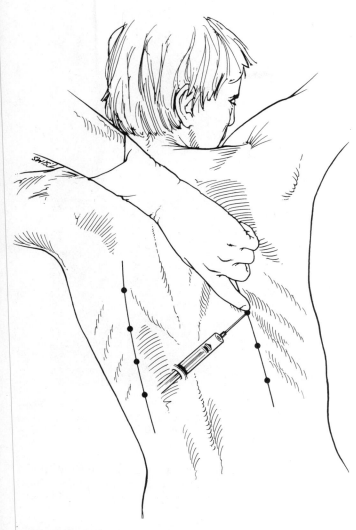

Fig. 19-4 Intercostal block. Figure shows correct placement of anesthetist's finger on the inferior edge of patient's rib. Note that the needle with syringe touches rib before slipping under it to touch intercostal nerve. Needle should be inserted obliquely under rib to prevent development of a pneumothorax. (From Raj PP, Pai U, Rawal N: Techniques of regional anesthesia in adults. In Raj PP, editor: *Clinical Practice of Regional Anesthesia.* New York, Churchill Livingstone, 1991.)

and learns the anatomy of the areas before trying the technique. Resuscitative equipment and skilled personnel should be nearby.

Contraindications

An intercostal nerve block is contraindicated if pneumothorax would be deleterious to the patient, if there is infection at the site of the injection, if the patient is on anticoagulant therapy, if the patient is allergic to local anesthetics, and if the patient is in shock.

Complications

Pneumothorax. Careful performance of the block will reduce the risk of development of pneumothorax. If it does

develop, it should be recognized and treated as necessary. The patient must be reassured.

Subarachnoid block. An inadvertent subarachnoid block should be treated as a spinal block. This complication has been reported and proven with dye studies. Because the dura occasionally extends out along the intercostal nerve a variable distance before it adheres to the nerve as the neurilemma or nerve sheath, an anesthetic drug deposited in this potential space can dissect back into the subarachnoid space and result in spinal anesthesia (Fig. 19-5). Therefore all of the devices necessary to support the patient should be present (e.g., airway equipment, breathing bag, intravenous [IV] fluids, vasopressors).

Intravascular injection leading to systemic toxicity. Treat the toxicity. Intravascular absorption is much more problematic. Since the intercostal space is supplied by a rich network of vascular anastomoses because of the high metabolic activity of the intercostal muscles, there is a much greater absorption of the local anesthetic, leading to high plasma levels. Blood anesthetic levels are higher here and peak sooner than when the same amount of local anesthetic is injected elsewhere, such as axillary sheath or other nerve blocks. This may lead to toxic reactions. Pay careful attention to the maximum dosage allowed, and add a vasoconstrictor in small concentrations (i.e., a 1:200,000 to 1:400,000 concentration is useful).

Interpleural Block

Placement of an interpleural catheter for use in postoperative pain was first performed by Dr. Fin Reiestad and Dr. K.E. Strömskag in 1986 in Molde, Norway.[1-3] The interpleural catheter placement is accomplished by insertion of an epidural catheter into the pleural space, through which is administered intrapleural local anesthetics. The mechanism of this method of analgesia is unknown. It is thought that possible reverse diffusion of local anesthetics from pleural spaces back into the subpleural space and then through thin muscles to reach a larger number of intercostal spaces, subsequently blocking the intercostal nerves, is the mechanism of action. The advantages of this procedure are that it is not complex to perform, there is no risk of hypotension or central nervous system (CNS) depression, and the patient does not suffer from itching or urinary retention.

Indications

It is indicated for cholecystectomy, renal surgery, unilateral breast procedure, thoracotomy, subcostal or flank incisions, multiple rib fractures, flail chest, thoracic herpes zoster, and pancreatic pain.

Technique

The patient lies on the unoperated side or in a sitting position. Insert a 16- to 18-gauge Tuohy needle with the bevel cephalad at a 30° to 40° angle through the eighth intercostal space, and advance it along the superior border of the rib. Insert the needle 8 to 10 cm from the posterior midline (*line 1,* Fig. 19-6), then introduce it in a medial direction

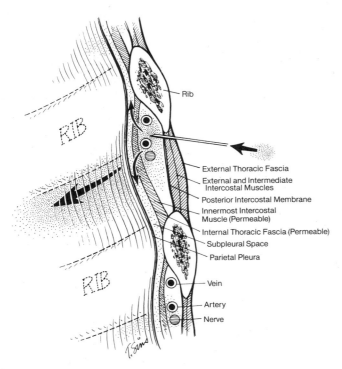

Fig. 19-5 Intercostal block. Figure shows potential spaces that injected solution can traverse. (From Raj PP, Pai U, Rawal N: Techniques of regional anesthesia in adults. In Raj PP, editor: *Clinical Practice of Regional Anesthesia.* New York, Churchill Livingstone, 1991.)

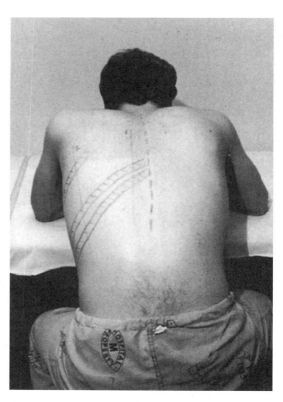

Fig. 19-6 Needle placement for intrapleural catheter. (From Neumann MM, Reynolds LM: Somatic nerve blocks B. In Raj PP, editor: *Practical Management of Pain,* ed 2. St Louis, Mosby, 1992.)

with the cutting edge upwards. After perforating the internal intercostal membrane, a distinct resistance is felt. At this point remove the stylet, and connect a glass syringe with 3 to 4 ml of air (Fig. 19-7). Advance the needle slowly with continuous pressure on the syringe. A "clicking" perforation of the parietal pleura will be encountered. This indicates a loss of resistance. Disconnect the syringe and cover the needle to prevent aspiration of air. Immediately thereafter, introduce the catheter 5 to 6 cm into the pleural space, and withdraw the needle. Secure the catheter on the skin with plastic dressing.

If the patient is on a ventilator, disconnect the ventilator before the pleural puncture is performed and until the needle is removed. If the patient is breathing spontaneously, have the patient hold his or her breath during this period. If the patient has an open chest, place the catheter at the postero-medial aspect of the incision and loosely anchor it with absorbable suture.

After a test dose is performed, a loading dose of 20 ml of 0.5% bupivacaine with epinephrine 1:200,000 is administered via the catheter. For continuous infusion, after the loading dose, 0.25% to 0.5% bupivacaine should be run at 5 to 10 ml/hr.

For the performance of this procedure on a closed-chest pediatric patient, one can use a dose of 0.5 ml/kg of 0.25% bupivacaine with epinephrine 1:200,000 as a bolus. For infusion one can use as little as 0.1 to 0.5 mg/kg/hr to 0.25 to 2.5 mg/kg/hr bupivacaine.

Precautions and contraindications include pleural fibrosis, pleural effusion, allergy to local anesthetics, hemothorax or pneumothorax, local or systemic infection, and bleeding diathesis.

Upper Extremity

Anatomy

The brachial plexus is formed by ventral rami of C_5, C_6, C_7, C_8, and T_1, with minor contributions from C_4 and T_2. From above as it transverses distally, the brachial plexus divides into roots, trunks, divisions, cords, and branches (Fig. 19-8).

The roots enter the interscalene groove between the scalenus anterior and the scalenus medius muscles. C_5 and C_6 nerve roots form the upper trunk. The C_7 nerve root continues as the middle trunk, and the C_8 and T_1 nerve roots unite to form the lower trunk at the lateral part of the scalenus anterior muscle. The lower trunk is ensheathed by the prevertebral fascia and lies in the same plane as the subclavian artery. The upper and middle trunks lie above the subclavian artery; the lower trunk lies posterior to the subclavian artery close to the first rib.

Each trunk divides into the anterior and posterior divisions. The posterior divisions of all the trunks unite to form the posterior cord. The anterior divisions of the upper and middle trunks form the lateral cord, and the anterior division of the lower trunk forms the medial cord. The cords

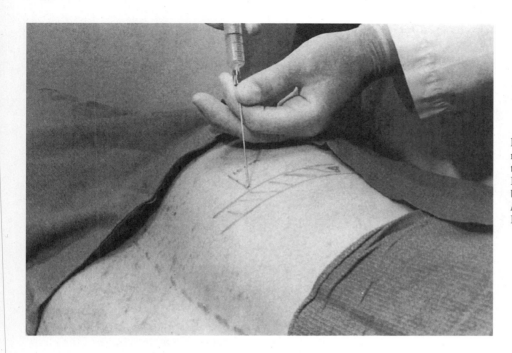

Fig. 19-7 Needle and syringe placement for loss of resistance when entering pleural space. (From Neumann MM, Reynolds LM: Somatic nerve blocks B. In Raj PP, editor: *Practical Management of Pain,* ed 2. St Louis, Mosby, 1992.)

are designated as posterior, lateral, or medial according to their relationship to the second part of the axillary artery, behind the pectoralis minor muscle.

Branches of the brachial plexus given at the roots are (1) C_5 contribution to the phrenic nerve, (2) C_5-C_7 nerve to the serratus anterior, and (3) nerve to rhomboids and levator scapulae (C_5). The branches given at the trunks are at the upper trunk (1) nerve to subclavius and (2) suprascapular nerve to supraspinatus and infraspinatus. The branches given at the cords are the (1) lateral cord (lateral pectoral nerve, musculocutaneous nerve, and lateral head of the median nerve, (2) medial cord (medial pectoral nerve, medial cutaneous nerve of the arm and forearm, medial head of the median curve, and lumbar nerve), and (3) posterior cord (upper and lower subscapular nerve, nerve to latissimus dorsi, axillary nerve to shoulder joint and to deltoid and teres minor, and radial nerve).

Except for the innervation of the skin over the upper part of the shoulder (C_3-C_4) and the upper part of the medial arm (T_2), all of the motor and sensory innervation of the upper extremity is derived from the brachial plexus. The sympathetic innervation is derived from the T_1 to T_5 spinal segments. The T_1 and T_2 postganglionic fibers traverse the brachial plexus via the stellate ganglion, and the T_3 to T_5 postganglionic fibers join the vascular branches of the subclavian artery to the arm.

Indications

A brachial plexus block is indicated for anesthesia of the upper extremity during surgery, pain relief after trauma, relief of postoperative pain, and chronic pain relief in patients with certain medical conditions. A brachial plexus block is indicated if pain relief is not adequate after stellate ganglion blocks for causalgia, reflex sympathetic dystrophy, peripheral neuropathies, or Raynaud's disease. Catheters can be placed on the brachial plexus at all sites if prolonged pain

relief is required. Neurolytic blocks can also be done for cancer pain involving the brachial plexus.

Using 10 ml of a local anesthetic produces a consistently good block of each trunk, division, or the mixed peripheral nerve. Since the brachial plexus block involves four major nerves, a total of 40 ml is required for surgical anesthesia. Lesser volumes of 10 to 20 ml are required for pain relief. The site of needle entry does not change the volume requirement. A high needle entry in the brachial plexus sheath, such as that used for the interscalene, supraclavicular, or infraclavicular blocks, causes the motor block to appear earlier than the sensory block. A more distal needle entry such as that used for an axillary block is associated with greater sensory block and poor motor block.

For a consistent brachial plexus motor block the recommended agents are 0.5% bupivacaine, 3% chloroprocaine, 1% etidocaine, 1.5% lidocaine, 1.5% mepivacaine (Carbocaine), or 2% prilocaine. For a sensory block alone lesser concentrations of a local anesthetic such as 2% chloroprocaine or 1% lidocaine may be used. For brachial plexalgia involving the nerve trunks, divisions, or cords secondary to cancer, neurolytic blocks can be tried. Phenol 6% to 10% may be injected, up to a maximum volume of 10 ml at any one time.

INTERSCALENE APPROACH[4]

The brachial plexus in the interscalene region consists of roots and trunks covered by the prevertebral fascia and enclosed between the fasciae of the anterior and middle scalene muscles (Fig. 19-9).

Technique

The patient lies supine with the head turned to the opposite direction. One arm rests on the side, extending to the knee. The physician stands on the side to be blocked at the level of the neck.

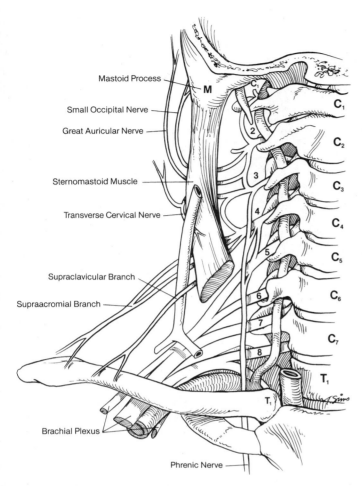

Fig. 19-8 Anatomy of cervical plexus and its relationship to brachial plexus. (From Raj PP, Pai U, Rawal N: Techniques of regional anesthesia in adults. In Raj PP, editor: *Clinical Practice of Regional Anesthesia*. New York, Churchill Livingstone, 1991.)

Landmarks

To identify landmarks, palpate the cricoid cartilage (C_6 level) and the posterior border of sternocleidomastoid muscle. Then roll the fingers posteriorly to the posterior border of the sternomastoid and onto the interscalene groove. The interscalene groove can be accentuated if the patient raises the head against resistance. The point of entry of the needle is where the external jugular vein crosses the sternomastoid (C_6 level) (Fig. 19-10).

Procedure

After a sterile preparation, stand on the side to be blocked at the level of the neck, and palpate the interscalene groove at the C_7 level. Infiltrate any local anesthetic intracutaneously with a 27-gauge needle. Then take in hand a 20-ml syringe attached to an extension set and a 22-gauge needle. Insert the needle through the landmark, perpendicular to the skin and in a caudal direction. At this point a nerve stimulator could be attached to the needle, with the ground electrode in the opposite shoulder. As the needle enters the interscalene groove, a paresthesia should be elicited in the

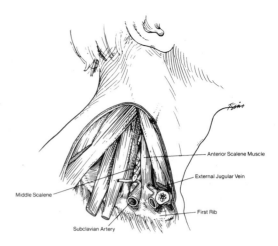

Fig. 19-9 Regional anatomy of brachial plexus in interscalene groove. (From Raj PP, Pai U, Rawal N: Techniques of regional anesthesia in adults. In Raj PP, editor: *Clinical Practice of Regional Anesthesia*. New York, Churchill Livingstone, 1991.)

shoulder, elbow, or thumb. When paresthesia of the elbow or thumb is obtained, stop the needle advancement. As the nerve stimulator current is applied, the biceps, forearm muscles, or wrist and hand muscles will contract. The needle is in a correct position if the paresthesia is in the thumb or contractions are seen in the wrist or fingers. If paresthesia of the shoulder or elbow is present or the biceps are contracting, the needle may be at the C_5-C_6 nerve root. If the diaphragm is contracting unilaterally, the phrenic nerve has been stimulated; the needle is too anterior and medial.

A brachial plexus block performed via the interscalene approach provides anesthesia of the shoulder, elbow, forearm, and hand; usually there is no anesthesia of the inner aspect of the upper arm and the elbow. The ulnar nerve is blocked in about half of the cases.

Precautions

Before injection the aspiration test is done to prevent vascular or cerebrospinal fluid (CSF) spread. Administer a test dose of 1 to 3 ml of local anesthetic solution to test for CNS toxicity or total spinal block. Stop the injection as soon as signs of toxicity appear.

Complications

A total spinal block may be prevented by performing the aspiration test before injection. A high epidural block is managed by airway control, oxygen administration, and maintenance of blood pressure.

CNS toxic reactions causing unconsciousness are managed with oxygen administration and the maintenance of respiratory, cardiac, and CNS functions. Cardiac toxic reactions causing cardiac arrhythmias are managed with oxygen administration and the maintenance of respiratory, cardiac, and CNS functions.

An inadvertent stellate ganglion block requires no treatment. Similarly, an inadvertent laryngeal nerve block requires no treatment; however, there should be no oral in-

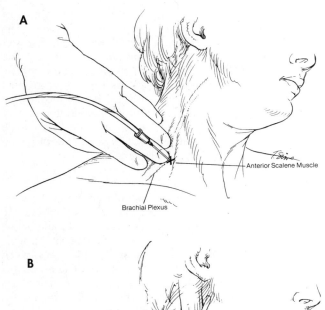

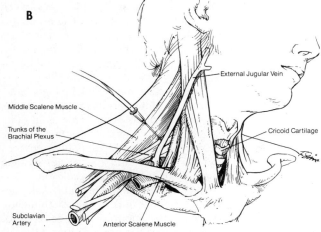

Fig. 19-10 A, Superficial landmarks, site of entry, and position of needle for interscalene approach to brachial plexus block. **B,** Note that needle usually contacts upper trunk. (From Raj PP, Pai U, Rawal N: Techniques of regional anesthesia in adults. In Raj PP, editor: *Clinical Practice of Regional Anesthesia.* New York, Churchill Livingstone, 1991.)

take until the patient can sip water. An inadvertent phrenic nerve block is managed by maintaining adequate ventilation.

The treatment of a pneumothorax depends on the size of the pneumothorax. A chest x-ray film must be made and a pulmonary physician consulted for further management.

SUPRACLAVICULAR APPROACH[5]
Anatomy

The trunks of the brachial plexus form divisions and cords at this level. The medial cord lies posterior to the third part of the subclavian artery. The lateral and posterior cords lie posterolateral to the artery.

Drugs

For a procedure of short duration (<1 hour), 40 ml of 2% to 3% 2-chloroprocaine is appropriate. For a procedure of medium duration (2 hours), 40 ml of 1% to 1½% lidocaine is appropriate. For a procedure of long duration (>3 hours),

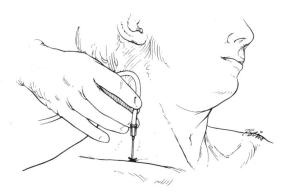

Fig. 19-11 Subclavian perivascular approach of brachial plexus. Note the point of entry is at interscalene groove, where subclavian artery pulsation is felt. (From Raj PP, Pai U, Rawal N: Techniques of regional anesthesia in adults. In Raj PP, editor: *Clinical Practice of Regional Anesthesia.* New York, Churchill Livingstone, 1991.)

40 ml of 0.5% or 0.75% bupivacaine or 1% etidocaine or 20 ml of 2% lidocaine plus 20 ml of 0.5% bupivacaine may be used. For neurolytic procedures, 6% phenol in diatrizoate is recommended.

Technique

The patient is positioned supine with a roll between the scapulae. The arms rest on the side, extended toward the knee. The patient's head is turned to the opposite side. For accentuation of the sternomastoid and scalene muscles, the head may be lifted 30° off the table.

Landmark

The landmark is the midpoint of the clavicle midway between the prominence of the top of the shoulder (acromial end of the clavicle) and the sternal end of the clavicle. The point of needle entry is on the lateral border of the anterior scalene muscle at the midpoint of the clavicle.

Alternative technique

For a perivascular subclavian approach[6] the needle entry site is the C_7 level in the interscalene groove, with the needle directed caudad and the needle hub in line with the ear (Fig. 19-11).

Procedure

After a sterile preparation of the region, insert the needle at the point of entry above the midpoint of the clavicle in the backward, inward, and downward direction. The needle appears to be at right angles to all planes at this level of the neck (Fig. 19-12). Even though the needle is directed toward the first rib, it need not touch the rib. Paresthesia of the digits of the hand or wrist is sought. If it is obtained and an aspiration test is negative for air or blood, inject 1 to 3 ml of local anesthetic as a test dose, followed by injection of the total calculated volume of the local anesthetic after 5 minutes if there are no systemic effects. If paresthesia is not obtained and the needle touches the first rib, it usually touches it at the subclavian groove. Walk the needle

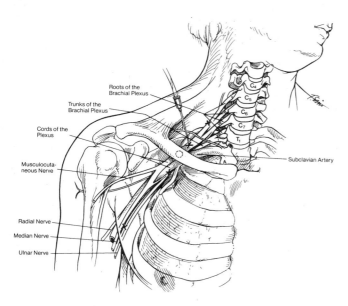

Fig. 19-12 Anatomy of brachial plexus and four sites where brachial plexus can be performed. (From Raj PP, Pai U, Rawal N: Techniques of regional anesthesia in adults. In Raj PP, editor: *Clinical Practice of Regional Anesthesia*. New York, Churchill Livingstone, 1991.)

posteriorly to elicit paresthesia. If paresthesia is not obtained, contact with the rib will be lost. Make contact with the rib again, and walk the needle toward the vertebra. If no paresthesia is obtained at this point, repeat the procedure. The nerve stimulator can be used as described earlier in this section to aid in the location of the brachial plexus.

A brachial plexus block by the supraclavicular approach provides anesthesia of the whole arm up to the shoulder, except the inside of the upper third of the upper arm. A sympathetic block is also produced at the same regions.

Precautions

Avoid puncturing the subclavian artery or the lung and entering the epidural or subarachnoid space.

The stellate ganglion may be blocked, especially with large volumes. The vagus nerve and its branches in the neck may also be blocked.

Complications

Possible complications include pneumothorax and a hematoma in the neck. A hematoma in the neck is treated by reassuring the patient, watching, and aspirating or evacuating the hematoma, if necessary. The hematoma will disappear spontaneously in 2 to 3 weeks. A pneumothorax of less than 10% may be treated conservatively; a pneumothorax of more than 20% requires chest tube placement.

INFRACLAVICULAR APPROACH[7]
Anatomy

The axilla occupies the pyramid-shaped infraclavicular space between the upper lateral part of the chest and the medial side of the arm. It consists of an apex, base, and four walls. The apex faces the root of the neck and is lim-

ited by the out border of the first rib, the superior border of the scapula, and the posterior surface of the clavicle. The base is formed by the skin and the axillary fascia. The pectoralis major and minor muscles form the anterior wall. The subscapularis teres major and the latissimus dorsi complete the posterior wall. The medial wall is formed by the first four ribs, and the lateral wall is formed by the medial side of the arm. The contents of the axilla include the axillary vessels, the brachial plexus with its branches, some branches of the intercostal nerves, a large number of lymph glands, fat, and loose areolar tissue.

Indications

Deposition of a local anesthetic solution inside the brachial plexus sheath in the infraclavicular regional blocks the cords and branches of the brachial plexus above and below the level of formation of the musculocutaneous and axillary nerves. Thus an infraclavicular approach is useful when anesthesia from hand to shoulder is desired. In addition, this technique allows easy blocking of the ulnar segment of the medial cord and the intercostobrachial nerve, which helps to prevent tourniquet pain without requiring additional infiltration.

The infraclavicular approach to the brachial plexus block provides adequate anesthesia of the entire arm. Although the danger of penetrating blood vessels is the same as in other approaches, the risk of pneumothorax is less because the needle is directed laterally from the midpoint of the clavicle. The lung lies behind the medial third of the clavicle and hence escapes potential damage from the needle tip.

For consistently good results with the infraclavicular approach it is necessary to use a peripheral nerve stimulator. The neurostimulator technique simplifies the process of locating the brachial plexus, which is deeper in the infraclavicular regional than at other sites, and improves the success rate of the infraclavicular block.

Technique

The patient lies supine and the physician stands opposite the arm to be blocked. Although the patient's arm is usually abducted 90° and the head is turned away from the arm, the block can be performed with the patient's arm and head in any position.

Landmarks

A line drawn from the C_6 tubercle to the brachial artery in the arm and which crosses the midpoint of the clavicle provides the surface marking of the brachial plexus in the infraclavicular region.

Before cleansing, the whole length of the clavicle and the subclavian artery where it dips under the clavicle should be identified by palpation and marked. If the artery cannot be felt, the midpoint of the clavicle should be identified. The point of needle entry is 1 inch below the midpoint of the clavicle (Fig. 19-13).

Procedure

After the field has been sterilized and draped, test the stimulator and the leads and attach the ground electrode to the patient's shoulder opposite the site of needle entry. Infil-

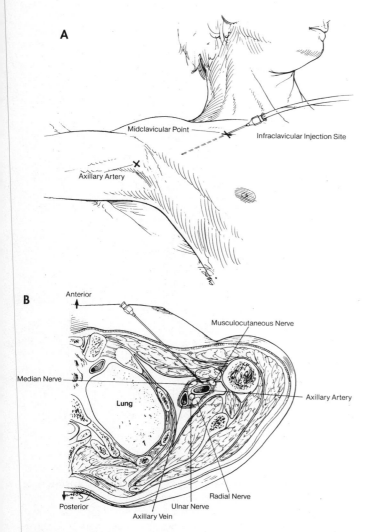

A,

Midclavicular Point — Infraclavicular Injection Site

Axillary Artery

B

Anterior

Musculocutaneous Nerve

Median Nerve

Lung

Axillary Artery

Posterior

Radial Nerve

Ulnar Nerve

Axillary Vein

Fig. 19-13 A, Technique of brachial plexus block by infraclavicular approach. A 22-gauge, 3½-inch needle is directed from 1 inch below midpoint of clavicle toward brachial artery in upper arm. **B,** Horizontal section of axilla showing the relationship of axilla and the direction of needle laterally from point of entry. (From Raj PP, Pai U, Rawal N: Techniques of regional anesthesia in adults. In Raj PP, editor: *Clinical Practice of Regional Anesthesia.* New York, Churchill Livingstone, 1991.)

trate the skin with a small amount of local anesthetic 1 inch below the inferior border of the clavicle at its midpoint. Introduce a 22-gauge, unsheathed standard 3½-inch spinal needle through the skin wheal with the needle point directed laterally toward the brachial artery. When the needle has just penetrated the skin, attach the exploring electrode to either the stem or the metal hub of the needle with a sterile alligator clip. Set the voltage control of the peripheral nerve stimulator to deliver 6 to 8 V at 1 or 2 impulses per second, and advance the needle at an angle of 45° to the skin. The pectoralis group of muscles will contract and adduct the shoulder. When that occurs, reduce the voltage until the patient is comfortable. When the needle tip is past the muscles, the contraction should stop.

As the needle approaches the fibers of the brachial plexus, the muscles supplied by the musculocutaneous, median, ulnar, and radial nerves will move. Carefully observe the forearm and hand for these movements. When flexion or extension of the elbow, wrist, or digits is observed, the needle point is close to nerve fibers of the brachial plexus. At this point decrease voltage to the lowest level (2 to 4 V) that still allows muscle movement to be observed. Advance the needle again until maximum muscle movements are seen than then begin to diminish. The diminution in muscle movement signals that the needle tip has passed the nerve. Then withdraw the needle slowly until maximum muscle movements are again observed at the lowest voltage. Hold the needle in that position for the injection. It is preferable to use extension tubing so that the needle is not displaced when the syringe is attached.

After negative aspiration for blood, inject 2 ml of local anesthetic solution. If the needle is correctly located, within 0.5 cm of nerve fibers, muscle movements will cease within 30 seconds. If muscle movement continues, the needle tip may have passed the nerve; in this case, withdraw the needle until best muscle movements are seen, and then repeat the test dose.

When the needle is in position on the nerve fibers, inject an adequate volume and concentration of local anesthetic solution.

If another nearby nerve is to be located, withdraw the needle and immediately advance it toward the nerve. A delay may result in the disappearance of helpful muscular movement, since the first injection may block adjacent nerves. If that occurs, repeat the procedure at a higher voltage to locate and block the second nerve.

After successful injection, anesthesia and weakness spread from the shoulder to the wrist. The outer fibers are anesthetized first. The anesthetic takes longer to reach the core bundles, which supply the distal parts, so that hand is anesthetized last.

Confirm the block by clinical examination and by using the peripheral nerve stimulator to confirm that no muscle movements appear at higher voltages.

Contraindications

This technique is not indicated if there is an infection in the skin, chest wall, or axilla.

AXILLARY APPROACH[8]

Anatomy

In the axilla the nerves from the brachial plexus and the axillary artery are enclosed in a fibrous neuromuscular fascial sheath. The median and musculocutaneous nerves are anterior or anterolateral (i.e., above and beyond the artery). The ulnar nerve is medial. The radial nerve is posterolateral, or below and behind the vessel.

Technique

The patient should be supine with the arm abducted 90° at the shoulder joint; the forearm should be placed in the supine position. Some physicians prefer to hyperabduct the arm at the shoulder joint with external rotation and flexion at the elbow joint; this position should be avoided, because

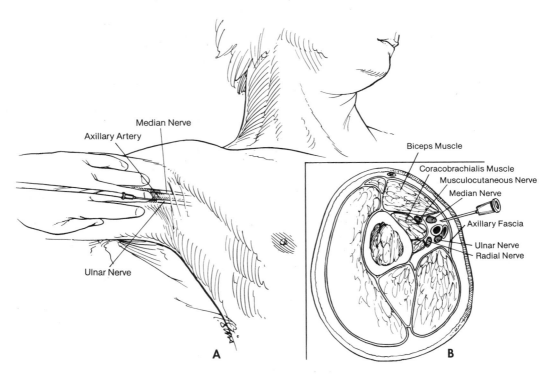

Fig. 19-14 Axillary approach to brachial plexus block. Middle finger of the anesthetist's nondominant hand is on axillary artery. The 25-gauge, 1-inch needle is directed toward axilla. Inset shows needle in neurovascular bundle close to brachial artery. Musculocutaneous nerve in coracobrachialis muscle, outside brachial plexus sheath at this site. (From Raj PP, Pai U, Rawal N: Techniques of regional anesthesia in adults. In Raj PP, editor: *Clinical Practice of Regional Anesthesia.* New York, Churchill Livingstone, 1991.)

abduction beyond 90° will impede the proximal spread of local anesthetic to the origin of the musculocutaneous nerve. However, hyperabduction may be necessary to palpate the artery in a difficult case.

Landmarks

Palpate the axillary artery at the border of the anterior axillary wall and the upper arm, and mark it up to a distance of 2 cm.

Procedure

After the area has been sterilized and draped, the physician stands on the side of the arm to be blocked and palpates the axillary artery, with the palm of one hand lying comfortably over the upper arm. Next, insert the needle just proximal to the palpating finger and within the borders of the finger (the envisioned size of the brachial sheath at that level) (Fig. 19-14).

As the needle is inserted, three different methods can be used to confirm the needle's position in the brachial plexus sheath: (1) when or if the needle penetrates the axillary artery, withdraw the needle until the needle pulsates over the artery and blood can no longer be aspirated; (2) paresthesia can be elicited in the distribution of the ulnar, median, or radial nerve; (3) with the use of a peripheral nerve stimulator, muscular movements of the hand will be seen at the

lowest voltage (2 V) and will be abolished by injection of 2 ml of a local anesthetic solution.

Once the needle position is confirmed, compress the axillary artery, and inject an adequate volume and concentration of anesthetic solution. Compression of the axillary artery during injection facilitates the proximal spread of the anesthetic solution to block the musculocutaneous nerves.

If signs of toxicity are seen after injection, indicating that inadvertent intravascular injection has occurred, it is essential to stop the injection, withdraw the needle, and stabilize the patient. If the axillary block must be done, repeat the procedure when the patient is stable.

After injection remove the needle, massage the area, and bring the arm down to the side while the operator continues to compress the axilla for a few minutes.

Limitations

Although the axillary approach is the approach most commonly used today, it has several limitations. It can be performed only when the arm is abducted to 90° or more. Anesthesia proximal to the elbow progresses slowly and may not reach the mid to upper arm. Furthermore, an axillary approach makes it difficult to block the musculocutaneous and axillary nerves, which supply the shoulder and the lateral arm region. When a tourniquet is used, additional infiltration is necessary to block the intercostobrachial nerve.

Contraindications

Axillary block is contraindicated if the patient has infected glands or the arm cannot be abducted to 90° at the shoulder joint.

COMPLICATIONS OF THE BRACHIAL PLEXUS BLOCK

Since most major nerves occupy a neurovascular bundle, inadvertent intraarterial injection is always a risk. Even an extremely low dose of local anesthetic (e.g., a "test" dose) may precipitate a seizure if injected into an artery under high pressure and if reverse flow occurs.

Although direct IV injection is more likely to occur than intraarterial injection, the volume or total dose of local anesthetic required to produce a seizure is much greater. This provides the opportunity for the physician to observe preseizure symptoms such as dizziness.

Because a toxic response to intravascular injection occurs immediately, resuscitation equipment and drugs (including IV diazepam and barbiturates) must be available before the block is begun. Injections resulting in CNS toxicity are treated the same way.

Hematoma may occur after any nerve block. Although most hematomas are not serious, they may cause complications. The early effect of a hematoma is to compress the neurovascular bundle, rendering ischemic the area distal to the hematoma. The hematoma should be decompressed before irreversible neurologic damage occurs. Calcification of a hematoma is a theoretic and late complication.

NERVE BLOCKS AT THE ELBOW

A single nerve or a combination of nerves can be blocked to reinforce the brachial plexus block or for diagnostic or therapeutic purposes. Nerve blocks at the elbow by themselves can produce anesthesia of the hand and wrist and are indicated for surgery at those sites when a tourniquet is not required or the procedure is short. Neurolytic blocks can be done for cancer patients if pain relief has been provided by previous local anesthetic diagnostic blocks.

Anatomy

The median nerve is situated on the medial side of the brachial artery and on the biceps tendon, underneath the deep fascia. The radial nerve is located between the brachioradialis and brachialis muscles, lateral to the tendon of the biceps. It lies in front of the lateral condyle of the humerus. The ulnar nerve lies in the groove posterior to the medial condyle of the humerus, midway between the olecranon and the medial epicondyle. The musculocutaneous nerve lies superficially lateral to the biceps tendon at the crease of the elbow. At this point it lies superficial to the deep fascia (Fig. 19-15).

Drugs

For each nerve 5 ml of a local anesthetic and 1 to 2 ml of 6% phenol in diatrizoate are required. For a short procedure (up to 1½ hours), 1% to 1.5% lidocaine with or without 1:200,000 epinephrine may be used. For a long procedure (3 to 3½ hours), 0.5% or 0.75% of bupivacaine or 1% etidocaine may be used. For prolonged anesthesia, 6% phenol in diatrizoate is appropriate.

Technique

For a block of the median, radial, or musculocutaneous nerves, the patient lies supine with the arm in slight flexion at the elbow to accentuate the crease. Flexion also makes the biceps tendon and brachioradialis muscle prominent. For a block of the ulnar nerve, the elbow should be flexed a little more than 90°, with the hand angled toward the contralateral shoulder.

Landmarks

For a block of the median nerve, locate the biceps tendon at its insertion by the pulsation of the brachial artery. The point of needle entry is medial to the brachial artery. For a block of the radial nerve, locate a point 1 cm lateral to the biceps tendon medial to the brachioradialis. For a block of the ulnar nerve, locate a point between the medial epicondyle and the olecranon process in the ulnar groove. For a block of the musculocutaneous nerve, locate a point 1 cm lateral to the biceps tendon.

Procedure

After a sterile preparation, insert the 22-gauge needles at each nerve. Paresthesia of the ulnar, median, and radial nerves is obtained. A nerve stimulator can be attached and appropriate muscle contractions identified.

Complications

Possible complications include infection, bruising, and postblock dysthesia. Avoid too many paresthesias. Postblock dysthesia is treated by a stellate ganglion block. It usually subsides in 3 weeks.

WRIST BLOCK

Anatomy

The median nerve is situated medial to the flexor carpi radialis tendon deep in the palmaris longus tendon under the deep fascia at the palmar crease of the wrist. The ulnar nerve is situated lateral to the flexor carpi ulnaris tendon and medial to the ulnar artery under the deep fascia at the palmar crease of the wrist. A superficial branch of the radial nerve is situated as branches in the superficial fascia at the lateral aspect of the distal end of the radius.

Indications

A wrist block is indicated for surgery or to provide analgesia distal to the metacarpophalangeal joint. It is useful for suture of a laceration or fracture of the digits, and for incision of paronychia or abscesses of the digits.

Drugs

For each nerve, 5 ml of a local anesthetic is injected, as follows. For a short procedure (up to 1½ hours), lidocaine is injected with or without 1:200,000 epinephrine. For a long procedure, 0.5% or 0.75% of bupivacaine or etidocaine is injected. For neurolytic procedures, 1 to 2 ml of 6% phenol in diatrizoate is recommended.

Technique

The patient is positioned supine with the hand resting on the table for the block of the median and ulnar nerves. For a block of the radial nerve, the patient's hand should be in a midprone position.

Landmarks

The ulnar nerve is located by identifying the flexor carpi ulnaris tendon, pisiform bone, and ulnar artery. The median nerve is located by identifying the palmaris longus tendon and the flexor carpi radialis tendon with the wrist flexed. The radial nerve transverses the anatomic snuffbox at the lateral aspect of the wrist, bounded by abductor pollicis longus, extensor pollicis brevis, and extensor pollicis longus overlying the styloid process of the radius.

Procedure

After a sterile preparation, insert the 22-gauge needles at each nerve, as shown in Figs. 19-16 and 19-17. Paresthesia of the ulnar, median, and radial nerves is obtained. A nerve stimulator can be attached and appropriate muscle contractions identified.

Complications

Possible complications include infection, bruising, and postblock dysesthesia. Postblock dysesthesia is treated by stellate ganglion block. It usually subsides in 3 weeks.

In addition, because of the close proximity of the synovial sheaths of the space of the hand and forearm, special precautions must be taken to prevent sepsis. Epinephrine should *not* be used.

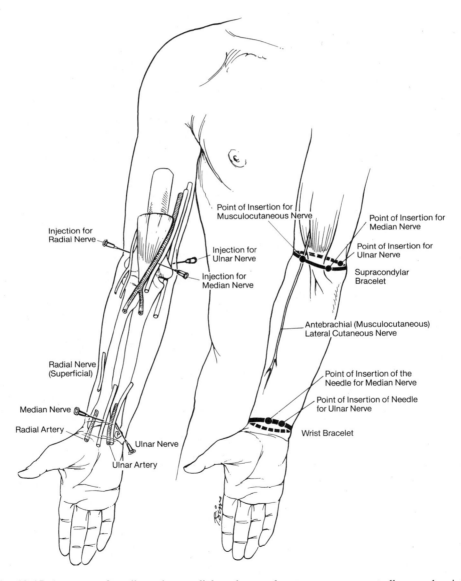

Fig. 19-15 Anatomy of median, ulnar, radial, and musculocutaneous nerves at elbow and wrists. Note landmarks at wrist and elbow for blocks of these nerves. (From Raj PP, Pai U, Rawal N: Techniques of regional anesthesia in adults. In Raj PP, editor: *Clinical Practice of Regional Anesthesia.* New York, Churchill Livingstone, 1991.)

DIGITAL BLOCK
Anatomy

Palmar digital nerves are the branches of the median nerve for the thumb, index, middle, and one half of the ring fingers, and the ulnar nerve supplies the little finger and the medial side of the ring finger. Dorsal digital nerves arise from radial nerve to the lateral supply of the thumb, index, and middle fingers, and the ulnar nerve supplies one half of the ring and little fingers.

Common digital nerves in the palm are located proximal to the metacarpal heads and deep to the palmar aponeurosis.

Indications

A digital block is indicated for minor procedures on the finger and for neurolysis of a digital nerve for pain relief.

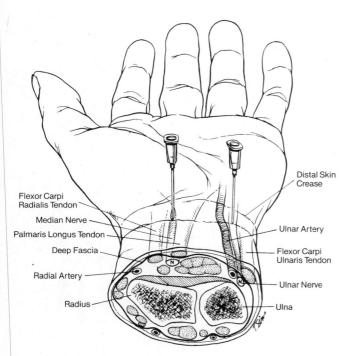

Fig. 19-16 Technique of blocking median and ulnar nerves at wrists. (From Raj PP, Pai U, Rawal N: Techniques of regional anesthesia in adults. In Raj PP, editor: *Clinical Practice of Regional Anesthesia*. New York, Churchill Livingstone, 1991.)

Drugs

The block is achieved with 1% mepicavaine or lidocaine or 6% phenol in diatrizoate.

Technique

The hand and fingers are extended.

Landmarks

Landmarks are the heads of the metacarpal bones and the bases of the proximal phalanx.

Procedure

The patient's fingers are extended and abducted from each other. Raise a skin wheal on the dorsal surface of the inter-metacarpal space of the hand at the level of the head of the metacarpal bone. Introduce a No. 23 1½-inch needle deep into the hand along the axis of the fingers until the resistance of the palmar aponeurosis is felt. Inject local anesthetic, 1 to 2 ml, as the needle is withdrawn. Through the same skin wheal subcutaneous infiltration at the bases of fingers on either side is done to block the dorsal digital branches.

Complications

Injection of a large volume of the local anesthetic is to be avoided because it may cause pressure on the blood vessels and ischemia of the digit. Epinephrine is contraindicated because the vasoconstriction may jeopardize the blood supply to the digit.

SUPRASCAPULAR NERVE BLOCK
Anatomy

The suprascapular nerve is a branch of the level of the trunk of the brachial plexus from the fifth and sixth cervical nerves. After leaving the brachial plexus, it enters the scapular region through the suprascapular notch on the cephalic border of the scapula and then is distributed to the suprascapular and infrascapular muscles. It supplies a large sensory component to the shoulder joint, with a variable cutaneous branch to the cephalic and lateral aspects of the upper extremity just below the deltoid insertion.

Landmarks

Identify the spine of the scapula, and draw a line vertically through the midpoint of the spine and parallel to the vertebral column. Bisect the upper and outer quadrants so formed, and insert a needle at a distance of 2 cm along this

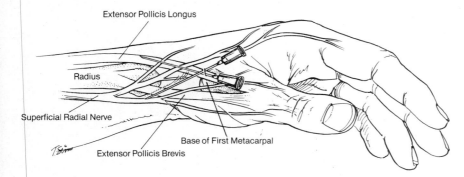

Fig. 19-17 Technique of blocking superficial branches of radial nerve at wrist. (From Raj PP, Pai U, Rawal N: Techniques of regional anesthesia in adults. In Raj PP, editor: *Clinical Practice of Regional Anesthesia*. New York, Churchill Livingstone, 1991.)

line (Fig. 19-18). Insert the needle at a right angle to the skin, and advance it until the dorsal surface of the scapula is located. Then walk the needle along this dorsal surface until the suprascapular notch is identified. If a nerve stimulator is used, contractions of the supraspinatus and infraspinatus muscles will confirm placement. At this location inject 5 ml of local anesthetic. It is not always possible to ascertain any dermal analgesia as a result of this block. The success of a block can be determined if motor-blocking concentrations of drug are used when abduction of the arm will be compromised for the first 15° before the deltoid muscle takes over.

Indications

The suprascapular nerve is blocked diagnostically for pains around the shoulder in an attempt to see if the pain is arising from within the shoulder joint. Therapeutically, repeated blocks can be performed for arthritic shoulder pain, although this is usually not a satisfactory long-term solution.

Difficulties

The main concern with this block is the risk of pneumothorax if the needle passes over the superior border of the scapula and enters the thoracic cavity between the ribs during its initial advancement. Also, if and when the needle is walked into the suprascapular notch, it should not be advanced because pleural puncture with subsequent pneumothorax could occur. The nerve is accompanied by the corresponding suprascapular vessels, and intravascular injection is a risk.

Lower Extremity

Indications

For chronic pain relief or for operations on the lower extremity, the subarachnoid block and the epidural block are still the most common nerve block procedures performed. Although conduction anesthesia has a high success rate and is relatively easy to perform, spinal or epidural procedures may not be indicated in certain groups of patients, including the elderly, debilitated, arthritic, obese, or critically ill, or for those with neurolysis of the nerves. In these patients, branches of the lumbosacral plexus can be blocked. The common branches of the lumbosacral plexus include the sciatic nerve, the femoral nerve, the obturator nerve, and the lateral femoral cutaneous nerves (Fig. 19-19, *A*).

SCIATIC NERVE
Anatomy

The sciatic nerve (L_4-L_5, S_1-S_3), the largest nerve in the body, measures 1.5 to 2 cm in width and 0.3 to 0.9 cm in thickness as it leaves the pelvis. After leaving the pelvis it passes through a tunnel between the greater trochanter and the ischial tuberosity. At this point the greater sciatic nerve passes posterior to the gemelli, obturator internus, and quadriceps femoris and anterior to the gluteus maximus muscles (Fig. 19-19, *B*).

The posterior femoral cutaneous branch (S_1-S_3), which innervates the posterior aspect of the thigh, varies in prox-

imity to the sciatic nerve and may either travel with it or separate from it cephalad. Blood vessels accompanying the sciatic nerve at this point of blocking are the sciatic artery, a branch of the inferior gluteal artery, and the inferior gluteal veins. However, in this region both arteries and veins are relatively small.

Technique

In the posterior approach of Labat,[9] place the patient in the Sims' position. Identify the superior iliac spine and the greater trochanter. Draw a line between the two, and drop a second perpendicular line at its midpoint. The point of entry is 1 to 1½ inches along this line. This point should lie on a line drawn from the sacral diatus to the greater trochanter (Fig. 19-20).

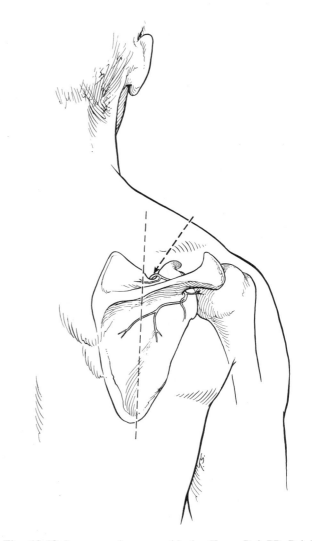

Fig. 19-18 Suprascapular nerve block. (From Raj PP, Pai U, Rawal N: Techniques of regional anesthesia in adults. In Raj PP, editor: *Clinical Practice of Regional Anesthesia*. New York, Churchill Livingstone, 1991.)

Procedure

Posterior approach (Labat). After preparation and infiltration of the skin, insert a 3½-inch, 22-gauge needle perpendicular to the skin at the chosen landmark. After the needle passes through the muscle (piriformis), it contacts the sciatic nerve (2½ inches deep), which at this point is traversing the leg from the greater sciatic notch. Paresthesia is obtained toward the foot, or dorsiflexion or plantar flexion is noted with the nerve stimulator.

Anterior approach (Beck).[10] With the patient supine, draw a line from the anterior superior iliac spine to the public tubercle. It is divided into three parts: draw a parallel line to the above at the level of the greater trochanter; drop

a perpendicular line from the top line to the bottom at the junction of the medial and middle one third; and the point of entry is at the bottom line where the perpendicular line meets the lesser trochanter (Fig. 19-21).

Insert a 6-inch, 22-gauge needle through the landmark perpendicularly until bone is contacted (lesser trochanter). Note the depth of needle entry. Place a marker 1 inch proximally and the needle is slipped past the bone medially until either it touches the sciatic nerve or until it goes 1 inch deeper than the first insertion. Inject local anesthetic in the neurovascular space between the muscles.

Supine sciatic approach (Raj).[11] Place the patient supine. Flex the extremity to be blocked at the hip as far as pos-

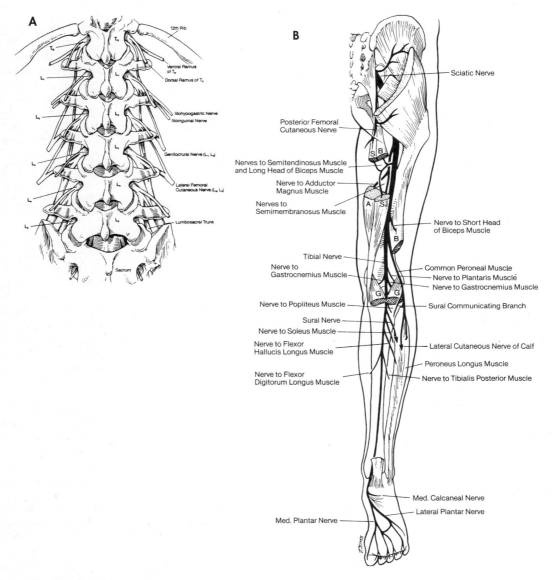

Fig. 19-19 A, Formation of lumbosacral plexus and its branches. The important branches of plexus include sciatic nerve, femoral nerve, obturator nerve, and lateral femoral cutaneous nerves. **B,** Anatomy of lower extremity and course of sciatic nerve and its branches. (From Raj PP, Pai U, Rawal N: Techniques of regional anesthesia in adults. In Raj PP, editor: *Clinical Practice of Regional Anesthesia.* New York, Churchill Livingstone, 1991.)

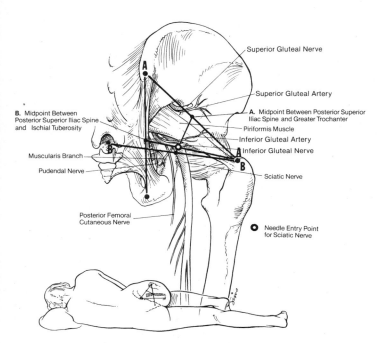

Fig. 19-20 Position for Labat technique of sciatic nerve block. Point of entry of needle can be arrived at in various ways: *A*, by drawing a line between posterior superior iliac spine and greater trochanter and dropping a line from its midpoint 1½ inches sacral coccygeal membrane and greater trochanter: or *B*, by taking a midpoint between posterosuperior iliac spine and ischial tuberosity. Point of entry is where a line drawn from this point horizontally meets line dropped between posterior iliac spine and greater trochanter. (From Raj PP, Pai U, Rawal N: Techniques of regional anesthesia in adults. In Raj PP, editor: *Clinical Practice of Regional Anesthesia.* New York, Churchill Livingstone, 1991.)

sible (90° to 120°) (Fig. 19-22). The extremity may be supported by the use of a Mayo table, an assistant, the patient, or by placing it in the lithotomy position. In this position, the sciatic nerve is stretched tightly in the hollow between the greater trochanter and the ischial tuberosity and the gluteus maximus muscles are thinned, making the sciatic nerve more superficial.

Locate the midpoint of a line drawn between the greater trochanter and the ischial tuberosity. Raise a skin wheal, and inject 1% lidocaine through a 25-gauge, 1.588-cm needle. Use a 22-gauge, 8.89-cm spinal needle attached to a peripheral nerve stimulator as a probing electrode.[12] Insert the needle perpendicular to the skin, and activate the nerve stimulator after the needle has penetrated the skin. Advance the needle slowly until the best plantar flexion or dorsiflexion of the foot is noted. Inject a 2-ml test dose of 2% lidocaine; it should abolish this movement. Deposit an additional 18 to 20 ml of anesthetic solution if the test is positive (i.e., if the movements previously noted disappear).

This supine approach is practical for repeat blocks, moribund patients, and patients with multiple trauma who cannot be positioned otherwise. If the patient has had a hip prosthesis so that the greater trochanter may be absent, probing by the nerve stimulator allows identification of the sciatic nerve without difficulty.

Indications/Contraindications

A sciatic nerve block provides analgesia and anesthesia in the lower extremity in the area of the sciatic nerve distribution. It also provides sympathetic block in the same distribution. It is indicated for surgical procedures of the leg and foot and for diagnostic and therapeutic nerve blocks for acute or chronic pain in the leg and foot. It has been useful for poor healing ulcers because of poor peripheral circulation, for treating traumatic pain, and for providing pain relief for exercises during rehabilitation of limb trauma.

Contraindications are relative and include local infection and recent injury at the site of injection to the nerve.

FEMORAL NERVE[13]
Anatomy

The femoral nerve (L_2, L_3, L_4) arises from the lumbar plexus and runs downward between the psoas major and iliacus muscles, covered by the iliopsoas fascia. The psoas facia separates the nerve from the femoral artery. The femoral nerve lies lateral to the artery and deep to the inguinal ligament. About 1 inch below the inguinal ligament, the nerve divides into muscular and cutaneous branches. Muscular branches supply the muscles of the front of the thigh. The cutaneous branches are the medial and intermediate cutaneous nerves of the thigh, which supply the skin of the front of the thigh, and the saphenous nerve. The saphenous nerve innervates the medial side of the leg up to the middle of the medial border of the foot (Fig. 19-23).

Indications

A femoral nerve block is indicated for superficial surgery on the anterior aspect of the thigh, such as skin grafting, saphenous vein tripping, and saphenous vein harvesting. It is also included as one of the multiple lower extremity blocks used for arthroscopy, knee surgery, amputations, and ankle surgery. For the relief of postoperative knee pain, a catheter can be placed on the femoral nerve for prolonged analgesia and for healing of ischemic ulcers on the medial aspect of the leg.

Technique

The patient is positioned supine with the thigh on the flat surface, slightly abducted from midline (Fig. 19-24).

Landmarks

Landmarks are the anterior superior iliac spine, the pubic symphysis, the pulsation of the femoral artery, and the inguinal ligament. The point of entry is one finger breadth lateral to the femoral artery at the midinguinal point.

Procedure

After local infiltration at the point of entry, place the nondominant hand on the front of the patient's thigh with the middle finger on the femoral artery. Insert the needle on a line with the finger and lateral to the artery (see Fig. 19-24). Direct it cephalad at an angle of 30° until paresthesia of the knee is elicited. If a nerve stimulator is used, elicit patellar movement. Once the position of the

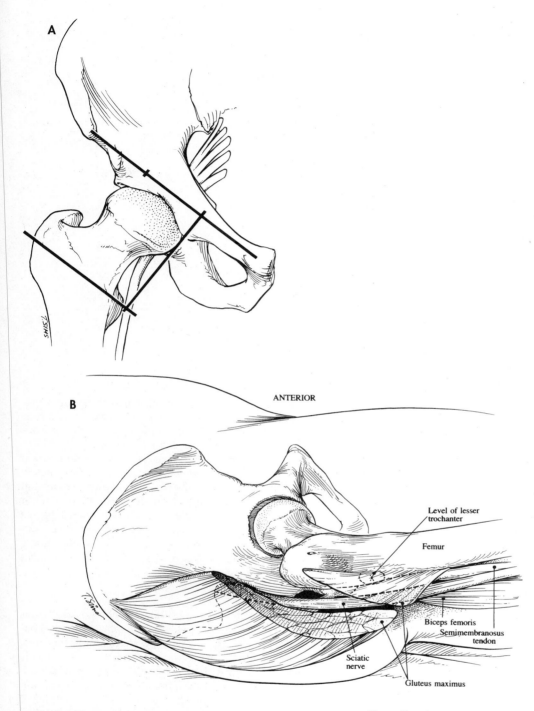

Fig. 19-21 A, Anterior approach to sciatic nerve as described by Beck. **B,** Anatomy of sciatic nerve with patient in supine position as viewed from side. Note course of sciatic nerve behind femur and anterior to gluteus maximus. (From Raj PP, Pai U, Rawal N: Techniques of regional anesthesia in adults. In Raj PP, editor: *Clinical Practice of Regional Anesthesia.* New York, Churchill Livingstone, 1991.)

needle has been confirmed, perform an aspiration test for blood, and inject the calculated volume of the local anesthetic.

A femoral nerve block provides sensory anesthesia of the anteromedial thigh, the medial aspect of the leg, and the proximal foot. There is loss of extension of the knee and some loss of the flexion at the hip joint.

Contraindications

Contraindications include ulceration in the groin, glandular infection, and septicemia.

Complications

Complications include infection, hematoma, femoral neuritis, and prolonged block.

OBTURATOR NERVE
Anatomy

The obturator nerve (L_2, L_3, L_4) is the motor nerve to the abductor muscles of the thigh. It innervates a small segment of the medial side of the thigh in the lower third. It also gives articular branches to the hip and knee joint. The obturator nerves arise from the lumbar plexus in common with

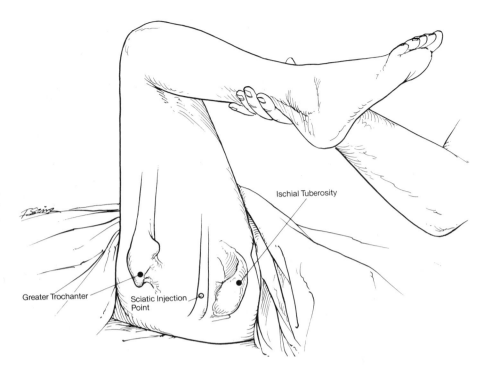

Fig. 19-22 Position of patient and landmark for supine approach to sciatic nerve. (From Raj PP, Pai U, Rawal N: Techniques of regional anesthesia in adults. In Raj PP, editor: *Clinical Practice of Regional Anesthesia.* New York, Churchill Livingstone, 1991.)

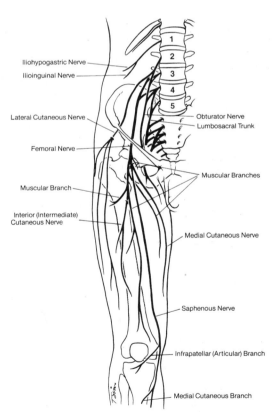

Fig. 19-23 Anatomy of lumbar plexus and its branches. Note especially formation of femoral nerve, obturator nerve, and lateral femoral cutaneous nerve. (From Raj PP, Pai U, Rawal N: Techniques of regional anesthesia in adults. In Raj PP, editor: *Clinical Practice of Regional Anesthesia.* New York, Churchill Livingstone, 1991.)

the femoral nerve and within the substance of the psoas major muscle. The nerve emerges out at the medial border, runs along the lateral pelvic wall, exits through the obturator foramen, and reaches the medial thigh (Fig. 19-25).

The obturator nerve has a variable sensory contribution to the medial part of the thigh, about a handbreadth below the perineum. It can, however, extend down the medial thigh to the level of the knee. Its main distribution is motor to the adductor muscles of the thigh, and it does supply a geniculate branch to the knee joint. Because of its large motor supply, this nerve is readily identifiable when a nerve stimulator is used; contracts in the adductor muscle mass of the thigh are readily seen.

Indications

Along with the femoral and lateral femoral cutaneous nerves, the obturator nerve is blocked for acute pain control intraoperatively and for postoperative pain in this area. The main indication for nonoperative blockade is a spastic condition associated with spinal cord damage in which adductor spasm interferes with rehabilitation or personal toilet and hygiene. Neurolytic blockade of this particular nerve is often indicated, and diagnostic nerve blocks ahead of time can be used to ascertain how much of the persistent adduction is due to muscle tension, as opposed to contracture, which would require surgical tenotomy for relief. Blockade of this nerve is effected with 5 to 10 ml of a local anesthetic or neurolytic agent.

Drugs

For a short-duration block, 1% lidocaine or mepivacaine is used. For a block of longer duration, 0.5% bupivacaine is used. For a neurolytic block, 6% phenol is used.

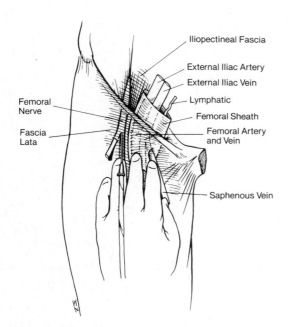

Fig. 19-24 Femoral nerve block technique. Note that femoral nerve is separated from artery by a sheath. (From Raj PP, Pai U, Rawal N: Techniques of regional anesthesia in adults. In Raj PP, editor: *Clinical Practice of Regional Anesthesia.* New York, Churchill Livingstone, 1991.)

Procedure

Place the patient in a supine position with the thigh abducted to make the adductor longus tendon prominent at its attachment to the pubic bone. Stand on the opposite side to be blocked, facing the patient.

Make a skin wheal 1 cm lateral and inferior to the pubic tubercle. Introduce a 22-gauge, 3½ inch needle through the wheal in a direction perpendicular to the skin until the inferior pubic ramus is contacted. Withdraw the needle, and direct it laterally 2.5 cm deeper in a slightly superior and posterior direction. After the needle placement is confirmed by fluoroscopy or by a nerve stimulator situated in the obturator foramen, inject 10 ml of the anesthetic solution. Paresthesia is not usually obtained. An effective block will result in loss of adduction and external rotation of the thigh.

Difficulties

It is often difficult to locate the obturator nerve because of its deep location. Because the block is often performed on individuals with spinal cord injury, spasticity, and contracture, it is not feasible to place the thigh in the optimal laterally rotated position for this block.

Complications

Intravascular injection or hematoma may occur because of the close proximity of the obturator vessels to the nerve.

LATERAL FEMORAL CUTANEOUS NERVE BLOCK
Anatomy

The lateral femoral cutaneous nerve arises from L_2 and L_3 and lies on the iliac muscle at the lateral border of the psoas major muscle. After running on the medial side of anterosuperior iliac spine, it pierces the fascia lata 1½ to 2 inches below the inguinal ligament to innervate the lateral side of the skin of the thigh.

Indications

The lateral femoral cutaneous block is indicated primarily for the control of acute pain in operative procedures involving this anatomic distribution. It has been used for the diagnosis and treatment of chronic pain states. The chronic pain state most often associated with this particular nerve distribution is *meralgia paresthetica,* a neuritic type of pain in the distribution of this nerve that is usually due to ongoing trauma to the nerve such as that caused by a heavy belt riding low on the hip. A temporary nerve block can be diagnostic in this condition. The permanent solution is usually correction of the precipitating cause.

Technique

Position the patient supine with the thigh in a neutral position on the bed (Fig. 19-26, *A*).

Landmarks

Landmarks are the anterosuperior iliac spine and the inguinal ligament.

Procedure

A skin wheal is made at a point 2 to 3 cm below and medial to the anterosuperior iliac spine with a No. 27 needle. Introduce a No. 22 1½-inch needle attached to a 10-ml syringe upward and laterally through the skin wheal and toward the iliac crest just posterior to the anterosuperior iliac spine until it touches the inner side of the shelving iliac crest (Fig. 19-26, *B*). Inject local anesthetic, 5 ml, as the needle is withdrawn. Repeat the process at another angle, and inject another 5 ml of local anesthetic.

The lateral femoral cutaneous nerve can also be blocked in conjunction with the femoral nerve component of the lumbar plexus by injecting a large volume in a cephalad direction when doing a femoral nerve block.

Difficulties

Because this nerve is strictly a sensory nerve, blockade is not associated with any motor weakness and is well tolerated, although the permanent numbness that can follow both trauma and/or permanent blocks to the nerve can become a source of chronic pain.

Because this nerve is not in immediate relation to any important structures at the injection site described above, there are no significant complications.

TIBIAL NERVE BLOCK AT THE KNEE
Anatomy

The tibial nerve is the medial of the two terminal branches of the sciatic nerve that are given off in the upper part of the popliteal fossa. It descends vertically in the middle of the popliteal fossa from the upper angle to the lower angle. The popliteal artery is related medially to the nerve in the upper part, laterally to the nerve in the lower part, and deep to the nerve in the middle. Pulsation of the popliteal artery

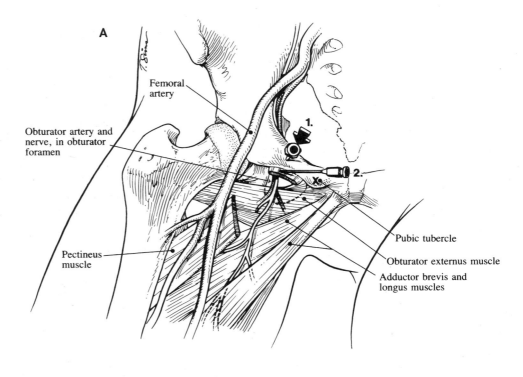

Fig. 19-25 Anatomy of technique of obturator nerve block. Obturator nerve is shown to exit from obturator foramen. *1* shows needle position on superior ramus. *2* shows needle position in obturator foramen. (From Raj PP, Pai U: Somatc nerve blocks C. In Raj PP, editor: *Practical Management of Pain.* ed 2, St Louis, Mosby, 1992.)

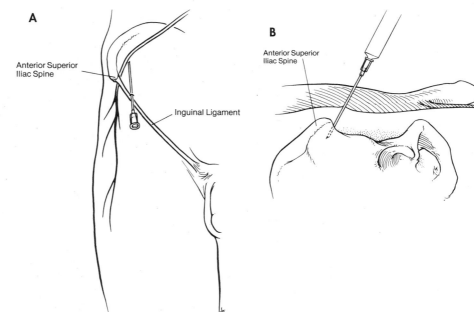

Fig. 19-26 A, Approach to lateral femoral cutaneous nerve block. **B,** Direction of needle in lateral view. (From Raj PP, Pai U: Somatc nerve blocks C. In Raj PP, editor: *Practical Management of Pain.* ed 2, St Louis, Mosby, 1992.)

at the joint line of the knee is a good landmark for the nerve. The tibial nerve descends down the back of the leg to innervate the muscles of the posterior compartment of the leg. At the medial side of the ankle it divides into medial and lateral plantar branches, which traverse toward the respective sides of the foot. The tibial nerve gives off the medial calcanean branches before dividing into plantar nerves at the ankle (Fig. 19-27).

Indications

This block can be useful for pain in the ankle and the foot, during surgery or postoperatively. It may also be used to relieve the severe pain of intractable reflex sympathetic dystrophy, decubitus ulcers of the heel, and trauma.

Technique

The patient may be positioned either prone, with the knee extended, or laterally, with the leg extended.

Landmarks

Landmarks are the pulsation of the popliteal artery at the bend of the knee and the vertical line in the middle of the popliteal fossa.

Procedure

Raise a skin wheal in the middle of the popliteal fossa over the midline, and insert the needle vertically toward the popliteal artery. Paresthesia of the leg and the sole of the foot is sought. A nerve stimulator can be used to objectively confirm placement of the needle on the nerve because there will be visible plantar flexion on the foot. Inject analgesic solution, 5 to 10 ml, at the appropriate site.

Complications

Vascular injection is possible because of proximity of the popliteal artery to the tibial nerve.

ANKLE BLOCK
Indications

An ankle block is indicated for surgery or relief of pain in the sole or the dorsum of the foot.

Anatomy

An ankle bock involves five nerves that innervate below the ankle. These are described below.

1. *Tibial nerve.* Continuing from the leg, the tibial nerve runs about the midpoint between the medial malleolus and calcaneus muscles on the medial side of the ankle under the flexor retinaculum. It lies posterior to the pulsation of the posterior tibial artery. It innervates the skin and the muscle of the plantar aspect of the foot.
2. *Deep peroneal nerve.* As a continuation of the nerve in the front of the leg, the deep peroneal nerve lies deep to the extensor retinaculum with the anterior tibial artery on the anterior surface of the distal end of the tibia. It lies lateral to the tendon of the extensor hallucis longus. It innervates the extensor hallucis muscle, some neighboring joints and skin, and the adjacent sides of the great toe and second toe (Fig. 19-28).
3. *Sural nerve.* The sural nerve is formed at the back of the calf muscles in the midline by contributions from the tibial and common peroneal nerves. It runs on the lateral aspect of the ankle midway between the lateral malleolus and calcaneus muscles toward the lateral side of the little toe.
4. *Saphenous nerve.* The only branch of the femoral nerve below the knee, the saphenous nerve runs in the superficial fascia in front of the medial malleolus with a great saphenous vein. It innervates up to the middle of the medial side of the foot.
5. *Superficial peroneal nerve.* The superficial peroneal nerve pierces the deep fascia in the lower third of the lateral aspect of the leg, then lies in the superficial fascia to divide into branches to supply the dorsum of the foot and the toes not innervated by the sural and deep peroneal nerves.

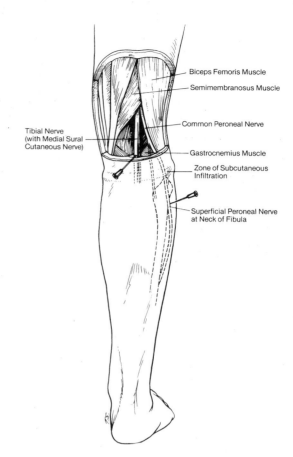

Fig. 19-27 Course of tibial and common peroneal nerves at knee and technique of blocking them. (From Raj PP, Pai U, Rawal N: Techniques of regional anesthesia in adults. In Raj PP, editor: *Clinical Practice of Regional Anesthesia.* New York, Churchill Livingstone, 1991.)

Drugs

One of the local anesthetics listed below is injected, 5 ml per nerve. For a procedure of short duration, 1% to 1.5% lidocaine with or without 1:20,000 epinephrine is injected. For a procedure of longer duration (3 to 3½ hours), 0.5% to 0.75% bupivacaine or 1% etidocaine is injected.

Technique

The foot is placed on the bed with the knee flexed.

Landmarks

Landmarks are the medial malleolus, the lateral malleolus, the posterior tubercle of the calcaneus, the tendocalcaneous, the pulsation of the tibial artery, and the extensor hallucis longus tendon.

Procedure

1. *Tibial block.* After a skin wheal has been made with a 27-gauge needle midway between the medial malleolus and calcaneus and posterior to the pulsation of the posterior tibial artery, introduce a 23-gauge needle to elicit paresthesia in the foot (or twitching of sole of

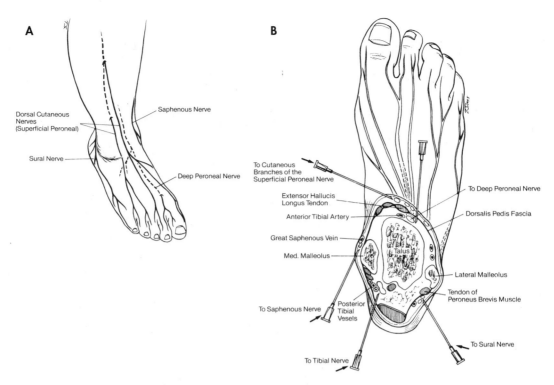

Fig. 19-28 A, Anatomy of tibial and peroneal nerves and their branches at ankle. **B,** Sites of block. (From Raj PP, Pai U, Rawal N: Techniques of regional anesthesia in adults. In Raj PP, editor: *Clinical Practice of Regional Anesthesia.* New York, Churchill Livingstone, 1991.)

foot, with the nerve stimulator). Inject then 5 to 6 ml of local anesthetic.

2. *Deep peroneal nerve.* Raise a skin wheal on the front of the ankle lateral to extensor hallucis longus tendon at about the anterior tibial artery, and insert a 23-gauge needle to hit the bone. Then inject 5 ml of local anesthetic.

3. *Sural nerve.* After a skin wheal is raised, inject 5 ml of local anesthetic deep to the point midway between the lateral malleolus and the calcaneus.

4. *Saphenous nerve.* Inject 5 ml of local anesthetic around the great saphenous vein in front of the medial malleolus.

5. *Superficial peroneal nerve.* Raise a skin wheal on the lower third of the leg just lateral to the anterior border of the tibia at the upper part of the lateral malleolus. Infiltrate the subcutaneous tissue just superficial to the deep fascia. The depth of needle insertion depends on the amount of subcutaneous fat. It is done as a field block over an area 2 to 3 inches wide and lateral to the anterior border of the tibia to block all of the branches of the superficial peroneal nerve as they go on to the dorsum of the foot.

Complications

Complications include neuropathy, prolonged block, infection, and hematoma.

COMMON PERONEAL NERVE BLOCK
Anatomy

The common peroneal nerve usually arises about the upper part of the back of the thigh as one of the two terminal branches of the sciatic nerve. After descending obliquely downward and laterally across the lateral angle of popliteal fossa, it runs toward the lateral aspect of the neck of the fibula to divide into the superficial and deep peroneal nerves.

The superficial peroneal nerve traverses toward the lateral compartment of the leg to innervate the perineal muscles and then becomes cutaneous at the lower third of the leg. The deep peroneal nerve goes toward the anterior compartment of the leg and finally ends at the dorsum of the foot (see Fig. 19-27).

Indications

The common peroneal nerve block is performed in conjunction with tibial nerve and saphenous nerve blocks at the knee for surgery below the knee not involving the use of a tourniquet.

Technique

The common peroneal nerve block may be performed with the patient in one of two positions: supine, with the thigh flexed at the hip joint, the leg flexed at the knee, and the foot flat on the bed; or in a lateral position, with the down leg extended and the upper leg flexed at the knee.

Landmark

The landmark is the head of the fibula below the lateral condyle of the tibia in the posterior part. The neck of the fibula lies below the head, where the common peroneal nerve can be felt on deep pressure.

Procedure

After a skin wheal has been made at a point in the region of the anterior part of the neck of the fibula (below the head), insert a 23-gauge needle posteriorly and medially to touch the bone. Paresthesia can be elicited, or nerve stimulation will cause twitching of the leg muscles and dorsiflexion of the ankle. Inject 5 to 6 ml of local anesthetic.

Complication

Neuritis of the common peroneal nerve can be produced if the anesthetic is injected into the nerve because the nerve lies directly against the neck of the fibula.

PUDENDAL NERVE BLOCK
Anatomy

The pudendal nerve (S_2, S_3, S_4) arises from the sacral plexus. After crossing the ischial spine and the sacrospinous ligament, it enters the lesser sciatic foramen and runs on the medial side of the ischium with the pudendal vessels in the pudendal canal (Alcock's canal). At the anterior end of the canal it sends branches to the perineal region. The inferior hemorrhoidal nerve innervates the anal region, and other anterior branches innervate the urogenital region.

Indications

A pudendal nerve block is indicated for obstetric vaginal procedures (e.g., vaginal delivery and forceps delivery) and for somatic perineal pain.

Equipment

Iowa trumpet
12- to 14-cm, 20-gauge needle

Technique

Place the patient in the lithotomy position.

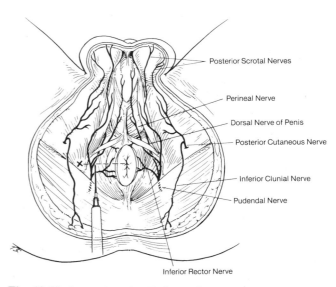

Fig. 19-29 Anatomy and technique of pudendal block (perineal route). (From Raj PP, Pai U, Rawal N: Techniques of regional anesthesia in adults. In Raj PP, editor: *Clinical Practice of Regional Anesthesia.* New York, Churchill Livingstone, 1991.)

Landmarks

Landmarks are the ischial spine, sacrospinous ligament, and the ischial tuberosity.

Procedure

In the transvaginal approach, guide the needle within the Iowa trumpet along the operator's index and middle finger; the needle progresses transvaginally toward the ischial spine after piercing the sacrospinous ligament. Inject local anesthetic in the pudendal canal.

In the perineal route approach raise a skin wheal 2 to 3 cm posteromedially to the ischial tuberosity. Introduce a 12- to 15-cm, 22-gauge needle through the skin wheal in a posterior and lateral direction (Fig. 19-29); it is guided by the operator's finger in the rectum or vagina toward the ischial spine. After the needle pierces the sacrospinous ligament, inject 10 to 15 ml of local anesthetic around the ligament.

B. LESS COMMON SOMATIC NERVE BLOCKS

Less common nerve blocks in the management of pain can be categorized as those which are usually performed rarely for specific pain syndromes by a physician who is especially trained in performing such procedures. These blocks are rarely performed because either the pain syndromes affecting the region of those nerves are not common (such as trigeminal neuralgia) or the nerve to be blocked is located close to other vital structures which when blocked can cause significant side effects (e.g., vagus and glossopharyngeal nerve blocks). Three less common nerve blocks have been chosen that are essential for a pain practitioner to perform in his or her clinical practice. These blocks are: (1) lumbar plexus block, (2) psoas compartment block, and (3) trans-

sacral nerve block. Other less common nerve blocks such as trigeminal ganglion block, superior and inferior hypogastric blocks, and interpleural block are described elsewhere in this book.

1. LUMBAR PLEXUS BLOCK

Unlike those of the upper arm, nerves of the lower extremity travel widely separate courses from their origins, making it impossible to block them all with a single approach.

History

Winnie described the lumbar plexus block in the early 1980s.[14]

Indications

Lumbar plexus block is useful for painful conditions of the lower extremity. If conduction anesthesia or peripheral inguinal paravascular or sciatic nerve blocks are contraindicated, the combined lumbosacral plexus block may be an alternative.

Anatomy

The lumbar plexus is formed by the union of ventral primary of upper four lumbar nerves. The ventral primary division of first lumbar nerve splits into an upper and lower branch. The upper branch joins a branch of the twelfth thoracic nerve to form the common trunk of the iliohypogastric and ilioinguinal nerves, whereas the lower branch joins the branch of the second lumbar nerve to form the genitofemoral nerve. The ventral primary division also splits into an upper and lower branch. The lower branch gives rise to femoral, lateral femoral cutaneous, and obturator nerves. The ventral division of the second, third, and fourth lumbar nerves join to form the obturator nerve. The larger branches of the dorsal divisions of the second, third, and fourth lumbar nerves join to femoral nerve, and smaller branches of the dorsal, second, third, and fourth lumbar nerves form the lateral femoral cutaneous nerve. The lumbar plexus is formed by the anterior primary rami of the second, third, and fourth lumbar nerves as they emerge from the intervertebral foramina ventral to the quadratus lumborum and dorsal to the psoas major muscles. As the three major constituent branches of the lumbar plexus, femoral, obturator, and lateral femoral cutaneous nerves descend to the leg, they are sandwiched between these muscles and their fasciae. The lumbar nerves are approachable at this site. It is usually combined with a sacral plexus block to cover the whole lower extremity. The sacral plexus is formed by the lumbosacral trunk from the fourth and fifth lumbar nerves and by the first, second, and third sacral nerves.

Technique

Place the patient in the lateral position, lying on the side opposite the one to be blocked. Draw a line connecting the superior borders of both iliac crests. This indicates the L_3-L_4 or L_4-L_5 interspace. Draw a second line through the posterior superior iliac spine, parallel to the spinous processes. The point where the intercristal line crosses the paraspinous line is the needle entry site. Insert a 22-gauge 9-cm needle perpendicular to the skin but in a slightly medial direction. When the transverse process is encountered, redirect the needle slightly more caudad, and advance it until paraesthesia is obtained. This usually occurs at a depth of 5 to 6 cm beneath the skin. Immobilize the needle at that point. After a test dose, inject 30 to 40 ml of local anesthetic solution.

Confirmation of block

A block of the lower extremity is achieved when there is anesthesia in the distribution of the femoral, obturator, and lateral femoral cutaneous nerves.

Practical aspects

A large volume is needed to cover both the lumbar and sacral plexuses. The sciatic nerve is usually inadequately blocked. A peripheral nerve stimulator is helpful in the objective evaluation of nerve stimulation and hence in the placement of the needle tip on the nerve.

Complications

A block of the lumbar and sacral plexuses can result in complications such as subarachnoid or epidural block, intravascular injection causing CNS and CVS toxicity, lumbar sympathetic block, and neuropathy.

2. PSOAS COMPARTMENT BLOCK

History

Chayen et al. described the psoas compartment block in 1976.[15]

Indications

The psoas compartment block provides adequate analgesia for surgery of the hip and the anterolateral thigh. When combined with a sciatic nerve block, analgesia of the whole leg is achieved. The combined approach is a useful alternative to conduction blocks.

Anatomy

See discussion of anatomy for lumbar plexus block in the previous section.

Technique

The patient is placed on his or her side with the hips flexed and the side to be operated on facing upward. The fourth lumbar spine is identified by the intercristal line. Mark the site of injection 2 cm cephalad and 5 cm lateral to this point. After a sterile prep and infiltration, insert a 20-gauge, 15-cm needle perpendicular to the skin, and advance it until it contacts the transverse process of L_5. Then redirect the needle slightly cephalad, and advance it 1 to 2 cm deeper. Attach a glass syringe filled with 20 ml air to the needle. With light tapping on the plunger, advance the needle until resistance to the tapping disappears. The needle passes through the quadratus lumborum muscle into the psoas compartment at this point, usually at a depth of 12 cm. After aspiration to test for blood, CSF, or air, inject 20 ml of air to dilute the psoas compartment. This is followed by 30 ml of anesthetic solution. For a combined psoas-sciatic block, use a volume of 25 ml for the psoas compartment block and 15 ml for sciatic nerve block.

Alternative techniques

The psoas compartment can also be reached by the lateral technique of Reid described for lumbar sympathetic block. When the needle touches the side of the vertebral body, the operator retracts the needle by 2 to 4 mm instead of pushing it forward to slip it off of the body. Testing for blood, air, or CSF should then be carried out, and if negative, the same procedure as explained in the original description of the technique by Chayen et al. should be followed from this point.

Confirmation of block

Anesthesia of the distribution of the lumbar plexus is a sign of successful block.

Practical aspects

More accurate placement of the needle can be achieved with a nerve stimulator. When the needle tip is on the femoral nerve, there will be contractions of the quadriceps femoris muscle with every stimulation.

Complications

Complications possible with the psoas compartment block are similar to those for the lumbar somatic nerve root or combined lumbosacral plexus blocks.

3. TRANSSACRAL NERVE BLOCK
History

Transsacral block was first performed by Pauchet and Läwen in 1909.[16]

Indications

The transsacral block is indicated for diagnostic, prognostic, or therapeutic purposes in pain syndromes of the pelvis and perineum, especially those caused by malignancy. Hypertonic bladder in paraplegics can be treated with a bilateral block of S_2-S_3.

Anatomy

The five pairs of sacral and one pair of coccygeal nerves arise at the level of T_{12} and L_1, course downward within the cauda equina, and, after reaching the sacral canal, exit at their respective intervertebral foramina. At that point they immediately divide into anterior and posterior primary divisions.

The posterior primary divisions of the upper four sacral nerves pass posteriorly through the posterior sacral foramina, and that of the fifth sacral and the coccygeal nerves emerge through the sacral hiatus. The upper three posterior divisions then divide into medial branches, which supply the multifidi muscles, and into lateral branches, which form the posterior sacral plexus supplying the skin on the medial part of the gluteus maximus. The posterior primary divisions of the lower two sacral nerves and that of the coccygeal nerve unite to form the posterior anococcygeal nerve, which supplies the skin over the coccyx.

The anterior primary divisions of the upper four sacral nerves pass anteriorly into the pelvis through the anterior sacral foramina; that of the fifth emerges from the sacral hiatus and passes anteriorly. The anterior division of the coccygeal nerve also passes anteriorly below the rudimentary transverse process of Col. The anterior primary divisions then take part in the formation of the sacral plexus.

Technique

The patient is in a prone position, usually with a pillow under the pelvis. Locate the posterior superior iliac spine, the most posteromedial point of the iliac crest. Then identify the sacral cornua. These landmarks are situated at the level of the second and fifth sacral foramina respectively. After a sterile prep, identify the above landmarks. Raise a skin wheal 1 cm medial and inferior to the posterior superior iliac spine. This overlies the second sacral foramen. Raise a second skin wheal 1 cm medial and inferior to the sacral cornua, which overlies the fifth sacral foramen. The distance between the two wheals is then divided into three equal parts by raising two intermediate wheals overlying the third and fourth sacral foramina. Then locate the first foramen by raising a wheal 2 cm superior to the second sacral foramen. All five should form a straight line parallel to the midline.

For injections involving the first and second sacral foramen, 8-cm, 22-gauge needles are used, whereas 5-cm, 22-gauge needles are used for the other sacral foramina. At each of the five foramina, introduce a needle perpendicularly with a slight medial and inferior direction. After the posterior surface of the sacrum is contacted, mark each needle by measuring off a depth of 1.5 cm for the first sacral nerve, 1 cm for the second sacral nerve, and 0.5 cm for the remaining nerves from the skin at each respective point. Then withdraw the needle slightly, and reinsert it with a controlled fanwise movement until it advances to the measured depth. Paresthesia can be elicited at that point.

If the needles have been properly placed, they will be in a straight line. After negative aspiration for blood, CSF, or a dose of air, 5 to 10 ml of local anesthetic for the first sacral nerve and 5 ml for the other nerves is injected at each site. For neurolytic block, inject 1 to 3 ml at each sacral foramen. Fluoroscopy may be employed to locate the foramina by taking anteroposterior and lateral views with the needles in place.

Complications

Possible complications are intravascular injection, subarachnoid or epidural injection, or perforation of the pelvic viscera.

REFERENCES

1. Reiestad F, Strömskag KE: Interpleural catheter in the management of postoperative pain. *Reg Anesth* 11:89-91, 1986.
2. Rocco A, Reiestad F: Intrapleural administration of local anesthetics for pain relief in patients with multiple rib fractures. *Reg Anesth* 12:10-14, 1987.
3. Gomez MN et al: Intrapleural bupivacaine for intraoperative analgesia—A dangerous technique? *Anesth Analg* 67:S78, 1988.
4. Winnie AP: Interscalene brachial plexus block. *Anesth Analg* 49;455-466, 1970.
5. Kulenkampff D: Anesthesia of the brachial plexus. *Zentralbl Chir* 38:1337-1350, 1911.
6. Winnie AP, Collins VJ: The subclavian perivascular technique of brachial plexus anesthesia. *Anesthesiology* 25:353-363, 1964.
7. Raj PP et al: Infraclavicular brachial plexus block: A new approach. *Anesth Analg* 52:897-904, 1973.
8. DeJong RH: Axillary block of the brachial plexus. *Anesthesiology* 22:215-225, 1961.
9. Labat G: *Regional Anesthesia*. Philadelphia, WB Saunders, 1930.
10. Beck GP: Anterior approach to sciatic nerve block. *Anesthesiology* 24:222-224, 1963.
11. Raj PP et al: New single position supine approach to sciatic femoral nerve block. *Anesth Analg* 54:489, 1975.
12. Raj PP, Rosenblatt R, Montgomery SJ: Use of the nerve stimulator for peripheral blocks. *Reg Anesth* 5:19, 1980.
13. Winnie AP, Ramamurthy S, Durrani Z: The inguinal paravascular technic of lumbar plexus anesthesia: The "3-in-1 block." *Anesth Analg* 52:989-996, 1973.
14. Winnie AP: Plexus anesthesia: upper and lower extremity surgery. Presentation at Regional Anesthesia update, Boston, Mass, October 1983.
15. Chayen D, Nathen H, Chayen M: The psoas compartment block. *Anesthesiology* 45:95, 1976.
16. Blocks of the trunk and perineum. In Raj PP, Nolte H, Stanton-Hicks M, editors: *Illustrated Manual of Regional Anesthesia*. Heidelberg, Germany, Springer-Verlag, 1988.

QUESTIONS: PERIPHERAL NERVE BLOCKS

1. The 12 pairs of thoracic nerve roots can be blocked:
   A. As they emerge from thoracic intervertebral foramina
   B. In the thoracic epidural space as the anterior and posterior nerve roots unite
   C. After the anterior primary rami of the thoracic nerve roots have been given off
   D. At the level of thoracic sympathetic ganglion
2. The intercostal nerve block is commonly done at all of the following EXCEPT:
   A. At the angle of the rib posteriorly
   B. At the posterior axillary line
   C. At the midaxillary line
   D. At the head of the rib posteriorly
3. A successful brachial plexus by the interscalene approach will provide analgesia of all of the following EXCEPT:
   A. Shoulder
   B. Inner aspect of the upper arm and elbow
   C. Forearm
   D. Hand
4. The landmark for supraclavicular approach to brachial plexus block are all of the following EXCEPT:
   A. Midpoint of the clavicle
   B. Point of entry 1 cm superior to midpoint of clavicle
   C. Lateral border of the anterior scalene muscle
   D. Midway between sternal and clavicular head of the sternomastoid

5. The following is true about the lumbar plexus:
   A. Formed by the union of anterior primary divisions of L_1-L_4 nerve roots
   B. Does not join the T_{12} to form a common trunk of iliohypogastric and ilioinguinal nerves
   C. Formed by the union of both anterior primary divisions of L_1-L_4 nerve roots
   D. Formed by the union of posterior division of L_1-L_4 nerve roots

ANSWERS

1. A
2. D
3. B
4. D
5. A

20   Autonomic Nerve Blocks

P. Prithvi Raj, Richard L. Rauck, and Gabor B. Racz

A. Sphenopalatine Ganglion Block

Indications

Greenfield Sluder first described the syndrome known as lower half headache, or sphenopalatine neuralgia, in 1909. The syndrome includes unilateral pain at the root of the nose spreading to the maxilla mastoid and occiput, with possible extension to the shoulder and even down to the fingertips. Associated features may include salivation, lacrimation, and rhinorrhea. The syndrome overlaps other pain syndromes of vasospastic cause, including cluster headache and migraine variants.

Comments

The claims for therapeutic effectiveness of sphenopalatine ganglion block have ranged from headaches, facial pain, neck pain, tennis elbow, sciatica, etc. The more recent trend is to use the procedure in frontal headaches and cluster headaches and first and second division mediated pains of the trigeminal nerve. The original application of topical local anesthetics to the posterior nasal pharynx just behind the middle turbinate has now been supplemented by the development of radiofrequency lesioning of the sphenopalatine ganglion.

Anatomy

The sphenopalatine ganglion, also called the pterygopalatine and nasal or Meckel's ganglion, is one of four autonomic ganglia inside the head. The sphenopalatine ganglion is located posterior to the middle turbinate and is 1 to 9 mm deep to the lateral nasal mucosa. Because of the close proximity, topical anesthetic readily diffuses through the mucosa if applied locally. The ganglion is a 5- to 7-mm triangular structure and is a large collection of cells that communicates with the first and second division of the trigeminal nerve, the facial nerve, and the carotid plexus, through which there is a direct communication with the cervical sympathetic ganglion chain. Thus there are sympathetic, parasympathetic (via the superficial petrosal nerve), and somatic connections through the cervical spinal cord. The sphenopalatine ganglion, by its anatomic location, is interposed in the sympathetic reflex arc between the spinal cord and the head.

Techniques

Technique one: topical application of cocaine or local anesthetic. Dip a 3½-inch cotton tipped applicator in an-

esthetic solution. Pass the applicator parallel to the zygomatic arch that corresponds to the middle turbinate to the back of the nasal pharynx, and gently push the applicator laterally as the ganglion is just posterior to the middle turbinate and beneath the lateral nasal mucosa. Apply a second applicator similarly just slightly posterior and superior to the first one. Evidence of successfully reaching the sphenopalatine ganglion by the local anesthetic solution is ipsilateral tearing. The sphenopalatine communicates with the lacrimal glands. Leave the applicators in place for 30 to 45 minutes, then evaluate the patient for effectiveness of therapy. Patients often mention numbness in the back of the throat, a bitter taste that may also be associated with lightheadedness that resolves within 30 minutes of the treatment. Our self-imposed limit is to repeat the procedure but, if and when the pain returns, not to exceed 4 to 5 nerve blocks. If the duration of pain relief is sustained, the block may not have to be repeated. On the other hand, if there is no resolution of the problem after the 4 to 5 blocks, use a training mirror and the culture sticks to instruct the patient on self-application of 2% viscous lidocaine. If the effectiveness that the patient desires is not achieved yet there was clear evidence of interrupting the pain with the procedure, proceed to radiofrequency thermocoagulation (RFTC) after an initial 1-ml block of the sphenopalatine ganglion while directly aiming for the ganglion.

Technique two: local anesthetic block of sphenopalatine ganglion. Place the patient in the supine position with the head resting on a special head piece on the procedure table. Direct the C-arm fluoroscopy from the head of the table with the patient's head inside the C of the fluoroscopy arm. The first view is a lateral view, visualizing the cervical spine and the overlying mandible. Gently rotate the head so that both mandible rami are superimposed. Move the unit toward the head when the pterygopalatine fossa is visualized. Insertion of the needle is under the zygoma and anterior to the mandible. The needle direction is medial and cephalad slightly posteriorly. Visualize the course of the needle on the C-arm as it enters the pterygopalatine fossa. There may be paresthesia elicited, usually to the teeth, from contact with the maxillary nerve. Then rotate the fluoroscopy to give anteroposterior visualization so that the needle tip is seen just beneath the lateral nasal mucosa. If the needle is advanced medially, it will enter the nasal cavity as evidenced by aspirating air. Stimulate the insulated needle, and if the needle is over the sphenopalatine ganglion, a tingling sensation or buzzing sensation is felt just behind the nose in the midline. If stimulation is felt to the hard palate, then the needle is beneath the sphenopalatine ganglion and is stimulating the palatine branch that originates from the ganglion. If the stimulation elicits sensation in the posterior upper teeth, then the needle is anterior or lateral to the ganglion. Make appropriate adjustments in order to get stimulation and tingling behind the nose. At this point 1 ml of local anesthetic with or without steroids can be administered to evaluate the effectiveness of distractive procedures that may be carried out at a later date.

Technique three: radiofrequency thermocoagulation of sphenopalatine ganglion. Again, place the patient in the supine position on the table with the head extended. Position the C-arm exactly as described for the block. The target for visualization and needle placement for the sphenopalatine ganglion is a dimple in the pterygopalatine fossa that usually lies near the upper end of the pterygopalatine fossa and plate. Once the pterygopalatine fossa is identified, gently rotate the head from left to right to bring into view the two pterygopalatine plates being superimposed so that the ipsilateral pterygopalatine fossa can be visualized. The double lines should become a single line when the head is rotated just appropriately. The needle that is used is a 10-cm SMK (Radionics needle) with a 5-mm uninsulated tip that is placed just in front of the mandible beneath the zygomatic arch, and it passes posteromedially and cephalad until it just enters the pterygopalatine fossa. This corresponds to the small depression in the bony structure of the pterygopalatine plate and fossa. At this point connect the needle to the Radionics or other lesioning unit stimulator on a 1-V scale at 75 pulses per second and 0.25 to 0.5 msec pulse width. Slowly increase the voltage until a buzzing sensation is elicited. It usually occurs at about 0.5 to 0.7 V. If stimulation is in the hard palate, reposition the needle proximally; otherwise the lesioning will be followed by a numbness of the hard palate. Similarly, if stimulation of the teeth occurs, then the needle is close to the maxillary nerve and numbness of the posterior upper molars will result. To assure that the needle tip is sufficiently medial, where the ganglion is located just beneath the mucosa, the C-arm must be rotated in an anteroposterior direction, and the bony structures of the nose show the needle tip to be close to the lateral wall of the nasal pharynx. If the needle tip is not close enough to the lateral nasal wall, then it must be advanced more medially. Anatomic location of the needle is important to proceed with lesioning. After appropriate stimulation inject local anesthetic, (1 ml of any local anesthetic) and follow this with lesioning at 80° C for 70 seconds. The needle, after the lesioning is advanced more medially, may perforate nasal mucosa when the lesioning is repeated. It is common to have bleeding if the mucosa is perforated, which usually is self-limited. Follow and observe the patient to make sure that no bleeding is taking place. If bleeding is present, apply topical cocaine with the application as described earlier. The informed consent should include possible complications, nosebleed, infection, numbness of the hard palate, numbness of the teeth, and possibly no therapeutic effectiveness from the procedure.

Equipment

A radiofrequency lesion generator and a 10-cm insulated (SMK) 22-gauge needle with a 5-mm uninsulated active tip are used. The patient needs to be sedated, have any intravenous line, pulse oximetry, blood pressure, and electrocardiogram monitored.

SUGGESTED READINGS

Amster JL: Sphenopalatine ganglion block for the relief of painful vascular and muscular spasm with special reference to lumbosacral pain. *NY State Journal of Medicine* 48:475-489, 1948.

Byrd H, Byrd W: Sphenopalatine phenomena—Present status of knowledge. *Arch Intern Med* 46:1036-1038, 1930.

Chase WD: Sphenopalatine ganglion treatment of certain nose conditions. *Atlanta Medical Journal* 30:779-780, 1927.

Dock G: Sluder's nasal ganglion syndrome and its relation to internal medicine. *JAMA* 93:750-753, 1929.

Evans TH: Nerve branch at superior orbital fissure connecting sixth cranial with component of sphenopalatine ganglion. *Am J Ophthalmol* 27:645-646, 1944.

Frazier CH: A surgical approach to the sphenopalatine ganglion. *Ann Surg* 74:328-330, 1921.

Gundrum LK: Migraine controlled through the nasal ganglion. *Arch Otolaryngol* 8:564-566, 1928.

Higbee D: Functional and anatomic relations of sphenopalatine ganglion to the autonomic nervous system. *Archives of Otolaryngology* 50:45-58, 1949.

Poe DL: Transantral approach for excision of sphenopalatine ganglion for intractable facial pain. *Archives of Otolaryngology* 51:891-900, 1950.

Pollack HL: Difficulties and complications of sphenopalatine ganglion injections. *Ann Otolaryngology Rhinoplasty and Laryngology* 25:958-966, 1089-1096, 1916.

Ruskin SL: Contributions to the study of the sphenopalatine ganglion. *Laryngoscope* 35:87-108, 1925.

Ruskin SL: Herpes zoster oticus relieved by sphenopalatine ganglion treatment. *Laryngoscope* 35:301-302, 1925.

Ruskin SL: The surgical aspect of the nasal ganglion. *NY State Journal of Medicine* 25:929-932, 1925.

Sluder G: Further clinical observations on the sphenopalatine ganglion (motor, sensory, and gustatory). *Bulletin of the St. Louis Medical Society* 4:64-65, 1910.

Sluder G: The anatomical and clinical relations of the sphenopalatine (Meckel's) ganglion to the nose and its accessory sinuses. *NY Medical Journal* 90:293-298, 1909.

Sluder G: The syndrome of sphenopalatine ganglion neurosis. *Am J Med Sci* 3:868-878, 1910.

Stewart D, Lambert V: Sphenopalatine ganglion. *J Laryngol Otol* 45:753-771, 1930.

B. Stellate Ganglion Block

Anatomy

Cell bodies for preganglionic nerves originate in the anterolateral horn of the spinal cord. Fibers destined for the head and neck originate in the first and second thoracic spinal cord segments, whereas preganglionic nerves to the upper extremity originate at segments T_2-T_8 and occasionally T_9. Preganglionic axons to the head and neck exit with the ventral roots of T_1 and T_2, then travel as white communicating rami before joining the sympathetic chain and passing cephalad to synapse at either the inferior (stellate), middle, or superior cervical ganglion. Postganglionic nerves will either follow the carotid arteries (external or internal) to the head or integrate as the gray communicating rami before joining the cervical plexus or upper cervical nerves to innervate structures of the neck (Fig. 20-1). To achieve suc-

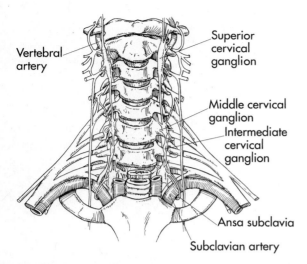

Fig. 20-1 Cervical sympathetic ganglia and stellate ganglion. Note the relationship of structures to the respective ganglia. (From Rauck RL: Sympathetic nerve blocks A. In Raj PP, editor: *Practical Management of Pain,* ed 2. St Louis, Mosby, 1992.)

cessful sympathetic denervation of the head and neck, block the stellate ganglion, since all preganglionic nerves either synapse here or pass through on their way to more cephalad ganglia. Blockade of the middle or superior ganglia misses the contribution of sympathetic fibers traveling from the stellate ganglion to the vertebral plexus and ultimately to the corresponding areas of the cranial vault supplied by the vertebral artery.[1]

Sympathetic nerves to the upper extremity exit T_2-T_8 through ventral spinal routes, travel as white communicating rami to the sympathetic chain, then pass cephalad to synapse at the second thoracic ganglion, first thoracic or inferior cervical ganglion (stellate), and occasionally middle cervical ganglion. Most postganglionic nerves leave the chain as gray communicating rami to join the anterior divisions at C_5-T_1, nerves that form the brachial plexus. Some postganglionic nerves pass directly from the chain to form the subclavian perivascular plexus and innervate the subclavian, axillary, and upper part of the brachial arteries.[2]

Most individuals have the inferior cervical ganglion fused to the first thoracic ganglion forming the stellate ganglion. Although the ganglion itself is inconstant, it commonly measures 2.5 cm long, 1.0 cm wide, and 0.5 cm thick. It usually lies in front of the neck of the first rib and extends to the interspace between C_7 and T_1. When elongated, it may lie over the anterior tubercle of C_7; in individuals with unfused ganglia the inferior cervical ganglion rests over C_7 and the first thoracic ganglion over the neck of the first rib. From a three-dimensional perspective the stellate ganglion is limited medially by the longus colli muscle, laterally by the scalene muscles, anteriorly by the subclavian artery, posteriorly by the transverse processes and prevertebral fascia, and inferiorly by the posterior aspect of the pleura (Fig. 20-2). At the level of the stellate ganglion the vertebral artery lies anterior, having originated from the subclavian artery. After passing over the ganglion, the artery enters the vertebral foramen and is located posterior to the anterior

tubercle of C_6 (Fig. 20-3). Since the classic approach to blockade of the stellate ganglion is at the level of C_6 (Chaussignac's tubercle), the location of the needle is positioned anterior to the artery. Other structures posterior to the stellate ganglion include the anterior divisions of the C_8 and T_1 nerves (inferior aspects of the brachial plexus). The stellate ganglion supplies sympathetic innervation to the upper extremity through gray communicating rami of C_7, C_8, T_1, and occasionally C_5 and C_6. Other inconstant contributions to the upper extremity include contributions from the T_2 and T_3 gray communicating rami. These latter fibers do not pass through the stellate ganglion but join the brachial plexus and ultimately innervate distal structures of the upper extremity. These fibers have sometimes been implicated in inadequate relief of sympathetically mediated pain, despite evidence of a satisfactory stellate block.[3]

These anomalous pathways have been termed Kuntz's nerves and can be reliably blocked only by a posterior approach.[3] Although technically more difficult than the classically taught anterior approach, the use of nerve imaging techniques (e.g., computerized tomography) can help prevent the major risk of pneumothorax. If a local anesthetic block is successful using this approach, neurolysis can be performed using low volumes of either aqueous phenol or alcohol (2 to 3 ml). Since most if not all sympathetic fibers to the upper extremity pass through these upper thoracic ganglia, the results of this neurolytic block can be quite successful.

Other efferent fibers from the stellate ganglion follow the major vascular structures including the subclavian and common carotid arteries. The subclavian arterial plexus also receives contributions from the ansa cervicalis (originating from the stellate ganglion) and the intermediate cervical ganglion.

Indications

The following clinical conditions have been treated with sympathetic block of the cervicothoracic chain:

Pain
    Reflex sympathetic dystrophy
    Causalgia
    Herpes zoster (shingles)
    Postherpetic neuralgia, early
    Phantom limb pain
    Paget's disease
    Neoplasm
    Postradiation neuritis
    Pain from central nervous system (CNS) lesions
    Intractable angina pectoris
Vascular insufficiency
    Raynaud's disease
    Frostbite
    Vasospasm
    Occlusive vascular disease
    Embolic vascular disease
    Scleroderma
Other
    Hyperhidrosis
    Ménière's disease

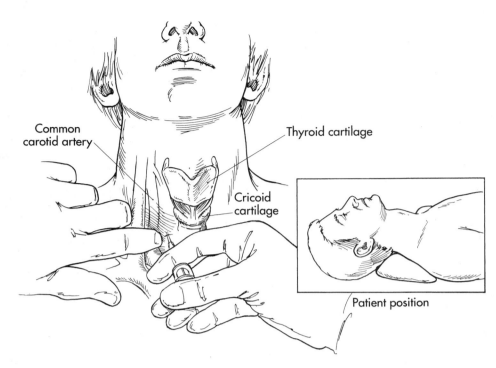

Fig. 20-2 Stellate ganglion block. C_6 anterior tubercle is directly beneath the operator's index finger. Carotid artery is retracted laterally when necessary. Needle is perpendicular to all skin planes and is inserted directly posterior. *Inset,* Patient positioned for stellate ganglion block. Pillow or roll should be between shoulders to extend neck, bring esophagus midline, and facilitate palpation of Chaussignac's tubercle. (From Rauck RL: Sympathetic nerve blocks A. In Raj PP, editor: *Practical Management of Pain,* ed 2. St Louis, Mosby, 1992.)

Common carotid artery

Thyroid cartilage

Cricoid cartilage

Patient position

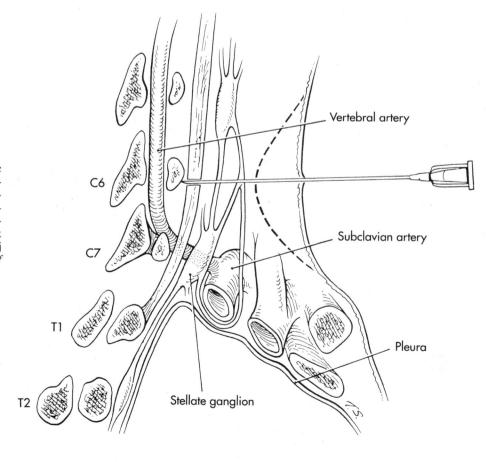

Fig. 20-3 Sagittal view of sympathetic chain. Note that stellate ganglion is positioned directly posterior to vertebral artery. Longus colli muscle separates ganglia from bone at C_6 level. Needle is superior to stellate ganglion. (From Rauck RL: Sympathetic nerve blocks A. In Raj PP, editor: *Practical Management of Pain,* ed 2. St Louis, Mosby, 1992.)

Vertebral artery

Subclavian artery

Pleura

Stellate ganglion

C6

C7

T1

T2

Shoulder/hand syndrome
Stroke
Sudden blindness
Vascular headaches

Many of the above indications are addressed in other chapters of this book. Some remain controversial, and reports of efficacy are based largely on case reports instead of large studies with good study design. In particular, treatment with stellate ganglion block for phantom limb pain, postherpetic neuralgia, vascular occlusion of large vessels, stroke, and Ménière's disease has yielded questionable results. Others such as angina pectoris require blockade of the upper five thoracic sympathetic ganglia, in addition to the stellate ganglion, to provide relief.[3]

Technique

Patient preparation. Proper preparation of the patient for the initial block ideally begins at the visit before the procedure. Patients are much more likely to remember discharge instructions and expected side effects if these are explained during a visit when they are not apprehensive about an impending procedure. A booklet explaining the procedure in detail, side effects that may be expected, and potential complications allay the fears of most patients. Conversations about the realistic expectations of sympathetic blockade should be held before any procedures. The goals of blockade and the number of blocks in a given series differ with each specific pain syndrome, and these should be discussed when possible at visits before the blockade. Patients are much less likely to experience frustration or despair if they understand beforehand what can be expected. If the cause of pain is unclear and the intended block is considered diagnostic, a complete explanation will allow the patient to record valuable information concerning the effectiveness of the procedure.

Informed consent must be obtained whenever sympathetic blockade is anticipated. Potential risks, complications, and side effects that may occur should be explained in detail. The patient should share the responsibility for decision making and must understand that risks are present and that complications do occur.

An intravenous (IV) line placed before the block is not considered mandatory at all pain clinics. Its placement does facilitate the use of IV sedation when indicated and provides access for the administration of resuscitative drugs should a complication occur. Skilled physicians can perform a stellate ganglion block quickly and relatively painlessly. In these situations an IV may not be necessary, although all standard resuscitative drugs, suction, oxygen, cardiac defibrillators, and instruments for endotracheal cannulation need to be readily accessible. Preblock sedation through an IV is recommended in procedures involving anxious patients and in certain teaching situations, such as where the operator is inexperienced or "hands-on" teaching is expected.

Anterior approach. The patient lies supine with the head resting flat on the table, without the use of a pillow. Place a folded sheet or thin pillow under the shoulders of most patients to further facilitate extension of the neck and make palpation of bony landmarks easier (see Fig. 20-2). Keep the head midline with the mouth slightly open to relax the tension on the anterior cervical musculature. Hyperextension of the neck also causes the esophagus to become midline, away from the transverse processes on the left.

The site of needle entry is the C_6 level, Chaussignac's tubercle, and can be most readily identified by first locating the cricoid cartilage (see Fig. 20-3). For most individuals this is approximately 3.0 cm cephalad to the sternoclavicular joint. Palpation of the tubercle can be expected at the medial border of the sternocleidomastoid muscle, approximately 1.5 cm lateral to the midline. Location of the carotid artery should be noted, its position most commonly lateral to the C_6 tubercle. In some individuals it is necessary to retract the common carotid artery lateral, away from the site of entry.

To ensure proper needle location, the C_6 tubercle must be correctly identified. This is most easily performed using firm pressure with the index finger. In either a left- or right-handed stellate ganglion block, the nondominant hand should be used for palpating landmarks. The patient does not tolerate a jabbing motion well; rather, gentle but firm probing can easily define the borders of the tubercle. A single finger, the index finger, relays the most specific tactile information. An alternative approach traps the tubercle between the index and middle fingers.[4]

Antiseptically prep the skin, and insert the needle posteriorly, penetrating the skin at the tip of the operator's index finger. A prior skin wheal with local anesthetic is rarely necessary, except in some teaching situations or in the case of patients with obese necks, in which repeated punctures may be anticipated. Use a 23-gauge needle, 4 to 5 cm long, and puncture the skin directly downward (posterior), perpendicular to the table in all planes. Although a smaller gauge (e.g., 25-gauge) needle can be used, its added flexibility and smaller caliber make it more difficult to reliably ascertain when bone is encountered and then to maintain the proper location for injection.

The needle passes through the underlying tissue until it contacts either the C_6 tubercle or the junction between the C_6 vertebral body and the tubercle. The depth of these structures differs, with the tubercle itself being more anterior than the junction between body and tubercle. Regardless of the specific location encountered at C_6, if the skin is being properly displaced posteriorly by the nondominant index finger, the depth is rarely beyond 2.0 to 2.5 cm. The important difference between medial and lateral location of bone at C_6 relates to the presence of the longus colli. It is located over the lateral aspect of the vertebral body and medial aspect of the transverse process. It does not cover the C_6 tubercle; only the prevertebral fascia that invests the longus colli also covers the C_6 tubercle. Therefore if the needle contacts the medial aspect of the transverse process at a depth somewhat greater than expected, be prepared to withdraw the needle 0.5 cm to avoid injection into the longus colli muscle. Injection into the muscle belly can prevent caudad diffusion of local anesthetic to the stellate ganglion. Location of the needle on the superficial tip of the C_6 anterior tubercle requires only withdrawal of the needle from periosteum before injection.

The procedure is most easily performed if the syringe is attached before needle placement. This prevents accidental dislodgement of the needle from the bone if attachment is attempted after needle placement. Once bone is encountered, maintain pressure with the palpating finger, withdraw the needle 2 to 5 mm, and inject the medication. Alternatively, once bone is met, the palpating hand can release and fix the needle by grasping its hub. The dominant hand is now free to aspirate and inject.

Injection of medication must be performed in a routine and systematic fashion. An initial test dose must be injected in all cases. Less than 1 ml of solution injected intravascularly has resulted in loss of consciousness and seizure activity. Before any injection careful aspiration must be performed, either for blood or cerebrospinal fluid (CSF). If the aspiration is negative, administer 0.5 to 1.0 ml of solution, and ask the patient to raise the thumb to indicate he or she is having no adverse symptoms. It should be explained to the patient before the block and repeated during the procedure that talking will result in movement of the neck musculature and can dislodge the needle from its proper location. To maintain verbal contact with the patient, ask the patient to point a thumb or finger upward during the procedure. After the initial test dose inject the remainder of the solution, carefully aspirating after each 3 to 4 ml.

During injection or needle placement a paresthesia of the arm or hand may be elicited. This should uniformly be interpreted to mean that placement of the needle is deep to the anterior tubercle, adjacent to the C_6 or C_7 nerve root. Repositioning of the needle is necessary. Any aspiration of blood or CSF also necessitates repositioning of the needle.

The total volume of solution necessary depends on the block desired.[3] If placed properly, 5 ml of solution will block the stellate ganglion. This does not reliably block all fibers to the upper extremities, since contributions from T_2 and T_3 may be present. Injection of 10 ml of solution more reliably blocks all sympathetic innervation to the upper extremity, even in patients with the anomalous Kuntz nerves. If blockade is being performed for sympathetically mediated pain of the thoracic viscera including the heart, administer 15 to 20 ml of solution.

Evidence of block

Sympathetic interruption to the head, supplied by the stellate ganglion, can be easily documented by the presence of a Horner's syndrome: myosis (pinpoint pupil), ptosis (drooping of the upper eyelid), and enophthalmos (sinking of the eyeball). Associated findings include conjunctival injection, nasal congestion, and facial anhidrosis. These signs can be present without complete interruption of the sympathetic nerves to the upper extremity.

Evidence of sympathetic blockade to the upper extremity includes visible engorgement of the veins on the back of the hand and forearm, psychogalvanic reflex, plethysmography, thermography, and a sweat test. A rise in skin temperature also occurs, provided the preblock temperature does not exceed 33° to 34° C.

Side effects and complications

Side effects from a stellate ganglion block should be distinguished from complications. Most unpleasant side effects result from Horner's syndrome and include ptosis, myosis, and nasal congestion.

Common complications from a stellate ganglion block occur from the diffusion of local anesthetic onto nearby nervous structures. These include the recurrent laryngeal nerve with complaints of hoarseness, feeling of a lump in the throat, and sometimes a subjective shortness of breath. Bilateral stellate blocks are rarely advised, since bilateral blocking of the recurrent laryngeal nerve can result in respiratory compromise and loss of laryngeal reflexes. Block of the phrenic nerve results in temporary paralysis of the diaphragm and can result in respiratory embarrassment in patients whose respiratory reserve is already severely compromised. Partial brachial plexus block can also result secondary to spread along the prevertebral fascia[5] or if the needle location is too posterior. Discharge the patient with a sling and careful instructions on how to care for a partially blocked arm if this occurs.

The two most feared complications from a stellate ganglion block include an intraspinal injection and seizures from an intravascular injection. Respiratory embarrassment and the need for mechanical ventilation can result from either injection into the epidural (if high concentrations of local anesthetic are used) or intrathecal space. If this occurs, patients need continual reassurance that everything is being appropriately managed and that they will recover without sequelae. Some sedation is required while the local anesthetic wears off. No drugs are necessary for endotracheal cannulation, since profound anesthesia of the larynx can be expected.

Intravascular injection most commonly occurs in the vertebral artery. Small amounts of local anesthetic will result in unconsciousness, respiratory paralysis, seizures, and sometimes severe arterial hypotension. Increased IV fluids, vasopressors if indicated, oxygen, and endotracheal intubation may be necessary. If the amount of drug injected into the artery is small (less than 2 ml), the above sequelae will be short-lived and self-limiting, with oxygen and increased fluid administration often being the only needed therapy. Be careful when performing a stellate ganglion block that no air is injected from the syringe. Cerebral air embolisms have been reported from this procedure and are preventable.[3,6,7]

The risk of pneumothorax also exists with the anterior approach. If the C_7 tubercle is used and the needle is inserted caudally, the dome of the lung can be penetrated. This occurs more easily in thin, tall individuals whose dome can extend more cephalad.

Alternative approaches

C_7 anterior approach. The anterior approach to the stellate ganglion at C_7 is similar to the approach described at C_6. Unlike the C_6 tubercle, C_7 has only a vestigial tubercle, which is very difficult to palpate. To identify C_7 one must usually first find Chaussignac's tubercle (C_6), then move one finger breadth caudad from the inferior tip. The patient

must be positioned with a pillow under the shoulders to extend the cervical spine and help make the tubercle more superficial.

The advantage to blockade at C_7 is that a lower volume of local anesthetic is necessary to provide complete interruption of the upper extremity sympathetic innervation. Solution, 6 to 9 ml, will suffice. The bothersome side effect of a recurrent laryngeal nerve block is less frequent with this approach. The technique carries two disadvantages: The less pronounced landmarks make needle positioning less reliable, and the risk of pneumothorax increases, since the dome of the lung is in close proximity.

Posterior approach. The ease of performing a stellate ganglion block by the anterior approach has rendered the posterior approach unnecessary except for specific indications.[3,8] The posterior approach should be used for the patient who develops a Horner's syndrome with an anterior approach but fails to show other signs of sympathetic denervation to the upper extremity. Should this occur despite repetitive, well-placed blocks, the patient may have a fascial tissue barrier preventing caudad diffusion of the drug.

The posterior approach at the T_2 or T_3 level provides sympathetic interruption to the upper extremity.

Patients chosen for chemical sympathectomy of the upper extremity also should be blocked with the posterior approach. Although dilute solutions of phenol have been injected by the anterior approach at C_6, the smaller volume used may prevent reliable diffusion to the stellate ganglion.[9] If the volume is increased, the risk of spread to the recurrent laryngeal nerve, phrenic nerve, or brachial plexus would be unacceptably high. Also, the development of a Horner's syndrome would be invariably achieved if complete neurolytic destruction occurred by the anterior approach. The posterior approach can often avoid a Horner's syndrome. The patient must understand and accept this potentially permanent complication before neurolysis.

A major disadvantage to sympathetic block by the posterior approach is the high risk of pneumothorax (Fig. 20-4). The apex of the lung lies near the sympathetic chain at T_2 and can be difficult to avoid by even the most experienced of operators. With the recent advent of computed to-

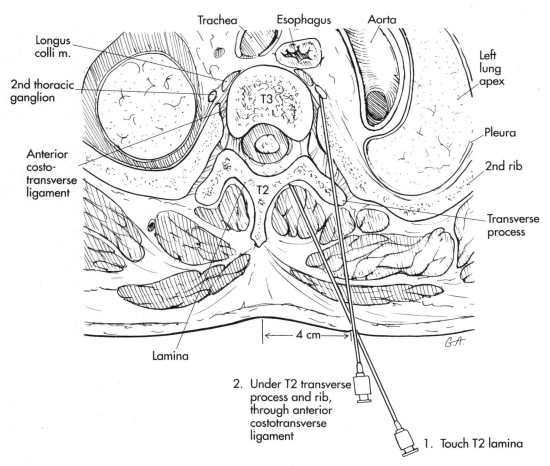

Fig. 20-4 Posterior approach to upper thoracic sympathetic chain block. Needle is introduced 4 cm from midline, then walked off T_2 lamina. Needle should always be directed medially. (From Rauck RL: Sympathetic nerve blocks A. In Raj PP, editor: *Practical Management of Pain,* ed 2. St Louis, Mosby, 1992.)

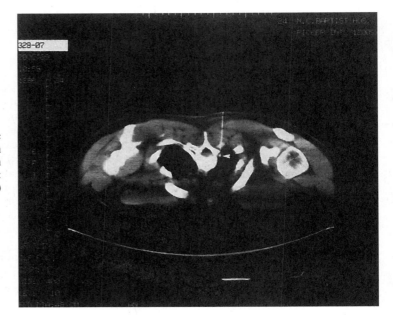

Fig. 20-5 CT radiograph of upper thoracic sympathetic block. Arrow shows contrast held close to vertebral column by endothoracic fascia and costrotransverse ligament. (From Rauck RL: Sympathetic nerve blocks A. In Raj PP, editor: *Practical Management of Pain,* ed 2, St Louis, Mosby, 1992.)

mography (CT), precise needle location can be more readily achieved.[8] Whenever neurolysis is anticipated, CT-guided placement should be employed.

Anatomy. The sympathetic chain lies close to the neck of the ribs in the thoracic space. Unlike the cervical and lumbar regions where the longus colli muscle and psoas muscles respectively separate the sympathetic chain from somatic nerves, no muscular separation exists in the thoracic region. The risk of intravertebral diffusion of drug during this block must be closely monitored. The pleura also abuts the sympathetic chain in the thoracic region, making precise needle location essential to avoid a pneumothorax. The risk of pneumothorax approaches 4% when this approach is employed.[4]

Technique. The posterior approach can be performed with the patient either in the prone position or lateral with the side to be blocked uppermost.[1,4] With the advent of new imaging techniques (e.g., fluoroscopy and CT), the prone position provides more useful information. This block was classically taught with needles inserted 6.0 cm from the midline. Entry at this point makes it extremely difficult to localize the needles properly along the vertebral body without passing through the pleura or parenchymal tissue (Fig. 20-5). Bonica later described a technique in which the needle was inserted 2.0 cm from the midline and advanced adjacent to the vertebral body. However, in many patients 2.0 cm will not allow the needle to pass off lamina without using an undesirable lateral direction, ultimately leading to a pneumothorax. Rather, a distance of 3 to 4 cm from the midline allows proper alignment; the needle shaft should pass from the lamina and be parallel with the sagittal plane. The needle should never be directed laterally, beyond the perpendicular plane. If the needle continues to contact lamina after repositioning to the perpendicular plane, raise a new skin wheal 1.0 cm lateral to the original wheal and retrace the process.

The space lateral to the T_1 spinous process can be used if local anesthetic is injected. If a neurolytic procedure is anticipated, identify either the T_2 or T_3 spinous process. After prepping and draping the area, raise a skin wheal 3 to 4 cm lateral to the spine. Use a 22-gauge, 8- to 10-cm needle to contact the ipsilateral lamina. Then position the needle laterally off the lamina until it passes through the anterior costotransverse ligament. This can be done by loss-of-resistance technique, similar to that described for epidural location. Alternatively, a skin marker can be placed after contact with the lamina, requiring a depth of 2.0 cm once the needle passes from the lamina. At this point inject 2 to 3 ml of radiocontrast material. Proper spread is characteristically seen (Fig. 20-6). If dye cannot be visualized, pleural or intravascular injection is likely. If neurolysis is anticipated, the intraspinal space must also be closely inspected for any back diffusion of dye before the injection of a neurolytic agent. Once proper location is verified with contrast, inject 2 to 3 ml of local anesthetic or neurolytic slowly with repeated aspiration.

Neurolysis. Neurolysis of the upper thoracic sympathetic chain by the posterior approach should only be performed when one of the image intensifiers is used, preferably CT. Needles can be positioned erroneously (Fig. 20-7) with disastrous results if a neurolytic agent is injected.

For neurolysis, use the T_2 or T_3 spinous process. Although a Horner's syndrome may be avoided by this approach, the risk remains, and the patient must understand and accept this possible occurrence. Once the needle is positioned, contrast material must be injected to check for either interpleural spread, intraspinal diffusion, or intravascular injection. If good spread of dye is visualized, slowly inject 2 to 3 ml of 10% aqueous phenol.

Complications. The two main complications to this approach are pneumothorax and intraspinal injection (see Fig. 20-7). A third complication, when neurolysis is performed,

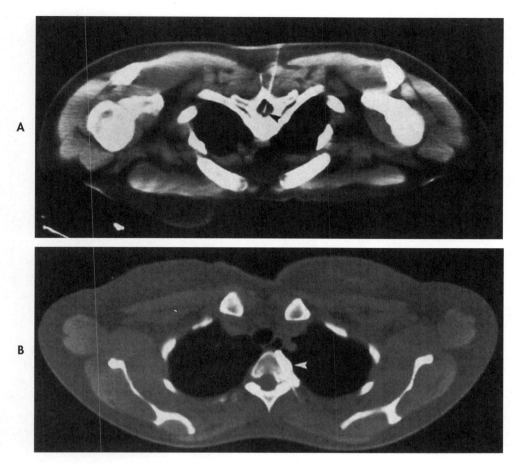

Fig. 20-6 A, Potential complication of thoracic sympathetic block. Inadvertent placement of 22-gauge needle into thoracic spine *(see arrow)* during upper thoracic sympathetic block. A leg and chest paresthesia were elicted but no neurologic sequelae resulted. **B,** Placement of needle into pleura *(see arrow)*. No pneumothorax was found on postblock chest x-rays. (From Rauck RL: Sympathetic nerve blocks A. In Raj PP, editor: *Practical Management of Pain,* ed 2. St Louis, Mosby, 1992.)

concerns the possibility of a persistent Horner's syndrome. A pneumothorax can be avoided with careful placement of the needle, making sure the needle angulation is never lateral and the advancement through the costotransverse ligaments (posterior and anterior) is controlled, slow, and uses the loss-of-resistance technique. Intraspinal injection most commonly occurs by diffusion through the intervertebral foramen and can be avoided by initially injecting a water-soluble contrast dye and checking location by x-ray. The optimal method for checking location and solution spread employs CT.[8]

To check for a possible subsequent Horner's syndrome, first inject local anesthetic into the region and inspect the patient after 15 to 30 minutes. This does not always preclude a Horner's syndrome developing with neurolytic injection, and prior local anesthetic injection may not be considered optimal in all situations.

REFERENCES

1. Bonica JJ: *The Management of Pain.* Philadelphia, Lea & Febiger, 1953.
2. Moore DC: *Stellate Ganglion Block.* Springfield, Ill, Charles C Thomas, 1954.
3. Bonica JJ: *Sympathetic Nerve Blocks for Pain Diagnosis and Therapy.* New York, Breon Laboratories, 1984.
4. Bridenbaugh PO, Cousins MJ: *Neural Blockade in Clinical Anesthesia and Management of Pain.* Philadelphia, JB Lippincott, 1988.
5. Carron H, Litwiller R: Stellate ganglion block. *Anesth Analg* 54:567-570, 1975.
6. Moore DC: *Regional Block,* ed 4. Springfield, Ill, Charles C Thomas, 1975.
7. Adelman MH: Cerebral air embolism complicating stellate ganglion block. *Journal of Mt Sinai Hospital* 15:28-30, 1948.
8. Dondelinger RF, Kurdziel JC: Percutaneous phenol block of the upper thoracic sympathetic chain with computed tomography guidance. *Acta Radiol* 28:511-515, 1987.
9. Racz G: *Techniques of Neurolysis.* Boston, Kluwer Academic Publishers, 1989.

C. Thoracic Sympathetic Block

Anatomy

The thoracic sympathetic chain lies near somatic nerves as they emanate from the intervertebral foramen. Their poste

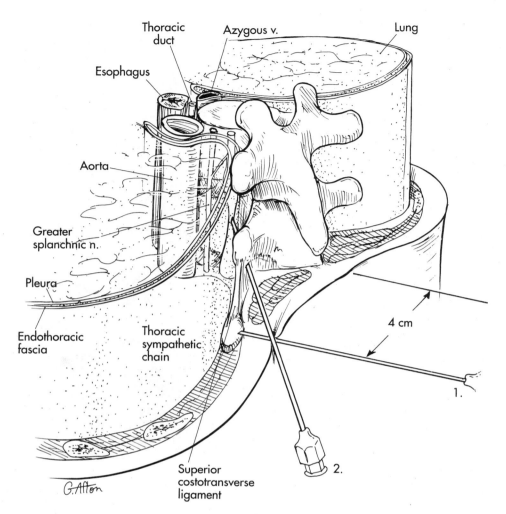

Fig. 20-7 Midthoracic sympathetic block. (From Rauck RL: Sympathetic nerve blocks A. In Raj PP, editor: *Practical Management of Pain,* ed 2. St Louis, Mosby, 1992.)

rior orientation on the vertebral bodies is constant throughout the thoracic space. Ten pairs of ganglia (occasionally 11) can be found as the chain courses through the thoracic cavity. The pleura is directly anterior to the ganglia, separated in most places by only the thin endothoracic fascia (Fig. 20-8).

Indications

Few indications exist for thoracic sympathetic block. Thoracic epidural block can provide similar results without the high risk of pneumothorax. Some oncologic processes can produce a relatively specific sympathetic pain of the thoracic viscera, which can be alleviated by a neurolytic injected onto the thoracic sympathetic chain. This avoids potential complications of a neurolytic intraspinal block.

Technique

Position the patient prone, and outline the spinous processes. Image intensification should be employed whenever possible. Raise a skin wheal 4 to 5 cm lateral to the spi-

nous process. Direct the needle to the lamina, and then walk it laterally. Place a skin marker 1.0 cm above the skin, and use the loss-of-resistance technique as the needle passes from the lamina. The needle should never be advanced in a lateral direction, as this invariably results in a pneumothorax. If lamina is still contacted with the needle in a perpendicular plane, raise a skin wheal 2.0 cm lateral to the original and repeat the above steps. After a needle passes from the lamina, it will engage the costotransverse ligament, and immediately upon piercing the ligament a loss of resistance is encountered. Solution of 2 to 3 ml should anesthetize the chain at this point, although posterior diffusion to the corresponding somatic nerve can occur. A more complete description of this technique was described earlier in the chapter.

Complications

Pneumothorax must be considered the main reason this block is not performed more frequently. The risk of pneumothorax exceeds 4% with experienced physicians; punc-

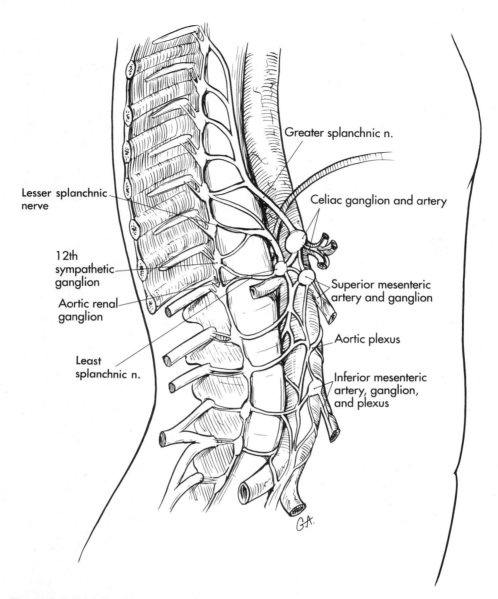

Fig. 20-8 Splanchnic nerves; greater, lesser, and least. Formation of the respective abdominal plexuses are noted. (From Rauck RL: Sympathetic nerve blocks A. In Raj PP, editor: *Practical Management of Pain,* ed 2. St Louis, Mosby, 1992.)

ture of the pleura no doubt occurs much more frequently.[1] The risk of neurolysis also includes the likelihood of medicine diffusing to the nearby somatic nerves and producing neuralgic pain. The needle can also be inadvertently placed into the intraspinal space or adjacent to the intervertebral foramen, with resultant injection of medicine onto the spinal cord.

REFERENCE

1. Dondelinger RF, Kurdziel JC: Percutaneous phenol block of the upper thoracic sympathetic chain with computed tomography guidance. *Acta Radiol* 28:511-515, 1987.

D. Celiac Plexus Splanchnic Nerve Block

Anatomic considerations

Sympathetic innervation of the abdominal viscera originates in the anterolateral horn of the spinal cord. Preganglionic axons from T_5 to T_{12} leave the spinal cord with the ventral spinal routes to join the white communicating rami en route to the sympathetic chain. In contradistinction to other preganglionic sympathetic nerves, these axons do not synapse in the sympathetic chain; rather, they pass through the chain to synapse at distal sites including the celiac, aortico

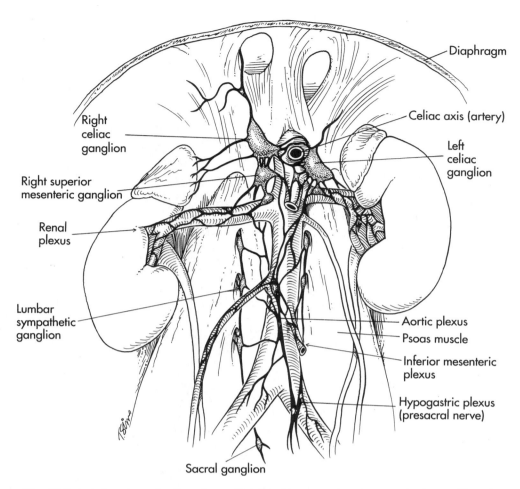

Fig. 20-9 Anterior view of celiac plexus. Relationship to nearby structures is shown. Note the dense, diffuse intertwining network of nerves which form plexus. (From Rauck RL: Sympathetic nerve blocks A. In Raj PP, editor: *Practical Management of Pain,* ed 2. St Louis, Mosby, 1992.)

renal, and superior mesenteric ganglia. Postganglionic nerves accompany blood vessels to their respective visceral structures (Fig. 20-9).

Preganglionic nerves from T_5-T_9 and occasionally T_4 and T_{10} travel caudally from the sympathetic chain along the lateral and anterolateral aspects of the vertebral bodies. At the level of T_9 and T_{10} the axons coalesce to form the greater splanchnic nerve, pierce the diaphragm, and end as numerous terminal endings in the celiac plexus. Most travel ipsilaterally, although a few cross and synapse with contralateral postganglionic cell bodies.

Sympathetic nerves from T_{10}-T_{11}, and occasionally T_{12}, combine to form the lesser splanchnic nerve. Their course parallels the greater splanchnic nerve in a posterolateral position and ends in either the celiac plexus or aorticorenal ganglion. The least splanchnic nerves arise from T_{12}, parallel posteriorly the lesser splanchnic nerve, and synapse in the aorticorenal ganglion.

The above-mentioned sympathetic nerves are efferent nerves that maintain important characteristics in reflexive sympathetically medicated pain. Nociceptive information from abdominal viscera occurs in afferent nerves that are part of the spinal nerves but accompany the sympathetic nerves. Cell bodies exist in the posterior roots of the spinal nerves, with proximal axons synapsing in the dorsal horn of the spinal cord. Distal axons pass with this posterior spinal nerve but then join the sympathetic nerves and continue through the white communicating rami, the sympathetic chain, the respective splanchnic nerve and ganglion, and finally to the walls of the abdominal viscera.

The celiac plexus lies anterior to the aorta and epigastrium (see Fig. 20-9). It is also located just anterior to the crus of the diaphragm and becomes an important consideration in deciding the approach to blockade. The plexus extends for several centimeters in front of the aorta and laterally around the aorta (Fig. 20-10). Fibers within the plexus arise from preganglionic splanchnic nerves, parasympathetic preganglionic nerves from the vagus, some sensory nerves from the phrenic and vagus nerves, and sympathetic postganglionic fibers. Afferent fibers concerned with nociception pass diffusely through the celiac plexus and represent the main target of celiac plexus blockade.

The above fibers coalesce to form a dense, intertwining network of autonomic nerves. Three pairs of ganglia exist

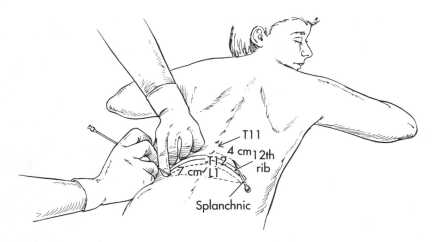

Fig. 20-10 Surface landmarks for splanchnic nerve block or celiac plexus block. The diagram drawn resembles a flat isosceles triangle. (From Rauck RL: Sympathetic nerve blocks A. In Raj PP, editor: *Practical Management of Pain,* ed 2. St Louis, Mosby, 1992.)

within the plexus: the celiac ganglia, the superior mesenteric ganglia, and the aortic renal ganglia. Postganglionic nerves from these ganglia will innervate all of the abdominal viscera with the exception of part of the transverse colon, the left colon, rectum, and pelvic viscera. Pelvic viscera ultimately have nociceptive synapse from T_{10}-L_1 spinal levels and include the uterus and cervix.[1]

Indications

Any pain originating from visceral structures and innervated by the celiac plexus can be effectively alleviated by blockade of the plexus, which includes the pancreas, liver, gallbladder, omentum, mesentery, and the alimentary tract from the stomach to the transverse portion of the large colon (Fig. 20-11). The particular disease state determines the effectiveness of a celiac plexus block in producing sustained pain relief beyond the duration of the local anesthetic solution. The pain syndrome involved should dictate whether a local anesthetic block, neurolytic injection, catheter placement, or steroid injection should be anticipated.

The best indication for neurolytic celiac plexus block is upper abdominal malignancy, in particular pancreatic cancer. This was initially described by Kappis in 1914.[2] The pain is described as severe and unremitting, narcotics often poorly alleviate the pain, and the progression of the disease makes the time course from diagnosis to death short, often less than 6 months. These factors, together with the excellent analgesia achieved with neurolytic blockade, make celiac plexus block the treatment of choice for pancreatic cancer pain.

An additional benefit in these patients may be the effect of celiac plexus block on gastric motility. Complete sympathetic denervation of the gastrointestinal tract allows unopposed parasympathetic activity and increased peristalsis. Although diarrhea has been reported in a few patients, a concomitant decrease in the incidence of nausea and vomiting has also been reported. The presence of severe nausea and vomiting has been cited as a primary indication in pa-

tients with pancreatic cancer whose pain might otherwise be reasonably managed with oral narcotics (personal communication, D. Brown, 1989).

An alternative to neurolysis for patients who have had multiple abdominal surgeries and continue to complain of pain involves the addition of a corticosteroid preparation to the local anesthetic solution. Best results can be expected in patients who have an inflammatory component involving the celiac plexus. Betamethasone (Celestone) has dual properties of excellent tissue dispersion, essential for the diffuse celiac plexus, and depot characteristics that would help to prolong the effect from blockade. Good controlled studies are lacking.

The cause of some patients' abdominal pain cannot be clearly elucidated at initial evaluation, especially in patients who have undergone multiple abdominal surgeries. In these patients it can be difficult to differentiate abdominal wall pain from underlying visceral pain. Either a local anesthetic celiac plexus block or an intercostal nerve block should be considered a pain-specific block and will differentiate visceral from somatic pain.

The long-term benefit of a neurolytic celiac plexus block in patients with nonmalignant abdominal pain has been conflicting.[3-7] Often regeneration of new pathways or development of a deafferent pain syndrome has occurred in these patients at a 6- to 12-month follow-up.

Nonetheless, some patients' symptoms include intractable, intolerable abdominal pain. Although long-term success with neurolytic celiac blocks has not been encouraging, short-term relief may allow some patients to gain coping skills and learn to manage their pain. This alternative may prove superior to unmerited surgical reexploration. A candidate for neurolytic celiac plexus block may be the person whose pain is uncontrolled, who has required repeated pain-related hospital admissions, who has had multiple surgical procedures for pain without benefit, and who is debating further surgical explorations. If pain relief can be achieved with a local anesthetic celiac plexus block but not maintained and the addition of steroids in the celiac plexus

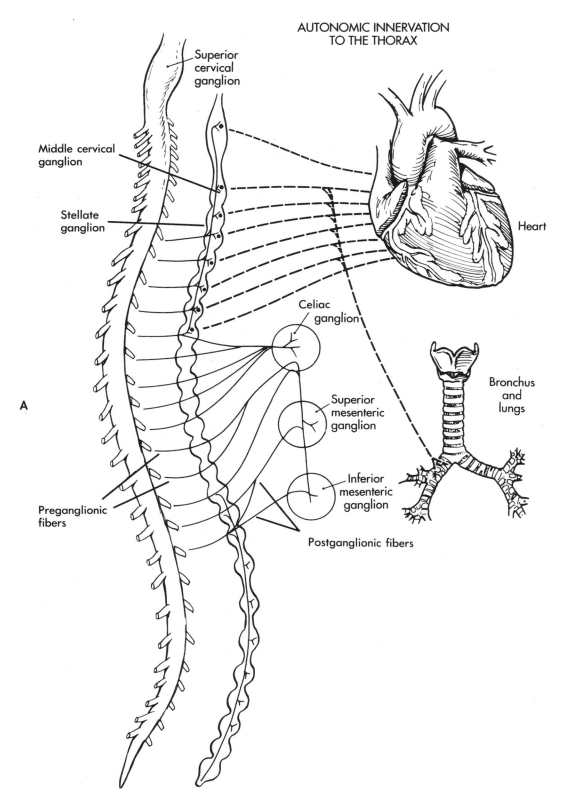

Fig. 20-11 Innervation of the sympathetic nervous system. Preganglion and postganglion fibers are distinguished. (From Rauck RL: Sympathetic nerve blocks A. In Raj PP, editor: *Practical Management of Pain,* ed 2. St Louis, Mosby, 1992.)

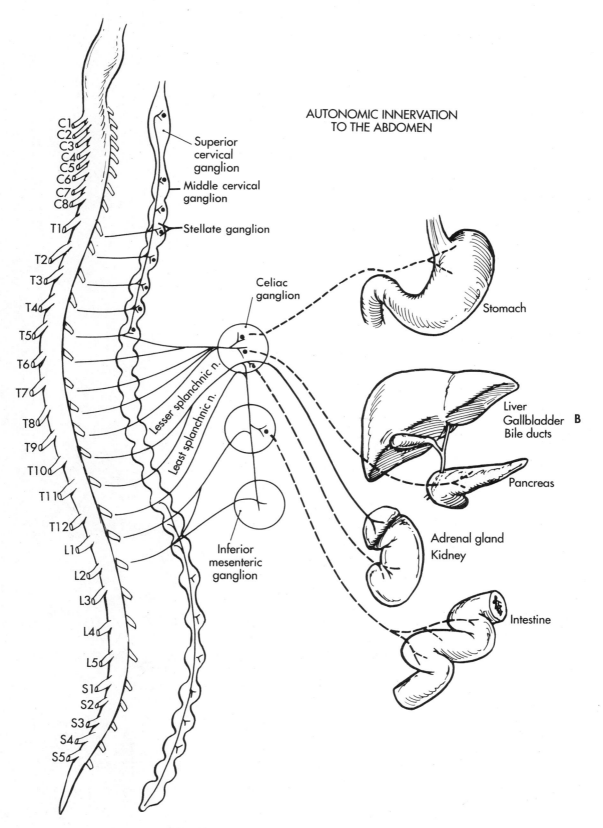

Fig. 20-11, cont'd. For legend see opposite page.

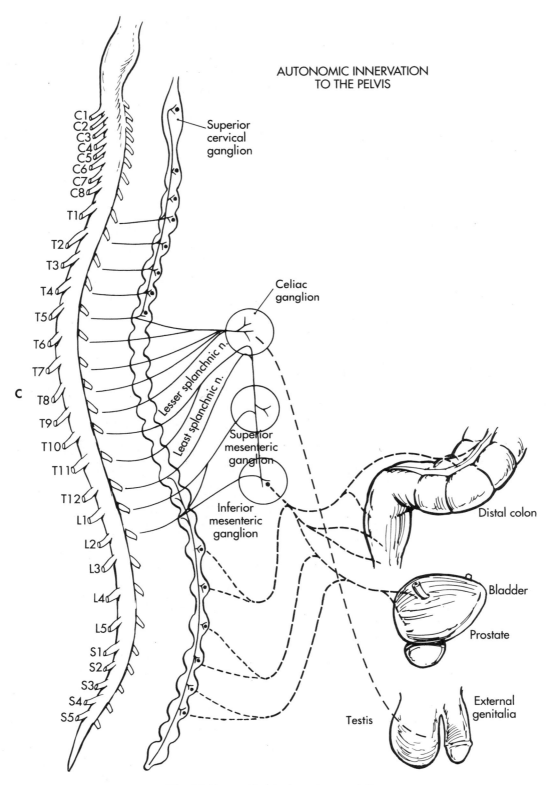

AUTONOMIC INNERVATION
TO THE PELVIS

Superior
cervical
ganglion

C1
C2
C3
C4
C5
C6
C7
C8
T1
T2
T3
T4
T5
T6
T7
T8
T9
T10
T11
T12
L1
L2
L3
L4
L5
S1
S2
S3
S4
S5

C

Celiac
ganglion

Lesser splanchnic n.

Least splanchnic n.

Superior
mesenteric
ganglion

Inferior
mesenteric
ganglion

Distal colon

Bladder

Prostate

Testis

External
genitalia

Fig. 20-11, cont'd. For legend see p. 240.

block is ineffective, a neurolytic celiac plexus block should be considered.

Lateral technique

Before blockade, obtain informed consent and insert an IV catheter. Position the patient with a pillow under the lower abdomen to remove the lumbar lordosis and allow easier palpation of the spinous processes. In patients whose pain does not allow them to lie prone or in highly anxious patients, give premedication through the IV. In situations when the block is performed for diagnostic purposes, premedication should be avoided. Also, the block can be performed in the lateral position, although technical considerations make needle placement more difficult.

Landmarks drawn with an indelible skin marker greatly facilitate needle placement, even for those experienced with the procedure (Fig. 20-12). This may be done before prepping and draping the patient or with a sterile marker after prepping. Landmarks to be drawn include the spinous processes of T_{12} and L_1 and the inferior border of the twelfth rib. The T_{12} spinous process needs to be correctly identified and should be marked by following the twelfth rib medially and counting cephalad from the L_5 spinous process.

Mark the site for needle entry 7 to 8 cm lateral from the spinous process. Use either 20- or 22-gauge needles, 12 to 18 cm long. The exact length depends on body habitus. The insertion point should be immediately inferior to the border of the twelfth rib. Entry site should not exceed 8 cm from midline (7 cm in thin individuals) to avoid the risk of placing the needle through renal parenchymal tissue. Likewise, it is extremely important that the needles not be immediately placed beneath the T_{11} rib because a pneumothorax can result.

The ultimate directional positioning of the needle toward midline will depend on whether the splanchnic nerves or celiac plexus are to be blocked (Fig. 20-13). Classically, needles have been directed to the L_1 spinous process for block of the celiac plexus. Splanchnic nerves are blocked by positioning the needles more cephalad toward the eleventh or twelfth thoracic spinous process. If the L_2 spinous process is mistaken for the L_1 process, inadequate cephalad spread of solution may result.

Anatomically, the crus of the diaphragm determines whether the block performed represents a true celiac plexus block or a splanchnic nerve block. If the tip of the needle lies posterior to the crus, the nerves blocked will belong to the splanchnic nerves. When the needles are advanced anteriorly, they pass transcrurally and the solution injected blocks nerves to the celiac plexus. Needles placed at the T_{11} vertebral body are always located posteriorly to the crus. Below this level the crus migrates posteriorly to attach to the T_{12}[8] vertebral bodies. At the T_{12} or L_1 level the needles can be placed either anterior or posterior to the crus. The classically taught needle placement at the anterior border of the vertebral body most often results in placement posterior to the crus. For reliable placement anterior to the crus, the needle needs to be placed transcrurally, often through the abdominal aorta.

Infiltration with local anesthetics of deep muscular structures and periosteum lessens the need for sedation. Heavy sedation should especially be avoided whenever a diagnostic block is being performed. With advancement of the needle, two bony landmarks, the twelfth rib and the transverse process of L_1, can be mistaken for the vertebral body. Both are superficial to the vertebral body; the twelfth rib is quite superficial, but the transverse process can sometimes be misleading. If any question remains after bone is encountered, the needle should be removed and redirected cephalad. Caudad redirection can create a final placement at L_2, the results of which are less than optimal.

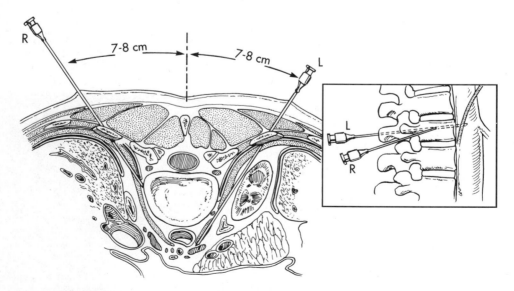

Fig. 20-12 Retrocrural and transcrural needle placement for celiac plexus block. *Inset, R,* Needle is retrocrural and will result in solution to spread and block the splanchnic nerves. *Inset, L,* Needle is transcrural and will block the celiac plexus directly. (From Rauck RL: Sympathetic nerve blocks A. In Raj PP, editor: *Practical Management of Pain,* ed 2. St Louis, Mosby, 1992.)

Once the vertebral body has been reached, place a skin marker on the needle 2 to 3 cm from the skin. Then walk the needle laterally until it just slips from the lateral surface of the vertebral body (Fig. 20-14). To make accurate small adjustments in the needle placement, it must first be withdrawn to superficial, subcutaneous structures. If adjustments with the smaller 22-gauge needle are attempted while the needle is deep, either they will be unsuccessful or the degree of change will be unpredictable. The needle should be first withdrawn to the skin, then a small increase in the angle made before reinsertion. The skin may be considered a fulcrum, with the celiac plexus being quite far from this point. Anything greater than small changes in the needle angle at the skin result in much larger changes in position at the ultimate destination (i.e., celiac plexus).

Once the lateral aspect of the vertebral body has passed, a pop is often felt when the needle passes through the psoas fascia. At this point the needles approach the great vessels and should be advanced slowly. The aorta is encountered from the left and the inferior vena cava from the right. Pancreatic or other intraabdominal masses often distort these structures laterally and posteriorly along the vertebral column. Optimal location of the needle can be checked by feeling for arterial pulsations. These pulsations can be transmitted through a needle to the aorta. These pulsations can also be observed visually if the needle approximates the

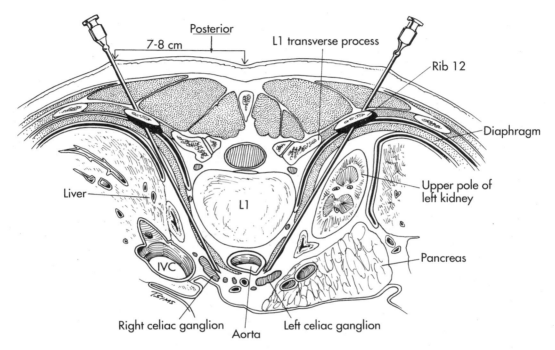

Fig. 20-13 Cross-section of celiac plexus block. Note proximity of renal parenchymal tissue necessitating needles placed no further than 7 to 8 cm from midline. (From Rauck RL: Sympathetic nerve blocks A. In Raj PP, editor: *Practical Management of Pain,* ed 2. St Louis, Mosby, 1992.)

Fig. 20-14 X-ray taken under direct fluoroscopic control. Spread of solution is monitored. No lateral diffusion is seen, and good confluence of contrast is seen anterior to the vertebral body. This is further confirmed by lateral cross-table x-ray. (From Rauck RL: Sympathetic nerve blocks A. In Raj PP, editor: *Practical Management of Pain,* ed 2. St Louis, Mosby, 1992.)

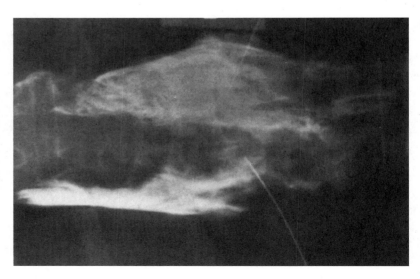

aorta. These checks should be performed as the needle passes its final 2 to 3 cm past the lateral part of the vertebral body.

After proper placement of the needles, carefully aspirate both needles before injection. If blood is encountered, slowly withdraw the needle until negative aspiration is achieved. Alternatively, on the aortic side, the needle can be advanced through the aorta until no blood is returned, and injection can be made at this location.

Initially, inject 2 to 3 ml of a local anesthetic solution containing epinephrine to further test for either intravascular or intraspinal placement. If negative, inject 15 ml bupivacaine 0.5% with epinephrine 1:200,000 through each needle.

Image intensification

Image intensification techniques can aid the performance of celiac plexus blocks; they include x-rays, fluoroscopy, and CT.[9-11] Since many pain clinics do not have these facilities on site, these blocks have to be performed in the radiology suite. This is rarely necessary when diagnostic blocks are performed or whenever local anesthetic injections are the sole agents used. The potential seriousness and permanency of complications with neurolytic solutions make image intensification preferable.

Fluoroscopy and CT-guided placement each have advantages.[5,12,13] Fluoroscopy yields a real-time display during the injection of solutions. Verification of needle placement can be performed before injection. Intravascular, intraspinal, lateral spread of solution into the psoas muscle or along the diaphragm can easily be seen. Proper, diffuse spread can be monitored as the total volume is injected (Fig. 20-15).[5]

The advantage of CT-guided placement rests with the precision of needle location (Fig. 20-16). If anatomic variations are expected secondary to extensive disease, CT can easily identify these before placement and aid technically difficult placement conditions. Once positioned, needle tips can be discretely seen in relation to all nearby structures. Installation of small volumes of air through the needles

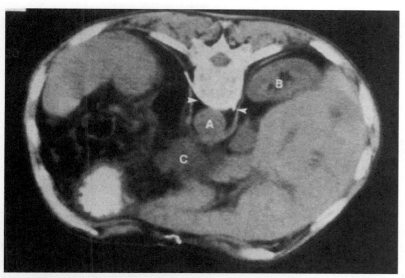

A

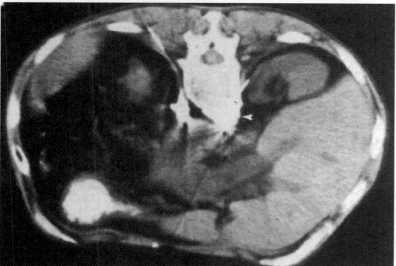

B

Fig. 20-15 CT radiograph of celiac plexus block. **A,** Precise needle location *(see arrow)* is observed with respect to surrounding structures. *A,* Aorta; *B,* kidney; *C,* pancreas. **B,** Contract material fills the periaortic space *(see arrow).* (From Rauck RL: Sympathetic nerve blocks A. In Raj PP, editor: *Practical Management of Pain,* ed 2. St Louis, Mosby, 1992.)

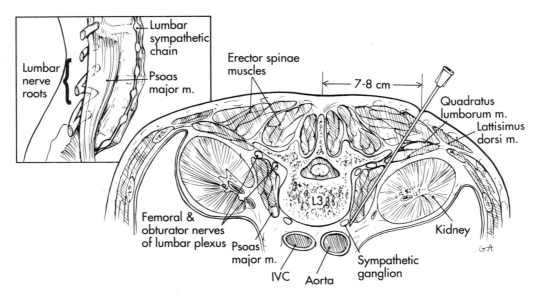

Fig. 20-16 Anatomy of lumbar sympathetic chain. Sympathetic chain has migrated to anterolateral border of vertebral bodies. Chain is separated from somatic nerve roots by large psoas muscle. (From Rauck RL: Sympathetic nerve blocks A. In Raj PP, editor: *Practical Management of Pain,* ed 2. St Louis, Mosby, 1992.)

clearly shows where the spread of subsequent solution can be expected.

The use of CT also provides a good teaching instrument, demonstrating the close proximity of above-mentioned structures, including the kidneys, great vessels, and diaphragmatic crus. The high cost of CT, however, precludes its use in routine cases, especially when fluoroscopy is available.

Alternative approaches

Single-needle approach. A single-needle approach using the left side has been reported with good results.[14,15] The technique for needle placement is similar to that previously described for bilateral placement. Final location of the needle has been reported both posterior to the aorta and anterior by a transaortic approach.

Adequate volume must be used, since only one needle is used and the celiac plexus is a diffuse network. The use of 20 ml, and possibly 30 ml, should be considered whenever feasible.

Anterior approach. An anterior approach to the celiac plexus has been employed with the needle inserted through the abdominal wall at the T_{12} level. A thin 22-gauge needle should be used, since bowel will often be perforated. This has not been a problem in other abdominal percutaneous radiologic procedures (personal communication, N. Karstaedt, 1989). The needle tip locates anterior to the aorta at the exact position of the celiac plexus. For patients who cannot lie prone, this approach may have applicability. However, since patients undergoing this procedure will have either a large pancreatic mass or another intraabdominal tumor anterior to the plexus, a needle through these often vascular masses would be contraindicated.

Catheter placement. Patients with nonmalignant abdominal pain often fare poorly after neurolytic blockade of

the celiac plexus, yet many derive temporary benefit from local anesthetic blockade. Since this pain is sympathetically mediated and reflexively perpetuated, continuous denervation of the plexus by local anesthetic infusion may provide prolonged analgesia.

The technique for placement is similar to that described previously.[4] Instead of 22-gauge needles, use a 6- or 8-inch catheter system made by Becton and Dickinson (Longdwel Catheter), placed bilaterally. Once placed, secure it at the skin with either a 2.0-cm silk skin suture or benzoin and Steri-strips. Then place a sterile, clear dressing over the catheters, which are connected to local anesthetic solutions of bupivacaine 0.1% and run at 6 to 8 ml/hour. These catheters can be maintained for 4 to 7 days if placed sterilely and the sites checked daily.

REFERENCES

1. Bonica JJ: *Sympathetic Nerve Blocks for Pain Diagnosis and Therapy.* New York, Breon Laboratories, 1984.
2. Kappis M: Ertahrungen mit Localanasthesia des Bauchuperationen. *Verhandl der Deutsch Gesellsch 1 Chir,* pp 43, 87, 1914.
3. Bell S, Cole R, Robert-Thomason IC: Coeliac plexus block for control of pain in chronic pancreatitis. *BMJ* 281:1604, 1980.
4. Gorbitz C, Leavens ME: Alcohol block of the celiac plexus for control of upper abdominal pain caused by cancer and pancreatitis. *J Neurosurg* 34:575-579, 1971.
5. Hegedus V: Relief of pancreatic pain by radiography-guided block. *AJR Am J Roentgenol* 133:1101-1103, 1979.
6. Leung JW et al: Coeliac plexus block for pain in pancreatic cancer and chronic pancreatitis. *Br J Surg* 70:730-732, 1983.
7. Owitz S, Koppolu S: Celiac plexus block: An overview. *Mt Sinai Journal of Medicine* 50:486-490, 1983.
8. Mitchell GAG: *Anatomy of the Autonomic Nervous System.* New York, Churchill Livingstone, 1953.
9. Jackson SH, Jacobs JB, Epstein RA: A radiographic approach to celiac plexus block. *Anesthesiology* 31:373-375, 1969.
10. Jacobs JB, Jackson SH, Doppman JL: A radiographic approach to celiac ganglion block. *Radiology* 92:1372-1373, 1969.

11. Moore DC, Bush WH, Burnett LL: Celiac plexus block: A roentgenographic, anatomic study of technique and spread of solution in patients and corpses. *Anesth Analg* 60:369-379, 1981.
12. Buy JN, Muss AA, Singler RC: CT guided celiac plexus and splanchnic nerve neurolysis. *J Comput Assist Tomogr* 6:315-319, 1982.
13. Singler RC: An improved technique for alcohol neurolysis of the celiac plexus. *Anesthesiology* 56:137-141, 1982.
14. Filshie J et al: Unilateral computerized tomography guided coeliac plexus block: A technique for pain relief. *Anaesthesia* 38:498-503, 1983.
15. HanKemeier V: Neurolytic celiac plexus block for cancer-related upper abdominal pain using the unilateral puncture technique and lateral position. *Pain* 4:S135, 1987.

E. Lumbar Sympathetic Block

Anatomic considerations

The lumbar sympathetic chain lies at the anterolateral border of the vertebral bodies. Unlike the more cephalad portions, the lumbar chain has many inconstant findings. The chain rarely appears in the same size or shape or in the same location within a given individual. The ganglia are also quite variable, with four sets being more common than five, a result of fusion of the T_{12} and L_1 ganglia.[1] Their position also varies; they can be segmentally located or closely grouped between the second and fourth lumbar vertebrae. The size of the ganglion also varies from 3 to 5 mm wide and from 10 to 15 mm in length.

The lumbar sympathetic chain consists of preganglionic axons and postganglionic neurons. The cell bodies of the preganglionic nerves arise from T_{11}, T_{12}, L_1, and L_2 and occasionally T_{10} and L_3. Their axons leave the spinal canal with the corresponding anterior spinal nerves, join the chain as white communicating rami, and then synapse in the appropriate ganglia.

Postganglionic axons depart the chain either directly to form a diffuse plexus around the iliac and femoral arteries, or, more commonly, as gray communicating rami to combine with spinal nerves of the lumbar and lumbosacral plexuses. They join all the major nerves of the lower extremity and ultimately end with the corresponding vessels. Most fibers traveling this network pass through the second and third lumbar sympathetic ganglia; blockade of these ganglia results in near complete denervation of the lower limb.

Preganglionic efferent axons for visceral structures synapse most commonly in the inferior three thoracic and first lumbar ganglia. They join hypogastric and aortic plexuses en route to the pelvic viscera. Afferent, nociceptive fibers in this region accompany the sympathetic fibers and relay pain sensations from kidney, ureter, bladder, distal portion of transverse colon, left (descending) colon, rectum, prostate, testicle, cervix, and uterus.

The anatomic positioning of the lumbar sympathetic chain at the anterolateral border of the vertebral border differs from more cephalad portions of the chain and allows it to be removed from somatic nerves (Fig. 20-17). The aorta is positioned anteriorly and slightly medial to the chain on the left side. The inferior vena cava is more closely approximated to the chain on the right in an anterior plane. Many other small lumbar arteries and veins are positioned near the sympathetic chain. The psoas muscle is situated posteriorly and lateral to the sympathetic chain.

Indications

Lumbar sympathetic blocks are used extensively in the treatment of reflex sympathetic dystrophy and causalgia. Blockade of the sympathetic nerves can also be performed with a spinal, epidural, or peripheral nerve block, but relief of pain after a lumbar sympathetic block will most clearly delineate the cause of pain as sympathetically mediated. Most fibers headed for the lower extremity pass through the second and third lumbar ganglia, so that a sympathetic block placed at this level provides almost complete sympathetic denervation to the lower extremity. The pain relief obtained is usually immediate and can be long lasting, although a delay of several hours can be seen in some patients.

Peripheral vascular insufficiency represented the initial indication for lumbar sympathetic block, performed in 1926 by Mandl.[2] This continues to be a major reason for sympathetic block, although vascular bypass techniques have partially supplanted its use. Although proximal, fixed lesions are more amenable to surgical correction, diffuse distal disease often responds better to sympathectomy. Local anesthetic blocks provide sufficient evidence concerning the efficacy of sympathetic denervation. If pain relief or signs of vascular improvement are observed, most patients will require a chemical sympathectomy for prolonged relief of symptoms.

Patients with acute herpes zoster and possibly postherpetic neuralgia can benefit from lumbar sympathetic blockade. Improved circulation to the vasa nervosum and peripheral structures can decrease inflammation and prevent further neuronal damage caused by the virus. Sympathetic blockade alone should not be viewed as sufficient treatment in most cases of acute herpes zoster; epidural placement of local anesthetics and corticosteroids in combination with intralesion injections peripherally are necessary for effective early resolution of symptoms.

Deafferented pain syndromes, in particular, phantom limb pain, have had inconsistent results with sympathetic blocks. Truly deafferented pain would not be expected to benefit from sympathetic block, yet many deafferented syndromes do have a component of sympathetically mediated pain. A recent study involving patients after traumatic myelopathy with symptoms of sympathetic pain demonstrated good relief with lumbar sympathetic blocks.[3] Pain from cancer of the lower extremity, gastrointestinal tract distal to the transverse colon, or visceral structures within the pelvis can often be relieved by sympathetic block. The pain often has a neurogenic cause, involving the lumbar or lumbosacral plexuses in particular, with a component of resulting sympathetically mediated pain. Other space-occupying lesions of the pelvis often produce pain, relieved in part by sympathetic block. Acute radiation neuritis and some chronic postradiation neuralgias can be partially relieved from sympathetic blocks.

Many of the above-mentioned cancer pain syndromes have a mixed somatic-visceral cause. Narcotics, whether oral, parenteral, or intraspinal, often inadequately relieve visceral pain. Thus, although sympathetic denervation may not provide complete relief of pain, it can make management with narcotics acceptable to patients. A local anesthetic sympathetic block should be initially performed to

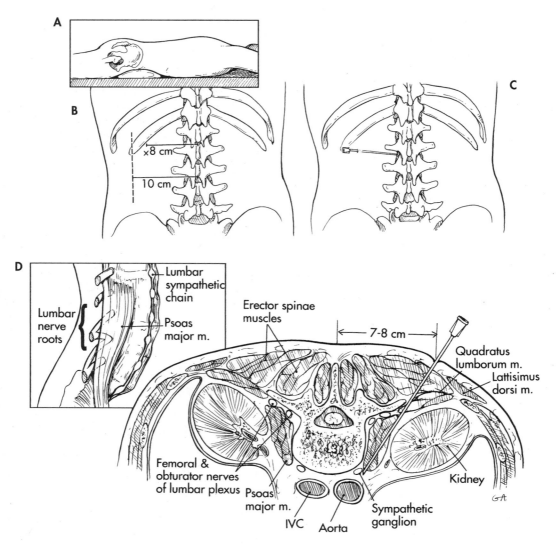

Fig. 20-17 Lateral approach to lumbar sympathetic nerve block. **A,** Patient is positioned prone with pillow beneath anterior iliac spine. **B,** Skin landmarks include twelfth rib, posterior iliac crest, and cephalad tip of L_2 spinous process. **C,** Insert needle 7-8 cm from midline, perpendicular to spinal canal at L_2. **D,** Cross-sectional view of final needle placement. (From Rauck RL: Sympathetic nerve blocks A. In Raj PP, editor: *Practical Management of Pain,* ed 2. St Louis, Mosby, 1992.)

demonstrate therapeutic efficacy. If it is initially effective but symptoms recur, serious consideration should be given to permanent neurolysis.

Finally, patients who suffer from chronic, ill-defined pelvic pain can derive benefit from sympathetic blockade, which can be helpful in patients whose pain presents a diagnostic dilemma. Repeated local anesthetic blocks have broken the pain cycle in some patients. Unfortunately, the results from neurolysis have been disappointing.

Technique

Two techniques are described: a lateral approach first described by Reid[4] and a classic prone position initially reported by Mandl.[1] Obtain informed consent before block, and place an IV line. Sedation is not essential and can be avoided in specific diagnostic cases if sufficient local anes-

thetic is infiltrated along the proposed needle course. Too much local anesthetic can result in partial blockade of the lumbar plexus, resulting in partial blockade of the lower extremity and a false rise in the temperature of the measured extremity. Since the needles pass through many muscular structures of the low back and result in a transient back pain, sedation can effectively alleviate this discomfort associated with needle placement and prevent patients from being afraid of the needles or block.

Lateral approach. Position the patient prone with one or two pillows placed under the lower abdomen across the anterior iliac crest (Fig. 20-18). This allows flexion of the lower lumbar spine, making skin landmarks easier to palpate and opening the spaces between respective transverse processes. Mark and outline the spinous processes of L_2, L_3, and L_4. This can be further checked by marking the in-

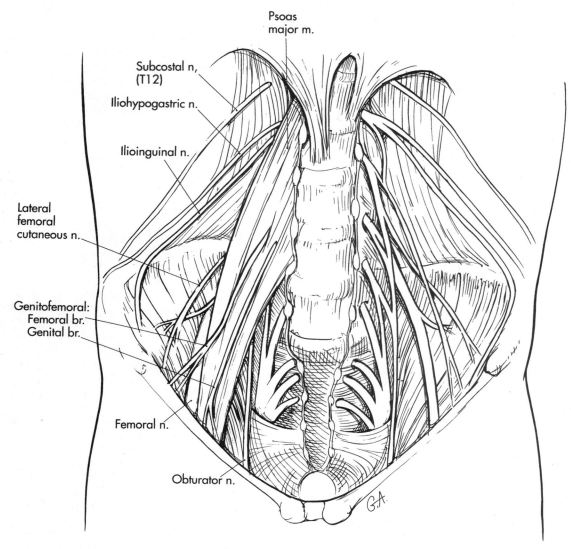

Fig. 20-18 Anterior view of nerves from lumbar plexus as they exit masculature of back. Note genitofemoral nerve on psoas major muscle. (From Racz GB et al: Sympathetic nerve blocks B. In Raj PP, editor: *Practical Management of Pain,* ed 2. St Louis, Mosby, 1992.)

ferior border of T_{12} and the posterior iliac crest. The midpoint between these two lines, 7 cm from the midline, will place the mark at the L_2-L_3 region. This mark should be adjusted to be perpendicular to the caudad aspect of the L_2 vertebra. This corresponds to the interspace between the respective transverse processes of L_2-L_3.

The optimal distance from midline for needle insertion is reported anywhere from 4 to 10 cm.[5,6] Any of these distances has been used successfully by different operators. Distances beyond 8 cm may subject the kidney to possible puncture. Distances of 4 to 5 cm, described in the classical approach, do not allow much cross-sectional area of the vertebral body for projection of the advancing needle tip. For inexperienced operators, this can make identification of the vertebral body more difficult. Reid described the optimal distance as 7 cm from midline to provide easy identifica-

tion of the vertebral body and avoid puncture of renal parenchymal tissue.[4]

Classically, two or three needles have been individually placed at the L_2, L_3, and L_4 levels. Contrast material injected with subsequent x-ray or image-intensification has repeatedly demonstrated good longitudinal spread of solution along the anterolateral border of the vertebral bodies with a single-needle technique. This single-needle technique was used by Reid. Clinical verification has consistently reported temperature rises of the distal extremity. The use of multiple-needle techniques can be reversed for situations when a temperature increase does not occur despite adequate placement or when pain relief is not achieved despite good location in patients with known sympathetic pain.

Once a skin wheal is raised, inject deeper infiltration of local anesthetic solution along the anticipated tract for subsequent needle placement. Too much solution should be avoided, since spillover onto the lumbar plexus can occur and result in some distal temperature rise of the measured extremity.

Advance a 22-gauge, 12- to 18-cm needle slowly until it comes in contact with the vertebral body. Initially, the needle is inserted directly toward the vertebral column. The angle of the needle with respect to the skin can be as shallow as 45° in thin individuals, somewhat steeper in more obese patients. The classic approach advocated locating the transverse process on insertion of the needle, then redirecting either cephalad or caudad to find the intertransverse space and vertebral body.[6] This step, however, is not essential; if the transverse process is not encountered during the initial pass, further insertion of the needle will locate the vertebral body. If the transverse process is bypassed, it is important to recognize that the bone felt is vertebral body. Also, do not confuse the transverse process for vertebral body whenever shallow bone is encountered. This distinction may seem intuitively easy considering the difference in depths of these two structures, but in obese patients the increased adiposity most often exists between skin and transverse process, making that distance longer and shortening the relative discrepancy between transverse process and vertebral body.

Once the vertebral body has been appropriately identified, place a rubber skin marker on the needle 2 to 3 cm from the skin. Remove the needle toward the skin, and then redirect it at a slightly steeper angle. The length of the needles necessitates small-angle changes at the skin to prevent large changes at the distal end. With correct repositioning, the needle passes just lateral to the vertebral body and rests at the anterolateral border. If the needle is placed in the proper location, it will lie anterior to the vertebral insertion of the psoas fascia.

Before injection, carry out careful aspiration in two planes. The aorta on the left and the inferior vena cava on the right both lie reasonably near the sympathetic chain. Test-dose injections of an epinephrine-containing local anesthetic solution protect against both inadvertent intraspinal placement and intravascular injection.

Most preservative-free local anesthetics at commercially prepared concentrations block the sympathetic chain. If a single-needle technique is used, inject 15 ml of volume to insure proper cephalad and caudad spread of solution. Initial injection with 2-chloroprocaine yields a faster onset of block, as manifested by a recorded temperature rise of the distal extremity. A short-lasting agent injected initially will also prevent 18 to 24 hours of quadriceps weakness if the needle is in the psoas muscle and the lumbar plexus inadvertently blocked. After a temperature rise is noted (which can take 15 to 20 minutes in some individuals) and no weakness is found, 15 ml of bupivacaine 0.5% with epinephrine 1:200,000 can be instilled.

Classic "paramedian" approach. Place the patient prone, and outline the spinous processes of L_2, L_3, and L_4. Raise skin wheals 4 to 5 cm lateral to the midline. Insert shorter 8- to 12-cm, 20-gauge needles at a 70° to 80° angle toward the midline. Advance the needle until it makes contact with the transverse process; at a depth of 4 to 6 cm,

place a skin marker 3 to 5 cm from the skin. Then reposition the needle inferiorly and medially to slip off the transverse process and pass to the vertebral body, approximately 2 cm deep to the transverse process. Reposition the needle further to slip off the vertebral body, and advance it to the previously positioned skin marker. The needle should now lie anterior to the psoas fascia at the anterolateral border of the vertebral body. Repeat the process with the other two needles, and inject the solution as previously described.

Neurolytic block

Neurolysis of the lumbar sympathetic chain is easily performed and one of the most useful neurolytic procedures.[7] It can be indicated for recalcitrant reflex sympathetic dystrophy, causalgia, peripheral vascular disease, pelvic malignancies, and deafferentation pain syndromes. Neurolysis should only be considered after local anesthetic blocks of the lumbar sympathetic chain have documented efficacy but have failed to produce long-lasting relief.

Prior screening and preparedness will select those patients suitable for blockade. Possible complications must be adequately explained and informed consent obtained. Place an IV line and give sedation as indicated.

Needle placement for neurolysis does not differ from a local anesthetic lumbar sympathetic block. Image intensification, in particular, fluoroscopy, greatly facilitates placement, allows real-time visualization of drug diffusion, and helps prevent possible complications by ill-placed needles or neurolytic solution. When a single-needle technique is used, fluoroscopy documents adequate cephalad spread to the upper limits of L_2 and caudad diffusion of drug to L_4. Check needle placement before the injection of contrast. This can be done in both anteroposterior and lateral planes. C-arm fluoroscopy is ideal and allows real-time visualization of both planes. Myelography suites commonly image in only one plane but allow spot films to be taken in the lateral position.

Monitor distal skin temperatures during neurolysis for further documentation of block. If any questions remain after the placement of needles, inject a local anesthetic solution before neurolysis and evaluate for signs of efficacy such as a temperature rise and relief of symptoms.

The spread of contrast is characteristic and reproducible. The dye confines itself to the anterolateral border of the vertebral body in a tight, linear fashion. Movement of contrast is cephalad and caudad with no lateral diffusion of drug to the vertebral bodies. Contrast that diffuses laterally most often is being deposited either in the psoas muscle or on the fascia; this appears either as a roundish, poorly circumscribed picture or bandlike with muscular striations visibly present. In either situation, neurolytic agents should not be injected.

Phenol is the agent of choice for neurolysis. It has been shown to have a lower incidence of neuralgias than equivalent injections with alcohol.[8] Although volumes as small as 2 ml through each of three needles have been used, larger volumes (15 ml) through a single needle have been equally efficacious. Concentrations of 6% phenol have been replaced with 10% and 12% solutions with evidence in cat sciatic nerves that higher concentrations do provide more permanent neurologic destruction.[9] After the neurolytic agent has been injected, place 1 ml of saline through the needle to prevent any neurolytic agent from spilling onto somatic nerves during withdrawal.

Catheter placement

Longdwell catheters (Becton & Dickinson), 6- or 8-inch, 16-gauge extracatheters with stylet, are easily placed on the lumbar sympathetic chain for short-term infusions of local anesthetics. If effective and if the clinical situation dictates, a neurolytic solution can then be injected without need for further blockade.

The technique for catheter placement is best performed with the lateral approach as described above. Image intensification, although not mandatory, should be used whenever possible, since precise location allows infusion of lower volumes of solution. If neurolysis is planned after a period of local anesthetic infusion, image intensification can verify that the catheters have not been dislodged since initial placement.

The length of infusion necessary varies with each clinical situation. Infusions lasting 7 days or longer have been managed with a single catheter. Strict sterile technique must be used during placement, and the exit site should be kept sterile and visible for daily checks.

The most common long-term management problem with a catheter system is posterior dislodgement into the psoas muscle, manifested by decreased sensation and weakness of the quadriceps muscles. Nurses must be adequately educated and patients warned to prevent any falls. Dislodgement occurs most often in obese or very active patients and results from excessive movements of the underlying tissues.

Bupivacaine is the agent used for infusions. Initial doses and infusion settings are 0.1% at 6 ml/hr. Both the concentration and rate can be increased if an adequate block cannot be maintained. Rates of 20 ml/hr have been necessary in refractory cases. Concentrations of 0.25% have been used near the end of the infusion period if tachyphylaxis has developed.

A catheter system and infusion of local anesthetics can provide continuous denervation of the sympathetic nervous system. Patients with recalcitrant reflex sympathetic dystrophy, who derive only temporary benefit from a routine lumbar sympathetic block, can respond in the long term to catheter placement. Concomitant, aggressive physical therapy should be prescribed and is tolerated much better by a patient while the catheter is in place.

Complications

The most common side effect from a lumbar sympathetic block is a backache, which results from the placement of the needles through the paravertebral muscles of the back. Carefully explain this to patients before blockade, and the use of a heating pad and ice packs along with rest and occasional muscle relaxants may be necessary.

Intravascular injections of larger volumes of local anesthetics can produce serious, systemic, toxic reactions. This is best avoided using test doses, repeated aspiration, and epinephrine-containing solutions in combination with electrocardiograph monitoring.

Inadvertent subarachnoid injections occur rarely if the needle is mistakenly repositioned from bone into a dural cuff. The length of the needle and its small diameter hinder free flow of CSF. The high pressure generated during aspiration of the small, 22-gauge needle often sucks the arachnoid against the bevel, resulting in no flow of CSF. An initial, small injection of local anesthetic and test for spinal effect will avoid the subsequent total spinal seen if 15 ml of local anesthetic is injected into the subarachnoid space.

Not uncommonly, the needle passes through the intervertebral disk. The sensation of passing through Swiss cheese is easily noted, necessitating removal of the needle and repositioning. Medication cannot be easily injected into a disk. No sequelae have been reported from this occurrence, and any extrusion of disk material would be lateral, away from the spinal canal, and not of any clinical significance.

Renal trauma or puncture of a ureter can occur if proper technique is not followed. Most importantly, the needle should not be inserted more than 7 to 8 cm from the midline. Sequelae would be minimal unless a neurolytic agent were injected, resulting in possible ureteral stricture or extravasation of urine.

Blockade of the genitofemoral nerve or lumbar plexus within the psoas muscle can occur if the needle is placed too far laterally or posteriorly. If a local anesthetic solution is used, a resulting numbness or weakness can occur in the groin, anterior thigh, or quadriceps. To avoid the 18- to 24-hour weakness seen with bupivacaine, inject a short duration agent (2-chloroprocaine) initially and test the strength of the quadriceps.

Lateral spread of neurolytic solution from the lumbar sympathetic chain can result in genitofemoral neuralgia and, less often, lumbar plexus involvement.[8,10,11] Neurolysis can result despite appropriate technique and the appearance of good spread within the proper fascial plane.

Boas et al. report a 6% incidence of genitofemoral neuralgia in their patients.[12] Cousins et al. reported on 35 patients receiving 100% alcohol using a technique without image intensification.[8] Mild neuralgia (less than 1 week) occurred in 14% and severe neuralgia (greater than 1 week) in 26%. Use of a similar technique with phenol resulted in a respective incidence of 6% and 16%. Sensory loss was reported in 5% of patients and motor weakness in 6%.[8]

The genitofemoral nerve is most susceptible at the L_4-L_5 vertebral level, after it has emerged from the psoas major muscle, and lies anterior to the fascia near the sympathetic chain. Most mild neuralgias can be treated with nonnarcotic analgesics and reassurance that this complication is transient. For severe cases Boas has reported success using IV lidocaine 1 to 2 mg/kg over two to three minutes, sufficient to produce light toxicity symptoms. The pain disappears, and normal cutaneous sensation returns. In refractory cases, transcutaneous electrical nerve stimulation, tricyclic antidepressants, and antiepileptic agents may be necessary.

REFERENCES

1. Bonica JJ: *Sympathetic Nerve Blocks for Pain Diagnosis and Therapy.* New York, Breon Laboratories, 1984.
2. Mandl F: *Die paravertebral injection.* Vienna, Springer-Verlag, 1926.
3. Cremer SA, Maynard F, Davidoff G: The reflex sympathetic dystro-

phy syndrome associated with traumatic myelopathy: Report of 5 cases. *Pain* 37:187-192, 1989.

4. Reid W, Watt JK, Gray TG: Phenol injection of the sympathetic chain. *Br J Surg* 57:45-50, 1970.
5. Bonica JJ: *The Management of Pain.* Philadelphia, Lea & Febiger, 1953.
6. Bridenbaugh PO, Cousins MJ: *Neural Blockade in Clinical Anesthesia and Management of Pain.* Philadelphia, JB Lippincott, 1988.
7. Boas RA, Hatangdi VS, Richards EG: Lumbar sympathectomy: A percutaneous chemical technique. *Advances in Pain Research and Therapy* 1:685, 1976.
8. Cousins MJ et al: Neurolytic lumbar sympathetic blockade: Duration of denervation and relief of rest pain. *Anaesth Intensive Care* 7(2):121-135, 1979.
9. Gregg R et al: Electrophysiologic and histopathologic investigation of phenol in renografin as a neurolytic agent. *Anesthesiology* 63:A239, 1985.
10. Dam WH: Therapeutic blockades. *Acta Chirurgica Scandinavia* 343(suppl):89-101, 1965.
11. Raskin NH et al: Postsympathectomy neuralgia amelioration with diphenylhydantoin and carbamazepine. *Am J Surg* 128:75-78, 1974.
12. Boas RA: Sympathetic blocks in clinical practice. In Stanton-Hicks M, editor: *International Anesthesia Clinics, Regional Anesthesia—Advances in Selected Topics, vol 16,* ed 4. Boston, Little, Brown & Co, 1978.

F. Hypogastric Plexus Block

The autonomic nervous system clearly is involved in painful syndromes; nerve blocks and destructive procedures by surgical means and injections of neurolytic substances (i.e., alcohol and phenol) have resulted in successful therapies. However, the hypogastric plexus has not been used in the less invasive block therapies that can readily be repeated and carry less complications than the surgical procedures of presacral neurectomies. Because the pain fibers that travel through the hypogastric plexus bypass the lower spinal cord, usual spinal and epidural nerve blocks are ineffective, commonly failing to give adequate pain relief.

Credit for bringing hypogastric plexus block to the attention of the physician belongs to Ricardo Plancarte and his group in Mexico City.[1,2]

Racz describes his experience with this procedure. His patient had cancer of the rectum followed by abdominal-perineal reaction. Hypogastric plexus anesthetic (0.5% bupivacaine) block gave 8 to 10 hour pain relief, and the following day, phenol injection (6% 10 ml) resulted in 16 months of pain relief. The block had to be repeated on the opposite side 2 years later, by which time there was significant metastases.

Racz's patient population includes the cancer patient and also the intractable noncancer pain sufferer (Table 20-1).

Pelvic pain may travel through a number of pain pathways, including the sympathetics through the celiac ganglion and splanchnic nerves, in addition to the lower spinal

Table 20-1 Patient profile

	Number of patients	Average age	Age range
Male	18	50.2	32-75
Female	16	54.2	30-82
Total	34	52.4	30-82

cord, which in turn explains the failure of lumbar epidural nerve blocks.

Especially in patients with pelvic pain that tends to respond favorably to superior hypogastric plexus block, tenderness can be elicited by putting pressure on the ischial tuberosity (Racz sign), and the patient commonly complains while sitting.

Technique

There are several approaches to the block. For purely pelvic pain, the target is the inferior hypogastric plexus. The needle tip needs to be in front of the promintory (i.e., junction of L_5-S_1). Injection of contrast will spread from the midline L_5-S_1 to lateral pelvic wall and inferiorally to the S_1 nerve root.

If pain involves the ilium (pain or ischial tuberosity pressure—Racz sign), the needle placement needs to be on the lower end of L_5. The contrast will spread in front of L_5 on the surface of the vertebra and the psoas muscle, down into the pelvis towards the S_1 nerve root and laterally towards the pelvic brim.

Needle placement

Place the needle with the patient in the face-down position (Fig. 20-19), under fluoroscopic control. After appropriate sterile prep and draping, follow either the lateral or median approach for the puncture site.

Lateral approach. Draw a line lateral to the L_4-L_5 interspace and measure 7 cm. Use a 15-cm, 20-gauge needle. Direct the needle approximately 45° medial and caudad to miss the transverse process of L_5 and the sacral ala. In the lateral x-ray view, the needle tip needs to be at the anterior junction of L_5-S_1. In the anterior-posterior view, the needle must be at least 1 cm within the bone outline of L_5-S_1.

Medial approach. Rotate the fluoroscopy C-arm 15° laterally and 15° caudally so that the x-ray beam looks into the pelvis. This view enlarges the space between the L_5 transverse process, sacral ala, and the posterior superior iliac spine. Under fluoroscopy using the 15-cm, 20-gauge needle, mark the most inferior and lateral part of this bone-free space. Place the needle and direct it medially and slightly caudad. Rotate C-arm to lateral view and observe needle pass below the transverse process and through the superior part of the L_5 neural foramen. When the anterior edge of L_5 vertebral body at its lower third is reached, aspirate; and if negative for blood, inject 4 to 5 ml of water-soluble contrast material. The contrast should be within the lateral bony edge and the spread as described.

Common problems

Problem	Solution
1. Touching L_5 nerve root	Redirect needle
2. Intravascular spread of contrast even in face of negative aspiration	Redirect; if problem not solved, abort procedure and repeat another day
3. Needle tip is too lateral	Withdraw and redirect

The injection must be in the posterior retroperitoneal space (Fig. 20-20), which is condensed by thin line spread of contrast in the lateral x-ray view. A unique problem is when good pain relief is obtained from one or more local anesthetic injections; but when the neurolytic injection is attempted, the contrast injection is intravascular. We solved this problem by switching to an epidural needle. Position this down to the neural foramen and place a soft-tipped Racz catheter (Tunnel-Cath) with stylet under fluoroscopy. Advance it past the L_5 nerve root through the psoas muscle until the catheter tip is in the appropriate location in both x-ray views without evidence of intravenous spread.

Anatomy

The superior hypogastric plexus lies anterior to the fifth lumbar vertebra, left to the midline, just inferior to the aortic bifurcation. The plexus branches left and right and descends into the pelvis as the inferior hypogastric plexus, which gives rise to the pelvic, middle rectal, vesicle, prostatic, and uterovaginal plexus.[3] The superior hypogastric plexus is often just left of midline and sometimes condenses into several bundles; it has acquired the name *presacral nerve* for this reason. This plexus contains postganglionic sympathetic fibers and afferent pain fibers. Many preganglionic parasympathetic fibers run independently and to the left of the superior hypogastric plexus. The inferior hypogastric plexus receives more parasympathetic fibers from the second, third, and fourth sacral levels.

Three main divisions of the hypogastric plexus are the superior hypogastric plexus, the right and left inferior hypogastric plexus, and the pelvic plexus. The inferior hypogastric plexus gives rise not only to the pelvic plexus but also to the middle rectal plexus, the vesicle plexus, the uterovaginal plexus, and the prostatic plexus. Innervates of the hypogastric plexus include the vagina, rectum, bladder, perineum, vulva, prostate, and uterus. The hypogastric plexus is composed of postganglionic sympathetic fibers, preganglionic parasympathetic fibers, visceral afferent fibers, and C-fibers.

Discussion

A report by Plancarte et al.[2] on 20 patients using 10% phenol, 8 ml volume, resulted in 70% improvement of pain for 3 to 12 months. They also supplemented the somatic component of the pain with epidural steroids and dilute (2% to 3%) phenol. These patients all had advanced carcinoma: cervical, prostatic, testicular, and rectal. The only significant complication was vascular puncture. They did bilateral injections for the midline pelvic pain.

Racz's experience carries the technique to other intractable pelvic pains where multiple diagnostic blocks confirm the pain to be mediated through the hypogastric plexus. All of his neurolytic injections were unilateral. The proximity of the ureter forces one to use not greater than 6% phenol because many injections have been done for noncancerous, sympathetically mediated pain in the vicinity of the ureter (lumbar sympathetic and celiac plexus blocks) without any significant complications.

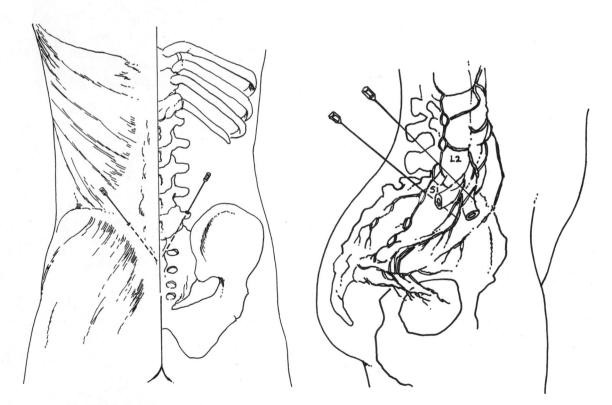

Fig. 20-19 Posterior, lateral, and anterior views of hypogastric plexus approach with reference to skeletal muscle, vessels, and position of needles. (From Plancarte R et al: Hypogastric plexus block: Retroperitoneal approach. *Anesthesiology* 71A:739, 1989.)

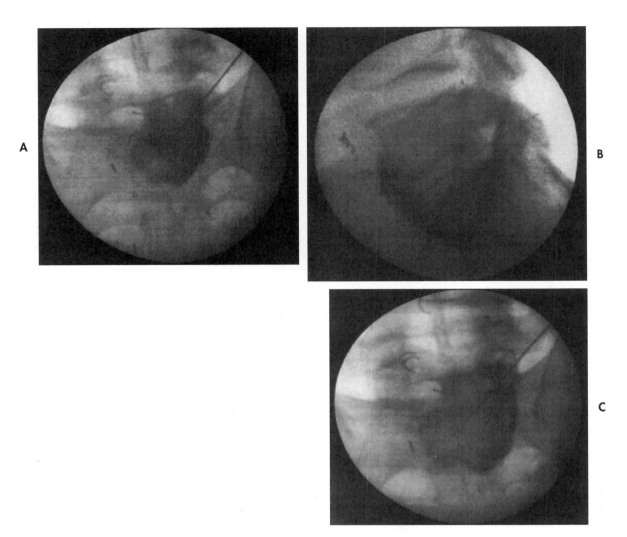

Fig. 20-20 A, Paramedian needle placement between transversal process of L_5 and sacral ala. Spread of 10 ml Omnipaque. **B,** Lateral view shows needle in front of L_5-S_1 disk and spread of contrast in retroperitoneal space. **C,** 10 ml of 6% phenol in saline injected and spread is indicated by displacement of contrast. (From Racz GB et al: Sympathetic nerve blocks B. In Raj PP, editor: *Practical Management of Pain,* ed 2. St Louis, Mosby, 1992.)

Table 20-2 Relief according to diagnosis

	Significant relief on discharge		Duration of relief (months)			
	Yes	**No**	**<1**	**1-3**	**3-6**	**Unspecified**
Pelvic pain	15 (83.33%)	3 (16.67%)	—	5 (33.33%)	7 (46.67%)	3
Vaginal pain or dyspareunia	3 (60%)	2 (40%)				1
			33.33%	66.67%		
Scrotal/perineal pain	2 (40%)	3 (60%)	100%			
Coccydinia	4	2				2
Buttock/ischial pain	19 (63.33%)	11 (36.67%)		6	2	38
			31.58%	10.53%	15.70%	42.10%
Iliac/inguinal pain	5	10	20%	1	20%	13
	33.33%	66.67%				60%
Thigh pain	—	6				
	—	100%				

Many patients had two or more complaints or areas of pain for which hypogastric block was performed. The total, therefore, will exceed the actual number of blocks performed.

Surgical presacral neurectomy is remarkably trouble free in terms of serious secondary bladder and sexual dysfunction complications. One should not attempt bilateral neurolytic hypogastric blocks in male patients because of the possibility of sexual dysfunction. However, the technique is safe in intractable noncancer-caused pelvic pain, but so far experience is limited to unilateral procedures both in male and female patients.

Conclusion

Hypogastric plexus block offers a new technique for relieving pelvic pain for patients suffering from cancer-caused autonomic pain originating from the pelvis (Table 20-2). In addition, noncancer-origin intractable pain also responds to local anesthetic as well as neurolytic injection of 6% phenol into the superior hypogastric plexus and into the presacral nerves. Patient selection is still a problem, but diagnostic hypogastric plexus block is safe using the technique described.

REFERENCES

1. Plancarte R: Personal communication, 1994.
2. Plancarte R et al: Hypogastric plexus block: Retroperitoneal approach. *Anesthesiology* 71:A739, 1989.
3. Renaer M: *Chronic Pelvic Pain in Women.* New York, Springer-Verlag, 1981.

QUESTIONS: AUTONOMIC NERVE BLOCKS

1. The ganglion that is located posterior to the middle turbinate, deep to the lateral nasal mucosa is called:
   A. Geniculate ganglion
   B. Sphenopalatine ganglion
   C. Otic ganglion
   D. Gasserian ganglion

2. In this approach for stellate ganglion block, the patient lies supine, with the head hyperextended. The C_6 tubercle is palpated and confirmed by locating the cricoid cartilage. The common carotid artery is retracted laterally. Then a 4- to 5-cm long needle is inserted between the trachea and the finger retracting the carotid vessel towards the anterior surface of the transverse process:
   A. Anterolateral approach
   B. Anterior approach
   C. Posterior approach
   D. Posterolateral approach

3. The preganglionic sympathetic nerves that are destined to end in the celiac, aorticorneal, and superior mesenteric ganglia come from these sites of anterolateral horn of the spinal cord:
   A. T_1-T_4
   B. T_5-T_{12}
   C. T_{12}-L_2
   D. L_2-L_5

4. The celiac plexus is located just anterior to the crux of the diaphragm and extends several centimeters:
   A. Anterolaterally around the aorta
   B. Posterolaterally around the aorta
   C. Anteromedial to lumbar sympathetic ganglia
   D. Posteromedial to lumbar sympathetic ganglia

5. For patients with large abdominal mass and difficulty in lying prone, this approach is indicated for celiac plexus block:
   A. Lateral approach
   B. Anterior approach
   C. Sitting approach
   D. Surgical open approach

ANSWERS

1. B
2. B
3. B
4. A
5. B

256

PART FOUR

Special Techniques

21 Epidural Steroids

Honorio T. Benzon

NONORGANIC PHYSICAL SIGNS IN LOW BACK PAIN

Waddell et al.[1] described five types of nonorganic physical signs in low back pain: nonorganic tenderness, stimulation tests, distraction test, regional disturbances, and overreaction (Box 21-1). Nonorganic tenderness can be superficial (tenderness to light pinch in the back) or nonanatomic. Stimulation tests include axial loading and trunk rotation. Axial loading is positive when radicular pain is precipitated by vertical loading on the patient's head, while positive trunk rotation test is characterized by back pain on passive rotation of the shoulders and pelvis. An example of distraction is a discrepancy of the straight leg raising on distraction as compared to formal testing. Regional disturbances include sensory and motor abnormalities that cannot be explained on a neuroanatomic basis. Overreaction is disproportionate verbalization, facial expression, muscle tension and tremor, collapsing, or sweating. Although isolated positive signs are ignored, three or more of the five signs is clinically significant.

CAUSES OF BACK PAIN FROM MECHANICAL PROBLEMS

Back pain can be due to several causes[2] (Box 21-2). Back and radicular leg pain secondary to a mechanical problem such as herniated disc can be due to compression and deformation of the nerve[3] or secondary to inflammatory changes in the nerves.[4] Mechanical factors cannot solely explain the occurrence of pain for the following reasons. First, clinical symptoms and signs are not necessarily present in patients with disc herniation.[5-7] Second, improvement with nonsurgical therapy may not be associated with a change in the pathologic anatomy.[7] Lastly, clinical improvement after chymopapain or epidural steroid injections precedes any observable structural change.[4]

Inflammatory changes in the nerves had been proposed as a significant contributor to the production of back pain. Nerve roots appear swollen and inflamed on myelography and during surgery.[8,9] Persistent altered fibrinolytic activity in patients with chronic back pain suggests a possible role for chronic inflammation.[10] Nucleus pulposus induces marked inflammatory responses in the dura, nerve roots, and the spinal cord.[4] High levels of inflammatory phospholipase A_2 activity has been recorded in lumbar disk herniations. The phospholipase A_2 activity in extracts from human lumbar disk is 20 to 10,000 times more than the phospholipase A_2 activity from any other human source.[4]

The occurrence of back pain in patients without demonstrable disk pathology has been ascribed to tears in the an-nulus, without nuclear herniation, and loss of nuclear fluid, especially the protoglycans.[11]

MECHANISM OF ANALGESIC EFFECT OF STEROIDS

Steroids relieve pain by reducing inflammation and by blocking transmission of nociceptive C fiber input. Steroids decrease inflammation by inhibiting the action of phospholipase A_2.[12,13] Phospholipase A_2 has been found to induce membrane injury and edema in animals by generating membrane perturbants, unsaturated fatty acids, and lysoderivatives.[14] More importantly, phospholipase A is the enzyme responsible for the liberation of arachidonic fatty acids from cell membranes at the site of inflammation.[13,15] This is the rate-limiting step in the production of prostaglandins and leukotrienes. Prostaglandins and leukotrienes sensitize small neurons and enhance pain generation.[16-18] Altered permeability in response to inflammatory mediators results in venous congestion and intraneural edema. Abnormal conduction by nerve fibers and generation of pain follow.[4]

Steroids also produce analgesia by blocking transmission of nociceptive input. Corticosteroids prevent the development of ectopic neural discharges from experimental neuromas and suppress ongoing discharge in chronic neuromas.[19] This suppression of neuroma discharge has been attributed to a direct membrane action and not to an antiinflammatory effect of the steroid. Local application of methylprednisolone acetate has been found to block transmission in C fibers but not in A beta fibers.[20] The effect was reversible, suggesting direct membrane action of the steroid.

TRIGGER POINT INJECTIONS

Back pain may be due to musculoskeletal myofascial problems resulting in myofascial syndrome or fibromyalgia syndrome.[3] The presence of a trigger point is a diagnostic feature of myofascial pain syndrome. Trigger points are identified by subjective and objective findings.[21] Subjective complaints include easy fatigability, stiffness, referred pain predictable for that trigger point, and deep tenderness at the trigger point. Referred pain patterns from trigger points in the sternocleidomastoid,[21] facial, cervical, and scapular regions, and upper and lower extremities[22] have been described. The pain-reference zone of a trigger point is predictable from one patient to another. The following characteristics are observed in these pain-reference zones: diffuse deep tenderness and cutaneous hyperalgesia; skeletal muscle spasm; and vasomotor, secretory, and other autonomic changes.[21] Objective trigger point findings include a

Box 21-1 NONORGANIC PHYSICAL SIGNS IN LOW BACK PAIN

Tenderness
    Superficial
    Nonanatomic
Stimulation
    Axial loading
    Rotation
Distraction
    Straight leg raising
Regional disturbances
    Weakness
    Sensory disturbances
Overreaction

Adapted from Waddell G et al: Nonorganic physical signs in low back pain. *Spine* 5:117-125, 1980.

Box 21-2 DIFFERENTIAL DIAGNOSIS OF LOW BACK PAIN

Bone disease
Circulatory disorders
Congenital disorders
Degenerative disease/bony structural changes
Infections
Inflammatory diseases
Mechanical problems
Metabolic disorders
Musculoskeletal/myofascial problems
Neuropathy
Neuropathic changes secondary to neural scarring, fibrosis, mechanical causes, metabolic conditions, heavy metal toxicity
Psychologic problems
Referred visceral pain from pulmonary, gastrointestinal, genitourinary, or gynecological sources
Trauma—strains, sprains, fractures
Tumors—benign, malignant

Adapted from Rowlingson J: Low back pain and pain of the lower extremity. In Raj PP, editor: *Practical Management of Pain,* ed 2. St Louis, Mosby, 1992.

palpably firm, tense band in the muscle; production of a local twitch response; restricted stretch range of motion; weakness without atrophy; and no neurologic deficit.[21] When the muscle is placed under moderate passive tension and the band is snapped briskly with the palpating finger, the "jump sign" is elicited, which is caused by visible shortening of the muscle that contains the band.[23]

The mechanisms for development of trigger points have been proposed.[24] Trauma locally tears the sarcoplasmic reticulum and releases calcium. The calcium, together with the available adenosine triphosphate, continuously activates local contractile activity. The intense muscle metabolic activity produces substances that sensitize sensory nerve endings. Reflex, localized vasoconstriction is stimulated to control the runaway metabolic activity.[23] To restore normal function, stretching of the locked actin and myosin filaments has been recommended to terminate the runaway contracture activity.[24] This allows enough adenosine triphosphate to accumulate and restore normal sarcoplasmic reticulum function and also allows circulation to remove the noxious metabolic products.

The spray-and-stretch technique and trigger point injection are effective treatments for myofascial trigger points. These are followed by deep massage, specific manual resistive exercises, and an exercise program.[22] Travell has described the spray-and-stretch technique.[21,23] Trigger point injection involves the injection of a local anesthetic with or without a steroid. Procaine,[23] lidocaine,[25] bupivacaine,[26] etidocaine,[26] and mepivacaine[27] have been used.

A study that compared mepivacaine to saline trigger point injections showed no difference in results.[27] In this study, the effect of the benzyl alcohol preservative in the saline, which has a local anesthetic property, cannot be excluded. Another study showed bupivacaine or etidocaine to have better results than preservative-free saline.[26] A randomized, double-blind evaluation compared lidocaine, lidocaine with steroid, dry needling or acupuncture, and vapocoolant spray with acupressure, and showed that therapy without medication was as good as therapy with medication.[25] The improvement with acupuncture and vapocoolant/acupressure therapy was 63% versus 42% for the local anesthetic/steroid combination. The investigators concluded that the injected substance was not a critical factor, since dry needling gave equal symptomatic relief.[25] Relief with dry needling or acupuncture, termed *hyperstimulation analgesia,* can be explained by the gate-control theory of pain[28] or by the release of endorphins.[29]

The advantage of a local anesthetic-containing solution is that the injection is not painful. The local anesthetic also reverses the muscle spasm and induces vasodilation, which are processes that contribute to the production of trigger points. The steroid is added because of histologic evidence of mild inflammatory reaction in the muscle.[30] The steroid may be dexamethasone sodium phosphate (4 mg/50 ml of local anesthetic)[30] or triamcinolone hexacetonide (0.75 ml/0.75 ml of local anesthetic).[25] Repeating the trigger point injection every 4 to 7 days has been recommended until long-lasting diminution of the pain is achieved.[30]

Myofascial trigger point syndrome should not be confused with fibromyalgia syndrome. Instead of trigger points, fibromyalgia is characterized by tender points which are areas of excessive tenderness that do not exhibit the "jump sign." In fibromyalgia, there are usually many tender points, depression is a prominent component, disturbed sleep patterns are frequent, and women are mostly affected.[31,32] Fibromyalgia usually responds to antidepressants, muscle relaxants, patient counseling, and local anesthetic spray or injection.[31]

Steroid injections for low back pain of mechanical cause

Steroids for low back pain can be administered by intramuscular (IM), epidural, and intrathecal routes. The rationale for steroid use is its antiinflammatory effect[33] and its ability to block nociceptive C fiber input.[19,20] The IM injection of decreasing doses of dexamethasone was found effective in relieving back pain secondary to herniated disk. Of the 80 patients given this treatment, 66 (73%) either had no pain or only mild pain, whereas 11 (12%) required surgery.[34]

Epidural steroid injections

Epidural steroid injections have been recommended to deliver the drug to the area of the affected nerve roots, thereby decreasing the systemic effect of the administered steroid. White and colleagues showed that epidural steroid injection was most effective in the presence of nerve root irritation[35] (Table 21-1). Signs of nerve root irritation include radicular pain, dermatomal hypesthesia, weakness of muscle groups innervated by the involved nerve roots, decreased deep tendon reflexes, and diminished straight leg raising.

Kepes and Duncalf reviewed the literature on epidural steroid injection and concluded that its use was not scientifically proven.[36] On the other hand, I have concluded that its use is warranted.[33,37,38] There are seven prospective, randomized, controlled studies on the use of epidural steroid injection in patients with disk pathology.[39-45] Four of these studies are discussed in detail (Table 21-2); three studies have limitations. In one study, Vent injected the steroid into the epidural and intrathecal spaces during laminectomy.[39] In the Breivik et al. study, the patients had chronic pain, and one third of them had had a previous laminectomy.[40] In the Yates study, no diagnostic criteria for inclusion was stated, and it was not clear whether the patients had acute or chronic low back pain or had previous back surgery.[41]

Beliveau gave caudal injections of methylprednisolone, procaine, and saline to 18 patients.[42] The same number of patients had caudal injections of procaine and saline. He noted that the two groups responded equally to the injections.

In another study, Cuckler and colleagues gave epidural methylprednisolone in water and procaine to their treatment group and gave saline and procaine to their control group.[43] They found that the success rate was the same in the two groups. Their study has several shortcomings. The cause of their patients' back pain was not uniform. Some had herniated disk, others had spinal stenosis, and a few patients had had a laminectomy. In addition, their control solution con-

Table 21-1 Effectiveness of epidural steroid injections on different causes of back pain

Causes of back pain	Effect of steroid injection
Annulus tear ("back sprain")	Hastens recovery
Chronic lumbar degenerative disk disease	Transient relief
Herniated nucleus pulposus without neurologic deficit	Transient relief
Herniated nucleus pulposus with nerve root irritation	Therapeutic
Herniated nucleus pulposus with nerve root compression	Therapeutic
Spondylolysis	Rarely of value
Spondylolisthesis	Therapeutic if nerve root irritation is present
Facet arthropathy	Steroid injection into the apophyseal joint may be successful
Scoliosis	May be effective if nerve root entrapment is present
Ankylosis spondylitis	Ineffective
Spinal stenosis	Transient relief
Functional low back pain	Ineffective

Adapted from Benzon HT: Epidural steroid injections for low back pain and lumbosacral radiculopathy. *Pain* 24:277-295, 1986.

Table 21-2 Results of controlled studies on epidural steroid injections*

Type of study	Cause of back pain	Duration of symptoms	Treatments studied, route	Number of injections	Success rate (%), steroid vs. control
P,R†	Disk lesion	Not specified	MP + procaine vs. procaine, caudal	1-2	18/24 (75%); 75% vs. 67%
P,R,DB‡	Herniated disk, spinal stenosis, status post laminectomy	13 weeks to 36 months	MP + sterile water + procaine vs. saline + procaine, lumbar	1	25/42 (61%); 61% vs. 62.5%
P,R,DB§	Degenerated disk	<1 year	MP + saline vs. saline, lumbar	1-2	21/35 (60%); 60% vs. 31%
P,R,DB‖	Herniated disk	1 to 3 weeks	MP vs. saline, lumbar	1	Same results (25%-70%)

Adapted from Benzon HT: Epidural steroid injections for low back pain and lumbosacral radiculopathy. *Pain* 24:277-295, 1986.
*P, prospective; R, randomized; DB, double blind; MP, methylprednisolone.
†Beliveau P: A comparison between epidural anesthesia with and without corticosteroid in the treatment of sciatica. *Rheumatol Phys Med* 11:490-493, 1971.
‡Cuckler JM et al: The use of epidural steroids in the treatment of lumbar radicular pain. *J Bone Joint Surg Am* 67:63-66, 1985.
§Dilke TDW, Burry HC, Grahame R: Extradural corticosteroid injection in management of lumbar nerve root compression. *BMJ* 2:635-637, 1973.
‖Snoek W, Weber H, Jorgensen B: Double-blind evaluation of extradural methylprednisolone for herniated lumbar discs. *Acta Orthop Scand* 48:635-641, 1977.

tained procaine, instead of a placebo. Coomes[44] showed that caudal injections of procaine gave better results (60% versus 25%) and patients had shorter recovery periods (11 versus 31 days) than with bed rest alone. Cuckler[43] also evaluated patients 1 day after epidural injection, which is not an adequate time for the steroid to exert its effect.

Two studies have similar patient populations. Dilke and co-workers[45] found significantly better results in the steroid group, whereas Snoek et al.[46] did not find statistical significance, probably because of the numerous criteria that they employed. Snoek and colleagues could have gotten better results if they had diluted their steroid, which would have provided a better spread and also would have decreased the concentration of the polyethylene glycol vehicle in the steroid preparation.

Although the steroid is usually diluted in saline or local anesthetic, relief is mainly due to the steroid.[47] The diluent spreads the steroid better to the various nerve roots inflamed in the presence of a herniated disk[9] and also decreases the concentration of the polyethylene glycol vehicle. Polyethylene glycol caused degenerative lesions in rat sciatic nerves,[48] and at 40% concentration, can temporarily block conduction of the A, B, and C nerve fibers.[49] However, the concentration of the polyethylene glycol in most commercial steroid preparations is 2.8% to 3.0%.

Methylprednisolone or triamcinolone can also be used and, although there has been no study that directly compares the two drugs, they seem to be equally effective. The epidural injection of triamcinolone[50] or methylprednisolone[51] does not cause significant inflammatory changes in the spinal nerve roots and meninges.

Most patients take several days to respond to epidural steroid injection. Green and co-workers noted that 37% of their patients responded to the steroid within 2 days, 59% noted relief between 4 and 6 days, and 4% improved after 6 days.[52] It is therefore advisable to wait at least a week before deciding on a subsequent injection. If there is no response to the initial injection, some investigators recommend against further injections. Others recommend one or two more injections. Warr et al. noted that 84 of 144 previously unresponsive patients improved after one or two more epidural steroid injections.[53] Usually, three injections of steroids is the maximum number given, since Brown noted no further benefit after three injections.[54]

Response to the epidural steroid injection is related to the duration of symptoms (Table 21-3). Patients who have had symptoms less than 3 months have response rates of 83% to 100%.[52,55,56] When radiculopathy has been present for 6 months or less, response decreases to between 67% and 81%[55,57] and to 46% in patients who have had symptoms over 1 year.[53] Patients with shorter duration of symptoms also have a more sustained relief than those with chronic pain. Patients with chronic back pain have better response if they have a symptom-free interval (i.e., new radiculopathy), if their new symptoms have a recent onset, and if their radicular symptoms involve a different nerve root.

Studies that prospectively followed patients after epidural steroid injection had different results, probably because the patients studied had different causes and different durations

of their back pain (Table 21-4). Green and colleagues and Snoek and co-workers studied patients with herniated disk. In Green's study,[52] 41% of the patients who responded had sustained relief for at least a year. In Snoek's study,[45] 45% of the patients ultimately underwent a laminectomy. The patients that Cuckler and colleagues[43] studied either had herniated disk or spinal stenosis. At follow-ups, from 13 to 30 months, 26% of the patients with herniated disk and 22% of the patients with spinal stenosis were still improved. White and colleagues[35] studied patients with different causes of back pain (see Table 21-1). They noted success rates at 6 months for 34% of their patients with acute pain and for 12% of their patients with chronic pain, whereas their patients' overall success rate at 2 years was 1.3%.[35]

Table 21-3 Success rate of epidural steroids related to duration of back pain[a]

Duration of symptoms (months)	Success rate
≤3	83%-100%[b,c,d]
3-6	67%-81%[c,e]
6-12	44%-69%[c,e,f]
>12	46%-58%[c,f]

[a]Results in postlaminectomy patients not included.
[b]Green PWB et al: The role of epidural cortisone injection in the treatment of discogenic low back pain. *Clin Orthop* 153:121-125, 1980.
[c]Harley C: Extradural corticosteroid infiltration. A follow-up study of 50 cases. *Ann Phys Med* 9:22-28, 1967.
[d]Brown FW: Management of discogenic pain using epidural and intrathecal steroids. *Clin Orthop* 129:72-78, 1977.
[e]Heyse-Moore G: A rational approach to the use of epidural medication in the treatment of sciatic pain. *Acta Orthop Scand* 49:366-370, 1978.
[f]Warr AC et al: Chronic lumbosciatic syndrome treated by epidural steroid injection and manipulation. *Practitioner* 209:53-59, 1972.

Table 21-4 Follow-up results of epidural steroid injections*

Duration of pain	Duration of follow-up	Follow-up success rate
≤ 6 mos	1.5 yrs (6 mos to 5 yrs)	41%†
1 to 3 wks	14 ± 6 mos	(52% had laminectomy)‡
13 wks to 36 mos	20.8 mos (13 to 30 mos)	26% (HNP); 22% (SS)§
1 day to 6 mos	6 mos	34% (acute); 12% (chronic)
	24 mos	1.3%‖

HNP, herniated nucleus pulposus; SS, spinal stenosis.
*Only studies that followed their patients for at least 6 months are included.
†Green PWB et al: The role of epidural cortisone injection in the treatment of discogenic low back pain. *Clin Orthop* 153:121-125, 1980.
‡Dilke TDW, Barry HC, Grahame R: Extradural corticosteroid injection in management of lumbar nerve root compression. *BMJ* 2:635-637, 1973.
§Cuckler JM et al: The use of epidural steroids in the treatment of lumbar radicular pain. *J Bone Joint Surg Am* 67:63-66, 1985.
‖White AH, Derby R, Wynne G: Epidural injections for the diagnosis and treatment of low back pain. *Spine* 5:78-86, 1980.

The epidural administration of steroids can have a systemic effect; cases of Cushing's syndrome have been published.[58] The suppression of the hypothalamic-pituitary-adrenal system has occurred in patients up to 3[59] to 5 weeks[60] after an epidural administration of steroids.

Epidural steroid injection is just another modality in the treatment of low back pain. Other treatments include bed rest, analgesics, and muscle relaxants during the acute stage;[61] physical therapy exercises; training in proper body mechanics; and identification and management of any psychologic, financial, marital, and work-related problems. The proper role of some of these treatments has been addressed by Deyo and co-workers.[62,63]

Patients whose herniated disks are conservatively managed can have prolonged improvement. Long-term follow-up showed that 68% to 82% of patients treated with IM dexamethasone,[34] bed rest,[64] or bed rest with back support[65] had either no pain or only mild pain; only 7% to 12% of the patients needed laminectomy.[34,64,65]

Intrathecal steroid injections

The intrathecal administration of steroids had been contraindicated because of the possible development of arachnoiditis.[33] Because arachnoiditis developed in patients who had numerous intrathecal steroid injections,[49] its cautious use has been recently recommended.[66] Intrathecal steroid injection does not seem to be effective; a study showed that patients who did not respond to an epidural steroid injection did not respond to a subsequent intrathecal steroid injection.[67]

Facet joint injections

Facet joints are true synovial joints that connect adjacent vertebrae posteriorly. The synovial membrane contains a rich supply of blood vessels and nerves. The capsule blends with the ligamentum flavum medially and superiorly, which prevents the capsule from protruding into the spinal foramen or between the articular surfaces of the joint. Abnormalities of the facet joint such as inflammation, arthritis, or segmental instability can result in the painful so-called *facet syndrome*.

Facet joint involvement predominantly causes back pain without nerve root irritation. The classic symptoms of a facet syndrome are hip and buttock pain; cramping leg pain, primarily above the knee; low back stiffness; and absence of paresthesia.[68] Signs include local paralumbar tenderness, pain on hyperextension of the spine; absence of neurologic deficit; absence of nerve root tension signs; and hip, buttock, or back pain on straight leg raising.[68]

Several prospective studies did not find significant improvement with facet joint injections. In one study, improvement was noted to be independent from the injected solution, including saline.[69] In another study, mean pain relief was only 29%, and the authors concluded that the facet joint was usually not the cause of pain in a majority of low back pain patients.[70] In a third study, no statistical difference was noted between methylprednisolone and saline injection regarding pain relief or improvement in back flexion or functional status.[71]

REFERENCES

1. Waddell G et al: Nonorganic physical signs in low back pain. *Spine* 5:117-125, 1980.
2. Rowlingson J: Low back pain and pain of the lower extremity. In Raj PP, editor: *Practical Management of Pain,* ed 2. St Louis, Mosby, 1992.
3. Howe JF, Loeser JD, Calvin WH: Mechanosensitivity of dorsal root ganglia and chronically injured axons: A physiological basis for the radicular pain of nerve root compression. *Pain* 3:25-41, 1977.
4. Saal JS et al: High levels of inflammatory phospholipase A$_2$ activity in lumbar disc herniations. *Spine* 15:674-678, 1990.
5. Hitselberger WE, Witten RM: Abnormal myelograms in asymptomatic patients. *J Neurosurg* 28:204-206, 1968.
6. Wiesel SW et al: A study of computer assisted tomography: I. The incidence of positive CAT scan in an asymptomatic group of patients. *Spine* 9:549-551, 1984.
7. Saal JA, Saal JS: The nonoperative treatment of herniated nucleus pulposus with radiculopathy: An outcome study. *Spine* 14:431-437, 1989.
8. Berg A: Clinical and myelographic studies of conservatively treated cases of lumbar intervertebral disc protrusion. *Acta Chir Scand* 104:124-129, 1953.
9. Murphy RW: Nerve roots and spinal nerves in degenerated disc disease: An outcome study. *Spine* 14:431-437, 1989.
10. Klimiuk PS et al: Serial measurements of fibrinolytic activity in acute low back pain and sciatica. *Spine* 12:925-928, 1987.
11. McCarron RF et al: The inflammatory effect of nucleus pulposus. A possible element in the pathogenesis of low back pain. *Spine* 12:760-764, 1987.
12. Hirata F et al: A phospholipase A$_2$ inhibitory protein in rabbit neutrophils induced by glucocorticoids. *Proc Natl Acad Sci USA* 77:2533-2536, 1980.
13. Franson RC, Weir DC: Inhibition of a potent phospholipase A$_2$-activity in the synovial fluid of patients with arthritis by nonsteroidal antiinflammatory agents. *Clin Res* 31:650A, 1983.
14. Vishwanath BS, Fawzy AA, Franson RC: Edema inducing activity of phospholipase A$_2$ purified from human synovial fluid and inhibition by aristocolochic acid. *Inflammation* 12:549-561, 1988.
15. Famaey JP: Phospholipases, eicosanoid production and inflammation. *Clin Rheumatol* 1:84-94, 1982.
16. Levine LD et al: Leukotriene F$_4$ produces hyperalgesia that is dependent on polymorphonuclear leukotrienes. *Science* 225:743-745, 1984.
17. Levine LD, Taiwo Y: Hyperalgesic properties of 15 lipoxygenase products of arachidonic acid. *Proc Natl Acad Sci USA* 83:5331-5334, 1986.
18. Pateromichelakis S, Rood JP: Prostaglandin E$_2$ increases mechanically evoked potentials in the peripheral nerve. *Experientia* 37:282-284, 1981.
19. Devor M, Govrin-Lippman R, Raber P: Corticosteroids suppress ectopic neural discharge originating in experimental neuromas. *Pain* 22:127-137, 1985.
20. Johansson A, Hao J, Sjolund B: Local corticosteroid application blocks transmission in normal nociceptive C-fibres. *Acta Anaesthesiol Scand* 34:335-338, 1990.
21. Travell J: Identification of myofascial trigger syndromes: A case of atypical facial neuralgia. *Arch Phys Med Rehabil* 62:100-106, 1981.
22. Rubin D: Myofascial trigger point syndromes: An approach to management. *Arch Phys Med Rehabil* 62:107-110, 1981.
23. Travell J: Myofascial trigger points: Clinical view. In Bonica JJ, Albe-Fessard D, editors: *Advances in Pain Research and Therapy.* New York, Raven Press, 1976.
24. Simon DG: Myofascial trigger points: A need for understanding. *Arch Phys Med Rehabil* 62:97-99, 1981.
25. Garvey TA, Marks MR, Wiesel SW: A prospective, randomized double-blind evaluation of trigger point injection therapy for low back pain. *Spine* 14:962-964, 1989.
26. Hameroff SR et al: Comparison of bupivacaine, etidocaine, and saline for trigger-point therapy. *Anesth Analg* 60:752-755, 1981.
27. Frost FA, Jesen B, Siggaard-Anderson J: A controlled, double-blind comparison of mepivacaine injection versus saline injection for myofascial pain. *Lancet* 1:499-501, 1980.
28. Melzack R: Myofascial trigger points: Relation to acupuncture and mechanism of pain. *Arch Phys Med Rehabil* 62:114-117, 1981.
29. Sjolund B, Terenius L, Erickson M: Increased cerebrospinal fluid lev-

els of endorphins after electroacupuncture. *Acta Physiol Scand* 100:382-384, 1977.

30. Brown BR: Diagnosis and therapy of common myofascial syndromes. *JAMA* 239:646-648, 1978.

31. Goldenberg DC: Fibromyalgia syndrome. An emerging but controversial condition. *JAMA* 257:2782-2787, 1987.

32. Boissevain MD, McCain GA: Toward an integrated understanding of fibromyalgia syndrome. I. Medical and pathophysiologic aspects. *Pain* 45:227-238, 1991.

33. Benzon HT: Epidural steroid injections for low back pain and lumbosacral radiculopathy. *Pain* 24:277-295, 1986.

34. Green LN: Dexamethasone in the management of symptoms due to herniated lumbar disc. *J Neurol Neurosurg Psychiatry* 38:1211-1217, 1975.

35. White AH, Derby R, Wynne G: Epidural injections for the diagnosis and treatment of low back pain. *Spine* 5:78-86, 1980.

36. Kepes ER, Duncalf D: Treatment of backache with spinal injections of local anesthetics, spinal and systemic. *Pain* 22:33-47, 1985.

37. Benzon HT: Epidural steroid injections. *Pain Digest* 1:271-280, 1992.

38. Benzon HT: Epidural steroids. In Raj PP, editor: *Practical Management of Pain*, ed 2. St Louis, Mosby, 1992.

39. Vent J: Eine prospektive randomisierte studie zur beeinflussung der beschwerden nach lumbaler diskotomie durch intraoperative cortisoneaapilkation in die wurzeltaschen sowie in den periduralraum. *Z Orthop Ihre Grenzbeg* 119:284-286, 1981.

40. Breivik H et al: Treatment of chronic low back pain and sciatica: Comparison of caudal epidural steroid injections of bupivacaine and methylprednisolone with bupivacaine followed by saline. In Bonica JJ, Albe-Fessard D, editors: *Advances in Pain Research and Therapy.* New York, Raven Press, 1976.

41. Yates DW: A comparison of the types of epidural injection commonly used in the treatment of low back pain and sciatica. *Rheumatol Rehab* 17:181-186, 1978.

42. Beliveau P: A comparison between epidural anesthesia with and without corticosteroid in the treatment of sciatica. *Rheumatol Phys Med* 11:490-493, 1971.

43. Cuckler JM et al: The use of epidural steroids in the treatment of lumbar radicular pain. *J Bone Joint Surg Am* 67:63-66, 1985.

44. Coomes EN: A comparison between epidural anesthesia and bed rest in sciatica. *BMJ* 1:20-24, 1961.

45. Dilke TDW, Burry HC, Grahame R: Extradural corticosteroid injection in management of lumbar nerve root compression. *BMJ* 2:635-637, 1973.

46. Snoek W, Weber H, Jorgensen B: Double-blind evaluation of extradural methylprednisolone for herniated lumbar discs. *Acta Orthop Scand* 48:635-641, 1977.

47. Swerdlow M, Sayle-Creer W: A study of extradural medication in relief of the lumbosciatic syndrome. *Anaesthesia* 25:341-345, 1970.

48. Wood MKM, Arguelles J, Norenberg MD: Degenerative lesions in rat sciatic nerves after local injections of methylprednisolone in aqueous solution. *Reg Anesth* 5:181-186, 1978.

49. Benzon HT et al: The effect of polyethylene glycol on mammalian nerve impulses. *Anesth Analg* 66:553-559, 1987.

50. Delaney TJ et al: Epidural steroid effects on nerves and meninges. *Anesth Analg* 59:610-614, 1980.

51. Cicala RS et al: Methylprednisolone acetate does not cause inflammatory changes in the epidural space. *Anesthesiology* 72:556-558, 1990.

52. Green PWB et al: The role of epidural cortisone injection in the treatment of discogenic low back pain. *Clin Orthop* 153:121-125, 1980.

53. Warr AC et al: Chronic lumbosciatic syndrome treated by epidural steroid injection and manipulation. *Practitioner* 209:53-59, 1972.

54. Brown FW: Protocol for management of acute low back pain with or without radiculopathy, including the use of epidural and intrathecal steroids. In Brown FW, editor: *American Academy of Orthopaedic Surgeons Symposium on the Lumbar Spine.* St Louis, Mosby, 1981.

55. Harley C: Extradural corticosteroid infiltration. A follow-up study of 50 cases. *Ann Phys Med* 9:22-28, 1967.

56. Brown FW: Management of discogenic pain using epidural and intrathecal steroids. *Clin Orthop* 129:72-78, 1977.

57. Heyse-Moore G: A rational approach to the use of epidural medication in the treatment of sciatic pain. *Acta Orthop Scand* 49:366-370, 1978.

58. Knight CL, Burnell JC: Systemic side-effects of extradural steroids. *J Neurosurg* 48:1023-1025, 1978.

59. Burn JMB, Langdon L: Duration of action of methylprednisolone. A study in the patients with the lumbosciatic syndrome. *Arch Phys Med Rehabil* 53:29-34, 1974.

60. Kay J, Raff H, Findling JW: Epidural triamcinolone causes prolonged and severe depression of the pituitary-adrenal axis. *Anesthesiology* 75:A694, 1991.

61. Deyo RA, Diehl AK, Rosenthal M: How many days of bed rest for acute low back pain? A randomized clinical trial. *N Engl J Med* 315:1064-1070, 1986.

62. Deyo RA et al: A controlled trial of transcutaneous electrical nerve stimulation (TENS) and exercise for low back pain. *N Engl J Med* 322:1627-1634, 1990.

63. Deyo RA: Fads in the treatment of low back pain. *N Engl J Med* 325:1039-1040, 1991.

64. Pearce J, Moll JMH: Conservative treatment and natural history of acute lumbar discs. *J Neurol Neurosurg Psychiatry* 30:13-17, 1967.

65. Friedenberg ZB, Shoemaker RC: The result of non-operative treatment of lumbar discs. *Am J Surg* 88:933-935, 1954.

66. Wilkinson HA: Intrathecal depo-medrol: A review. *Clin J Pain* 8:49-56, 1992.

67. Abram SE: Subarachnoid corticosteroid injection following inadequate response to epidural steroids for sciatica. *Anesth Analg* 57:313-315.

68. Lippit AB: The facet joint and its role in spine pain. Management with facet joint injections. *Spine* 9:746-750, 1984.

69. Lilius G et al: Lumbar facet joint syndrome. *J Bone Joint Surg Am* 71:681-684, 1989.

70. Jackson RP, Jacobs RR, Montesano PX: Facet joint injection in low back pain. A prospective statistical study. *Spine* 13:966-971, 1988.

71. Carette S et al: A controlled trial of corticosteroid injections into facet joints for chronic low back pain. *N Engl J Med* 325:1002-1007, 1991.

QUESTIONS: EPIDURAL STEROIDS

1. The polyethylene glycol in depot steroids:
   A. Does not cause degenerative lesions in nerves of experimental animals
   B. Is present in methylprednisolone but not triamcinolone
   C. Is not concentrated enough in the commercial preparation to block nerve transmission
   D. Does not cause arachnoiditis when injected intrathecally

2. Intrathecal steroid injections:
   A. Should be given when there is no response to an epidural steroid injection
   B. Do not cause suppression of the hypothalamic-adrenal system
   C. May be given in cases of arachnoiditis
   D. May cause arachnoiditis

3. Facet joint syndromes:
   A. Are due to abnormalities such as inflammation, arthritis, or segmental instability of the facet joint
   B. Are characterized by pain that usually radiates below the knee
   C. Are usually characterized by nerve root tension signs such as limitation of straight leg raising
   D. Are treated with facet injection, and the relief is related to the use of a local anesthetic

4. A 30-year-old man had low back pain that radiated to the lateral aspect of his right leg. The pain was precipitated by the patient lifting a heavy object 3 days before onset. Which of the following statements is true?
   A. An EMG should be performed to localize the involved nerve root.
   B. A CT scan is of no value since the injury is recent.
   C. Physical examination will show decreased knee jerk.
   D. The patient will probably have a good response to an epidural steroid injection.

For question 5, choose from the following:
   A. 1, 2, and 3
   B. 1 and 3
   C. 2 and 4
   D. 4
   E. All of the above

5. Patients with chronic back pain may respond to epidural steroid injections if:
   1. A local anesthetic is added to the steroid
   2. They have a symptom-free interval
   3. Three epidural steroid injections are given
   4. Their new radiculopathy involves a nerve root different from the one they had before

ANSWERS

1. C
2. D
3. A
4. D
5. C

22 Facet Blocks

P. Prithvi Raj and Monica M. Neumann

The facet joints of the spine may be otherwise known as the apophyseal joints. The Greek word *apophysis* means "an offshoot"; the anatomic definition of the word is a natural outgrowth or process on a vertebra or other bone.[1] Ghormley[2] described the *facet syndrome* in 1933. Facet syndrome includes the degenerative changes and associated muscle spasms that develop when a facet joint is involved in a sprain from a forceful or violent twisting motion. The intraarticular facet joints at all levels are subject to trauma.

FACET SYNDROMES
Cervical facet syndrome

A cervical facet syndrome may result from the sudden stop of a vehicle, athletic or occupational injuries, sleeping with a twisted neck, or a sudden jerk of the neck that results in overriding the superior on the inferior articular facet. Degenerative changes include joint capsular hypertrophy, osteophyte formation, and increased fibrous layer formation, all of which may cause intense muscle spasms on the ipsilateral side. The patient has pain upon palpation of the transverse process and a decreased range of motion at the involved level. Rotating motion and hyperextension may particularly aggravate the pain, which is described as dull and aching, and most frequently radiates to the occipital region, shoulder, arm, and cervicoscapular area. The patient holds the head to one side and is unable to touch the ear to the shoulder on the affected side.[3]

Cervical facet syndrome is diagnosed by evaluating a patient's history, physical examination, and x-ray tests. Carrera et al.[4] suggested that computed tomography (CT) might have an important role in diagnosing lumbar facet syndrome; they also suggested that CT could prove beneficial in the diagnosis of cervical facet syndrome. Cervical facet arthrography may or may not indicate joint pathology; there appears to be no correlation between degree of symptoms experienced by the patient and possible joint pathology.

Conservative treatment of cervical facet syndrome includes local heat, traction, nonsteroidal antiinflammatory medications, local myofascial trigger point injections, and local injection in the paravertebral muscles. Manual manipulation may be required to reduce the subluxation. Arthrography, with local anesthetic and steroid injections performed using a fluoroscopy, may prove beneficial; some patients have experienced pain relief for up to 12 months.[5] Because subarachnoid and epidural injections are possible, cervical facet joint injections should be undertaken only with fluoroscopic control.

Thoracic facet joint syndrome

Thoracic facet joint syndrome is similar to cervical facet syndrome. It results from a sudden twisting motion, such as twisting while lifting overhead or from an unguarded rotating motion of the thoracic spine. The resultant pain may be a mild, dull, and aching pain that can radiate to encircle the chest, or it may be a sharp pleuritic-type pain that can affect functional vital capacity or become overwhelming to the patient. The patient usually experiences decreased motion in the portion of the spine involved, and examination may reveal a loss of the thoracic curve or muscle spasm, which can cause localized scoliosis.

Diagnosis is made after reviewing the patient's history, physical examination, and plain x-rays. Computed tomography may provide a more precise diagnosis of the area of involvement, but x-ray findings may not correlate with the clinical picture.

Treatment consists of local heat, nonsteroidal antiinflammatory medications, and/or local muscle (myofascial) injections. Intercostal nerve blocks may help splint and guard the affected area, especially if functional vital capacity is decreased.[3] Hydrotherapy, or swimming in warm water (95° F), may significantly improve the thoracic facet syndrome. If the involved articular facet is identified, the joint may be blocked indirectly by a paravertebral somatic nerve block using an adequate volume of local anesthetic and steroid solution. However, because of the anatomic location of the joint and the proximity of the joint to the rib and the epidural space, individual facet joint blocks in the thoracic spine are not described. Fluoroscopic control should be used when performing any thoracic nerve block procedure.

Lumbar facet syndrome

The lumbar facet joints frequently have the most problems of any facet joint of the spine. Patients primarily complain of low back pain with or without radiation. Etiologies such as degenerative disk disease, disk herniation, or trauma should be evaluated before diagnosing lumbar facet syndrome based on low back pain. An aggravated lumbar facet is distinguished by pain described as a dull ache radiating into the low back, buttocks, hip, and posterior or lateral thigh down to the knee. Hamstring pain, muscle spasm, decreased straight leg raising, and depressed deep tendon reflexes may be present.[6] The pain only occasionally radiates below the knee; when it does, it is usually associated with prolonged pathologic changes of the involved facet. The pain then may present as sciatica. During examination, the patient may complain of tenderness with deep palpation over the facet joint, sharp aching pain upon extending the lumbar spine, and pain with simultaneous rotation and flexion of the lumbar spine. Frequently there is muscle spasm of the ipsilateral paraspinous muscles.

Make a diagnosis based on the patient's history, physical examination, and any changes from the x-ray or CT scan examination.

Treatment consists of: application of local heat, nonsteroidal antiinflammatory medications, electroacupuncture therapy, local myofascial trigger point injections to the paraspinous muscles, and single or multiple level lumbar articular facet joint injections.

ANATOMY

The apophyseal articulations are formed by the joining of the superior articular facet of one vertebra with the inferior articular facet of the upper adjacent vertebra (Fig. 22-1). The articular surfaces of the facets are covered by hyaline cartilage. The joints are lined by synovium and, where the

surfaces of the facets are not in contact, tabs of synovial tissue project into the joint from the joint margins.[7] The fibrous joint capsule forms superior and inferior joint recesses that may contain small synovial villi.[8] The inferior and posterior portions of the recesses are larger to allow a wider range of motion. Medially and anteriorly, the capsule blends with the ligamentum flavum and is adjacent to the neural foramen and the nerve root.

The joint capsule is richly innervated.[6-9] Each dorsal ramus sends branches level to the facet joint and to the lower facet joint (Fig. 22-2). Consequently, each posterior ramus innervates two facet joints, and each facet joint has innervation from two levels.

The articular facets in the cervical spine extend laterally from the junction of the lamina and pedicles and are oriented in the coronal plane to permit flexion, extension, and lateral bending (Fig. 22-3). In the thoracic spine the facets extend superiorly and inferiorly from the junctions of the

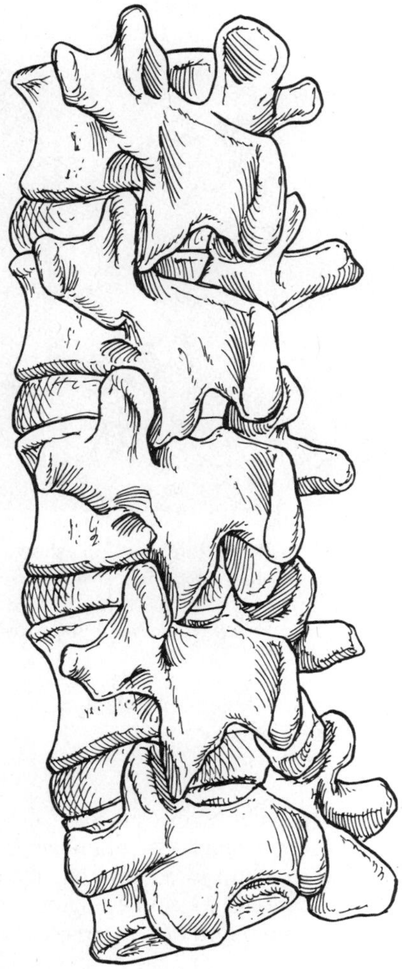

Fig. 22-1 The lumbar facet joints are best visualized with 30° to 45° obliquity. The inferior articular facet from the vertebra above and the superior articular facet from the vertebra below articulate to form the facet joint. (From Sauser DD, Neumann MM: Facet block. In Raj PP, editor: *Practical Management of Pain,* ed 2. St Louis, Mosby, 1992.)

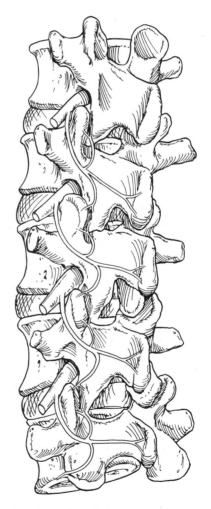

Fig. 22-2 Each articular facet is innervated by branches from the posterior ramus at the same level and the level above, resulting in a dual nerve supply. (From Sauser DD, Neumann MM: Facet block. In Raj PP, editor: *Practical Management of Pain,* ed 2. St Louis, Mosby, 1992.)

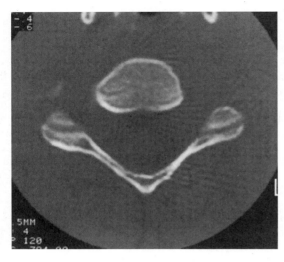

Fig. 22-3 CT through the midcervical region showing the facet joints oriented in the coronal plane. (From Sauser DD, Neumann MM: Facet block. In Raj PP, editor: *Practical Management of Pain,* ed 2. St Louis, Mosby, 1992.)

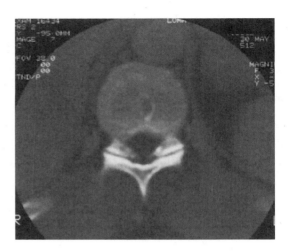

Fig. 22-4 CT through the midthoracic region showing the facet joints oriented just off the coronal plane. (From Sauser DD, Neumann MM: Facet block. In Raj PP, editor: *Practical Management of Pain,* ed 2. St Louis, Mosby, 1992.)

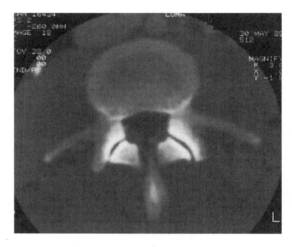

Fig. 22-5 CT through the lower lumbar region showing the curved facet joints oriented approximately 45° off the sagittal plane. (From Sauser DD, Neumann MM: Facet block. In Raj PP, editor: *Practical Management of Pain,* ed 2. St Louis, Mosby, 1992.)

lamina and pedicles, and the apophyseal joints are oriented approximately 20° off the coronal plane (Fig. 22-4). The superior facets in the lumbar spine are concave posteriorly, and the inferior facets are convex anteriorly. The lumbar facet joints are oriented approximately 45° off the sagittal plane, but because of the curvature of the joints, the posterior portion of the joint is much closer to the sagittal plane (Fig. 22-5).

INDICATIONS

Facet arthrography is a diagnostic procedure that is therapeutic in many cases when combined with an injection of a local anesthetic and an antiinflammatory agent. Relief of symptoms can last much longer than expected from the pharmacologic effects of the injected agents.[6,9,10,11]

The major indications for facet injection are: focal tenderness over a facet joint, chronic low back pain with or without radiation but with a normal radiographic workup, back pain with evidence of disk disease and facet arthritis, and postlaminectomy syndrome without arachnoiditis or recurrent disk disease.[11,12]

Local anesthetic injections can be used to determine the cause of back pain in patients with spondylolysis. The injection can demonstrate an abnormal communication between the facet joint and a defect in the pars interarticularis (Fig. 22-6). In patients with a transitional vertebra at the lumbosacral junction, an anesthetic injection can determine if there is a painful pseudoarthrosis between the transverse process and the sacrum (Fig. 22-7). In patients with posterolateral spine fusion and painful pseudoarthrosis, anesthetic injection may delineate the cause of the pain.

CONTRAINDICATIONS

The only *absolute* contraindication to facet block injection is infection in the overlying soft tissues. Allergy to contrast agents is a relative contraindication because facet injection can now be accomplished without injecting contrast, and the

newer nonionic contrast agents available also decrease the risk in allergic individuals.

COMPLICATIONS

Complications from facet blocks are rare and include infection, allergic reaction, and transient radicular pain. Theoretically, the subarachnoid space could be entered during a facet block. It is important to aspirate before any injection to be certain there is no return of cerebrospinal fluid (CSF). Use fluoroscopic visualization and proper technique when placing the needle to ensure against this possibility.

FACET BLOCK TECHNIQUES
Blind technique

The lumbar facet joint injection may be attempted by a "blind" technique. The L_5-S_1 facet joint is more difficult to

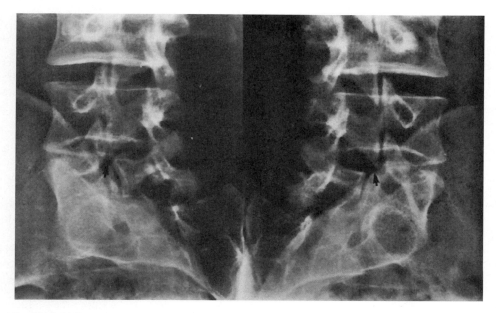

Fig. 22-6 Oblique radiographs of the lower lumbar spine showing spondylolysis with bilateral defects in the pars interarticularis at L5 *(arrows).* (From Sauser DD, Neumann MM: Facet block. In Raj PP, editor: *Practical Management of Pain,* ed 2. St Louis, Mosby, 1992.)

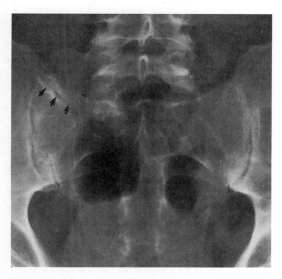

Fig. 22-7 Anteroposterior radiograph of the sacrum and lower lumbar spine showing partial sacralization of L_5 on the right, with pseudoarthrosis between the enlarged transverse process of L_5 and the superior margin of the sacrum *(arrows).* (From Sauser DD, Neumann MM: Facet block. In Raj PP, editor: *Practical Management of Pain,* ed 2. St Louis, Mosby, 1992.)

reach because of the overriding effect of the posterior superior iliac crest. Place the patient in a prone position and rotate the patient obliquely with a 30° angle pillow placed under the iliac crest of the side to be injected. This helps position the posterior facet joints in a vertical plane and allows the needle to advance perpendicular to the table at an approximate 60° angle to the skin. Place the needle about 6 to 8 cm lateral to the midportion of the spinous process.

After sterile prep and drape, advance a 22-gauge, 3½-inch spinal needle until bone is encountered. Aspirate for CSF or blood before injecting any local anesthetic or steroid solution. If an injection of 1 to 3 ml of hypertonic saline reproduces the pain, inject 2 to 5 ml of local anesthetic and steroid solution.

Radiographic technique

Radiographic localization of the facet joints can be used for needle insertion with arthrography to document the intraarticular position of the tip of the needle and to eliminate any question as to whether the response to the injection was technique related. Although arthrography and injection of the cervical facets using fluoroscopy has been described,[6] virtually all referrals for facet injection are for low back pain.

Facet joints can only be entered from a posterior approach. The patient is placed in the prone position on the x-ray table, and the symptomatic side is rotated up while visualizing the facet joint under fluoroscopy to determine the optimum obliquity. Because of the curvature of the facet joints in the lumbar spine, the 45° obliquity best shows the facet joints on plain radiographs but is demonstrating the anterior portion of the joint and not the portion of the joint accessible to puncture for facet injection. The minimum obliquity that allows visualization of the facet joint is usually best for facet injection. This may be close to the sagittal plane. At the L_5-S_1 level, carefully position the posterior ilium over the facet joint to avoid placing the patient in too steep an obliquity. After positioning the patient under fluoroscopy, place a wedge sponge under the abdomen, and flex the hip and knee on the symptomatic side to maintain the position and decrease lumbar lordosis. Mark the skin where the needles are to be inserted.

The tray for facet injection should include a 3-ml syringe and a 22-gauge, 3½-inch spinal needle for each facet to be injected. Fill a syringe with contrast solution and attach it to an extension tube used for arthrography. Fill a 10-ml syringe with 1% lidocaine to use for local anesthesia. Then fill each 3-ml syringe with 1.5 ml of 0.5% bupivacaine and 20 mg of methylprednisolone acetate (Depo-Medrol).

After anesthetizing the skin, vertically direct the 22-gauge spinal needle toward the facet joint. Inject lidocaine through the spinal needle while it is advanced to achieve local anesthesia in the soft tissues overlying the facet joint. Carefully pass the tip of the needle directly to the facet joint by observing its tip frequently with fluoroscopy. Sometimes puncture of the joint capsule can be felt. More often, however, the bone prevents further advance of the needle after entering the joint. When the tip of the needle is superimposed on the facet joint and the needle cannot be advanced any further, the needle tip should be in or very near the facet joint. Make small adjustments in needle position by retracting the needle 1 to 2 cm and readvancing. To prevent having to work around already positioned needles, start with the most cephalad joint and work caudally when injecting multiple joints.

When the needle tip is positioned within the joint, attempt aspiration to be certain the needle has not entered the subarachnoid space. If there is no return of CSF, attach the extension tubing with contrast, and inject 1 ml of iodinated contrast medium. Expose a spot film with each facet injection to document the intraarticular position of the needle tip. Once the needle position has been documented, inject 1.5 ml of 0.5% bupivacaine and 20 mg of methylprednisolone acetate into each joint, and remove the needles.

EFFICACY

Most patients experience little or no pain during injection of the facet joints. If the injected facet is the cause of the pain, there is frequently dramatic relief of pain immediately after the injection. The patient is asked to sit, climb off the table, and walk while still in the radiographic procedure room. Question the patient about any immediate change in symptoms, and instruct the patient to keep track of any change in pain over the next 24-hour period and the following weeks.

The immediate response to the injection and long-term relief of pain are significant. The test is considered positive if there is complete relief of low back pain and sciatica after intraarticular facet block, if the pain continues to be absent during the 24-hour period after the study, and if the patient's normal activities do not exacerbate the pain.[11-13]

Initial relief of pain has been reported in 54% to 65% of patients undergoing facet block. Between 20% and 30% of these patients had continued relief of pain for over 6 months.[9-11]

Raymond and Dumas reported that when maximum volumes of contrast, local anesthetic, and steroid injection were strictly controlled to prevent rupture of the joint capsule, the overall response rate in 25 patients dropped to 16%,

and there was no long-term therapeutic benefit.[14] Their findings suggested that many patients responding favorably to facet blocks were affected by an extraarticular disorder, and that the diffusion of the injected material into the tissues surrounding the facet joint after rupture of the joint capsule was the reason for the therapeutic effect of the injection.

SUMMARY

· The facet syndrome is a significant cause of back pain with or without radiation.

· Facet injection is a diagnostic procedure that is therapeutic in many cases.

· Facet injection is best done under fluoroscopic guidance.

· Arthrography is performed to document needle position before injection of anesthesia.

· Findings on plain radiographs and arthrography have little correlation with the patient's symptoms.

· With proper patient selection and technique, 54% to 65% of patients can gain immediate relief; 20% to 30% can have long-term relief (more than 6 months).

· The therapeutic effect in some patients may be related to rupture of the joint capsule and diffusion of the local anesthetic solution into the surrounding soft tissues.

· Local anesthetic injection to determine the cause of back pain may also be useful in patients with spondylolysis, in patients with a transitional vertebra, and in patients with persistent pain following posterolateral spine fusion.

REFERENCES

1. *Webster's New Collegiate Dictionary,* ed 9. Springfield, Mass, Merriam-Webster, 1985.
2. Ghormley RK: Low back pain. With special reference to the articular facets, with presentation of an operative procedure. *JAMA* 101:1773-1777, 1933.
3. Bonica JJ: *The Management of Pain.* Philadelphia, Lea & Febiger, 1953.
4. Carrera GF, Williams AL, Haughton VM: Computed tomography in sciatica. *Radiology* 137:433-437, 1980.
5. Dory MA: Arthrography of the cervical facet joints. *Radiology* 148:379-382, 1983.
6. Mooney V, Robertson J: The facet syndrome. *Clin Orthop* 115:149-156, 1976.
7. Hadley LA: Anatomico-roentgenographic studies of the posterior spinal articulations. *AJR* 86:270-276, 1961.
8. Lewin T, Moffett B, Viidik A: The morphology of the lumbar synovial intervertebral joints. *Acta Morphol Neerl Scand* 4:299-319, 1961.
9. Pederson HE, Blunck CFJ, Gardiner E: The anatomy of lumbosacral posterior rami and meningeal branches of spinal nerves (sinu-vertebral nerves). *J Bone Joint Surg Am* 38A:377-391, 1956.
10. Destouet JM et al: Lumbar facet joint injection: Indication, technique, clinical correlation, and preliminary results. *Radiology* 145:321-325, 1982.
11. Carrera GF: Lumbar facet joint injection in low back pain and sciatica: Preliminary results. *Radiology* 137:665-667, 1980.
12. Ghelman B, Goldman AB: Lumbar facet injection. In Goldman AB, editor: *Procedures in Skeletal Radiology,* ed 1. Orlando, Fla, Grune & Stratton, 1984.
13. Dory MA: Arthrography of the lumbar facet joints. *Radiology* 140:23-27, 1981.
14. Raymond J, Dumas J: Intra-articular facet block: Diagnostic test or therapeutic procedure? *Radiology* 151:333-336, 1984.

QUESTIONS: FACET BLOCKS

1. The diagnosis of facet syndrome is made by all of the following EXCEPT:
   A. History
   B. Physical examination
   C. Radiographic evaluation
   D. Blood chemistry

2. Best treatment of cervical facet syndrome is:
   A. Conservative management, with physical therapy, local trigger point injection, and nonsteroidal anti-inflammatory drugs
   B. Surgical management
   C. Use of systemic narcotics
   D. Psychotherapy

3. The diagnosis of lumbar facet syndrome can be made if all of the following are seen during history and physical examination EXCEPT:
   A. Dull ache that radiates into the low back, buttocks, hip, or posterior or lateral thigh up to the knee
   B. Tenderness to deep palpation over the facet joint
   C. Sharp aching pain on extensions of the lumbar spine
   D. Radiating pain of flexion of the lumbar spine

4. The apophysial joint is formed by all of the following EXCEPT:
   A. Superior articular facet of the lower vertebra
   B. Inferior articular facet of the upper vertebra
   C. Synovium and fibrous joint capsule
   D. Ligamentum flavum

5. Whereas the articular facets of the cervical spine are oriented in the coronal plane and thoracic facets are 20° off the coronal plane, the lumbar facets are oriented in a sagittal plane approximately:
   A. 35°
   B. 45°
   C. 55°
   D. 65°

ANSWERS

1. D
2. A
3. D
4. D
5. B

23 Epidural Infusion and Patient Controlled Epidural Analgesia

P. Prithvi Raj

Infusion techniques in the epidural space and on the peripheral nerves are now being commonly used for acute and chronic pain patients. In acute pain, it has been beneficial for trauma, postsurgery, and acute medical conditions. Similarly, in chronic pain the technique has been useful for rehabilitation of patients with chronic back pain, reflex sympathetic dystrophy, peripheral neuropathy, and cancer pain.

EPIDURAL ANALGESIA

Continuous epidural analgesia is not a new concept.[1,2,3] The first description of this technique was in 1949 and consisted of administering intermittent boluses of a local anesthetic for 1 to 5 days postoperatively.[4] Although effective analgesia was obtained, significant sympathetic blockade accompanied the pain relief with fluctuating levels of analgesia as the effect of the bolus began to regress. Continuous epidural analgesia with intermittent bolus injections is labor intensive and requires skilled personnel to reassess and rebolus the patient every few hours. Because of these shortcomings, continuous infusion (CI) of epidural local anesthetics has now become commonplace (Fig. 23-1).

Continuous infusion versus intermittent bolus

Continuous epidural infusion offers many therapeutic advantages over intermittent bolusing. The primary advantage of CI is continuous analgesia compared to intermittent dosing. Although single boluses of opioids, such as epidural morphine, may provide 12 hours of pain relief, there is a wide variability reported in the duration of effective analgesia, ranging from 4 to 24 hours.[5,6] Because of the wide variability, it was difficult to titrate uniform levels of pain relief. Continuous infusions provide for easier titration, particularly when employing shorter-acting opioids such as fentanyl or sufentanil. Epidurally administered fentanyl has an onset of action within 4 to 5 minutes and a peak effect within 20 minutes.[7,8,9] This rapidity in onset facilitates adjustment in dosage because the patient quickly appreciates the subjective pain relief.

Another disadvantage of the intermittent bolus technique is the need for action when pain relief subsides 4 to 6 hours after epidural administration of morphine. A decision must be made whether to inject a second dose of epidural opioid or supplement the bolus with systemic administration of an analgesic. Supplementation with parenteral narcotic or sedative drugs increases the risk of respiratory depression in a patient with previously administered epidural narcotic.

For intermittent bolus technique to be successful, longer-acting agents such as morphine and hydromorphone must be administered to provide a reasonable duration of analgesia. These opioids are associated with a higher risk of delayed-onset respiratory depression.[6]

A third disadvantage of the bolus epidural technique is the tachyphylaxis that develops with repeat boluses.[9,10] In contrast, continuous infusion of analgesia using the same dose actually increases the intensity of the block, thus the rate of infusion may have to be decreased to maintain the same degree of analgesia over time.

Continuous epidural infusions of analgesic agents, especially opioids, cause fewer fluctuations in the cerebrospinal fluid concentrations. However, it takes several hours to infuse enough of a long-acting agent such as morphine to provide adequate analgesia; this represents a major disadvantage. This drawback can be overcome by administering of a 5 to 10 ml loading bolus of epidural local anesthetic solution at the beginning of the infusion or by injecting a bolus of short-acting opioid such as fentanyl or sufentanil. It usually takes five half-lives of the infused drug to reach a steady state, which when calculated for morphine or bupivacaine is about 15 to 18 hours.

Catheter location

Segmental limitation of epidural analgesia mandates placing an epidural catheter at sites adjacent to dermatomes covering the field of pain. This reduces dose requirements while increasing the specificity of the spinal analgesia.[11,12] Suggested interspaces where catheters are mostly located for epidural infusion of analgesic solutions are as follows:

Thoracic surgery	T_2-T_8
Upper abdominal surgery	T_4-L_1
Lower abdominal surgery	T_{10}-L_3
Upper extremity surgery	C_2-C_8
Lower extremity surgery	T_{12}-L_3

ANALGESIC AGENTS

Epidural analgesia is commonly provided with a local anesthetic, an opioid, or an opioid and a local anesthetic combination.

Local anesthetic

Local anesthetic agents are best used to provide analgesia and anesthesia for patients undergoing surgery and to maintain postoperative pain relief. Lidocaine and bupivacaine are both effective to achieve and maintain adequate analge-

Infusion technique

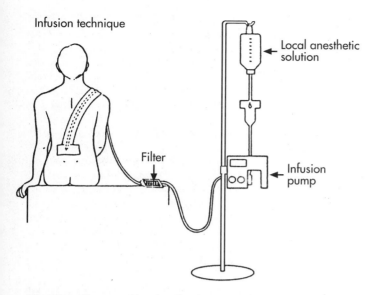

Fig. 23-1 The assembly of analgesic solution, infusion pump, and catheter connection with a filter for epidural infusion technique. (From Pither C, Hartrick C: Postoperative pain. In Raj PP, editor: *Handbook of Regional Anesthesia.* New York, Churchill Livingstone, 1988.)

sia.[9,10] In general, lidocaine use is limited to bolus form to establish or rescue a block, whereas bupivacaine can be used as an infusion. Development of tachyphylaxis is a problem inherent with bolus administration of a local anesthetic through the epidural catheter. Tachyphylaxis has not developed when bupivacaine is administered as an infusion.

Continuous infusion of dilute local anesthetic solutions has simplified maintenance and improved analgesic uniformity; however, concentrations sufficient to produce pain relief usually result in progressive sensorimotor blockade. Such deficits are undesirable, since the ability to ambulate is compromised.

Local anesthetic agents alone can accumulate in the systemic circulation.[9,13] This accumulation is more pronounced with the short acting amides such as lidocaine than the longer acting amides. The decrease in systemic effects with longer acting agents has been attributed to more nonspecific binding of the longer acting agents in the fat of the epidural space compared with the shorter acting amides. Even when bupivacaine was infused for 72 hours after abdominal surgery, the serum bupivacaine level increased and peaked at 48 to 60 hours.[14] The toxicity of local anesthetics is less pronounced when the agents accumulate slowly, but there is an ever present risk of central nervous system depression, convulsions, or cardiac arrest.

The concentration of local anesthetic will influence the analgesia and the profile of side effects. A constant-rate infusion of 0.25% and above of bupivacaine has been associated with hypotension, muscle weakness, sensory block, and possible accumulation of toxic systemic levels of bupivacaine.[9] Higher plasma levels of the agent may occur in the elderly and frail. Side effects may be attenuated by using lower concentrations. A low dose constant-rate infusion of epidurally administered bupivacaine (0.03% to 0.06%)

close to the dermatomal level desired for pain relief can decrease the incidence of side effects. Although the low dose of bupivacaine is effective, it provides a level of analgesia less profound than the combination of bupivacaine with low concentrations of epidurally administered morphine or the use of opioids alone.[9,15,16]

Opioid and local anesthetic combination

In an effort to combine the desirable analgesic properties of local anesthetics and epidural opioids, several investigators described the concomitant use of morphine-bupivacaine epidural infusions for pain relief.[17-20] These studies demonstrated either additive or synergistic analgesic activity between a variety of opioids and dilute concentrations of bupivacaine.[11,19,21] Such combinations provided pain relief of greater magnitude than the relief attained with either agent alone, and the incidence and severity of side effects were minimized. This advantage may be explained by the different analgesic properties of each class of agents and their ability to block pain at two different sites in the spinal cord. Opioids produce analgesia by specifically binding and activating the opiate receptors in the substantia gelatinosa, whereas local anesthetics provide analgesia by blocking impulse transmission at the nerve roots and dorsal root ganglia.

Bupivacaine, in concentrations of 0.03% to 0.125%, has been combined most often with morphine, fentanyl, or meperidine. Morphine and bupivacaine use has resulted in effective analgesia in the management of patients after thoracic, abdominal, and general surgery.[9,16,22,23] However, fentanyl combined with bupivacaine had a lower incidence of side effects than the morphine-bupivacaine combination. Bupivacaine, 0.03% to 0.125%, mixed with fentanyl 2 to 3 μg/ml and given at a rate of 8 to 10 ml/hour to a 70 kg patient, usually provides excellent analgesia with minimal respiratory depression and sensory motor blockade. Bupivacaine 0.03% combined with 0.005% morphine or 2 to 3 μg/ml fentanyl and infused at 8 to 10 ml/hour achieve similar results for chronic pain patients.

Specific concentrations of drugs and rates of infusion should be tailored to individual patients. For example, it is possible to treat or prevent significant hypotension by decreasing the local anesthetic concentration, eliminating the local anesthetic, decreasing the rate of a combined local anesthetic/opioid infusion, or infusing intravenous fluids. Sedation or carbon dioxide retention can be treated by changing the specific epidurally administered opioid, decreasing the concentration of the opioid, decreasing the overall infusion rate, or eliminating the opioid from the infusion.

Management of inadequate analgesia

Although continuous epidural infusion techniques provide excellent results in most patients, there are occasions when individuals experience inadequate pain relief. In these cases, evaluate and correct the causes of inadequate analgesia. The most common test is to review the placement of the catheter. Administer 5 ml of the epidural infusion solution, and reassess the patient's analgesia after 30 minutes. If analgesia remains inadequate, administer 5 to 10 ml of 2% lidocaine in two fractionated doses.

This test dose will generally yield one of three results. If bilateral sensory block occurs in a few segmental dermatomes, correct catheter placement is confirmed. In this case, insufficient volume of the infusion mixture was the likely cause of inadequate analgesia. This can be rectified by increasing the rate of infusion. A unilateral sensory block is probably indicative of a catheter tip placed too far lateral into the epidural space (i.e., at the foramina). The catheter can be withdrawn 1 to 2 cm and the test dose repeated. Finally, lack of any sensory block would indicate that the epidural catheter is no longer in the epidural space. Remove the catheter and replace with another epidural catheter or choose an alternative therapy.

Complications

Complications with a continuous epidural technique include accidental intrathecal administration of the analgesic drug, infection, epidural hematoma, and respiratory depression. To decrease the incidence of these complications, the following guidelines are advocated.

1. Use appropriate concentrations of local anesthetics (such as 0.03% to 0.125% bupivacaine). This can prevent serious hypotension and can aid the diagnosis of subarachnoid catheter migration more readily by providing progressive levels of sensory blockade where none would have been expected. For another safety feature, combine a diluted local anesthetic solution with half the usual dose of an opioid such as 0.005% to 0.01% of morphine or fentanyl 1 to 3 μg/ml.
2. Examine catheter insertion sites daily, monitor temperature, and periodically evaluate for neurologic signs of meningism. If symptoms of infection are present, remove the catheter and begin appropriate antibiotic therapy. We have experienced one case of epidural abscess in 2000 epidural infusion cases. This case promptly resolved in 6 weeks with aggressive antibiotic therapy. Infections limited to the cutaneous superficial and subcutaneous tissues can develop and resolve with local conservative therapy.
3. If epidural catheters are placed at least 1 hour before heparinization, the incidence of epidural hematoma is not significant. Epidural catheters may be inserted safely in patients who receive warfarin postoperatively, if coagulation status is normal at the time of catheter insertion.

Limitations of continuous epidural analgesia

There are limitations to epidural infusion analgesia. First, it cannot independently control pain occurring from multiple sites. Epidural analgesia normally can provide analgesia for 5 to 7 continuous dermatomal regions such as L_4 to S_5 or T_2 to T_8. Patients with multiple injuries may require other forms of pain control.

The site of the epidural catheter influences the adequacy of pain relief and maintenance of normal vital function. In general, place the epidural catheter within the dermatomal distribution of the pain to achieve the best results with the least amount of drug. For example, pain from a thoracotomy is best treated with a thoracic epidural infusion, and pain in the lower extremity requires a lumbar epidural infusion.

PATIENT CONTROLLED EPIDURAL ANALGESIA

Patient controlled epidural analgesia (PCEA) has been offered to patients recovering from intraabdominal, major orthopedic, or thoracic surgery and for chronic pain states such as cancer. The technique has several potential advantages. Patients have the ability to titrate analgesic doses in amounts proportional to individual levels of pain intensity. Because of large interindividual variations of pain relief,[24] this can optimize spinal opioid analgesia. Most of the published work describing PCEA comes from Europe.[24,25] Chrubasik and Wieners compared three different epidural opioids using PCEA technique.[25] These studies showed that the self-administered morphine dosage required for effective analgesia was much smaller than the amount used with continuous epidural opioid and intravenous patient-controlled analgesia (PCA) techniques.[26,27,28] They found that the patients' serum morphine levels were very low. Table 23-1 lists various investigators, the opioids they used in their studies, and the average hourly consumption.

Sjöström and colleagues[24] evaluated morphine PCEA and demonstrated efficacy. They employed 1 mg intermittent boluses with a 30-minute lockout period. The average consumption was about 0.5 mg/hr, and serum morphine levels were well below minimum effective plasma concentrations usually associated with parenteral delivery. Marlowe and co-workers[29] compared constant infusion epidural opioid to PCEA and found the self-administration technique to be superior because less opiate was required to provide similar levels of analgesia. Walmsley et al. reported high efficacy of PCEA in evaluating more than 4000 surgical patients.[30] The following advantages are stated for PCEA over CI epidural analgesia:

- Increased efficiency
- Increased satisfaction
- Decreased sedation
- Reduced opioid usage

The following are the advantages of PCEA compared to IV PCA:

- Self-adjustment by patient
- Self-satisfaction with a resulting decrease in anxiety
- Reduced opioid requirement

PCEA technique with morphine[29]

1. **Loading dose.** Place lower thoracic or upper lumbar catheters preoperatively or intraoperatively using standard techniques. Give patients a loading dose of 2 to 3 mg of preservative-free morphine and start a basal infusion of 0.4 mg/hr (0.02% solution). Allow patients to self-administer 0.2 mg morphine every 10 to 15 minutes with a maximum dose of 1 to 2 mg/hr. Administer the loading dose only after a local anesthetic test dose (2 to 3 ml of lidocaine 2%) has demonstrated that the catheter is not subarachnoid. The optimal size of the loading dose and the timing of administration have yet to be determined; however, because of morphine's latency to peak effect, the loading dose needs to be given as early as possible. Breakthrough pain is common in these patients during the first 6 to 8 hours postoperatively.

Table 23-1 Consumptions of opioids with PCEA mode

PCEA epidural opiates	Average consumption (mg/hour)
Morphine sulfate*	0.52
Demerol*	18.0
Hydromorphone†	0.1
Morphine sulfate‡,§	0.47
Morphine sulfate§,‖	0.25

*Sjöström S, Hartvig D, Tamsen A: Patient controlled analgesia with extradural morphine or pethidine. *Br J Anaesth* 60:358, 1988.
†Marlowe S, Engstrom R, White PF: Epidural patient-controlled analgesia (PCA): An alternative to continuous epidural infusions. *Pain* 37:97, 1989.
‡Walmsley PNH et al: A comparison of epidural and intravenous PCA after gynecological surgery. *Anesthesiology* 73(3A):A684, 1989.
§Infusion and PCEA.
‖Chrubasik J, Wieners K: Continuous-plus-on demand epidural infusion of morphine for postoperative pain relief by means of a small, externally worn infusion device. *Anesthesiology* 62:263, 1985.

Treat breakthrough pain with epidural morphine boluses of 0.5 to 1.0 mg/hr. If two doses are inadequate to provide analgesia, retest the catheter with local anesthetic to confirm epidural placement and to rule out dislodgement. The loading dose can be augmented with fentanyl 50 to 100 μg administered epidurally. This drug speeds the onset of the analgesia, possibly because of dual action (i.e., rapid vascular uptake) and epidural intense neuroaxial action. Residual levels of intraoperatively administered local anesthetics can augment initial epidural morphine analgesia and contribute to subsequent postoperative pain relief.

2. **Lockout.** The short lockout period is somewhat controversial in view of the longer latency of morphine's epidural effect. Sjöström and co-workers chose 30 minutes as the lockout period.[24] There have been few problems with morphine's longer latency to peak epidural effect, but a suitable loading dose should be administered 90 to 120 minutes before PCEA is begun. Patients may perceive early analgesic benefits from the small rise in serum morphine levels occurring soon after a PCA bolus. The faster latency of response to a single PCA bolus may be related to the "primed" or "loaded" state of spinal cord tissues during infusion and an optimal time interval between load and initiation of PCEA opioid. Alternatively, patients may be satisfied from the placebo effect associated with self-administration techniques.

The size of the intermittent PCEA dose should be limited to avoid excessive accumulations of morphine. Small boluses with short lockouts are safe and do not lead to excessive accumulation of the drug before the initial dose becomes effective.

3. **Continuous infusion.** A continuous infusion provides the major portion of epidurally administered morphine. Tolerance to morphine was not observed when continuous infusions were added to PCEA in the routine postoperative patient. Several authors[26,27] believe that continuous infusions, by avoiding peaks and valleys in cerebrospinal fluid levels, provide more uni-

form levels of analgesia while reducing the incidence of side effects.

Serum levels at 24 hours are low. Of 20 samples that were studied, 90% were less than 6.5 ng/ml.[30] This indicates that the systemic absorption of morphine provides minimal contribution toward the overall level of analgesia. Breakthrough pain is treated with small morphine boluses. Changing the rate of infusion has little effect in the short term because it requires five half-lives to reach the new equilibrium.

Alternative choice of analgesic agents with PCEA

Lipophilic opioids. Fentanyl, sufentanil, and hydromorphone can be used with a PCEA infusion technique; however, the amount of drug needed to provide effective analgesia appears to be much greater than with equivalent doses of morphine. Administration of lipophilic opioids by continuous infusions and/or PCEA has been questioned by several authors.[31,32] Estok and co-workers[32] showed that fentanyl administered by intravenous PCA or PCEA provided equivalent analgesia.

Epidurally administered lipophilic opioids may have special use in the following circumstances:

· When administered via thoracic epidural catheters
· To speed the onset of epidural opioid analgesia
· In large volumes of dilute solution or combined with local anesthetics. Cohen and co-workers[33,34] compared combinations of fentanyl bupivacaine and buprenorphine-bupivacaine for PCEA. The average hourly doses of opioid were minimized, presumably because of the effective analgesia provided by concurrently administered bupivacaine, so that 24-hour serum concentrations were low.

Lipophilic agents may be useful for breakthrough pain, especially in the first few hours postoperatively.

Local anesthetics. PCEA with local anesthetics has been reported to be safe and effective during labor. The technique was first described in 1988 by Gambling and co-workers,[35] who compared bupivacaine (0.125%) delivered as PCEA to continuous infusion. They found that PCEA was better than continuous epidural infusion of bupivacaine because patients in the PCEA group required significantly less bupivacaine to provide similar analgesia. The technique was believed to be safe, reliable, and not associated with excessive sensory blockade (Table 23-2).

Lysak et al.[36] evaluated 0.125% bupivacaine combined with three different concentrations of fentanyl and found the optimum regimen for PCEA. The control group received continuous infusion of plain bupivacaine. Their results suggested that PCEA provided greater safety for monitoring hemodynamics, sensory levels, and duration of labor. They concluded that the optimal concentration of fentanyl for a PCEA hourly dosage was 1 μg/ml.

Bupivacaine and fentanyl administered as PCEA with infusion also demonstrated increased safety and efficacy. Fewer top-ups and lower infusion rates were necessary in the PCEA group compared to the continuous infusion group. Naulty and co-workers[39] used bupivacaine-sufentanil combinations during labor and demonstrated no particular benefits of PCEA with this combination of drugs. In fact, total drug requirements were higher in the PCEA

Table 23-2 Efficacy of PCEA as reported by various authors

Analgesic drug	Additional drug	CI (ml/hr)	PCA dose (ml)	Lockout (minutes)	Comment
Bupivacaine 0.125%*	1:400,000 Epinephrine	—	4	20	Greater satisfaction with PCEA than continuous infusion
Bupivacaine 0.125%†	—	4	4	20	PCEA group used less local than CI group
Bupivacaine 0.125%‡	Fentanyl 1 μg/ml	6	4	10	Fewer boluses needed compared with CI group
Bupivacaine 0.125%§	Fentanyl 1μg/ml	4	4	10	Fewer boluses needed compared with CI
Bupivacaine 0.063%‖	Sufentanil 0.3 μg/ml	5	2	6	No advantage over CI

*Gambling DR et al: A comparative study of patient contolled epidural analgesia (PCEA) and continuous infusion epidural analgesia (CIEA) during labor. *Can J Anaesth* 35(3):249-254, 1988.

†Gambling DR et al: Comparison of patient controlled epidural analgesia and conventional intermittent "top-up" injections during labor. *Anesth Analg* 70:256-261, 1990.

‡Lysak SZ, Eisenach JC, Dobson CE: Patient-controlled epidural analgesia during labor: A comparison of three solutions with a continuous infusion control. *Anesthesiology* 72:4449, 1990.

§Viscomi C, Eisenach JC: Patient-controlled epidural analgesia during labor. *Obstet Gynecol* 77(3A):A685, 1989.

‖Naulty JS et al: Epidural PCA vs. continuous infusion of sufentanil-bupivacaine for analgesia during labor and delivery. *Anesthesiology* 73(3A):A963, 1990.

group. Whether this was attributable to the drugs employed or the PCEA regimen, i.e., small volumes of self-administered doses, remains to be seen.

Diluted local anesthetic solutions (0.03 to 0.06% bupivacaine) can be used in selected postoperative patients. However, local anesthetics should only be used in the first 12 to 24 hours postoperatively to avoid interference with ambulation. They are probably best employed with segmentally placed catheters in patients recovering from major upper abdominal or thoracic surgery. A small but definite incidence of hypotension and lower extremity weakness does occur with PCEA technique.

PCA is a relatively new technique that may offer adequate analgesia with lower opioid dosage than IV PCA while providing greater control and higher patient satisfaction than continuous infusion. There is a potential decrease in dose-dependent side effects. Its clinical advantages may outweigh the greater cost and invasiveness of the technique. However, more data needs to be analyzed before the optimum technique to control acute and chronic pain can be selected.

SUGGESTED READINGS

Lubenow TR: Epidural analgesia: Considerations and delivery methods. In Sinatra RS et al, editors: *Acute Pain: Mechanisms and Management.* St Louis, Mosby, 1992.

Walmsley Paul NH: Patient controlled epidural analgesia. In Sinatra RS et al, editors: *Acute Pain: Mechanisms and Management.* St Louis, Mosby, 1992.

REFERENCES

1. Green R, Dawkins CJM: Post operative analgesia: The use of continuous drip epidural block. *Anaesthesia* 21:372, 1966.
2. Sqoerel WE, Thomas A, Gerula GR: Continuous drip analgesia: Experience with mechanical devises. *Can J Anaesth* 17:37, 1970.
3. Rosenblatt RM, Raj PP: Experience with volumetric infusion pumps for continuous epidural analgesia. *Reg Anaesth* 4(1) Jan-Mar, 1979.
4. Cleland JG: Continuous peridural caudal analgesia in surgery and early ambulation. *Northwest Medicine* 48:266, 1949.
5. Akerman B, Arwenstrom E, Post C: Local anesthetics potentiate spinal morphine antinociception. *Anesth Analg* 67:943-948, 1988.
6. Bromage PR, Camporesi E, Chestnut D: Epidural narcotics for postoperative analgesia. *Anesth Anal* 59:473-480, 1980.
7. Cousins MJ, Mather LE: Intrathecal and epidural administration of opioids. *Anesthesiology* 61:276-310, 1984.
8. Rutler DV, Skewes DG, Morgan M: Extradural opioids for postoperative analgesia. *Br J Anaesth* 53:915-920, 1981.
9. Scott NB et al: Continuous thoracic extradural 0.05% bupivacaine with or without morphine: Effect on quality of blockade, lung function and the surgical stress response. *Br J Anaesth* 62:253-257, 1989.
10. Raj PP, Denson D, Finnason R: Prolonged epidural analgesia: Intermittent or continuous? In Meyer J, Nolte H, editors: *Die Kontinuerliche Peridural Anesthesia.* From the 7th International Symposium uber Die Regional An-Aesthesia AM, January 7, 1982, Minden, Germany. Stultgant, Germany, George Themaverlag, 1983.
11. Lubenow TR, Durrani Z, Ivankovish AD: Evaluation of continuous epidural fentanyl/butorphanol infusion for postoperative pain. *Anesthesiology* 69(3A):381, 1988.
12. Rosseel PMJ et al: Epidural sufentanil for intraoperative and postoperative analgesia in thoracic surgery: A comparative study with intravenous sufentanil. *Acta Anaesthesiol Scand* 32:193-198, 1988.
13. Tucker GT et al: Observed and predicted accumulation of local anesthetics during continuous extradural analgesia. *Br J Anaesth* 49:237, 1977.
14. Schweitzer SA, Morgan DJ: Plasma bupivacaine concentrations during postoperative continuous epidural analgesia. *Anaesth Intensive Care* 15:425-430, 1987.
15. Gregory MA et al: Morphine concentration in brain and spinal cord after subarachnoid morphine injection in baboons. *Anesth Analg* 64:929-932, 1985.
16. Rawal N, Sjöstrand U, Dahlström B: Postoperative pain relief by epidural morphine. *Anesth Analg* 60:726-731, 1981.
17. Chestnut DH et al: Continuous infusion epidural analgesia during labor: A randomized double-blind comparison of 0.0625% bupivacaine/0.0002% fentanyl versus 0.125% bupivacaine. *Anesthesiology* 68:754-759, 1988.
18. Cullen M et al: Continuous thoracic epidural analgesia after major abdominal operations: A randomized prospective double-blind study. *Surgery* 98:718-728, 1985.
19. Fisher R et al: Comparison of continuous epidural infusion of fentanyl-bupivacaine and morphine-bupivacaine in the management of postoperative pain. *Anesth Analg* 67:559-563, 1988.
20. Logas WG et al: Continuous thoracic epidural analgesia for postoperative pain relief following thoracotomy: A randomized prospective study. *Anesthesiology* 67:787-791, 1987.
21. Hjortsø NC et al: Epidural morphine improves pain relief and maintains sensory analgesia during continuous epidural bupivacaine after abdominal surgery. *Anesth Analg* 65:1033-1036, 1986.

22. Magora F et al: Observation on extradural morphine analgesia in various pain conditions. *Br J Anaesth* 52:247-252, 1980.

23. Rutberg H et al: Effects of extradural administration of morphine, or bupivacaine on the endocrine response to upper abdominal surgery. *Br J Anaesth* 56:233-238, 1984.

24. Sjöström S, Hartvig D, Tamsen A: Patient controlled analgesia with extradural morphine or pethidine. *Br J Anaesth* 60:358, 1988.

25. Chrubasik J, Wieners K: Continuous-plus-on demand epidural infusion of morphine for postoperative pain relief by means of a small, externally worn infusion devise. *Anesthesiology* 62:263, 1985.

26. Downing JE, Stedman PM, Busch EH: Continuous low volume infusion of epidural morphine for postoperative pain. *Reg Anesth* 13(suppl):84, 1988.

27. Planner RS et al: Continuous epidural morphine analgesia after radical operations upon the pelvis. *Surg Gynecol Obstet* 166:229, 1988.

28. Rauck R et al: Comparison of the efficacy of epidural morphine given by intermittent injection of continuous infusion for the management of postoperative pain. *Anesthesiology* 65:A201, 1986.

29. Marlowe S, Engstrom R, White PF: Epidural patient-controlled analgesia (PCA): An alternative to continuous epidural infusions. *Pain* 37:97, 1989.

30. Walmsley PNH et al: A comparison of epidural and intravenous PCA after gynecological surgery. *Anesthesiology* 73(3A):A684, 1989.

31. Loper KA, Ready LB, Sandler AN: Epidural and IV fentanyl infusions are clinically equivalent following knee surgery. *Anesthesiology* 71(3A):A1149, 1989.

32. Estok PM et al: Use of PCA to compare IV to epidural administration of fentanyl in the postoperative patient. *Anesthesiology* 67(3A):A230, 1987.

33. Cohen S, Amar D, Pantuck CB: Continuous epidural-PCA post-cesarean section: Buprenorphine-bupivacaine 0.03% vs. fentanyl-bupivacaine 0.03%. *Anesthesiology* 73(3A):A975, 1990.

34. Cohen S, Amar D, Pantuck CB: Continuous epidural-PCA cesarean section: Buprenorphine-bupivacaine 0.015% with epinephrine vs fentanyl-bupivacaine 0.015% with and without epinephrine. *Anesthesiology* 73(3A):A918, 1990.

35. Gambling DR et al: A comparative study of patient controlled epidural analgesia (PCEA) and continuous infusion epidural analgesia (CIEA) during labour. *Can J Anaesth* 35(3):249-254, 1988.

36. Lysak SZ, Eisenach JC, Dobson CE: Patient-controlled epidural analgesia during labor: A comparison of three solutions with a continuous infusion control. *Anesthesiology* 72:44-49, 1990.

37. Gambling DR et al: Comparison of patient controlled epidural analgesia and conventional intermittent "top-up" injections during labor. *Anesth Analg* 70:256-261, 1990.

38. Viscomi C, Eisenach JC: Patient-controlled epidural analgesia during labor. *Obstet Gynecol* 77(3A):A685, 1989.

39. Naulty JS et al: Epidural PCA vs. continuous infusion of sufentanil-bupivacaine for analgesia during labor and delivery. *Anesthesiology* 73(3A):A963, 1990.

QUESTIONS: EPIDURAL INFUSION AND PATIENT CONTROLLED EPIDURAL ANALGESIA

1. The therapeutic advantage of continuous epidural infusion over intermittent bolusing is all of the following EXCEPT:
   A. Ease of titration
   B. No tachyphylaxis
   C. Steady-state concentration
   D. Increased local anesthetic concentration

2. Segmental epidural analgesia mandates placement of an epidural catheter at sites adjacent to dermatomes covering the field of pain. This reduces dose requirements while increasing the specificity of spinal analgesia. Suggested interspaces for thoracic surgery are:
   A. T_9-T_{11}
   B. T_2-T_8
   C. C_6-T_1
   D. T_{12}-L_2

3. In comparison with each drug infused alone, combinations of local anesthetics and opioids provide pain relief:
   A. Of lesser magnitude
   B. Of greater magnitude
   C. With more side effects
   D. With lesser reliability

4. Patient controlled epidural analgesia is indicated for patients with all of the following EXCEPT:
   A. Intraabdominal surgery
   B. Major orthopedic surgery
   C. Major thoracic surgery
   D. Diagnostic arthroscopic surgery

5. A common technique of patient controlled epidural analgesia consists of bupivacaine 0.065% with fentanyl (μg/ml concentration) with a lockout interval of 20 minutes and running at a continuous infusion rate of:
   A. 2-4 ml/hr
   B. 4-6 ml/hr
   C. 8-10 ml/hr
   D. 10-12 ml/hr

ANSWERS

1. D
2. B
3. B
4. D
5. B

24 Implantable Drug-Delivery Systems

Steven D. Waldman

Intraspinal narcotics have dramatically influenced the way pain of malignant origin is managed; this is seen by the continued decline in the number of neurodestructive procedures performed to palliate cancer pain.[1] Recently, this powerful modality has been expanded to treat selected patients suffering from chronic benign pain.[2] In tandem, various implantable drug-delivery systems have been developed to complement and facilitate the delivery of opioids and other drugs to the neuraxis. This chapter reviews the practical considerations for selecting an implantable drug-delivery system and presents a simplified technique for the tunneling of epidural and subarachnoid catheters.

IMPLANTABLE DRUG-DELIVERY SYSTEMS
Classification

Box 24-1 describes the six basic types of implantable drug-delivery systems. The Type I system, a simple percutaneous catheter analogous to those used for obstetric pain control, is the type that anesthesiologists are most familiar with. The Type II system is simply a catheter suitable for percutaneous placement and tunneling. The Type III system consists of a totally implantable injection port that is attached to a Type II tunneled catheter. The Type IV system is a totally implantable, mechanically activated pump attached to a Type II tunneled catheter and is in principle a patient-controlled analgesia device. The Type V system is the totally implantable continuous infusion pump connected to a Type II tunneled catheter. The Type VI system is a totally implantable programmable infusion pump attached to a Type II tunneled catheter. The programmable feature of the Type VI implantable drug-delivery system allows a broad spectrum of delivery rates and modes, including occasional bolus injections.

Each of these drug-delivery systems has a unique profile of advantages and disadvantages.[3] The pain management specialist must be familiar with the particular merits of each system if optimal selection is to be made. In this time of increasing pressure to control the costs of health care, economic factors must also play a role in the selection of an implantable drug-delivery system. The cost of both the intended delivery system and the drugs to be administered through the delivery system must be considered before implantation. A perfectly functioning implantable drug-delivery system is of no value to the patient who is unable to pay for the drugs, special needles, and supplies needed to use the delivery system. Similarly, implanted systems may superimpose financial hardship upon a difficult terminal course. With prior planning, the financial issues can be individualized and resolved.

Issues to be considered before device placement

Appropriate patient selection is crucial if optimal results are to be achieved, in terms of pain palliation and patient satisfaction. Factors that must be considered before placement of an implantable drug-delivery system are summarized in Box 24-2.[1,3] These issues will be discussed further.

Preimplantation trial. The first responsibility to the patient being considered for an implantable drug-delivery system is to make a diagnosis of the pain problem and analyze the appropriateness of the patient's current analgesic regimen. If the diagnosis and therapy are correct, the extent of disease is defined, and oncologic and analgesic therapy have been optimized, it is appropriate to proceed to a trial of spinal opioids.[3,4] A preimplantation trial of spinal opioids is necessary to determine whether an implantable drug-delivery system can adequately relieve the patient's pain. Not all pain is relieved by spinal opioids.[5] An implantable drug-delivery system should never be implanted without first verifying the ability of the spinal drug being considered to relieve the patient's symptoms adequately on two separate occasions.[6] Extensive clinical experience suggests that implantation should not proceed unless the magnitude of relief is less than 50% of the preinjection intensity, with a duration of at least twice the half-life of the agent; for example, 8 to 12 hours in the case of morphine.[7]

Failure to provide pain relief during a preimplantation trial may occur for several reasons: test injections made in the wrong place; psychologic reasons such as depression; advanced tolerance to opioids; incorrect dose of spinal drugs; or a principal component of the patient's symptoms not being susceptible to spinal application of opioid, (e.g., some central pain syndromes).[5,6,8] If a question remains about the ability of spinal drugs to provide symptom relief after two trial doses, a placebo injection may help clarify the situation.

It is widely accepted that this response to acute drug administration is highly predictive of the long-term outcome of chronic drug administration. Failure to see adequate, long-lasting analgesia under these conditions is cause to reconsider placement of an implantable narcotic-delivery system.

Unless the efficacy of spinal opioids is clearly demonstrated during the preimplantation trial, the patient could be subjected to the implantation of a delivery system that will fail to achieve the desired pain relief. With the exception of electrical stimulation and spinal drugs, few invasive pain therapies allow the patient and physician to test the therapy before an irreversible result has occurred. Local anesthetic

Box 24-1 SPINAL DRUG DELIVERY SYSTEMS

Type I   Percutaneous epidural or subarachnoid catheter

Type II   Percutaneous epidural or subarachnoid catheter
             with subcutaneous tunneling

Type III   Totally implanted epidural or subarachnoid catheter
             with subcutaneous injection port

Type IV   Totally implanted epidural or subarachnoid catheter
             with subcutaneous injection port

Type IV   Totally implanted epidural or subarachnoid catheter
             with implanted manually activated pump

Type V   Totally implanted epidural or subarachnoid catheter
             with implanted infusion pump

Type VI   Totally implanted epidural or subarachnoid catheter
             with implanted programmable infusion pump

Box 24-2 PREIMPLANTATION CONSIDERATIONS

Results of preimplantation trials of spinal drugs
Infection
Clotting disorders
Behavioral abnormalities
Physiologic abnormalities
Cost of delivery system
Cost of drugs, needles, and supplies
Evaluation of support system
Concurrent therapy
Life expectancy

blocks are useful in educating the patient before neurodestructive procedures but cannot always predict the adequacy, extent, or complications of an irreversible destructive procedure.

Infection and local conditions. Infection, inflammation, or dermatitis at the proposed cutaneous site of implantation—and the presence of generalized sepsis—represent absolute contraindications to device implantation. The management of patients with lesions near the proposed implantation site is more difficult. For example, many cancer patients have infected pressure sores, colostomies or ileostomies, or chronic infections in areas of tumor necrosis. An implantable drug-delivery system may be placed if attention is given to sterile technique during implantation, injection, and refill of the implantable drug-delivery system. Prophylactic antibiotic use should also be considered during placement of implantable ports and pumps.

Anticoagulation and hematologic abnormalities. The fully anticoagulated patient represents a special problem when considering placement of an implantable drug-delivery system. Preimplantation trials of spinal drugs for relief of pelvic and lower body pain have been performed safely in the presence of anticoagulation by administering the opioid caudally with a 25-gauge, 1.5-inch needle.[9] Unfortunately, spinal opioids administered in the lumbar or caudal region may not relieve upper body pain without a

substantial increase in the dose. Carefully weigh the risk-to-benefit ratio of stopping anticoagulants in order to proceed with preimplantation trials of cervical or thoracic spinal drugs.

Coagulopathy caused by disease is also common, particularly in cancer patients. Platelet count and function and tests for procoagulant factor activity should be assessed in all cancer patients and in others whose history or physical examination suggests the possibility of coagulopathy. Efforts should be made to reverse the coagulopathy if possible. If this is not possible, assess the risk-to-benefit ratio of proceeding with preimplantation trials.

Physiologic abnormalities. Physiologic abnormalities, such as electrolyte imbalance and drug-induced organic brain syndrome, may impair the patient's ability to assess the adequacy of symptom relief.[5] Many abnormalities are reversible, and an effort should be made to correct them before a trial of spinal drugs is undertaken. It should be remembered that the confusion secondary to these physiologic abnormalities may be incorrectly interpreted as uncontrolled pain by the patient and the pain management specialist.[6]

Behavior abnormalities. Behavioral abnormalities that are often difficult to identify may affect the patient's ability to assess the adequacy of symptom relief.[10,11] These abnormalities may coexist with physiologic factors, but care must be taken not to attribute inadequate symptom relief solely to behavioral factors until all potential physiologic causes have been explored.[12]

Support system. An implantable drug-delivery system requires a level of commitment from patients, and their support systems. Someone must be available day and night to care for and inject the implantable drug-delivery system should the patient be unable to do so. Thus one or more persons must be designated as the patient's support system for the implantable drug-delivery systems, and these individuals must be acceptable to the patient. It should be remembered that the cancer patient who injects his own implantable drug-delivery system initially may be unable to do so later in the course of disease. Inability or unwillingness by the designated support system to care for the implantable drug-delivery system has significant implications when selecting the appropriate system.

Life expectancy. Although prediction of a cancer patient's life expectancy can be difficult, an estimate in terms of days, weeks, or months is essential to select the most appropriate implantable drug-delivery system.[1] Often the patient's general condition will improve when adequate symptom control is provided, and this must be taken into account when estimating life expectancy.

Types of implantable drug-delivery systems

Type I percutaneous catheters. Type I percutaneous catheters have gained wide acceptance for the short-term administration of spinal opioids and/or local anesthetics for the palliation of acute pain, including obstetric and postoperative pain. The Type I system also has three applications in cancer pain management. The first is in the acute setting, where delivery of opioids into the epidural or subarachnoid space can provide temporary palliation of pain postoperatively or until other concurrent treatments, such as radiotherapy, become effective. The second is in imminently dying patients too ill for more invasive procedures.[1,5,13] The third is the use of a percutaneous catheter to administer test doses of spinal opioids before placing a more permanent implantable drug-delivery system. In many centers the use of a Type I percutaneous catheter to deliver epidural and especially subarachnoid opioids is limited. Improved catheter fixation, reduced risk of infection, and the relative ease of tunneling[1,3,14] has led many pain specialists to tunnel the spinal catheter to the flank, abdomen, or chest wall, even for short-term administration of opioids. Despite several reports that the Type I system can be used for prolonged periods in immunocompromised patients without an increased risk of infection,[15] the validity of this observation has not been established. In view of the potentially devastating and life-threatening consequences of catheter-induced spinal infection, as well as the highly favorable risk-to-benefit ratio of the Type II tunneled catheter, the use of the Type I system should be limited solely to the acute setting.[1,3]

Type II subcutaneous tunneled catheters. The subcutaneous tunneled catheter is selected for patients with life expectancies of weeks to months. The low cost, ease of implementation, and ease of catheter care and injection make the Type II system the preferred delivery system at many centers. The Type II system can be implanted or removed in the outpatient setting and has a decreased incidence of infection when compared with the Type I system.

Type III totally implantable reservoir. The totally implantable reservoir is often chosen for patients with life expectancies of months to years who have had excellent relief of symptoms with trial doses of spinal drugs.[1,15] The Type III system has potentially less risk of infection than with the Type I and II systems, and a decreased risk of catheter failure. Injection of the Type III system is more difficult than with Type I and II systems; this can be significant when training lay people to inject and care for this system.[16] Furthermore, removal or replacement requires a surgical incision.

Type IV totally implantable mechanically activated pump. Poletti and colleagues created one of the earliest totally implantable systems for patient-activated drug delivery. This system consisted of an implantable sterile blood bag with a hydrocephalus shunt valve in series with the bag and spinal catheter. The valve could be activated by the patient to allow self-administration of an opioid from the implanted bag. This concept has now been extended by Cordis, through introduction of a totally implantable reservoir that is accessed percutaneously through a septum on the surface of the device. The device also has a mechanical valve system activated by a set of buttons on the pump surface. The patient delivers spinal drugs by depressing the buttons in the proper sequence.[1,17] The Type IV system has potentially less risk of infection than the Type I, II, and III systems. Subarachnoid delivery is more feasible with the Type IV system than with the Type I and II systems. The greatest advantage of this system is that the patient can titrate the dose of the drug based on symptoms and can pretreat symptoms before periods of increased activity.

Type V totally implantable infusion pump. The totally implantable infusion pump is also used in patients with life expectancies of months to years who obtained relief of symptoms after trial doses of spinal drugs.[1,18] Type V delivery systems may also be indicated in cancer patients with shorter life expectancies, who experience intermittent confusion secondary to metabolic abnormalities or systematically administered drugs. Clinical experience suggests that such patients may obtain analgesia with fewer side effects with low-dose continuous spinal opioid infusion than repeated bolus injections into a spinal catheter. Alternatively, an implanted port with an external infusion pump may suffice in this situation, although this may be more inconvenient and require more support.

Since Type V systems require infrequent refills and run continuously, they are ideal for patients with limited medical or nonmedical family support services. The Type V system is usually selected with an auxiliary bolus injection port to take advantage of potential drug options, such as local anesthetic injections.

Advantages of the Type V system include the minimal risk of infection after the perioperative period and the infrequent need to inject the pump relative to other implantable drug deliver systems where the pump reservoir needs to be refilled approximately every 7 to 20 days. The overall high cost of the Type V system is a disadvantage and may occasionally result in selecting a less effective or more inconvenient analgesic technique.

Type VI totally implantable programmable infusion pump. The Type VI totally implantable programmable infusion pump is implanted with the same ease as the Type V system.[19,20] This system allows a broad spectrum of delivery rates and modes, including occasional bolus injections. Its principal application to date has been intrathecal infusion, especially in the therapy of spasticity in multiple sclerosis and spinal cord injury patients.[4,20,21] There is yet no proven advantage of programmable systems over the simpler continuous infusion systems. However, there are several theoretic advantages for cancer pain patients, including the reduction of side effects that may occur with the bolus injections provided by Type I, II, III, and IV implantable drug-delivery systems, coupled with the added ability to pretreat symptoms associated with periods of increased activity.

SIMPLIFIED SUBCUTANEOUS PLACEMENT OF EPIDURAL CATHETERS FOR LONG-TERM ADMINISTRATION

In patients who require long-term administration of intraspinal narcotics, the subcutaneously implanted delivery systems offer the safest option. Silastic catheters are preferable to catheters made of other materials because they cause less tissue reaction when implanted on a long-term basis. Tissue reaction has been implicated in the development of tolerance to intraspinal narcotics.[22] A variety of silastic catheters small enough to allow placement through a 17 gauge Tuohy needle are now commercially available. Many of these catheters are sold with a malleable tunneling device. The malleability of the tunneling device also allows for tunneling the catheter around the flank without repeated in and out maneuvers that may increase the risk of infection or catheter damage.

The technique described here is suitable for the patient who is suffering from severe multisystem disease and may not be a candidate for more invasive procedures. The anesthesiologist may perform this technique on an outpatient basis, which avoids the inconvenience, risk, and expense of hospitalization. Subcutaneous placement of silastic catheters offers a simple, safe, and cost-effective approach to the long-term delivery of intraspinal narcotics.

Description of technique

Catheter placement may be carried out with the patient in the sitting, lateral, or prone position. Selection of position is based on the patient's ability to maintain the chosen position for the 15 to 20 minutes needed to place and tunnel the catheter subcutaneously. Since most catheters are placed on an outpatient basis, choosing the most comfortable position is important to minimize the need for adjunctive intravenous narcotics or sedation.

After septic preparation of the skin including the tunneling site and catheter exit site, place a 17 gauge Tuohy needle into the epidural space at the level of desired catheter placement. Then advance the silastic catheter through the Tuohy needle into the epidural space. Silastic catheters have a tendency to drag against the internal needle wall and fold back onto themselves. This can be avoided by wetting both the needle and catheter with saline before attempting to advance the catheter through the needle. After the catheter enters the epidural space, gently advance the catheter an additional 4 to 5 cm. A small incision is made with a No. 15 scalpel, extending cranially and caudally approximately 0.5 cm with the epidural needle still in place to avoid inadvertent damage to the catheter. Carefully and completely dissect all tissue away from the needle to allow the catheter to fall freely into the incision as the tunneling tool is advanced. The needle is then carefully withdrawn back along the catheter until the tip is outside the skin. Withdraw the catheter wire stylet, and remove the Tuohy needle from the catheter. Then attach the injection port to the distal end of the catheter. After aspiration, inject 4 to 5 ml of 1.5% lidocaine into the epidural space via the catheter to provide dense segmental sensory block for the subcutaneous tunneling. This approach avoids the need for painful subcutaneous infiltration at the tunneling site. Injection through the catheter at this point also allows for inspection for any leaks before subcutaneous tunneling.

Shape the malleable tunneling device to match the contour of the flank. Now lift the skin with thumb forceps, and introduce the tunneling device subcutaneously and guide it laterally. When the tip of the tunneling device reaches the exit point laterally, turn it away from the patient; this forces the tip against the skin. Use the scalpel to cut down onto the tip. Then advance the tunneling device through the incision. This approach allows for a straight catheter path and decreases the incidence of catheter failure secondary to subcutaneous catheter kinking.

If a one-piece catheter is used, remove the injection port, and thread the distal end of the catheter onto the stud on the proximal end of the tunneling device. Withdraw the tunneling device through the second incision, and bring the catheter with it through the subcutaneous tunnel. Then attach a subcutaneous reservoir or continuous-infusion pump to the distal end of the catheter after making a small subcutaneous pocket, or simply inject the catheter via the injection port. By repeating the tunneling procedure one or two times, the catheter can be advanced to an anterior position in the midsubcostal area if the patient is expected to inject his own catheter. If nursing staff or family members are expected to inject the catheter, it may be left posteriorly.

If a two-piece catheter is used, tunnel the distal portion of the catheter in an analogous manner and then attach to the proximal epidural portion.

Reinsert the injection port into the distal catheter, and inject a small amount of preservative-free saline to ensure catheter integrity. Close the wounds at each incision with one or two 4-0 nylon interrupted sutures, and apply a sterile dressing. Remove sutures in approximately 10 days. The catheter is now ready for injection with opioids.

SUMMARY

The administration of spinal drugs via implantable drug-delivery systems is a useful addition to the armamentarium of the pain management specialist. Proper selection of the patient and an appropriate delivery system are crucial if optimal results are to be achieved. The chronic administration of opioids and other drugs into the epidural or subarachnoid space is in its infancy. Future advances in the pharmacology of spinal drugs and development of new delivery-system technologies will expand the options available for the relief of cancer pain.

REFERENCES

1. Waldman SD, Coombs DW: Selection of implantable narcotic delivery systems. *Anesth Analg* 68:377-384, 1989.
2. Waldman SD, Cronen MC: Thoracic epidural morphine in the palliation of chest wall pain secondary to relapsing polychondritis. *J Pain Symptom Manage* 4:60-63, 1989.
3. Waldman SD: A simplified approach to the subcutaneous placement of epidural catheters for long-term administration of morphine sulfate. *J Pain Symptom Manage* 3:163-166, 1987.
4. Parke B et al: Functional outcome after delivery of intrathecal baclofen. *Arch Phys Med Rehabil* 70:30-33, 1989.
5. Waldman SD, Feldstein GS, Allen ML: Selection of patients for implantable spinal narcotic delivery systems. *Anesth Analg* 65:883-885, 1986.
6. Arner S, Arner B: Differential effects of epidural morphine in the treatment of cancer related pain. *Acta Anaesthesiol Scan* 29:32-36, 1985.
7. Coombs DW, Saunders RL, Schweberger CL: Epidural narcotic infusion reservoir: Implantation technique and efficacy. *Anesthesiology* 56:469-473, 1982.
8. Onofrio BM, Yaksh TL, Arnold PG: Continuous low-dose intrathecal morphine administration in the treatment of chronic pain of malignant origin. *Mayo Clin Proc* 56:516-520, 1981.
9. Waldman SD et al: Caudal administration of morphine sulfate in anticoagulated and thrombocytopenic patients. *Anesth Analg* 66:267-268, 1987.
10. Bond MR: Psychological and emotional aspects of cancer pain. In Bonica JJ, Ventafridda V, editors: *Proceedings of International Symposium on Pain of Advanced Cancer: Advances in Pain Research and Therapy*, vol 2. New York, Raven Press, 1977.
11. Sternbach RA: *Pain Patients: Traits and Treatment*. New York, Academic Press, 1974.
12. Zenz M: Epidural opiates for the treatment of cancer pain. In Zim-

merman M, Drugs P, Wagner G, editors: *Recent Results in Cancer Research.* Heidelberg, Germany, Springer-Verlag, 1989.

13. Crawford ME et al: Pain treatment on outpatient basis utilizing extradural opiates: A Danish multicenter study comprising 105 patients. *Pain* 16:41-46, 1983.

14. Peder C, Crawford M: Fixation of epidural catheters by means of subcutaneous tissue tunneling. *Ugeskr Laeger* 144:2631-2633, 1982.

15. Downing JE, Busch EH, Stedman PM: Epidural morphine delivered by a percutaneous epidural catheter for outpatient treatment of cancer pain. *Anesth Analg* 67:1159-1161, 1988.

16. Cousin M, Gourley G, Cherry D: A technique for the insertion of an implantable portal system for the long-term epidural administration of opioids in the treatment of cancer pain. *Anesth Intensive Care* 13:145-152, 1985.

17. Poletti CB et al: Cancer pain relieved by long-term epidural morphine with a permanent indwelling system for self-administration. *J Neurosurg* 56:581-584, 1981.

18. Gestin Y: A totally implantable multi-dose pump allowing cancer patients intrathecal access for the self-administration of morphine at home: A follow-up of 30 cases. *Anaesthesist* 36:391, 1987.

19. Coombs DW: *Continuous Spinal Morphine Analgesia for Relief of Cancer Pain,* ed 1. Monograph from Shiley Infusaid, Inc. Cambridge, MA, Shea Bros, 1985.

20. Waldman SD et al: Intraspinal opioid therapy. In Patt RB, editor: *Cancer Pain.* Philadelphia, JB Lippincott, 1993.

21. Waldman SD, Feldstein GS, Allen ML: A troubleshooting guide to the subcutaneous epidural implantable reservoir. *J Pain Symptom Manage* 1:217-222, 1986.

22. Feldstein GS, Waldman SD, Allen ML: Reversal of intraspinal narcotic tolerance by epidurally administered methylprednisolone. *Anesth Analg* 66:264-268, 1987.

QUESTIONS: IMPLANTABLE DRUG-DELIVERY SYSTEMS

1. There are currently _____ classifications of implantable drug-delivery systems in clinical use:
   A. 1
   B. 3
   C. 4
   D. 6
   E. 9

2. The preimplantation trial:
   A. Verifies that the drug administered will relieve the patient's pain
   B. Allows the patient to experience the anticipated results of drug administration before implantation
   C. Allows the patient to experience the side effects of drug administration before implantation
   D. Allows the patient to learn the mechanism of the pump

3. Contraindications of implantation of a drug-delivery system include all of the following EXCEPT:
   A. Sepsis
   B. Coagulopathy
   C. Bipolar personality
   D. Cancer pain

4. Physiologic abnormalities that may interfere with the patient's ability to assess pain relief during preimplantation trials include all of the following EXCEPT:
   A. Hyponateria
   B. Cerebral metastatic disease
   C. Drug-induced organic brain syndrome
   D. Normocalcemia

5. Behavioral abnormalities that may interfere with the patient's ability to assess pain relief during preimplantation trials include:
   A. Preexisting chemical dependence on opioid analgesics
   B. Preexisting psychiatric disease
   C. Compliance of the patient
   D. Patient desire for sedation and anxiolysis associated with systemic opioids

ANSWERS

1. C
2. A
3. D
4. D
5. C

25 Neurolytic Agents

James E. Heavner

Neurolytic agents are injected near neural structures involved in nociception to irreversibly destroy the structures and thereby provide permanent pain relief. Neurolytic agents are also used to treat spasticity. Phenol and ethyl alcohol (ethanol) are the neurolytic substances most commonly used. Hypertonic saline is used to a lesser extent. Neurolytic agents typically are used to relieve pain in patients with short life expectancies caused by advanced stages of malignancies. However, neurolytics sometimes are used to treat pain in nonterminal patients whose pain is not caused by cancer.

In 1993, Labat and Greene[1] reported that an injection of 33.3% alcohol produced satisfactory clinical results in the management of painful disorders. The first use of phenol by injection for the purpose of neurolysis was reported by Putnam and Hampton in 1936.[2] Hitchcock[3] first used intrathecal injection of supernatants of frozen saline to treat intractable pain. He later demonstrated that the solution was hypertonic and produced neurolysis.[4] A variety of other agents and combinations of agents have been tried, for example, distilled water and ammonium salt solutions.

PROPERTIES DESIRABLE IN NEUROLYTICS

The single most important property for a neurolytic to have is selective action on neural structures that transmit and process nociceptive information. Selective actions of phenol, hypertonic saline, and ethanol on A delta and C nerve fibers have been reported but were not substantiated.

Alcohol

Ethyl alcohol is miscible with water and with many organic liquids. The terms *95% alcohol* and *alcohol* refer to a binary azeotrope having a distillate composition of 95.57% ethyl alcohol. Alcohol, USP contains not less than 92.3% and not more than 93.8% ethyl alcohol by weight, corresponding to not less than 94.9% and not more than 96.0% by volume of ethanol.

Ethanol extracts phospholipid, cholesterol, and cerebroside from neural tissue and precipitates mucoprotein and lipoproteins. The minimum concentration of alcohol required for neurolysis has not been definitely established. Concentrations between 50% and 100% are usually used. Often the local anesthetic is used as the diluent.

Alcohol spreads quite rapidly from the injection site. Between 90% and 98% of the ethanol that enters the body is completely oxidized. This occurs chiefly in the liver and is initiated principally by alcohol dehydrogenase.[5]

Alcoholic neuritis is a potential complication associated with alcohol neurolysis.

Phenol

Phenol is a combination of carbolic acid, phenic acid, phenylic acid, phenyl hydroxide, hydroxybenzine and oxybenzene. One gram of phenol dissolves in about 15 ml water (6.67%), and it is very soluble in alcohol, glycerol, and a number of other organic substances. It oxidizes and turns red when exposed to air and light.

Phenol produces neurolysis via a protein-denaturing effect. Concentrations of 2% phenol in saline have a reversible, local anesthetic action and do not produce tissue destruction when applied to nerve bundles. A 2% solution of phenol is painted onto organs to denervate them. Equal amounts of nerve damage are produced by 3% phenol in saline and 40% ethanol solution.[6] The block produced by phenol tends to be less profound and of shorter duration than that produced by alcohol. Phenol is usually mixed with saline or glycerine and is also mixed with sterile water or material used for contrast radiography. Phenol is not available as a ready-to-use pharmaceutical preparation. It is prepared from analytical-grade phenol and, because of its protein-denaturing effect, is sterile. Phenol is highly soluble in glycerin and diffuses from it slowly. This is an advantage when injecting intrathecally because it allows for limited spread and highly localized tissue fixation. Phenol and glycerine must be free of water, or the necrotizing effect will be much greater than anticipated. Choice of vehicle clearly influences the amount of phenol delivered and determines how the phenol distributes. Because of solubility limitations, the maximum concentration of phenol in saline is about 6.6%. However, aqueous solutions of phenol are far more potent than glycerin solutions.

Phenol is metabolized by the liver. Principal pathways for phenol elimination include conjugation to glucuronides and oxidation to equinol compounds or to carbon dioxide and water; and a variety of conjugates are excreted via the kidneys.

Systemic reactions to phenol include central nervous system (CNS) stimulation, cardiovascular depression, and nausea, and vomiting.

Hypertonic saline

Sodium and chloride are natural components of the extracellular fluid. A 10% aqueous solution is most commonly used and is available as a pharmaceutical preparation. Little research has been reported to define the mechanism of action of hypertonic solutions.

Injections of hypertonic saline can be quite painful; therefore local anesthetics are generally injected before saline. Intrathecal injection of hypertonic saline can produce a number of side effects, but the most notable adverse reaction is an increase in cerebrospinal fluid (CSF) pressure that triggers an increase in blood pressure (BP), heart rate, and respiration rate.

Precautions

Procedural-related complications similar to those that occur with regional anesthetic techniques can occur during the administration of neurolytic agents. These complications include: hypotension secondary to sympathetic block and systemic toxic reactions—heart rate and rhythm disturbances, blood pressure changes, and CNS excitation or depression that are produced by accidental intravascular injection. Neurolytics may also produce necrosis of nontarget tissue—blood vessels, muscle, and skin; and may interfere with bowel, urinary bladder, and sexual function.

REFERENCES

1. Labat G, Greene MB: Contributions to the modern method of diagnosis and treatment of so-called sciatic neuralgias. *Am J Surg* 11:435, 1931.
2. Putnam TJ, Hampton AO: A technique of injection into the Gasserian ganglion under roentgenographic control. *Arch Neurol Psych* 35:93, 1936.
3. Hitchcock E: Hypothermic subarachnoid irrigation for intractable pain. *Lancet* 1:1133, 1967.
4. Hitchcock E: Osmolytic neurolysis for intractable facial pain. *Lancet* 1:434, 1969.
5. Rall TW: Hypnotics and sedatives; ethanol. In Gilman AG et al, editors: *The Pharmacological Basis of Therapeutics,* ed 8. New York, Pergamon Press, 1990.
6. Moller JE, Helweg-Larson J, Jacobsen E: Histopathological lesions in the sciatic nerve of the rat following perineural application of phenol and alcohol solutions. *Dan Med Bull* 16:116, 1969.

QUESTIONS: NEUROLYTIC AGENTS

1. In terms of neurolytic activity, 40% ethanol is equal to approximately:
    A. 3% phenol in saline
    B. 3% phenol in glycerin
    C. 6% phenol in glycerin
    D. 6% phenol + 3% chloroprocaine
2. The mechanism whereby hypertonic saline produces neurolysis is:
    A. Hypoxia secondary to vasospasm
    B. Extraction of phospholipid from neural tissue
    C. Induction of cell death via repetitive discharge induced by excess sodium
    D. Not clearly established

For questions 3-5, choose from the following:
A: 1, 2, and 3
B: 1 and 3
C: 2 and 4
D: 4
E: All of the above

3. Which of the following statements about ethanol are true?
    1. The minimum concentration of ethanol required for neurolysis is 10%.
    2. Ethanol and local anesthetics are sometimes used together.
    3. Ethanol is sometimes mixed with glycerin.
    4. Alcohol spreads quite rapidly from the injection site.

4. Which of the following statements regarding phenol and alcohol are true?
    1. They are biotransformed by liver enzymes.
    2. They are excreted from the body essentially unchanged via the kidneys.
    3. They act by highly selective mechanisms.
    4. They cannot be used in patients with pancreatic cancer.
5. Procedural complications related to the use of neurolytics include:
    1. Systemic toxic reactions caused by accidental intravascular injection
    2. Hypotension secondary to sympathetic block
    3. Intense pruritus in the facial area
    4. High-output renal failure

ANSWERS

1. B
2. D
3. C
4. B
5. B

26 Peripheral Neurolysis

P. Prithvi Raj and *Richard B. Patt*

One option for prolonged interruption of the nociceptive pathway involves the neurolysis of peripheral nerves by chemical, thermal, cryogenic, or surgical means. It is indicated for patients with limited life expectancy and patients who have recurrent or intractable pain after a series of analgesic blocks. Peripheral neurolysis has not become commonplace because it

- Is impermanent
- Can cause neuritis and deafferentation pain
- Can produce motor deficit when mixed nerves are ablated
- Has the potential for unintentional damage to nontargeted tissue

The impact of each of these problems can be minimized by careful selection of patients and performance with great care and expertise. The following criteria should be considered before peripheral neurolysis:

- Determine and document that the pain is severe.
- Document that the pain is expected to persist with less invasive alternative techniques.
- Document that the pain is well localized and in the distribution of an identifiable nerve.
- Confirm that the pain is relieved with a prior local anesthetic block.
- Document that there is absence of undesirable deficits after the local anesthetic blocks.

ISSUES TO CONSIDER BEFORE NEUROLYSIS

The appearance of neuropathic (causalgic) pain is a feature common to most ablative procedures.[1,2] It can be minimized by limiting the selection of patients to those with short life expectancy and patients who are unlikely to survive the duration of pain relief. In the event that the patient does survive the duration of pain relief, the peripheral neurolysis should be repeatable at the same site or more proximally. The provision of neurolytic blockade in patients with chronic nonmalignant pain is controversial. Some believe that with proper informed consent this is an acceptable practice in carefully selected patients with pain that is otherwise benign but intractable.

The potential for damage to nontargeted tissue is of concern with any destructive procedure, but in general it is less likely to occur for peripheral neurolysis than when central or deep sympathetic neurolytic blocks are undertaken. This is particularly true when localization is facilitated by electrical stimulation, radiographic guidance, and/or test doses of a local anesthetic.[3-5]

Accurate localization and subsequent immobilization of the needle are critical to success. Most nerve blocks are performed percutaneously, without the benefit afforded by direct vision. A thorough knowledge of the pertinent regional anatomy is essential to help make the best use of surface, vascular, and deep bony landmarks. Paresthesia is usually a sensitive guide to the proximity of the needle to the targeted nerve, but it is subject to different techniques and interpretations by the physician and the patient. If paresthesia is to be relied upon, the patient must be coached in advance and maintained in a cooperative, lucid state; the technique must be slow and deliberate, with careful maintenance of verbal contact throughout. Localization can be facilitated further by electrical stimulation and radiographic guidance, with observation of the spread of radiologic contrast solution. These adjuncts are particularly useful when anatomy has been altered by tumor invasion, surgery, and radiotherapy. Unfortunately, it is often difficult to elicit the aid of a qualified radiologist. Although the above adjuvant techniques are useful, a preneurolytic test dose of local anesthetic should be regarded as essential to exclude aberrant placement, to guard against possible injury, and as a further confirmation of correct placement. Clearing the injecting needle with air or saline after the administration of the neurolytic agent is a further measure that may help avoid skin slough and tissue injury from drug spilled on tissue during withdrawal of the needle.

The reasons for the limited duration of analgesia are uncertain, but it has been postulated to be related to the creation by peripheral neurolysis of an incomplete lesion of the targeted nerve.[6] Whereas local anesthetic injected in the general vicinity of a nerve trunk may diffuse through neighboring soft tissue and often result in an effective neural blockade, neurolytic drugs spread poorly and require precise location of the needle on the targeted nerve. This means that best results are obtained when the neurolytic solution is deposed directly onto the nerve. To avoid complications the volume and the concentration of the injected neurolytic must also be carefully controlled. Controlled comparisons between different concentrations and volumes of neurolytic agents have not been carried out. Incomplete lesions and consequent return of partial function might be influenced by these factors.

Incomplete lesions may lead to the development of post-treatment neuritis.[6,7] An association between the creation of incomplete or inaccurate lesions and subsequent neuritis is supported indirectly by the work of Roviaro and colleagues, who injected three neighboring intercostal nerves with 6% phenol in glycerin (1 ml per segment) under direct vision at thoracotomy.[8] Of 32 patients treated, neither neuritis nor deafferentation pain were reported at the 1-year follow-up, a finding that is in marked contrast to results after percutaneous neurolytic intercostal blocks.[9]

SELECTION OF A NEUROLYTIC AGENT

Early investigators used either absolute alcohol or 5% to 7% phenol for peripheral neurolysis. In an effort to improve success rate, one used either absolute alcohol or higher than usual concentrations of phenol (10% to 12%).[10-14] Because of limits in physical properties, a maximum of 6.7% phenol can only be dissolved in water at room temperature, but the addition of small amounts of glycerin or water-soluble radiocontrast materials increase phenol's solubility to as much as 15%. Some workers are concerned that the use of higher concentrations of phenol might predispose to vascular injury.[15] It is well known that the effect of a neurolytic block is transient (2 weeks to 6 months). It is best to forewarn patients to expect that the neurolytic procedure may need to be repeated from one to three times. In most clinical series more than half of the patients receive more than one neurolytic procedure.

Although alcohol and phenol are commonly used for producing chemical neurolysis in contemporary practice, ammonium sulfate and chlorocresol have occasionally been advocated. Compared to sympathetic and central sites, peripheral neurolysis is unique in that neuritis and dysesthesias follow treatment in 2% to 28% of patients.[7,16] The incidence of neuritis after peripheral neurolysis with alcohol is widely held to be higher than when phenol is used, although this finding has not been documented in controlled studies.[17,18]

Alcohol

The perineural injection of alcohol is followed immediately by severe burning pain along the nerve's distribution, which lasts about a minute before giving way to a warm, numb sensation. Pain upon injection may be diminished by the prior injection of a local anesthetic. Some authors recommend against the injection of local anesthetic and neurolytic drug in succession because of theoretic concerns about dilution of the latter and because pain upon injection of alcohol serves to help confirm needle placement. To precede the injection of any neurolytic drug with an injection of local anesthetic optimizes comfort and serves as a "test dose" to exclude aberrant needle placement that may lead to irreversible side effects. Some burning or pain is still likely but well tolerated when patients are forewarned. Extreme care must be taken to brace the needle to avoid movement when syringes are changed.

Alcohol is commercially available in 1-ml and 5-ml ampules as a colorless solution that can be injected readily through small-bore needles and is hypobaric with respect to cerebrospinal fluid (CSF). Specific gravity is not of concern when injecting on the peripheral nerve because injection takes place in a nonfluid medium. In the periphery, alcohol generally is used undiluted. Denervation and pain relief accrue over a few days after injection, usually after 1 week. If no pain relief is present in weeks, then the neurolysis is incomplete and needs repetition.

Phenol

Injectable phenol requires preparation by a pharmacist. Various concentrations of phenol ranging from 3% to 15% prepared with saline, water, glycerin, and different radiocontrast solutions have been advocated. Phenol is relatively insoluble in water, and at room temperature, concentrations in excess of 6.7% cannot be obtained without the addition of glycerin. Phenol mixed in glycerin is hyperbaric with respect to CSF; but it is so viscid that even when warmed, injection is difficult through needles smaller in caliber than 20 gauge. Shelf life is said to exceed 1 year when preparations are refrigerated and not exposed to light. A biphasic action has been observed clinically, characterized by an initial local anesthetic effect producing subjective warmth and numbness that gives way to neurolysis. The hypalgesia that follows phenol injection generally is not as dense as that after alcohol. Quality and extent of analgesia may fade slightly within the first 24 hours of administration. This may be due to its local anesthetic action. The neurolytic action of phenol may be evident clinically only after 3 to 7 days. Similar to alcohol if pain relief is inadequate at 2 weeks, this may be due to incomplete neurolysis and needs repetition.

Although some authors have suggested that alcohol and phenol essentially are interchangeable, neuritis is more likely with injections of alcohol than phenol. Most physicians use phenol when a peripheral injection is indicated in patients with an unknown life expectancy, thus theoretically minimizing the chance of neuritis. Alcohol has been commonly selected for injections of the cranial nerves.[19]

Alternative techniques and agents

Although less commonly applied, other alternatives for interrupting nerve transmission warrant discussion here. Surgical interruption of peripheral nerves is rarely performed in part because percutaneous nerve ablation is preferable to surgery, which is generally more invasive. Glycerol, noted only serendipitously to have neurolytic properties and which is used to treat idiopathic trigeminal neuralgia,[20] is being investigated for efficacy in peripheral blocks. Butyl aminobenzoate, or butamben, is a substance that recently was reported to have neurolytic characteristics and is expected to be a subject of further research.[21-24] Cryoanalgesia has its proponents,[25] but results have been disappointing, despite theoretic advantages of producing reversible injury. Results of cryoanalgesia are often transient, probes are bulky, and the technique requires exquisitely precise placement, often necessitating the creation of lesions under direct vision. It probably should be reserved for patients with longer life expectancies, in whom it is essential to minimize the likelihood of neuritis. In contrast, thermal ablation by means of radiofrequency coagulation has numerous potential advantages over injection techniques and is increasing in popularity. Probes are superior to those used for cryogenic lesioning, and the discrete, controllable lesion that results avoids the uncertainties associated with the spread of injected solutions. A radiofrequency lesion is produced within seconds, so great care must be taken to assure that the probe is positioned properly. Unfortunately, equipment is costly, and training is poor or nonexistent before its use.

NEUROLYSIS OF THE NERVES IN THE HEAD AND NECK

The most common indication for neurolysis in the head and neck region is intractable pain resulting from cancer. Head and neck pain resulting from cancer remains a therapeutic challenge,[26] particularly if radiotherapy has proven ineffective or has already been maximized. Conventional analgesic therapy may prove inadequate because of the erosive nature of many tumors and the area's rich innervation. Further, physiologic splinting, ordinarily an important protective reflex, is often ineffective in cases of craniocervical pain because pain is aggravated by relatively involuntary motion produced by swallowing, eating, coughing, talking, and other movements of the head. Despite overlapping contributions from cranial nerves V, VII, IX, X, and the upper cervical nerves, pain relief often can be obtained with carefully planned nerve blocks. Treatment success may be affected adversely by anatomic distortion induced by previous surgery or radiotherapy and the potential for tumor invasion or radiation fibrosis to reduce contact between the neurolytic and targeted nervous tissue, a so-called "sheltering" effect. Typically there is considerable overlap among the sensory fields of neighboring nerves. For this reason, as well as the influence of the cranial nerves on swallowing and control of breathing, neurolytic blocks should be preceded by diagnostic/prognostic local anesthetic injections. Despite these considerations, blockade of the cranial and/or upper cervical nerves is of great value in selected patients.

Trigeminal ganglion and nerve neurolysis

Blockade of the trigeminal nerve within the foramen ovale at the base of the skull or of its branches may be adequate to relieve localized pain of the face (Fig. 26-1). Lysis of the second or third division usually is performed by the extraoral route. Maxillary nerve block is indicated for pain involving the middle third of the face (i.e., the maxilla, cheek, nasal cavity, hard palate, and tonsilar fossa) (Fig. 26-2). Mandibular nerve block is indicated for pain involving the jaw and anterior two thirds of the tongue (Fig. 26-3). Alcohol blocks of the mandibular nerve have occasionally caused skin slough.[9] Neurolytic blockade of the ophthalmic nerve is rarely used in contemporary practice.[27] If tumor progression is anticipated, it is preferable to extend the field of analgesia prophylactically by blocking the gasserian ganglion.[19]

Gasserian ganglion injection is considered for pain in the distribution of the second or third division when tumor growth or postsurgical changes prohibit access to the maxillary or mandibular nerve. When pain extends cervically or to the angle of the jaw, supplementary paravertebral blockade of the second or third cervical nerve roots may be necessary for more complete relief of pain.[28] Blockade of the smaller branches of the trigeminal nerve has been

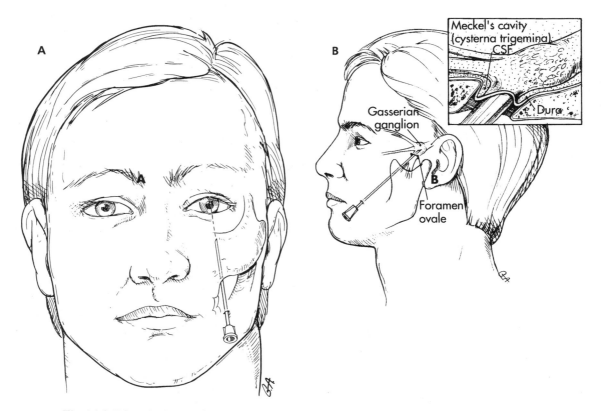

Fig. 26-1 Trigeminal (gasserian) ganglion block. **A,** Needle direction in anterior view where needle tip is in line with pupil. **B,** Lateral view illustrating posterosuperior direction of needle tip in front of ear and at superior edge of coronoid notch. (From Katz J: Somatic nerve blocks. In Raj PP, editor: *Practical Management of Pain,* ed 2. St Louis, Mosby, 1992.)

described[7] and may be undertaken for well localized pain in a confined distribution, particularly resulting from a lesion that is more likely to erode than spread, or when anatomic distortion precludes access to the parent nerves.

Glossopharyngeal and vagal neurolysis

In cases of pain that are less well localized or are concentrated near the base of the tongue, pharynx, or throat, blockade of the ninth or tenth cranial nerve may be required to achieve more complete relief.[29,30] The sensory field of the glossopharyngeal nerve includes the nasopharynx, eustachian tube, soft palate, uvula, tonsil, base of the tongue, and part of the external auditory canal (Fig. 26-4). The vagus nerve subserves the larynx and contributes fibers to the ear, external auditory canal, and tympanic membrane. Bilateral destruction of the glossopharyngeal and vagus nerves is not recommended because of potential interference with swallowing mechanisms and protective airway reflexes.[7,19] When available, radiofrequency coagulation is the preferred means of lesion generation. Blockade of the superior laryngeal nerves has been described for laryngeal pain of tabetic, tuberculous, and malignant origin.[14,29,31]

Phrenic neurolysis

Intractable hiccups (singultus) also is amenable to nerve-block therapy. Unilateral phrenic nerve block has been used under these circumstances with excellent results, although conservative measures should be exhausted first.[7,32] Before performing a neurolytic phrenic nerve block, evaluate the results of a prognostic block with local anesthetic to assure that ventilatory function will not be compromised by a more lasting procedure.

When intractable craniocervical pain is not amenable to nerve-block therapy, intraspinal opioid therapy by means of an implanted cervical epidural catheter[33] or intraventricular opioid therapy may be considered.[33,34] Numerous neurosurgical procedures have been devised to manage rostral pain but are of limited practical value because of their invasive nature and high morbidity and mortality.[1]

Efficacy

In a series of 70 pain patients treated with peripheral and cranial neurolysis with head and neck cancer, Bonica achieved complete relief of pain in 63% of the patients, in 31% moderate relief was obtained, and in 6% pain relief was slight or insignificant. Similar results were obtained by an earlier study by Grant.[35] McEwen et al.[36] reported good or fair relief in 70% of cancer patients treated with gasserian ganglion block. Using radiofrequency thermocoagulation techniques, Siegfried and Broggi reported lasting comfort in about 50% of 20 patients treated, with percutaneous ablation of the trigeminal ganglion.[37] The same authors reported good results in two patients treated with thermal ablation of the glossopharyngeal nerve.[38] Although one patient underwent a repeat procedure at 6 months for recurrence of pain and the other had temporary dysphagia and permanent twelfth nerve palsy, long-term results ultimately were gratifying. Using an anterior approach, Pagura et al. reported good to excellent results in 15 cancer patients treated with thermocoagulation of the glossopharyngeal nerve.[39] Treatment was supplemented by trigeminal

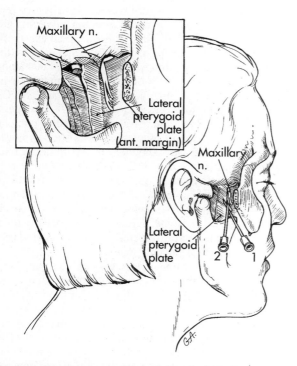

Fig. 26-2 Maxillary nerve block. *1,* Depth of needle entry to reach at lateral pterygoid plate; *2,* Anterior direction of needle required to slip off pterygoid plate to reach maxillary nerve. Inset shows magnification of pterygopalatine fossa in which maxillary nerve traverses. (From Katz J: Somatic nerve blocks. In Raj PP, editor: *Practical Management of Pain,* ed 2. St Louis, Mosby, 1992.)

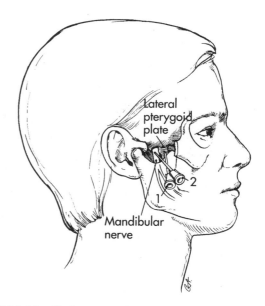

Fig. 26-3 Mandibular nerve block. *1,* Initial needle direction to reach lateral pterygoid plate; *2,* Posterior direction of needle required to reach mandibular nerve at base of skull as it exits foramen ovale. (From Katz J: Somatic nerve blocks. In Raj PP, editor: *Practical Management of Pain,* ed 2. St Louis, Mosby, 1992.)

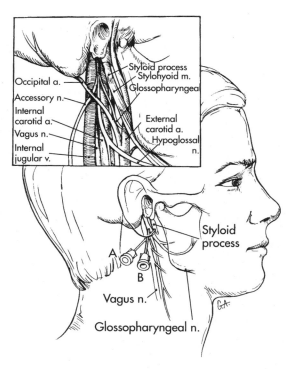

Fig. 26-4 Glossopharyngeal and vagus nerve block. *A* and *B* show the needle direction for either glossopharyngeal or vagus nerve block at level of styloid process. Inset magnifies relationships of important structures in that area. (From Katz J: Somatic nerve blocks. In Raj PP, editor: *Practical Management of Pain*, ed 2. St Louis, Mosby, 1992.)

thermoablation in eight patients because of overlapping pain.

NEUROLYSIS OF THE NERVES IN THE UPPER EXTREMITY

All neurolytic procedures that have the potential to relieve upper extremity pain are associated with a risk of producing weakness in the limb. Carefully performed, cervical subarachnoid neurolytic injections of phenol or alcohol are likely to relieve pain without affecting motor function. This is because the drug is deposited preferentially onto the sensory rootlets. Paravertebral somatic block is applicable for localized pain, and even then because of sensory overlap multiple nerves usually need to be blocked and some degree of motor dysfunction should be anticipated. Radiologic guidance is strongly recommended for neurolytic paravertebral block, as well as the careful observation of the effects of preneurolytic test doses of local anesthetic and fractionated administration to avoid subarachnoid or epidural spread. The brachial plexus (Fig. 26-5) has a high proportion of motor fibers and is therefore not to be injected unless motor strength is already deficient, as in some cases of Pancoast's tumor, or unless the arm already is rendered useless by intractable pain, as in the case of pathologic fracture. Relatively little experience has been reported with neurolytic block of the more peripheral nerves of the upper limb.

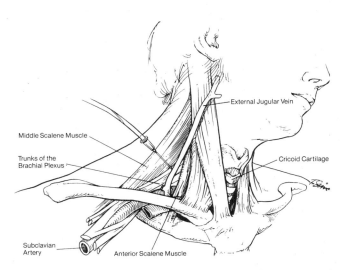

Fig. 26-5 Brachial plexus block. (From Raj PP, Pai U: Upper and lower extremity. In Raj PP, editor: *Practical Management of Pain*, ed 2. St Louis, Mosby, 1992.)

Efficacy

Bonica infiltrated 20 ml of 95% alcohol on the brachial plexus, which did paralyze the upper extremity but gave relief of pain until death. Pain relief lasted from 3.5 weeks to 3.5 months after injections of 5% aqueous phenol on the brachial plexus. Kaplan et al.[40] reported on a single but well-documented case of phenol brachial plexus block performed in a patient with recurrent sarcoma involving the humeral head. After a successful prognostic local anesthetic block, 12.5 ml of 6% phenol in water was injected by the supraclavicular route, resulting in a significant but incomplete level of pain relief. Residual pain was managed by supplementary paravertebral phenol blocks of C_5 and C_6, and later, in response to increased tumor growth, T_{1-3} paravertebral blocks (0.5 to 1.0 ml 6% aqueous phenol/segment) were performed. In a report of a single case, Neill achieved excellent palliation of pain secondary to a pathologic fracture of the humerus in a man with multiple myeloma with two successive interscalene injections of 20 ml of 50% alcohol.[41] In a report of five cases, Mullin et al. used an interscalene injection of 3% aqueous phenol to manage the pain of Pancoast's syndrome.[42] Excellent short-term relief of pain was obtained in all patients and was sustained for up to 7 months in three patients, but only at the expense of relatively frequent repetition at 3- to 6-week intervals. Neurologic sequelae were not observed, suggesting that dilute phenol, although its effects are short in duration, may be relatively safe in patients with normal motor function.

In response to concerns about reports of inadequate or short-lived analgesia after lytic brachial plexus block, Patt et al. elected treatment with a higher concentration of phenol than has been reported previously.[10,42] Four patients underwent brachial plexus block with 10 to 20 ml of 10% to 12% aqueous phenol mixed with 20% glycerin to maintain the phenol's solubility in water. The solution was mildly viscid and readily injectable through a 20- or 22-gauge needle. Three patients had pain and muscle weakness secondary to tumor invasion of the apex of the lung and brachial plexus, and one patient with breast cancer had painful metastases to the cervical spine. Pain persisted in the latter patient despite two cervical subarachnoid neurolytic blocks. One patient had a pathologic fracture of the humerus as well, and all four patients had a useless limb from either neurologic involvement or intractable pain.

Patt et al. used an axillary approach in all patients. A paresthesia or positive response to electrical nerve stimulation was relied on for verification of needle placement in all but one case, which was conducted under fluoroscopy through a catheter. Good to excellent pain relief was obtained in all patients until death occurred at 12 weeks in two patients, 8 weeks in one patient, and 5 weeks in another. No unexpected complications occurred. Increased motor weakness was observed in all cases but was well tolerated. Interestingly, in three of the four cases, relief of pain was not immediately forthcoming but accrued gradually over several days. An additional patient with shoulder and upper arm pain was referred for brachial plexus block but was found to have excellent upper limb strength. After a diagnostic/prognostic local anesthetic block, she instead was treated with a 4-ml injection of 10% phenol in the vicinity of the suprascapular nerve, which was localized with a nerve stimulator. No loss of motor power occurred, and she had excellent pain relief until her death 8 weeks later. Another preterminal patient with shoulder pain secondary to multiple myeloma received a suprascapular nerve block with 4 ml of absolute alcohol, which resulted in moderate relief of pain without complications until his death 4 weeks later. Another patient with pain resulting from a parascapular soft tissue mass secondary to lung cancer experienced good pain relief for 4 weeks after a phenol suprascapular nerve block with 5 ml of 10% phenol. Pain gradually returned, and the patient was persuaded to undergo radiotherapy, which provided pain relief that persisted until his death.

NEUROLYSIS OF THORACIC AND ABDOMINAL WALL NERVES

Pain originating in the thoracic or abdominal wall or parietal peritoneum can be treated with multiple intercostal[14,43,44,66] or paravertebral blocks.[7,45] Except after pneumonectomy, the risk of pneumothorax exists for blocks performed in the thoracic region, although when proper technique is observed it should occur infrequently.[44] The use of radiologic guidance has been reported for intercostal block (Fig. 26-6).[6] Most physicians "walk the needle off" the rib and look for the presence of a paresthesia as guides for placement. Localized bony pain associated with rib metastases also may respond to local infiltration around the bone with steroids, a technique that has produced good response in radiologic guidance and is strongly recommended for neurolytic paravertebral block, the careful observation of the effects of preneurolytic test doses of local anesthetic, and fractionated administration to avoid subarachnoid, epidural, or intrapleural spread, all of which have been documented.[46]

Efficacy

Doyle[43,47] reported on a series of 46 patients treated in a hospice environment with multiple phenol intercostal

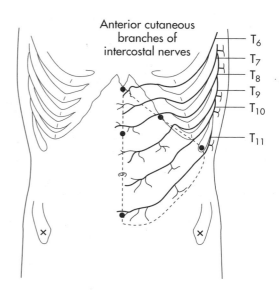

Fig. 26-6 Intercostal nerve block. Note distribution of intercostal nerves T_6-T_{11} in abdominal wall. They can be neurolysed for pain in somatic structures of abdomen. (From Raj PP, Pai U: Techniques of nerve blocking. In Raj PP, editor: *Hardbook of Regional Anesthesia.* New York, Churchill Livingstone, 1985.)

blocks. He used 1.0 to 1.5 ml of 6% phenol "in oil" per segment and obtained total relief of pain for a mean duration of 3 weeks (range, 1 to 6 weeks). Radiologic guidance was not used, and no complications occurred. To illustrate that radiologic confirmation is advisable, a patient with adhesions experienced acute bronchospasm after an unintentional presumed intrabronchial or intrapulmonary injection of small amount (0.5 ml) of 8% phenol in saline.[48]

Bonica reports favorable results subsequent to the paravertebral injection of 1 ml alcohol per involved segment in patients with abdominal and chest wall pain secondary to vertebral, paravertebral, and visceral neoplasms associated with peritoneal invasion.[7] In an anecdotal report, Vernon[45] noted good relief of back pain of metastatic origin and no untoward effects after paravertebral injection of alcohol in two patients, although little detail was provided.

Mehta and Ranger[49] report of blocks of the individual branches of the lumbar plexus in 103 patients with abdominal pain of unknown cause. The authors describe having blocked the iliohypogastric, ilioinguinal, and upper and lower intercostal nerves within the rectus sheath with 2 to 3 ml of aqueous phenol. Follow-up at 3 weeks revealed complete and partial relief of pain in 58% and 32% of patients, respectively, with no recurrence in 70% of respondents at 3-year follow-up.

NEUROLYSIS OF PERINEAL AND LOWER EXTREMITY NERVES

Treatment of intractable perineal and lower limb pain is difficult because pain is often bilateral or midline in distribution and the relevant neuroanatomy predisposes to paresis and incontinence when neurolytic techniques are applied. When bowel and bladder function are not of concern because of preexisting dysfunction and/or surgical diversions, neurolytic subarachnoid block should be considered. Decision-making is more difficult in the continent, ambulatory patient with intractable pain. Although neurolytic subarachnoid and epidural block can be performed in the thoracic region relatively safely, these techniques are hazardous when performed in the lumbosacral region, even with careful attention to technique.

Recently, blocks of the hypogastric plexus and ganglion impar have been introduced[50,51] and can be considered as options for pelvic or rectal pain that is sympathetically mediated.

The sacral roots are accessed readily as they emerge from the posterior plate of the sacrum, and injections here may relieve pelvic, rectal, and lower extremity pain. Selective sacral root block is preferable to spinal injections in this region in patients with normal urinary and bowel function because carefully executed nerve blocks here will not affect continence.[52] A single sacral nerve, most often the third[53] or sometimes the fourth sacral nerve,[54] usually exerts a dominant influence on bladder musculature, and as a result, blockade of the nondominant nerves, based on trials of local anesthetic injections, has little urodynamic effect. The radiologic guidance is a useful adjunct to sacral nerve block. The foramina are not well visualized on anteroposterior views, but the needle penetration of the posterior sacral plate is readily apparent on lateral views.

Neurolytic injections of other peripheral nerves subserving the lower extremity sometimes are attempted, but generally only after local anesthetic injection has confirmed that reduction in pain is possible without much effect on motor function.

Efficacy

Robertson[52] described a series of nine patients with intractable perineal pain secondary to carcinoma of the rectum. After a test block with local anesthetic of the sacral nerves, he injected 2.5 ml of 6% aqueous phenol at the S_4 foramen on the side of predominant pain. Satisfactory analgesia was obtained in all cases and persisted in two cases for 202 and 414 days, respectively, after a single block. Duration was inadequate in the other cases, but pain relief was maintained uniformly by second or third injections until death. In seven of the nine patients duration of relief from the first neurolysis was less than 10 days, suggesting that most patients require repeated treatment, but this limitation was mitigated by ease of repetition. Motor and autonomic function was unaffected, and no other complications occurred. In a similar study on patients with bladder pain secondary to spasticity, Simon et al.[53] obtained an average of 26.5 months of pain relief in patients after sacral injections of 2 ml of 6% aqueous phenol. Most patients obtained relief with unilateral blockade of the third sacral nerve, although preliminary local anesthetic blocks identified some patients whose pain was mediated by S_2 and S_4. Several patients required repeat treatment, and no lasting complications were observed.

An isolated report of bladder atony after otherwise successful S_3 and S_4 alcohol block[56] emphasizes the need for careful observation of the results of preneurolytic prognostic blocks with local anesthetic. A recent well-designed

study[52] assessed the spread of a mixture of radiocontrast solution and local anesthetic injected in 1- and 2-ml aliquots for sacral block. The authors demonstrated a wider spread of solution in the latter group and concluded that 1 ml of anesthetic is sufficient to produce a selective sacral nerve root block. They were also able to demonstrate that reflux into the sacral canal was much less likely when the needle tip was positioned at the anterior border of the sacrum rather than in the midportion of the sacral foramen. It is uncertain how these results apply to the spread of neurolytic solutions.

Successful treatment of penile pain and malignant priapism secondary to venous obstruction from bladder cancer was reported anecdotally with injections of 5% aqueous phenol near the dorsal nerves of the penis close to the symphysis pubis.[57]

Feldman and Yeung[58] treated 26 patients for intractable claudication with paravertebral injections of lumbar somatic nerve with 5 to 10 ml of 7.5% phenol in myodil and reported good long-term improvement without negative sequelae. Doyle[43,47] mentions performing two femoral nerve blocks with phenol in a patient with invasion of the femoral sheath area, but provides no other details. Patt et al. performed an alcohol injection of the sciatic nerve in a patient with preexisting motor weakness from invasion of the nerve by pelvic tumor with good short-term results.[10] They observed heightened distress and poor tolerance of resulting foot drop in other patients with less complete motor deficit even though they had prognostic local anesthetic sciatic nerve blocks. Rastogi and Kumar make a brief mention of "successful" alcohol block of the sciatic nerve in three patients with cancer.[5] Singler reported on a single case of successful sciatic and femoral neurolysis performed with 75% alcohol for intractable spasticity. A few reports have appeared documenting the injection of the lumbar somatic nerves with phenol within the psoas sheath for the relief of ischemic pain.[58,59] That 5 to 10 ml of 7% phenol[55] and 5 ml of 10% phenol[59] dissolved in contrast medium were injected without significant neurologic side effects is surprising but suggests potential applications in patients with cancer.

NEUROLYSIS FOR SPASTICITY

Peripheral nerve blocks with phenol have been advocated in spastic patients to improve balance, gait, self-care, and global rehabilitation. An important distinction between peripheral neurolytic blocks for pain versus spasticity is that in the latter, motor or mixed nerves are targeted preferentially. Nevertheless, given the paucity of data of peripheral neurolytic blocks for the management of pain, it is worthwhile to try to extrapolate information obtained from work with spastic patients.

Moritz[60] reported on a series of 50 spastic patients who received a total of 90 peripheral nerve blocks (musculocutaneous, median, ulnar, tibial, obturator, femoral, and superior gluteal nerves) performed with either 2% phenol in saline or 3% aqueous phenol. A nerve stimulator was used for needle localization. Focal motor weakness lasted only about 1 week in 15% of patients, but the average duration of effect was 8 months. He noted incidence of transient dysesthesias (10%), which usually resolved in days or weeks, and no sensory disturbances; these findings are not surprising given the dilute solutions used. Reporting on 521 blocks of peripheral nerves performed with 6% aqueous phenol, Gibson[47] noted one serious complication, a 69-year-old hemiplegic patient who, after five successful blocks, underwent a brachioradialis and musculocutaneous block; the patient subsequently developed an arterial occlusion in the upper limb that required a high amputation.

LOCAL NEUROLYTIC INJECTION

Local anesthetic and/or steroid injections of *trigger points* is a well-accepted means of managing chronic myofascial pain. The clinical effects of locally injected neurolytics are unknown, and local infiltration generally is avoided because of concerns about skin slough and worsening of pain because of local ischemia or necrosis. Cousins[17] refers to the practice of injecting persistent trigger points with 5% to 6% aqueous phenol but cautions that further research is needed to determine its safety and efficacy.

Ramamurthy et al.[2] mention having performed three "myoneural" blocks with 6% aqueous phenol but provide no further detail. In a study of patients with painful palpable peripheral neuromas, local injections of 0.1 to 0.5 ml of 5% phenol in glycerin were performed.[61] Fifteen neuromas were treated in 10 patients, with a total of 20 blocks. Complete relief was obtained and maintained in all but one patient for the 8- to 22-month follow-up period, and no complications or neuritis were reported. In another series of patients with poststernotomy pain presumably resulting from scar neuroma,[62,63] 17 patients were treated with multiple, serial local neurolytic injections of 2 to 3 ml of 6% aqueous phenol or 1.5 to 2.0 ml of absolute alcohol. Complete relief was obtained in most patients, and no complications referable to neurolysis were observed. Finally, Defalque[64] obtained complete relief in 63 of 69 patients by performing repeated trigger-point injections near surgical scars with 1.0 ml of absolute alcohol and noted no complications other than localized numbness. The implications for this treatment modality in patients with cancer pain are uncertain.

Patt et al. wrote of experiences with periosteal injections of dilute aqueous phenol (3% to 5%) for persistent refractory bone pain, a technique mentioned by Swerdlow.[65] The two patients they treated had minimal relief with periosteal injections of local anesthetic and steroid. They ultimately achieved lasting relief after two neurolytic injections.

The use of local subcutaneous infiltration with absolute alcohol for intractable anal and vulvar pruritus has been reported by several authors.[66-68] Although the relevance to patients with carcinomatous pain is uncertain, these techniques deserve mention because of their apparent safety in patients with nonmalignant pain and itch. In one series[67] over two thirds of patients experienced complete symptomatic relief that persisted for 1 to 5 years. Complications were limited to local skin reactions that, although initially distressing, subsided over a period of 2 to 3 weeks.

SUMMARY

Peripheral neurolysis has specific but important indications in the management of intractable cancer pain. It is inappropriate and inadequate for benign intractable nonmalignant pain. Careful attention needs to be paid to the applicability of more conservative alternative techniques before the use of peripheral neurolysis.

SUGGESTED READING

Patt R, editor: *Peripheral Neurolysis and the Management of Cancer Pain.* Philadelphia, JB Lippincott, 1993.

REFERENCES

1. Patt R: Neurosurgical interventions for chronic pain problems. *Anesthesiology Clinics of North America* 5:609, 1987.
2. Ramamurthy S et al: Evaluation of neurolytic blocks using phenol and cryogenic block in the management of chronic pain. *J Pain Symptom Manage* 4:72, 1989.
3. Pender JW, Pugh DG: Diagnostic and therapeutic nerve blocks: Necessity for roentgenograms. *JAMA* 146:798, 1951.
4. Raj PP, Rosenblatt R, Montgomery S: Uses of the nerve stimulator for peripheral block. *Reg Anesth* 5:14, 1980.
5. Rastogi V, Kumar R: Peripheral nerve stimulator as an aid for therapeutic alcohol blocks. *Anesthesiology* 38:163, 1983.
6. Moore DC: Intercostal nerve block and celiac plexus block for pain therapy. In Benedetti C et al, editors: *Advances in Pain Research and Therapy, vol 4.* New York, Raven Press, 1984.
7. Bonica JJ: *Management of Pain.* Philadelphia, Lea & Febiger, 1953.
8. Roviaro GC et al: Intrathoracic intercostal nerve block with phenol in open chest surgery. *Chest* 90:64, 1986.
9. Moore DC: *Regional Block,* ed 4. Springfield, Ill, Charles C Thomas, 1965.
10. Patt RB, Millard R: A role for peripheral neurolysis in the management of intractable cancer pain. *Pain* (Suppl 5):S358, 1990.
11. Szalados J, Patt R: Management of a patient with displaced orthopedic hardware. *J Pain Symptom Manage* 6:934-937, 1991.
12. Takagi Y, Kayama T, Yamamoto Y: Subarachnoid neurolytic block with 15% phenol glycerin in the treatment of cancer pain. *Pain* (Suppl 4):133, 1987.
13. Ischia S et al: Lytic saddle block: Clinical comparison of the results, using phenol at 5, 10, and 15 percent. In Benedetti C et al, editors: *Advances in Pain Research and Therapy, vol 7.* New York, Raven Press, 1984.
14. Chrucher M: Peripheral nerve blocks in the relief of intractable pain. In Swerdlow M, Charlton JE, editors: *Relief of Intractable Pain,* ed. 4. Amsterdam, Elsevier, 1989.
15. Swerdlow M: Spinal and peripheral neurolysis for managing Pancoast syndrome. In Bonica JJ, Ventafridda V, Pagni C, editors: *Advances in Pain Research and Therapy, vol 4.* New York, Raven Press, 1982.
16. Mandl F: *Paravertebral Block.* New York, Grune and Stratton, 1947.
17. Cousins MJ, Dwyer B, Gibb D: Chronic pain and neurolytic neural blockade. In Cousins MJ, Bridenbaugh PO, editors: *Neural Blockade,* ed 2, Philadelphia, JB Lippincott, 1988.
18. Katz J: Current role of neurolytic agents. *Adv Neurol* 4:471, 1974.
19. Madrid JL, Bonica JJ: Cranial nerve blocks. In Bonica JJ, Ventafridda V, editors: *Advances in Pain Research and Therapy, vol 2.* New York, Raven Press, 1979.
20. Hakanson S: Trigeminal neuralgia treated by the injection of glycerol into the trigeminal cistern. *Neurosurgery* 9:638, 1981.
21. Shulman M: Treatment of cancer pain with epidural butyl-aminobenzoate suspension. *Reg Anesth* 12:1, 1987.
22. Shulman M: Intercostal nerve block with 10% butamben suspension for the treatment of chronic noncancer pain. *Anesthesiology* 71:A737, 1989.
23. Shulman M, Joseph NJ, Haller CA: Local effects of epidural and subarachnoid injections of butylaminobenzoate suspension. *Reg Anesth* 12:23, 1987.
24. Shulman M: Epidural butamben for the treatment of metastatic cancer pain. *Anesthesiology* 67:A245, 1987.
25. Evans PJD, Lloyd JW, Jack TM: Cryoanalgesia for intractable pain. *J R Soc Med* 74:804, 1981.
26. Wilson PJEM: Neurosurgery and relief of pain associated with head and neck cancer. *Ear Nose Throat J* 62:250, 1983.

27. Pitkin GP: Blocking the trigeminal nerve. In Southworth JL, Hingson RA, Pitkin WM, editors: *Conduction Anesthesia,* ed 2. Philadelphia, JB Lippincott, 1953.

28. Patt R, Jain S: Management of a patient with osteoradionecrosis of the mandible with nerve blocks. *J Pain Symptom Manage* 5:59, 1990.

29. Bonica JJ et al: Neurolytic blockade and hypophysectomy. In Bonica JJ, editor: *Management of Pain,* ed 2. Philadelphia, Lea & Febiger, 1990.

30. Montgomery W, Cousins MJ: Aspects of the management of chronic pain illustrated by ninth cranial nerve block. *Br J Anaesth* 44:383, 1972.

31. Labat G: *Regional Anesthesia.* Philadelphia, WB Saunders, 1922.

32. Twycross RG, Lack SA: *Therapeutics in Terminal Care.* New York, Churchill Livingstone, 1986.

33. Waldman SD et al: Cervical epidural implantable narcotic delivery systems in the management of upper body pain. *Anesth Analg* 66:780, 1987.

34. Lobato RD et al: Intraventricular morphine for intractable cancer pain. Rationale, methods, clinical results. *Acta Anaesthesiol Scand* 31:68, 1987.

35. Grant FC: Surgical methods for relief of pain. *Bull NY Acad Med* 19:373, 1943.

36. McEwen BW et al: The pain clinic. A clinic for the management of intractable pain. *Med J Aust* 1:676, 1965.

37. Siegfried J, Broggi G: Percutaneous thermocoagulation of the gasserian ganglion in the treatment of pain in advanced cancer. In Bonica JJ, Ventafridda V, editors: *Advances in Pain Research and Therapy, vol 2.* New York, Raven Press, 1979.

38. Broggi G, Siegfried J: Percutaneous differential radiofrequency rhizotomy glossopharyngeal nerve in facial pain due to cancer. In Bonica JJ, Ventafridda V, editors: *Advances in Pain Research and Therapy, vol 2.* New York, Raven Press, 1979.

39. Pagura JR, Schnapp M, Passarelli P: Percutaneous radiofrequency glossopharyngeal rhizotomy for cancer pain. *Applied Neurophysiology* 46:154, 1983.

40. Kaplan R, Aurellano Z, Pfisterer W: Phenol brachial plexus block for upper extremity cancer pain. *Reg Anesth* 13:58, 1988.

41. Neill RS: Ablation of the brachial plexus. *Anaesthesia* 34:1024, 1979.

42. Mullin V: Brachial plexus block with phenol for painful arm associated with Pancoast syndrome. *Anesthesiology* 53:431, 1980.

43. Doyle D: Nerve blocks in advanced cancer. *Practitioner* 226:539, 1982.

44. Moore D, Bridenbaugh DL: Intercostal nerve block in 4333 patients: Indications techniques, complications. *Anesth Analg* 41:1, 1962.

45. Swerdlow M: Role of chemical neurolysis and local anesthetic infiltration. In Swerdlow M, Ventafridda V, editors: *Cancer Pain.* Lancaster, MTP Press, 1987.

46. Conacher ID, Kokri M: Postoperative paravertebral blocks for thoracic surgery: Radiological appraisal. *Br J Anaesth* 59:155, 1987.

47. Gibson JM II: Phenol block in the treatment of spasticity. *Gerontology* 33:327, 1987.

48. Atkinson GL, Shupack RC: Acute bronchospasm complicating intercostal nerve block with phenol. *Anesth Analg* 68, 1989.

49. Mehta M, Ranger I: Persistent abdominal pain. *Anaesthesia* 26:330, 1971.

50. Plancarte R et al: Superior hypogastric plexus block for pelvic cancer pain. *Anesthesiology* 73:236, 1990.

51. Plancarte R, Amescua C, Patt RB: Presacral blockade of the ganglion impar ganglion of Walther. *Anesthesiology* 73:A751, 1990.

52. Robertson DH: Transsacral neurolytic nerve block: An alternative approach to intractable perineal pain. *Br J Anaesth* 55:873, 1983.

53. Clark AJ, Awad SA: Selective transsacral nerve root blocks. *Reg Anesth* 15:125, 1990.

54. Rockswold GL, Bradley WE, Chou SN: Effect of sacral nerve blocks on the function of the urinary bladder in humans. *J Neurosurg* 40:83, 1974.

55. Simon DL, Carron H, Rowlingson JC: Treatment of bladder pain with transsacral nerve block. *Anesth Analg* 61:46, 1982.

56. Goffen BS: Transsacral block. *Anesth Analg* 62:623, 1982.

57. Wilson F: Neurolytic and other locally acting drugs in the management of pain. *Pharmacol Ther* 53:431, 1991.

58. Feldman SA, Yeung ML: Treatment of intermittent claudication: Lumbar paravertebral somatic block with phenol. *Anaesthesia* 30:174, 1975.

59. Jack ED: Regional anaesthesia for pain relief. *Br J Anaesth* 47:278, 1975.

60. Moritz U: Phenol block of peripheral nerves. *Scand J Rehabil Med* 5:160, 1973.

61. Kirvel, Nieminen S: Treatment of painful neuromas with neurolytic blockade. *Pain* 41:161, 1990.

62. Defalque RJ, Bromley JJ: Poststernotomy neuralgia: A new pain syndrome. *Anesth Analg* 69:81, 1989.

63. Todd DP: Poststernotomy neuralgia: A new pain syndrome. *Anesth Analg* 69:691, 1989.

64. Defalque RJ: Painful trigger points in surgical scars. *Anesth Analg* 61:518, 1982.

65. Swerdlow M: Role of chemical neurolysis and local anesthetic infiltration. In Swerdlow M, Ventafridda V, editors: *Cancer Pain.* Lancaster, MTP Press, 1987.

66. Stone HB: A treatment for pruritus ani. *Bulletin of Johns Hopkins Hospital* 27:242, 1916.

67. Woodruff JD, Babkinia A: Local alcohol injection of the vulva: Discussion of 35 cases. *Obstet Gynecol* 54:512, 1979.

68. Woodruff JD, Thompson B: Local alcohol injection in the treatment of vulvar pruritus. *Obstet Gynecol* 40:18, 1972.

27 Cryolysis

Jeff M. Arthur and Gabor B. Racz

In 1938 the interest of the medical profession was re-awakened to the therapeutic use of low temperatures when Fay and Smith reported finding tumor regression following localized freezing, a finding similarly observed 87 years earlier by Arnott.[1-5] During the next half century, many technologic developments that occurred led to a new interest in *cryoanalgesia,* the term for creating a nerve injury by freezing. Cryoanalgesia developments include freezing carbon dioxide and fashioning into dry ice pencils for topical application; and cooling metal rods (cryoprobes) in baths of dry ice and acetone or ether, and pressing the rods against the tissue to be frozen.[6]

It was not until liquid air and liquid nitrogen became available, however, that another generation of more powerful cryoprobes was developed. In 1961 Cooper and colleagues developed the first cryoprobe.[1,7] The probe employed the principle of phase change using liquid nitrogen to produce a temperature of $-196°$ C. Later, Amoils developed a smaller, more easily controlled probe for ophthalmic surgery and introduced the enclosed gas expansion cryoprobe.[1,8] This probe used the Joule-Thompson principle, was driven by liquid carbon dioxide, and was capable of reaching temperatures of $-50°$ C. Since that time, numerous probes have been developed using this principle and nitrous oxide as the primary refrigerant, which is capable of achieving minimal temperatures of approximately $-70°$ C. Currently, these probes are available in many sizes and shapes and have incorporated thermocouples and nerve stimulators. Many probes can be inserted through the skin for localization and freezing of nerves percutaneously.[1,9,10]

In the 1960s physicians in pain control became more involved with the new types of precision cryoprobes, and in the early 1970s the concept of therapeutic peripheral nerve freezing was reintroduced. Nelson and colleagues[6,11] Brain,[6,12] and Lloyd and colleagues[9] applied cryoprobes to various nerves including the intercostal, pharyngeal, trigeminal, sacral, and others in the treatment of various chronic neuralgias and pain. Lloyd and colleagues are credited with naming the technique cryoanalgesia, and have demonstrated that prolonged analgesia can be obtained after a single freezing of a peripheral nerve. They particularly stressed the safety of the procedure and reported that nerve function always returned and neuroma formation did not occur.[1,9]

HISTOLOGIC BASIS OF CRYONEUROLYSIS

The mechanism of cold-induced nerve injury is still unknown. Many explanations have been suggested, including: hypertonicity of intracellular and extracellular fluids,[13,14] physical destruction by large cellular ice crystals,[1,15,16] minimal cell volume,[1,17] damage to proteins,[1,18] membrane rupture caused by rapid water loss,[1,19] ischemic necrosis,[1,20-22] and the production of autoantibodies.[1,21,23] Many of the studies have been conducted in vitro, and subsequent interpretation in main is difficult. However, freezing represents nothing more than the removal of pure water from a solution and isolating it as ice crystals into an inert foreign body. All subsequent biochemical, anatomic, and physiologic consequences of freezing are directly or indirectly the consequence of this single event.[1] Many have closely studied the mechanism of freeze injury: Joy and Finean, Menz, Carter and co-workers, and Whittaker; they all agreed that the major factors in freeze injury were the development of intracellular and extracellular ice crystals.[24] The formation of ice either causes gross shifts in tissue osmolarity and cell wall permeability or produces physical disruption of the myelin sheath and Schwann's cell.[24] Myers et al[22] suggested that freezing an injury also caused extensive vascular damage and permitted plasma and extracellular extravasation, which increased endoneural fluid pressure. Subsequently, they found that the nerve fiber underwent wallerian degeneration, a process associated with elevated endoneural fluid pressure.[22] Nevertheless, once the ice crystal formation produced destruction of the nerve, no additional benefit was achieved by decreasing the temperature of the cell. However, it was found that the size of the lesion created and the length of the nerve involvement were temperature dependent to a point.[24]

Southerland described categories or "degrees" of peripheral nerve injury based on histology and prognosis.[6,25] The degree of injury sought by a peripheral cryolesion is that of a second-degree injury, which occurs when a short length of peripheral nerve is frozen to $-20°$ C or lower.[6,25,26] In this injury, there is a "loss of axonal continuity without breaching of the endoneurium." The axons of nerve are damaged at the site of injury. The fibrous architecture (endoneurium, perineurium, epineurium) of the nerve, however, is preserved. The axon and myelin sheaths degenerate from the point of freezing distally to the nerve's termination (wallerian degeneration). Regeneration begins immediately from the proximal stump. The growing tips of individual axons (growth cones) advance distally within the lumen of their still-intact endoneurial tubes at a rate of approximately 1.0 to 1.5 mm per day. After a period of time and a distance directly proportional from the point of injury to the distal end of the nerve, axon sprouts reach their end organs. Nerve histology after regrowth is restored to normal. However, maximum nerve conduction velocity remains reduced an average of 35 days, even after new myelin sheaths have fully matured.[6,27] However, normal sensory and motor functions do return, provided that (in the case of limbs) regrowth occurs before irreversible endoneural fibrosis, muscle wasting, or contractures can occur.[6]

Third-, fourth-, and fifth-degree nerve injuries occur with more permanent forms of neurolytic lesions, such as use of radiofrequency thermocoagulation, alcohol, phenol, and surgical resection. These types of nerve injuries are prone to neuritis and the formation of neuromas. Because of the disruption of the endoneural and perineural fiber sheaths, respectively, there is a more erratic and disorganized reformation of the nerve between the nerve stump and its end organ. Useful regeneration does not occur with fifth-degree injuries; the nerve is completely transected, and the two ends are separated. Neuromas, however, can still form.[6]

In contrast, a cryolesion is reversible and has not been associated with neuromata. In several studies on animals, there was no evidence of neuroma formation at necropsy, and the degree of fibrosis and scarring at the site of injury was minimal. The extent of cell destruction by a cryolesion will be dependent on several factors, but the rate of freezing and thawing and the temperature attained by the tissue in proximity to the cryoprobe are the most important.[24] Evans and co-workers showed that when a rat sciatic nerve was directly exposed to cryolesion, the time for regeneration of the nerve was independent of the duration of freezing and the application of a repeat freeze cycle.[24] However, the temperature attained by the nerve was important. Evans concluded that where the temperature remained greater than −20° C, the results were unpredictable. Below this temperature, the interruption was prolonged and uninfluenced by greater reductions in temperature.[24]

This contrasted data presented by Gill et al.,[28] which showed that repeated freeze-thaw cycles greatly enhanced the size of the cryolesion. Generally, repeat freeze-thaw cycles in vivo will in fact increase the freeze zone or size of the cryolesion. Evans supported this theory in his study and explained that, in a clinical setting, the cryoprobe may not be directly abutting the nerve but only approximating it; and the tissue surrounding the probe may not reach the critical temperature of −20° C. Repeated freeze-thaw cycles, as demonstrated by Gill and colleagues, will decrease the temperature at a more distal site from the cryoprobe and can increase the freeze zone by as much as 70%.[24,28] In 1955 Douglas and Malcolm showed that it was possible for nerve impulses to jump an inactivated area of the axon. In cats, they demonstrated that an injury 3 to 6 mm long was sufficient to stop salsitory conduction.[29] Evans et al, found that in a laboratory, a 4-mm lesion was always an effective lesion of rat sciatic nerve.[24] Therefore the size of the cryolesion seems to be one of the important factors governing the success of treatment.

When using a percutaneous cryoprobe, the rate of cooling the tissue depends on the geometry of the cryoprobe and its capacity for heat extraction. The *iceball* (probe tip to ice interface with tissue) shows a sharp temperature gradient across its radius of approximately 10° C/ml.[1,30] The tissues closest to the probe attain the maximum sub-zero temperature, whereas the remaining tissues show a rapid rise toward 0° C. The central zone undergoes rapid cooling while the peripheral zone is influenced by the heat generated as the surrounding tissue slowly cools. Extending the duration of freezing will produce some increase in the size of the iceball and the central zone until a plateau is reached, whereby heat extraction by the probe balances the heat production by the surrounding tissue. Here again, Gill and co-workers[28] showed that repetitive freezing could increase the amount of tissue frozen and the rate of freezing tissue surrounding the probe. Despite debate in the literature, there is uniform agreement that temperatures below −20° C cause cellular freezing, and cells do not recover.[1,31]

STRUCTURE OF THE CRYOPROBE

Many designs of cryoprobes currently exist that incorporate several different refrigerating principles. Currently, however, only two types are powerful and practical enough to be used for clinical cryoanalgesia: those that refrigerate by expansion of a compressed gas such as nitrous oxide, and those that refrigerate using a change-of-phase liquified gas such as nitrogen. The most popular cryoprobes currently employed are modified versions of the cryoprobe designed by Amoils in 1967, which use the Joule-Thompson effect where gas is expanded through an orifice and thereby reduces the temperature of the gas.[6,32] Figure 27-1, *A*, depicts the construction of a modern Joule-Thompson-type cryoprobe. This illustration shows nitrous oxide gas being cooled by expansion at the probe tip and then being exhausted through a port in the center of the probe shaft. Nitrous oxide is an extremely convenient gas to use because it can easily be stored under pressure as a liquid at room temperature. Gas-expansion cryoprobes usually produce temperatures −70° to −80° C and work at full nitrous oxide cylinder pressures of 750 lb/sq in. However, other gases including carbon dioxide have been used for this probe.[6]

Modern versions of the cryoprobe also use a temperature thermocouple imbedded in the tip to measure probe temperature. A nerve stimulator is incorporated to help freeze pinpoint nerves and to avoid those nerves not intended to be lysed. The typical freeze-zone diameter for a gas expansion cryoprobe set at −60° C is two to three times the probe's diameter, as compared with 3.5 to 5 times the diameter of a liquid nitrogen probe at −180° C (see below). The standard freeze zone that could be created at equilibrium was approximately 10 mm with the 14-gauge gas expansion cryoprobe, and approximately 6 mm with the 16 gauge cryoprobe, as measured by the author in vitro.

Currently manufactured cryoprobes have insulation around them, but using a standard intravenous (IV) catheter (12- and 14-gauge catheters for 14- and 16-gauge cryoprobes, respectively) provides additional insulation, that protects the tissues not intended to be frozen. Insulation around cryoprobes can leak and freeze tissue other than that at the tip of the probe. This can be very hazardous if the lesion to be frozen is in close proximity to other important structures. With an IV cannula surrounding the cryoprobe, freezing at the insulated area does occur; however, the temperature is unlikely to reach the critical −20° C mark, and therefore tissue in this area is unlikely to be permanently

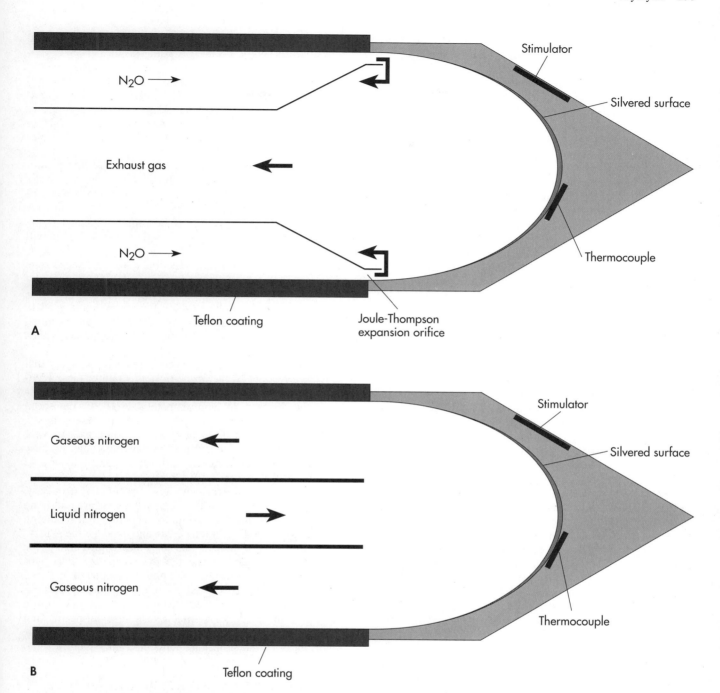

Fig. 27-1 A, Diagrammatic cross section of gas expansion (Joule-Thompson) and **B,** liquid nitrogen cryoprobe tips. (Modified from Lloyd JW, Barnard JDW, Glynn CJ: Cryoanalgesia; a new approach to pain relief. *Lancet* 2:932-934, 1976.)

damaged. In addition to insulation safety, the IV needle with a cannula can be used to easily pierce the skin and act as a guide in directing the cryoprobe to the site intended for lesioning. This is important because cryoprobes tend to be delicate and are easily damaged by bending. There are many components to the cryoprobe that can be easily disrupted by bending (see Fig. 27-1). This is especially true in the smaller (18-gauge) probe that is currently available.

The second type of cryoprobe uses a change of phase to produce refrigeration. The original model was designed in 1951 by Irving Cooper and Arnold Lee, and that basic design continues to be followed today. Their design consisted of a long insulated metal tube through which a stream of liquid nitrogen could enter and evaporate (Fig. 27-1, *B*).

Temperatures $-196°$ C can be attained with a liquid nitrogen cryoprobe. Freezing capacity is proportional to the rate at which liquid nitrogen is delivered to the surface area of the probe tip and the rate at which latent heat evaporates the liquid nitrogen.[6,7]

Liquid nitrogen is difficult to store; it must be stored in large thermos bottles called *Dewar flasks,* from which it evaporates, whether it is used or not. Fortunately liquid nitrogen is inexpensive and readily obtainable. It is also potentially hazardous to handle. This type of cryoprobe and the instrumentation required to operate it are far more expensive than the Joule-Thompson gas-expansion cryoprobe apparatus.[6] Nevertheless, the greater freezing capacity of the liquid nitrogen probe may prove useful and necessary for certain percutaneous uses.

Recently a helium gas cryoprobe has been described. The construction is similar to the liquid nitrogen probe, but it uses helium gas that has been precooled to −80° C by liquid nitrogen. This cold gas is delivered at a high velocity to impinge on the spherically shaped probe tip. The gas is then redirected back through the annulus surrounding the supply tube.[33,34] Bald reported that an 8 mm probe tip created an iceball of 28 mm after 10 minutes of freezing with a gas flow of 42 L/min and a tip temperature of −138° C. The clinical utility for this probe remains to be seen.

TYPICAL USE OF THE GAS-EXPANSION CRYOPROBE

The key to the successful use of the gas-expansion cryoprobe is placing the tip of the probe as close as possible and preferably abutting the nerve to be lysed. As previously stated, it is critical for a minimum length of 4 mm of the nerve to reach a temperature of −20° C or below in order to stop nerve conduction.[24] Therefore, the cryoprobe must be very close to the area to be lysed. Typically the nerve to be frozen is blocked with a local anesthetic; this also proves that the cryolysis will provide adequate results. After this block has been allowed to resolve, the patient can be treated with a cryolesion. This is essential because patients with existing local anesthetic blocks cannot give accurate reports about the motor or sensory stimulation provided by the cryoprobe; and therefore close proximity of the cryoprobe to the nerve cannot be ascertained.

After preparing the skin thoroughly with a bactericidal substance, a skin wheal of local anesthetic can be injected to lessen the pain when inserting the cryoprobe. Then insert the IV "catheter over needle" through the skin and direct it toward the area to be frozen. Do not get the tip of the needle too close to the area to be lysed, because the tip of the needle is very sharp and cutting, and further nerve damage may occur. Once the IV cannula is in place, remove the needle and leave the cannula behind. The cryoprobe can be easily inserted through the IV cannula and directed toward the area for lesioning. Once the desired area has been reached, position the cryoprobe and check using fluoroscopy. Using fluoroscopy to check position is strongly advised for many types of lesions being performed percutaneously, because the probe tip needs to be in the exact location for success. Once the tip of the probe has been positioned, the nerve stimulator in the cryoprobe can be used. First a 2-Hz motor stimulus is given to the patient using the entire range of voltage from 0 to approximately 5 volts.

This is done slowly, and, if any motor component is seen, reposition the probe because freezing motor nerves is generally unwanted. Once the motor stimulus shows a negative reading, the sensory stimulator is activated; start at 0 volts and increase as necessary. Unlike with motor stimulation, the desire is to provoke sensory stimulation and to specifically recreate pain in the distribution corresponding to the patient's complaints. After this is done, the cryolesioning can begin.

The typical duration for a cryolesion is 1.0 to 1.5 minutes. Flow through the probe will depend on the size of the probe. The typical nitrous oxide gas-expansion probe will reach a temperature of −60 to −70° C at the tip; the zone of maximum freezing occurs at 1.5 minutes. Longer freezing may increase the freeze zone slightly, but the effect will be minimal.

A much more useful technique to expand the freeze zone is to use the freeze-thaw-refreeze cycle (previously described). Once the 1.5-minute freezing cycle has been performed, allow the probe to thaw for approximately 20 to 30 seconds. Do not move the probe. After this thawing time, freeze again for another 1.5 minutes. This approach yields maximum freeze zone and benefits.

Some cryoprobes are equipped with thermocouples that provide a readout of the probe-tip temperature; these readings can be used to extend the freeze time until a steady-state temperature of approximately −60° C has been reached. This technique, compared to a pure time technique, is sometimes useful in situations where high heat transfer may occur. It is also useful for the thawing cycle, because it measures the temperature of the tissue and allows it to rise above 0° C before refreezing.

Multiple sites of freezing are occasionally necessary. However, the probe must thoroughly thaw before removing it from one area and proceeding to the next. After removing the probe and the IV cannula, clean and bandage the skin.

Severe pain can indicate that the probe is proximal to the nerve to be lesioned during the first freezing cycle. This pain should stop when the lesioning is completed at 1 to 2 minutes. Refreezing is usually painless. If pain is present, it usually means that the electrode moved or was never close enough to the nerve for complete lesioning during the first freezing. Patients need to be warned regarding the possible painfulness of the procedure, and they may require sedation.

SPECIFIC LESIONS WITH PERCUTANEOUS CRYOPROBE

Percutaneous cryoprobe application has been used for many types of neural lesioning. In fact, any nerve that can be isolated by percutaneous or direct vision cryoprobe can undergo cryoneurolysis. The following is a review of some of the more popular uses for the cryoprobe. However, despite the lack of neuroma formation and low incidence of neuritis with a cryolesion, it is not a benign procedure, and cryoneurolysis of motor nerves should be avoided.

Facial pain

Treatment of postherpetic and nonherpetic trigeminal neuralgia by cryoneurolysis has been described throughout the literature. When treating the trigeminal nerve or its branches, the most commonly described method of cryoneurolysis is to expose the nerve with a surgical incision after administering a local anesthesia. Once the nerve is isolated, it is frozen, thawed, and refrozen. Using this technique, Barnard et al. found in a 4-year study that 67% of patients with nonherpetic neuralgia experienced pain relief a median of 93 days; this exceeded the duration of sensory loss of a median 60 days.[35] In addition, Zakrzewska studied the management of paroxysmal trigeminal neuralgia in 29 patients over 5 years; 41% of the patients in the study were pain free for over 1 year, and there was no permanent sensory loss in any of the patients.[36] Barnard et al. also described the use of cryoneurolysis for posttraumatic neuralgia, malignant disease causing facial pain, and neuralgia of unknown ideology. They used the cryoprobe to lyse supraorbital, supratrochlear, infraorbital, mental, and lingual nerves in 21 patients. In these patients, they compared freezing followed by sectioning to freezing alone. They found that the median time of pain relief was 116 days for cryoneurolysis alone and only 38 days for freezing and subsequent sectioning. However, sensory loss lasted 49 days for cryoneurolysis and 131 days for freezing and sectioning. They concluded that cryoanalgesia was a useful therapeutic tool to manage intractable facial pain because it provided a reliable, prolonged, and reversible nerve block that could be achieved by a simple technique that did not appear to aggravate symptoms.[37] Goss described using cryoneurotomy for intractable temporomandibular joint pain. In his review of six patients with intractable neurogenic pain of the auricular nerves, cryoneurolysis was performed percutaneously, and all six patients had excellent pain relief for 1 year after the procedure. Four of the six had recurrent pain. He also found that repeat cryoneurolysis had decreasing effectiveness.[38] Cryoprobes have also been described for use in oral surgery and pituitary cryoablation.[39,40]

Thoracic pain

Chronic and acute thoracic pain have been treated with cryoneurolysis, intraoperatively at the end of thoracotomy for acute pain and percutaneously for chronic thoracic pain. A vast array of literature exists on this subject. Classically, the lesion is formed intraoperatively by placing the cryoprobe beneath the rib of the appropriate dermatome to be frozen and performing the lesion. Percutaneously, the lesion can be performed by placing the cryoprobe through the paraspinous musculature until the tip of the probe comes to rest at the thoracic spine foramen, which is associated with the dorsal root ganglion of the appropriate dermatome. Results of pain control with this technique vary from poor to excellent. Lloyd et al. found in 17 patients that the median duration of pain relief was 14 days, the range of relief was from 0 to 147 days, and two patients had no relief.[9] More recently Green and colleagues reported that in 41 patients studied, 50% had significant pain relief for 3 months after cryoneurolysis. They also did not see neuritis in any of these patients after this procedure. They concluded that cryoanalgesia was an appropriate technique for chest pain caused by intercostal neuralgia, and that subsequent pain relief could outlast motor and sensory blockade.[41]

Spinal pain

The use of percutaneous cryoprobe for facet rhizotomy has been described in the literature for the treatment of low back pain and lumbar disk syndrome. This procedure has been used to block the articular nerve of Luschka at the junction of the pedicle with transverse process. At this site, the nerve has not yet branched into ascending, lateral, and medial branches; therefore a single lesion can produce analgesia. However, in this technique, the nerve must be lysed at the level in question, at one level above, and one level below the facet of pathology. This is due to the branching nature of the nerves innervating the facets. Schuster used this technique for facet pain in 52 patients and found that 47 of these patients had significant relief from back pain. Of these 47, only one had to be retreated for recurrent pain after 9 months without pain.[42] In a like study, Brechner reported significant pain relief continuing for 3 months in 40% of patients treated by percutaneous cryogenic neurolysis of the articular nerve of Luschka.[43]

Pelvic pain

Sacral foramenal cryolesions have been used to treat cancer, coccydynia, and sciatic pain. A bilateral S_4 block is useful for treating coccydynia and perineal pain from cancer of the rectum; and, reportedly, this avoids bladder denervation. Also, S_1 and S_2 cryolesions can treat pain in sciatic distribution. However, multiple bilateral sacral block is best avoided when bladder dysfunction is a possible complication.[44] Evans et al. reported treating intractable perineal pain by inserting the cryoprobe through the sacral hiatus into the sacral channel to produce analgesia over the lower sacral nerve roots. In one study they found that 78% of patients treated by this method had pain improvement with a median duration of 30 days. Also, successful treatment was reported in patients suffering from pelvic cancer and coccydynia; best results were obtained in patients who received numerous freeze applications or prolonged freezing.[45] Using the technique described by Evans et al. where the cryoprobe is inserted through the sacral hiatus, Glynn found that patients had excellent pain relief in diastasis of the symphysis pubis during pregnancy.[46] In the cases studied by Glynn, the average duration of pain relief was greater than 6 weeks. He further reported that the results suggested that the pain of these patients originated from the pelvic floor and not from the symphysis pubis. Patients who underwent this treatment stated that they could feel the movement of the symphysis pubis without pain.[46]

Cryoneurolysis of the iliohypogastric and ilioinguinal nerves has also been described. In a study by Khiroya et al., cryoneurolysis of the ilioinguinal nerve was performed for postoperative pain relief after herniorrhaphy. They compared patients who had their ilioinguinal nerves frozen during surgery to those who did not, and they concluded that cryoanalgesia of the ilioinguinal nerve alone did not produce significant early postherniorrhaphy pain relief.[47] Treatment of iliohypogastric and ilioinguinal nerve entrapment by cryoneurolysis has also been reported by Racz and Hagstrom.[48] In their study, 25 patients had several causes of pain, including pregnancy. Of the patients treated with cryotherapy, none reported side effects of neuritis, and 46% had good-to-excellent pain relief. Of the 25, 5 were pregnant and had spontaneous onset of ilioinguinal or iliohypogastric neuralgia. All 5 patients experienced complete pain relief after diagnostic blockade and permanent relief after one or two cryotherapy procedures. This syndrome occurs spontaneously in pregnancy at the rate of 1:3,000 to 1:5,000 and is important to recognize because it can easily be treated by this cryotherapy. According to observations by Racz and Hagstrom, many pregnant patients had exploratory laparotomies to rule out acute abdominal diseases which might have been avoided if a simple diagnostic block with local anesthetic had been used instead to rule out the syndrome.[48]

Peripheral nerve pain

Blocking peripheral nerves by cryotherapy has been used for neuroma, causalgia, flexion contractures, and nerve entrapment syndromes. The nerves to be frozen must not have a significant motor component unless motor destruction is the goal, for example, in the later stages of multiple sclerosis. The reversibility of the nerve block, however, allows for return of motor function after normal regeneration.[44] Wang reported that, in patients treated for chronically painful peripheral nerve lesions, 50% of the patients treated in one study had pain relief for 1 to 12 months.[49] He also reported that the pain eventually returned. However, during the period of remission, patients returned to normal activities. Wang concurred with the concept that it is especially important when freezing peripheral nerves to have precise localization of the nerves in order to obtain adequate neurolysis.

Complications of cryotherapy

Many of the complications reported in the literature pertain to how the use of cutaneous cryosurgical techniques affect nerves that lie subcutaneously. However, some complications do exist for the use of the percutaneous cryoprobe. Cryosurgical equipment must be tested thoroughly before using to ensure that there are no leaks. A significant leakage of refrigerant can cause freezing along the shaft of the cryoprobe and subsequent freezing of structures other than those intended (as previously stated). Marsland et al. studied peripheral nerves and blood vessels damaged by cryogenics and reported that significant vascular damage could occur during cryotherapy.[50] The possible complications of this should be considered.

The most common problem is frostbite of the skin at the entry site, which can usually be prevented by an introducer sheath. Unattended motor damage can occur, but the patient very often recovers. A frustrating aspect of cryoneurolysis is that therapeutic effectiveness can not be predicted; pain relief can last from 3 to 1000 days.

CONCLUSION

In conclusion, cryoanalgesia and cryoneurolysis by percutaneous cryoprobe are safe and effective methods that can produce neuroblockade of moderate to long duration.

REFERENCES

1. Evans PJD: Cryoanalgesia. The application of low temperatures to nerves to produce anaesthesia or analgesia. *Anaesthesia* 36:1003-1013, 1981.
2. Fay T: Observation on prolonged human refrigeration. *NY St J Med* 40:4, 1940.
3. Smith LW, Fay T: Temperature factors in cancer and embryonal cell growth. *JAMA* 113:60, 1939.
4. Barnard JDW, Lloyd JW: Cryoanalgesia. *Nursing Times* 165:7-9, 1977.
5. Arnott J: *On the Treatment of Cancer by the Regular Application of an Anaesthetic Temperature.* London, G Churchill, 1851.
6. Riopelle JM et al: Cryoanalgesia: Present day status. *Sem in Anesth* IV, 305:12, Dec 4, 1985.
7. Garamy G: Engineering aspects of cryosurgery. In Rand RW, Rinfret A, von Leden H editors: *Cryosurgery.* Springfield, Ill, Charles C Thomas, 1968.
8. Amoils SP: The Joule Thompson cryoprobe. *Arch Ophthalmol* 78:201-207, 1967.
9. Lloyd JW, Barnard JDW, Glynn CJ: Cryoanalgesia, a new approach to pain relief. *Lancet* 2:932-934, 1976.
10. Hannington-Kiff JG: A "cryoseeker" for percutaneous cryoanalgesia. *Lancet* 2:816-817, 1978.
11. Nelson KN et al: Intraoperative intercostal nerve freezing to present postthoracotomy pain. *Ann Thorac Surg* 18:280-285, 1974.
12. Brain D: Non-neoplastic conditions of the throat and nose. In Holden HB, editor: *Practical Cryosurgery.* St Louis, Mosby, 1975.
13. Lovelock JE: The haemolysis of human red bloodcells by freezing and thawing. *Biochemica et Biophysica Acta* 10:414-426, 1953.
14. Farrant J: Mechanism of cell damage during freezing and thawing and its prevention. *Nature* 205:1284-1287, 1965.
15. Asahina E, editor: Cellular injury and resistance to freezing organisms. In: *Proceedings of the International Conference on Low Temperature Science, vol 2.* Hokkaido, Japan, Hokkaido University, 1967.
16. Meryman HT: Physical limitation of the rapid freezing method. *Pro Soc,* Lond [BIOL] 147:452-459, 1957.
17. Meryman HT: Modified model for the mechanism of freezing injury in erythrocytes. *Nature* 218:333-336, 1968.
18. Levitt J, Dean J: The role of membrane proteins in freezing injury and resistance. In Wolstenholme GEW, O'Connor M editors: *The Frozen Cell: A Cibu Foundation Symposium.* London, Churchill Livingstone, 1970.
19. Litvan GG: Mechanisms of cryoinjury in biological systems. *Cryobiology* 9:182-191, 1972.
20. Zacarian SA: Histopathology of skin cancer following cryosurgery, Preliminary report. *In Surg* 54:255-261, 1970.
21. Rothenborg HW: 125 I-serum albumin assay of edema in rat skin with and without vasoconstriction after cryosurgery type freezing. *Cryobiology* 9:1-8, 1972.
22. Myers RR et al: Biophysical and pathological effects of cryogenic nerve lesion. *Ann Neurol* 20:5-7, 1981.
23. Shulman S: Cryo-immunology: The production of antibody by the freezing of tissue. In Ran RW, Rinfret A, von Leden H editors: *Cryosurgery.* Springfield, Ill, Charles C Thomas, 1968.
24. Evans PJD, Lloyd JW, Green CJ: Cryoanalgesia: The response to alterations in freeze cycle and temperature. *Br J Anaesth* 53:1121-1127, 1981.
25. Sunderland S: *Nerves and Nerve Injuries,* ed 2. London, Churchill Livingstone, 1978.
26. Carter DC et al: The effect of cryosurgery on peripheral nerve function. *J R Coll Surg Edinb* 17:25-31, 1972.
27. Kalichman MW, Myers RR: Behavioral and electrophysiological recovery following cryogenic nerve injury. *Exp Neurol* 96:692-702, 1987.
28. Gill W, Frazier J, Carter D: Repeated freeze-thaw cycles in cryosurgery. *Nature* 219:410-413, 1968.
29. Douglas WW, Malcolm JL: Effect of localized cooling on conduction in cat nerves. *J Physiol Lond* 130:63-71, 1955.
30. Evans PJD: Cryoanalgesia, the application of low temperatures to nerves to produce anaesthesia or analgesia. *Anaesthesia* 36:1003-1013, 1981. and Spembly LTD: Manufacturer's specifications for gas expansion cryoprobes.
31. Williams KL, Holden HB: Cryosurgery in general and ENT surgery. *Br J Hosp Med* 14:14-25, 1975.
32. Barron RF: Cryoinstrumentation. In von Leden H, Cahan WG editors: *Cryogenics in Surgery.* Flushing, NY, Medical Examination Publishing Co, 1971.

33. Bald WB: A helium gas probe for use in cryosurgery. *Cryobiology* 21:570-573, 1984.
34. Abreu O, Kellner K: Heat transfer coefficients within the cavity formed by the tip of cryosurgical probes. *Cryogenics* 19:567-570, 1979.
35. Barnard J, Lloyd JW, Evans PJD: Cryoanalgesia in the management of chronic facial pain. *J Maxillofac Surg* 9:101, 1981.
36. Zakrzewska JM: Cryotherapy in the management of paroxysmal trigeminal neuralgia. *J Neurol Neurosurg Psychiatry* 50:485-487, 1987.
37. Barnard JDW, Lloyd JW, Glynn CJ: Cryosurgery in the management of intractable facial pain. *Br J Oral Maxillofac Surg* 16:135-141, 1978-79.
38. Goss AN: Cryoneurotomy for intractable temporomandibular joint pain. *Br J Oral Maxillofac Surg* 26:26-31, 1988.
39. Leopard PJ: Cryosurgery and its application to oral surgery. *Br J Oral Maxillofac Surg* 13:128-152, 1975.
40. Duthie AM: Pituitary cryoablation. *Anaesthesia* 38:495-497, 1983.
41. Green CR et al: Long term follow up of cryoanalgesia for chronic thoracic pain. *Reg Anaesth* 18:25 (Suppl) March-April 1993.
42. Schuster GD: The use of cryoanalgesia in the painful facet syndrome. *Neural Orthop Surg* 3(4):271-274, 1982.
43. Brechner T: Percutaneous cryogenic neurolysis of the articular nerve of Luschka. *Reg Anesth* 6:18-22, 1981.
44. *Pain Management.* Neurostat Clinical Information. San Diego, Westco Medical Corp, 1981.
45. Evans PJD, Lloyd JW, Jack TM: Cryoanalgesia for intractable perineal pain. *J R Soc Med* 74:804-809, 1981.
46. Glynn CJ: Cryoanalgesia to relieve pain in diastasis of the symphysis pubis during pregnancy. *BMJ* 290:1-2, 1985.
47. Khiroya RC, Davenport HT, Jones JG: Cryoanalgesia for pain after herniorrhaphy. *Anaesthesia* 41:73-76, 1986.
48. Racz G, Hagstrom D: Iliohypogastric and ilioinguinal nerve entrapment: Diagnosis and treatment. *Pain Digest* 2:43-48, 1992.
49. Wang JK: Cryoanalgesia for painful peripheral nerve lesions. *Pain* 22:191-194, 1985.
50. Marsland AR, Ramamurthy S, Barnes J: Cryogenic damage to peripheral nerves and blood vessels in the rat. *Br J Anaesth* 55:555-558, 1983.

QUESTIONS: CRYOLYSIS

1. Below what temperature does cell death occur?
   A. 0° C
   B. −10° C
   C. −20° C
   D. −60° C
2. What degree of nerve injury is produced with a cryolesion?
   A. First
   B. Second
   C. Third
   D. Fourth
3. Evans and colleagues showed in vitro that the rate of nerve regeneration after a cryolesion, i.e., cell death, was independent of all of the following EXCEPT:
   A. Duration of freezing
   B. Repeat freeze cycle
   C. Nerve cell temperature
   D. Size of the freeze zone

For questions 4-5, choose from the following:
A. 1, 2, and 3
B. 1 and 2
C. 2 and 4
D. 4
E. All of the above

4. Which of the following types of cryoprobes are currently in clinical use?
   1. Gas expansion
   2. Helium gas
   3. Change of phase
   4. Joule-Thompson
5. Which of the following are indications for percutaneous cryoneurolysis?
   1. Treatment of neuromas
   2. Treatment of flexion contractures
   3. Treatment of chest wall pain
   4. Treatment of nerve entrapment pain

ANSWERS

1. C
2. A
3. C
4. E
5. E

28 Radiofrequency

Carl E. Noe and *Gabor B. Racz*

Electrical current has been used to produce neural lesions in patients for a hundred years. Modern radiofrequency thermocoagulation has been used to ablate pain pathways in the trigeminal ganglion, spinal cord, dorsal root entry zone, dorsal root ganglion, sympathetic chain, and peripheral nerve. Unfortunately, the long-term effects of ablative techniques on clinical pain syndromes are incompletely known.

The radiofrequency lesion is formed when neural temperatures exceed 45° C. These temperatures are a result of frictional heat that is generated by molecular movement in a field of alternating current at radio wave frequency. Frequencies above 250 kHz produce an electromagnetic field around an active electrode. An active electrode is placed in the desired anatomic location, and an indifferent electrode is placed to minimize current passage across the myocardium. The current disperses via the second electrode, which is usually a high area contact plate. Wattage is gradually increased and heat develops in the tissue, which conducts to the active probe. Heat is generated as current flows through a probe with a built-in thermocouple. Thus the thermocouple needle combination allows lesioning, monitoring, and injecting without moving the appropriately positioned device. The temperature of the probe itself assumes equilibrium with the temperature of the tissue surrounding it. The heat is not emitted from the probe itself but from the current movement which generates the heat as it passes through the tissues. The temperature is monitored, and wattage is adjusted to a target temperature, which is a primary determinant of lesion size. For low-power procedures such as facet denervation, 10 to 20 watts are used. For hypophyseal destruction, more energy is used. Other factors such as active electrode diameter and length, contribute to wattage requirements. Tissue blood flow is important because significant heat convection can occur, with significant blood flow in the area of the lesion. Homogenous tissue is necessary for a lesion shape that is symmetric.[1]

Lesion size has a near-linear relationship with temperature. The advantage of using the radiofrequency technique for neurolytic procedures is the ability to monitor temperature during lesion formation. Lesion size plateaus with time. After 60 seconds at a certain temperature, lesion growth is minimal; therefore the time of lesion creation can be limited once the target temperature is reached. Lesions may extend a few millimeters beyond the active electrode tip, but the majority of the lesion volume surrounds the axis of the active electrode. Commercially available electrodes are insulated to expose a relatively short tip that acts as the active electrode. Stimulation can be performed at frequencies from 5 to 100 Hz and 0.1 to 10.0 V to assist placement and ensure safety. Higher frequencies and lower voltages are used to reproduce pain while localizing the target structure, whereas low frequency and higher voltages are used to assess neuromuscular activity before lesion generation.

A temperature of 45° C produces irreversible neuronal injury, but temperatures as high as 90° C have been used clinically to produce lesions of adequate size. In homogeneous tissue, lesions have smooth borders along the 45° C isotherm. Blood flow will convect heat away from the lesion area and reduce predicted lesion size. Earlier direct current radiofrequency lesions were associated with irregular borders and less control. Avoid lesion temperatures above 90° C to prevent boiling and tissue tearing with electrode removal.

Lesion shape is spheroidal around the active electrode and tapers at the tip so that minimal lesion formation occurs beyond the tip of the active electrode. In clinical implication, the placement of the active electrode should be oriented in an axis that will produce a spheroidal lesion along the desired location for neurolysis.[2]

Wilkinson introduced sympatholysis using radiofrequency energy at the upper thoracic chain.[3,4] Rocco in one study and Haynsworth and Noe in two studies described results of using the lumbar sympathetic chain.[5,6,7] Horner's syndrome and pneumothorax are the primary complications from the upper thoracic technique, and postsympatholysis neuralgia and incomplete sympatholysis are the remaining problems with lumbar radiofrequency sympatholysis. Although the active radiofrequency electrode may be placed radiographically, the location of the sympathetic chain has proven to be variable. This variability and the consequences of sympathetic destruction have limited the widespread use of these techniques. A recently introduced technique by Racz, using a blunt-tip, 10-mm active electrode, has simplified the procedure to one lesion per lumbar level. In 132 consecutive lesions, no cases of postsympathectomy neuralgia occurred.

AN EXAMPLE: LUMBAR LESIONING

The lumbar technique is performed in the prone position with the dispersal plate on the thigh. A 15-cm Radionics, 5-mm bare tip, and Sluyter-Mehta cannulae are placed 6 to 8 cm lateral to the midline at the second, third, and fourth lumbar vertebrae. Skin entry is made just inferior to the transverse process so that the probe can be passed under the transverse process but over the exiting nerve root. This approach is simplified by oblique fluoroscopy along the axis from the skin entry site and the anterolateral surface of the vertebral body.[8] Once the probe has reached the psoas muscle, use a lateral fluoroscopic image to avoid advancement anterior to the vertebral body. Since the sympathetic chain lies just anterior to the psoas muscle, lesions should be placed when the probe tip penetrates the psoas. This can be determined with contrast injection, after aspiration to exclude intravascular placement; and by fluoroscopy in the lateral and anterior-posterior (AP) placement, and in the lateral and AP views. The lateral view will frequently reveal contrast spread in a thin ribbon superiorly and inferiorly. The AP view will show the contrast spreading laterally into the psoas muscle if the tip has failed to penetrate the anterior psoas fascia. Once radiographic placement is satisfactory, aspiration is repeated and stimulation at 5 Hz and 4 V is performed. No neuromuscular activity should be experienced by the patient or observed. Administer 1 ml of 0.5% lidocaine for analgesia, and initiate lesion formation; 80° C for 60 seconds is desirable. The probe can be advanced in 0.5 cm increments until lesions have been placed to the anterior aspect of the vertebral body as viewed by lateral fluoroscopy. Aspiration, contrast injection, and stimulation should be repeated before each lesion placement. This process can be repeated from the anterior psoas muscle to the anterior aspect of the vertebral body. Injecting methylprednisolone (20 ml) in 3 ml 0.5% bupivacaine after lesion production may reduce the severity of postsympatholytic neuralgia.

DISCUSSION

Radiofrequency lesioning is a neurodestructive procedure. Therefore it has to be considered an end-of-the-line procedure when conservative therapeutic modalities have failed. The physician performing radiofrequency procedures must have appropriate training and experience before beginning such neurodestructive procedures. All of these procedures should be done under fluoroscopic guidance after appropriate test stimulation and verification of the tissues about to be destroyed has been accomplished. Different temperatures have various levels of neurodestructive capabilities. Numbness or motor paralysis occurs very rarely as a consequence of the lesioning. The tissues can be injured anywhere along the passing of the needle probe if there is a break in the insulation. Therefore supermaximal motor stimulation is always part of the procedure before lesioning is performed, in the event that the insulated portion of the needle passes near a motor nerve such as in lumbar sympathetic lesioning. If there is a break in insulation, not only the lumbar sympathetic ganglion but also the lumbar nerve root may be neurodestructed, which is definitely not the desired outcome. Kline[9] describes the essential information for trainees and others interested in radiofrequency techniques.

Radiofrequency lesioning can have definite advantages over alternative neurodestructive procedures, primarily because the lesion is controlled. The complications associated with neurolytic solutions, resulting from intravasular injection and spread along tissue planes, can be avoided. The proximal and distal spread of the lesion beyond the uninsulated tip of the probe is only 1 mm, and the cross-sectional diameter of the lesion is 5 to 6 mm. The advantages include[9]:

1. Well-controlled lesion size
2. Temperature is monitored in the core of the lesion by the built-in thermal couple
3. Electrode placement can be verified by fluoroscopic guidance using electrical stimulation and impedance monitoring
4. Procedure can be performed without general anesthetics.
5. Procedure can be performed on an outpatient basis, and effectiveness can be recognized in approximately 4 weeks
6. There is a low morbidity and mortality associated with the lesioning itself; however, potential complications include major neurologic injury, and extreme care must be taken when injecting local anesthetics and steroids, as well as during probe placement, location verification, and lesion formation.
7. Procedure can be repeated

Monitor patients because radiofrequency equipment can interact with pacemakers and spinal cord stimulators. The equipment used in the procedure must be safe, precise, and must yield reproducible results. The equipment[9] must be able to:

1. Measure impedance
2. Stimulate a wide range of frequencies
3. Accurately time the duration of the lesion for a precise temperature measurement in the core of the lesion tissue
4. Accurately measure and indicate amperage and voltage
5. Gradually increase temperature with time

Patients should be selected based on the following criteria[9]:

1. Other noninvasive conservative measures have failed.
2. Substance abuse has been identified and dealt with, such as opioids, sedatives, and alcohol; and patient has entered a program to resolve the issues in addition to symptom control.
3. Appropriate psychologic assessment and therapy has been performed for depression, anxiety, anger, and secondary gain. The patient has been entered into an appropriate behavioral management program.
4. The patients accept their lifestyle changes, address psychologic issues, and interact with physicians, therapists, and psychologists in an appropriate manner.
5. Fully informed consent, including recognition of realistic expectations and procedural risks, must be obtained.

Procedural considerations must be preceded by full awareness of the anatomy, pain pathways, anticipated outcomes, and the need to have a multidisciplinary team carrying out such procedures.

The most commonly used procedures include neurodestructive procedures around facet joints in the neck, thoracic, lumbar, and lumbar cervical areas. Anterior compartment pain from lumbar disease can be solved by lesioning the anterior communicating branch.[10] Radiofrequency lumbar ganglionotomy, partial rhizotomy, sacral ganglionotomy, thoracic ganglionotomy, cervical ganglionotomy, cervical facets, disks, nerve roots, myofascial tissues, sphenopalatine ganglion, and radiofrequency lesioning of the stellate ganglion via the interior approach have been useful at C_6, C_7, and T_1 areas.

Radiofrequency lesioning of the trigeminal ganglion, as described by Sweet et al., has been an important experience in neurosurgical circles.[11] Percutaneous cordotomy is probably the most studied and indicated procedure, especially in the treatment of cancer pain. This procedure has resulted in excellent unilateral pain relief, especially affecting the torso on the contralateral side of the lesioning. The hazards of the procedure include worse pain when the patient outlives the duration of the lesioning and the possibility of Ondine's curse if bilateral lesioning is carried out. The incidence of radiofrequency cordotomies, even in patients with cancer pain, seems to have decreased since the introduction of spinal opioids, other neuroaugmentation procedures such as spinal cord stimulation, and in patients who respond favorably to more modern forms of cancer therapies. It is especially tragic when complications of therapy such as permanent numbness or, in rare instances, development of neuropathic pain persist when the cancer is no longer a problem. As a general rule, deafferentation pains do not respond to radiofrequency lesioning.

As a consequence of radiofrequency lesioning, patients who have sensing pacemakers may have a period of asystole unless their pacemakers have an override. Pacemaker features should be determined before radiofrequency procedures, and continous electrocardiographic monitoring is indicated during radiofrequency procedures. An additional problem that has not been fully documented but merits a word of caution concerns close-distance radiofrequency lesioning, such as in stellate ganglion radiofrequency thermocoagulation, with patients who have cervical spinal cord stimulators. The current may actually pass in the direction of the spinal cord stimulator and involve the spinal cord. There is no information regarding long-term effect, but data need to be gathered.

At this time there are ongoing double-blind studies to determine the appropriate location for facet lesioning in the cervical area. These studies will very likely positively influence the practice of radiofrequency lesioning for cervical facet joint disease. Clinically, radiofrequency lesioning is a very useful technique that needs to be substantiated by outcome studies. The equipment that has been used by most centers is the Radionics RFG-B and the newer RFG-F3C.

Because all radiofrequecy procedures should be carried out under fluoroscopic control, the physician should exercise caution by minimizing radiation exposure and injury to the patient and thereby to the physician.

REFERENCES

1. Cosman ER, Nashold BD, Ovelmann-Levitt J: Theoretical aspects of radiofrequency lesions in the dorsal root entry zone. *Neurosurgery* 15:945-950, 1984.
2. Bogduk N, Macintosh J, Marsland A: Technical limitations to the efficacy of radiofrequency neurotomy for spinal pain. *Neurosurgery* 20:529-535, 1987.
3. Wilkinson HA: Radiofrequency percutaneous upper-thoracic sympathectomy. *N Engl J Med* 311:34-36, 1984.
4. Wilkinson HA: Percutaneous radiofrequency upper thoracic sympathectomy: A new technique. *Neurosurgery* 15:811-814, 1984.
5. Rocco AG: Radiofrequency lumbar sympathectomy for sympathetically-maintained pain. *Reg Anesth* 15 (suppl):24, 1991.
6. Haynsworth RF, Noe CE: Percutaneous lumbar sympathectomy: A comparison of radiofrequency denervation versus phenol neurolysis. *Anesthesiology* 74:459-463, 1991.
7. Noe CE, Haynsworth RF: Radiofrequency lumbar sympatholysis. *J Vasc Surg* 17:801-806, 1993.
8. Sluyter ME, Mehta M: Percutaneous thermal lesions in the treatment of back and neck pain. In Lipton S, Miles J, editors: *Persistent Pain. Modern Methods of Treatment, vol 3.* London, Academic Press, 1981.
9. Kline MT: *Stereotactic Radiofrequency Lesions as Part of the Management of Pain.* Orlando, Fla, Paul M. Deutsch Press, 1992.
10. Sluyter ME, Racz GB, editors: *Techniques of Neurolysis.* Boston, Kluwer Academic Publishers, 1989.
11. Sweet WH: The treatment of trigeminal neuralgia (tic douloureux). *N Engl J Med* 315:174-177, 1986.

QUESTIONS: RADIOFREQUENCY

For questions 1-2, choose from the following:

A: 1, 2, and 3
B: 1 and 3
C: 2 and 4
D: 4
E: All of the above

1. During a lumbar facet radiofrequency denervation procedure, stimulation at 5 Hz before lesion formation produces neuromuscular activity in a lower extremity. The next action should be:
    1. Abandon the procedure
    2. Insert 2% lidocaine
    3. Reposition the probe
    4. Produce a large lesion

2. Radiofrequency thermocoagulation has been successfully used for:
    1. Dorsal root entry zone lesions
    2. Cordotomy
    3. Peripheral nerve block
    4. Celiac plexus block

3. Radiofrequency thermocoagulation produces a lesion characterized by:
    A. Charred tissue
    B. Tissue vaporization
    C. Hematoma formation
    D. Spheroid shape

4. Radiofrequency thermocoagulation employs what type of energy?
    A. Ultrasound
    B. Direct current
    C. Laser
    D. Alternating current

5. Heat develops in tissue during radiofrequency thermocoagulation by:
    A. Convection
    B. Conduction
    C. Friction
    D. The tip of the probe heat

ANSWERS

1. B
2. A
3. D
4. D
5. C

29 Acupuncture

P. Prithvi Raj and David Evans

Acupuncture is one of the oldest forms of medical therapy; its history goes back at least 2000 years. Literally millions of patients have received this form of treatment for acute and chronic pain, but the method is still controversial; in fact, most clinics that treat chronic pain do not consider it "mainstream" medical therapy and certainly do not use it as a frontline method of treatment.

Acupuncture has recently been extensively reviewed,[1] and it would appear that it can now be based more scientifically. Whether this satisfies the critics remains to be seen. One of the most difficult aspects of acupuncture to accept is the location of the needle points, which, in the traditional Chinese literature, seem to have no relationship to any anatomic structures directly relating to the nervous system. The *Nei Ching,* an ancient Chinese text that first described acupuncture, describes 361 classical acupuncture points. These points lie along specific pathways, or meridians, which extend in a network throughout the body. The *Ching* meridians are the vertical tracts from which branch the horizontal, or *Lo,* meridians. All of the points for needle insertion in classical Chinese acupuncture are located on the vertical (Ching) meridians. There are 14 meridians, 12 double and 2 single. The concept of the yin and the yang plays an important part in the way that the meridians relate to solid and hollow organs, depending on whether the organ has Tsang (solid) or Fu (hollow) properties. These meridians are also supposed to connect the internal organs with points that are related in a very proximate way to nerves and blood vessels.

A measurement called the *cun* is also important in Chinese acupuncture. The cun is roughly the distance between the distal skinfold of the third phalanx and the proximal fold of the first phalanx of the middle finger, measured in the relaxed or partially bent position. The meridians and their points and how they relate to prominent anatomic landmarks are measured in terms of the cun. The crucial question, of course, is whether these acupuncture points are any different from any other points where an acupuncturist may insert a needle.

Traditional Chinese literature describes sensations, or *techi,* produced by the introduction of needles at various points in the skin, specifically those related to the acupuncture site. These techi are variously described but can be grouped into four main categories: *Suan* (ache), *Ma* (numbness), *Chang* (pressure) and *Chung* (heaviness). To a great extent these sensations are located around the site of the needle insertion. These sensations may radiate for short distances in about 20% of patients; and in a very small number of patients, this radiation may extend extensively along the tract or meridian. This more extensive radiation is known as *propagated sensation along channels* (PSAC).[2] PSAC can be blocked remotely along the course of the radiation by local anesthetics, cooling, and pressure.[3] PSAC is of some importance and has come under considerable critical analysis because it supports a principal tenet held by traditional acupuncturists: Stimulation produced by the insertion of acupuncture needles is conveyed to the target sites by channels hitherto undiscovered by modern science. Thus the peripheral and central nervous systems are not necessarily the only conduits of impulses (electrical or otherwise) that affect nociception. For instance, stimulation at a point on the medial side of the wrist may produce sensations in the lateral side of the arm, head, and abdomen. This implies that special conducting channels are in effect. However, the fact that stimulation can produce sensations in a phantom limb would suggest that the central nervous system must be involved in some way.[4]

Much work has been done on the differences in skin potential and electrical resistance that occur between acupuncture and nonacupuncture sites. By probing the skin with electrodes in the upper limb, Brown et al.[5] found points on the skin that demonstrated differences in electrical activity when compared with other areas. These loci correlated with the insertion sites of acupuncture needles. There is also some evidence that these loci corresponded to points where the peripheral nervous system was especially accessible.[6]

The effect of acupuncture on the central nervous system is critically important. Extensive research has been done in this area that has contributed to our understanding of neurophysiology, but it has not definitively explained the effects of acupuncture. The discovery of endorphins stimulated a great deal of interest in acupuncture analgesia. Although nalaxone has been shown to block acupuncture analgesia in animals and humans,[7-9] the role of opioids has not been settled; in fact, their general relationship to chronic pain is very obscure. There seems to be no doubt that acupuncture increases the endorphin level in various parts of the central nervous system. The type of endorphin produced varies with the intensity of the stimulation. Enkephalins are produced at 4 Hz, whereas dynorphins are found at 100 Hz.[10] The injection of enkephalin, dynorphin A, or dynorphin B antisera reduces acupuncture analgesia at different intensity levels of stimulation.[11] At 2 Hz, metaenkephalin analgesia is reduced; at 15 Hz, dynorphin A is reduced; and at 100 Hz, dynorphin B is diminished. It has also been demonstrated that the messenger RNA involved with the production of endorphins is elevated after electrical acupuncture.[12,13] Others[8] have shown that acupuncture blocked the effects of single nociceptive cell stimulation, and this was reversed by narcotic antagonists. However, many other neurotransmitters have been shown to be affected by acupuncture[14,15]: 5-hydroxytryptamine (5-HT), acetylcholine, norepinephrine, dopamine, and enkephalins. Competitive 5-HT blockers such as cyproheptadine reduce acupuncture analgesia, whereas drugs such as chlomipramine (a drug that blocks 5-HT inactivation), enhance acupuncture analgesia.

The class of peripheral nerve fibers that responds to acupuncture has been investigated,[16] and generally, the evidence suggests that the smaller fibers produce the greater degree of analgesia. However, there is also evidence[17] that shows that stimulation of the larger fibers has the greater effect. Other experiments[16] have suggested that the pain from unmyelinated C fibers may be more easily suppressed than the myelinated delta A fibers.

Investigation[18] of the changes in the electroencephalogram (EEG) and sensory evoked potentials have shown that acupuncture influences the electrical profile of these parameters. A comparison of needles placed in specific and nonspecific loci showed marked attenuation of delta and beta waves in the EEG with point-specific stimulation. With sensory evoked potentials there were changes in the latency periods and the timing of some of the peaks of the electrical activity.

Acupuncture points may be labile[19] as they relate to the disease process, not as they relate to their location. In patients who were examined as they developed various disease processes, tenderness of the acupuncture points increased as the disease progressed. In most healthy people, this tenderness cannot be demonstrated; however, in a small percentage of otherwise healthy individuals, tender points can be found. There is a theory that the acupuncture site exists in three states: latent (no disease), passive (asymptomatic), and active (symptomatic); this theory has not been proven.

In fact, the pathology of tender areas is poorly understood and controversial. Acupuncture also produces other physiologic changes that are not necessarily related to its analgesic properties. In 1982 an acupuncture-like stimulus produced generalized vasodilation.[20-22] The increased flow through the microcirculation was reflected in the increase in skin temperature. This vasodilation was not affected by narcotic antagonists or cholinergic or adrenergic blockers. It has been suggested that the chemical mediator is a vasoactive intestinal polypeptide. This response to acupuncture is not immediate but appears after a latent period of about 30 minutes, and the effect may persist for many hours. The clinical implications are significant, particularly in those patients who have chronic skin ulceration, because healing proceeds with an attendant reduction in the pain level. It is interesting that the rise in skin temperature in the affected area may be several times that in normal skin.

It has been suggested[23-25] that the effects of acupuncture are not related to any specific effects of the technique itself but are related to the psychologic relationship between the therapist and the patient. Indeed, some therapists may have such a charismatic personality that merely talking to the patient decreases the anxiety level, which can have a considerable ameliorating effect on the patient's pain level. However, studies in experimental pain have demonstrated that there is a difference between hypnosis and acupuncture.[26] This difference was found in one well-conducted study that compared the effects of cold baths on the pain level using hypnosis, true and false acupuncture sites, morphine, and placebo. Another study found that hypnotic suggestibility did not predict success with acupuncture. This study also indicated that acupuncture-responsive patients have a higher level of pain tolerance and perceive it less than the average population. It has been shown[27] that narcotic antagonists revised acupuncture analgesia, although they had no effect on the analgesia produced by hypnosis.

Although a great deal of data about acupuncture is anecdotal or the result of uncontrolled clinical trials, there is a body of information that supports the effects of acupuncture, especially when compared with narcotics and placebo. The only area where there is apparently an element of doubt is when sham acupuncture is compared with true acupuncture.

TECHNIQUE
Positioning

Almost any position that allows adequate access is suitable. However, patients should not be placed in positions that are uncomfortable or tend to distort the anatomy. The elderly, very obese, frail, or rheumatoid may be particularly difficult to position adequately; and at times this may lead to abandoning the procedure.

A lateral recumbent position is preferred for those points that are located on the lateral side of the body, and the lithotomy position is prefered for the perineum. The sitting position is used for most other sites.

Needles

Although many types of needles have been described in modern practice, stainless steel or presterilized aluminum are the most suitable needles. These needles come in numerous lengths and gauges; the most common have a gauge of about 30 and are between 20 to 100 mm long. The shorter needles are used where shallow penetration is needed, such as around the face; the longer needles are used for the penetration of deeper structures, and especially in the limbs.

After proper sterilization of the skin, the needles should be inserted as rapidly as possible. The skin should be stretched over the acupuncture site and the needle firmly inserted to the required depth. For increased accuracy, especially for those with a discernible tremor, the wrist or forearm should be rested against the patient's body.

Various angles have been described for the insertion of the needle. In principle, the deeper the penetration of the needle the more perpendicular the needle should be angled. In the face, therefore, an angle of about 10 to 20° is recommended; for deep structures of the limbs, close to 90°.

The insertion of the needle may cause the patient to experience *techi*. However, most patients do not experience these sensations but respond positively to acupuncture.

Once the needles are inserted, they may be manipulated either by hand or by electrical stimulation. If the hand is used, there are basically three kinds of movements employed:

1. A rotatory motion between the first finger and the thumb. Rotation should not be more than 180°; more than this apparently causes tissue damage.
2. An oscillating movement may be employed by gently moving the needle back and forth.
3. A twirling or up and down movement. This movement produces a much higher level of stimulation than the other motions.

Currently, electrical stimulation is the preferred method of manipulation of acupuncture needles for several reasons. The hand method is extremely labor intensive and can fatigue the therapist if a treatment is lengthy. Some evidence has shown that electrical stimulation is more effective; this may be because the stimulation is more uniform and better controlled, with better standardization. Also, with electrical stimulation, the strength of the stimulus can be changed accurately within a wide range and can be varied between weak and strong.

COMPLICATIONS

Acupuncture appears to be remarkably free of complications. One of the most common reactions is fainting or syncope, which can usually be treated adequately by conservative measures. Pneumothorax is a rare complication that can occur when needles are inserted into the thoracic area. To avoid this complication, insert needles at a shallow angle and avoid deep insertion. Infection is an obvious hazard but can be minimized by applying standard sterile techniques. With the use of disposable needles, the incidence of hepatitis and acquired immunodeficiency syndrome should be nil.

Needles may break, especially if there is a rapid, severe movement such as during a grand mal seizure. A needle may occasionally become difficult to remove and appear to be "frozen" in the tissues.

The electrical current may burn and damage tissues such as nerves and muscles. Battery-powered units are probably safer than those connected to wall outlets; faulty connections and unit malfunction could conceivably lead to electrocution.

CONTRAINDICATIONS

There are very few absolute contraindications for acupuncture use. There have been anecdotal reports of acupuncture causing abortion, so it should be avoided in the first 3 months of pregnancy. Bacterial endocarditis has also been reported in patients with rheumatic heart disease, and localized hemorrhage has occurred with patients on anticoagulants. Acupuncture should be avoided in the thoracic region in patients who have severe chronic obstructive pulmonary disease where the production of pneumothorax would be catastrophic.

LOCATION AND FUNCTION OF ACUPUNCTURE POINTS

Although over 300 acupuncture points have been described, only about 100 are used by practitioners in the West. Each point has a name, serial number, and meridian number. For example, a point on the lateral side of the thigh has the des-

ignation feng shih, 218, GB 31; feng shih is the name, 218 the serial number, and GB 31 the meridian number. In breakdown of the general location of points, the head and neck have 21, the back 12, the thorax and abdomen 11, the arm and shoulder 18, and the leg 22.

Head and neck

Feng Chih, 207, GB 20 (Fig. 29-1) is located in the depression between the sternomastoid and trapezius muscles. It is the spot indicated for occipital headaches and neck pain.

Hsia Kuan, 149, ST 7 (Fig. 29-2) is located in the angle between the mandibular notch and the inferior border of the zygomatic arch, anterior to the condyloid process. This area is indicated for trigeminal neuralgia and temporomandibular arthritis.

Shang Hsing, 5, VG 23 (Fig. 29-3) is located at the midpoint of the forehead about 5 cun above the nose and is supplied by the ophthalmic branch of the trigeminal nerve. It is the site indicated for frontal headache.

Ya Men, 13, VG 15 (see Fig. 29-1), which is located between the spinous processes of the first and second vertebra, is supplied by the posterior ramus of the third cervical nerve and is indicated for occipital headache and neck pain.

Back (Fig. 29-4)

Ta Chui, 14, VG 14 is located between the spinous processes of the seventh cervical and first thoracic vertebra; it is supplied by the posterior ramus of the eighth cervical nerve. This area is indicated for neck pain, and the needle should be inserted perpendicularly to 1.5 cun.

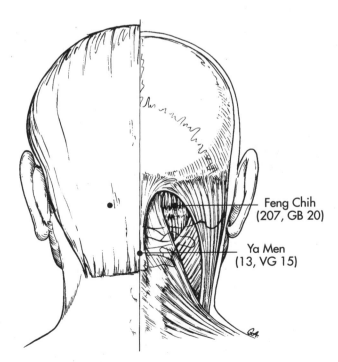

Fig. 29-1 Feng Chih and Ya Men points. (From Evans D: Acupuncutre. In Raj PP, editor: *Practical Management of Pain,* ed 2. St Louis, Mosby, 1992.)

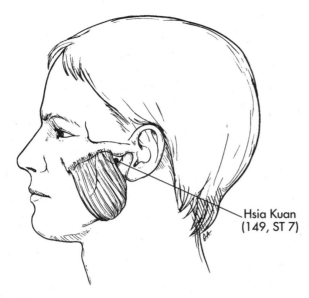

Fig. 29-2 Hsia Kuan point. (From Evans D: Acupuncture. In Raj PP, editor: *Practical Management of Pain,* ed 2. St Louis, Mosby, 1992.)

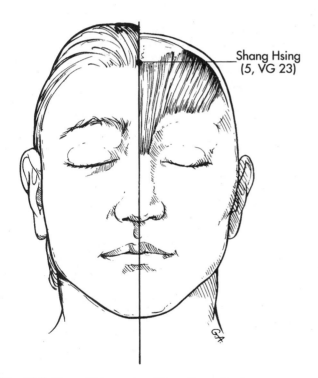

Fig. 29-3 Shang Hsing point. (From Evans D: Acupuncture. In Raj PP, editor: *Practical Management of Pain,* ed 2. St Louis, Mosby, 1992.)

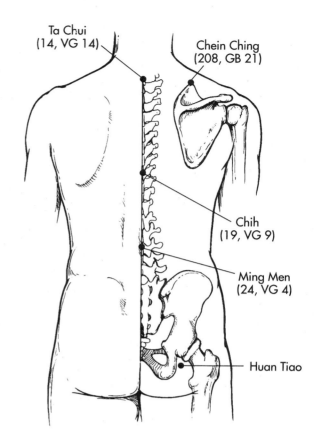

Fig. 29-4 Ta Chui, Chein Ching, Chih, Ming Men, and Huan Tiao. (From Evans D: Acupuncture. In Raj PP, editor: *Practical Management of Pain,* ed 2. St Louis, Mosby, 1992.)

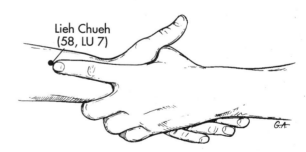

Fig. 29-5 Lieh Chueh point. (From Evans D: Acupuncture. In Raj PP, editor: *Practical Management of Pain,* ed 2. St Louis, Mosby, 1992.)

Chih, 19, VG 9 is situated in the midline just below the spinous process of the seventh thoracic vertebra. It is supplied by the posterior ramus of the seventh thoracic nerve and is indicated for chest and back pain.

Ming Men, 24, VG 4 is located in the midline between the spines of the second and third lumbar vertebra, supplied by the posterior ramus of the first and second lumbar nerves. This spot is indicated for low back pain; needles should be inserted perpendicularly to 1.0 cun.

Chien Ching, 208, GB 21 is located in the upper part of the trapezius muscle between the first thoracic spine and the acromion. It is supplied by the supraclavicular nerve and accessory nerve. This site is indicated for neck, shoulder, and back pain.

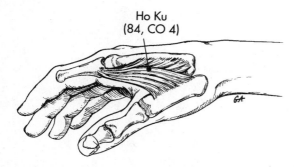

Fig. 29-6 Ho Ku point. (From Evans D: Acupuncture. In Raj PP, editor: *Practical Management of Pain,* ed 2. St Louis, Mosby, 1992.)

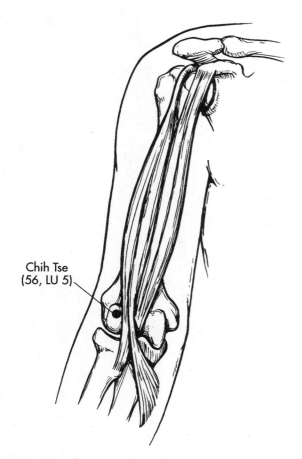

Fig. 29-7 Chih Tse point. (From Evans D: Acupuncture. In Raj PP, editor: *Practical Management of Pain,* ed 2. St Louis, Mosby, 1992.)

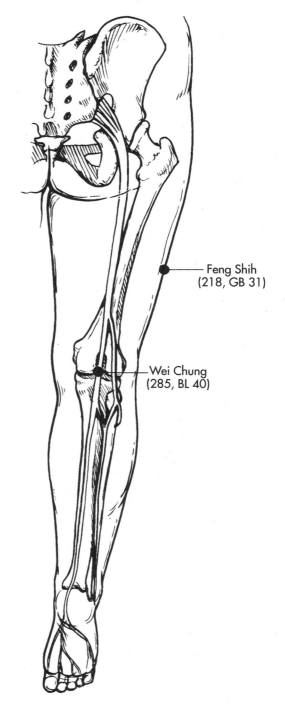

Fig. 29-8 Feng Shih and Wei Chung points. (From Evans D: Acupuncture. In Raj PP, editor: *Practical Management of Pain,* ed 2. St Louis, Mosby, 1992.)

Upper limb

Lieh Chueh, 58, LU 7 (Fig. 29-5) is 1.5 to 2.0 cun proximal to the transverse crease, just above the styloid process of the radius. This area is supplied by branches of the radial nerve and is indicated for headache and neck pain.

Ho Ku, 84, CO 4 (Fig. 29-6), located between the first and second metatarsal bones in the web, is supplied by the radial nerve. It is indicated for headache.

Chih Tse, 56, LU 5 (Fig. 29-7) is located in the antecubital fossa on the lateral side of the biceps tendon and medial to the brachioradialis. The area is supplied by the antebrachial and median nerves and is indicated for painful elbow.

Chien Chen, 132, SI 9 (Fig. 29-7) is located on the lateral border of the scapula just above the posterior fold of

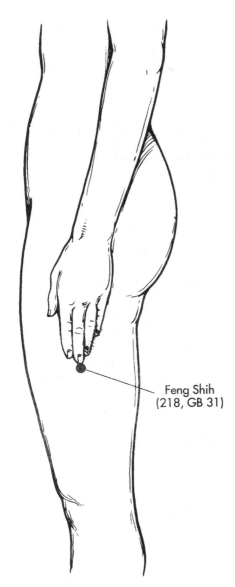

Fig. 29-9 Feng Shih point. (From Evans D: Acupuncture. In Raj PP, editor: *Practical Management of Pain,* ed 2. St. Louis, Mosby, 1992.)

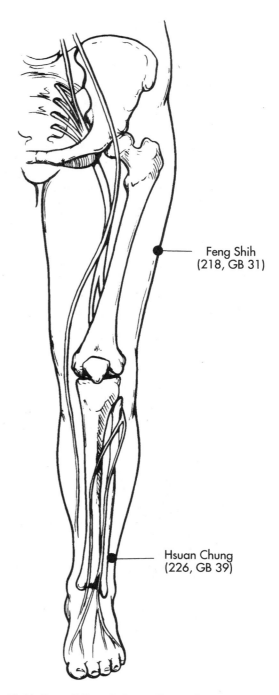

Fig. 29-10 Feng Shih and Hsuan Chung sites. (From Evans D: Acupuncture. In Raj PP, editor: *Practical Management of Pain,* ed 2. St Louis, Mosby, 1992.)

the axilla; it is supplied by branches of the brachial cutaneous and axillary nerves. This site is indicated for shoulder pain.

Lower limb

Huan Tiao, 217, GB 30 (see Fig. 29-4) is an area located at the junction of the middle and lateral third of a line drawn between the greater trochanter and the sacral hiatus. It is supplied by branches of the sciatic nerve and inferior gluteal nerve. Huan Tiao is indicated for sciatica and back pain.

Wei Chung, 285, BL 40 (Fig. 29-8), which is located in the center of the popliteal fossa, is supplied by the tibial and posterior femoral cutaneous nerves. This site is indicated for sciatica and painful knees.

Feng Shih, 218, GB 31 (Figs. 29-8 to 29-10) is a site located on the lateral aspect of the thigh about 8 cun above a line drawn laterally from the superior border of the patella, between the biceps femoralis and vastus lateralis. It is supplied by the lateral femoral cutaneous nerve of the thigh; it is indicated for sciatica, back, and hip pain.

Hsuan Chung, 226, GB 39 (Fig. 29-10) is a location 3 cun above the lateral malleolus between the posterior border of the fibula and the tendons of peroneus brevis and longus. This site is supplied by the superficial and deep peroneal nerves and is indicated for painful ankles and migraine.

Thorax and abdomen

Shan Chung, 35, VC 17 is a location in the midline of the sternum midway between the nipples at the level of the fourth intercostal space. It is supplied by branches of the fourth intercostal nerve and is indicated for chest pain.

Ju Ken, 160, ST 18 can be located below the nipples in the sixth intercostal space. It is supplied by branches of the fifth and sixth intercostal nerves and is indicated for chest pain.

Chung Wan, 40, VC 12 is a site located in the linea alba at the midpoint between the xyphoid and the umbilicus. It is supplied by the seventh and eighth intercostal nerves and is indicated for epigastric pain.

Chung Chi, 49, VC 3 is located in the linea alba about 4 cun below the umbilicus and is supplied by the iliohypogastric nerve. It is indicated for lower abdominal pain.

CLINICAL INDICATIONS

The literature is particularly confusing regarding the use of acupuncture. Some pain problems seem to respond better than others. Musculoskeletal pains caused by such diverse conditions as osteoarthritis (not rheumatoid), bursitis, tenosynovitis, and fibrositis seem to respond well. The acute pain and spasm caused by injury also respond well. There have been good results with various forms of headache, such as migraine, which seems to respond well.

Those who practice acupuncture believe that it has to be performed correctly to get good results. A thorough knowledge of the anatomy of the acupuncture points is essential. Placement has to be extremely accurate, and stimulation must be applied correctly. At times it may be more appropriate to stimulate by hand than electrically. Periodically, an increased or decreased level of stimulation may be necessary. As stated previously, there is no substitution for experience and clinical acumen.

REFERENCES

1. Pomeranz B, Stux G: *Scientific Bases of Acupuncture.* New York, Springer-Verlag, 1988.
2. Cooperative Group of Investigation of PSC. In *Advances in Acupuncture and Acupuncture Anesthesia.* Beijing, The People's Medical Publishing House, 1980.
3. Research Group of Acupuncture Anesthesia, Peking Medical College Institute of Medicine and Pharmacology of Fujian Province: *Studies of Phenomenon of Blocking Activities of Channels and Collaterals.* Beijing, Science Press, 1986.
4. Xue CC: The phenomenon in propagated sensation along channels (PSC) and the cerebral cortex. In Zhang X, editor: *Research on Acupuncture, Moxibustion and Acupuncture Anesthesia.* Beijing, Science Press, 1986.
5. Brown ML, Ulett GA, Stern JA: Acupuncture loci: Techniques for location. *Am J Chin Med* 2:67-74, 1974.
6. Liu YK, Varela M, Oswald R: The correspondence between some motor points and acupuncture. *Am J Chinese Med* 3:347-358, 1975.
7. Mayer DJ, Price DD, Raffi A: Antagonism of acupuncture analgesia in man by the narcotic antagonist naloxone. *Brain Res* 121:368-372, 1977.
8. Pomeranz B, Chiu D: Naloxone blocks acupuncture analgesia and causes hyperalgesia: Endorphin is implicated. *Life Sci* 19:1757-1762, 1976.
9. Fan SG, Tang J, Han JS: Naloxone blockade of acupuncture analgesia in the rat. *Kexue Tongbao* 34:1149-1152, 1979.
10. Han JS et al: High and low frequency electro-acupuncture analgesia are mediated by different opioids. *Pain Suppl* 2:543, 1984.
11. Han JS et al: Acupuncture mechanisms in rabbits studied with microinjection of antibodies against β-endorphins, enkephalin, and substance P. *Neuropharmacology* 23:1-5, 1984.
12. Zheng M, Yang SL, Tsou K: Electro-acupuncture markedly increases proenkephalin mRNA in rat striatum and pituitary. *Sci China, B* 31:81, 1987.
13. Zheng M et al: Electro-acupuncture increases propiomelanocortin mRNA in the pituitary and the proenkephalin mRNA in the adrenal gland in the rat. *Clin J Physiol Sci* 3:106, 1987.
14. Kanada B: Mechanisms of acupuncture analgesia. *Tidsskr Nor Laegeforen* 94:422-431, 1974.
15. Han JS, Terenius L: Neurochemical basis of acupuncture analgesia. *Ann Rev Pharmacol Toxicol* 22:193-220, 1982.
16. Chen L et al: An analytical study of afferent fibres for impulses of acupuncture. In Zhang X, editor: *Research on Acupuncture, Moxibustion, and Acupuncture Anesthesia.* Beijing, Science Press, 1986.
17. Lu G et al: Analysis of afferent fibres transmitting needling sensations of acupoint. In Zhang X, editor: *Research on Acupuncture, Moxibustion, and Acupuncture Anesthesia.* Beijing, Science Press, 1986.
18. Saletu B et al: Hypno- and acupuncture analgesia: A neurophysiological reality? *Neuropsychobiology* 1:242-281, 1975.
19. Dung HH: Characterization of the three functional phases of acupuncture points. *Chin Med J (Engl)* 97:751-754, 1984.
20. Kanada B: Vasodilation by transcutaneous nerve stimulation in peripheral ischemia. *Eur Heart J* 3:303-314, 1982.
21. Kanada B, Eielsen O: In search of mediators of skin vasodilation induced by transcutaneous nerve stimulation: Failure to block the response by antagonists of endogenous vasodilators. *Gen Pharmacol* 14:623-633, 1983.
22. Kanada B, Eielsen O: In search of mediators of skin vasodilation induced by transcutaneous nerve stimulation: 11, Serotonin implied. *Gen Pharmacol* 14:635-641, 1983.
23. Spiegal H, Spiegal D: *Trance and Treatment.* New York, Basic Book, 1978.
24. Kroger WS: Hypnotism and acupuncture. *JAMA* 220:1012, 1972.
25. Ulett GA, Peterson D: *Applied Hypnosis and Positive Suggestion.* St Louis, Mosby, 1963.
26. Ulett GA: Acupuncture is not hypnosis. Recent physiological studies. *Am J of Acupuncture* 11:5-13, 1983.
27. Goldstein A, Hilgard EF: Failure of the opiate antagonist naloxone to modify hypnotic analgesia. *Proc Natl Acad Sci USA* 72:2041-2043, 1975.

QUESTIONS: ACUPUNCTURE

1. Acupuncture points are located on meridians. How many meridians are there?
   A. 3
   B. 6
   C. 8
   D. 14
2. The following sensation is essential for a successful acupuncture treatment:
   A. Cun
   B. Techi
   C. Suan
   D. Ma
3. The peripheral nerve fibers that respond to acupuncture are generally:
   A. Smaller fibers
   B. Larger fibers
   C. Medium sized fibers
   D. Motor fibers
4. During the performance of acupuncture, once the needles are inserted they may be manipulated by hand or by electrical stimulations. If the hand is used, there are three kinds of movements. Of the movements listed below, which one is NOT employed?
   A. Rotating motion
   B. Oscillating movement
   C. Twirling or up-and-down movement
   D. Scratching movement

5. The acupuncture point located between the first and second metatarsal bones in the web is called:
   A. Lieh Chuch
   B. Ho Ku
   C. Chih Tse
   D. Chien chen

ANSWERS

1. D
2. B
3. A
4. D
5. B

30 Analgesia with Intravenous Local Anesthetics

P. Prithvi Raj and James C. Phero

Since 1908 there have been many reports published that describe the analgesic effect of intravenous (IV) local anesthetics. Local anesthetics administered IV may be useful to patients with chronic pain states when other therapeutic modalities have been ineffective.

Local anesthetics have effects on the central nervous system (CNS). Animal studies showed that local anesthetics produced changes in the states of consciousness in animals.[1] In humans, local anesthetics have sedative and central analgesic effects.[2]

Various theories have described the pharmacodynamics of local anesthetics. In 1938 Leriche proposed that injury to tissue caused reflex vasoconstriction, which resulted in anoxia, capillary dysfunction, and increased permeability.[3,4] Leriche theorized that this physiologic process led to the accumulation of nociceptive metabolites and consequently caused irritation of the peripheral nerve endings. Leriche believed that procaine acted directly on the arteriolar, metaarteriolar, and capillary endothelia, produced widespread vasodilation, and thereby anesthetized the irritated endothelial nerve endings and interrupted the reflex pain arc.

Lundy observed several jaundiced patients with pruritus who received a slow injection of 20 ml of 0.1% procaine solution and experienced 4 hours of analgesia.[5] His results supported Leriche's theory that peripheral irritation may be accompanied by capillary hyperpermeability, which allows transudation of procaine into the tissues resulting in nerve-ending anesthesia.

In 1943 Gordon used procaine to produce analgesia in burn patients, but only in the burned region and tissues affected by edema.[6] One year later Bigelow and Harrison subcutaneously injected 4 to 50 ml of 2% procaine solution into the arms of normal subjects.[7] They noted a marked increase in the pain threshold in the forehead and therefore asserted that the change resulted from a systemic action of procaine after circulatory absorption, rather than from a direct action of the agent.

In 1946 Allen et al. used IV procaine in burn patients and discovered six to eight times more procaine in the transudate of the injured area than in normal tissue.[8] Using the data from the studies performed by Gordon, and Bigelow and Harrison, Allen et al. postulated that analgesia resulted both from procaine's local anesthetic action in the inflamed and traumatized tissue and from central action in the nervous system. They also found that procaine partially blocked the sympathetic nervous system and neutralized the abnormal vasoconstriction from the pain.

Graubard and Peterson combined these theories in 1950 and attributed the resulting relief of pain to the direct anesthetic action on irritated nerve fibers, and to the indirect action of the procaine metabolite, diethylaminoethanol, on the vascular endothelium.[9]

Rowlingson et al. used IV lidocaine in normal volunteers and observed that blood levels below 3 μg/ml did not produce analgesia to ischemic pain produced by a tourniquet.[10]

Boas et al. used IV lidocaine, 1.5 to 2 μg/ml serum level, in patients with neuralgia and deafferentation syndrome to produce pain relief.[11] Anderson et al. and Loeser et al. hypothesized that pain associated with neurologic deafferentation may have a spinal electrogram pattern characterized by spontaneous high frequency burst-discharge activity in the CNS.[12,13] In 1985 Cassuto et al. reported that a continuous low dose IV infusion of lidocaine administered postoperatively was effective in alleviating postoperative pain.[14] Straussman et al. showed that pretreatment of trigeminal neurons with IV lidocaine abolished neuron response to bradykinins.[15] Since pain may be mediated by several pathways or substances, the lack of neuron response to bradykinins may explain why local anesthetics are successful in relieving pain in some patients but not in others.

CHOICE OF DRUG

Procaine has been the classic local anesthetic agent used for IV administration because of its potency and low toxicity. However, its short action, even at maximum dosages, has been its major disadvantage.

Bonica advocated IV tetracaine as being particularly beneficial "in painful states, pruritus, and in other conditions in which a reflex pattern must be broken" because of its potency and long duration.[16] Horan[17] reported that in 80% to 90% of patients receiving IV tetracaine, pain relief lasted two to three times longer than the relief achieved with procaine.

Interest has arisen concerning the efficacy of IV lidocaine in managing painful conditions such as neuralgia, deafferentation syndrome, and paroxysmal attacks associated with postherpetic neuralgia. For postherpetic neuralgia, Hatangdi et al. used IV lidocaine, 1.0 to 1.5 mg/kg.[18] Generally there was complete relief of lancinating pain within seconds after injection. In addition, the degree of success with IV lidocaine often indicated patient response to oral antiepileptic drugs. Boas, Covino, and Shahnarian used this local anesthetic agent in patients with deafferentation syndrome and noted that significant pain relief occurred within 15 to 20 minutes after starting the infusion.[11] In 1982 Atkinson advocated IV lidocaine for the management of intractable pain of adiposis dolorosa and administered a 0.1% solution of lidocaine IV to equal a total dose of 200 mg over 35 minutes.[19]

IV lidocaine has been effective in the treatment of chronic diabetic neuropathy, vascular headaches, and tinnitus.[20-22] Edwards et al. treated 211 patients in various chronic pain conditions with an infusion of IV lidocaine, in doses ranging between 1 and 5 mg/kg administered over 5 to 35 minutes.[23] These authors concluded that repeated infusions of lidocaine may be helpful in treating radicular low back pain and various peripheral neuropathies.

For the treatment of some painful disorders, IV chloroprocaine may have advantages over lidocaine because of its rapid hydrolysis by plasma cholinesterase.

Schnapp et al. used IV chloroprocaine to treat chronic intractable pain.[24] Of the patients, 43% reported more than 50% relief that lasted longer than 30 days. Phero et al. considered IV chloroprocaine to be safe and possibly efficacious in managing certain chronic intractable pain problems, particularly in patients with musculoskeletal pain.[25]

TECHNIQUE OF ADMINISTRATION

Two techniques have been used to administer IV local anesthetics in pain management: a single bolus dose or continuous infusion. Leriche was the first to use a single dose of 5 to 10 ml of 1% procaine solution.[4] Lundy used a 0.1% solution of procaine infused over several hours for pruritus.[5] Graubard and Peterson devised the procaine unit, which was 4 mg/kg of 0.1% procaine infused over 20 minutes via flowmeter.[9] Half of this dose was initially given as a bolus; then the rest of the dose was adjusted according to the incidence of side effects. In 500 patients, Bonica substituted Graubard's procaine unit with tetracaine, delivering a total dose of 3 mg/kg (not exceeding 250 mg) over 2 to 3 hours.[16] The onset of analgesia occurred within 30 minutes and lasted longer than the procaine.

Boas et al. administered lidocaine with an infusion pump at a rate of 4 mg/min for 1 hour in patients with deafferentation syndrome. These patients reported pain relief with serum lidocaine levels of 1.5 to 2.0 μg/ml.[11] Foldes and McNall compared procaine, chloroprocaine, tetracaine, and lidocaine at conventional comparable concentration ratios as used for regional anesthesia techniques and found no significant differences between these agents in the time of onset and the signs and symptoms of toxicity.[26] However, the signs and symptoms of local anesthetic toxicity disappeared faster with 2-chloroprocaine, which was hydrolyzed four times faster than procaine. Investigators noted that the faster an agent was hydrolyzed in the serum, the larger the dosage required to maintain toxicity. Conversely, the slower an agent was hydrolyzed, the smaller the dosage required to produce a toxic plasma level.

In 1981 Schnapp et al. delivered 3% 2-chloroprocaine without preservatives via a 30 ml syringe at a rate of 30 to 120 mg/min until the pain had subsided or 900 mg had been injected.[24] In that study, 44 patients were given a series of four 2-chloroprocaine IV injections 1 to 14 days apart, and 43% had pain relief that lasted more than 30 days. Patients with allodynia or chronic pain responded favorably to this treatment.

CONTROLLED INFUSION OF IV 2-CHLOROPROCAINE FOR PAIN RELIEF

The infusion pump is used to minimize the incidence of side effects. All patients receiving this treatment have exhibited chronic pain problems refractory to conventional therapeutic modalities (surgery, nerve blocks, physical therapy, analgesics, etc.). These patients had ASA I or II status, no known allergies to ester compounds, and normal serum pseudocholinesterase levels.

A 1% chloroprocaine solution was administered at a rate of 1 to 1.5 mg/kg/min until a total dose of 10 to 20 mg/kg had been delivered. All infusions were conducted in a controlled environment where resuscitative equipment and drugs were immediately available. In addition, the patient's vital signs (electrocardiogram [ECG], blood pressure, and heart rate), and mentation were monitored. If there was evidence of CNS toxicity besides mild symptoms of tinnitus, metallic taste, and lightheadedness, the rate of infusion was decreased by one half; or if the symptoms persisted or worsened the infusion was discontinued. Patients were required to rest for 1 hour after conclusion of the treatment, and then if in satisfactory condition were discharged home in the company of an escort.

Monitoring

Monitoring the patient during IV infusion of a local anesthetic is essential. Evaluate the patient's ECG, blood pressure, and heart rate every 5 minutes, and monitor mentation continuously. In over 108 treatments at the pain control center, no serious untoward sequelae were noted.

Evaluation

Patients initially receive a series of four or five IV chloroprocaine infusions to evaluate efficacy of the modality. Pain relief scores are obtained before, during, and after the infusion. For the period between treatments (usually 1 to 3 weeks) in the diagnostic series, patients are required to evaluate pain relief, function, and psychologic scores on a visual analogue scale in the morning, afternoon, evening, and night. In addition, the amount of oral medication consumed per day is documented.

SIDE EFFECTS

The side effects of IV local anesthetics have long been documented and are associated with CNS toxicity.[23-26] Early signs and symptoms include metallic taste, tinnitus, lightheadedness, agitation, and drowsiness. Moderate signs of CNS toxicity include difficulty with ocular focusing, nystagmus, slurred speech, dysarthria, numbness in the lips and tongue, and tingling or a heavy feeling in the extremities. Untoward effects of late CNS toxicity include hypotension or hypertension, bradycardia or tachycardia, seizure, anaphylaxis, and unconsciousness. Cardiac and respiratory failure, coma, and death may occur in the very late stages of CNS toxicity. On rare occasions, patients may experience anxiety and/or psychosis after the IV administration of lidocaine or chloroprocaine.[28,29]

REFERENCES

1. Wagman IH, de Jong RN, Prince DA: Effects of lidocaine on the central nervous system. *Anesthesiology* 28:155, 1967.
2. Gold HG, Cahell M: The sedative, central analgesic and anticonvulsant actions of local anesthetics. *Am J Med Sci* 244:646-654, 1962.
3. Leriche R: Intra-arterial therapy of infections and other diseases. *Memoires de l'Academie de Chirugie* 64:220, 1938.
4. Leriche R: Simple methods of easing pain in the extremities in arterial diseases and in certain vasomotor disorders. *Presse Med* 49:799, 1941.
5. Lundy JS: *Clinical Anesthesia.* Philadelphia, WB Saunders, 1941.
6. Gordon RA: Intravenous novocaine for analgesia in burns. *Can Med Assoc J* 49:478, 1943.
7. Bigelow N, Harrison I: General analgesic effects of procaine. *J Pharmacol Exp Ther* 81:368, 1944.
8. Allen FM, Grossman LW, Lyons LV: Intravenous procaine analgesia. *Anesth Analg* 25:1, 1946.
9. Graubard DJ, Peterson MC: *Clinical Uses of Intravenous Procaine.* Springfield, Ill, Charles C Thomas, 1950.
10. Rowlingson JC et al: Lidocaine as an analgesic for experimental pain. *Anesthesiology* 52:20, 1980.
11. Boas RA, Covino BG, Shahnarian A: Analgesic responses to IV lignocaine. *Br J Anaesth* 54:501, 1982.
12. Anderson LS et al: Deafferentation neuronal hyperactivity: A possible etiology of paresthesias following retrogasserian rhizotomy. *J Neurosurg* 35:444, 1971.
13. Loeser JD, Ward AA, White DE: Chronic deafferentation of human spinal cord neurons. *J Neurosurg* 29:48, 1968.
14. Cassuto T et al: Inhibition of postoperative pain by continuous low-dose intravenous infusion of lidocaine. *Anesth Analg* 64:971, 1985.
15. Straussman A et al: Responses of trigeminal nucleus caudalis neurons to mechanical and chemical stimulation of cranial blood vessels. *Society of Neurosciences Abstracts* 13:116, 1987.
16. Horan JS: The intravenous administration of local anesthetic agents in the management of pain. In Bonica JJ, editor: *The Management of Pain.* Philadelphia, Lea & Febiger, 1953.
17. Bonica JJ: Regional anesthesia with tetracaine. *Anesthesiology* 11:606-716, 1950.
18. Hatangdi VS, Boas RA, Richards EG: Post-herpetic neuralgia: Management with anti-epileptic and tricyclic drugs. In Bonica JJ, Albe-Fessard DG, editors: *Advances in Pain Research and Therapy, vol 1.* New York, Raven Press, 1976.
19. Atkinson RL: Intravenous lidocaine for the treatment of intractable pain of adiposis dolorosa. *Int J Obes* 6:351, 1982.
20. Kastrup Y et al: Intravenous lidocaine infusion—A new treatment of chronic painful diabetic neuropathy. *Pain* 28:69, 1987.
21. Maciewicz R et al: Relief of vascular headache with intravenous lidocaine: Clinical observations and a proposed mechanism. *Clin J Pain* 4:11, 1988.
22. Duckert LG, Reas TS: Treatment of tinnitus with intravenous lidocaine: A double-blind randomized trial otolaryngology. *Head Neck* 91:550, 1983.
23. Edwards WT et al: Intravenous lidocaine in the management of various chronic pain states. A review of 211 cases. *Reg Anaesth* 10:1-6, 1985.
24. Schnapp M, Mays KS, North WC: Intravenous chloroprocaine in the treatment of pain. *Anesth Analg* 60:844-845, 1981.
25. Phero JC et al: Controlled intravenous administration of chloroprocaine for intractable management. *Reg Anaesth* 9:50-51, 1984.
26. Foldes FF, McNall PG: 2-chloroprocaine: A new local anesthetic agent. *Anesthesiology* 13:287-296, 1981.
27. Parris WCV, Gerlock AJ, MacDonnell RC: Intra-arterial chloroprocaine for the control of pain associated with partial splenic embolization. *Anesth Analg* 60:112-115, 1981.
28. Backon T: Hoigne's syndrome and doom anxiety. *Am J Psychiatry* 145:1041, 1988.
29. Saravay SM et al: "Doom anxiety" and delirium in lidocaine toxicity. *Am J Psychiatry* 144:159, 1987.

QUESTIONS: ANALGESIA WITH INTRAVENOUS LOCAL ANESTHETICS

1. There is controversy as to the mechanisms of faction of IV local anesthetic agents. Earlier theories suggest peripheral site of action at the arteriolar and capillary endothelia. The later theory suggests CNS activity because:
   A. Spinal electrogram of deafferentation is changed with IV local anesthetics
   B. IV local anesthetics effects the low frequency discharge activity in the CNS
   C. IV local anesthetic causes numbness in the periphery
   D. Patient experiences hypotension with the use of IV local anesthetics

2. The choice of drug for IV local anesthetic currently is lidocaine. It is indicated for all of the following conditions EXCEPT:
   A. Peripheral neuralgia
   B. Deafferentation syndrome
   C. Paroxysmal attacks associated with postherpetic neuralgia
   D. Acute low back pain without radiculopathy

3. The side effects of IV local anesthetics are related to CNS toxicity. Early signs are all of the following EXCEPT:
   A. Metallic taste
   B. Tinnitus
   C. Agitation
   D. Increased appetite

ANSWERS

1. A
2. D
3. D

31 Ablative Techniques

Ronald P. Pawl

Ablative neurosurgical procedures were designed to interrupt sensory pathways to the brain or in the brain and brain stem. These procedures were originally contrived because pain was thought to be purely nociceptive; pain was a peripheral phenomenon that could be reduced to mechanical, chemical, or thermal phenomena at nerve endings. Therefore it was believed that interruption of specific sensory neural pathways would eliminate pain in the affected structure.

Health care workers who deal daily with patients and their pain describe pain as a perception; an integrated peripheral and central (or brain and mind) phenomenon. Pain is not merely a peripheral neural alarm monitoring the integrity of body tissues.

John Mullan, past chairman of the Department of Neurosurgery at the University of Chicago, pioneered the development of percutaneous cordotomy and promptly recognized the frustration of surgeons who treat intractable pain. He pointed out in the 1960s that cordotomy alleviated pain in patients with cancer if their lives did not extend far beyond 6 to 12 months. However, the same procedure had little effect on pain when applied to patients with intractable pain in the same parts of the body but not caused by cancer and when the patient survived for years. In fact, cordotomy often led to more disagreeable dysesthesias in the numbed area.

Neurosurgeons who interrupt the sensory path in the trigeminal nerve for facial pain quickly learn that numbing the face can cure the pain in patients with tic or trigeminal neuralgia when the pain is related to neural irritation by a blood vessel. However, the same procedure is ineffective and often exacerbates the painful condition of patients with nontic facial pains or atypical facial pain, a disorder now recognized to have central origins. Occipital nerve excision was taught as a method of surgical neurectomy to cure intractable headaches in the 1950s, but has been largely abandoned as ineffective. Current research on pain mechanisms has not defined the exact mechanisms of neuropathic or deafferentation pain, and considerable debate exists on which clinical syndromes represent neuropathic pain.[1-5]

Trigeminal neuralgia responds well to various ablative techniques that interrupt the nerve, root, or nucleus in the brain stem, and is not accompanied by clinical evidence of deafferentation. However, sensitive electronic testing has demonstrated loss of some sensibility in the distribution of the affected nerve in some patients. Postherpetic trigeminal neuralgia often leads to intractable pain with clear evidence of deafferentation, but does not respond to ablative techniques. Indeed, if deafferentation plays a role in the pro-

duction of chronic pain syndromes, then ablative techniques would seldom work, and when performed on peripheral nerves, would always exacerbate pain.

Even medical personnel who are experts in treating intractable pain argue the roles of nociception versus perception and motivation in patients reporting persistent pain. It is clear that a simplistic approach to the treatment of any intractable pain (including application of surgical procedures to ablate sensorineural pathways), without considering the involved psychologic, social, and motivational factors will alleviate pain only in a very select group of patients.

The "Yo Mama" rule of David Leak should be used when applying ablative procedures to patients with intractable pain: Don't do anything to the patient that you wouldn't do to "yo mama." But Leak adds the critical corollary to the rule: You have to *like* "yo mama."[6] The other rule is to never try to take away a patient's pain when the pain is accomplishing some important end or secondary gain, without you and the patient knowing that that is your goal.

An important factor that has reduced the number and type of ablative surgical procedures is a renewed interest in stimulating the nervous system to treat pain. Miniaturized electrodes with a multiple array of stimulating contacts can be introduced percutaneously to many parts of the nervous system, spinal cord, and brain stem to treat pain, even though rather dismal results were reported through the middle of the 1980s.[7] Neurostimulation is more attractive than ablating neural tissue if pain can be relieved significantly because there is no loss of neural function. The controversy on stimulation procedures is far from over, and there are enough conflicting results reported to make the role of stimulation for pain treatment uncertain.

Finally, it is important to realize the placebo effect of any surgical procedure that is intended to relieve pain. Surgical procedures have not been subjected to the same critical scrutiny of blind prospective studies that are the standard for pharmacologic treatments. Gybels addressed this issue after reviewing the world literature in writing a book on the role of neurosurgery in pain treatment and pain relief. He said,

Reports of results range from anecdotal accounts, through studies reporting the percentages of patient responses in several response categories, to evaluations taking into account on a semiquantitative basis the consumption of analgesics and activity levels, and also making (sic) distinctions between short-term and long-term results. Almost all of these reports can be described as presenting retrospective, uncontrolled and incomplete data from a group of selected patients. It is striking that some operations have been done on too few comparable patients, adequately examined and followed, to reach a decision as to their utility. Others have been performed on tens of thousands of patients; for example, facet rhizolysis for the relief of back pain; but the literature does not allow us to make a clear statement as to the indications for and the result of this operation.[8]

Patients with chronic pain syndromes, especially those with pain of benign origin, have associated serious psychologic and motivational problems. It is unwise to use ablative surgical procedures in treating patients with chronic pain unless the source of pain is of cancerous origin. Fields, and Gildenberg and Devaul, in their texts on chronic pain, have recommended against using ablative surgical procedures to treat chronic benign pain.[9,10]

Patients with cancer and pain resulting from tissue destruction benefit from certain selective ablative procedures discussed in the following paragraphs.

NEURECTOMY
Cranial nerves

Trigeminal neuralgia. Trigeminal neuralgia, or tic douloureux ("tic" for short), is a disorder of the elderly or those with multiple sclerosis. Patients have specific shooting pain with a defined irritative cause such as a blood vessel compressing the root of the nerve or a demyelinating plaque in the brain stem. The pain may respond to chemical therapy with anticonvulsants; if it doesn't, it responds well to ablative surgical therapy.

Surgical treatment of trigeminal neuralgia was greatly simplified and the hazards of invasive therapy reduced with the introduction of a glycerol injection into the cistern of the gasserian ganglion or into the ganglion. Older surgical techniques injured the ganglion or the root by a direct incision or compression and were accompanied by the hazards of open craniotomy. In the 1920s the nerve branches or the ganglion were ablated by an alcohol injection, but the procedure often damaged other intracranial structures because the flow of the alcohol was uncontrolled. Phenol was introduced in the 1960s. It was mixed with glycerin, a thick and slow-moving substance, and the resultant combination reduced the chances of the chemical moving through the cerebrospinal fluid (CSF) to other intracranial structures. A serendipitous discovery occurred when the phenol was left out of the glycerin/phenol mixture and only glycerol was injected, which relieved the patient's pain. In most cases, glycerol injections cause little if any clinically detectable loss of sensibility, even though electronic monitoring may detect the presence of sensory impairment. The technique is quick and can be performed as an outpatient procedure. Few side effects have been reported, except for some facial anesthesia. However, damage to the nerve could lead to corneal numbness and susceptibility to ulceration and abrasion. Of patients receiving one injection, 65% reported relief, and 85% experienced relief after two injections. These numbers compare favorably with radiofrequency thermocoagulation of the ganglion, which produces relief in 85% to 90% of patients at the expense of possible permanent appreciable numbness in the face, and often only after a second procedure is performed.[11] The recurrence rate of the tic pain after glycerol rhizotomy is 10% in the first 2 years. Of patients with multiple sclerosis who develop tic pain from lesions in the brain stem, 85% to 90% gain relief from glycerol rhizolysis, but nearly 40% have a recurrence in the first 2 years.[12]

In both techniques the ganglion is accessed via the foramen ovale in the base of the skull by needle penetration through the cheek under fluoroscopic control. Radiofrequency lesioning is done in increments to limit numbness to the trigger zone of the face or mouth. The patient will need general anesthesia in the form of short-acting intravenous barbiturates, usually several times. In spite of incremental lesioning, the patient may awaken after a single radiofrequency coagulation with half of the face including the cornea, completely numb. This complication has been reported in 7% of cases. Both percutaneous techniques provide excellent relief of pain for patients with trigeminal neuralgia, and can be used safely in people who have high-risk medical problems, such as the elderly.

Percutaneous ablation of the trigeminal ganglion or root can also reduce or eliminate facial pain of cancerous origin, as long as the pain is confined to the distribution of the fifth cranial nerve. Cancerous facial pain that extends to the ear or behind, or into the neck and pharyngeal regions, is less affected by trigeminal lesioning because of the overlapping pain fibers that traverse the seventh, ninth, and tenth cranial nerves, and the upper cervical roots.

Cluster headache. Both the trigeminal nerve and the nervus intermedius have been sectioned in attempts to treat intractable cluster headache for patients refractory to pharmacologic treatment. Resection of the trigeminal nerve has been ineffective, as in cases of atypical facial pain; but interruption of the greater superficial petrosal nerve in the nervus intermedius has been successful in selected cases. Sectioning the nervus intermedius interrupts nociceptive sensory fibers and interferes with the parasympathetic fibers that may play a role in the autonomic components of cluster headache. The disadvantage is that the procedure requires craniectomy in the posterior fossa and carries the risks of that surgery, especially hearing loss. Cochlear monitoring techniques during surgery reduce the hearing loss hazard.[13]

Interruption of the pain fibers in the nervus intermedius and geniculate ganglion via craniotomy have also been performed for intractable ear pain in selected cases. The disorder is rare, and few reports on the topic exist. Complications include CSF leak, meningitis, hearing loss, and vertigo.[14]

Glossopharyngeal neuralgia. Glossopharyngeal neuralgia is a ticlike pain involving the ninth cranial nerve with a trigger zone in the oropharynx and pain mainly in the throat. This neuralgia can also be treated by radiofrequency thermocoagulation of the nerve. The target is the portion of the nerve just outside the jugular foramen. Percutaneous anterior and lateral approaches to the nerve have been described. Complications include injury to the vagal nerve, hoarseness, blood pressure instability, and difficulty swallowing.[15] There are not enough case reports to give an accurate estimate of outcome of the procedure.

Peripheral neurectomy

Peripheral nerves are rarely severed in the current treatment of pain.[16] Traditionally, interruption of peripheral nerves to alleviate chronic pain have been limited to nerves that are exclusively sensory or have little motor function. Occipital neurectomy is one example, and has been largely abandoned. Occasionally percutaneous radiofrequency lesioning of the occipital nerves still occurs; but the indications are unclear, and the outcome results make the procedure unattractive.

Resection of painful traumatically induced peripheral neuromas has given significant relief to a minority of patients. Selection criteria are vague, except that the pain should be specific to the neuroma and the locale of the nerve. Particular surgical techniques, such as burying the resected nerve end in fat, muscle, or bone, do not enhance pain relief.[17]

Sympathectomy

Lumbar sympathectomy or stellate ganglionectomy was introduced as pain treatment because of the vascular effects of the procedures. Since many patients suffered vascular ischemia caused by arteriosclerosis, and the ischemic pain in lower extremities was often alleviated by lumbar sympathectomy, temporary or permanent sympathectomy was performed in other painful conditions where the vascular system played a significant role, particularly headache syndromes.

In the 1960s Winnie and Collins noted that patients with some intractable pain syndromes gained temporary relief from epidural or paraspinal sympathetic blockade.[18] Since that time sympathetic blocks have been studied extensively, and the procedure has evolved to include several techniques. In spite of a great deal of literature on the subject, there is still confusion about the role of temporary or permanent sympathetic blocks in the treatment of patients with chronic pain syndromes. Currently, the terminology concerning sympathetic blocks for pain treatment has been obfuscated. For example, the term *reflex sympathetic dystrophy syndrome,* is a causalgia-like chronic pain syndrome with specific observable abnormalities.[19] Another term, *sympathetically maintained pain,* describes pain that is somewhat relieved by a sympathetic anesthetic block. These two terms are used in part interchangeably. The result has been a plethora of clinical diagnoses and extensive block therapy of purported cases of reflex sympathetic dystrophy syndrome in patients with chronic pain complaints; but with no evidence of actual reflex sympathetic dystrophy syndrome.

Also since the 1960s, there is little mention of surgical sympathectomy as treatment; although in practice occasional cases are performed. The issue is so controversial that recommendations must await further study; but it is clear that surgical or chemical sympathectomy has little value in the treatment of chronic pain, even in those situations where a temporary block with local anesthetic has produced temporary relief.[20] In the treatment of spinal-cord–injury pain, surgical sympathectomy is not of value.[21]

Rhizotomy and dorsal ganglionectomy

In the past, sensory ablative surgery was frequently used on the nerve root or dorsal root ganglion at single or multiple levels to treat intractable thoracic, trunk, and extrem-

ity pain. In 1984 Pawl reported on the use of surgical extirpation of dorsal root ganglia for the treatment of intractable sciatica after multiple spinal surgeries.[22] In general, the technique failed to give significant long-term relief, and often added a new dimension of sensory problems, including dysesthesia, paresthesia, and numbness. A long-term follow-up study by North and colleagues confirmed this observation.[23] Recently, radiofrequency lesioning of the dorsal root ganglia has been used to treat chronic pain syndromes. Although the technique is relatively safe with few motor side effects, long-term relief was not obtained.[24] Gildenberg and DeVaul also noted the lack of success in relieving sciatic pain by rhizotomy.[10]

Postthoracotomy and postherpetic neuralgia were previously treated by surgical rhizotomy proximal to the rib. Initial reports of success were later replaced by reports of failure, and the procedure has been generally abandoned.[25]

CORDOTOMY

Cordotomy ranks with neurectomy as one of the oldest ablative surgical techniques used to treat intractable pain. Early in this century an autopsy was performed on a patient who was clinically numb on one side of the body. A tuberculoma was found in the spinothalamic sensory path on the opposite side of the body from the numbness. The tract thereafter became a surgical target to numb patients' painful parts. In the past performing the procedure was done via laminectomy to expose the spinal cord, and there was disagreement whether the patient should have local or general anesthesia for the procedure. Under local anesthesia, the patient could directly report the degree of numbness and pain relief. However, patient movement and anxiety during the surgery under local anesthesia frustrated surgical attempts. Rigorous rules of measurement were developed on how much of the spinal cord to cut so that the procedure could be performed with general anesthesia. These rules were not very reliable, however, since the spinal cord size varied with the size of the patient. Therefore the surgeon and patient had to wait for the return of the patient's consciousness after the procedure to determine the effectiveness of the cut in the cord. Additionally, the patient had to deal with the pain and disability of a laminectomy, and the complication of damage to the anterior spinal artery during the procedure at times led to disastrous neurologic consequences.

Mullan et al.[26] pioneered the development of a percutaneous technique, which resolved the guesswork of the open surgical cordotomy, but unfortunately added new complications. The only ready access to the spinal cord for a needle electrode is at the craniovertebral border or C_1-C_2 laterally, where the bony structures are separated for cranial rotation. That part of the spinal cord is where decussation of the corticospinal motor pathway from the pyramids (located ventrally in the medulla oblongata) to the corticospinal tracts (located dorsolaterally in the spinal cord) occurs, and the crossing of the ventrolateral spinothalamic sensory path in the cord moves toward the dorsal part of the medulla. This intermingling of the motor and sensory paths varies from person to person. After introduction of this technique, the percutaneous procedure often resulted in weakness or paralysis, as well as pain relief. As technology improved, monitoring techniques during the procedure directed appropriate placement of the electrode tip into sensory fibers, and motor complications in extremities were markedly reduced.

However, another problem emerged. When patients with bilateral or midline pain from cancer were treated with bilateral cordotomy, they often suffered sleep apnea, referred to as Ondine's curse. (Ondine was a mythologic character who was punished by the gods for some miscreant activity. If he fell asleep, he would die, so he had to remain awake all of the time.) Patients who underwent bilateral upper cervical cordotomy would stop breathing in their sleep and die because the motor pathways for respiration travel in the same quadrant of the spinal cord as the ventrolateral spinothalamic tracts. Consequently, percutaneous high cervical cordotomy is a treatment limited to those whose pain is unilateral. Additionally, because of the decussations of the sensory tracts and the location of the sensory pain fibers near motor tracts, treatment of upper extremity pain was more hazardous and difficult to accomplish. Therefore high cervical cordotomy provides the most effective pain relief in patients with unilateral lower extremity or flank pain.

To obviate these problems, a percutaneous method was developed to ablate the spinothalamic tract lower in the spinal cord below C_4 where the respiratory paths exit the cord.[27] However, this procedure had to be performed transdiscally because there was no ready access to the cord laterally. Proper placement of the needle was difficult transdiscally; the needle had to be repeatedly adjusted through the entire disk, which was painful for the patient. In addition, most patients who had cancer were in an older age group who also had degenerative narrowing and osteophyte formation in the disks that interfered with needle placement; thus the procedure was largely abandoned. Currently, cordotomy is rarely used; it has been supplanted by superior methods of oral or parenteral pain control, including intraspinal morphine pumps. High cervical cordotomy is effective in alleviating unilateral lower extremity or flank pain in a patient with a life expectancy of less than 1 year.[28]

In some centers, cordotomy and cordectomy are still used to treat the pain occurring after spinal cord lesions that are usually traumatic.[29] These procedures and the root entry zone lesions described later offer little hope of altering steady pain, which improves in only 26% of cases. Cordotomy, cordectomy, and root zone lesions do alter shooting pains and evoked pains, (i.e., allodynia or hyperpathia), in 85% to 90% of reported cases. However, long-term follow-up was not reported.[26] Other reports note little efficacy in the relief of spinal cord injury pain with cordotomy and cordectomy.[21]

Burst firing in the second-order neurons of the dorsal grey matter on the spinal cord was found in experimental animals. The burst firing occurred where the cord level had been surgically deafferented, and this led to the development of ablative surgical technique of the dorsal root entry zone lesioning.[30,31] This procedure is still quite controversial and performed in only a few centers. Root entry zone technique has been recommended for patients with brachial plexus avulsions, postherpetic neuralgia, and traumatic paraplegia with intractable pain. Although the original au-

thors have reported pain relief of 65% to 80%, others have reported considerably less success, especially in long-term follow-up. Furthermore, motor weakness may develop in 50%, and new pain may develop in 40% of patients after the procedure.[32] Complications also include CSF leak; loss of additional sensory function; exacerbation of bowel, bladder, and sexual dysfunction; and epidural and subcutaneous hematomas.[21]

Facial pain caused by vascular lesions of the brain stem has been treated successfully with dorsal root entry zone lesions in the descending nucleus caudalis of the trigeminal nerve, high in the cervical spinal cord. Of the two patients reported, one achieved 50% relief and the other had complete relief, but no long-term follow-up was reported.[33]

Commissurotomy

Commissurotomy was introduced to treat bilateral or midline pain of cancerous origin. The anterior commissure of the spinal cord, which is largely made up of nerve fibers passing from the dorsal grey matter to the contralateral spinothalamic tracts, is interrupted. The tract is located just anterior to the central canal of the cord and can be reached surgically by splitting the posterior columns of the cord or by introducing a radiofrequency needle into the tract percutaneously. Although successful in relieving pain, especially in the pelvic and rectal regions, the procedure causes a fairly high incidence of paresis and ataxia, and has largely been abandoned in favor of oral or intraspinal opiate therapy.[20]

MESENCEPHALOTOMY

Stereotactically guided lesioning of the dorsal mesencephalon in the region of the medial lemniscus and spinothalamic tract is used to treat patients with cancer pain, primarily in European centers. Relief of pain has been variable, ranging from 60% of patients in one study to 84% in another.[19] The procedure appears to have no value in treating patients with deafferentation pain, including spinal cord injury pain.[21,34,35]

THALAMOTOMY

Although thalamotomy was used more extensively in the treatment of pain before the 1980s, there are now fewer reports in the current literature.

When thalamotomy at multiple sites is compared to mesencephalotomy in the relief of cancer-originating pain, mesencephalotomy is superior because it produces a relief rate of about 85% after surgery compared to 50% for thalamotomy. However, mesencephalotomy has a higher mortality rate of 2% and a higher morbidity rate, which includes anesthesia dolorosa and gaze palsies.[35]

CINGULOTOMY

Stereotactic lesioning in the frontal lobe cingulum was devised to interrupt the cortical projections of the thalamic nuclei thought to be responsible for the unpleasant quality of pain perception. Complications of the procedure include significant alteration in effect and attention. The procedure has not been found effective in relieving spinal cord injury pain[21] and is not regularly performed at present.

SUMMARY

Ablative neurosurgical procedures have been tested and used to treat every chronic painful human condition, but are limited in success to a few disorders.[36] In patients with cancer, oral and parenteral intraspinal opiate analgesia provide adequate pain relief in most cases; rarely is the surgeon called upon to interrupt sensory pathways to control a patient's pain. When surgery becomes necessary, percutaneous cordotomy can be effective in controlling unilateral lower extremity or flank pain, and unilateral or bilateral stereotactic mesencephalotomy can be effective for more generalized control of pain. The latter procedure has more serious complications neurologically and is only performed in a few specialized centers.

When chronic pain stems from benign origins, ablative procedures are fraught with high failure rates and neurologic complications, especially additional uncomfortable sensory phenomena, and are not recommended in general. Dorsal root entry zone lesions, to control pain in brachial plexus avulsion cases or in postherpetic and spinal-cord–injured patients, remain controversial with regard to pain relief outcome, and have a relatively high complication rate. The use of these lesions awaits further investigation. Ablative lesions to control reflex sympathetic dystrophy syndromes and sympathetically maintained pain have not been demonstrated to be of any value. Furthermore, until the taxonomy of these disorders is clarified and the origins of the disorders determined, ablative procedures of any kind should be avoided.

Lesioning of the trigeminal nerve ganglion or root to control trigeminal neuralgias is the notable exception to using ablative procedures in chronic pain. The high degree of success and low morbidity rates in the percutaneous techniques make them highly useful.

REFERENCES

1. Fromm GH: Physiological rationale for the treatment of neuropathic pain. *APS Jour* 2(1):1, 1993.
2. Dubner R: Neuropathic pain: New understanding leads to new treatments. *APS Jour* 2(1):8, 1993.
3. Burchiel K: Is trigeminal neuralgia a neuropathic pain? *APS Jour* 2(1):12, 1993.
4. Sessle B: Neural mechanisms implicated in the pathogenesis of trigeminal neuralgia and other neuropathic pain states. *APS Jour* 2(1):17, 1993.
5. Fromm GH: Commentary on the commentaries: Physiologic rationale for the treatment of neuropathic pain. *APS Jour* 2(1):21, 1993.
6. Leak WD: Home care therapy. In Raj PP, editor: *Practical Management of Pain*. St Louis, Mosby, 1992.
7. North RB et al: Spinal cord stimulation for chronic intractable pain: Superiority of "multi-channel" devices. *Pain* 44:119, 1991.
8. Gybels J: Analysis of clinical outcome of a surgical procedure. *Pain* 44:103, 1991.
9. Fields HL: *Pain*. New York, McGraw-Hill, 1987.
10. Gildenberg PL, DeVaul RA: *The Chronic Pain Patient. Evaluation and Management*. Basel, Switzerland, S Karger, 1985.
11. Sanders M, Henny CHP: Results of selective percutaneous controlled radiofrequency lesions for treatment of trigeminal neuralgia. *Clin J Pain* 8:23, 1992.
12. Dieckman G et al: Five-and-a-half years' experience with percutaneous retrogasserian glycerol rhizotomy in treatment of trigeminal neuralgia. *Appl Neurophysiol* 50:401, 1987.
13. Rowed DW: Chronic cluster headache managed by nervus intermedius section. *Headache* 30(7):401, 1990.
14. Rupa V, Saunders RL, Weider DJ: Geniculate neuralgia: The surgical management of primary otalgia. *J Neurosurg* 75:505, 1991.
15. Salar G et al: Selective percutaneous thermolesions of the ninth cranial nerve by lateral cervical approach: Report of eight cases. *Surg Neurol* 20:276, 1983.
16. Dubuisson A, Kline DG: Indications for peripheral nerve and brachial plexus surgery. *Neurol Clin* 10(4):935, 1992.
17. Burchiel KJ, Johans TJ, Ochoa J: The surgical treatment of painful traumatic neuromas. *J Neurosurg* 78:714, 1993.
18. Winnie AP, Collins VJ: The pain clinic. I. Differential neural blockade in pain syndromes of questionable etiology. *Med Clin North Am* 52:123-129, 1968.
19. Gibbons JJ et al: Interscalene blocks for chronic upper extremity pain. *Clin J Pain* 8:264-269, 1992.
20. Tasker R: Surgical approaches to the primary afferent and the spinal cord. In Fields HL, Dubner R, Cerveno F, editors: *Advances in Pain Research and Therapy vol 9*. New York, Raven Press, 1985.
21. Balazy TE: Clinical management of chronic pain in spinal cord injury. *Clin J Pain* 8:102, 1992.
22. Pawl RP: Ganglionectomy for the relief of intractable sciatica. *Contemporary Neurosurgery* 5(26):1, 1984.
23. North RB et al: Dorsal root ganglionectomy for failed back surgery syndrome: A five year follow-up study. *J Neurosurg* 74:236, 1991.
24. van Kleef M et al: Effects and side effects of a percutaneous thermal lesion of the dorsal root ganglion in patients with cervical pain syndrome. *Pain* 52:49, 1993.
25. Tasker R: Deafferentation. In Wall PD, Melzack R, editors: *Textbook of Pain*. Edinburgh, Churchill Livingstone, 1984.
26. Mullan S et al: Percutaneous intramedullary cordotomy utilizing the unipolar anodal electrolytic lesion. *J Neurosurg* 22:548-553, 1965.
27. Lin PM, Gildenberg PL, Polakoff PP: An anterior approach to percutaneous lower cervical cordotomy. *J Neurosurg* 25:553-560, 1966.
28. Sundaresan N, DiGiasinto GV, Hughes JE: Neurosurgery in the treatment of cancer pain. *Cancer* 63(11 supp):2365, 1989.
29. Tasker RR, DeCarvalho GTC, Dolan EJ: Intractable pain of spinal cord origin: Clinical features and implications for surgery. *J Neurosurg* 77:373, 1992.
30. Loeser JD, Ward AA: Some effects of deafferentation on neurons of the cat spinal cord. *Arch Neurol* 17:629, 1967.
31. Alexander E III, Nashold BS, Rossitch E: Dorsal root entry zone surgery for pain management. *Pain Management* 4:15, 1991.
32. Kumagai Y et al: Problems related to dorsal root entry zone lesions. *Acta Neurochir (Wein)* 115:71, 1992.
33. Sampson JH, Nashold BS: Facial pain due to vascular lesions of the brain stem relieved by dorsal root entry lesions in the nucleus caudalis. *J Neurosurg* 77:473, 1992.
34. Bosch DA: Stereotactic rostral mesenchephalotomy in cancer pain and deafferentation pain. *J Neurosurg* 75:747, 1991.
35. Frank F et al: Stereotactic mesencephalotomy versus multiple thalamotomies in the treatment of chronic cancer pain syndromes. *Appl Neurophysiol* 50:314, 1987.
36. Pawl RP: Surgery for pain. *Semin Neurol* 9(3):257, 1989.

QUESTIONS: ABLATIVE TECHNIQUES

1. If trigeminal neuralgia fails to respond to oral medication, the most appropriate next step is to:
   A. Refer to patient for psychologic counseling and biofeedback
   B. Inject the trigger zone with local anesthetic
   C. Prescribe a combination of tricyclic mood elevators and phenothiazines
   D. Refer the patient for rhizolysis of the nerve root or ganglion
2. Cordotomy is a surgical procedure that:
   A. Severs the spinal cord
   B. Selectively severs the spinothalamic tract
   C. Selectively severs the corticospinal tract
   D. Severs the spinal terminale cord
3. Cordotomy is best suited to treat:
   A. Cancerous, unilateral pain in the lower extremity
   B. Benign, unilateral pain in the lower extremity
   C. Cancerous, bilateral pain in the upper extremities
   D. Benign, bilateral pain in the upper extremities
4. Mesencephalotomy is a:
   A. Procedure done in the midmenstrual cycle
   B. Lesion in the middle of the cerebral hemispheres
   C. Stereotactic lesion not often used today
   D. Special procedure with limited pain treatment
5. Cingulotomy affects which part of the brain?
   A. Primary sensory cortex
   B. Thalamic projection for disagreeable sense
   C. Secondary sensory cortex
   D. Thalamic projection for primary sensation

ANSWERS

1. D
2. B
3. A
4. C
5. B

32 Neural Stimulation: Spinal Cord and Peripheral Nerve Stimulation

W. David Leak and A. Elizabeth Ansel

Neural stimulation has been a significant part of medical history. Advances in today's technology and physiologic research have helped define avenues where this tool, when properly used, can afford society outstanding clinical and economic benefits.

HISTORY

"For any type of gout, a live black torpedo should, when pain begins, be placed under the feet. The patient must stand on a moist shore by the sea, and he should stay like this until his whole foot and leg up to the knee, is numbed. This takes away present pain and prevents pain for coming on if it has not already arisen" (Scribonius Largus, c.e. 46).[1] Sensory stimulation for pain relief, even if performed with electric fishes, is an ancient technique.[1]

A classical textbook of Oriental medicine, *Nei Ching,* from about 2600 B.C., described acupuncture techniques, where different pathologic conditions were claimed to be healed by inserting and manipulating sharp, thin objects (bamboo sticks, fish bones) into certain points of the body tissues. Later on bronze needles were inserted into very well-defined points along a number of lines (meridians) on the body surface. An alternative was to heat the tissue by burning certain weeds (moxa) on the skin.[1]

In France at the beginning of the nineteenth century, needles were used as electrodes for discharging Leyden bottle condensers into the tissues to achieve pain relief. With the development of devices generating and storing electricity in the eighteenth and nineteenth centuries, "electroanalgesia" became widely used in Western countries to alleviate low-back pain, arthritis, acute pain from tooth extraction, and other surgical procedures. However, with the appearance of effective volatile anesthetic agents and oral analgesics, the stimulation methods were gradually forgotten, probably because they gave a varying and unpredictable therapeutic response. Moreover, the equipment used was nonportable and often insufficient.

In the 1700s Benjamin Franklin invented an electrostatic generator and used a method of passing current across painful areas known as "Franklinization." Subsequent to Franklin's invention, the violet ray was developed. This modality applied diathermal heat to painful areas through glass electrodes.

In 1901 Bayliss systematically studied how areas of skin would develop flushing when the dorsal roots of animals were stimulated electrically. The work of Bayliss was expanded by Forester, who in 1933 stimulated peripheral nerves to cause vasodilation in medical students. These efforts were used to define the concept of dermatomes. They also established definite neural control of skin blood flow.

In 1965 Melzack and Wall described the gate control theory of pain by as an ability to suppress transmission of pain signals in small diameter fibers (A-delta and C) by activity in large diameter, nonnoxious fibers (A-beta).[2]

Shealy et al., and Wall and Sweet published the first clinical reports of pain relief by direct spinal cord stimulation in 1967. Access to the cord generally required a significant surgical intervention to place the electrode. Initially there was an overenthusiastic use of the primitive simulators available. They were implanted in many inappropriate patients, which resulted in a large number of failures. Unresolved reimbursement issues also prompted a number of centers to abandon spinal cord stimulation.

In the 1970s, described as the dark ages of neurostimulation, technology was primitive, and treatable conditions and patients were not well identified. Failure was more common than success. Patient selection criteria had not been fully established. Some progress was made, however. In 1973 Cook initially published a favorable response in multiple sclerosis patients who had been implanted for pain. Shimoji developed a catheter type of electrode in 1974, and Waltz developed a laminotomy type of electrode for clinical application. In 1979 quadrapolar electrode catheters were introduced. In that same year, the Health Care Finance Administration adopted selection criteria for reimbursement.

In the 1980s treatable conditions and patients were identified by implanting physicians. The technology advanced to where product failure was no longer a consideration. With the advent of more refined percutaneous instruments including needles and lead arrays in conjunction with better radiologic imaging equipment, the procedure has become widely used by many physicians. The first multiprogrammable electronics were introduced in 1980, and totally implantable neural stimulator systems were introduced in 1981. Eight-channel multiprogrammable electronics and the first eight-electrode catheter were developed in 1986. 1988 signalled the introduction of the noninvasive programmable implantable pulse generator that also had radiofrequency capabilities. In the 1990s successful adaptation of multilead electrode arrays, implantable programmable pulse generators, implantable radio frequency receivers, and more sophisticated objective patient screening methods has led to very high success rates.

PHYSIOLOGY

Excitable cells, such as in nerves and muscles, can be simply described as a uniform-conducting intracellular region separated from the extracellular space by a very thin (-100A) plasma membrane. The excitable cell properties arise from the unequal intracellular and extracellular ionic composition ([Na]o > [Na]i and [K]o < [K]i) and the selectively permeable membrane properties. At rest the concentration gradients cause ion movements that establish a resting potential. Upon stimulation the membrane undergoes a phasic change in permeability that results in ion movement and characteristic action potential.[3]

Sensitivity of neural tissue to frequency and amplitude variations significantly alters the physiologic response in the living organism. High frequency, low amplitude stimulation silences most dorsal horn cells, including presumably noxious ones, which are active only during strong pinching or clamping. The inhibition is dramatic.[3] Conversely, low frequency, high amplitude stimulation is much less effective. This may explain part of the efficacy of spinal cord stimulation or peripheral nerve stimulation for peripheral vascular disease and reflex sympathetic dystrophy, since sympathetic fibers are normally recruited more with this type of stimulation. Therefore inhibition of the sympathetic system is more likely by high frequency, low amplitude stimulation.

Stimulation recruits A-beta fibers; paresthesia is frequency dependent. If a patient is stimulated at higher frequencies, A-delta fibers are recruited and the frequency dependency is diminished. Excessive A-delta fiber stimulation causes the patient to report unpleasant paresthesia, which might feel prickling or even epicritic (sharp, well localized). However, if such a paresthesia was better able to suppress C fiber activity, then pain would be less protopathic (agonal, diffuse).

Stimulating large diameter afferents with nonnoxious stimuli could close down or inhibit messages from the ascending small diameter nociceptive fibers and interneurons. Subsequent theories include inhibitory pathways being stimulated by spinal descending tracts. Spinal cord stimulation physiologically may be affected by a number of mechanisms. The basics include electrical contact with a cathode (negative electrode), which causes excitation of nervous tissue. The inside of living neural cells is negatively charged. Thus the exposure of an external negative charge causes depolarization to a positive potential on the inside of the cell, which therefore causes an action potential and thus a nonnoxious message.

Neurohumoral responses have been documented. Chronic pain sufferers have demonstrated lower levels of endorphin and serotonin in the cerebral spinal fluid when compared to subjects who did not complain of chronic pain. Both chemicals show demonstrative increases that are subject to neural stimulation, although the analgesic effects of spinal cord stimulation have not been reversible by naloxone.[4] Other physiologic responses include increases in transcutaneous oxygen pressures ($TcpO_2$), and decreases in carbon dioxide ($TcpCO_2$), and patients with significant peripheral vascular disease. The clinical significance is substantial reduction in pain, suffering, and foot amputation.[5]

Stimulation methods may be either bipolar or unipolar. The difference is based on proximity of the anode to the cathode. When the anode (positive lead) and the cathode (negative lead) are very close, this is called *bipolar stimulation*. This occurs when an electrode array is activated on a spinal cord stimulator lead with at least one negative electrode and one positive. The electric field will be very close and will remain very near the electrical contacts.

Where the cathode is very remote from the anode (for example, when a pulse generator case is positive and the spinal cord stimulator lead has a cathode that is activated) this is termed *unipolar stimulation*. This leads to very broad fields as the current runs from the cathode to the anode.

The major factor in successful stimulation is electrode positioning. Successful stimulation demands topographic coverage of the electrical field of paresthesia over the area of the pain (Fig. 32-1).

INDICATIONS

The general indications for spinal cord stimulation are for suppression of chronic, intractable pain of the trunk or limbs.[6] Examples of specific diseases where spinal cord stimulation may be indicated include: arachnoiditis,[7] spastic torticollis,[8] intercostal neuralgia,[9] peripheral neuropathy,[10] reflex sympathetic dystrophy,[11] phantom limb pain,[12] radicular pain associated with intraspinal fibrosis,[13] peripheral pain associated with ischemic vascular disease,[14] or peripheral pain associated with postherpetic neuralgia.[9]

Certain conditions that are specifically amenable to peripheral nerve stimulation include reflex sympathetic dystrophy, causalgia, direct nerve injury, and plexus avulsion. The pathologies that respond best to peripheral stimulation are deafferentation or neuropathic conditions.[15]

CONDITIONS FOR IMPLANTATION

Guidelines have been established by the Health Care and Finance Administration (HCFA) on implantation of spinal cord and peripheral nerve simulators. Spinal cord simulators should be used only:

1. As a late resort for patients with chronic, intractable pain
2. When other treatment modalities (pharmacologic, surgical, physical, or psychologic therapies) have been tried and do not prove satisfactory, have been judged unsuitable, or contraindicated for the patient
3. When patients have undergone careful screening and diagnosis by a multidisciplinary team before implantation
4. When all the facilities, equipment, and professional support personnel required for the proper diagnosis, treatment, training, and follow-up of the patient are available
5. When demonstration of pain relief with a *temporarily implanted* electrode precedes permanent implantation[9]
6. With demonstrated pathology (an objective basis for the pain)
7. With documentation of no drug addiction

The screening criteria for peripheral nerve stimulation including the previous guidelines should also include pain confined or related to a specific nerve branch, and pain that can be ablated by a peripheral nerve block. This will be discussed in more detail later.

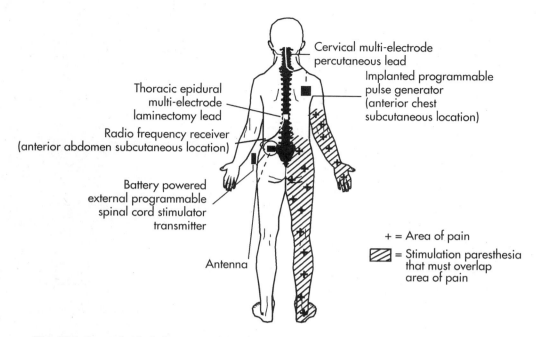

Fig. 32-1 Area of pain being covered by the paresthesia created by electronic stimulation of the spinal cord.

CONTRAINDICATIONS

There are a few contraindications to spinal cord stimulation as a therapeutic option:

1. Patient fails the screening
2. Patient is adverse to electrical stimulation
3. Patient is adverse to an implant as a modality of treating their pain
4. An active and uncontrolled coagulopathy at the time of procedure
5. Localized or disseminated infection at the time of the planned implantation
6. Physician's lack of experience or training in implanting stimulator devices
7. Patient has a demand cardiac pacemaker
8. Patient needs magnetic resonance imaging in the immediate foreseeable future
9. Untreated and unresolved serious drug habituation
10. Absence of an objectively documented cause for the pain

THE DIAGNOSTIC WORKUP

To comply with indications and the relative contraindications, proper diagnosis is essential. For the proper diagnosis procedure, see Chapters 3 and 5.

FAILED TREATMENT

It is extremely important to document, within the confines of the history and physical, what medications and therapeutic interventions have not been successful for the patient. Specifically indicate the medical, neurosurgical, orthopedic, vascular, behavioral medicine, or other consultants who have been involved. Determine that there are no contrain-

dications to spinal cord implantation and that no better alternatives exist.

IMPLANTATION PROCEDURES
Precautions

The screening stimulator lead array is implanted in a sterile operatory. Determine that adequate stimulation has been achieved on the operating room table. The stimulator paresthesia must cover the area of pain if possible. The entire system is not implanted in a single setting. The possible exception to this is in cases of objective documentation of clinical improvement in peripheral vascular disease. Operating room screening and immediate full system implantation is discouraged for the following reasons:

1. The patient is usually under the influence of a preoperative or intraoperative sedative administered to ease their discomfort during the placement of the intraspinal lead.
2. The patient is not bearing weight during the time of lead implantation and is not participating in activities of daily living. Thus using a stimulator system is an unrealistic test of pain relief.
3. The transient changes in body chemistry and position may remove the pain generator. Therefore the physician may not have the opportunity to see the pain in its most exaggerated form during the brief tenure in the operating room.

Ambulation after temporary placement of the lead in the prone or lateral position may cause migration of a percutaneously placed lead, thus altering the area of stimulation. Be certain that the system to be implanted can withstand changing positions from recumbent to ambulatory, and

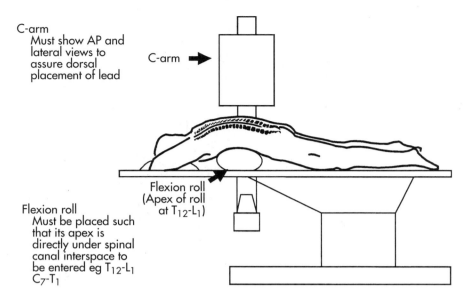

C-arm
  Must show AP and
  lateral views to
  assure dorsal
  placement of lead

C-arm

Flexion roll
(Apex of roll
at T_{12}-L_1)

Flexion roll
  Must be placed such
  that its apex is
  directly under spinal
  canal interspace to
  be entered eg T_{12}-L_1
  C_7-T_1

Fig. 32-2 Prone positioning of the patient with the level of entry of the spinal cord stimulator at the apex of the spinal flexion. Fluoroscopy assures proper level of implantation.

make sure that the paresthesia coverage does not vary significantly with ambulation.

It is recommended that the patient receive intravenous prophylaxis antibiotics approximately 30 minutes before the percutaneous implantation of the lead array. It is also recommended that, without exception, all leads be placed with fluoroscopic guidance. A mild sedative should be available to patients to help detraumatize the experience of having a spinal cord stimulating electrode placed into the spinal canal and to diminish the probability of sudden dangerous movement.

Procedure

The prone position is preferred. This allows for maximal spine flexion without depending on the patient's muscle strength when the apex of the flexion is the site selected for entry of the lead. Table 32-1 illustrates desired levels of lead placement. The patient in the prone position also facilitates easy direction to either side of the spinal canal with fluoroscopic guidance, without having to contend with gravity if the patient is in the lateral position (Fig. 32-2).

Once the lead is in the spinal canal and paresthesia is achieved, the lead is tunneled from the supraspinous ligament to a flank exit site. The screening wires are attached to the lead, which allows for multiweek screening. The patient is allowed to return to activities of daily living to determine the efficacy of the system. This system allows the implanter to alter and monitor results of changes in the following electronic parameters: polarity, electrode selection, pulse width, rate, and cycle.

Document via visual analog scales and pain maps. Determine areas of stimulation versus areas of pain, and amount of relief of pain prestimulation and poststimulation. If the patient demonstrates increased activities of daily living, and 50% or greater relief of their pain is from the stimu-

Table 32-1 Lead placement

Pain distribution	Entry level	Lead tip level
Foot only	L_2-L_3	T_{11}-L_1
Lower extremity with hip and back involvement	T_{12}-L_1	T_9-T_{10}
Upper chest wall (intercostal)	T_4-T_6	T_1-T_2
Upper extremity	T_1-T_2	C_2-C_5

lation alone (without adjunct narcotic analgesics above their usual level of analgesic consumption), permanent implantation may be indicated.[15]

The patient should be maintained on antibiotics as long as the percutaneous lead is present and for a brief period subsequent to total system implantation. The decision whether to place an implantable programmable neurologic stimulator power source or a radiofrequency receiver with external transmitter and antennae is based on a number of variables. The first and foremost is whether the physics of the implanted system are exceeded during the screening period. Other factors to consider include the use of the external power source depending somewhat on the patient being able to place their antenna, if the system is guided by an audible signal. This may cause problems with patients who have impaired hearing. The problem can be overcome by teaching patients to find their radiofrequency receiver by using a shrinking concentric circle motion until they reach maximal stimulation from the antennae.

Once the patient has demonstrated capability of properly operating the system, they are discharged, usually within 12 to 24 hours of their final implant.

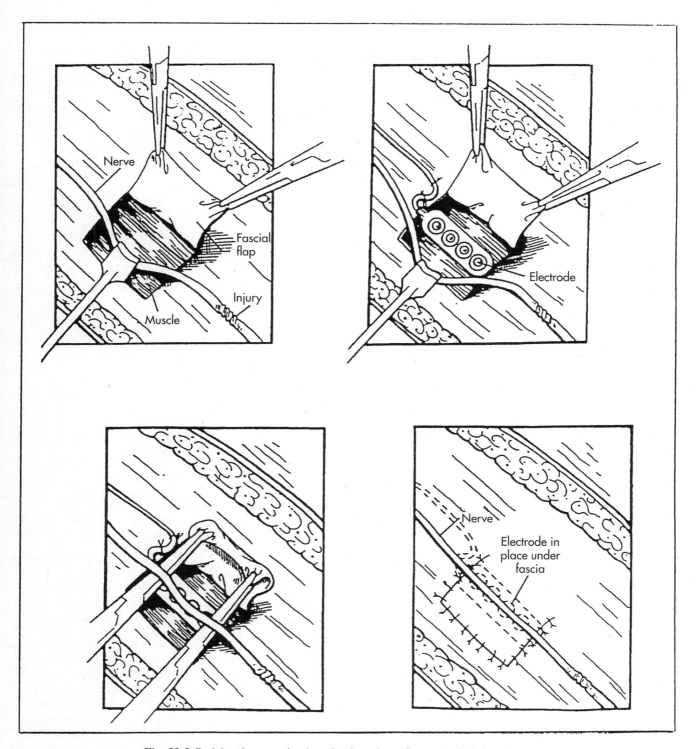

Fig. 32-3 Peripheral nerve stimulator implantation. (Courtesy of Medtronic, Inc.)

PERIPHERAL NERVE STIMULATION
History

Peripheral nerve stimulation has been used since 1965. Peripheral nerve stimulation was initially performed with cuffs containing stimulation electrodes. Technical and clinical complications were significant. Electrode migration and equipment malfunction created the need for more stable equipment design to be developed. Scar formation caused by direct contact between the nerve and the cuff led to nerve constriction. Flat electrode arrays with a thin panel of fas-

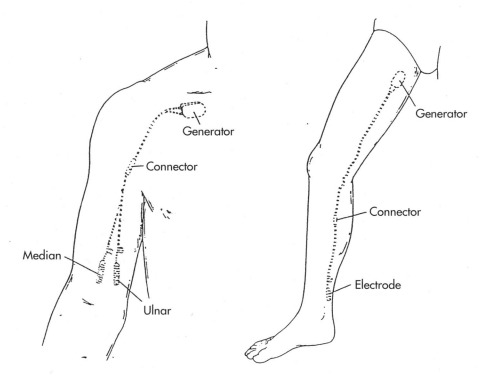

Fig. 32-4 A, Implantation sites for generator and stimulation electrode: ulnar or median nerve. **B,** Implantation sites for generator and stimulator electrode: Tibialis nerve. (From Racz GB, Browne T: Peripheral stimulator implant for treatment of causalgia caused by electrical burns. *Tex Med* 84:45-50, 1988.)

cia between the nerve and the stimulator proved to be much more stable and clinically effective.[16]

Peripheral nerve stimulation has been used successfully to treat pain of neurogenic origin in upper extremities, lower extremities, and intercostal nerves. As equipment design improved so did the clinical selection and screening procedure.

Selection criteria for peripheral nerve stimulation

Patients with single nerve pathology are the best peripheral nerve stimulator candidates. Patients with multiple nerve lesions have been successfully screened and implanted. Clinical syndromes that have responded favorably to peripheral nerve stimulation include:

· Reflex sympathetic dystrophy
· Causalgia
· Plexus avulsion
· Operative trauma
· Entrapment neuropathies
· Injection injuries

Clinical selection criteria include:

· Chronic intractable pain, recalcitrant to other therapies
· Temporary relief from local anesthetic injection
· No psychologic contraindications
· Objective evidence of pathology, (e.g., electromyography, somatosensory evoked potential, or selective tissue conductance studies)

· No drug habituation
· Relief from temporary screen

Surgical technique

Anesthetize the patient. Prep and drape the hand and arm. Do not use a tourniquet. The site for placement of electrode stimulation must be proximal to the injury.

Make a longitudinal incision on the medial aspect of the arm, centered between the elbow and axilla. Dissect down to the neurovascular bundle to free the nerve (median or ulnar) and to isolate an area approximately 4 cm long for placing of the electrode. Place the electrode underneath the nerve with multiple peripheral sutures to hold it securely in place. Then create a flap of fascial tissue, usually from intermuscular septum, and fold over the electrode to prevent its direct contact with the nerve. Allow the nerve to return to its normal position and for it to pass over the full length of the electrode, which is separated by the fascial flap. Suture several soft tissue elements loosely to hold the nerve over the electrode. Percutaneously bring the lead to a small wound in the shoulder area and attach it to a temporary connector brought through the skin. Close the wounds and dress them with transparent barrier dressings so that they can be observed postoperatively. Connect the temporary leads to the battery pack and adjust electrical stimulation over the next 3 days after evaluating the electrode requirements for best results. Assess the temporary stimulation to determine whether stimulation will work, and if it does, which electrode combination will work best. This way, the physician can determine whether to implant the more permanent and expensive (more than $5,000) stimulator unit[17] (Figs. 32-3 and 32-4).

Complications

As indicated per the discussion on consent, complications can occur. Patient-related complications might include infection, bleeding, adverse drug reaction, injury to the spinal cord, nerve injury, cerebrospinal fluid leak, poor pain relief, fibrosis at the tip of the stimulator, and/or motor stimulation. Mechanical problems that may occur include lead fracture, lead shearing and shortage, intraoperative or postoperative lead movement, extension cable fracture, battery malfunction or depletion, or transmitter malfunction or depletion.

Efficacy

Spinal cord stimulation has been effective in 53% to 70% of patients over 2.2 to 5 years.[18] Reports to measure the effectiveness of spinal cord stimulation included: good to excellent pain relief, decreased consumption of narcotics and other analgesias, improved tissue oxygenation, decreased incidence of amputation in peripheral vascular disease, increased activities of daily living, and return to work.

SUMMARY

Spinal cord and peripheral nerve stimulation are effective alternatives to suppress recalcitrant intractable pain of the extremities and trunk. The reported incidence of mechanical failures and dysfunction was 2.2 revisions required in the first 8 months of implantation. This incidence has dropped dramatically to fewer than 5% of implanted patients needing mechanical revision of their systems. This may be attributed to refinement of the equipment and better training and maturation of the learning curve of physician implanters. Careful follow-up and education of the patients is essential.

REFERENCES

1. Sjolund BH, Eriksson MBE: Stimulation techniques in the management of pain. In Kosterlist HW, Terenius LY, editors: *Pain Society.* Dahlan Konferenzen, 1980.
2. Melzack R, Wall PD: Pain mechanisms: A new theory. *Science* 150:971-979, 1965.
3. Plonsey R: Neural stimulation. In Myklebust JB, Cusick JF, editors: *Electrical Field Modeling.* Boca Raton, Fla, CRC Press, circa 1981.
4. Meyerson BA: Electrical stimulation of the spinal cord and brain. In Bonica JJ, editor: *The Management of Pain,* ed 2. Philadelphia, Lea & Febiger, 1990.
5. Bunt TJ, Holloway GA: Experience with epidural spinal stimulation in the treatment of end-stage peripheral vascular disease. *Seminars in Vascular Surgery* 4:216-220, 1991.
6. North R et al: Failed back surgery syndrome: Five year follow-up after spinal cord stimulator implantation. *Neurosurgery* 28:692-699, 1991.
7. Siegfried J, Lazorthes Y: Long term followup of dorsal cord stimulation for chronic pain syndromes after multiple lumbar operations. *Applied Neurophysiology* 45:201-204, 1982.
8. Waltz JM: Computerized percutaneous multi-level spinal cord stimulation in motor disorders. *Applied Neurophysiology* 45:73-92, 1982.
9. Leak WD: Intercostal neuralgia. History of over 100 spinal cord stimulator implants. Unpublished manuscript.
10. Long DM et al: Electrical stimulation of the spinal cord and peripheral nerves for pain control. *Applied Neurophysiology* 44:207-217, 1981.
11. Racz GB et al: Percutaneous dorsal column stimulator for chronic pain control. *Spine* 14:1-4, 1989.
12. North RB: Spinal cord stimulation for intractable pain: Indications and technique. *Current Therapy in Neurological Surgery* 2:297-301, 1989.
13. De La Porte C, Siegfried J: Lumbosacral spinal fibrosis (spinal arachnoiditis). *Spine* 8, 1983.
14. Jacobs M et al: Foot salvage and improvement of microvascular flow as the result of epidural spinal cord electrical stimulation. *J Vasc Surg* 12:354-360, 1990.
15. FDA approval of the Itrel totally implantable Spinal Cord Stimulation System: Department of Health and Human Services letter to Product Regulation Manager. Medtronic, Inc: *Spinal Cord Stimulation: Background and Efficacy.* August 1989.
16. Waisbrod H, Panhans CH: Direct nerve stimulation for painful peripheral neuropathies. *J Bone Joint Surg* 67-B:470-472, 1985.
17. Racz GB, Browne T: Peripheral stimulator implant for treatment of causalgia caused by electrical burns. *Tex Med* 84:45-50, 1988.
18. Health Care and Finance Administration: *Guidelines for Spinal Cord Stimulation Implantation.* Washington, DC, 1979.

QUESTIONS: NEURAL STIMULATION: SPINAL CORD AND PERIPHERAL NERVE STIMULATION

1. Inconsidering spinal cord stimulation, which of the following types of stimulation silences most dorsal horn cells?
   A. Low-frequency, low-amplitude stimulation
   B. High-frequency, low-amplitude stimulation
   C. High-frequency, high-amplitude stimulation
   D. Mid-frequency, mid-amplitude stimulation
2. Spinal cord stimulation has been demonstrated to produce the following neurohumoral changes:
   A. An increase in CSF endorphin and serotonin
   B. An increase in CSF endorphin and a decrease in serotonin
   C. A decrease in CSF endorphin and a decrease in CSF endorphin
   D. An increase in serotonin and a decrease in CSF endorphin
3. When referring to electrical stimulation, which of the following terms properly describes the electrode polarity used in spinal cord stimulation?
   A. The anode is a negative lead.
   B. The cathode is a positive lead.
   C. The anode is a neutral lead
   D. The anode is a positive lead.

4. The major factor in successful spinal cord stimulation is:
   A. Electrode positioning
   B. Electrode combination
   C. Size of electrode
   D. Amount of current passed between electrodes
5. Spinal cord stimulation has been demonstrated to be somewhat effective in which of the following disease states?
   A. Spasmodic torticollis
   B. Mixed-migraine headaches
   C. Temporal arteritis
   D. Cluster headaches

ANSWERS

1. B
2. A
3. D
4. A
5. A

33 Physical Therapy

Elise A. Trumble and Margaret P. Krengel

The role of rehabilitation services in treating pain has expanded significantly in the past several years. The rehabilitation team now includes physical, occupational, and exercise therapists who contribute to the rehabilitation program in unique yet complementary ways.

The emphasis of rehabilitation has shifted from applying pain-relieving modalities to developing pain-relieving behaviors. The patient should be educated in anatomy, body mechanics, and work ergonomics that will enable the individual to return to a previous lifestyle and employment with new and improved postures and body mechanics. Pain remains a symptom that must be treated in some very specific ways acutely. Later, pain can be considered a signal that alerts the patient to less than optimal posture, position, or movement rather than the problem. Rehabilitation should treat both pain symptoms and behaviors. Rehabilitation therapists have learned that early and effective application of pain-relieving modalities, education, and behaviors can reduce or alleviate many problems associated with pain.

Every discipline in the rehabilitation team has better, more objective measurement tools at its disposal than were available 5 years ago. These tools reduce the subjective component of the evaluation and improve the validity of the results.

Instead of viewing the rehabilitation treatments as general techniques that can be applied at any time in a patient's program, we present the techniques appropriate for the stage of tissue healing from the onset of injury. Thus we can determine the status of the tissue structures involved. Clinicians should be aware of the stages of tissue healing when evaluating, managing, and predicting the patient's future condition.

The purpose of this chapter is to update the reader about the current services in evaluation and treatment available through the rehabilitation therapies.

PHYSICAL THERAPY MODALITIES AND OTHER FUNCTIONAL RESTORATION PROGRAMS
Heat therapy

The major factors determining the number and intensity of the physiologic reactions to heat are:
1. The level of tissue temperature (therapeutic range is 43° C [109.4° F] to 45° C [113° F]
2. The duration of tissue temperature elevation, which is 3 to 30 minutes
3. The rate of temperature rise in tissues
4. The size of the area treated

Superficial heat. The types of superficial heat are listed. Even though the physical properties differ, none of these agents can overcome the combination of skin tolerance, tissue thermal conductivity, and the body's response to produce localized temperature elevations of more than a few degrees at depths of a few centimeters.

Conduction

Hot (hydrocollator) packs

1. Provides a clinically useful temperature for 30 minutes
2. Advantages include low cost, minimal maintenance, long life, patient acceptance, and easy to use
3. Alternatives include electric heating pads, hot water bottles, and circulating water heating pads
4. Exposure time: 20 minutes

Paraffin baths

1. A mixture of mineral oil and paraffin (1:7)
2. Temperatures of 52° to 54° C are well tolerated because the mixture has a low heat capacity and an insulating layer of wax builds up on the treated area
3. Dip method versus continuous immersion

Conversion. Heat lamps are inexpensive, versatile, and an easy way to warm superficial tissues. The lamps use a 250-watt bulb that the therapist positions 40 to 50 cm from the patient.

Convection. Convection is based on hydrotherapy (whirlpool baths and hubbard tanks). Pumps agitate water and provide convective heating, massage, and gentle debridement. Hydrotherapy can be effective for mobilization of joints, as an adjunct in the treatment of rheumatoid arthritis, and for muscle spasm. Temperatures of 33° to 36° C are considered neutral; hubbard tank temperatures should be limited to 39° C. Single extremity treatments can be more rigorous, and in a healthy individual, temperatures from 43° to 46° C are possible. Hydrotherapy is well suited for burn and treatment at neutral temperatures.

Contrast baths are thought to be effective because of reflex hyperemia produced by the alternating exposure to heat (43° C) and cold (16° C).

Deep-heat modalities (conversion).

Ultrasound. Ultrasound is arbitrarily defined as sound at frequencies above the limits of human hearing (more than 17,000 Hz). Ultrasound machines use ceramic and quartz piezoelectric crystals to produce ultrasonic energy. Intensities of 0.5 to 2 W/cm^2 are used. Phonophoresis includes the addition of a steroid, which is theoretically forced into the tissue to potentiate treatment effectiveness. Precautions and contraindications include fluid-filled cavities and ultrasound over metal implants.

Short wave diathermy. Short wave diathermy uses radio waves to heat tissue by conversion.

Microwave. Microwave is electromagnetic radiation at frequencies of 915 and 2456 MHz.

Cold therapy (cryotherapy)

Superficial cold therapy is used to reduce blood flow, decrease metabolic activity, lessen muscle tone, decrease swelling, and inhibit spasticity and clonus. It can also increase gastrointestinal motility, slow nerve conduction, and produce analgesia.

Cryotherapy is restricted to superficial agents that are inexpensive but effective. These include ice, cold water, refrigerated units, vaporizing liquids, and chemical packs. Chilling causes an initial period of vasoconstriction until subcutaneous tissues reach 15° C. Thereafter, vessels dilate. Temperatures of 13° to 15° C for 20 to 30 minutes are used.

Transcutaneous electrical nerve stimulation

Transcutaneous electrical nerve stimulation (TENS) produces analgesia in a wide range of medical conditions, but its usefulness is questioned by recent studies. TENS units are small simple devices consisting of a power source (rechargeable battery), one or more signal generators, and a set of electrodes. Typically, output currents are less than 100 mA, pulse rates are between 0.5 and 200 Hz, and pulse widths are from 10 to several hundred microseconds. Pulse and wave train shape vary widely. All TENS units allow adjustment of the stimulus intensity. Electrode placement and stimulation parameter choice remain more art than science.

Iontophoresis

Iontophoresis is a process in which electrically charged molecules or atoms (ions) are driven into tissue with an electrical field. Voltage provides the driving force. Iontophoresis delivers high concentrates of polar substances into the skin, but to questionable depths.

Vibration

Vibration is used for muscle facilitation and reeducation, and for acute and chronic pain conditions.

Biofeedback

Biofeedback has been used successfully for a variety of pain states, including headaches and generalized muscle tension.

Traction

Indications. Traction is indicated for injuries of the cervical and lumbar spine.

Application Techniques. The following techniques can be applied in traction:

1. Manual
2. Mechanical
3. Motorized: continuous, intermittent
4. Gravity

Parameters

1. Positioning
2. Continuous versus intermittent
3. Weight:
   Cervical—25 to 30 lbs
   Lumbar—50 to 100 lbs

Failures. Failures have been generally related to inadequate weight, poor positioning, or stretching of pain-sensitive tissues.

Contraindications. Contraindications to traction include instability, vertebrobasilar disease with improper positioning, signs of myelopathy, significant osteopenia, spine tumors, lumbar traction in pregnant women, spine infections, extreme anxiety, and lumbar traction in patients with restrictive lung disease.

Compression

The following are types of compression:

· Elevation
· String wrapping
· Ace wraps
· Garments
· Gradient pumps

Massage

Indications. Massage can be used in any condition to relieve pain, reduce swelling, or mobilize contracted tissue.

Contraindications. The contraindications of massage are: infections, thrombophlebitis, malignancies, burns, and skin diseases.

Reflex effects. Stimulation of peripheral receptors in the skin produce centrally mediated sensations of pleasure and peripherally cause muscle relaxation.

Mechanical effects. The mechanical effects of massage consist of measures to assist the return flow and circulation of blood and lymph, to produce intramuscular motion to stretch adhesions, and to mobilize fluid accumulation.

Techniques. Massage techniques include stroking (effleurage), compression (pétrissage), and percussion (tapotement).

Electrical stimulation

Electrical stimulation does not strengthen normal muscles more rapidly than traditional approaches. For immobilized and injured muscles, electrical stimulation maintains isometric strength; when there is splinting and pain, it may supplement volitional movements and speed of recovery. In the patient with upper motor neuron spinal cord injury, functional electrical stimulation (FES) may increase strength, normalize blood pressure, allow for limited ambulation, and lead to a sense of well-being.

Orthotics

1. Braces, corsets, collars, slings, and supports
2. Cushioning devices and pads
3. Shoes: lifts and inserts
4. Splints: static and dynamic
5. Mobility aids: canes, crutches, walkers, wheelchairs

Therapeutic exercise

Therapeutic exercise is defined as the prescribed body movement to correct an impairment, improve musculoskeletal function, or maintain a state of well-being. For example, aerobic exercise reduces pain complaints while developing and maintaining cardiovascular conditioning.

Aquatics therapy

Pool therapy can be extremely beneficial because the buoyancy allows aerobic exercise, range of motion, and weight bearing that would not be possible out of water. Water can be soothing, relaxing, and particularly helpful to an anxious and fearful patient. Short-term individual treatment should be followed by group classes; and thereafter the patient should work independently.

PHYSICAL AND OCCUPATIONAL THERAPY Rx GUIDELINES

The physician ordering physical or occupational therapy should realize that the therapist is a trained professional who should be recognized as an equal member of the treatment team. Communication between physician and therapist is key to achieving a successful outcome for the chronic pain patient. The therapist sees the patient more frequently than the physician and may be able to provide important insights into physical and psychosocial factors affecting the patient's presentation.

The therapy prescription should include a general order to evaluate and treat plus any limitations or specifics requested by the physician. The prescription should include the diagnosis, frequency and length of recommended treatment, and most importantly, any precautions or contraindications.

Physical and occupational therapy should be active and not passive. Modalities may be useful early in treatment, but in general should be discouraged in favor of therapy that is functionally oriented and encourages patient independence.

MANUAL THERAPY

Manual therapy refers to specific skills by the therapist in muscle, joint, and somatic dysfunction. As with any discipline, some therapists have exceptional skills in this area. Manual therapy is best used as an integrated part of a comprehensive pain management program.

FUNCTIONAL RESTORATION PROGRAMS

Between formal one-on-one physical therapy and an independent fitness center program is a functional restoration type of program. This cost-effective approach involves a structured physical conditioning program in a group setting. Individuals may attend three to five times a week for 2 to 4 hours each visit and engage in stretching, strengthening, and aerobic conditioning plus educational activities and work simulation. Dependency on the therapist is discouraged, and the program is geared towards healthy behaviors and return to leisure and work activities. The group setting provides friendship among patients and encourages mutual support.

GYM PROGRAMS AND FITNESS CENTERS

There are two levels of these types of programs. Ideally, the physical therapy center has a supervised low-cost gym program available so that the patient can be weaned early from one-on-one physical therapy and use the gym facility. In such an arrangement the insurer is not paying physical therapy rates for an exercise program, yet the patient is still in a protected and supervised environment. Usually, as formal therapy is winding down, the independent gym program begins. By the time individual therapy is over, the patient is independently continuing in the gym or fitness center program.

The second level of the program is the private gym or YMCA, where there is some supervision, but the patients are generally on their own. To prevent reinjury, patients should not start this type of program without specific directions from the physician or physical therapist.

WORK HARDENING VERSUS WORK CONDITIONING

Work hardening is a specific return to work program where the injured worker is expected to be able to return to a particular job. Work hardening involves 2 to 6 weeks of specific simulated work activities before returning to employment.

Work toughening or conditioning, where the individual exercises in a gym, is not work hardening. Although work hardening may include gym exercise activities, the program is task specific for the particular job and involves both emotional and physical reactivation to meet job demands.

ERGONOMICS

Ergonomics is the study of how people interact with their physical environment, and how that interaction might be modified to prevent or reduce musculoskeletal disorders. For instance, tools might be redesigned to prevent wrist tendinitis and carpal tunnel syndrome. The ergonomic system model consists of four parts: the task, the operator, the environment, and the equipment. The objective is to maximize system performance and minimize mismatches between system elements.

Basic ergonomic principles include keeping the wrists straight and the elbows down, minimizing spine twisting and bending, and providing adjustable chairs or work surfaces. More specifically, ergonomic redesign requirements include reduction of forces, frequency of activities, holding time, and extreme postural deviations. The costs of ignoring ergonomic principles include lower productivity and performance, higher absenteeism, increased risk of worker injuries, and more worker compensation claims.

VOCATIONAL REHABILITATION AND VOLUNTEER ACTIVITIES

For chronic pain patients whose goal is to return to gainful employment, vocational rehabilitation efforts should be an integral part of pain management and should be started early in the rehabilitation process. Resources such as workers' compensation or state vocational rehabilitation services should be identified. Employers should be encouraged to make reasonable accommodations and to consider the patient returning to work in a modified or part-time position.

Volunteer activities allow many individuals to have meaningful interactions with other people, stay busy, get out of the home, and make a worthwhile social contribution.

AVOCATIONAL AND RECREATIONAL ISSUES

Recreational activities can be pleasurable, time filling, socially reinforcing and physically and mentally therapeutic.

PM&R GUIDING PRINCIPLES

- Do no harm
- Cost-effective care
- Pain control
- Patient empowerment
- Functional restoration
- Return to work and leisure activities

QUESTIONS: PHYSICAL THERAPY

1. The principles of physical therapy and rehabilitation of pain patients include all of the following EXCEPT:
   A. Development of pain-relieving behaviors
   B. Work ergonomics
   C. Education of body mechanics
   D. Limit the previous life-style and work
2. The contraindication for heat therapy is:
   A. Pain
   B. Muscle spasm
   C. Edema
   D. Bursitis
3. Ultrasound machines use ceramic and quartz piezo-electric crystals to produce ultrasonic energy. The sound produced by these machines is above the frequencies of human hearing. Their frequencies range more than:
   A. 1000 Hz
   B. 5000 Hz
   C. 13,000 Hz
   D. 17,000 Hz
4. A process in which electrically charged molecules (ions) are driven into the tissue with an electrical field is known as:
   A. Vibration
   B. Compression
   C. Biofeedback
   D. Iontophoresis

5. In functional restoration programs, the aim is to provide all of the following EXCEPT:
   A. Aerobic conditioning
   B. Group therapy
   C. Dependency on the physical therapist
   D. Cost-effective approach

ANSWERS

1. D
2. C
3. D
4. D
5. C

PART FIVE

Pain Syndromes

34 Taxonomy

P. Prithvi Raj

The word *taxonomy* means the systematic classification of subjects, sorted into groups to reflect similarity, with generally broader groups residing over those that are more restricted. An orderly arrangement in chronic pain is an immense task, and many systems have been proposed. Whatever system is created needs to have a wide enough application to cover both clinical practice and research and not just some bureaucratic regulations. It is reasonable to ask why a taxonomy is necessary. The reason is that physicians face problems in dealing with complex and chronic pain, and a clear understanding of pain syndromes is needed in order to treat them effectively and reliably.

Some of the problems faced with pain include:

1. Inexact definition of pain
2. Difficult and unreliable method to measure or quantify pain
3. Observer bias in assessing a patient's behavior, which quantifies the intensity of pain

DEFINITION OF PAIN

The International Association for the Study of Pain's (IASP) definition of pain is "an unpleasant sensory and emotional experience associated with actual or potential tissue damage or described in terms of such damage."[1-3] From this definition, it is important to emphasize that pain is always subjective, a sensation, and unpleasant; and we are urged to evaluate *both* the physical and the nonphysical components of the experience called *pain*. Pain is actually a construct or concept.[2] It is a function of a personal theoretic orientation. For instance, a neurosurgeon who sees pain only as a neuroanatomic or neurophysiologic event will not see the psychologic aspects of pain as significant. On the other hand, the psychologist will understand pain to be an integration of physical, psychologic, and social factors and will apply emotional, environmental, and psychophysiologic questions to patients in search of variations within these realms. Thus two qualified specialists can come up with very different impressions of a patient's pain.

Chronic pain really means that the pain is not acute.[3] This is pain that persists in spite of good therapy and sometimes extraordinary treatment. The problem with chronic pain is that it can interfere with the patient's attitude about health and recovery, behaviors, and lifestyle. Furthermore, these patients suffer. In fact, the emotional/psychosocial influence on pain has been highlighted by Twycross.[4] He assessed factors that affected the pain threshold (the point at which a given stimulus provokes the report of pain from a patient)

in hospice patients in England. He listed conditions such as discomfort, insomnia, fatigue, anxiety, fear, anger, and depression as factors that would tend to lower a patient's threshold. On the other hand, the threshold could be raised by relief of pain, restful sleep, relaxation, sympathy and understanding, elevation of mood, and diversion from the pain.

Pain is clearly a multidimensional experience. It is neurophysiologic, biochemical, psychologic, ethnocultural, religious, cognitive, affective, and environmental. Thus its classification can be understandably complex and its management elusive at worst and difficult at best. It results in physiologic, anatomic, and behavioral changes that persist even when the original pathology is removed.

ACUTE VERSUS CHRONIC PAIN

Table 34-1 characterizes the differences between acute and chronic pain based upon clinical features. These two entities are different diseases; each are characterized by the knowledge base required to evaluate and manage them. The knowledge base is derived from the clinical experience gained by healthcare professionals who choose to deal with pain patients. They consider the extent of the patient's body involvement with pain and the time it takes for the chronic pain syndrome to develop; the nervous system responses to either the acute or the ongoing pain; the possibility that adverse behavioral consequences will develop; and that all treatments done for acute pain may make chronic pain worse.

Chronic pain

Feuerstein presented the components of an operational definition for chronic pain.[2] In this categorization, he found the following important:

1. Pain sensation
2. Pain behavior
3. Functional status at work (this basically involves the traditional ergonomic considerations)
4. Functional status at home (this includes not just the physical environment, but evaluation of the family interaction system based upon roles that each member plays, the communications that occur, and the problem-solving skills that are available to individuals and within the family unit)
5. The emotional state of the patient (this plays a significant role in the initiation, exacerbation, and maintenance of chronic pain; again, pain is not all physical and this important component must be evaluated)

Table 34-1 Acute versus chronic pain

Acute pain	Chronic pain
Ample training and opportunity	Less so
Evaluation and R_x takes less time	Time consuming
Pain is a useful signal	Pain is a disease affecting attitudes, lifestyles, and behavior
Pain plus anxiety	Pain plus frustration
Usually self-limiting/short R_x	Persists/long R_x
Individual problem	Pain is more than the patient
Priority of R_x options	Different than for acute
Patient *needs* to be in.tune with R_x goals	Less so
Likelihood of success with proper R_x	Less so
Expectations of R_x are high	Less so

Table 34-2 Axis I: Regions*

Region	Code
Head, face, and mouth	000
Cervical region	100
Upper shoulder and upper limbs	200
Thoracic region	300
Abdominal region	400
Lower back, lumbar spine, sacrum, and coccyx	500
Lower limbs	600
Pelvic region	700
Anal, perineal, and genital region	800
More than three major sites	900

From Merskey H: Classification of chronic pain. Descriptions of chronic pain syndromes and definitions of pain terms. *Pain Supp* 3:S10, 1986.
*Record main site first. If there are two important regions, record separately. If there is more than one site of pain, separate coding will be necessary.

Table 34-3 Axis II: Systems

System	Code
Nervous system (central, peripheral, and autonomic) and special senses; physical disturbance or dysfunction	00
Nervous system (psychologic and social)	10
Respiratory and cardiovascular systems	20
Musculoskeletal system and connective tissue	30
Cutaneous and subcutaneous, and associated glands (breast, apocrine, etc.)	40
Gastrointestinal system	50
Genitourinary system	60
Other organs or viscera (e.g., thyroid, lymphatic, hemopoietic)	70
More than one system	80

From Merskey H: Classification of chronic pain. Descriptions of chronic pain syndromes and definitions of pain terms. *Pain Suppl* 3:S10, 1986.

Box 34-1 THE IASP FIVE AXIS PAIN TAXONOMY: OVERVIEW

Axis I: Region
Axis II: System
Axis III: Temporal characteristics of pain: pattern of occurrence
Axis IV: Patient's statement of intensity: time since onset of pain
Axis V: Etiology

---

6. Somatic preoccupation (this reflects the patient's ability to focus on bodily symptoms, almost to the exclusion of the ability to function)

TAXONOMY AND CLASSIFICATION OF PAIN

Single axis classification systems based on the previous components merely distinguish acute from chronic pain or describe cancer pain syndromes. These systems generally become inadequate when descriptors and qualifiers are needed beyond the simple, primary designation for purposes of exacting exchange of information.[5,6] The IASP Subcommittee on Taxonomy created the first multiaxial system, based upon the region of the body involved in chronic pain, the organ systems affected, the temporal characteristics and pattern of the pain, the duration and intensity, and the etiology.[1,3,5,6]

Box 34-1 reveals the five axis pain taxonomy. Axis I deals with the regions where the pain occurs (Table 34-2). Axis II details the systems of the body which are involved in the pain (Table 34-3). Axis III relates the temporal charac-

teristics of the pain with attention to the pattern of occurrence (Table 34-4). Axis IV is based on statements of intensity provided by the patient, which indicate the time since onset of the pain (Table 34-5). Table 34-6 demonstrates the components of Axis V, which is based on the etiology of the patient's pain.

Advantages

The advantages of the IASP five region system are[1,3]:

1. This was developed by a multidisciplinary association that is widely diversified in geography and expertise
2. IASP publishes a respected and well-circulated journal so taxonomy is well distributed
3. The system should be easy to adopt because it is based on five axes already used in medicine
4. It is a starting point for a complex task

The IASP system is provisional, yet it is a framework and a place to begin. Using the system should improve spoken and written communication by standardizing recording

Table 34-4 Axis III: Temporal characteristics of pain

Pattern of occurrence	Code
Not recorded, not applicable, or not known	0
Single episode, limited duration (e.g., ruptured aneurysm, sprained ankle)	1
Continuous or nearly continuous, nonfluctuating (e.g., low back pain)	2
Continuous or nearly continuous, fluctuating severity (e.g., ruptured intervertebral disk)	3
Recurring, irregularly (e.g., headache, mixed type)	4
Recurring, regularly (e.g., premenstrual pain)	5
Paroxysmal (e.g., tic douloureux)	6
Sustained with superimposed paroxysms	7
Other combinations	8
None of the above	9

From Merkey H: Classification of chronic pain. Descriptions of chronic pain syndromes and definitions of pain terms. *Pain Suppl* 3:S10, 1986.

Table 34-5 Axis IV: Statement of intensity: Time since onset of pain

Time	Code
Not recorded, not applicable, or not known	.0
Mild: 1 month or less	.1
1 month to 6 months	.2
More than 6 months	.3
Medium: 1 month or less	.4
1 month to 6 months	.5
More than 6 months	.6
Severe: 1 month or less	.7
1 month to 6 months	.8
More than 6 months	.9

From Merskey H: Classification of chronic pain. Descriptions of chronic pain syndromes and definitions of pain terms. *Pain Suppl* 3:S11, 1986.

symptoms, complaints, and observations; reporting and relevance of research; exchange of information; and improvement in the management of pain throughout the world.

Disadvantages

It is clearly hard to be mutually exclusive and completely exhaustive with any system. The IASP system uses some natural breakouts and some that are artificial but convenient.

Ventafridda and Caraceni criticized the IASP system for shedding little light on the classification issue. They felt that the system was just a list of diseases and lesions that cause pain.[7] They cautioned that physicians should be aware of using terms that deny the physical component of pain, and would thereby influence treatment choices.

Procacci and Maresca noted in trying to deal with international populations of patients that linguistic and philologic issues, and the operative applicability of the taxonomy would need to be addressed.[8] There also would be epistemologic issues. One of their fundamental points is that the physician needs to be able to use the system, and their criti-

Table 34-6 Axis V: Etiology

Etiology	Code
Genetic or congenital disorders (e.g., congenital dislocation)	.00
Trauma, operation, burns	.01
Infective, parasitic	.02
Inflammatory (no known infective agent) immune reactions	.03
Neoplasm	.04
Toxic, metabolic (e.g., alcoholic neuropathy, anoxia, vascular, nutritional, endocrine) radiation	.05
Degenerative, mechanical	.06
Dysfunctional (including psychophysiologic)	.07
Unknown or other	.08
Origin is psychologic* (e.g., conversion hysteria, depressive hallucination)	.09

From Merskey H: Classification of chronic pain. Descriptions of chronic pain syndromes and definitions of pain therapy. *Pain Suppl* 3:S11, 1986.
*No physical cause should be held to be present nor any pathophysiologic mechanism.

cism of the IASP system was that is was too elaborate and difficult for the ordinary physician to use.

Controversy

Turk and Rudy suggested that the lack of a universally accepted classification system has resulted in a lot of confusion, and that investigators and physicians are unable to compare observations and results of research.[9] They noted that an infinite number of classification systems can be developed deductively, depending upon the rationale behind common factors believed to discriminate diagnoses. Their data suggested that the psychosocial and behavioral responses associated with chronic pain are common to a diverse sample of pain patients despite the differences in demographic characteristics and medical diagnoses. They have proved that taxonomy is still an issue and that there is yet no universal system.

REFERENCES

1. Merskey H: Classification of chronic pain. Descriptions of chronic pain syndromes and definitions of pain terms. *Pain Suppl* 3, 1986.
2. Feuerstein M: Definitions of pain. In Tollison CD, editor: *Handbook of Chronic Pain Management*. Baltimore, Williams & Wilkins, 1989.
3. Bonica JJ: Definitions and taxonomy of pain. In Bonica JJ, editor: *The Management of Pain*. Philadelphia, Lea & Febiger, 1990.
4. Twycross RG: The relief of pain in far-advanced cancer. *Reg Anesth* 5(3):2-11, 1980.
5. Boyd DB: Taxonomy and classification of pain. In Tollison CD, editor: *Handbook of Chronic Pain Management*. Baltimore, Williams & Wilkins, 1989.
6. Longmire DR: Tutorial 7: The classification of pain and pain syndromes. *Pain Digest* 2:229-233, 1992.
7. Ventafridda V, Caraceni A: Cancer pain classification: A controversial issue. *Pain* 46:1-2, 1991.
8. Procacci P, Maresca M: Considerations on taxonomy of pain. *Pain* 45:332-333, 1991.
9. Turk DC, Rudy TE: The robustness of an empirically derived taxonomy of chronic pain patients. *Pain* 43:27-35, 1990.

35 Trauma

Richard L. Rauck

Traumatic injuries rank as the leading cause of death in the United States for persons under the age of 40.[1,2] Overall, trauma ranks third in listed causes of mortality.[3] Two major causes contribute to the high mortality associated with trauma in this country. First, the advent of the high-speed automobile, coupled with an increasing population, has resulted in a steady and dramatic rise in automobile-related deaths over the past 50 years. Second, the rapid and continuing escalation of violent crimes in the past decade has produced many trauma victims.

Chest trauma accounts for 25% of the 100,000 annual traumatic deaths, with blunt thoracic injuries from automobile accidents being more common than penetrating injuries.[4,5] Accidental falls and crush injuries are distant second and third causes of blunt trauma. Violent crimes account for nearly all the penetrating chest trauma seen in the United States.

Management of trauma victims requires a multidisciplinary team.[2,6-9] Pain and the associated stress response observed in trauma patients should always be viewed as detrimental, and attempts at alleviating the pain need high priority. However, other issues such as monitoring cerebral function can sometimes be viewed as conflicting with pain management. In reality, effective optimal pain management should consider the entire clinical condition and tailor an approach which addresses all concerns.

Pain management in trauma victims has focused on the acute setting. Unfortunately, too many trauma patients develop chronic pain syndromes. More focus in the acute period should center on prevention of long-term pain syndromes. The costs of long-term pain management of both treatment and disability far outweigh the short-term cost of acute pain management in trauma care. We are just beginning to understand the value of certain acute pain management techniques which will decrease the likelihood and severity of long-term pain.[3]

HISTORY

For centuries the classical management for chest wall injuries involved external traction and stabilization.[10,11] Work in the 1950s by Avery and co-workers led to the use of mechanical ventilation and hyperventilation as a mechanism to provide "internal pneumatic stabilization" of the chest wall.[12] Many reports described lower morbidity and mortality with this technique, particularly when compared with

the previous techniques of external stabilization and fixation.[10,11,13-20]

It became evident, however, that mechanical ventilation did not affect all trauma patients in the same way.[21] Some patients did well and recovered uneventfully, whereas others continued to die from what was often considered "stiff lung." Many studies during the 1960s continued to demonstrate mortality figures in 20% to 70%. Relihan and Litwin, for example, studied 58 mechanically-ventilated patients via tracheostomies and found a pulmonary infection rate of 87% and a mortality rate of 30%.[19]

These studies did not try to segregate out pulmonary parenchymal disease from chest wall disease. Also, associated traumatic injuries were rarely accounted for, nor were they classified. Attention to pain and its role in the trauma patient was never addressed nor considered important for the healing process.

As mechanical ventilation became more sophisticated, reports demonstrated the benefit of certain types of ventilatory patterns such as intermittent mandatory ventilation with positive end-expiratory pressure versus standard controlled mechanical ventilation.[22,23]

Trinkle and co-workers were among the earliest to recognize analgesia as important in the traumatically-injured patient.[24,25] These researchers advocated the use of spontaneous ventilation whenever possible and the aggressive management of any underlying pulmonary pathology. They acknowledged the need for good chest wall analgesia to maximize the patient's ability to ventilate spontaneously. Intercostal nerve blocks and appropriate use of morphine sulfate were employed.

As the trend changed to spontaneous ventilation, research supported the idea that the critical pathophysiologic derangement in thoracic trauma was due to the underlying damage to pulmonary parenchyma.[26] To appropriately manage this and prevent adult respiratory distress syndrome, strict maintenance of intravascular fluids, chest physiotherapy, and pain relief became more important.

Richardson et al. examined 427 patients prospectively and classified them as: (1) flail chest; (2) pulmonary contusion; (3) pneumothorax; or (4) multiple rib fractures without a flail segment.[21] Endotracheal intubation for blunt chest trauma occurred only if patients: had hypoxemia ($PO_2 < 55$ mmHg on room air, or 60 mmHg on supplemental O_2); respiratory distress ($PCO_2 > 55$ mmHg); shock, severe neurologic injury, or other major associated injuries; general anesthesia; or airway obstruction. Intercostal nerve blocks were performed for patients with significant pain.

Results indicated 77% of patients were managed without endotracheal intubation. For the group not initially intubated, 96.9% were successfully managed without significant pulmonary complications or mechanical ventilation. The termination of 4 of the 10 patients who failed conservative management was felt to have been preventable had better pulmonary care been provided.

Although the gains and understanding of pain management techniques are slowly evolving for patients with chest trauma, less enlightenment is still frequently witnessed for patients with other trauma. Multitrauma patients will always require resuscitative efforts as the utmost priority. However, once the initial resuscitation has occurred and patients have stabilized, attention to pain management should be viewed as more than just a luxury. Pain relief, itself, should be one goal, because the benefits of effective pain management extend well beyond initial relief. Earlier, more effective rehabilitation will occur in patients who are optimally pain managed. The prevention of chronic pain syndromes such as causalgia, reflex sympathetic dystrophy, nerve entrapments, chronic posttraumatic headaches, and other syndromes would undoubtedly be cost-effective.

PATHOPHYSIOLOGY

It is beyond the scope of this chapter to describe all the pathophysiologic events involved in different types of traumatic injuries. However, the pain physician should have a working knowledge of the important processes involved and their relationship to pain management techniques. For instance, certain head injuries may necessitate frequent mental function monitoring and render some pain management techniques less desirable. Other injuries will predispose patients to significant blood dyscrasias which would tend to contraindicate certain pain-relieving techniques.

Thoracic injuries represent a major area of interest and problem to trauma specialists; and this is an area where pain practitioners can provide a valuable resource beyond simple pain relief. The following discussion will therefore be limited to the pathophysiology of chest wall lesion.

Chest wall lesion

The role of pain management in the trauma patient depends on the injuries involved and the underlying pathophysiology. Uncontrolled pain should never be considered beneficial in any trauma patient. Circulating catecholamines and other neuroendocrine peptides have repeatedly been shown to be deleterious in animals and humans.[27,28] All trauma patients should be provided with optimal pain management that is tailored to the injuries sustained.

A commonly injured area in trauma is the chest region. Injuries to the chest can be classified as either nonpenetrating or penetrating, which is an important distinction since survival for nonpenetrating injuries has not shown the dramatic improvement recorded for penetrating injuries.[15,20,29] This reflects the increasing severity of nonpenetrating injuries, most commonly the automobile accident, where kinetic energy from deceleration injuries transmits tremendous force and ultimate disruption of the bony thorax and underlying tissues, in particular to the pulmonary parenchymal tissue.[30]

Rib fractures are the most common injury to the bony thorax.[20] In healthy individuals, a simple nondisplaced rib fracture is viewed merely as a painful inconvenience. In severely compromised pulmonary patients a rib fracture can prevent them from breathing effectively or clearing secretions adequately, with resulting serious morbidity. Elderly or compromised patients must be watched carefully and their pain effectively managed to prevent atelectasis or pneumonia.

When more than one rib has been fractured in two locations, or if the fractures occur posteriorly with concomitant sternochondral dislocation, a flail chest segment can result.[31-35] The flailed segment enlarges with the number of ribs involved; if greater than six ribs are fractured, the entire hemithorax can move paradoxically, making the flail difficult to detect. With a flail segment the chest wall becomes unstable, and ventilation is impaired. Mortality for patients with greater than six fractured ribs is twice that of patients with fewer fractures.[15,17,36,37]

Another diagnostic consideration concerns the patient with fractures of the upper four ribs.[38] These flailed segments can be difficult to detect but must be carefully looked for since the integrity of the upper rib cage is essential for adequate ventilation.

The ability to control the pain occurring from derangements of the chest wall has greatly improved, as described in the section on treatment.[39] Unfortunately, the same cannot be said for underlying derangements to the pulmonary parenchyma.[40-44] Pulmonary contusion describes the physiologic and anatomic lesion which occurs most frequently after nonpenetrating, compression-decompression injuries. Pain does not represent a major limiting problem in this setting, since lung tissue itself has few primary nociceptive afferents.

Trauma to the lung causes a disruption at the alveolar-capillary interface, resulting in both hemorrhage and edema in the alveolar and interstitial spaces.[45,46] Alveolar tissue may also shear from the bronchial tree, secondary to interstitial forces and airway distention from sudden pressure changes. Increased capillary permeability with blood leaking into the bronchial tree, and changes in alveolar surfactant resulting in atelectasis, result in generalized edema of the lung, which is also frequently seen in the undamaged contralateral lung. These pathophysiologic derangements have many similarities to those in patients with adult respiratory distress syndrome.[47-49]

Associated thoracic injuries

Box 35-1 lists the common thoracic injuries associated with patients sustaining rib fractures. Enhanced morbidity should be feared with the coexistence of these injuries.[50-53] The first rib lies in a coronal rather than vertical plane; is protected by the scapula, clavicle, humerus, and related soft tissues, and therefore withstands most applied forces. A fracture of the first rib demands special attention and a search for more serious injuries.[20,43,50]

Box 35-1 ASSOCIATED THORACIC INJURIES

Pulmonary contusion
Cardiac contusion
Aortic disruption
Pneumo/hemothorax
Other great vessel disruption
Neural injury
   Intercostal
   Lung thoracic
   Thoracodorsal
   Brachial plexus disruption
Orthopedic injuries
   Clavicular fracture
   Scapular fracture
   Sternal fracture: displaced or nondisplaced
Bronchial/tracheal disruption
Esophageal perforation
Diaphragmatic rupture

Sternal fractures are often associated with other thoracic trauma including cardiac injuries, tamponade, and disruption of the great vessels in the thorax.[54] Patients with fractured clavicles must be evaluated for any compromise to the subclavian vessels or brachial plexus.[51] Scapular fractures occur more infrequently but must be considered serious.[52] In one series of 53 patients with scapular fractures, only 10 had no other significant injuries and 22 had coexisting head injuries along with a variety of other organ system dysfunction.[37]

NONTHORACIC TRAUMA

Injuries to the extremities can often benefit from pain management techniques. Because the severity of these injuries will vary greatly, the need for specific pain management techniques may not always be considered when deciding on the importance and relevance of any technique.[6,55]

Patients who have brachial plexus injuries often suffer from multisystem trauma.[56] They can have direct trauma to the plexus, avulsion of the plexus at the dorsal horn in the spinal cord, or stretch of the plexus without evidence of avulsion. Direct nerve injury to the plexus can either be complete or incomplete. While the pain complaints may be similar in both situations, the distinction can have important therapeutic considerations.

Patients who have documented injury to a major nerve of an extremity will be vulnerable to the development of causalgia. Causalgia should be considered in any patient with a partial nerve injury to a major somatic nerve, particularly the sciatic nerve or brachial plexus (classically, the median nerve).[57] Primary symptoms include exquisite burning pain and intense allodynia. These symptoms will appear out of proportion to the injury.

The symptoms of causalgia may often not be readily apparent immediately after the injury. They can occur several days or, uncommonly, weeks after the injury. The practitioner must be prepared to reexamine the patient frequently for the development of the syndrome. The underlying pathophysiology of this syndrome accounts for the intense pain complaints and centers on hyperactivity of the sympathetic nervous system. While treatment focuses on interrupting the sympathetic activity, restoration of nervous function depends on other factors.

Patients with major vascular disruption in their extremities will often benefit from pain management endeavors. Sympathetic hyperactivity occurs reflexively in patients with vascular disruption. With vascular reanastomosis, the sympathetic activity may remain elevated, which further compromises flow. Techniques to diminish sympathetic overactivity and provide pain relief will augment blood flow to the extremity in question.[57]

Patients who suffer traumatic amputations are at risk of developing phantom limb pain. Traumatic amputations will elicit a barrage of nociceptive activity which cannot easily be turned off in the early posttraumatic period. The increased afferent activity makes the patient susceptible to more permanent changes in the dorsal horn of the spinal cord.

Epidural anesthesia or analgesia can minimize the severity and decrease the incidence of phantom limb pain.[58,59] This has been demonstrated in the perioperative period but not the posttraumatic period. In elective procedures, the epidural catheter has been placed prior to surgery, which produces a preemptive effect. Whether this is necessary to provide adequate analgesia has not been researched. In a trauma setting, a catheter cannot be placed preemptively; but theoretically, it may still provide excellent analgesia and prevent the N-methyl D-aspartate receptor or other receptors from producing chronic intraspinous changes that lead to chronic pain and long-term phantom pain. If no contraindications exist, these catheters should be placed as soon as the patient has stabilized, either preoperatively, postoperatively, or in the intensive care unit. Epidural catheters can be managed for 5 to 7 days with local anesthetic and low-dose opiates. Early psychological intervention, teaching imagery, and telescoping techniques can also aid in pain relief.

Soft-tissue injuries occur with all penetrating lesions and most nonpenetrating or blunt trauma. The degree of injury, the treatment rendered, and the patient characteristics will determine whether the acutely-injured trauma patient will develop a chronic pain syndrome such as myofascial pain syndrome, reactive fibromyalgia, chronic low back pain, sympathetically maintained pain, phantom limb pain, or posttraumatic headache.[3,60-62]

Traumatic injuries do not always occur as a single event. Cumulative trauma disorders account for 50% of all occupational illnesses in the United States.[63] These result from performance of repetitive tasks and are listed in Box 35-1. Risk factors include: repetition, high force, awkward joint posture, direct pressure, vibration, and prolonged constrained posture.[63] Rest, job alterations, physical therapy, nonsteroidal antiinflammatory drugs and/or other adjuncted medications, and nerve blocks may be indicated. Early recognition and treatment help prevent long-term derangement and chronic pain syndromes.

Pediatric trauma claimed 8000 lives during 1989, which is more than any childhood disease.[64] The incidence of head trauma is more frequent in children than adults, partly because of anatomical differences in a child. Rib fractures and flail chest occur less frequently in a child because of increased elasticity in the incompletely ossified bony structure.[65] Many of the pain management techniques used in the adult population can also be employed in children. These include epidural analgesia, intercostal nerve blocks, interpleural catheters, brachial plexus blocks or catheters, and stellate ganglion blocks.[66] Patient-controlled analgesia (PCA) has also been utilized effectively, although an age of 5 to 6 years is required; most younger children experience difficulty with the concept of PCA.

DELAYED SEQUELAE

With the advent of trauma centers and specialized trauma teams, more patients survive the immediate effects of severe multitrauma. As a result a larger group of patients have emerged with long-term sequelae from their trauma.[14,16] In a review of patients who sustained flail chest injuries, only 12 of 32 questioned were employed full-time, 1 year after their injury. Of the 32, 25% had subjective chest tightness, 49% complained of thoracic wall pain, and 38% complained of moderate-to-severe changes in their activity level. Objective dyspneic indices measured 50% of patients with mild dyspnea, and 20% suffered moderate dyspnea. Abnormal spirometry was observed in 57% of the patients.[67]

In a separate study, 8 of 12 flail-chest patients had permanent sequelae. In addition, 6 of these 8 patients had extrathoracic injuries and associated long-term morbidity. Persistent chest wall pain, chest wall deformity, and dyspnea were the most common complaints.[68]

Associated trauma and long-term morbidity are frequently observed with rib fractures. Intercostal nerves are often implicated in part, because of their close proximity to the rib. Damage can occur secondary to entrapment from the caudad edges of the rib fragments, hematoma, or direct laceration.[50] During the healing process, the rib will form a callus which can either engulf the intercostal nerve or distend the nerve if the callus is large enough. Neuromas can also develop if the intercostal nerve has been completely transected.[50] Iatrogenic intercostal nerve damage can also occur during thoracostomy tube placement or during surgery from retractors.

In these patients, the pain will be neuralgic in origin and will follow the dermatomal pattern of the injured intercostal nerve. Numbness may or may not be present, depending on the extent of the injury. Treatment is discussed in a later section.

Long-term sequelae from peripheral somatic nerve injuries often result and can be particularly difficult to treat. Whenever possible, these pain syndromes should be recognized during the acute injury phase, and treatment should be instituted early. The best way to prevent long-term sequelae in this group is to prevent the perpetuation of the pain into a long-term problem. Early and aggressive treatment is essential.

Myofascial pain problems represent a major long-term problem in the trauma patient. Fibromyalgia was reportedly initiated by trauma event in 11% of 127 diagnosed patients.[60] This syndrome does not always correlate with the severity of the trauma. Minor trauma can render patients subject to severe, debilitating conditions. Litigation and other issues can complicate treatment. Again, the best treatment outcomes will occur in patients who are accurately diagnosed early and receive appropriate, aggressive treatment.

Whiplash injuries and posttraumatic headaches constitute a major long-term problem following trauma.[69,70] Whiplash injuries most commonly involve the muscular and ligamentous tissues of the posterior neck. In the acute phase, symptomatic treatment suffices with nonsteroidal antiinflammatory drugs, ice, and a short course of physical therapy, when indicated. Chronic pain, which too commonly results after an acute injury that is not adequately managed or in susceptible patients, can require prolonged treatment. Avoiding disability and disability life-style can be difficult.

Whiplash injuries can often produce headaches.[71,72] These headaches most commonly are posterior in location and are in contradistinction to other posttraumatic headaches. Posttraumatic headaches have been classified into three types: Type 1 results from excessive muscle contraction, Type II occurs after scarring and scalp tissue with entrapment of sensory nerves at the site of injury, and Type III is vasodilatory in nature. These headaches can become chronic and difficult to treat. Studies suggest that posttraumatic headaches continue to improve over the initial 6 months after trauma but then tend to plateau.[73]

Another sequela of head and face trauma includes disorders of the temporomandibular joint.[74] Unless la Forte fractures are also present, many chronic temporomandibular disorders will not be readily apparent at the initial injury. Chronic degenerative temporomandibular disorders often arise from traumatic injuries, although the inciting event may be temporally removed from the development of symptoms.

Severe orthopedic injuries can require many months to heal. Many of these patients can be expected to have significant pain during this process. External fixators in place for protracted periods can provide ongoing afferent nociception for some patients. These patients should be viewed as having subacute pain, rather than chronic pain, if the healing process is continuing. Many will not require further treatment once the offending device has been removed and the lesions have healed.

Other patients will develop chronic pain syndromes from these severe orthopedic injuries, in part, as a result of the anatomic abnormality that will alter gait and/or function. The compensatory mechanisms of the body can either be incomplete or lead to their own pain problems. For example, the patient whose leg is shortened from a severe tibial, fibular fracture has ongoing pain and develops a limp and subsequent compensatory pelvic asymmetry and myofascial hip pain.

Pain as a long-term sequela in the spinal cord-injured patient is beyond the scope of this chapter. Whether specific pain techniques during the acute phase will alter long-term outcome has not been well investigated. Instrumentation of spinal cord-injured patients during the acute injury phase is considered a relative contraindication by most. Chronically, many of these patients will develop pain syndromes in the transitional zone near the site of injury. Pain distal to the injured cord occurs most commonly in patients whose spinal cord level is not complete. Inhibition of C fiber activity through descending inhibitory modulation is often interrupted, allowing ongoing nociception. Alternatively, central pain develops in many of these patients following traumatic transection of the cord.

PAIN MANAGEMENT

Early evaluation of the trauma victim by the pain management team allows an individual treatment regimen tailored to the specific injuries of each patient. Full assessments may not always be feasible in the more seriously-injured patient. However, awareness of the injuries sustained, and a knowledge of the common acute and chronic pain syndromes that can result, leads to a more proactive course of pain therapy. Timing of therapies is also important and must be coordinated with all aspects of the patient's care.

With the frequent use of mechanical ventilation in the 1950s and 1960s, analgesia was not believed to help decrease morbidity and mortality; thus it did not aid recovery. Little attention was given a report in 1961 which demonstrated that six cases treated with epidural analgesia and local anesthetics obtained excellent analgesia and avoided mechanical ventilation.[75]

In 1973, Gibbons et al. reported on 30 chest injury patients treated with intercostal blocks and/or parenteral narcotics, and 27 patients who received thoracic epidurals and repeated injections of local anesthetics.[76,77] Thirteen of the intercostal/parenteral narcotic group ultimately required mechanical ventilation compared to six of the thoracic epidural group.

Present concepts in the management of the thoracic trauma patient began to gain widespread acceptance after the principles of Trinkle gained popularity.[20] These concepts demonstrated that mechanical ventilation was not required in most chest-injured patients and actually added significantly to patient morbidity and mortality. A central tenet in this conservative management stated that pain must be aggressively managed to allow patients to effectively breathe deep, cough, and avoid deleterious splinting.[78] The intermittent administration of intramuscular narcotics was recognized as extremely inadequate in achieving these goals.[24]

REGIONAL TECHNIQUES

Excellent analgesia can be provided through the use of regional anesthetic techniques. The decision to employ these techniques must involve the trauma team, the pain management team, and the patient or patient's family. The indications and contraindications discussed previously, must be considered within the context of each patient's clinical situation. Different specialists working in concert will also minimize any legal risk which may exist in this group of sick patients.

Management of the thoracic injury

Intercostal nerve blocks have been used for many years to treat rib fractures.[79] They can be combined with parenteral opiates to improve deep breathing and coughing. When the fractured ribs are unilateral, the patient can be positioned with the affected side up. If the fractures are bilateral or associated injuries preclude lateral positioning, the patient should be prone and pillows should be used as wedges.

Because of overlap in innervation of the intercostal nerves, one level above and below the fractured ribs should be blocked whenever possible.[57,80] The interspace should be marked prior to starting the procedure. The location for blockage depends on the fracture site; success necessitates blocking the nerve proximal to the fracture site. Also, a knowledge of where the different branches exit from the intercostal nerve and intercostal groove is necessary to ensure success. Blocking the rib posterior to the mid axillary line will reliably block the lateral cutaneous and anterior branches of the nerve.

Several reports have documented the benefits of intercostal nerve blocks for thoracic injuries. In a small series, Pedersen et al. demonstrated significantly better maximum respiratory flow rates at 1 hour after an intercostal nerve block, with the effect subsiding within 6 hours.[79] Other investigators have reported 8 to 12 hours of benefit from intercostal nerve blocks.[57,80]

The quality of analgesia is unquestioned with the intercostal technique. However, the duration of effect of 6 to 12 hours makes patient selection important. In patients with severe injuries, repeating the block two to three times a day for 5 to 7 days will demand significant manpower. Iatrogenically inducing a pneumothorax may also be a risk. In the future, longer-lasting local anesthetics may render this concern inconsequential.

Our group has found intercostal nerve blocks particularly helpful in patients who will be discharged home from an emergency department but whose pain is not expected to be well relieved with narcotics, and/or patients who return either to their local physician or emergency department during the early posttraumatic period with intractable pain not relieved with analgesics. In these situations, a single set of intercostal nerve blocks can often break a particularly difficult pain problem and allow subsequent opiates to provide sufficient analgesia. The importance of follow-up care and the possible risks of this procedure must be outlined for the patient.

A different approach to the intercostal nerve is through the interpleural space. This was first described by Reiestad for postoperative pain but it has since been described in the management of thoracic trauma.[9,81-84] Unlike the original description of placing these catheters at the T_7-T_8 interspace, an interpleural catheter placed for thoracic pain will perform better when positioned at the midpoint of the fractured ribs. Alternatively, it has been recommended to place these catheters close to the apex of the lung.[84]

Similar to an intercostal nerve block, the catheter will work best when positioned proximal to the fracture site. When thoracostomy tubes are present, the risk of having substantial amounts of local anesthetic sucked from the site of action exists and must be guarded against.[85] This can be best achieved by either placing the catheter distant from the thoracostomy tube or delaying suction for 15 to 20 minutes after instillation of drug. The decision to do the latter should only be made after a surgical consult and with appropriate monitoring of the patient.

Intermittent injections or continuous infusions through an interpleural catheter can be used. Some patients respond better to intermittent injections, although continuous infusions appear to work well later in the course of the healing process. Intermittent doses that provide adequate analgesia range from 20 to 30 ml of 0.5% bupivacaine. If bilateral catheters are employed, the concentration of bupivacaine should be halved to prevent toxicity from the local anesthetic. The need to decrease the local anesthetic concentration was demonstrated in 10 posttraumatic patients receiving lidocaine who demonstrated rapid peak plasma levels and relatively high plasma concentrations.[81]

Excessively high plasma levels of local anesthetics must be watched for in these patients with bilateral catheters, especially if damage to the pleura has occurred. A damaged pleura can result in altered pharmacokinetics and uptake of the drug from pleura into plasma.[83]

One advantage with intercostal nerve blocks or interpleural analgesia is the ability to use concomitant small doses of opiates. It does not represent a failure of the technique to employ narcotics because they can bridge the time to future blocks or reinjections, or can supplement a block that may not be complete. Also, opiates can provide analgesia for associated injuries not covered by the intercostal nerve.

Epidural analgesia

Epidural analgesia for traumatic injuries has been used for several decades. Its use was sporadic until physicians became aware that many trauma victims could be managed conservatively if their pain was adequately controlled. This change in treatment ideology was coupled with the discovery in 1979 of opiate receptors at the spinal cord. Subsequently, very effective opiate administration and subsequent analgesia could be achieved with minute doses.[86,87]

Before opiates, Dittmann et al. advocated in three articles the use of local anesthetics through epidural catheters for patients with traumatic rib fractures.[88-90] The authors were able to demonstrate a marked improvement in vital capacity and dynamic lung compliance after local anesthetics via epidural catheters. An increase in functional residual capacity and a decrease in airway resistance were also noted. Subsequent work by Worthley using thoracic epidurals and local anesthetics validated the efficacy of conservative management of thoracically-injured patients.[91]

Intraspinal narcotics were first employed in the trauma setting in 1980, shortly after their initial clinical application in cancer patients in 1979.[86] Johnston and McCaughey reported on six patients with multiple rib fractures and elevated PCO_2. The patients felt unable to breathe deep or cough effectively secondary to inadequate pain relief from systemic narcotic analgesics.[92] They were given 2 mg morphine sulfate through epidural catheters positioned dermatomally at the site of the fractures. Analgesia ranged from 3 to 50 hours, and there was a lack of side effects, particularly the hypotension seen with higher concentrations of local anesthetics, which made this technique appealing.

The effect of thoracic epidural analgesia on ventilatory mechanics in postthoracotomy patients was well described by Schulman and colleagues in 1984.[93] The effects of epidural analgesia in thoracic trauma have also been evaluated.[94,95] In a study by Cicala and co-workers, a more dramatic improvement in pulmonary function tests was seen with thoracic epidural bupivacaine when compared to lumbar epidural morphine sulphate. The bupivacaine group received a 10 ml bolus of 0.25% bupivacaine and a continuous infusion of 0.125% bupivacaine at 8 to 10 ml per hour. The opiate group received 5 mg epidural every 6 hours increased to a 7.5 mg dose if pain relief was deemed inadequate.

Aggressive physiotherapy represents a routine practice for many thoracic trauma victims and has been enhanced with the use of epidural morphine and bupivacaine.[93,96] Bupivacaine was given 30 minutes before physiotherapy, and the resultant decreased sensation allowed intensive physiotherapy. Ongoing morphine sulfate maintained analgesia when treatments were not being administered.

Continuous infusion of epidural morphine sulfate and fentanyl has been used in the trauma patient.[97,98] The dose of epidural fentanyl approached systemic fentanyl requirements (average 75 to 100 μg/hr), although the quality of analgesia may have been superior. Improvements in the vital capacity and maximum inspiratory pressures were demonstrated with epidural fentanyl.

Ullman et al. administered continuous morphine after an initial epidural bolus of fentanyl 100 μg and morphine 5 mg. Patients receiving continuous epidural had less ventilator-dependent time, decreased intensive care unit stays, shorter hospitalizations, and decreased incidence of tracheostomies when compared to a control group that was matched historically and by injury for severity indices. All patients receiving epidural analgesia reported excellent pain relief.

The last two decades have greatly enhanced our understanding of the pathophysiology of thoracic trauma and, consequently, the outcome of seriously-injured patients. The heterogeneity of the trauma patient can make it difficult to compare the results of different studies. An example includes the presence or absence of an associated pulmonary contusion, which may not be readily present at the initial presentation.

To successfully manage this group of patients, several key points must always be remembered: (1) It is important to recognize and treat the underlying pulmonary contusion. (2) Conservative, nonventilatory management should be used whenever clinically possible. (3) Aggressive pain management should be attempted to facilitate deep breathing, coughing, and respiratory physiotherapy and to avoid splinting, atelectasis, and respiratory failure.[24]

Pain management of intraabdominal injuries

Blunt or penetrating injuries of the abdominal cavity will often require surgical intraabdominal exploration and repair. Splenic rupture, liver lacerations, and great vessel lacerations are some of the many injuries which require intervention. Outcome studies comparing pain relief measures have not been performed for this group of trauma patients, in contrast to the data for the thoracic patient. However, it is well known from the surgical literature that patients undergoing upper abdominal procedures will splint, guard, and show significant decreases in functional respiratory capacity, vital capacity, and maximum inspiratory pressure.[99]

Extrapolation from the surgical literature indicates that trauma patients who have required upper abdominal surgical exploration can benefit from aggressive pain management techniques. This would be especially true for high-risk patients that have been identified by the American Society of Anesthesiologists' preoperative classification. Multiple studies have identified these patients at high risk following abdominal surgical procedures.[100,101]

The treatment of choice for trauma victims who require abdominal operations should be low or midthoracic epidurals, dependent on the procedure performed. As with the thoracic patient, some factors may preclude the use of this technique, and these include:

1. Emergent or unstable presentation, which may not allow sufficient time for placement before surgery
2. Spinal cord injuries, which in most situations will be considered a contraindication to epidural placement
3. Impending disseminated intravascular coagulation is also a contraindication to epidural instrumentation. This may be impossible to predict, but clinical indices such as massive intraoperative transfusions can alert a physician to its probability. The total patient must be assessed and discussed with the trauma team before proceeding with any epidural instrumentation.

Compression fractures and other vertebral abnormalities may not preclude the use of an epidural but a consultation with the trauma team and sometimes a neurosurgeon will be required before placement.

When epidural analgesia is contraindicated, blockade of the intercostal nerves, either by intercostal nerve block or interpleural analgesia, can often provide excellent analgesia, improved pulmonary dynamics, and probably many of the other benefits that are found with an epidural technique.

Pain management of extremity injuries

Extremity injuries can involve bony disruption, major somatic nerves, vascular injury, or extensive soft-tissue injury as seen in crush injuries.[102] Injuries can be classified as either blunt or penetrating and can disrupt a variety of systems. Appropriate pain management depends on the injuries sustained and the need for functional restoration. Many useful techniques can be employed which can not only provide pain relief but also improve outcome.

Sympathetic denervation during and after extremity reanastomosis can greatly benefit blood flow to the involved extremity. Whenever possible, this should be provided in a continuous manner for the period deemed necessary. Brachial plexus catheters, either axillary or infraclavicular, are particularly well-suited for this situation and can be left in place for a week or longer if necessary.[57] If prolonged catheterization is used, closely watch for signs and symptoms of infection.

Dilute solutions of local anesthetics (0.076% to 0.15% bupivacaine) will usually suffice. The application of narcotics is not indicated since opiate receptors have not been shown to exist along axonal sheaths of somatic nerves. Tachyphylaxis to the local solution can occur but can usually be managed by increasing the concentration of the solution. Total milligram dose of bupivacaine should not exceed 0.4 mg/kg/hour.[57]

Brachial plexus catheters may be contraindicated most commonly when the surgeon wishes to monitor neurological recovery and feels the potential for prolonged somatic blockade should be avoided. In these situations, a stellate ganglion block can be performed for upper-extremity situations. For lower-extremity cases a lumbar sympathetic catheter can be placed. Stellate ganglion catheters have been used but are difficult to keep in place, and the potential for catheter migration into an unwanted space must be considered. A cervical epidural catheter with dilute local anesthetic solutions can be used when continuous sympathetic denervation is desired.

Crush injuries are particularly prone to developing reflex sympathetic dystrophy. Because this will not occur in the majority of patients, pain out of proportion to the injury or pain that is not responsive to standard opiates should be closely examined for reflex sympathetic dystrophy. Effective management of reflex sympathetic dystrophy, when it is diagnosed early, mandates that treatment occur as soon as the diagnosis is suspected. Sympathetic blockade remains the treatment of choice in early, posttraumatic reflex sympathetic dystrophy.

Neurologic injuries to peripheral somatic nerves will almost always produce significant pain.[102] A partial nerve injury to a major somatic nerve with resultant burning pain should be considered causalgia and treated as such until proven otherwise. Sympathetic interruption should be obtained and maintained continuously whenever possible. Throughout the patient's hospitalized convalescence, (to the practical extent possible) an appropriate catheter should be maintained to prevent the barrage of primary afferent nociception from reaching the dorsal horn of the spinal cord where permanent changes in the architecture of the dorsal horn can produce the terrible pain of chronic causalgia.

Catheters which can be considered appropriate for causalgia or other nerve injuries include epidurals (lumbar, thoracic, or cervical); brachial plexus (predominantly axillary or infraclavicular); sciatic; or lumbar sympathetic catheters.

Head-injured patients and pain management

The head-injured patient can pose significant and unique problems for appropriate and aggressive pain management. In severe head injuries, pain management that interferes with neurological monitoring should be avoided. Individual patient tailoring should be done in concert with the trauma team and any neurosurgical consultants. The fear of neurologic side effects with opiates (e.g., sedation, respiratory depression) has classically led to the underutilization of opiates in these patients. Particularly, in the patient who is experiencing significant pain from extensive injuries and who is often combative, the use of sedatives and other drugs is inferior to good pain medication. Epidural administration can decrease the total amount of drug necessary and may be preferred in some situations.

Pain management paradigm for the trauma patient

Whenever possible, a member of the acute pain management team should be available 24 hours a day as part of the trauma team. Deciding what type of pain relief technique will be needed must be based on a complete knowledge of the patient. A complete history, physical exam, laboratory values, and other pertinent tests must be obtained. Discuss the pain management technique with the trauma team and any other consultants who will be affected before instituting.

We have designed a paradigm to use when deciding how to manage a trauma patient's pain (Figs. 35-1 and 35-2). Keep a current list of the injuries sustained as they become disclosed. Appropriate pain treatment can only be delivered after all injuries are understood and assessed.

Patients discharged home from the emergency department are most commonly treated with oral analgesics. Occasionally a patient will benefit from a set of intercostal nerve blocks with subsequent oral analgesics. If these patients will be discharged, they should be given written instructions about the risk of pneumothorax and who they should contact if they develop shortness of breath.

Patients admitted to the hospital usually go immediately to surgery, to an intensive care unit or other monitored unit, or to a general ward. Except for the patient who must be taken directly to surgery, a full assessment of the patient can be performed in the emergency department or shortly thereafter.

Patients who require early intubation and mechanical ventilation should be evaluated for the long-term necessity of such assistance. No clinical studies support the use of a regional technique during a prolonged mechanical ventilatory period. Since it can often be difficult initially to judge the length of time a patient will require ventilation, we feel it is best to wait until the patient stabilizes and then decide to wean from the ventilator. Once that decision has been made, often within 24 to 48 hours, we place a thoracic epidural nearest the involved dermatomes.

Contraindications to epidurals in trauma patients are clotting abnormalities, septicemia, and/or severe mental status changes. Clotting abnormalities can be easily determined with prothrombin/partial thromboplastin and platelet determinations.

Early bacteremia is common in many of these patients. Whenever possible, it is best to place epidurals before any temperature elevations. However, early temperature rises are often seen secondary to atelectasis. Epidural catheters can help prevent atelectasis from becoming a more severe pneumonia. Our policy states not to remove epidural catheters early in a patient's fever course if there is a known cause of the fever and the epidural catheter is deemed necessary by the trauma team. The epidural site must be monitored carefully for signs of infection; and examine the patient for any other signs of epidural abscess or meningitis. The decision to leave an epidural catheter in a patient who is at relative high risk should be a joint one with the trauma team. The trauma team should document that the benefits from the catheter outweigh the risk. We have followed these guidelines for over 7 years in our trauma population with no serious infections (epidural or intrathecal) to date.

Patients with severe mental status changes will most commonly be intubated, and an epidural catheter may be contraindicated. Head-injured patients who are extubated, have associated painful lesions, and require frequent mental status checks need not be excluded from epidural analgesia. Lower-dose opiates will be required through the epidural catheter to allow the patient clearer mental activity, if other factors are equal. In certain situations, the opiates can be completely removed and the patient managed solely with epidural local anesthetics.

Patients who have not sustained thoracic injuries but have abdominal, pelvic, or significant extremity pathology should be considered for pain management techniques. The options include epidural analgesia, peripheral nerve catheters, or sympathetic nerve blocks/catheters. The decision to use these techniques versus PCA depends on the severity of the lesions and the goals of the team. Excellent pain relief can often be achieved by any of the techniques. However, PCA cannot improve blood flow like regional anesthetic techniques with local anesthetics, and will also usually require larger amounts of opiates.

PCA is less invasive to the patient and can provide very adequate analgesia when pain relief is considered the primary goal. An example would be a young person involved in a motor vehicle accident who requires an exploratory laparotomy. If the patient is otherwise healthy, an epidural catheter may not have any added benefit over PCA. However, the same patient who has sustained other injuries, or a patient who has other known medical risk factors such as coronary artery disease, can have less morbidity and mortality if managed with an epidural catheter.

Where the epidural catheter is positioned in multitrauma patients can be a difficult decision. Our feeling is that thoracic lesions take precedence over other injuries. Patients with significant thoracic injuries should have a catheter inserted dermatomally, appropriate to the thoracic lesions. Other injuries may require systemic opiates to cover pain which cannot be controlled with the epidural. If this becomes necessary, remove the opiate from the epidural and use local anesthetics alone. Supplement the patient with systemic opiates, by PCA or intermittent intravenous bolus.

During placement of an epidural catheter in trauma patients, sterile technique must have top priority. Many of these patients will have catheters placed in an intensive care unit where nosocomial infection rates are high. Associated injuries and resuscitative measures often compromise the patient's immune system. These situations are compounded by the fact that positioning and inadequate help can make sterile technique difficult and challenging. Once the catheter has been placed and tested, secure in a sterile fashion. Use a combination of benzoin, steri-strips, and a sterile opsite for a sterile dressing and easy visibility to the catheter and insertion site. A complete description of the sterile technique is beyond the scope of this chapter and can be found elsewhere.[57]

How long an epidural catheter can be left in place without changing has never been adequately addressed. Our policy has been to leave catheters in place for 7 days if no signs of septicemia are present. In rare cases when a specific indication exists, we have left catheters in place for

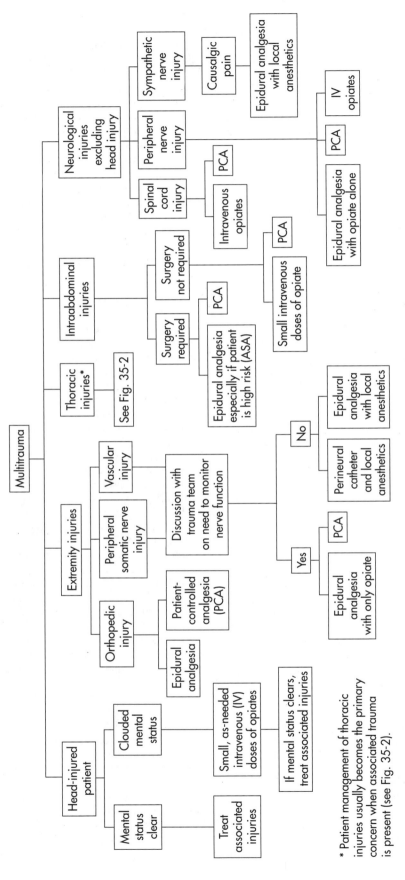

Fig. 35-1 Flow chart illustrating management of trauma patients.

* Patient management of thoracic injuries usually becomes the primary concern when associated trauma is present (see Fig. 35-2).

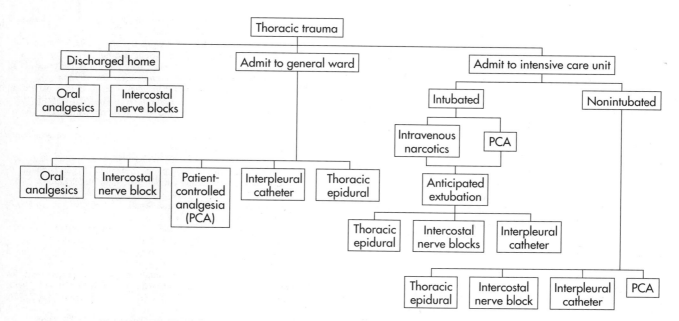

Fig. 35-2 Flow chart illustrating pain management techniques for thoracic trauma patients.

14 days. Many physicians feel, as we do, that reinstrumentation may represent a greater risk to infection than careful monitoring of an existing catheter. In contrast to vascular catheters, the epidural space has certain characteristics which safeguard against infection. The high concentration of macrophages in the epidural space aids in infection control, and local anesthetics exhibit bacteriostatic properties.

Fortunately, few catheters need to be kept in place for more than 5 days, and many can be removed within 72 hours. In our practice, the mean duration of epidural catheters in place has been 4.3 days (Table 35-1). Regardless of how long an epidural catheter is in place, monitor the site and the patient's infectious status daily. Clear sterile dressings which can be examined without breaking sterility are advised. If the site becomes erythematous or tender, or the patient develops an ongoing fever with an elevated white blood cell count, replacing the catheter or changing technique must be considered.

In patients whose respiratory condition deteriorates and for whom prolonged mechanical ventilation is predicted, removal of the catheter is often advocated with reinsertion later after the patient is actively weaned. This helps to keep the number of prolonged catheters to a minimum while providing optimal care.

Recommendations for epidural agents and dosing schedules should only be considered as guidelines since each patient will require individual tailoring for a specific set of injuries. Morphine sulfate has been used successfully and remains the prototypical opiate. The risk for respiratory depression with morphine sulfate is much less than the respiratory failure often seen with inadequate analgesia. Whereas fentanyl may have theoretical advantages over morphine sulfate with regard to respiratory depression, the doses necessary for analgesia approach systemic doses and offset many of its advantages as an epidural agent. Meperidine, with its definitive local anesthetic action, has been our sec-

Table 35-1 Data on trauma patients receiving epidural catheters*

Duration of epidural catheter (n = 74)	43 days
	(1 to 9 days)†
Intensive care unit stay	5.7 days
	(0 to 19 days)†
Associated injuries	
Rib fractures (number)	7
	(2 to 12)†
Pulmonary contusion	46
Pneumothorax	24
Hemothorax	14
Flail symptoms	19
Other fractures	1.3
	(0 to 6)†

*Based on personal experience.
†Range.

ond choice in patients who cannot tolerate morphine sulfate. Hydromorphone (Dilaudid) has similar hydrophilicity to morphine sulfate and can be dosed at one fifth the morphine dose.

Choosing the mode of opiate delivery is as important as choosing an epidural narcotic. Patients need continuous analgesia, not intermittent analgesia, which allows for splinting, atelectasis, pneumonias, and respiratory failure. Continuous analgesia can be done by intermittent injection, continuous infusion, or a patient-controlled design. If intermittent injection techniques are used, reinject in a timely fashion. This can be very difficult and require many manpower hours unless nursing will reinject. If nursing does reinject, teach strong precautions and provide inservice training to prevent inadvertent injections of other medications, which is a circumstance potentially catastrophic and possibly more likely in an intensive care unit, because so much activity is ongoing at the bedside.

Continuous infusions easily provide continuous analgesia and can be maintained with fewer manpower hours. Tubing with no sideports, such as nitroglycerin tubing, should always be employed. Continuous infusions also allow for the combination of different agents. Local anesthetics cannot be practically administered by intermittent bolus to trauma patients whose cardiovascular reserves often do not tolerate any significant sympathetic blockade.

Patients who are managed by a brachial plexus catheter should also have the catheter and site sterilely covered. These catheters will often require continuous infusion for 3 to 7 days, depending on the injury sustained. Dilute local anesthetic solutions, (e.g., bupivacaine 0.10% to 0.20%) usually suffice, although higher concentrations (0.25% to 0.375%) may be necessary in refractory cases or if tachyphylaxis results.

SUMMARY

Trauma patients, particularly complex multitrauma individuals, require a highly specialized team to provide optimal care and outcome. Effective, appropriate pain management should be an integral part of this team. The pain management team should work as part of the trauma team, and should manage the analgesic requirements in these patients. Specifically, the anesthesiologist has the training and expertise to offer regional techniques often necessary in the early posttraumatic period. Pain physicians must assume active roles in trauma patient therapy because they know the pain to expect from different lesions and the associated morbidity. The ability to tailor an individual analgesic regimen specific to the injuries sustained requires knowledge of all regional techniques available and how they may affect the individual in question. A thorough knowledge of efficacy, outcome effects, risks, and potential complications must exist. Once a pain management course is undertaken, the pain physician must stay an active, daily participant in the patient's care. Other members of the trauma team are not in a position to manage the complex pain relieving techniques presently employed. Monitoring the patient's progress demands daily attention to detail. Recovery from a traumatic event is a dynamic process which requires alterations to an initial plan. Flexibility should be available in any plan should the initial situation change. With the present emphasis on conservative management for many trauma patients, providing optimal analgesia becomes even more important. That ability exists and should be afforded to the trauma patient whenever possible.

REFERENCES

1. National Safety Council: *Accident Facts: Preliminary Condensed Edition.* March 1983.
2. Mackersie RC, Karagianes TG: Pain management following trauma and pain. *Crit Care Clin* 6:433-449, 1990.
3. Ashburn MA, Fine PG: Persistent pain following trauma. *Mil Med* 154:86-89, 1989.
4. Shorr RM et al: Blunt thoracic trauma. *Ann Surg* 206:200-205, 1987.
5. Wilson RF, Murray C, Antonenko DR: Nonpenetrating thoracic injuries. *Surg Clin North Am* 57:17-36, 1977.
6. Baker SP et al: The injury severity score: A method for describing patients with multiple injuries and evaluating emergency care. *J Trauma* 14:187-196, 1974.
7. Williams WG, Smith RE: Trauma of the chest. *The Coventry Conference.* Bristol, England, John Wright & Sons, 1977.
8. Kaiser KS: Assessment and management of pain in the critically ill trauma patient. *Critical Care Nursing* 15:14-34, 1992.
9. Mlynczak B: Assessment and management of the trauma patients in pain. *Critical Care Nursing Clinics of North America* 1:55-65, 1989.
10. Lindskog GE: Some historical aspects of thoracic trauma. *J Thorac Cardiovasc Surg* 42:1, 1961.
11. Thomas AN et al: Operative stabilization for flail chest after blunt trauma. *Thorac Cardiovasc Surg* 75:793-801, 1978.
12. Avery EE, Morch ET, Benson DW: Critically crushed chests (a new method of treatment with continuous mechanical hyperventilation to produce alkalotic apnea and internal pneumatic stabilization). *J Thoracic Surg* 32:291-308, 1956.
13. Ashbaugh DG et al: Chest trauma: Analysis of 685 patient. *Arch Surg* 95:546-555, 1967.
14. Christensson P et al: Early and late results of controlled ventilation in flail chest. *Chest* 75:456-460, 1979.
15. Conn JH et al: Thoracic trauma: Analysis of 1022 cases. *J Trauma* 3:22-40, 1963.
16. Hanning CD, Ledingham E, Ledingham I: Late respiratory sequelae of blunt chest injury: A preliminary report. *Thorax* 36:204-207, 1981.
17. Howell JF, Crawford ES, Jordan GL: The flail chest. *Am J Surg* 106:628-635, 1963.
18. Hughes RK: Thoracic trauma. *Ann Thorac Surg* 1:778, 1965.
19. Relihan M, Litwin MS: Morbidity and mortality associated with flail chest injury: A review of 85 cases. *J Trauma* 13:663-670, 1973.
20. Trinkle JK: Management of major thoracic wall trauma. *Current Surgery* 42:181-183, 1985.
21. Richardson JD, Adams L, Flint LM: Selective management of flail chest and pulmonary contusion. *Ann Surg* 196:481, 1982.
22. Cullen P et al: Treatment of flail chest: Use of intermittent mandatory ventilation and positive end-expiratory pressure. *Arch Surg* 110:1099-1103, 1975.
23. Pinilla JC: Acute respiratory failure in severe blunt chest trauma. *J Trauma* 22:221-226, 1982.
24. Trinkle KJ et al: Management of flail chest without mechanical ventilation. *Ann Thorac Surg* 19:355-362, 1975.
25. Trinkle KJ et al: Pulmonary contusion: Pathogenesis and effect of various resuscitative measures. *Ann Thorac Surg* 16:568-573, 1973.
26. Taylor GA et al: Symposium on trauma 1. Controversies in the management of pulmonary contusion. *Can J Surg* 25:167-170, 1982.
27. Davis RF, DeBoer LWV, Maroko PR: Thoracic epidural anesthesia reduces myocardial infarct size after coronary artery occlusion in dogs. *Anesth Analg* 65:711-717, 1986.
28. Klassen GA et al: Effect of acute sympathectomy by epidural anesthesia on the canine coronary circulation. *Anesthesiology* 52:8-15, 1980.
29. Moseley RV, Vernick JJ, Doty DB: Responses to blunt chest injury: A new experimental model. *J Trauma* 10:673-683, 1970.
30. Newman RJ, Jones IS: A prospective study of 413 consecutive car occupants with chest injuries. *J Trauma* 24:129-135, 1984.
31. Duff JH et al: Flail chest: A clinical review and physiological study. *J Trauma* 8:63-73, 1968.
32. Lewis F, Thomas AN, Schlobohm RM: Control of respiratory therapy in flail chest. *Ann Thorac Surg* 20:170-176, 1975.
33. Parham AM, Yarbrough DR, Redding JS: Flail chest syndrome and pulmonary contusion. *Arch Surg* 113:900-903, 1978.
34. Sankaran S, Wilson RF: Factors affecting prognosis in patients with flail chest. *J Thorac Cardiovasc Surg* 60:402-410, 1970.
35. Shackford SR et al: The management of flail chest. A comparison of ventilatory and nonventilatory treatment. *Am J Surg* 132:759-762, 1976.
36. McDougall AM et al: Chest trauma-current morbidity and mortality. *J Trauma* 17:547-553, 1977.
37. Mulder DS: Chest trauma: Current concepts. *Can J Surg* 23:340-342, 1980.
38. Perry JF, Galway CF: Factors influencing survival after flail chest injuries. *Arch Surg* 91:216, 1965.
39. Cordice J, Cabazon J: Chest trauma with pneumothorax and hemothorax. *J Thoracic Cardiovasc Surg* 50:316-333, 1965.

40. Daughtry DC: *Thoracic Trauma*. Boston, Little, Brown, 1980.
41. Hankins JR et al: Differential diagnosis of pulmonary parenchymal changes in thoracic trauma. *Am Surg* 39:309-318, 1973.
42. Johnson JA, Cogbill TH, Winga ER: Determinants of outcome after pulmonary contusion. *J Trauma* 26:695-697, 1986.
43. Keen G: *Chest Injuries*. Bristol, England, John Wright & Sons, 1975.
44. Kirsh MM, Sloan H: *Blunt Chest Trauma*. Boston, Little Brown, 1977.
45. Rutherford RB, Valentia J: An experimental study of "traumatic wet lung." *J Trauma* 11:146-166, 1971.
46. Schaal MA, Fischer RP, Perry JF: The unchanged mortality of flail chest injuries. *J Trauma* 19:492-496, 1979.
47. Blaisdell FW, Schlobohm RM: The respiratory distress syndrome, a review. *Surgery* 74:251, 1973.
48. Craven D, Oppenheimer L, Wood CD: Effects of contusion and flail chest on pulmonary perfusion and oxygen exchange. *J Appl Physiol* 47:729-737, 1979.
49. Fleming WH, Bowen JC, Petty C: The use of respiratory compliance as a guide to respiratory therapy. *J Trauma* 8:63-73, 1968.
50. Hix WR, Aaron BL: *Residual of Thoracic Trauma*. New York, Futura Publishing, 1987.
51. Howard FM, Shafer HJ: Injuries to the clavicle with neurovascular complications: A study of fourteen cases. *J Bone Joint Surg Am* 47A:2335, 1965.
52. Imatini RJ: Fractures of the scapula: A review of 53 fractures. *J Trauma* 15:473, 1975.
53. Iverson LI et al: Injury to the phrenic nerve resulting in diaphragmatic paralysis with special reference to skeletal trauma. *Am J Surg* 132:263, 1976.
54. Hills MW, Delprado AM, Deane SA: Sternal fractures: Associated injuries and management. *J Trauma* 35:55-60, 1993.
55. Greenspan L, McLellan BA, Greig H: Abbreviated injury scale and injury severity score: A scoring chart. *J Trauma* 25:60-64, 1985.
56. Werken C, de Vries LS: Brachial plexus injury in multitraumatized patients. *Clin Neurol Neurosurg* 95:S30-32, 1993.
57. Hartrick C: Pain due to trauma, including sports. In Raj PP, editor: *Practical Management of Pain*. Chicago, Mosby, 1986.
58. Wesolowski JA, Lema MJ: Phantom limb pain. *Reg Anesth* 18:121-127, 1993.
59. Bach S, Noreng MF, Tjellden NU: Phantom limb pain in amputees during the first 12 months following limb amputation, after preoperative lumbar epidural blocks. *Pain* 33:297-301, 1988.
60. Greenfield S, Fitzcharles M, Esdaile JM: Reactive fibromyalgia syndrome. *Arthritis Rheum* 35:678-681, 1992.
61. Elkind AH: Headache and facial pain associated with head injury. *Otolaryngol Clin North Am* 22:1251-1271, 1989.
62. Walsh K, Cruddas M, Coggon D: Risk of low back pain in people admitted to hospital for traffic accidents and falls. *J Epidemiol Community Health* 46:231-233, 1992.
63. Rempel DM, Harrison RJ, Barnhart S: Work-related cumulative trauma disorders of the upper extremity. *JAMA* 267:838-842, 1992.
64. Mazurek A: Pediatric trauma: Overview of the problem. *Journal of Post Anesthesia Nursing* 6:331-335, 1991.
65. Dickenson CM: Thoracic trauma in children. *Critical Care Nursing Clinics of North America* 3:423-432, 1991.
66. Tobias JD: Indications and application of epidural anesthesia in a pediatric population outside the perioperative period. *Clin Pediatr* 32:81-85, 1993.
67. Landercasper J, Cogbill TH, Lindesmith LA: Long-term disability after flail chest injury. *J Trauma* 34:410-414, 1984.
68. Beal SL, Oreskovich MR: Long-term disability associated with flail chest injury. *Am J Surg* 150:324-326, 1985.
69. Evans RW: Some observations on whiplash injuries. *Neurol Clin* 10:975-997, 1992.
70. Radanov BP et al: Role of psychosocial stress in recovery from common whiplash. *Lancet* 338:712-715, 1991.
71. Vijayan N, Watson C: Site of injury headache. *Headache* Sept:502-506, 1989.
72. Packard RC, Ham LP: Impairment ratings for posttraumatic headache. *Headache* 33:359-364, 1993.
73. Packard RC, Ham LP: Posttraumatic headache: Determining chronicity. *Headache* 33:133-134, 1993.
74. Pullinger AG, Seligman DA: Trauma history in diagnostic groups of temporomandibular disorders. *Oral Surg, Oral Med, Oral Pathol* 71:529-534, 1991.
75. Trahan M: Continuous epidural anaesthesia in multiple fractures of the ribs. *Can Anaesth Soc J* 8:512, 1961.
76. Gibbons J, Quail OJ, Quail A: Management of 130 cases of chest injury with respiratory failure. *Br J Anaesth* 45:1130-1135, 1973.
77. Gibbons J, James O, Quail A: Relief of pain in chest injury. *Br J Anaesth* 45:1136, 1973.
78. Shackford SR, Virgilio RW, Peters RM: Selective use of ventilator therapy in flail chest injury. *J Thoracic Cardiovasc Surg* 81:194, 1981.
79. Pedersen VM et al: Air-flow meter assessment of the effect of intercostal nerve blockade on respiratory function in rib fractures. *Eur J Surg* 149:119-120, 1983.
80. Cousins MJ, Bridenbaugh PO: Neural blockade. In: Cousins MJ, Bridenbaugh PO, editors: *Clinical Anesthesia and Management of Pain*. Philadelphia, JB Lippincott, 1988.
81. Carli PA et al: Intrapleural administration of lidocaine for treatment of post traumatic thoracic pain. *Anesthesiology* 87:A241, 1987.
82. Reiestad F, Stromskag KE, Holmqvist E: Intrapleural administration of bupivacaine in postoperative management of pain (abstract). *Anesthesiology* 65:A204, 1986.
83. Wulf H et al: Intrapleural catheter analgesia in patients with multiple rib fractures. *Anaesthesist* 40:19-24, 1991.
84. Iwama H et al: Intrapleural regional analgesia in pain management after chest trauma. *Masui* 42:669-676, 1993.
85. Knottenbelt JD, James MF, Bloomfield M: Intrapleural bupivacaine analgesia in chest trauma: A randomized double-blind controlled trial. *Injury* 22:114-116, 1991.
86. Behar M et al: Epidural morphine treatment of pain. *Lancet* 1:527-529, 1979.
87. Cousins MJ, Mather LE: Intrathecal and epidural administration of opioids. *Anesthesiology* 61:276-310, 1984.
88. Dittmann M et al: Epidural analgesia or mechanical ventilation for multiple rib fractures? *Intensive Care Med* 8:89, 1982.
89. Dittmann M, Keller R, Wolff G: A rationale for epidural analgesia in the treatment of multiple rib fractures. *Intensive Care Med* 4:193, 1978.
90. Dittmann M, Ferstl A, Wolff G: Epidural analgesia for the treatment of multiple rib fractures. *European Journal Intensive Care Medicine* 1:71-75, 1975.
91. Worthley LIG: Thoracic epidural in the management of chest trauma. *Intensive Care Med* 11:312-315, 1985.
92. Johnston JR, McCaughey W: Epidural morphine (a method of management of multiple fractured ribs). *Anaesthesia* 35:155-157, 1980.
93. Shulman M et al: Post thoracotomy pain and pulmonary function following epidural and systemic morphine. *Anesthesiology* 61:569-575, 1984.
94. Cicala RS, Voeller GR, Fox T: Epidural analgesia in thoracic trauma: Effects of lumbar morphine and thoracic bupivacaine on pulmonary function. *Crit Care Med* 18:229-231, 1990.
95. Koh SO et al: Epidural morphine on ventilatory function in chest trauma and thoracotomy patients. *Yonsei Med J* 32:250-254, 1991.
96. Rankin APN, Comber REH: Management of 50 cases of chest injury with a regimen of epidural bupivacaine and morphine. *Anaesth Intensive Care* 12:311-314, 1984.
97. Mackersie RC et al: Continuous epidural fentanyl analgesia: Ventilatory function improvement with routine use in treatment of blunt chest injury. *J Trauma* 27:1207-1212, 1987.
98. Ullman DA et al: The treatment of patients with multiple rib fractures using continuous thoracic epidural narcotic infusion. *Reg Anesth* 14:43-47, 1989.
99. Rauck RL et al: Comparison of the efficacy of epidural morphine given by intermittent injection or continuous infusion for the management of postoperative pain. *Reg Anesth* 19:316-324, 1994.
100. Tuman KJ et al: Effects of epidural anesthesia and analgesia on coagulation and outcome after major vascular surgery. *Anesth Analg* 73:696-704, 1991.
101. Yeager MP et al: Epidural anesthesia and analgesia in high-risk surgical patients. *Anesthesiology* 66:729-736, 1987.
102. Nulsen F, Klein DG: Acute injuries of peripheral nerves. In Yomanms JR editor: *Neurologic Surgery*. Philadelphia, WB Saunders, 1973.

QUESTIONS: TRAUMA

For questions 1-5, choose from the following:
A. 1, 2, and 3
B. 1 and 3
C. 2 and 4
D. 4
E. All of the above

1. A 7-year-old involved in a multitrauma is evaluated by the pain management team. Appropriate options to be considered, dependent on the injuries sustained, might include:
   1. Epidural analgesia
   2. PCA
   3. Brachial plexus catheter
   4. Interpleural catheter

2. A patient involved in an automobile accident is treated in the emergency department. More extensive injuries are ruled out, and the patient is diagnosed with a whiplash injury. Appropriate management considerations include:
   1. Immobilization in a soft collar for 4 weeks, which will rest the strained cervical muscles, allowing them to heal
   2. Performance of early cervical manipulations, Grade 2, to prevent microadhesions from developing after the trauma
   3. Alternate ice and heat for 4 weeks and avoidance of other physical therapy modalities while the neck muscles heal
   4. Administration of nonsteroidal antiinflammatory drugs, ice, and physical therapy early to prevent long-term sequela from developing

3. Injury of the long thoracic nerve will result in a deficit of the ipsilateral:
   1. Scapula
   2. Chest wall sensation between T_4-T_6
   3. Sensation of the underneath side of the upper arm
   4. Decreased respiratory effect secondary to block of the intercostalis muscles

4. One advantage of interpleural analgesia over epidural analgesia in the trauma patient is:
   1. Improved respiratory parameters with interpleural analgesia
   2. Decreased risk of infection with interpleural catheters
   3. Lower plasma local anesthetic concentrations after a bolus injection through an interpleural catheter
   4. The ability to concomitantly administer systemic opiates with an interpleural technique

5. A patient with a flail chest and lower-extremity fractures is consulted by the trauma team to provide pain management. The most appropriate plan would be:
   1. Small intravenous doses of opiates
   2. Lumbar epidural with a hydrophilic opiate to promote cephalad distribution to thoracic dermatomes
   3. Thoracic epidural with opiate and local anesthetic
   4. Thoracic epidural with local anesthetic alone and systemic PCA

ANSWERS

1. E
2. D
3. A
4. D
5. D

36 Postsurgical Pain

Honorio T. Benzon

VARIABILITY OF BLOOD LEVELS AND ANALGESIC RESPONSES FROM MULTIPLE INTRAMUSCULAR OPIOID INJECTIONS

The traditional technique of intramuscular (IM) opioid injections at fixed intervals is associated with variable blood levels and inconsistent analgesic responses. A study showed that 100 mg meperidine injected every 4 hours resulted in highly variable blood demerol concentrations. Intrapatient and interpatient meperidine blood concentrations varied between twofold and fivefold, and the time to reach peak blood concentrations varied by threefold and sevenfold, respectively.[1] This variability, secondary to unpredictable absorption from the site of injection, resulted in inadequate or transient analgesia. Erratic absorption and the relationship between variations in blood meperidine concentration and analgesic response[2] are the major reasons for the variable pain control after IM injections.

PREEMPTIVE ANALGESIA

Injury to nociceptive nerve fibers induces neural and behavioral changes that persist long after the injury has healed or the offending stimulus has been removed. This postinjury pain hypersensitivity can be due to posttraumatic changes in the peripheral nervous system (hyperalgesia) or in the central nervous system (CNS) (hyperexcitability). The noxious stimulus-induced neuroplasticity can be preempted by administration of analgesic agents or by regional nerve blockade.[3] These treatments are less effective when administered after the injury or when the prolonged central excitability has already been established.[4] For example, one study showed that the dose of morphine given to prevent central hyperexcitability was one tenth the dose needed to abolish the activity once it developed.[4]

Recent clinical studies support preemptive analgesia. Tverskoy and colleagues showed that preincisional infiltration with a local anesthetic significantly decreased pain after herniorrhaphy.[5] The time to first analgesic request was significantly longer in the patients who had preincisional lidocaine (515 ± 39 minutes) than the patients who had spinal (212 ± 21 minutes) or general (64 ± 8 minutes) anesthesia. Another study showed that fewer patients (58% versus 94%) required postoperative analgesics when lidocaine infiltration was given before a herniorrhaphy incision.[6] In addition, their demand for postoperative analgesics occurred significantly later (225 minutes versus 165 minutes).[6] A third study showed that the administration of epidural fentanyl before a thoracotomy incision decreased analgesic requirements (12 mg morphine versus 26 mg at 12

to 24 hours postoperatively) and resulted in lower visual analogue scores (VAS) (2.6 versus 4.7 at 6 hours postoperatively) compared to when the epidural fentanyl was given after the thoracotomy incision.[7]

PATIENT-CONTROLLED ANALGESIA

Patient-controlled analgesia (PCA) eliminates the variable absorption of the opioid from the injection site and bypasses the unavoidable delays that occur when an opioid is requested. These delays include the response of a very busy nurse; screening by the nurse of the appropriateness of the request; signing out and preparation of the drug; and, finally, injection of the opioid.[8] Patient-controlled analgesia is unique in that patients titrate their analgesic needs against sedation and other side effects of the opioid.

The attributes of an ideal analgesic for PCA use include a rapid onset of analgesic action, high analgesic efficacy (i.e., no ceiling effect) and an intermediate duration of effect for better controllability.[9] Morphine and meperidine satisfy most of these characteristics and are therefore the most widely used drugs. Fentanyl is too short acting, whereas methadone and buprenorphine have very long durations of action. The agonist-antagonist drugs have ceiling analgesic effects limiting their effectiveness. Recommended bolus doses and lockout intervals[10] for the various analgesics are shown in Table 36-1.

Studies that compared different analgesics for PCA use showed that movement-associated pain is least with morphine[11,12] and highest with meperidine.[12] Morphine and meperidine have slow onset of resting analgesia, but the pain intensity declines after 4 hours with morphine and within 16 hours after meperidine.[12] Oxymorphone has a rapid analgesic onset and little variability in rest and movement pain scores. However, it was found not to be as effective as morphine at later observations and was also associated with a higher degree of nausea.[12]

The use of a basal morphine infusion to the PCA, which was recommended to decrease the trough in morphine plasma concentrations during PCA, was found not to decrease resting pain but to reduce movement-associated pain scores.[13] The addition of a basal oxymorphone infusion to the oxymorphone PCA significantly reduced the VAS associated with rest and movement but resulted in a significantly higher incidence of nausea and vomiting.[13]

The addition of a nighttime basal opioid infusion did not improve the patients' ability to sleep or rest comfortably. Their postoperative scores for pain, sedation, fatigue, discomfort, and anxiety were the same whether a nighttime basal infusion was added or not.[14] The number of patient

Table 36-1 Guidelines regarding the bolus doses, lockout intervals, and continuous infusions for various parenteral analgesics when using a PCA system

Drug	Bolus dose (mg)	Lockout interval (min)	Continuous infusion (mg/hr^{-1})
Agonists			
Fentanyl citrate	0.015-0.05	3-10	0.02-0.1
Hydromorphone hydrochloride	0.10-0.5	5-15	0.2-0.5
Meperidine hydrochloride	5-15	5-15	5-40
Methadone hydrochloride	0.50-3.0	10-20	—
Morphine sulfate	0.50-3.0	5-20	1-10
Oxymorphone hydrochloride	0.20-0.8	5-15	0.1-1
Sufentanil citrate	0.003-0.015	3-10	0.004-0.03
Agonist-Antagonists			
Buprenorphine hydrochloride	0.03-0.2	10-20	—
Nalbuphine hydrochloride	1-5	5-15	1-8
Pentazocine hydrochloride	5-30	5-15	6-40

Note: The addition of a basal infusion to the PCA is controversial (see text).
Adapted from Lubenow TR, McCarthy RJ, Ivankovich AD: Management of acute postoperative pain. In Barash PG, Culen BF, Stoelting RK editors: *Clinical Anesthesia,* ed 2. Philadelphia, JB Lippincott, 1992.

Table 36-2 Epidural opioids: latency and duration of postoperative analgesia

Agent	Bolus dose	Analgesic effect			Continuous infusion	
		Onset (min)	Peak (min)	Duration (hr)	Concentration	Rate (ml/hr^{-1})
Meperidine	30-100 mg	5-10	12-30	4-6	—	—
Morphine	5 mg	24±6	30-60	12-24	0.01%	1-6
Methadone	5 mg	12±2	17±3	7±5	—	—
Hydromorphone	1 mg	13±4	23±8	11±6	0.005%	6-8
Fentanyl	100 μg	4-10	20	3±6	0.001%	4-12
Diamorphine	5 mg	5	9-15	12±6	—	—
Sufentanil	30-50 μg	7±6	26±8	4±7	0.0001%	10
Alfentanil	15 μg/kg^{-1}	15		1-2	—	—

Adapted from Cousins MJ, Mather LE: Intrathecal and epidural administration of opioids. *Anesthesiology* 61:276, 1984.

demands, supplemental bolus doses, opioid usage, and side effects were also the same in both groups. In addition, numerous programming errors were noted with the addition of a basal infusion.[14]

The VAS of patients who used PCA were found to be similar to those who had IM injections. The incidence of sedation, however, was significantly lower in the PCA group.[15] The decreased sedation, together with the control that the patients have over their analgesic needs, explains why more patients rate their pain relief to be superior with PCA and preferable over the IM route.

Studies that directly compared PCA with the IM and epidural routes of opioid administration showed significantly lower VAS with the epidural technique.[16,17] However, the significantly higher incidence of pruritus with epidural morphine made several patients prefer other modes of analgesic therapy for their next surgery.[16] In comparison, 90% of the patients who had the PCA preferred to receive the same treatment the next time they had surgery.[16]

EPIDURAL OPIOID INJECTIONS

Intraspinal opioid injections are based on the existence and pharmacology of spinal opiate receptors that provide an at-

tractive means to achieve regional anesthesia with minimal central effects. Initially, the opioid was injected intrathecally; but the higher incidence of respiratory depression with this approach led to the popularity of the epidural technique.

The latency and duration of postoperative analgesia with the different epidural opioids[18] are listed in Table 36-2. Morphine was the opioid initially employed, and Ready and co-workers established their safety and efficacy. In their 2 year experience with 11,089 individual morphine injections in 1106 patients, they had no death, neurologic injury, or infection.[19] Catheter-related problems occurred in 5% of their parents. Their treatment, including morphine strength, interval between injections, and duration of treatment, is shown in Table 36-3.

Complications of intraspinal opioid administration include pruritus, nausea and vomiting, urinary retention, and respiratory depression[20] (Table 36-4). The incidence of respiratory depression ranges from 0.09%[19] to 0.2%,[21] which is not different from the respiratory depression that occurs after oral or parenteral use, which is 0.9%.[19]

Randomized, double-blind studies showed the superiority of intermittent epidural morphine injections over IM or intravenous (IV) morphine injections. In a study of patients

Table 36-3 Treatment of postoperative pain with intermittent epidural morphine

	Surgical site			
	Thorax	**Abdomen**	**Lower extremity**	**Perineum**
Patients (number)	146	584	322	54
Morphine (mg)	4±1	4±1	4±1	3±1
Injection interval (hr)	8±3	9±3	11±5	12±6
Morphine (total mg/24 hr) (calculated)	13	10	8	7
Rest pain	1(3)	1(2)	1(3)	0(1)
Incident pain	5(4)	4(4)	4(4)	3(6)
Duration of treatment (days)	5±3	4±3	3±2	2±1

Morphine, injection interval, and duration of treatment, mean ± standard deviation.
Rest pain and incident pain, median and interquartile range (in parentheses).
Adapted from Ready LB et al: Postoperative epidural morphine is safe on surgical wards. *Anesthesiology* 75:452, 1991.

Table 36-4 Complications of the use of intraspinal narcotics

	Reported incidence (%)*		
Complication	**Spinal**	**Epidural**	**Treatment**
Respiratory depression	5-7	0.1-2	Support ventilation; naloxone
Pruritus	60	1-100	Antihistamine; naloxone
Nausea and vomiting	20-50	20-30	Antiemetic; transdermal scopolamine; naloxone
Urinary retention	50	15-25	Catheterize; naloxone

*Reported incidences vary widely, appear to be related to dose, and are higher with spinal than with epidural administration.
From Ready LB: Regional anesthesia with intraspinal opioids. In Bonica JJ, editor: *The Management of Pain,* ed 2. Philadelphia, Lea & Febiger, 1990.

who underwent gastroplasty, the use of epidural morphine resulted in earlier ambulation, earlier recovery of pulmonary and bowel function, and a shorter hospital stay.[22] In patients who had thoracotomy, epidural morphine provided significantly better analgesia and better pulmonary function than IV morphine.[23] This advantage of the epidural over the IV route was not seen after cesarean section,[24] a less painful operation than thoracotomy or gastroplasty.

Continuous infusions of epidural morphine, in contrast to intermittent epidural morphine injections, effectively reduce postoperative pain with minimal side effects.[25] Epidural fentanyl infusions, compared to morphine infusions, provide comparable analgesia with a lower incidence of nausea and pruritus.[26]

Inordinately high infusion rates of epidural fentanyl maintained adequate pain relief. Some have theorized that the predominant mechanism of analgesic effect of the fentanyl infusion is systemic in nature. Recent studies have supported this impression. Studies that compared epidural versus IV opiate infusions in patients who underwent knee surgery,[27] cesarean section,[28] and hysterectomy[29] showed the two techniques to be equally effective. The infusion rates that produced the same levels of analgesia were found to be comparable, and the plasma opioid concentrations were similar in both the epidural and IV groups.[27] Although the conclusions reached by the authors are correct, these studies were limited by gender distribution[28,29] and by operations that do not produce severe postoperative pain.[27-29] When investigators looked at operations that cause severe postoperative pain (gastroplasty,[22] major abdominal surgery,[30] or thoracotomy[23,31-35]) the results, though not uni-

form, were more supportive of epidural opioid injections (Table 36-5).

The conflicting results of the studies that compared epidural with IV opioid infusions after thoracotomy are partly attributable to the vertebral level of insertion of the epidural catheter. Sandler and co-workers[31] found the analgesia from the two techniques comparable and the time course for the plasma fentanyl concentrations similar, whereas Salomaki and his colleagues[32] noted significantly lower infusion rates and significantly lower plasma fentanyl concentrations with the epidural technique. Sandler and co-workers placed their epidural catheter at the L_2-L_3, L_3-L_4 interspace, and Salomaki and colleagues inserted their epidural catheter at the T_4-T_5 interspace. Another study[33] compared fentanyl infusions via epidurals in the lumbar L_4-L_5 and thoracic T_4-T_5, and IV routes. The investigators found no differences in the quality of analgesia and the amounts of fentanyl delivered between the three groups. However, patients who had the thoracic epidural fentanyl infusion had earlier bowel movements, better postoperative forced vital capacity and forced expiratory volume in 1 second, and shorter hospital stays than the patients in the other two groups. Taken collectively, these three studies[31-33] showed that thoracic epidural fentanyl infusions provided comparable analgesia and superior postoperative recovery when compared to either lumbar epidural or IV fentanyl infusions.

Studies that compared the epidural technique to IV PCA showed superiority of the epidural technique in more painful and extensive operations. Patients who had thoracotomy either had lower VAS[35] or required lower infusion rates to

Table 36-5 Comparison of epidural with parenteral opioids for postoperative pain

Authors	Type of study	Type of surgery	Routes compared	Drugs used	Superior technique
Rawal et al[a]	R, DB	Gastroplasty	TE vs IM	Morphine	Epidural
Shulman et al[b]	R, DB	Thoracotomy	LE vs IV	Morphine	Epidural
Camann et al[c]	R, DB	C-section	LE vs IV	Butorphanol	Equal
Loper et al[d]	R, DB	Knee surgery	LE vs IV	Fentanyl	Equal
Ellis et al[e]	R, DB	C-section	LE vs IV	Fentanyl	Equal
Camu et al[f]	R	Hysterectomy	LE vs IV	Alfentanil	Equal
Geller et al[g]	R, DB	Abdominal	LE vs IV	Sufentanil (LE,IV) Fentanyl (LE)	Epidural
Sandler et al[h]	R, DB	Thoracotomy	LE vs IV	Fentanyl	Equal
Salomaki et al[i]	R, DB	Thoracotomy	TE vs IV	Fentanyl	Epidural
Guinard et al[j]	R	Thoracotomy	LE vs TE vs IV	Fentanyl	TE
Grant et al[k]	R, DB	Thoracotomy	LE vs PCA	Fentanyl	Epidural
Benzon et al[l]	R, DB	Thoracotomy	TE vs PCA	Fentanyl (TE) Morphine (PCA)	Epidural
Allaire et al[m]	R	RRP	LE vs PCA	Fentanyl (LE) Morphine (PCA)	Epidural
Chauvin et al[n]	R	Abdominal	LE PCA vs IV PCA	Alfentanil	Equal[o]
Glass et al[p]	R,DB,C	Lower extremity, abdominal	LE PCA vs IV PCA	Fentanyl	Equal

R, randomized; DB, double-blind; C, cross over; TE, thoracic epidural; LE, lumbar epidural; IV, intravenous; IM, intramuscular; PCA, patient-controlled analgesia; RRP, radical retropubic prostatectomy.

[a]Rawal N et al: Comparison of intramuscular and epidural morphine for postoperative analgesia in the grossly obese: Influence on postoperative ambulation and pulmonary function. *Anesth Analg* 63:583, 1984.

[b]Shulman M et al: Postthoracotomy pain and pulmonary function following epidural and systemic morphine. *Anesthesiology* 61:569, 1984.

[c]Camann WR, Loferski BL, Fanciullo GJ: Does epidural administration of butorphanol offer any clinical advantage over intravenous route? *Anesthesiology* 76:216, 1992.

[d] Loper KA et al: Epidural and intravenous fentanyl infusions are clinically equivalent after knee surgery. *Anesth Analg* 70:72, 1990.

[e]Ellis DJ, Millar WA, Reisner LS: A randomized double-blind comparison of epidural versus intravenous fentanyl infusion for analgesia after cesarean section. *Anesthesiology* 72:981, 1990.

[f] Camu F, Debucquoy F: Alfentanil infusion for postoperative pain: A comparison of epidural and intravenous routes. *Anesthesiology* 75:171, 1991.

[g]Geller E et al: A randomized, double-blind comparison of epidural sufentanil versus intravenous sufentanil or epidural fentanyl analgesia after major abdominal surgery. *Anesth Analg* 76:1243, 1993.

[h] Sandler AN et al: A randomized, double-blind comparison of lumbar epidural and intravenous fentanyl infusions for postthoracotomy pain relief. *Anesthesiology* 77:626, 1992.

[i]Salomaki TE, Laitinen JO, Nuutinen LS: A randomized double-blind comparison of epidural versus intravenous fentanyl infusion for analgesia after thoracotomy. *Anesthesiology* 75:790, 1991.

[j]Guinard JP et al: A randomized comparison of intravenous versus lumbar and thoracic epidural fentanyl for analgesia after thoracotomy. *Anesthesiology* 77:1108, 1992.

[k]Grant RP et al: Patient-controlled lumbar epidural fentanyl compared with patient-controlled intravenous fentanyl for postthoracotomy pain relief. *Can J Anaesth* 39:214, 1992.

[l]Benzon HT et al: A randomized double-blind comparison of epidural fentanyl infusion versus patient-controlled analgesia with morphine for postthoracotomy pain. *Anesth Analg* 76:316, 1993.

[m]Allaire PH et al: A prospective randomized comparison of epidural infusion of fentanyl and intravenous administration of morphine by patient-controlled analgesia after radical retropubic prostatectomy. *Mayo Clin Proc* 67:1031, 1992.

[n]Chauvin M, Hongnat JM, Mourgeon E: Equivalence of postoperative analgesia with patient-controlled intravenous or epidural alfentanil. *Anesth Analg* 76:1251, 1993.

[o]Total alfentanil dose was higher in the IV PCA group.

[p]Glass PSA et al: Use of patient-controlled analgesia to compare the efficacy of epidural to intravenous fentanyl administration. *Anesth Analg* 74:345, 1992.

attain the same degree of analgesia.[34] Patients who underwent radical retropubic prostatectomy had better pain relief,[36] whereas patients who underwent major abdominal surgery required significantly less alfentanil.[37] Contradictory findings were noted in patients who underwent either a lower-extremity surgery or an abdominal surgery.[38]

Studies that directly compared lumbar with thoracic epidural catheter placement in thoracotomies found conflicting results. A retrospective study found lumbar placement to be as effective as thoracic placement.[39] Coe and colleagues[40] and Hurford and co-workers[41] found similar data.

Coe and colleagues used fentanyl alone, whereas Hurford and his colleagues employed infusions of fentanyl with bupivacaine. Both groups of investigators found lower, but not statistically significant, pain scores in the thoracic group. To achieve comparable analgesia, however, patients in the lumbar group required significantly higher rates of fentanyl infusion.[41] As previously stated, another study[33] showed equivalent analgesia and similar fentanyl requirements between thoracic and lumbar epidural placements. However, patients in the thoracic epidural group had earlier recovery of gastrointestinal (GI) and pulmonary functions and shorter hospital stays. A summary of these results is shown in Table 36-6.

OUTCOME STUDIES ON EPIDURAL OPIOID INJECTIONS

Most studies showed improved pain relief, decreased postoperative morbidity, and a shortened hospital stay after the postoperative administration of epidural opioids. Epidural morphine, compared to IM morphine, decreased the hospitalization stay after gastroplasty from 9 to 7 days.[22] A shorter hospital stay was also noted after thoracotomy when a thoracic epidural fentanyl infusion was used.[33] Two outcome studies showed significantly lower complication rates after epidural anesthesia and postoperative epidural analgesia in high-risk patients[42] and in patients undergoing major vascular surgery.[43] A recent outcome study confirmed better pain relief and postoperative pulmonary function with postoperative epidural opioid analgesia, but showed no reduction of pulmonary complications or diminution of hospital stays.[44]

TRANSDERMAL FENTANYL

Transdermal fentanyl can be administered in doses of 25, 50, 75, and 100 μg/hr. Doses of 75 and 100 μg/hr are the most commonly used dosages for postoperative analgesia. In a double-blind, placebo-controlled study, the analgesia from a 75 μg/hr transdermal therapeutic system of fentanyl was found to be significantly better than placebo.[45] Patients in the fentanyl group required significantly less morphine during the 24 hours that the systems were in place and for the first 12 hours after removal of the patch.[45] A transdermal therapeutic system of fentanyl at 100 μg/hr compared favorably with a continuous IV infusion of fentanyl of 100 μg/hr, in terms of total 24 hour morphine requirements (14 $\pm$ 6 mg versus 16 $\pm$ 13 mg) and steady-state mean serum fentanyl concentrations (2.2 $\pm$ 0.9 ng/ml^{-1} versus 1.4 $\pm$ 0.1 ng/ml^{-1}).[46]

There was a mean delay of 12.7 $\pm$ 9.6 hours before minimum effective blood fentanyl concentration was reached, and the pseudosteady state was reached between 36 and 48 hours.[47] These delays indicate that the patch should be administered several hours before the surgery. If applied immediately after surgery, parenteral opioids can be administered until the patch is effective. There was a decay time of 16 $\pm$ 7 hours after the patch was removed for the blood fentanyl concentration to decrease below the mean minimum effective analgesic concentration.[47] Supplemental opiates should therefore not be given until several hours after the patch has been removed.

INTRAARTICULAR MORPHINE

The existence of opiate receptors in the periphery led to clinical trials testing the analgesic effect of opioids injected in the vicinity of peripheral sensory nerve terminals. Stein and co-workers[48] showed that 1 mg of morphine injected intraarticularly after knee arthroscopy lowered postoperative VAS and reduced analgesic consumption. They also found that the concurrent administration of naloxone reversed the analgesic effect of the intraarticular morphine. However, their results were not confirmed by Raja and col-

Table 36-6 Lumbar versus thoracic epidural placement for postthoracotomy epidural analgesia

Type of study	Drug used	Comparative efficacy
Retrospective[a]	Morphine, intermittent	Equal
Randomized, blind[b]	Fentanyl, infusion	Equal[c]
Randomized[d]	Fentanyl, infusion	Equal[e]
Randomized[f]	Fentanyl with bupivacaine, infusion	Equal[g]

[a]Fromme GA, Steidl LJ, Danielson DR: Comparison of lumbar and thoracic epidural morphine for relief of postthoracotomy pain. *Anesth Analg* 64:454, 1985.
[b]Coe A et al: Pain following thoracotomy: A randomized, double-blind comparison of lumbar versus thoracic epidural fentanyl. *Anaesthesia* 46:918, 1991.
[c]Total fentanyl requirement was higher in the lumbar group.
[d]Guinard JP et al: A randomized comparison of intravenous versus lumbar and thoracic epidural fentanyl for analgesia after thoracotomy. *Anesthesiology* 77:1108, 1992.
[e]Patients in the thoracic group had earlier recovery of GI and pulmonary functions, and had shorter hospital stay.
[f]Hurford WE et al: Comparison of thoracic and lumbar epidural infusions of bupivacaine and fentanyl for postthoracotomy analgesia. *J Cardiothorac Vasc Anesth* 7:521, 1993.
[g]Higher infusion rates were needed in the lumbar group to attain comparable analgesia.

leagues.[49] In addition, Raja and colleagues, in contrast to Stein and co-workers, and Khoury and co-workers,[50] did not observe any delayed and prolonged analgesic effects of intraarticular morphine. The difference in their results may be due to differences in their methodology. Raja and colleagues[49] employed epidural anesthesia, whereas Stein and co-workers[48] used general anesthesia for their patients' surgeries. Raja and colleagues also added epinephrine to their injectate, which may have altered the perioperative inflammatory process within the knee.

Studies that compared intraarticular morphine with intraarticular bupivacaine showed slightly different results, depending on the dose of morphine. Khoury and co-workers[50] showed that 0.25% bupivacaine gave better analgesia than 1 mg morphine for the first hour after surgery. Both drugs gave equivalent analgesia between the second and third postoperative hours, and thereafter morphine gave significantly better analgesia from the third hour to the second postoperative day.[50] On the other hand, Raja and colleagues[49] found significantly better analgesia with bupivacaine compared to 3 mg of intraarticular morphine. When 5 mg morphine were used, significantly lower VAS were noted, especially at 8 and 24 hours after surgery.[51]

AGENCY FOR HEALTH CARE POLICY AND RESEARCH CLINICAL PRACTICE GUIDELINES

The Agency for Health Care Policy and Research (AHCPR) of the U.S. Department of Health and Human Services published clinical practice guidelines for the management of acute pain.[52] They stated that, unless contraindicated, pharmacologic management of mild-to-moderate postoperative pain should begin with a nonsteroidal antiinflammatory drug. Nonsteroidal antiinflammatory drugs decrease levels of inflammatory mediators at the site of tissue injury, do not cause sedation or respiratory depression, and do not interfere with bowel or bladder function. Ketorolac, 30 mg IV, provided equivalent analgesia compared to 50 μg fentanyl.[53] Compared to 60 mg codeine plus 600 mg acetaminophen, oral ketorolac 10 mg was associated with equivalent analgesia, lower incidence of nausea and somnolence, and earlier return of bowel function.[53] Nonsteroidal antiinflammatory drugs also have an opioid dose-sparing effect. In patients who underwent radical retropubic prostatectomy, the addition of IM ketorolac to an epidural fentanyl infusion resulted in lower fentanyl usage, less bladder spasm, and earlier recovery of GI function.[54]

Moderately severe to severe pain should be treated initially with an opioid. The opioid should be withheld if the patient is sedated or when the respiratory rate is less than 10 per minute. As soon as the patient tolerates oral intake, he or she should be switched to the oral route.

For patients who are known or suspected drug abusers, the AHCPR recommended the following:[52]

1. The mechanism of the pain should be defined and treated. Infection, ischemia, or a new surgical diagnosis should be treated accordingly.
2. Clinicians should distinguish between the temporal characteristics of abuse behavior. A history of drug abuse behavior may predispose to reemergence of the abuse behavior but does not require treatment approaches different from nonaddicted patients.
3. Pharmacologic principles of opioid use should be followed.
4. Nonopioid treatments such as nonsteroidal antiinflammatory drugs, nerve blocks, or transcutaneous electrical nerve stimulation should be given concomitantly with or to replace opioids.
5. Drug abuse behavior should be recognized and dealt with firmly.
6. Limits should be set to avoid excessive negotiations about drug selections or choices.

REFERENCES

1. Austin KI, Stapleton JV, Mather LE: Multiple intramuscular injections: A major source of variability in analgesic response to meperidine. *Pain* 8:47, 1980.
2. Austin KI, Stapleton JV, Mather LE: Relationship between blood meperidine concentrations and analgesic response. A preliminary report. *Anesthesiology* 53:460, 1980.
3. Gonzalez-Darder JM, Barbera J, Abellan MJ: Effects of prior anaesthesia on autonomy following sciatic transection in rats. *Pain* 24:87, 1986.
4. Woolf CJ, Wall PD: Morphine sensitive and morphine-insensitive actions of C-fibre input on the rat spinal cord. *Neurosci Lett* 64:221, 1986.
5. Tverskoy M et al: Postoperative pain after inguinal herniorrhaphy with different types of anesthesia. *Anesth Analg* 70:29, 1990.
6. Ejlersen E et al: A comparison between preincisional and postincisional lidocaine infiltration and postoperative pain. *Anesth Analg* 74:495, 1992.
7. Katz J et al: Preemptive analgesia. Clinical evidence of neuroplasticity contributing to postoperative pain. *Anesthesiology* 77:439, 1992.
8. Graves DA et al: Patient-controlled analgesia. *Ann Intern Med* 99:360, 1983.
9. White PD: Patient-controlled analgesia: A new approach to the management of postoperative pain. *Sem Anesth* 4:255, 1985.
10. Lubenow TR, McCarthy RJ, Ivankovich AD: Management of acute postoperative pain. In Barash PG, Cullen BF, Stoelting RK, editors: *Clinical Anesthesia,* ed 2. Philadelphia, JB Lippincott, 1992.
11. Bahar M, Rosen M, Vickers MD: Self-administered nalbuphine morphine and pethidine. Comparison by intravenous route, following cholecystectomy. *Anaesthesia* 40:529, 1985.
12. Sinatra RS et al: A comparison of morphine, meperidine, and oxymorphone as utilized in patient-controlled analgesia following cesarean delivery. *Anesthesiology* 70:585, 1989.
13. Sinatra R et al: An evaluation of morphine and oxymorphone administered via patient-controlled analgesia (PCA) or PCA plus basal infusion in postcesarean-delivery patients. *Anesthesiology* 71:502, 1989.
14. Parker RK, Holtmann B, White PF: Effects of a nighttime opioid infusion with PCA therapy on patient comfort and analgesic requirements after abdominal hysterectomy. *Anesthesiology* 76:362, 1992.
15. Ferrante FM et al: A statistical model for pain in patient-controlled analgesia and conventional intramuscular opioid regimens. *Anesth Analg* 67:457, 1988.
16. Eisenach JC, Grice SC, Dewan DM: Patient-controlled analgesia following cesarean section: A comparison between epidural and intramuscular narcotics. *Anesthesiology* 68:444, 1988.
17. Harrison DM et al: Epidural narcotics and patient-controlled analgesia for post-cesarean section pain relief. *Anesthesiology* 68:454, 1988.
18. Cousins MJ, Mather LE: Intrathecal and epidural administration of opioids. *Anesthesiology* 61:276, 1984.
19. Ready LB et al: Postoperative epidural morphine is safe on surgical wards. *Anesthesiology* 75:452, 1991.
20. Ready LB: Regional anesthesia with intraspinal opioids. In Bonica JJ, editor: *The Management of Pain,* ed 2. Philadelphia, Lea & Febiger, 1990.
21. Rawal N et al: Present state of extradural and intrathecal opioid analgesia in Sweden. A nationwide follow-up survey. *Br J Anaesth* 59:791, 1987.
22. Rawal N et al: Comparison of intramuscular and epidural morphine for postoperative analgesia in the grossly obese: Influence on postoperative ambulation and pulmonary function. *Anesth Analg* 63:583, 1984.
23. Shulman M et al: Postthoracotomy pain and pulmonary function following epidural and systemic morphine. *Anesthesiology* 61:569, 1984.
24. Camann WR, Loferski BL, Fanciullo GJ: Does epidural administration of butorphanol offer any clinical advantage over intravenous route? *Anesthesiology* 76:216, 1992.
25. El-Baz NM, Faber P, Jensik RJ: Continuous epidural infusion of morphine for treatment of pain after thoracic surgery; A new technique. *Anesth Analg* 63:757, 1984.
26. Fisher RL et al: Comparison of continuous epidural infusion of fentanyl-bupivacaine and morphine-bupivacaine in management of postoperative pain. *Anesth Analg* 67:559, 1988.
27. Loper KA et al: Epidural and intravenous fentanyl infusions are clinically equivalent after knee surgery. *Anesth Analg* 70:72, 1990.
28. Ellis DJ, Millar WA, Reisner LS: A randomized double-blind comparison of epidural versus intravenous fentanyl infusion for analgesia after cesarean section. *Anesthesiology* 72:981, 1990.
29. Camu F, Debucquoy F: Alfentanil infusion for postoperative pain: A comparison of epidural and intravenous routes. *Anesthesiology* 75:171, 1991.
30. Geller E et al: A randomized, double-blind comparison of epidural sufentanil versus intravenous sufentanil or epidural fentanyl analgesia after major abdominal surgery. *Anesth Analg* 76:1243, 1993.
31. Sandler AN et al: A randomized, double-blind comparison of lumbar epidural and intravenous fentanyl infusions for postthoracotomy pain relief. *Anesthesiology* 77:626, 1992.
32. Salomaki TE, Laitinen JO, Nuutinen LS: A randomized double-blind comparison of epidural versus intravenous fentanyl infusion for analgesia after thoracotomy. *Anesthesiology* 75:790, 1991.
33. Guinard JP et al: A randomized comparison of intravenous versus lumbar and thoracic epidural fentanyl for analgesia after thoracotomy. *Anesthesiology* 77:1108, 1992.
34. Grant RP et al: Patient-controlled lumbar epidural fentanyl compared with patient-controlled intravenous fentanyl for postthoracotomy pain relief. *Can J Anaesth* 39:214, 1992.
35. Benzon HT et al: A randomized double-blind comparison of epidural

fentanyl infusion versus patient-controlled analgesia with morphine for postthoracotomy pain. *Anesth Analg* 76:316, 1993.

36. Allaire PH et al: A prospective randomized comparison of epidural infusion of fentanyl and intravenous administration of morphine by patient-controlled analgesia after radical retropubic prostatectomy. *Mayo Clin Proc* 67:1031, 1992.

37. Chauvin M, Hongnat JM, Mourgeon E: Equivalence of postoperative analgesia with patient-controlled intravenous or epidural alfentanil. *Anesth Analg* 76:1251, 1993.

38. Glass PSA et al: Use of patient-controlled analgesia to compare the efficacy of epidural to intravenous fentanyl administration. *Anesth Analg* 74:345, 1992.

39. Fromme GA, Steidl LJ, Danielson DR: Comparison of lumbar and thoracic epidural morphine for relief of postthoracotomy pain. *Anesth Analg* 64:454, 1985.

40. Coe A et al: Pain following thoracotomy: A randomized, double-blind comparison of lumbar versus thoracic epidural fentanyl. *Anaesthesia* 46:918, 1991.

41. Hurford WE et al: Comparison of thoracic and lumbar epidural infusions of bupivacaine and fentanyl for postthoracotomy analgesia. *J Cardiothorac Vasc Anesth* 7:521, 1993.

42. Yeager MP et al: Epidural anesthesia and analgesia in high-risk surgical patients. *Anesthesiology* 66:729, 1987.

43. Tuman KJ et al: Effects of epidural anesthesia and analgesia on coagulation and outcome after major vascular surgery. *Anesth Analg* 73:696, 1991.

44. Jayr C et al: Epidural analgesia using bupivacaine and opioids versus parenteral opioids. *Anesthesiology* 78:666, 1993.

45. Caplan RA et al: Transdermal fentanyl for postoperative pain. *JAMA* 261:1036, 1989.

46. Holley FO, Van Stennis C: Postoperative analgesia with fentanyl: Pharmacokinetics and pharmacodynamics of constant-rate I.V. and transdermal delivery. *Br J Anaesth* 60:608, 1988.

47. Gourlay GK et al: The transdermal administration of fentanyl in treatment of postoperative pain: Pharmacokinetics and pharmacodynamics. *Pain* 37:1193, 1989.

48. Stein C et al: Analgesic effect of intra-articular morphine after arthroscopic knee surgery. *N Engl J Med* 235:1123, 1991.

49. Raja SN, Dickstein RE, Johnson CA: Comparison of postoperative analgesic effects of intra-articular bupivacaine and morphine following arthroscopic knee surgery. *Anesthesiology* 77:1143, 1992.

50. Khoury GF et al: Intra-articular morphine, bupivacaine, and morphine/bupivacaine for pain control after knee videoarthroscopy. *Anesthesiology* 77:263, 1992.

51. Joshi GP et al: Intra-articular analgesia following knee arthroscopy. *Anesth Analg* 76:333, 1993.

52. Clinical Practice Guidelines. Acute pain management: Operative or medical procedures and trauma. US Department of Health and Human Services Agency for Health Care Policy and Research, 1992.

53. Wong HY et al: A randomized, double-blind evaluation of ketorolac tromethamine for postoperative analgesia in ambulatory surgery patients. *Anesthesiology* 78:6, 1993.

54. Grass JA et al: Assessment of ketorolac as an adjunct to fentanyl patient-controlled epidural analgesia after radical retropubic prostatectomy. *Anesthesiology* 78:642, 1993.

QUESTIONS: POSTSURGICAL PAIN

1. Respiratory depression from epidural opioids is characterized by:
   A. A respiratory rate that is an adequate indicator of ventilatory status
   B. A pattern of respiratory depression that is slow and progressive rather than sudden apnea
   C. Sedation is not a significant indicator in its development
   D. Increased incidence unrelated to the vertebral level of opioid injection

2. A 52-year-old man who just had a gastrectomy complained of severe pain in the recovery room. His vital signs include a blood pressure of 90/50, heart rate of 110, and respiratory rate of 26/minute. What is the most appropriate next step?
   A. Patient-controlled analgesia should be started with morphine 2 mg as a bolus dose, and a lockout interval of 10 minutes.
   B. Fentanyl 100 μg in 5 ml saline should be injected through the epidural catheter and the epidural infusion started.
   C. Intravenous morphine should be given in 2 mg increments until there is pain relief.
   D. Bupivacaine 0.1% should be added to the epidural infusion.

For questions 3-5, choose from the following:
A: 1, 2, and 3
B: 1 and 3
C: 2 and 4
D: 4
E: All of the above

3. Rational use of opioids in postoperative pain includes the following:
   1. They should be used in the treatment of moderately severe to severe postoperative pain.
   2. Meperidine should never be used because of accumulation of normeperidine.
   3. The oral route should be used as soon as the patient tolerates oral intake.
   4. They should not be withheld even with respiratory rates of less than 8/min.

4. Preemptive analgesia refers to:
   1. Prevention of neuroplasticity changes in the peripheral or CNS after injury
   2. Prevention of pain that can be accomplished by regional nerve blockade or analgesic agents before surgical trauma
   3. The effectiveness of preincisional lidocaine in decreasing the pain after herniorrhaphy
   4. Equal doses of morphine prescribed before or after the injury

5. Intermittent epidural morphine injections for hospitalized wards are acceptable because:
   1. Respiratory depression is extremely rare, predictable, and easily treated
   2. The incidence of urinary retention is not higher than intermittent IM injections
   3. Nurses do not mind giving epidural injections
   4. There is low incidence of respiratory depression, and catheter-related problems are minimal

ANSWERS

1. B
2. C
3. B
4. A
5. D

37 Obstetric Pain

James C. Eisenach and *P. Prithvi Raj*

Labor pain is among the most severe pain experienced, and lack of treatment of labor pain can result in severe psychologic effects that can last throughout life. Treatment of pain in the obstetric patient differs significantly from treatment of pain in other patients. During labor, analgesic therapy affects two patients rather than one, and after delivery, women wish to interact with their newborn and prefer to avoid the sedation that commonly accompanies traditional analgesic therapy. This chapter focuses on treatment of labor pain, specifically: (a) the physiology of pregnancy and the physiology of pain during labor; (b) the pharmacology of commonly used drugs in obstetric analgesia; (c) techniques available for the treatment of pain relief during labor; and (d) treatment of labor pain in the setting of acute fetal stress.

PHYSIOLOGY OF PREGNANCY AND LABOR PAIN

Physiologic changes of pregnancy alter the response to and toxicity of analgesic therapy. These changes and their anesthetic implications are discussed in textbooks of obstetric analgesia[1,2] and are not detailed here. In general, side effects and toxicity from general and regional anesthesia are more common and severe during pregnancy. Pregnant patients are considered to be at greater risk than nonpregnant patients for pulmonary aspiration of gastric contents after loss of protective laryngeal reflexes. Sympathetic blockade accompanying epidural or spinal injection of local anesthetics may produce profound hypotension in pregnant women because of aortocaval compression by the gravid uterus and may adversely affect placental blood flow and fetal well-being. Cardiotoxicity from bupivacaine is more severe during pregnancy, and its treatment is more difficult. Epidural or spinal opioid therapy produces a higher incidence of nausea and pruritus in pregnant women and is associated with activation of herpes simplex labialis, which may raise concerns regarding newborn infection.[3] Because of these and other changes, analgesic therapy must be closely titrated and monitored.

The understanding of visceral pain and especially labor pain has lagged behind the understanding of acute somatic pain. Labor pain is real, severe, and universal over time and across societal and ethnic divisions.[4] Despite being the most commonly occurring and commonly treated form of severe visceral pain, the neurophysiologic mechanisms and neuromodulation of labor pain remain largely unknown.

Labor pain shares many characteristics with other types of visceral pain. However, as labor progresses, stretching, tearing, and cutting of perineal structures provides increasing somatic input. Therefore the pain of the second stage of labor and delivery includes pain with somatic components. This pain is no less real or intense than the visceral pain, but for the purposes of this review, the focus will be on the visceral components of labor pain that dominate the majority of labor.

Labor pain serves a biologic function

Unlike somatic pain, visceral pain is usually not linked to internal injury. As is true of other visceral organs, pain is produced by stretch or distension of the uterus or cervix, but incision of the human uterus is painless.[4] Unlike most forms of noxious somatic stimuli, these stimuli produce pain but not direct injury. However, like cardiac ischemic pain, labor pain warns of impending physical danger and beneficially alters behavior. In primates, labor pain results in concealment and suppression of vocalization at a time of increased vulnerability to predators.[5] In humans, labor pain usually causes the woman to seek shelter and aid from others. As argued by Scott,[6] short, painless labor may be associated with dramatic increases in perinatal mortality, perhaps because of the precipitant delivery. However, once labor pain has alerted the woman that the delivery process has begun, it no longer serves a useful purpose; the stress it produces may be detrimental to the fetus and should be treated.

During early labor, pain is felt over the T_{11}-T_{12} dermatomes, extending during active phase of the first stage of labor to T_{10} and L_1. Interestingly, pain is frequently not uniform within these dermatomes, but often described in patches, occasionally on one side only, and frequently predominating in the back. The neural correlates of this non-uniform localization are unknown but may relate to the innervation of the lower uterine segment and cervix.

Unlike contraction pain, which is usually localized diffusely over the lower abdomen, low back pain during labor is often continuous. Melzack and Blanger observed an association between low back pain during menstruation, labor pain scores during contractions, and continuous back pain during labor.[7] This suggests that continuous low back pain may be more resistant to psychoprophylactic coping techniques but more responsive to counterstimulation with transcutaneous electrical nerve stimulation, which perhaps reflects different neural mechanisms of tonic and phasic pains. The etiology of continuous pain in labor not associated with uterine contractions, and neurophysiologic differences between tonic and phasic labor pain and their response to extrinsic modulation have not been examined.

In early labor (cervical dilatation less than 5 cm), labor pain is described as discomforting, whereas labor at cervical dilatation greater than 5 cm is described as distressing, horrible, or excruciating. In addition, variability in perceived pain and analgesic requirements is great among parturients. Whereas differences in labor characteristics (e.g., fetal size, presentation, frequency of uterine contractions) are obvious causes of variability, patient characteristics are also important.

Labor pain stimulates an intense and complex autonomic response. These responses are particularly important in the obstetric setting because they adversely affect the fetus. Hyperventilation during contractions may impair maternal fetal oxygen transfer, and resultant maternal hypoventilation between contractions may cause maternal and fetal hypoxemia.[4] Sympathetic nervous system excitation and increasing circulating catecholamines may produce maternal tachycardia, hypertension, uterine artery constriction, and fetal asphyxia.[8] Effective maternal analgesia abolishes these responses and may improve fetal well-being.

There is a complex relationship between perceived pain intensity and behavior, anxiety, and their effect on labor progression. Pain scores during labor are lowered by the presence of a support person[9] but not consistently by psychologic training. However, psychologic training does reduce anxious states and pain behaviors during labor.[10] Racial, cultural, and ethnic factors alter behavior during labor pain, but not the patient's report regarding the intensity of perceived pain.[4] Both anxiety and perceived pain intensity[11] have been correlated with increased complications of labor and duration of labor. Interestingly, the pain intensity and

distress of a very early, latent labor has the most effect on labor and obstetric outcomes. The more distress the woman perceives in latent labor, the longer the labor and the greater the risk of abnormal fetal heart rate tracings and cesarean section. Providing epidural analgesia later in labor relieves pain but not distress,[12] leading to the speculation that some women may benefit from effective analgesia early in labor.

Afferent fibers supplying the uterus and cervix are primarily unmyelinated A-delta and C fibers traveling with sympathetic nerves. Anatomical studies demonstrate that these fibers pass sequentially through the uterine and cervical plexus; the inferior, middle, superior, and hypogastric plexuses; and the lumbar and lower thoracic sympathetic chain; thus entering the cord via the 10th, 11th, and 12th thoracic and first lumbar nerve roots. Pain relief during the first stage of labor can be achieved by local anesthetic injection near these fibers by paracervical, lumbar sympathetic, lumbar epidural, or spinal blocks (Fig. 37-1). In rats the receptive fields of these afferents in the hypogastric nerve are concentrated in the lower uterine body and cervix, most commonly ipsilateral to the recorded nerve.[13] All receptive fields cover less than 25% of the uterus and may extend to other pelvic viscera. Neuronal labeling studies demonstrate that left and right hypogastric nerves supply both sides of the uterine body with an ipsilateral predominance.

In labor pain the role of afferent fibers running with parasympathetic nerves is less certain. Clinical studies by Bonica and Chadwick suggested that the sensory fibers ac-

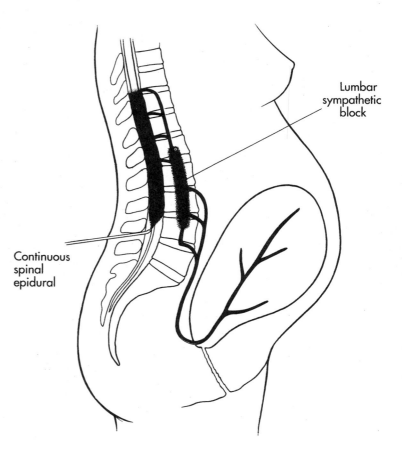

Fig. 37-1 Regional anesthetic techniques for obstetric analgesia-anesthesia. Lumbar sympathetic block is rarely used but is highly effective in relieving pain of the first stage and may be preferable to paracervical block, especially in high risk pregnancies. (Modified from Bonica JJ: An atlas on mechanisms and pathways of pain in labor. *What's New* 217:16, 1960.)

Lumbar sympathetic block

Continuous spinal epidural

companying the parasympathetic pelvic nerves in women played no role.[4] Vagal afferents, excited by cardiac ischemia, activated a spinal pain-suppressing system, which lead to painless, "silent" myocardial ischemia.[14] Whether or not recently demonstrated vagal afferents from the uterus[15] also modulate pain intensity of labor (which could explain the proportion of labors experienced without pain) has not been explored.

Noxious stimuli occurring during labor may activate spinal antinociceptive systems that could release antinociceptive mediators (norepinephrine[16] or enkephalins[17]) in cerebrospinal fluid (CSF), and could increase the pain threshold. In humans this system may not be tonically active but is activated by pain.[18] Labor pain in humans doubled CSF norepinephrine, which suggested that the descending noradrenergic inhibitory system may be activated by pain.[19] In contrast, CSF enkephalins were unchanged during labor. In the same study, women who experienced painful labor required less analgesic medication postoperatively than those without previous pain,[19] which supports the hypothesis that a pain inhibitory system is activated.

The pain of the first stage of labor is visceral in origin, emanating from the stretching and distention of the cervix and lower uterine segment and referred to lumbar and lower thoracic dermatomes. Neurophysiologic studies demonstrated that primary uterocervical afferents activated by mechanical and possibly ischemic and chemical stimuli enter the spinal cord via sympathetic nerves. Although precise spinal cord neurophysiologic studies of labor pain have not been performed, observations of the changes in the pain threshold during labor and clinical efficacy of spinally applied receptor selective agents suggest that the effect of primary uterine afferents on dorsal horn neurons is under powerful modulatory control.

ANALGESIA IN OBSTETRICS
Inhalation analgesics

Inhalation analgesia has been used since 1847 to relieve obstetric pain. Although the use of nitrous oxide, methoxyflurane, and trichloroethylene is widespread internationally, their use in the United States is fairly uncommon. This is due in part to concern over the toxicity of these agents when given in a poorly monitored setting and to the popularity of regional anesthetic techniques.

Nitrous oxide analgesia is commonly used in obstetric patients where regional analgesia is not available or is unwanted. Typically the patient self-administers the anesthetic using an approved apparatus that delivers no more than 70% nitrous oxide in oxygen by holding the face mask or mouthpiece. The physical properties of nitrous oxide are such that accumulation over time is negligible and elimination of the gas in the newborn is virtually completed within a few minutes of birth.

Volatile agents are administered via a face mask and demand-flow, draw-over vaporizer, using room air as the vehicle. Several commercial inhalers are available in other countries and are relatively inexpensive, robust, and easily portable. Whereas labor analgesia may be provided by trichloroethylene, methoxyflurane, enflurane, or isoflurane by such devices, concern over drug toxicity, drug overdose, and drug effects on the fetus have resulted in little use of these agents.

Opioids

Systematically administered opioids effectively relieve labor pain and are the most commonly used analgesics for this purpose. Extensive use attests to the safety and efficacy of opioids for treatment of labor pain. As with use of these compounds for other forms of acute pain, their efficacy is often limited by concern over side effects, inappropriate prescription, and education of medical and lay personnel. Additionally, opioids produce both maternal and fetal side effects such as maternal sedation, respiratory depression, delayed gastric emptying, postural hypotension, fetal and neonatal respiratory depression, and altered heart rate pattern. Although most of these effects are reversible with naloxone (0.1 to 0.4 mg to mother or 0.01 to 0.04 mg/kg to newborn), concern over these side effects has rightfully limited the amount of opioids prescribed during labor.

Epidural-spinal opioids

Since the description of spinal opioid receptors mediating analgesia and clinical application of intraspinal opioid therapy for acute and chronic pain, a number of studies have examined the use of epidural opioids during labor. In general, epidural opioids as sole analgesics during labor have been disappointing. A notable example is epidural morphine: Large doses are required, onset of analgesia is delayed, analgesia is not comparable to epidural local anesthetics during first stage and is inadequate during second stage, and the incidence of bothersome side effects, such as nausea and vomiting, is high.[20] More highly lipid-soluble drugs provide better analgesia. However, in agreement with animal data,[21] there is an inverse relationship between lipid solubility and apparent potency for pain relief. For example, morphine is more potent epidurally than systemically, whereas sufentanil and fentanyl are approximately equipotent by both routes.[22-24] The rationale for injecting epidurally large doses of sufentanil alone for labor analgesia is unclear. Additionally, respiratory depression from accidental IV injection of these lipid-soluble drugs and delayed respiratory depression from epidural injection may occur.[25] For these reasons, opioids are infrequently used alone but are commonly combined with local anesthetics for epidural analgesia.

Experience with intrathecal injection of opioids for labor analgesia is relatively new. Leighton[26] demonstrated that effective analgesia for prolonged periods during the first stage of labor followed a single intrathecal injection of 0.25 mg morphine and 25 μg fentanyl (Fig. 37-2). Similarly, recent experience with continuous spinal catheter techniques that use intermittent or continuous infusion of very small doses of lipid soluble opioids (3 to 5 μg sufentanil, 5 to 10 μg fentanyl, 10 to 20 mg meperidine) have been quite favorable.[27-29] However, the incidence of side effects in this population may be quite high with this technique. Experience is extremely limited at this time, and the ultimate utility of intrathecal opioids for labor analgesia is unclear.

Of clinically available opioids, only morphine and fentanyl have undergone extensive preclinical testing for in-

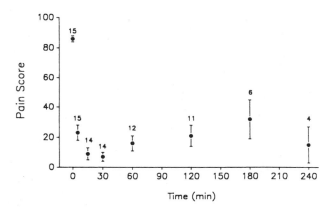

Fig. 37-2 Mean ± SEM pain scores (0=no pain, 100=worst imaginable pain) after intrathecal injection of fentanyl 26 μg and morphine 0.25 mg for pain relief during labor. The number of patients still laboring under intrathecal narcotic analgesia appears above each value. (From Leighton BL et al: Intrathecal narcotics for labor revisited: The combination of fentanyl and morphine intrathecally provides rapid onset of profound, prolonged analgesia. *Anesth Analg* 69:122-125, 1985.)

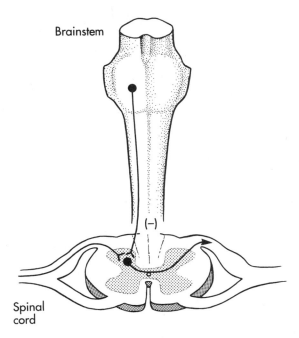

Fig. 37-3 Descending noradrenergic inhibition of spinal cord dorsal horn neurons. Norepinephrine is released, acting primarily on postsynaptic α_2-adrenergic receptor to produce analgesia. Intraspinal injection of α_2-adrenergic agonists produces analgesia by mimicking this system.

traspinal use, and only morphine is FDA approved for this indication. Other opioids have been reported to produce analgesia without serious side effects in humans but have not undergone such testing. Experience with neurotoxicity from approved local anesthetics and recent reports suggesting neurotoxicity from intrathecal injection of opioids (butorphanol, sufentanil, dynorphin)[30,31] suggest caution in using intraspinal opioids other than morphine or fentanyl in the absence of a definite indication.

Epidural-spinal α_2-adrenergic agonists

A$_2$-Adrenergic agonists produce analgesia by action within the spinal cord[32] (Fig. 37-3), and epinephrine, a preferential α_2-agonist, produces complete analgesia during labor and for forceps delivery when injected intrathecally.[33] Epidural administration of the more specific adrenergic agonist clonidine produces complete analgesia after cesarean section, although of relatively brief duration.[32] Continuous infusion of clonidine after cesarean section produces analgesia of prolonged duration. Sedation and, rarely, bradycardia may limit bolus clonidine administration. Animal data suggest that clonidine and other α_2-adrenergic agonists, injected in doses epidurally or intrathecally adequate to produce analgesia, will likely produce decreases in resting fetal heart rate because of placental transfer to the fetus.[34,35] Although no evidence of fetal distress has been associated with this pharmacologic effect, it would interfere with fetal heart rate monitoring. Therefore the use of such agents alone for analgesia in labor is unlikely.

Local Anesthetics

Local anesthetics may be administered by infiltration, peripheral nerve block, and intraspinally for analgesia during labor and after cesarean section. The three most commonly employed local anesthetics in obstetrics are lidocaine, 2-chloroprocaine, and bupivacaine. They differ in onset of action, duration of action, and incidence and type of toxic

side effects. In general, choice of agent should be based on desired onset and duration of activity. The major toxic side effects of these drugs relate to high systemic concentrations, which most commonly follow accidental intravascular injection. All local anesthetics may produce seizures and cardiovascular collapse. Bupivacaine is particularly toxic in pregnant patients. This toxicity is avoided by using small amounts of drugs in dilute concentrations during labor and by effective testing of epidural catheter tip location injection. Direct neurotoxicity of local anesthetics may also occur. The combination of 2-chloroprocaine and metabisulfite injected intrathecally can result in permanent neurologic damage.[36] Newer formulations of 2-chloroprocaine for epidural use do not contain metabisulfite but do contain EDTA, a calcium chelator. Recent animal data questions the safety of EDTA injected into the intrathecal space,[37] and accidental intrathecal injection of large doses of 2-chloroprocaine with EDTA should be avoided by appropriate catheter tip testing dosing.

ANALGESIA TECHNIQUES DURING LABOR
Hypnosis

Hypnosis by classical techniques effectively reduces the sensation of pain during labor in some women, and in a few may provide acceptable anesthesia for cesarean section. Compared with traditional regional or systemic analgesia regimens, hypnosis has been reported to shorten labor[38] and results in better fetal and neonatal acid-base status.[39] This technique has not been commonly applied to labor pain. Although hypnosis has many advantages over pharmacologic intervention (i.e., reversibility, no drug or equipment cost, no effect on fetus), the technique is time consuming, requires multiple training sessions during the last weeks of pregnancy, and requires the presence of a hypnotist during labor.

Psychoprophylaxis

Psychoprophylaxis entails education about the labor and delivery process and teaching techniques for coping with pain. Whether these methods truly prevent pain or provide coping mechanisms is not clear.[40] For example, some have reported that psychoprophylaxis does not decrease the woman's evaluation of pain, but does decrease anxiety and pain behavior during labor.[10] Others have reported a reduction in pain intensity scores in early, but not late labor, in women who had attended childbirth classes.[9] By improving coping, psychoprophylaxis may have beneficial effects on the progress of labor,[11] particularly during early stages.

Most commonly, psychoprophylaxis is provided by a method similar to that described by Lamaze.[41] Major ingredients include educating the patient on normal physiology of labor and delivery; the importance of having a "coach" present to aid in focusing attention during painful labor; and using visual focusing and breathing patterns to provide distraction during painful contractions. Since most women receiving Lamaze training request systemic or regional anesthesia during labor,[42] education usually includes discussions of other options of analgesia. In the psychoprophylaxis classes, the undesirability of prolonged maternal stress and pain and the resultant dangers to the fetus as demonstrated in animal models should be discussed.[8,43] Women who have a support person present during labor report less pain,[9] and distraction techniques provide a coping strategy.

Counterstimulation techniques

The efficacy of counterstimulation techniques is supported by two theoretic constructs. Stimulation of afferent nerves subserving the same dermatomes as the noxious stimulus may decrease perception of pain according to the gate control theory.[44] This is the rational basis for the use of transcutaneous electrical nerve stimulation (TENS). Additionally, noxious stimuli at dermatomal regions removed from the labor pain stimulus may decrease perception of pain according to the concept of diffuse noxious inhibitory controls.[17] Both constructs are the rational bases for the use of acupuncture.

Acupuncture, either by insertion of needles alone or with electrical stimulation of inserted needles, produces profound analgesia and anesthesia in certain individuals. In China acupuncture is employed alone or in conjunction with systemic opioids to provide anesthesia for a few surgical procedures. However, it has not been commonly applied to the treatment of labor pain.

TENS is a method of applying pulses of electrical current to the skin, and produces analgesia by an unknown mechanism. Although there are few studies of TENS used during labor, it has been reported effective in nearly 90% of women,[45] and decreases the usage of opioids.[46] TENS has been reported to be particularly effective for back pain during labor;[47] back pain is typically continuous and less

effectively dealt with by psychologic techniques.[7] For labor analgesia, surface TENS electrodes are placed on the back on each side of the midline over the T_{10}-L_1 dermatomes and over the sacrum. Baseline low level stimulation of the upper electrodes plus patient-controlled increases in stimulation levels during contractions produces a tingling sensation accompanied by some pain relief. Sacral electrodes are activated as labor progresses and pain intensity increases. TENS does not appear to affect the fetus, and commercially available units have been shown to be safe.[48] However, use of TENS during labor is limited by an interference with electronic fetal heart rate monitoring, a relative inefficacy during later stages of labor, an inability of some women to tolerate the stimulation, and the relatively expensive cost of the equipment.

Local anesthetic infiltration

Local anesthetic infiltration, usually with 0.5% to 1% lidocaine or 1% to 2% 2-chloroprocaine, produces local surgical anesthesia, typically for episiotomy and repair. Although effective for superficial repair, the quality of anesthesia is poor for deep repair (fourth degree lacerations) perhaps because of increased vascularity of this tissue and rapid drug uptake. As with any injection of local anesthetic, the patient should be monitored for signs of accidental IV injection.

Paracervical block

Paracervical block, which is typically performed by the obstetrician, involves injection of 5 to 10 ml of local anesthetic bilaterally into the submucosa adjacent to the cervix. This block produces excellent analgesia for the first stage of labor. However, paracervical block is associated with a high incidence of fetal bradycardia and distress[49] and is rarely performed. If paracervical block is chosen for labor analgesia, 2-chloroprocaine is probably the safest drug, although it only provides short lasting analgesia. Fetal heart rate should be continuously monitored, and personnel should be available for expeditious delivery in case of prolonged fetal distress.

Patient-controlled analagesia

Opioids are commonly administered IV for analgesia during labor. Their doses and side effects were reviewed previously. Unlike most surgical patients, many parturients have a desire to minimize the number and amount of medications they receive and to be alert for childbirth. Patient-controlled analgesia (PCA) may treat the pain of labor better than standard techniques in part because of the large and unpredictable variability in analgesic requirements among parturients (Fig. 37-4). In addition to large interpatient variation, the need for analgesics increases as labor progresses, which is demonstrated by increased rate of demands in patients using PCA (Fig. 37-5).[50] PCA should allow more immediate close and efficient titration of analgesic delivery during this period of changing pain intensity.

A major concern with IV meperidine for PCA during labor is fetal meperidine exposure and subsequent behavioral depression. Maternal use of meperidine averages 30 to 60

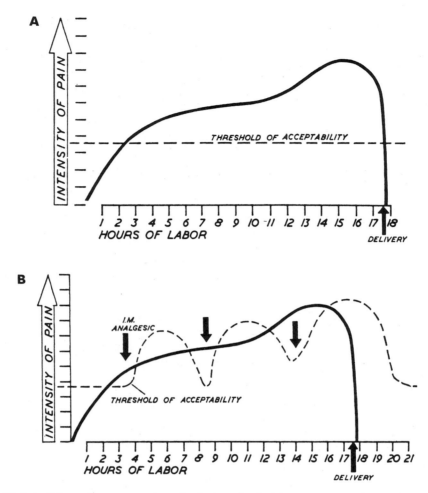

Fig. 37-4 A, Schematic representation of pain intensity in labor *(continuous line)* rising to cross the threshold of acceptability *(broken line)* in absence of analgesia. **B,** Similar representation of effect of intramuscular analgesia. The threshold of acceptability is intermittently raised above the pain level. A considerable amount of the analgesic action is wasted and there are periods when it is inadequate. (From Scott JS: Obstetric analgesia: A consideration of labor pain and a patient-controlled technique for its relief with meperidine. *Am J Obstet Gynecol* 106:970, 1970.)

mg/hr[6,51,52] during labor, which may lead to large fetal exposure during prolonged labor. Although cord blood levels of meperidine at delivery are lower in patients receiving PCA than "Please repeat as necessary" (PRN) dosing,[52] this does not necessarily mean less fetal exposure. To limit fetal effects, most authors discontinue IV PCA when full cervical dilatation is reached. Another method to limit opioid-induced newborn depression yet provide effective analgesia is to employ agonist/antagonist opiates. For example, both nalbuphine[53] and pentazocine[54] provide as good or better analgesia as meperidene with fewer maternal side effects, particularly nausea and vomiting. When compared with PRN IV nalbuphine, PCA improves analgesia and satisfaction, and decreases total dose and sedation during labor.[55] However, as with meperidine, relatively large doses of nalbuphine are required (5 to 12 mg/hr), which may affect the interpretation of the fetal heart rate and thus may render a difficult interpretation.

Continuous lumbar epidural analgesia

Lumbar epidural analgesia is now the standard by which other analgesic regimens during labor are compared. Details of lumbar epidural catheter insertion are covered elsewhere in this text. This review focuses on the aspects of epidural analgesia important in obstetrics.

Testing for accidental subarachnoid or intravascular cannulation of epidural catheters improves the safety of the technique and speeds the recognition of the need to reposition catheters. Although there is little controversy over selection of solutions or testing subarachnoid location (approximately 5 mg bupivacaine, 50 mg lidocaine, or 2-chloroprocaine suffice), the appropriate solution for testing IV location is less certain. Some advocate 15 μg epinephrine to provide objective evidence for IV injection (increased maternal heart rate and blood pressure). The increased heart rate is transient and may require sophisticated monitoring for reliable detection in the laboring parturi-

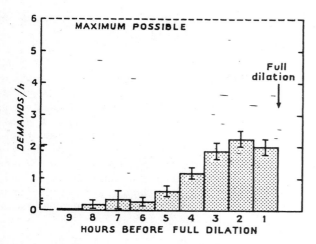

Fig. 37-5 Demand-rate *(demands/h)* of 42 patients in labor (mean ± SE). Each demand was 0.25 mg/kg meperidine. (From Evans JM et al: Apparatus for patient-controlled administration of intravenous narcotics during labor. *Lancet* i:17, 1976.)

Table 37-1 The epidural local anesthetic during labor

Solution	Dose
Bolus	
Bupivacaine 0.25%	6-10 ml
Bupivacaine 0.125%	12-15 ml
with fentanyl 5 μg/ml	8-10 ml
2-Chloroprocaine 2%	6-10 ml
Lidocaine 2%	6-10 ml
Infusion	
Bupivacaine 0.25%	6-10 ml/hr
Bupivacaine 0.125%	12-16 ml/hr
with fentanyl 1 μg/m	8-12 ml/hr
with epinephrine 1:800,000	8-12 ml/hr
2-Chloroprocaine 1%	12-16 ml/hr
Lidocaine 1%	10-14 ml/hr

ent.[56] In pregnant sheep, 15 μg epinephrine decreases uterine blood flow by 45%[57]; and in humans this dose is associated with fetal bradycardia.[56] Although this effect is transient and probably well tolerated in the normal patient, it may be less well tolerated in cases of decreased uteroplacental reserve.

For an alternative to epinephrine, a local anesthetic (2-chloroprocaine or lidocaine) can be injected in a dose (100 mg) that produces subjective symptoms if administered IV. The advantage of 2-chloroprocaine is rapid plasma hydrolysis that minimizes systemic or fetal effects and the lack of effect on uterine blood flow.[58] Advantages of lidocaine include lack of deleterious effect on the potency of subsequently injected bupivacaine or opioids (unlike 2-chloroprocaine which interferes with both), and more prolonged analgesia when injected in the epidural space. Although the sensitivity of these solutions in premedicated or laboring women is unknown, we routinely use them for catheter testing and believe that these solutions reliably and safely identify IV injections. Others have recommended injecting air into the epidural catheter while placing the fetal heart rate monitor over the maternal precordium to monitor for the presence of air.[59] Initial experience, although small, suggests that this is an extremely sensitive and specific test for intravascular cannulation.

Lumbar epidural analgesia for the first stage of labor is typically established by injecting of 10 ml of 2% lidocaine, 2% 2-chloroprocaine, or 0.25% bupivacaine. Subsequent analgesia may be maintained by intermittent injections of the local anesthetic in the same doses or by continuous epidural infusion (Table 37-1). Compared with intermittent doses, continuous infusion provides sustained and consistent analgesia with less fluctuation in degree of sympathetic blockade, incidence of hypotension, and maternal side effects. Typically, bupivacaine is infused at a rate between 10 and 16 ml/hr in concentrations between 0.0625% and 0.125%.

Opioids are frequently combined with local anesthetics. Studies have shown that including a lipid-soluble opioid by bolus (50 μg fentanyl or equivalent) or infusion (10 to 30 μg/hr fentanyl or equivalent) decreases the amount of bupivacaine required for equivalent pain relief by 20% to 40%.[60,61] A decreased bupivacaine dose leads to a less intense motor blockade and could theoretically reduce hemodynamic instability from sympathetic blockade. These benefits should be weighed against the cumulative opioid exposure to the fetus. Epidural fentanyl 75 μg does not affect fetal heart rate monitoring,[62] and 150 μg does not alter neonatal behavior.[63] However, the effects of larger doses are unknown, and animal work suggests that at least one of these potent opioids (alfentanil) may have prolonged affects on cognitive development.[64]

Combination therapy with epidural local anesthetic, opioid, and epinephrine has been the subject of few studies for labor analgesia. Inclusion of epinephrine enhances intraspinal fentanyl or sufentanil analgesia after surgery.[65,66] Whether such a combination would be effective for labor analgesia while avoiding use of local anesthetic and resultant sympathetic blockade is unknown. Similarly, addition of both fentanyl and epinephrine to bupivacaine dramatically prolongs analgesia from a single injection,[60] and this potentiation is abolished when even small doses of 2-chloroprocaine are used.

Patient-controlled epidural anesthesia

Providing safe and effective pain relief during labor requires titration of analgesics to treat a pain stimulus that varies greatly both between individuals and within each individual as labor progresses. Continuous epidural infusions are commonly employed during labor and, compared with intermittent injection, may enhance both analgesia and maternal and fetal safety.[67] However, no single set infusion rate will accommodate the great variation in individual requirements during labor. Some have addressed this issue by applying PCA technology to epidural drug delivery during labor.[68-70]

The ideal PCA agent would be rapid acting and highly effective without adverse side effects. Rapid onset improves patient feedback and allows close titration of drug requests to changes in pain intensities. Of combinations of bupivacaine, fentanyl, and epinephrine in one study,[68] the most appropriate combination was bupivacaine and fentanyl according to the machine settings shown in Box 37-1. Using this and similar protocols, patient-controlled epidural anesthesia (PCEA) decreased bupivacaine usage during labor when compared with continuous infusion. Two advantages of PCEA became apparent when this technique was clinically applicated. First, the need for physician-administered boluses decreased, which saved 15 to 30 minutes of monitoring time for a typical labor epidural.[69] Second, women decreased their local anesthetic usage with PCEA as they neared complete cervical dilatation and administered appropriate levels of analgesia for pushing during second stage without the need for physician-administered "pushing doses."

Spinal analgesia during labor

Administering opioids close to their site of action in the spinal cord allows for extremely small doses to produce analgesia. Leighton et al. demonstrated prolonged and profound analgesia for labor pain after an injection of a morphine and fentanyl intrathecal combination.[26] With the advent of catheters designed to pass through small gauge spinal needles, attention is being focused on continuous spinal analgesia (CSA) during labor. Advantages possible with CSA over an epidural technique include reliability (clear endpoint during placement, unilateral block unlikely), speed (rapid onset of local anesthetic effect), and decreased drug dose with less fetal exposure. Most importantly, by injecting drug near the spinal site of action, it may be possible to provide labor analgesia without risk of hypotension or motor blockade by injecting lipid-soluble opioids.

Initial experience with CSA during labor is just beginning to be reported.[27-29] Technical problems with insertion, maintenance, and removal of the ultrafine catheters have been common. As might be expected, injection of local anesthetic frequently leads to hypotension. Unfortunately, initial experience with fentanyl at doses up to 30 μg for CSA demonstrated inadequate analgesia in many patients.[29] However, combination drug use and CSA may yet produce excellent analgesia and minimal side effects.

The incidence of postdural puncture headache is probably not decreased by insertion of a catheter and may be prohibited in this patient group. The risk of infection after intrathecal catheterization may be greater than that after epidural, although experience is not yet wide enough to determine this. Finally, anecdotal reports of neurotoxicity associated with CSA suggest using with caution until there is wider experience with this technique.

Caudal anesthesia

Caudal epidural anesthesia, a common form of providing labor analgesia in the past, is infrequently used today. Although caudal epidural anesthesia provides excellent sacral analgesia for the second stage of labor, providing analgesia during the first stage of labor, which requires sensory blockade to lower thoracic dermatomes, requires large doses of local anesthetic. In addition, extremely large doses may be needed to provide adequate anesthesia for cesarean section. For these reasons, and the technical difficulty in placing continuous caudal catheters in laboring parturients, caudal anesthesia is infrequently used today.

Ilioinguinal nerve block

Ilioinguinal nerve block after cesarean section can provide analgesia.[71,72] Initial experience suggests that ilioinguinal nerve block dramatically decreases the dose of systemic opioid required for analgesia following cesarean section,[71] and produces analgesia comparable to intraspinal opioids but with fewer side effects.[72] The role of ilioinguinal nerve block following cesarean section is currently under debate.

REFERENCES

1. Shnider SM, Levinson G: *Anesthesia for Obstetrics,* ed 2. Baltimore, Williams & Wilkins, 1987.
2. James FM III: *Obstetric Anesthesia: The Complicated Patient,* ed 2. Philadelphia, FA Davis, 1988.
3. Crone L-AL et al: Recurrent herpes simplex virus labialis and the use of epidural morphine in obstetric patients. *Anesth Analg* 67:318-323, 1988.
4. Bonica JJ, Chadwick HS: Labour pain. In Wall PD, Melzack R, editors: *Textbook of Pain.* New York, Churchill Livingstone, 1989.
5. Lefebvre L, Carli G: Parturition in non-human primates: Pain and auditory concealment. *Pain* 21:315-327, 1985.
6. Scott JS: Obstetric analgesia: A consideration of labor pain and a patient-controlled technique for its relief with meperidine. *Am J Obstet Gynecol* 106:959-978, 1970.
7. Melzack R, Blanger E: Labour pain: Correlations with menstrual pain and acute low-back pain before and during pregnancy. *Pain* 36:225-229, 1989.
8. Shnider SM et al: Uterine blood flow and plasma norepinephrine changes during maternal stress in the pregnant ewe. *Anesthesiology* 50:524-527, 1979.
9. Brown ST, Campbell D, Kurtz A: Characteristics of labor pain at two stages of cervical dilation. *Pain* 38:289-295, 1989.
10. Bonnel AM, Boureau F: Labor pain assessment: Validity of a behavioral index. *Pain* 22:81-90, 1985.
11. Wuitchik M, Bakal D, Lipshitz J: The clinical significance of pain and cognitive activity in latent labor. *Obstet Gynecol* 73:35-42, 1989.
12. Wuitchik M, Bakal D, Lipshitz J: Relationships between pain, cognitive activity and epidural analgesia during labor. *Pain* 41:125-132, 1990.
13. Berkley KJ, Robbins A, Sato Y: Afferent fibers supplying the uterus in the rat. *J Neurophysiol* 59:142-163, 1988.
14. Foreman RD, Blair RW: Central organization of sympathetic cardiovascular response to pain. *Annu Rev Physiol* 50:607-622, 1988.
15. Ortega-Villalobos M et al: Vagus nerve afferent and efferent innervation of the rat uterus: An electrophysiological and HRP study. *Brain Res Bull* 25:365-371, 1990.
16. Tyce GM, Yaksh TL: Monoamine release from cat spinal cord by somatic stimuli: An intrinsic modulatory system. *J Physiol (Lond)* 314:513-529, 1981.

Box 37-1 PATIENT-CONTROLLED EPIDURAL ANESTHESIA

0.125% bupivacaine + 1 μg/ml fentanyl
Dose = 4 ml
Lockout = 10 min
Basal infusion = 6 ml/hr
Hourly limit = 20 ml
Typical hourly use: 10 ml

---

17. LeBars D et al: Noxious mechanical stimuli increase the release of Met-enkephalin-like material heterosegmentally in the rat spinal cord. *Brain Res* 402:188-192, 1987.

18. Talbot JD, Duncan GH, Bushnell MC: Effects of diffuse noxious inhibitory controls (DNICs) on the sensory-discriminative dimension of pain perception. *Pain* 36:231-238, 1989.

19. Eisenach JC et al: Effect of pregnancy and pain on cerebrospinal fluid immunoreactive enkephalins and norepinephrine in healthy humans. *Pain* 43:149-154, 1990.

20. Hughes SC et al: Maternal and neonatal effects of epidural morphine for labor and delivery. *Anesth Analg* 63:319-324, 1984.

21. McQuay HJ et al: Intrathecal opioids, potency and lipophilicity. *Pain* 36:111-115, 1989.

22. Eisenach JC, Grice SC, Dewan DM: Patient-controlled analgesia following cesarean section: A comparison with epidural and intramuscular narcotics. *Anesthesiology* 68:444-448, 1988.

23. Ellis DJ, Millar WL, Reisner LS: A randomized double-blind comparison of epidural versus intravenous fentanyl infusion for analgesia after cesarean section. *Anesthesiology* 72:981-986, 1990.

24. Cohen SE, Tan S, White PF: Sufentanil analgesia following cesarean section: Epidural versus intravenous administration. *Anesthesiology* 1:129-134, 1988.

25. Brockway MS et al: Profound respiratory depression after extradural fentanyl. *Br J Anaesth* 64:243-245, 1990.

26. Leighton BL et al: Intrathecal narcotics for labor revisited: The combination of fentanyl and morphine intrathecally provides rapid onset of profound, prolonged analgesia. *Anesth Analg* 69:122-125, 1989.

27. Naulty JS et al: Continuous subarachnoid sufentanil for labor analgesia. *Anesthesiology* 73:A964, 1990 (abstract).

28. Norris MC et al: Intrathecal meperidine for labor analgesia. *Anesthesiology* 73:A983, 1990 (abstract).

29. Arkoosh VA, Leighton BL, Norris MC: Continuous spinal analgesia for labor. Proceedings of the S.O.A.P. Annual Meeting 22:A2, Madison, Wis, 1990 (abstract).

30. Stewart P, Isaac L: Localization of dynorphin-induced neurotoxicity in rat spinal cord. *Life Sci* 44:1505-1514, 1989.

31. Rawal N et al: Histopathological effects of intrathecal sufentanil, butorphanol, and nalbuphine. *Pain Suppl* 5:S130, 1990 (abstract).

32. Mendez R, Eisenach JC, Kashtan K: Epidural clonidine analgesia after cesarean section. *Anesthesiology* 73:848-852, 1990.

33. Priddle HD, Andros GJ: Primary spinal anesthetic effects of epinephrine. *Anesth Analg* 34:156-161, 1950.

34. Eisenach JC et al: Epidural clonidine analgesia in obstetrics: Sheep studies. *Anesthesiology* 70:51-56, 1989.

35. Eisenach JC, Dewan DM: Intrathecal clonidine in obstetrics: Sheep studies. *Anesthesiology* 72:663-668, 1990.

36. Rosen MA et al: Evaluation of neurotoxicity after subarachnoid injection of large volumes of local anesthetic solutions. *Anesth Analg* 62:802-808, 1983.

37. Wang BC et al: Is EDTA harmless in the subarachnoid space? *Anesthesiology* 71:A1142, 1989 (abstract).

38. Flowers CE, Littlejohn TW, Wells HB: Pharmacologic and hypnoid analgesia. *Obstet Gynecol* 16:210-221, 1960.

39. Moya F, James LS: Medical hypnosis for obstetrics. *JAMA* 174:2026-2032, 1960.

40. Melzack R et al: Labour is still painful after prepared childbirth training. *Can Med Assoc J* 125:357-363, 1981.

41. Lamaze F: *Painless Childbirth: Psychoprophylactic method.* London, Burke, 1958.

42. Scott JR, Rose NB: Effect of psychoprophylaxis (Lamaze preparation) on labor and delivery in primiparas. *N Engl J Med* 294:1205-1207, 1976.

43. Morishima HO, Pedersen H, Finster M: The influence of maternal psychological stress on the fetus. *Am J Obstet Gynecol* 131:286-290, 1978.

44. Melzack R, Wall PD: Pain mechanisms: A new theory. *Science* 150:971-975, 1965.

45. Augustinsson L-E et al: Pain relief during delivery by transcutaneous electrical nerve stimulation. *Pain* 4:59-65, 1977.

46. Miller-Jones CMH: Transcutaneous nerve stimulation in labour (Forum). *Anaesthesia* 35:372-375, 1980.

47. Bundsen P, Peterson L-E, Selstam U: Pain relief in labor by transcutaneous electrical nerve stimulation: A prospective matched study. *Acta Obstet Gynecol Scand* 60:459-468, 1981.

48. Bundsen P, Ericson K: Pain relief in labor by transcutaneous electrical nerve stimulation. *Acta Obstet Gynecol Scand* 61:1-5, 1982.

49. Ralston DH, Shnider SM: The fetal and neonatal effects of regional anesthesia in obstetrics. *Anesthesiology* 48:34-64, 1978.

50. Evans JM et al: Apparatus for patient-controlled administration of intravenous narcotics during labour. *Lancet* i:17-18, 1976.

51. Robinson RO et al: Self-administered intravenous and intramuscular pethidine: A controlled trial in labour. *Anaesthesia* 35:763-770, 1980.

52. Bristow A, Wallace D, Jennings L: Parturient controlled infusion reduces meperidine in cord blood. Proceedings of the S.O.A.P. Annual Meeting 18:35, Salt Lake City, Utah, 1986 (abstract).

53. Frank M et al: Nalbuphine for obstetric analgesia: A comparison of nalbuphine with pethidine for pain relief in labour when administered by patient-controlled analgesia (PCA). *Anaesthesia* 42:697-703, 1987.

54. Erskine WAR et al: Self administered intravenous analgesia during labour. *S Afr Med J* 67:764-767, 1985.

55. Podlas J, Breland BD: Patient controlled analgesia with nalbuphine during labor. *Ostet Gynecol* 70:202-204, 1987.

56. Leighton BL et al: Limitations of epinephrine a marker of intravascular injection in laboring women. *Anesthesiology* 66:688-691, 1987.

57. Hood DD, Dewan DM, James FM III: Maternal and fetal effects of epinephrine in gravid ewes. *Anesthesiology* 64:610-613, 1986.

58. Chestnut DH, Weiner CP, Herrig JE: The effect of intravenously administered 2-chloroprocaine upon uterine artery blood flow velocity in gravid guinea pigs. *Anesthesiology* 70:305-308, 1989.

59. Leighton BL, Gross JC: Air: An effective indicator of intravenously located epidural catheters. *Anesthesiology* 71:848-851, 1989.

60. Grice SC, Eisenach JC, Dewan DM: Labor analgesia with epidural bupivacaine plus fentanyl: Enhancement with epinephrine and inhibition with 2-chloroprocaine. *Anesthesiology* 72:623-628, 1990.

61. Chestnut DH et al: Continuous infusion epidural analgesia during labor: A randomized, double-blind comparison of 0.0625% bupivacaine/0.0002% fentanyl versus 0.125% bupivacaine. *Anesthesiology* 68:745-759, 1988.

62. Viscomi CM et al: Fetal heart rate variability after epidural fentanyl during labor. *Anesth Analg* 71:679-683, 1990.

63. Capogna G et al: Neonatal neurobehavioral effects following maternal administration of epidural fentanyl during labor. *Anesthesiology* 67:A461, 1987.

64. Golub MS, Eisele JH Jr, Donald JM: Obstetric analgesia and infant outcome in monkeys: Infant development after intrapartum exposure to meperidine of alfentanil. *Am J Obstet Gynecol* 159:1280-1286, 1988.

65. Leicht CH et al: Prolongation of postoperative epidural sufentanil analgesia with epinephrine. *Anesth Analg* 70:323-325, 1990.

66. Malinow AM et al: Effect of epinephrine on intrathecal fentanyl analgesia in patients undergoing postpartum tubal ligation. *Anesthesiology* 73:381-385, 1990.

67. Li DF, Rees AD, Rosen M: Continuous extradural infusion of 0.0625% or 0.125% bupivacaine for pain relief in primigravid labour. *Br J Anaesth* 57:264-270, 1985.

68. Lysak SZ, Eisenach JC, Dobson CE II: Patient-controlled epidural analgesia during labor: A comparison of three solutions with a continuous infusion control. *Anesthesiology* 72:44-49, 1990.

69. Viscomi C, Eisenach JC: Patient controlled epidural analgesia during labor. *Obstet Gynecol* 77(3):348-351, March 1991.

70. Gambling DR, McMorland GH, Yu P: Comparison of patient-controlled epidural analgesia and conventional intermittent "top-up" injections during labor. *Anesth Analg* 70:256-261, 1990.

71. Bunting P, McConachie I: Ilioinguinal nerve blockade for analgesia after caesarean section. *Br J Anaesth* 61:773-775, 1988.

72. Witkowski TA, Leighton BL, Norris MC: Ilioinguinal nerve blocks: An alternative or supplement to intrathecal morphine. *Anesthesiology* 73:A692, 1990 (abstract).

QUESTIONS: OBSTETRIC PAIN

1. During early labor, pain is felt over the following dermatomes:
   A. T_5-T_9
   B. T_{11}-T_{12}
   C. L_2-L_3
   D. S_1-S_3
2. Afferent fibers supplying the uterus and cervix travel with sympathetic nerves. Before entering the spinal cord, these fibers pass sequentially through uterine and cervical plexus to all of the following regions EXCEPT:
   A. Inferior hypogastric plexus
   B. Superior hypogastric plexus
   C. Lumbar and lower thoracic sympathetic chain
   D. Anterior L_1 to L_5 spinal roots
3. The standard practice of providing analgesia during labor is:
   A. Paracervical block
   B. Continuous lumbar epidural analgesia
   C. Patient controlled analgesia
   D. Spinal block
4. Caudal anesthesia is not commonly used for labor analgesia today because:
   A. It is easy to provide analgesia from this site for the first stage of labor
   B. The first stage of labor requires blocking of lower thoracic dermatomes
   C. Small doses of local anesthetic are sufficient to provide adequate anesthesia for caesarean section
   D. It is technically easy to place a continuous caudal catheter in a laboring parturient

5. The most appropriate method of providing analgesia for labor by PCA technique is the following EXCEPT:
   A. Drugs 0.125% bupivacaine + 1 μ/ml fentanyl
   B. Lockout dose of 4 ml at 10 min.
   C. Basal infusion at 6 ml/hr
   D. Hourly limit of 4 ml

ANSWERS

1. B
2. D
3. B
4. B
5. D

38 Acute Medical Diseases

P Prithvi Raj

ACUTE VASCULAR DISORDERS

In patients who develop rather sudden, severe circulatory insufficiency of the limb from trauma, embolism, thrombosis, or chemical irritation, the local lesion initiates reflex spasm of the collateral vessels. The reflex spasm aggravates the circulatory insufficiency, which becomes much greater than if the collateral vessels were not so affected. Sympathetic block should be promptly initiated before changes occur that favor thrombosis in the endothelium of the vasospastic collateral vessels. The block reestablishes normal blood flow through the collaterals, and thus decreases or totally prevents tissue damage that might otherwise progress to gangrene.

After acute single injuries or repeated trauma, some patients develop segmentary vasospasm, which is manifested by a cold, cyanotic, painful, and edematous extremity. Although the vessels are not grossly injured, the degree of vasospasm may be so severe that it produces ischemia and consequent gangrene comparable with the results of intraluminal obstruction or section of the vessels. In such cases sympathetic blocks may determine whether the severe ischemia is a result of organic obstruction or actual division of the blood vessels or merely due to severe spasm. The blocks should be performed using long-lasting anesthetics. If the condition involves the lower limb, continuous epidural anesthesia is more useful because it provides uninterrupted sympathetic block and relief of somatic pain.

Interarterial injection of thiopental (Pentothal) or other very irritable agents often provokes very severe, intense spasm of the arteries and arterioles, which produces excruciating pain and often threatens the viability of the limb. In such patients sympathetic interruption by intravenous infusion of guanethidine may be more effective than regional sympathetic block; but even this will often not relieve the severe pain that can only be achieved with a block of the brachial plexus.[1,2]

Acute arterial occlusion

Acute arterial occlusion may be caused by thrombosis, embolism, or direct injury. The clinical picture varies depending on location of the obstruction, functional capability of the existent collateral circulation, and general condition of the patient. Pain develops rapidly as a result of tissue ischemia, which may be the product of the primary obstruction and reflex collateral vasospasm.[1,3] Treatment of an embolism consists of embolectomy, anticoagulant therapy, and concomitant sympathetic interruption to relieve the reflex spasm.

Before the advent of anticoagulant therapy, continuous epidural analgesia was administered immediately after the patient with sudden occlusion of major blood vessels in the lower limb entered the hospital. This was administered to relieve pain during the preoperative period and to anesthetize the patient for the surgical intervention. However, this is no longer practiced because of the risk of epidural hemorrhage consequent to anticoagulant therapy. On the other hand, for embolectomy in the upper limb, a brachial plexus block with bupivacaine (Marcaine) can provide preoperative and postoperative pain relief, sympathetic blockade, and anesthesia for the operation. The risk of serious sequelae from hemorrhage consequent to anticoagulant therapy is significantly less in the posterial triangle of the neck than the epidural space. An intravenous sympathetic block with guanethidine may relieve reflex spasm caused embolism in the upper or lower limb; but it does not provide the prompt pain relief and anesthesia for surgery as the aforementioned blocks.

Acute venous thrombosis

Acute venous thrombosis encompasses a spectrum of symptoms and signs usually considered under the diagnostic category of thrombophlebitis. Acute venous thrombosis is characterized by severe pain, marked edema, and excessive perspiration that is probably due to a sympathetic hyperactivity with consequent reflex spasm of the arterioles and venules, and increased sudomotor function.[1,3] Treatment should be largely supportive; apply heat and elevate to minimize swelling. If the thrombosis is localized to the superficial system, anticoagulants are not needed. However, if the deep venous system is also occluded, anticoagulants are definitely required.[4] In addition, sympathetic interruption may prove effective in decreasing the pain and edema. If anticoagulants are not being used, employ a cervicothoracic sympathetic block for the upper limb and a lumbar sympathetic block or continuous epidural analgesia for the lower limb. If anticoagulants are being used, achieve sympathetic interruption with the intravenous (IV) regional sympathetic block and guanethidine. Concomitant use of anticoagulants and regional anesthetic techniques, especially those that entail the injection into closed space such as the spinal canal, is contraindicated.

Cold injuries

Peripheral vascular disorders resulting from exposure to cold, such as trench foot and frostbite, are frequently characterized by initial and late vasospastic phases and an intermediate hyperemic phase.[3,4] Prompt institution of a continuous sympathetic block will probably relieve the symptoms of the first phase and may decrease the degree of tissue damage. In the late phase, vasospasm and the consequent coldness, pain, paresthesia, hyperhidrosis, and stiffness are chronic. Therefore although transient blocks are of diagnostic-prognostic value, the best therapeutic effects are produced by sympathectomy. However, even sympathectomy will not obviate amputation in severe cases with gangrene.

CHRONIC VASOSPASTIC DISORDERS
Raynaud's disease

Raynaud's disease is a relatively common clinical problem characterized by vasospasm of the microcirculation of the fingers unassociated with any other pathologic process.[1,3,4] The condition involves the digits of the upper extremity bilaterally, but there are patients who have the digits of all four extremities involved. The condition is manifested by intense whiteness of the fingers, which then turn blue and finally red during the rewarming process. With continuous precaution against exposure to cold, most of these patients can avoid tissue ischemia, which will eventually cause necrosis of the skin of the fingertips.

In Raynaud's disease and other chronic spastic disorders involving small arteries of the microcirculation, sympathetic blocks may be used as diagnostic and prognostic procedures (Fig. 38-1). Although prolonged improvement has been reported in some patients with these conditions after temporary sympathetic blocks, these blocks should be used primarily to determine the degree of vasospasm, especially if a sympathectomy is being considered. In unusual circumstances, chemical sympathectomy with phenol or alcohol

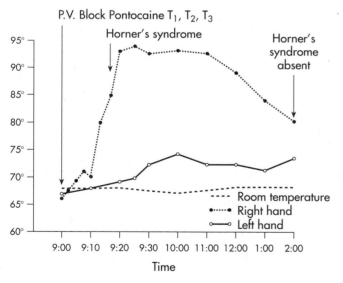

Fig. 38-1 Graph of skin temperature in a patient with Raynaud's disease in response to paravertebral sympathetic block. After the injection of 5 ml of 0.2% tetracaine (Pontocaine) through a needle placed at T_2 verterbral level, the patient developed Horner's syndrome and a maximal increase in skin temperature of the upper limb, which persisted for nearly 6 hours (indicating block of T_1-T_3).

has been substituted for surgery and has provided good results for several months. However, since most of these patients are relatively young and in good physical condition, they should be managed by either vasodilator drugs or by surgical sympathectomy.

Raynaud's phenomenon

Raynaud's phenomenon is characterized by the same symptomatology as Raynaud's disease but is caused by different underlying disorders. The condition usually is not bilateral, and primary therapy is directed toward the elimination of the underlying cause. If this is not possible and the vasospasm is intense and causes tissue necrosis, the patient should be treated with diagnostic sympathetic blocks. If these blocks produce adequate vasodilation and decrease or eliminate existing pain, then prolonged sympathetic interruption by chemical or surgical sympathectomy, or vasodilative drugs, should be considered.

Other disorders of microcirculation

Acrocyanosis is a vasospastic disorder manifested by persistent coldness, intense cyanosis, and frequently edema and hyperhidrosis. Some patients respond to repeated sympathetic blocks, but in persistent cases, sympathectomy will be necessary.

Livedo reticularis is characterized by marblelike mottling of the skin, that is aggravated by exposure to cold. Repeated sympathetic blocks may be tried to effect a cure. If these provide temporary relief, sympathectomy should be considered.

Erythromelalgia is almost the exact antithesis of Raynaud's disease and acrocyanosis. It is characterized by redness and burning pain in the extremities caused by abnormal vasodilation. Although the vessels are already abnormally dilated, sympathetic interruption may provide transient relief, and sympathectomy may produce prolonged benefits.[3] The basis for this beneficial effect is unknown.

Thromboangiitis obliterans (Buerger's disease)

Thromboangiitis obliterans was first described in 1908 by Buerger as a specific nonarteriosclerotic lesion involving arteries, veins, and nerves. This disease frequently leads to gangrene and tends to usually be limited to medium-sized arteries of the distal leg or arm. The condition occurs almost exclusively in young, cigarette-smoking males. It is usually bilateral and symmetric in involvement, and is manifested by instep claudication if the occlusion is in the leg, and hand claudication if the condition involves distal arteries of the arm and digits. At least half of the patients manifest sensitivity to cold. The most bothersome and most common pain problems are instep claudication and ischemic rest pain. Foot claudication is typical of the sequence of the walk → pain → rest → relief cycle. The ischemic rest pain, which involves the feet and toes or hands and fingers, is much more severe and unrelenting when it develops. It causes a very severe burning that is rarely helped by dependency.

The best therapy is total cessation of smoking, but unfortunately many of these patients are unable or unwilling to achieve this. Sympathetic interruption, particularly in the early stages of the disease, may indicate the degree of the reflex vasospasm associated with the obliterative process within the lumina of the vessels. For many of these patients, sympathetic block may give temporary relief of vasospasm and relief of pain, but it is of little or no value as a therapeutic measure in relieving claudication. On the other hand, chemical or surgical sympathectomy may be effective in relieving the rest pain and, for a small percentage of patients, in relieving the claudication. If sympathectomy is contemplated, several prognostic sympathetic blocks should be used to predict the effects of the prolonged interruption. In the past, skin temperature, oscillometric, and plethysmographic studies were used to select patients for sympathectomy; currently there has been more reliance on the walking tolerance test to establish the degree of increase in peripheral blood flow consequent to the sympatholytic procedure.

Arteriosclerosis obliterans

Occlusive arteriosclerotic disease of the lower limb vessels is the most common problem of patients seeking treatment for vascular insufficiency. This process produces a progressive decrease in tissue blood flow with consequent claudication, rest pain, incipient gangrene, or ulceration. In general, this condition is best treated by medical and surgical therapy. Vascular grafts that can bypass the obstruction of large- or medium-sized vessels in the limb have become important and widely used procedures and have decreased or postponed amputation. However, in patients for whom bypass graft surgery cannot be used because the obliterating vascular disorder is too extensive, sympathectomy is effective in relieving some of the symptomatology and postponing amputation.

Reid and associates,[5] Boas and co-workers,[6] and Cousins and Wright[7] found that chemical sympathectomy was preferred over surgical section, especially in debilitated patients suffering from severe cardiac or respiratory disease that would add a significant risk to anesthesia and surgical intervention. Moreover, since the results with chemical sympathectomy are very similar to those for surgical section, blocks are preferred even in patients in good physical condition. They can be administered on an outpatient basis, which allows the patient to rapidly return to the home environment, thus reducing postoperative morbidity (especially the risk of thrombosis associated with surgery and bed rest) and the duration and cost of hospitalization.

Clinicians who have had extensive experience with percutaneous chemical sympathectomy prefer using 7% or 10% phenol in Conray 420 and continuously monitoring the spread of the solution rather than 100% alcohol or 6% aqueous phenol because the incidence of severe neuralgia is significantly reduced. Best results have been achieved in patients whose primary complaint is rest pain not amenable to arterial reconstruction. In a series of 250 percutaneous chemical sympathectomies performed by Boas and associates,[6] 70% of the patients had rest pain; 30% had trophic changes with ulcerations, gangrenous changes, or both; and 25% had intermittent claudication. Long-term results included relieving rest pain in 75% of the patients (which they

stress was better than achieved with surgical sympathectomy), healing ischemic lesions in 60%, and improving claudication in only 30% of patients with this complaint. Transient lumbar neuralgia (presumably caused by involvement of somatic nerves) occurred in 7% of the patients. I have obtained similar results with lumbar chemical sympathectomy (Fig. 38-2).[1,3]

In a series of 386 patients reported by Cousins et al.,[8] rest pain was relieved completely in 49%, partially in 31%, and no relief was obtained in the remaining 20%. In those without preexisting gangrenous changes, 84% derived partial or complete pain relief compared to 56% with gangrenous lesions. The onset of pain relief coincided with the onset of sympathetic blockade (measured by cobalt sweat tests) and increased skin blood flow and temperature (as measured by thermocouples on both feet attached to a telethermometer and by occlusion plethysmography employed simultaneously in both feet before and after sympathetic block). Mean duration of pain relief (5.9 ± 0.6 months) was very similar to mean duration of sweat modification (6.0 ± 0 months). Two years after blockade 35% of the patients were alive and the skin was intact without evidence of ulcer or gangrene, 15% underwent reconstructive surgery, and 25% required either local debridement or major amputation within an average of 10 months after the block. Only 10% of the patients required repeat block on the same side within 3 to 12 months. The pain relief after the second block was always at least equal to the relief obtained after the first block.

SICKLE CELL DISEASE

Hemoglobin A, the predominant form of hemoglobin in red blood cells (RBCs), is composed of two α and two β subunits. Abnormal hemoglobins (Hb S) may result from an amino acid substitution in one of the chains. These hemoglobins can result in the formation of sickled RBCs under conditions of decreased oxygen tension. Homozygosity for Hb S occurs in 0.15% of black children and results clinically in sickle cell anemia.[9]

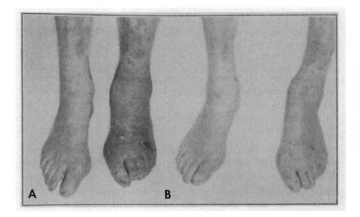

Fig. 38-2 Feet of a patient with arteriosclerosis obliterans and diabetes. **A,** Lesions of the left foot. **B,** 4 months after left lumbar sympathetic block with aqueous phenol. (From Bonica JJ: *The Management of Pain,* ed 2. Philadelphia, Lea & Febiger, 1990.)

Patients with sickle cell disease often manifest vasoocclusive phenomena, which are due to sludging in the microcirculation, with tissue hypoxia and infarction. These patients may experience episodic painful crises. The frequency and intensity of crises vary between patients with sickle cell disease, as well as in the same patient.[10] Factors associated with sickle crises include hypothermia, dehydration, exertion, hypoxemia, acidosis, and bacterial or viral infections.[9]

Acute pain may occur at multiple sites.[9] Abdominal pain in sickle crisis may be difficult to differentiate from causes of pain requiring acute surgical intervention (e.g., cholecystitis, appendicitis, bowel perforation). Patients may develop acute pleuritic chest pain with fever and occasionally infiltrates. Although thrombotic pulmonary infarction may occur, pneumonia in these immunocompromised patients must also be ruled out. Acute arthritis with synovial effusion can occur; this may be distinguished from a crystal or septic arthritis by joint fluid examination. Bone pain can be a frequent complaint. Rarely, males will develop painful priapism.

Patients with sickle cell disease may experience chronic pain, often related to recurrent vasoocclusive episodes.[9] Chronic hemolysis may lead to pigment gallstone formation with chronic cholecystitis. Pain related to orthopedic pathology may include vertebral compression fractures and aseptic necrosis of the femoral head. Osteomyelitis, often due to salmonella, can occur. Finally, chronic leg ulcers are frequently experienced by these patients.

Pain management of sickle cell disease can be quite difficult. Unfortunately, there is no specific treatment, and the lack of objective means to quantify disease activity requires the physician to treat the pain solely on the patient's report. Frequent encounters with health care providers often result in the impression that the patient is malingering or seeking drugs.[10]

Acute painful crises often require hospitalization. These patients are sometimes in so much pain that they are unable to move. Parenteral narcotics via intramuscular (IM) or subcutaneous routes should be given as needed, in addition to IV fluids, oxygen, and keeping the patient warm.[10] Continuous IV infusions of narcotics have also been successful, although close adjustment of the narcotic dose is necessary to decrease the incidence of problems.[11] Patient-controlled analgesia with narcotics can be effective, and in the future, may become standard therapy.[12]

Meperidine, for unclear reasons, is commonly given to patients with sickle cell disease.[10] Problems can arise with the use of meperidine in this population. The route of administration may be converted from parenteral to oral as the patient improves, but the low oral bioavailability is often not considered, and thus an inadequate dose of oral medication may be prescribed, which results in increased pain. Also, prolonged meperidine administration, particularly in the setting of sickle-associated renal dysfunction, can lead to agitation and even seizures from accumulation of the metabolite normeperidine.

Chronic pain, if not severe, can be managed with acetaminophen or nonsteroidal antiinflammatory drugs. Nonsteroidal antiinflammatory drugs, however, may cause renal failure in patients with borderline renal function. For more severe pain, narcotic analgesics are often necessary.[10] Hypertransfusion may prevent vasoocclusive crises but can expose the patient to the risks of iron overload and infections such as acquired immunodeficiency syndrome (AIDS) and hepatitis.[9]

HEMOPHILIA

Hemophilia is a congenital bleeding disorder. Hemophilia A, also known as classic hemophilia, is associated with a deficiency or abnormality of Factor VIII, whereas hemophilia B is related to a deficient or dysfunctional Factor IX. Both of these disorders are x-linked, and therefore occur almost exclusively in males. The incidence of classic hemophilia is one in 10,000 men.[13]

Hemophiliacs experience hemorrhages that can occur hours or days after trauma, involve any organ, and may persist for weeks. Patients often develop pain in a weight-bearing joint followed by swelling caused by a hemarthrosis.[13] Recurrent bleeding into the joint can lead to chronic hemophiliac arthropathy, which is characterized by osteoarthritis, articular fibrosis, joint ankylosis, and muscular atrophy.[13,14] Pain from an acute hemarthrosis can be severe but is otherwise similar to the pain associated with chronic arthropathy, and it can be difficult for adult hemophiliacs to distinguish.[14] Other sources of pain occurring in hemophiliacs include soft tissue and muscle hemorrhages that can result in compartment syndromes, pseudophlebitis, and ischemic neuropathy (e.g., occult retroperitoneal hematoma leading to a femoral neuropathy).

Primary therapy of hemorrhages consists of administering highly purified Factor VIII concentrates for classic hemophiliacs. Desmopressin can sometimes be helpful in hemophiliacs with mild disease because it elevates Factor VIII levels.[13] Narcotics may be necessary but should not be administered IM. Acetaminophen may be helpful, but nonsteroidal antiinflammatory drugs should be avoided because of antiplatelet effects that may increase bleeding. Joint aspiration after factor replacement occasionally may help to reduce pain and increase mobility.[15] Other therapies demonstrated to reduce pain in hemophiliacs include transcutaneous electrical nerve stimulation and relaxation techniques.[16,17]

In the past hemophiliacs were treated with pooled plasma products that were contaminated with human immunodeficiency virus (HIV). Consequently, a number of hemophiliacs developed AIDS. Hemophiliacs with AIDS are thus subject to developing the painful neurologic, rheumatologic, pulmonary, and gastrointestinal conditions seen in this disease.[18]

RHEUMATOID ARTHRITIS

Rheumatoid arthritis is a systemic illness that afflicts approximately 1% of the population.[19] It is usually insidious in onset, but it may occur with an acute presentation.[20] Onset of rheumatoid arthritis is more frequent in winter than summer. Most patients develop their initial symptoms between ages 30 and 50, and there appears to be an association between rheumatoid arthritis and the major histocompatibility antigen HLA-DR4.[19] Many patients tend to have a progressive, disabling, and destructive form of the disease, although some have an intermittent disease form, and rarely are there long remissions.[19] Diagnosis of rheumatoid arthritis is made on the basis of having four out of seven of the clinical criteria (Table 38-1). There is no benefit of early diagnosis because there is no evidence that early therapy improves prognosis. The small joints of the hand and wrist tend to be involved early. Other joints may become involved, including the cervical spine, temporomandibular joint, shoulder, elbow, hip, knee, ankle, and foot. There is an increased incidence of osteoporosis in rheumatoid arthritis; the role of low-dose glucocorticoids is unclear. Extraarticular manifestations of rheumatoid arthritis include rheumatoid nodules, anemia, eosinophilia, vasculitis involving multiple organs, pleuropulmonary nodules, interstitial pulmonary fibrosis, and pericarditis.[19,20]

The etiology of rheumatoid arthritis remains unknown.[20] Nevertheless, on pathologic examination, microvascular injury and an increase in the number of synovial lining cells appear early in rheumatoid arthritis. There is evidence of ongoing inflammation and immune activation. As the disease progresses, the synovium swells and villous projections protrude into the joint space. In time, the synovium erodes into bone and invades periarticular structures such as tendons and fascia.[21]

Patients with rheumatoid arthritis often have pain and stiffness involving multiple joints.[19] Pain appears to be due to stretching of the joint capsule from the accumulation of synovial fluid, hypertrophy of the synovium, and thickening of the joint capsule.[20] Pain in the affected joints typically worsens with movement, and the amount of pain from a given joint may not correlate with the degree of active inflammation. Stiffness usually occurs in the morning.[20] Joint tenderness may be present, particularly in the small hand and foot joints. The surrounding muscles may also be painful. Neck pain with radiation to the occiput and arm

paresthesias may be symptoms of atlantoaxial subluxation. Rotator cuff tears may lead to acute shoulder pain. Patients with rheumatoid arthritis may be prone to developing stress fractures of long bones, which can also cause acute pain. Rupture of a popliteal (Baker's) cyst can lead to calf pain that may mimic deep venous thrombosis.

The treatment of rheumatoid arthritis aims to relieve pain, reduce inflammation, preserve functional capacity, resolve the pathologic process, and facilitate healing.[20] A number of modalities besides drug therapy may be beneficial: rest and splinting; exercise can maintain muscle strength and joint mobility; and orthotic devices may decrease joint stress and therefore pain.

First-line drug therapy consists of using of salicylates and other nonsteroidal antiinflammatory drugs.[22] These agents can decrease pain and thus improve function; however, they do not interrupt disease progression. They should be taken in maximal doses. The nonsteroidal antiinflammatory drugs are no more effective than aspirin, but they may be better tolerated. If one agent is without effect, another nonsteroidal antiinflammatory drug, preferably of a different chemical class, should be tried. In addition, moderate doses of amitriptyline have also provided symptomatic relief, independent of its antidepressant effects.[23]

Patients on nonsteroidal antiinflammatory drugs who continue to have systemic and/or joint symptoms, evidence of joint or bone destruction on x-ray, loss of joint function, and persistent laboratory evidence of active inflammation may benefit from the addition of second-line agents.[22] These drugs are disease modifying because they may influence the progression of disease.[20] This class of medications includes gold compounds, antimalarials, D-penicillamine, and sulfasalazine, all of which have the potential for causing significant toxicity. In general, the less toxic drugs such as hydroxychloroquine or sulfasalazine should be tried ini-

Table 38-1 1988 Revised ARA criteria for classification of rheumatoid arthritis*

Criteria†	Definition
Morning stiffness	Morning stiffness in and around joints, lasting at least 1 hour before maximal improvement.
Arthritis of three or more joint areas	At least three joint areas simultaneously have soft tissue swelling or fluid (not bony overgrowth alone) observed by physician. The 14 possible joint areas are (right or left): PIP, MCP, wrist, elbow, heel, ankle, and MTP joints.
Arthritis of hand joints	At least one joint area swollen (see above) in wrist, MCP, or PIP joint.
Symmetric arthritis	Simultaneous involvement of the same joint areas (as in Item 2 above) on both sides of the body. (Bilateral involvement of PIP, MCP, or MTP joints is acceptable without absolute symmetry.)
Rheumatoid nodules	Subcutaneous nodules, over bony prominences, or extensor surfaces, or in juxtaarticular regions, observed by physician.
Serum rheumatoid factor	Demonstration of abnormal amounts of serum rheumatoid factor by any method that has been positive in less then 5% of normal control subjects.
Radiographic changes	Radiographic changes typical of rheumatoid arthritis on PA hand and wrist x-rays, which must include erosions or unequivocal bony decalcification localized to or most marked adjacent to involved joints (osteoarthritis changes alone do not qualify).

From Lewis MS, Hill S Jr, Warfield C: Medical diseases causing pain. In Raj PP, editor: *Practical Management of Pain,* ed 2. St Louis, Mosby, 1992.
PIP, posterior interphalangeal; MCP, metacarpophalangeal; MTP, metatarsophalangeal; PA, posteroanterior.
*For classification purposes, a patient is said to have rheumatoid arthritis if he or she has satisfied at least four of the above seven criteria.
†Criteria: Items 1 through 4 must be present for at least 6 weeks. Patients with two clinical diagnoses are not excluded. Designation as classic, definite, or probably rheumatoid arthritis is not to be made.

tially.[22] The effects of these agents may take months to occur; therefore nonsteroidal antiinflammatory drugs should be continued during this period.

It may be necessary to add low doses of oral glucocorticoids (e.g., < 7.5 mg daily of prednisone) for "bridge" therapy until the disease-modifying agent becomes effective.[22] If there is no significant response, long-term, low-dose therapy with glucocorticoid may be needed. Steroids can decrease pain and inflammation; however, they do not affect disease progression. An occasional acutely inflamed joint may also benefit from an intraarticular injection of depot steroid.

Patients with refractory disease may be candidates for immunosuppressive therapy.[20] Drugs that have been used include methotrexate, cyclophosphamide, and azathioprine. Low-dose methotrexate is sometimes used earlier in the course of rheumatoid arthritis because it appears to be well-tolerated. Gastrointestinal and hepatic toxicities are potential problems with weekly methotrexate administration.[22] The immunosuppressants do not appear to be more effective than disease-modifying groups.

Surgery may be a last resort for rheumatoid arthritis patients, with total joint replacement for structural joint damage.[24] Major indications include intolerable pain or prohibitive limitation of function, and the goals are to relieve pain, correct deformity, and improve function.[19,24] Surgery should not be taken lightly, because the risks include infection, prosthesis loosening with recurrence of pain, and possible cervical spinal cord damage if there is neck manipulation during intubation in a patient with atlantoaxial instability. Hand surgery can also be performed for joint instability or tendon rupture.

PANCREATITIS

Acute pancreatitis is associated with multiple causes (Box 38-1), although alcohol abuse and cholelithiasis account for most cases.[25] It is characterized by poorly localized, steady, dull or drilling epigastric or left upper quadrant pain that may radiate to the back and appears to lessen when sitting up and/or flexing the spine.[25,26] The pain reaches maximum intensity within 15 minutes to an hour and usually lasts 3 to 7 days. Physical examination may reveal epigastric discomfort with deep palpation but the absence of peritoneal signs because this is initially a retroperitoneal process. Nausea and vomiting, ileus, fever, shock, respiratory failure, disseminated intravascular coagulation (DIC), flank (Grey-Turner's sign) or periumbilical (Cullen's sign) hematomas, hyperglycemia, and hypocalcemic tetany from retroperitoneal saponification may ensue. The diagnosis of acute pancreatitis is based on the clinical history and examination, as well as possible elevated serum amylase and/or lipase levels. Radiologic studies that may be helpful include plain abdominal x-rays, ultrasound (possibly showing biliary or pancreatic duct pathology or peripancreatic edema), endoscopic retrograde (cholangiopancreatography), or CT scan.[25,27]

Acute pancreatitis is due to autodigestion by premature release of activated proteolytic pancreatic enzymes.[25] What causes the activation of these enzymes currently remains unknown. That the pancreas lacks a well-developed capsule

---

Box 38-1 CONDITIONS ASSOCIATED WITH ACUTE PANCREATITIS[25]

Cholelithiasis
Ethanol abuse
Idiopathic conditions
Medications
Abdominal operations
Hyperlipidemia
Injection into pancreatic duct
Trauma
Hypercalcemia
Pregnancy
Peptic ulcer
Outflow obstruction
Pancreas divisum
Organ transplantation
End-stage renal failure
Hereditary conditions (e.g., familial pancreatitis)
Scorpion bite
Miscellaneous: hypoperfusion, viral infections, mycoplasma pneumonia infection, intraductal parasites

---

and is located retroperitoneally explains why the destructive inflammatory process may also involve the duodenum, terminal common bile duct, splenic artery and vein, spleen, mesocolon, greater omentum, small bowel mesentery, the celiac and superior mesenteric ganglia, the lesser omental sac, the posterior mediastinum, the perirenal spaces, and the diaphragm.

Therapy for acute pancreatitis is largely supportive, as randomized, controlled trials have not demonstrated a decrease in morbidity or mortality for any specific type of therapy.[25] Indomethacin relieves pain but can possibly increase hemorrhage caused by the antiplatelet effects, so it may be relatively contraindicated. Narcotics should be administered if needed, although they are capable of inducing biliary spasm. In equianalgesic doses, morphine causes less of an increase in common bile duct pressures than meperidine or fentanyl.[28] A lower thoracic epidural block with a local anesthetic may also produce adequate analgesia.[29]

Chronic pancreatitis is characterized by recurrent or persistent abdominal pain, with evidence in some patients of pancreatic exocrine or endocrine insufficiency in the absence of pain.[30] Although the pathogenesis of chronic pancreatitis is not known, more than 90% of patients with this diagnosis have a history of associated alcohol abuse. Physical examination may reveal an underweight, malnourished individual with epigastric tenderness. Pathologically, chronic pancreatitis is characterized by irregular sclerosis of the gland; inflammation and destruction of exocrine tissue in a focal, segmental, or diffuse pattern with stricturing and dilatation of the pancreatic ducts; and intraductal protein plugs and calculi. Endocrine tissue (islets of Langerhan's) is destroyed slower than exocrine (acinar) tissue. These morphologic changes are usually progressive and irreversible and accompany the incurability of chronic pancreatitis.

Pain is the most common feature of chronic pancreatitis.[30] There is no correlation between morphology and the degree of pain experienced by the patient.[31] Theories to explain the pain of chronic pancreatitis include increased ductal pressure and pancreatitis-associated neuritis. Patients may experience recurrent bouts of acute pancreatitis and should be treated as mentioned previously.[30] Patients usually develop intermittent or persistent abdominal pain similar to that experienced in acute episodes. Pain may be precipitated by eating or lying supine. Drinking alcohol may also precipitate pain attacks, although the effects of long-term abstinence on severity and frequency of alcohol-related chronic pancreatitis are unclear. These patients should be treated with simple analgesics and if necessary, narcotics. Supplementation with trypsin-containing pancreatic enzymes may decrease pain (and malabsorption); this may be due to suppression of cholecystokinin-stimulated pancreatic secretion.[32] Some patients have derived long-term relief from neurolytic celiac plexus blocks, although studies have shown a lack of long-term benefit.[30,33] It is important to remember that the pain of chronic pancreatitis may "burn out" as endocrine and exocrine function diminish.[30]

Surgical management of pain may be considered for constant disabling pain that interferes with lifestyle, or several relapses of substantial pain per year, and failure to respond to the conservative medical program mentioned previously.[30] Patients with dilated pancreatic duct systems (demonstrated radiographically) may benefit from drainage procedures such as a longitudinal pancreaticojejunostomy. Patients who fail drainage procedures or patients with small pancreatic ducts may have good pain relief with resections. The nature of disease of the pancreas (diffuse versus localized) determines which type of operation to perform. Possible types of resection include limited resection, subtotal resection, total pancreatectomy, and partial pancreaticoduodenectomy (Whipple's procedure). Another approach that may offer promise is complete denervation of the pancreas by resection of the postganglionic nerves.[34]

REFERENCES

1. Bonica JJ: *The Management of Pain*. Philadelphia, Lea & Febiger, 1953.
2. Loh L, Nathan PW: Painful peripheral states and sympathetic blocks. *J Neurol Neurosurg Psychiatry* 41:664-671, 1978.
3. Bonica JJ: *Clinical Applications of Diagnostic and Therapeutic Nerve Blocks*. Springfield, Ill, Charles C Thomas, 1959.
4. Strandness DE Jr: *Peripheral Arterial Disease: A Physiologic Approach*. Boston, Little, Brown, 1969.
5. Reid W, Watt JK, Gray ThG: Phenol injection of the sympathetic chain. *Br J Surg* 57:45, 1970.
6. Boas RA, Hatangdi VS, Richards EG: Lumbar sympathectomy—A percutaneous chemical technique. In Bonica JJ, Albe-Fessard D, editors: *Advances in Pain Research and Therapy, vol 1*. New York, Raven Press, 1976.
7. Cousins MJ, Wright CJ: Graft, muscle, skin blood flow after epidural block in vascular surgical procedures. *Surg Gynecol Obstet* 133:59-64, 1971.
8. Cousins MJ et al: Neurolytic lumbar sympathetic blockade: Duration of denervation and relief of rest pain. *Anaesth Intensive Care* 7:2, 121-135, 1979.
9. Bunn HF: Disorders of hemoglobin. In Wilson JD et al, editors: *Harrison's Principles of Internal Medicine*, ed 12. New York, McGraw-Hill, 1991.
10. Benjamin LJ: Pain in sickle cell disease. In Foley KM, Payne RM, editors: *Current Therapy of Pain*. Philadelphia, BC Decker, 1989.
11. Cole TB et al: Intravenous narcotic therapy for children with severe sickle pain crises. *Am J Dis Child* 140:1255-1259, 1986.
12. Schecter NL, Berrien FB, Katz SM: The use of patient-controlled analgesia in adolescents with sickle cell pain crisis: A preliminary report. *J Pain Symptom Manage* 3:109-113, 1988.
13. Handin RI: Disorders of coagulation and thrombosis. In Wilson JD et al, editors: *Harrison's Principles of Internal Medicine*, ed 12. New York, McGraw-Hill, 1991.
14. Choiniere M, Melzack R: Acute and chronic pain in hemophilia. *Pain* 31:317-331, 1987.
15. Tyler DC: Pain in infants and children. In Bonica JJ, editor: *The Management of Pain*, ed 2. Philadelphia, Lea & Febiger, 1990.
16. Roche PA et al: Modification of haemophiliac haemorrhage pain by transcutaneous electric nerve stimulation. *Pain* 21:43-48, 1985.
17. Varni JW: Behavioral medicine in hemophilia arthritis pain management: Two case studies. *Arch Phys Med Rehabil* 62:183-187, 1981.
18. Lewis MS, Warfield CA: Management of pain in AIDS. *Hosp Prac (Off Ed)* 25(10A):51-54, 1990.
19. Harris ED: The clinical features of rheumatoid arthritis. In Kelley WN et al, editors: *Textbook of Rheumatology*, ed 3. Philadelphia, WB Saunders, 1989.
20. Lipsky PE: Rheumatoid arthritis. In Wilson JD et al, editors: *Harrison's Principles of Internal Medicine*, ed 12. New York, McGraw-Hill, 1991.
21. Bennett JC: Rheumatoid arthritis. In Wyndgaarden JB, Smith LH, editors: *Cecil Textbook of Medicine*, ed 17. Philadelphia, WB Saunders, 1985.
22. Harris ED: Management of rheumatoid arthritis. In Kelley WN et al, editors: *Textbook of Rheumatology*, ed 3. Philadelphia, WB Saunders, 1989.
23. Frank RG et al: Antidepressant analgesia in rheumatoid arthritis. *J Rheumatol* 15:1632-1638, 1988.
24. Docken WP, Warfield CA: Rheumatologic causes of pain: Rheumatoid arthritis. *Hosp Prac (Off Ed)* 23(1):57-66, 1988.
25. Soergel KH: Acute pancreatitis. In Sleisinger M, Fordtran JS, editors: *Gastrointestinal Disease: Pathophysiology, Diagnosis, Management*, ed 4. Philadelphia, WB Saunders, 1989.
26. Lankisch PG: Diagnosis of abdominal pain: How to distinguish between pancreatic and extrapancreatic causes. *Eur J Surg* 156:273-278, 1990.
27. Lunderquist A: Imaging in pancreatic pain. *Eur J Surg* 156:279-280, 1990.
28. Radnay PA et al: The effect of equi-analgesic doses of fentanyl, morphine, meperidine, and pentazocine on common bile duct pressure. *Anaesthesist* 29:26-29, 1980.
29. Mulholland MW, Debas HT, Bonica JJ: Diseases of the liver, biliary system, and pancreas. In Bonica JJ, editor: *The Management of Pain*, ed 2. Philadelphia, Lea & Febiger, 1990.
30. Grendell JH, Cello JP: Chronic pancreatitis. In Sleisinger M, Fordtran JS, editors: *Gastrointestinal Disease: Pathophysiology, Diagnosis, Management*, ed 4. Philadelphia, WB Saunders, 1989.
31. Ihse I: Pancreatic pain. *Br J Surg* 77:121-122, 1990.
32. Ihse I, Permeth J: Enzyme therapy and pancreatic pain. *Eur J Surg* 156:281-283, 1990.
33. Bengtsson M, Löfström JB: Nerve block in pancreatic pain. *Eur J Surg* 156:285-291, 1990.
34. Hiraoka T et al: A new surgical approach for control of pain in chronic pancreatitis: Complete denervation of the pancreas. *Am J Surg* 152:549-551, 1986.

QUESTIONS: ACUTE MEDICAL DISEASES

1. A sudden circulatory insufficiency in the limb caused by trauma or embolism can initiate:
   A. Reflex dilatation of the collateral vessels
   B. Reflex spasm of the collateral vessels
   C. Decreased afferent fiber nociceptive activity to the CNS
   D. Decreased efferent fiber activity to the periphery

2. Acute venous thrombosis (thrombophlebitis) encompasses a spectrum of signs or symptoms that include severe pain, marked edema, and excessive perspiration. If anticoagulants are being used for the treatment of this condition, the option available for increasing vascularity and pain relief to the effected limb is:
   A. Lumbar sympathetic block (lower extremity)
   B. Epidural local anesthetic infusion
   C. Oral narcotics
   D. Intravenous regional guanethidine injection

3. A specific nonarteriosclerotic lesion involving arteries, veins, and nerves that frequently leads to gangrene and confines itself to medium-sized arteries of the distal leg or the arm is due to:
   A. Thromboangiitis obliterans
   B. Thrombophlebitis
   C. Diabetic gangrene
   D. Frostbite

4. Patients with sickle cell disease can experience episodic painful crises, which are characterized by:
   A. Hypothermia
   B. Normoxemia
   C. Acidosis
   D. Dehydration

5. A congenital bleeding disorder that is X linked and occurs almost exclusively in men and is due to deficiency of Factor IX is known as
   A. Sickle cell disease
   B. Hemophilia B
   C. Hemophilia A
   D. Von Recklinghausen's disease

ANSWERS

1. B
2. D
3. A
4. B
5. B

39 Headache and Facial Pain

Steven D. Waldman

Headache is the most common medical complaint encountered in clinical practice. It has been estimated that more than 40 million Americans have headaches severe enough to require medical care. This chapter provides physicians with a practical approach to the evaluation and treatment of common headache and facial pain syndromes encountered in clinical practice. By gaining an understanding of each of these conditions, physicians can ease anxiety when evaluating and treating this group of patients.

TAKING A TARGETED HISTORY

The most important portion of the evaluation of the patient suffering from headache and facial pain syndromes is obtaining a targeted history. From responses to targeted questions, a specific constellation of symptoms should emerge, allowing the physician to make an accurate diagnosis. Failure to obtain a targeted history can lead to ill-advised treatment and, in some situations, failure to recognize life-threatening disease.

In simplistic terms, the targeted history allows physicians to determine sick from well. If it is determined that in all probability the patient is well (i.e., that no life-threatening illness exists), the workup and treatment plan may proceed at a more conservative pace. Obviously, if the targeted history points to a life-threatening disease process, an aggressive course of action is indicated.

The following areas of historical information should be explored, not only to distinguish sick patients from well ones, but also to try to ascertain the specific diagnosis.

Chronicity

The length of illness sets the direction of the initial history and carries much weight in determining sick from well. For this reason, it serves as the starting point of the targeted history. In general, headaches that have been present for 20 to 30 years are in and of themselves not associated with progressive and life-threatening neurologic disease. Instead, this would indicate a self-limited pain syndrome, and hence a well determination. Conversely, sudden onset of severe headache or a change in the character of a headache or facial pain syndrome that has been stable for many years must be considered to fall in the category of sick until proven otherwise. This type of pain manifestation has often been called the "first or worst" syndrome.[1] Patients who fall within this category deserve a high level of concern, and their pain should be viewed as a medical emergency (Box 39-1).

Age at onset

Headaches that begin in childhood through the second decade of life are most often vascular in nature. Statistically, headaches and facial pain that begin later in life are most commonly psychogenic ills, such as tension-type headache, nonneuralgic atypical facial pain, and fibromyalgia.[2] Two notable exceptions to this rule are trigeminal neuralgia (rarely seen before the third decade unless associated with multiple sclerosis) and temporal arteritis (the incidence of which increases markedly during the fifth and sixth decades).[3]

Duration and frequency of pain

Duration and frequency of pain provide the best clues to classification and diagnosis. In general, vascular headaches and trigeminal neuralgia tend to occur in an episodic fashion, with the duration of pain ranging from minutes in the case of cluster headache and trigeminal neuralgia to hours in the case of migraine. Cluster headache may be seasonal, with peak occurrences in the spring and fall.[4] Headaches and facial pain of organic origin (e.g., sinus disease, brain tumor) tend to be continuous and acutely can be exacerbated by exercise, change in position, and Valsalva's maneuver. These pain syndromes worsen over time if the underlying organic disease is not correctly diagnosed and treated or if the disease does not resolve spontaneously. Pain that is present on a daily basis and persists for months to years most likely falls under the category of tension-type headache or nonneuralgic atypical facial pain.

Onset-to-peak time

When coupled with the information obtained in the duration and frequency portion of the targeted history, the onset-to-peak time may help narrow the diagnostic possibilities (Fig. 39-1). A rapid onset-to-peak time (seconds to minutes) should increase suspicion of organic disease. Of particular concern are headaches that worsen with activities like exercise, Valsalva's maneuver, and bending forward (see Box 39-1). Notable exceptions to this rule are cluster headache and trigeminal neuralgia.

Migraine tends to evolve over several hours, with neurologic symptoms occurring early after onset in the migraine sufferer with aura. As mentioned earlier, cluster headache has a much more rapid onset to peak.

Box 39-1 FACTORS THAT CAUSE CONCERN

New headache of recent onset ("the first")
New headache of unusual severity ("the worst")
Headache associated with neurologic dysfunction
Headache associated with systemic illness (especially infection)
Headache that peaks rapidly
Headache associated with exertion
Focal headache
Sudden change in a previously stable headache pattern
Headache associated with Valsalva's maneuver
Nocturnal headache

Tension-type headache and nonneuralgic atypical facial pain evolve over a period of hours to days and then tend to remain constant.

Location

The location of headache or facial pain may provide additional information about the classification and diagnosis of the patient's pain syndrome. Pain localized to an anatomic structure should be evaluated in the context of common disease entities for that structure (e.g., otitis media, dental pain).

Vascular headache is usually unilateral, although the side may change from attack to attack. Cluster headache is usually localized to the ocular and retroocular region, whereas migraine tends to involve the entire hemicranium. Temporal arteritis is localized to the temple, but jaw claudication while chewing and generalized aching may confuse the presentation.

Tension-type headache is usually bilateral but can be unilateral, and it may be manifested as a band or caplike tightness in the the frontal, temporal, and occipital regions. Associated neck symptomatology often coexists.

Trigeminal neuralgia generally involves only one division of the trigeminal nerve (>98%).[5] If localization of pain overlaps anatomic distribution, nonneuralgic atypical facial pain, referred pain, or local pathology is a more likely explanation.

Character and severity of pain

Although there is considerable overlap in character and severity of pain, some generalizations can be made when taking a targeted history. Vascular headaches tend to be throbbing and pulsatile, with a pain intensity often described as intense. Cluster headache may have a deeper drilling and burning quality. This pain is reputed to be among the worst pains known. Trigeminal neuralgia is typically described as paroxysmal, jablike or shocklike pain, and nonneuralgic atypical facial pain is often described as a dull, nagging ache. Tension-type headache is described as a persistent dull ache, with a constant baseline level of pain and occasional severe exacerbations. Headache associated with lumbar puncture will worsen when the patient assumes the recumbent position.

Premonitory symptoms and aura

Premonitory symptoms and aura are usually associated with vascular headaches, specifically migraine. Premonitory symptoms usually precede the migraine attack by 2 to 48 hours and can include fatigue, elation, depression, changes in libido, craving for certain foods, or abnormal hunger. These premonitory symptoms occur before an attack of migraine without aura (previously called *common migraine*) or before the onset of aura in migraine with aura (previously called *classic migraine*).

Aurae are manifested by focal cerebral dysfunction. Most aurae are ocular symptoms originating in the visual cortex of the occipital lobe, and they are presumably due to localized ischemia of this region. Other examples of aurae include disturbances of smell, feeling, or motor function (Box 39-2).

Associated symptoms

The targeted history should include questions regarding other symptoms associated with the painful condition reported. Photophobia, sonophobia, nausea, vomiting, aversion to strong odors, and focal neurologic changes may be seen with migraine.[6] These symptoms may also be seen with other headache and facial pain syndromes. Cluster headache is frequently accompanied by symptoms of complete or partial Horner's syndrome: lacrimation, heavy rhinorrhea, and blanching of the face on the affected side.[2,4]

After the onset of subarachnoid hemorrhage, meningeal signs and the focal neurologic changes of stroke will occur rapidly. Tinnitus or hearing loss in patients with trigeminal neuralgia may indicate an underlying brainstem tumor.[7] Weakness, bowel or bladder difficulties, and sudden visual loss in patients suffering from trigeminal neuralgia may suggest coexisting multiple sclerosis (MS).

Precipitating factors

Migraine headache may be triggered by a change in diet or sleep habits, tyramine-containing foods, monosodium glutamate, nitrates, alcohol, hormones and/or oral contraceptives, fatigue, stress, menstruation, underlying tension-type headache, strong odors, and bright sunlight. Tension-type headache is usually triggered by underlying environmental or physiologic stress, depression, fatigue, and abnormalities of the cervical spine. Like migraine, cluster headache may be triggered by alcohol, high altitude, and, occasionally, vasodilating substances. Nonneuralgic atypical facial pain may be caused by stress, bruxism, prolonged dental work, and, occasionally, poorly fitting dental appliances.

Environmental factors

As mentioned previously, contact with vasodilating substances through diet, the skin, or the respiratory tract may precipitate vascular headache. Stress and pressure in the workplace, video display terminals, industrial fumes, carbon monoxide, high altitude, and airborne contaminants carried by heating and cooling systems also have been implicated as precipitating factors for headache.

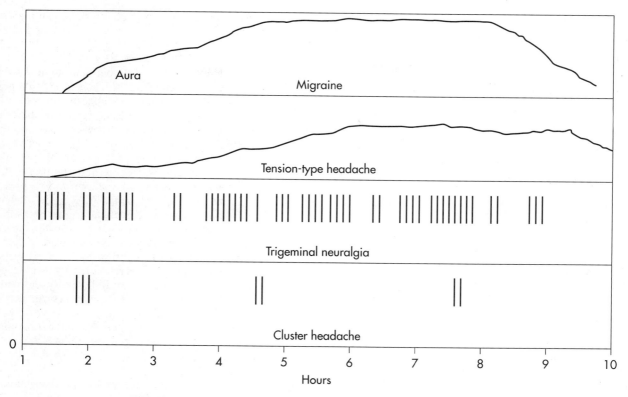

Fig. 39-1 Peak-to-onset profile in headache and facial pain syndromes.

Box 39-2 COMMONLY OCCURRING AURAE

Ocular symptoms
Fortification spectra (teichopsia)
Flashing lights (photopsia)
Scotomata
Hemianopia
Visual hallucinations

Auditory symptoms
Auditory hallucinations

Olfactory symptoms
Olfactory hallucinations

Motor and sensory symptoms
Weakness
Paresthesia

Family history

Migraine is a familial disease. If both parents suffer from migraine, there is a 70% to 75% chance that their children will have migraine.[3] If only one parent suffers from the disease, the incidence in offspring drops to 45%. Cluster headache, trigeminal neuralgia, and nonneuralgic atypical facial pain do not appear to be familial in nature.

Pregnancy and menstruation

Migraine may commonly occur with the onset of menses. Interestingly, it appears that pregnancy provides some amelioration of migraine headache after the first trimester. Menopause usually has the same effect; the migraine headache may disappear or decrease markedly in intensity and frequency. Hormone therapy at the time of menopause may prolong the headache syndrome.[8]

Some migraine headaches worsen with the initiation of oral contraceptives. There has been concern that the use of these drugs in migraine sufferers may increase the incidence of stroke, especially in patients who experience focal neurologic symptoms as part of an aura. This risk may be further increased if the patient is also a smoker.

Other forms of contraception usually provide a more favorable risk-to-benefit ratio in this group of patients. Therefore migraine sufferers should avoid oral contraceptives whenever possible.

Medical/surgical history

Headache can be a symptom of most systemic illnesses. Question the patient regarding infection; previous malignancy; medications that may cause headaches (including topical nitroglycerin); trauma; previous cranial surgery; recent lumbar puncture or myelogram; diseases of the eye, ear, nose, throat, and cervical spine; anemia; thyroid disease; travel out of the country; changes in food, sleep, workplace, and job; and, most important, environmental stress. The answers may offer important clues.

Past treatments

Many facial pain and headache sufferers have tried various treatment modalities in an effort to relieve pain. In evaluating the success or failure of each of these treatment techniques, the physician must decide what type of treatment will be beneficial and the probable diagnosis of the pain syndrome being treated.

Previous diagnostic tests

Physicians must evaluate adequacy, validity, age, and quality of previous testing when deciding whether additional testing is indicated. Factors that indicate additional testing include a change in a previously stable headache or facial pain problem, onset of a new headache or facial pain problem, discovery of a new systemic illness that may be contributing to or causing the pain problem, or new neurologic findings.

PERFORMING A TARGETED PHYSICAL EXAMINATION

As mentioned previously, the targeted history is the first and most important step in diagnosing the headache and facial pain patient. In the physical examination, the patient's history helps direct the pain management specialist to look for physical findings that could be associated with the pain syndrome being considered. Although in the vast majority of headache and facial pain patients the physical exam will be within normal limits, this can never be assumed. A careful examination for findings related to the pain problem or other systemic illness is mandatory for every patient being evaluated. Failure to carefully examine the patient or relying solely on history, laboratory, and radiographic findings will put the patient at extreme risk.

General appearance

The first step in the physical examination is to assess the general appearance of the patient. Evaluating the patient for depression, anxiety, and general physical appearance may yield valuable information about possible underlying psychopathology.

Examination of the head

Carefully examine the head for (1) previous surgical scars; (2) local infection; (3) occult tumor (especially intraoral and salivary gland); (4) hardened and tender temporal arteries; (5) sinus tenderness; (6) tenderness of the occipital nerves; (7) myofascial trigger points; (8) trigger areas of trigeminal and glossopharyngeal neuralgia; (9) dental and periodontal disease; (10) ocular anterior chamber disease; and (11) range of motion abnormalities of the temporomandibular joint.

Cervical spine

Abnormality of the cervical spine is probably a much more common etiologic factor in headache and facial pain than is recognized. Carefully examine the cervical spine for decreased or faulty range of motion, tenderness to palpation, presence of spasm and/or myofascial trigger points of the cervical paraspinous musculature, and evidence of occult infection or malignancy in all patients. Examine the extremities for radicular and myelopathic signs that may suggest cervical spine disease.

Cranial nerve evaluation

Examine all cranial nerves to rule out neurologic dysfunction in all patients suffering from headache and facial pain.[9] Specific areas to target include any abnormalities of olfaction, which may suggest tumor in the region of the cribriform plate or temporal lobe. Carefully evaluate the optic nerve for papilledema, loss of peripheral vision, and hypertensive or diabetic retinal changes. Palsies of the trochlear, oculomotor, and abducens nerves suggest significant intracranial pathology, and may also be present in low-pressure headache secondary to cerebrospinal (CSF) loss after myelography or lumbar puncture. Evaluate trigger areas in the distribution of the trigeminal nerve, and assess the presence of corneal anesthesia in all patients who were surgically treated for trigeminal pain. In addition, look for postherpetic scarring. Motor test the facial nerve to identify residual deficits secondary to previous stroke or Bell's palsy, or to eliminate intracranial pathology. Since the auditory nerve is frequently affected along with the trigeminal nerve in posterior fossa tumor, carefully evaluate for unilateral tinnitus and deafness to rule out acoustic neuroma.

Sensory examination

The presence of numbness after a radicular distribution in the upper extremity may suggest cervical spine disease that could be wholly or partly responsible for some headache syndromes.[2] Distal symmetric sensory deficit may suggest diabetic or ischemic neuropathy. Allodynia of the face and anterior triangle of the neck, especially in the presence of antecedent trauma, is suggestive of facial reflex sympathetic dystrophy.[10] Dysesthesias in the trigeminal distribution may suggest previous trigeminal herpes zoster. Trigger areas in the distribution of the trigeminal nerves are highly suggestive of trigeminal neuralgia. Exaggerated pain after application of hot or cold to a suspect tooth may ascertain the presence of dental pathology.

Motor examination

A motor deficit in the upper extremity after a radicular distribution suggests cervical spine disease, which may be wholly or partly responsible for some headache syndromes.[11] Poor fine motor coordination may suggest cerebellar dysfunction based on ischemia or tumor. Muscle wasting or atrophy may suggest lower motor neuron disease. Weakness of muscles of facial expression may indicate a painful Bell's palsy or previous stroke.

Reflexes

The pain management specialist should evaluate deep tendon and superficial reflexes to assess upper and lower motor neuron function. Reflex abnormalities may indicate radiculopathy, neuropathy, myelopathy, and demyelinating disease.

DIAGNOSTIC TESTING

The headache and facial pain patient may represent the most overtested group of patients in medicine today. Three important points must be stressed regarding testing in this group of patients:

1. Explain negative test results to the patient, negative findings are good in that they help rule out life-threatening disease.
2. Negative test results do not mean that the patient is not suffering from real pain.
3. Negative test results simply indicate that at the time the test was taken the findings were reported as negative. It is imperative that the pain management specialist understands this and immediately retests when new headache or facial pain symptoms occur in acute systemic illness (especially infection), or in changing or deteriorating neurologic findings.

Laboratory testing

Laboratory testing is generally ordered to rule out unsuspected systemic illness where headache or facial pain may be featured. A complete blood count (CBC) should be performed to rule out the presence of anemia associated with collagen vascular disease or other chronic illnesses.[12] Patients with primary or secondary polycythemia may present with headache as an initial complaint. White blood cell count with differential is important if acute or chronic infection is considered. Complete blood chemistries eliminate unsuspected renal or liver disease, diabetes, etc. Urinalysis may reveal occult renal pathology, glycosuria associated with diabetes, or proteinuria associated with collagen vascular disease, hypertension, or diabetes. Perform a sedimentation rate on any patient suspected of having temporal arteritis.[13] Order specific laboratory testing, such as thyroid function studies, if there is a clinical suspicion of abnormality.

Radiographic testing

Plain skull radiographs provide limited but useful information to evaluate the patient suffering from headache and facial pain. Skull radiographs can show bony abnormalities, including osteomyelitis, metastatic disease, occult fracture, temporomandibular joint disease, and erosion or enlargement of the sella turcica. Routine use of this test has been largely supplanted by computed tomography (CT) scan and, more recently, magnetic resonance imaging (MRI). Radiographs should be reserved for evaluating the previously mentioned problems and acute trauma.

Computed tomography

The CT scan has completely revolutionized the evaluation of the headache and facial pain patient. It rapidly identifies a wide variety of life-threatening conditions that previously could only be demonstrated by risky and highly invasive procedures such as pneumoencephalography and arteriography, or conditions that could only be diagnosed after significant CNS compromise had occurred.[9] Perform a CT scan on headache and facial pain patients when: (1) targeted history and physical examination suggest an intracranial lesion; (2) pain occurs in the presence of neurologic dysfunction, seizures, hemiplegia, loss of consciousness, personality change, or fever; (3) headache or facial pain is associated with trauma; (4) previously stable headaches or facial

pain have changed character; and (5) headaches or facial pain fail to respond to a rational treatment program. The pain management specialist should not hesitate to repeat CT scanning every 24 hours (or less if indicated) in the patient whose clinical condition continues to deteriorate, especially in those patients in whom infectious cause is a prime consideration.

Magnetic resonance imaging

The indications for MRI in headache and facial pain patients closely parallel the indications for CT scanning. The relative merits of each of these worthwhile diagnostic modalities have been greatly debated. Although there is considerable overlap in the information provided by CT scanning and MRI, MRI may be the test of choice in the following settings[9]:

1. MRI can demonstrate white matter plaque formation associated with MS that is not seen on CT scanning.
2. MRI provides superior imaging of the posterior fossa and brainstem relative to CT. Since tumors and demyelinating disease in this anatomic region are a consideration when evaluating patients with trigeminal neuralgia, MRI is probably the most useful test in this setting.
3. MRI produces better images of the cervical spine than CT.

Therefore MRI should be used when evaluating cervicogenic headache.

Because of the time and expense involved with this diagnostic modality, it should not be used as a routine screening tool for the chronic headache and facial pain sufferer.

Electroencephalogram and evoked potential testing

The electroencephalogram (EEG) and evoked potential are neurophysiologic tests that are useful in the evaluation of selected headache and facial pain patients. An EEG can evaluate the rare headache patient whose headaches appear to be related to seizure disorder; it is also indicated if an infectious cause is being considered.[14] The EEG may become positive quite early in viral encephalitis, long before the CT scan (a neuroanatomic test) reveals abnormality. The EEG may also reveal focal lesions, although the specificity in this indication is low.

Evoked potential testing is indicated as a confirmatory test in the patient with facial pain in whom MS is suspected.[9] Brainstem-evoked potentials may also be used in this group of patients to assess the integrity of brainstem function if tumor is suspected. Somatosensory-evoked potential testing may be used to assess the presence of myelopathy in the patient with cervical spondylosis who is suffering from cervicogenic headache. Visual-evoked response may add diagnostic information in the headache sufferer with visual disturbance, especially if neuroanatomic testing such as CT scanning suggests abnormality of the sella turcica.

Lumbar puncture

Lumbar puncture to obtain spinal fluid for analysis is indicated as an emergency diagnostic procedure in all patients with the acute onset of headache and facial pain in whom an infectious cause is considered likely.[9] The old adage that, "If you think you need to do a lumbar puncture, you had better do it," certainly applies in this life-threatening situation. The lumbar puncture is also indicated to ascertain if blood is present in the spinal fluid if a cerebral vascular accident is suspected.[14]

Lumbar puncture in the chronic headache and facial pain patient has minimal utility. It should be used to obtain spinal fluid to detect the presence of demyelinating proteins in the facial pain patient with suspected MS and to perform tests for fungal and tubercular infection in the chronic headache patient.

Lumbar puncture should not be performed in the presence of increased intracranial pressure evidenced by papilledema on funduscopic examination, findings on CT, or MRI scanning.[14,15] Lumbar puncture should be reserved for the previously mentioned indications because the addition of a superimposed postlumbar puncture headache along with a chronic headache complaint can further confuse efforts to diagnose and treat the patient.

Arteriography and digital subtraction angiography

Arteriography and digital subtraction angiography are neuroanatomic diagnostic tests indicated in patients suspected of having aneurysms, angiomas, arteriovenous malformations, and vascular tumors responsible for their headache or facial pain symptomatology.[9] They are also indicated when surgical excision of a tumor is being considered and the surgeon requires information regarding blood supply to the tumor. These tests have significant morbidity and occasional mortality, and should be used only in selected patients.

SPECIFIC HEADACHE AND PAIN SYNDROMES
Tension-type headache

The term *tension-type headache* refers to nonvascular headaches that can be episodic or chronic. Until recently, the condition was known as a muscle contraction headache. However, because many patients with this disorder have no demonstrable contraction of skeletal muscle associated with their pain, the Internal Headache Society has returned to calling this constellation of symptoms tension-type headache.

Patient profile. Tension-type headache is usually bilateral but can be unilateral. Patients may have a bandlike nonpulsatile ache or tightness in the frontal, temporal, and occipital regions.[16] There is often associated neck symptomatology. Tension-type headache evolves over a period of hours or days and then tends to remain constant without progressive symptomatology. There is no aura associated with this headache. Significant sleep disturbance is usually present. These headaches most frequently occur between 4:00 A.M. and 8:00 A.M. and 4:00 P.M. and 8:00 P.M.[2] Although both genders are affected, women predominate. There is no hereditary pattern to tension-type headache, but it may occur in family clusters because children mimic and learn the pain behavior of their parents.

Triggering factors. The triggering event for acute episodic tension-type headache is invariably either physical or psychologic stress. A worsening of preexisting degenerative cervical spine conditions, such as cervical spondylosis, can also trigger a headache.[17] The pathology responsible for the development of tension-type headache can also produce temporomandibular joint (TMJ) dysfunction. In some patients, the cause and effect sequence is reversed and TMJ dysfunction appears to trigger the headache.[17]

Tension headache therapy

Episodic treatment. In determining treatment, the physician must consider the frequency and severity of headaches, how the headaches affect the patient's life-style, the results of any previous therapy, and previous drug misuse and abuse. If the patient suffers from tension-type headache once every month or every two months, the condition can often be managed through teaching the patient to reduce or avoid stress. Analgesics or nonsteroidal antiinflammatory drugs can provide symptomatic relief during acute attacks.[18]

Combination analgesic drugs used concomitantly with barbiturates and/or narcotic analgesics have no place in the management of headache patients. The risk of abuse and dependence more than outweighs any theoretic benefit. These substances may contribute to the development of analgesic rebound headaches. The physician should also avoid an abortive treatment approach in patients with a prior history of drug misuse or abuse. Many abortive drugs, including simple analgesics and nonsteroidal antiinflammatory drugs, can produce serious consequences if abused.[19]

Prophylactic treatment. If the headaches occur more frequently than once every month or two, or are so severe that the patient repeatedly misses work or social engagements, then prophylactic therapy is indicated.

ANTIDEPRESSANTS. Antidepressants are generally the drugs of choice for prophylactic treatment of headaches.[2] They decrease the frequency and intensity of tension-type headaches, and they normalize sleep patterns and treat underlying depression.

Patients should be educated about the potential side effects of these drugs: sedation, dry mouth, blurred vision, constipation, and urinary retention. They should also be told that relief of headache pain generally takes 3 to 4 weeks. However the normalization of sleep that occurs immediately may be enough to noticeably improve the headache symptomatology.

Amitriptyline started at a single bedtime dose of 25 mg is a reasonable initial choice. The dose may be increased in 25 mg increments as side effects allow. Other drugs can be considered if the patient does not tolerate amitriptyline's sedation and anticholinergic effects, for example, trazodone 75 to 300 mg at bedtime or fluoxetine 20 to 40 mg at lunchtime. Because of the sedating nature of these drugs (with the exception of fluoxetine), they must be used with caution in the elderly or in patients who are at risk of falling. Exercise care when using these drugs in patients prone to cardiac arrhythmia because these drugs may be arrhythmogenic. Simple analgesics or the longer-acting nonsteroidal antiinflammatory drugs may be used with the antidepressant compounds to treat exacerbations of headache pain.

BIOFEEDBACK. Monitored relaxation training combined with patient education about coping strategies and stress-reduction techniques may be valuable in the motivated tension-type headache sufferer.[20] Appropriate patient selection is important if good results are to be achieved. If the patient is significantly depressed at therapy initiation, treat the depression before trying biofeedback. The skills learned in biofeedback training must be practiced on a regular basis in the home or work setting to achieve optimal results.

CERVICAL STEROID EPIDURAL NERVE BLOCKS. Cronen and Waldman have demonstrated the efficacy of cervical steroid epidural nerve blocks in providing long-term relief of tension-type headaches in a group of patients who failed all other treatment modalities.[21,22] Significant pain relief was noted by the majority of patients at the 3 month follow-up. Subsequent studies confirmed the safety of this technique to palliate a variety of painful conditions.[23] Cervical steroid epidural nerve blocks may be used early in the course of treatment on a daily basis or every other day while waiting for the antidepressant compounds to become effective.

Migraine headache

Migraine headache is defined as a periodic unilateral headache that may begin in childhood but almost always develops before age 30.[1] Attacks may occur every few days or only every 5 or 6 months. The headache may become generalized as the attack evolves. The pain is usually described as throbbing or pounding and may "settle" behind one eye. These headaches are usually associated with systemic symptoms of nausea and vomiting; diarrhea; photophobia; sonophobia; alterations in mood, libido, and appetite; and, occasionally, focal neurologic deficits. Migraine attacks usually last for more than 4 hours and frequently persist for 24 hours or longer. Approximately 60% to 70% of migraine sufferers are female, and many report a history of the disorder in family members.

Migraine headache may be triggered by change in diet or sleep habits, tyramine-containing foods, monosodium glutamate, nitrates, alcohol, hormones, oral contraceptives, fatigue, stress, menstruation, underlying muscle contraction headache, strong odors, and bright sunlight. Patients often unconsciously avoid these triggers.

Special forms of migraine. There has been confusion with the classification of headaches, particularly migraine.[16] Migraine without aura (previously called common migraine) is simply the migraine headache previously described. If the patient experiences painless preheadache focal neurologic symptoms (i.e., aura), it is migraine with aura. Most aurae are ocular symptoms that originate in the visual cortex of the occipital lobe and are presumably due to localized ischemia. Other examples of aura include disturbances of smell, feeling, or motor function.

Hemiplegic migraine and ophthalmoplegic migraine with aura. If the focal neurologic symptoms persist beyond the immediate headache period, this syndrome is termed *migraine with prolonged aura,* which was previously called complicated migraine.[6]

Migraine therapy. When deciding how to treat migraine, the physician should consider the frequency and severity of headaches, their effect on the patient's life-style, the presence of prolonged focal neurologic symptoms, the results of previous therapy and diagnostic testing, previous drug misuse and abuse, and the presence of other systemic diseases that might preclude the use of some treatments.[1]

If the patient's attacks occur only once a month or once every 2 months, a trial of abortive therapy to provide symptomatic relief of the acute attack may be warranted. This approach should be avoided in patients with a history of drug abuse because many abortive drugs can produce life-threatening consequences if abused.

If the headaches occur with greater frequency or cause the patient to miss work or be hospitalized, prophylactic treatment is indicated. Because migraine with prolonged aura can lead to permanent neurologic sequelae in rare cases, patients who report even infrequent episodes of these attacks should receive preventive therapy.

Abortive therapy. In order for abortive therapy to be effective, it must be initiated at the first sign of headache. This can often be difficult because of the short time between onset and peak experienced by many migraine sufferers. The route of administration should be appropriately tailored in patients with nausea, vomiting, or diarrhea.

ISOMETHEPTENE MUCATE. This drug should be considered first-line abortive therapy. It has stopped migraine headache in some patients,[15] and has an extremely favorable risk-to-benefit ratio, without the nausea, vomiting, rebound, or dependence seen with ergot alkaloids. The patient should take two capsules every hour until the headache is relieved. Total dose should not exceed five capsules in 24 hours.

ERGOT ALKALOIDS. This group of abortive agents was among the first used to treat migraine headache.[2] The ergots cause vasoconstriction of the extracranial vessels involved in the evolution of migraine. Ergotamine alone or in combination with caffeine is the most common and most effective oral form of this drug. Sublingual, rectal, and injectable forms are available for patients who cannot take medication orally because of nausea or vomiting.

Unfortunately, the ergot alkaloids have significant side effects. They constrict other vessels, including the coronary arteries and peripheral vasculature. For this reason, they should not be used in patients with preexisting vascular disease such as angina. Because of the high risk of complications with misuse or abuse, avoid these drugs when treating the patient with a history of drug abuse.

Some headache specialists feel that ergot alkaloids produce a physical dependence similar to opioids. Patients who have become dependent on ergotamines will generally experience severe headache when the drug is abruptly stopped. Tapering of this class of medications in the outpatient setting is difficult, and patients will generally require hospitalization.

Because of this unfavorable risk-to-benefit ratio, ergotamine cannot be considered first-line abortive therapy for most migraine patients. Ergotamine use should be restricted to select reliable patients in whom monitoring of drug usage is possible.

OXYGEN. Early inhalation of oxygen was first used in cluster headache, but it may abort or ameliorate migraine headache. It may be combined with other abortive drugs and treatment. Oxygen is delivered at 10 L/min with a close-fitting mask. Home use is worthwhile in some patients. Instruct the patient in the safe use of compressed gases and the need to avoid smoking when using this treatment.

SPHENOPALATINE GANGLION BLOCK. Blockade of the sphenopalatine ganglion can abort the acute attack of migraine. Its simplicity makes it useful in the pain center or emergency department,[24,25] and it may be safely used with oxygen and various other abortive treatments.

Use 2 ml of 2% viscous lidocaine or 10% cocaine on a daily basis to block the ganglion. Monitor the patient's vital signs after the procedure is completed because orthostatic hypotension occasionally occurs. This treatment can also help prevent migraine headache.

BIOFEEDBACK. Biofeedback combined with autogenic training has enabled some patients to abort or prevent attacks of migraine. The technique can be used alone or with other therapies.

INTRAVENOUS LIDOCAINE AND ANTIEMETICS. Several recent studies have reported that intravenous (IV) lidocaine alone or combined with antiemetics such as droperidol or promethazine relieved acute migraine attacks.[26] I have also found this technique favorable and it has helped me avoid using narcotic analgesics in this setting. Lidocaine (100 mg) combined with 25 mg of promethazine or 2.5 mg of droperidol is given IV over 5 minutes with careful observation for hypotension. This technique was combined with oxygen inhalation. In resistant cases, 1 ml of dihydroergotamine (DHE-45) IV may be combined with the previously-mentioned treatments.[26] Dihydroergotamine should not be used in any patient with preexisting vascular disease or migraine with prolonged aura.

NONSTEROIDAL ANTIINFLAMMATORY DRUGS. Several recent reports have described using naproxen sodium as an abortive agent for migraine.[27] The nausea and vomiting associated with acute migraine have limited the effectiveness of this approach in many patients. Our experience with this drug in the acute setting has been disappointing. The injectable nonsteroidal antiinflammatory drug ketorolac may play a useful role and could allow the physician to avoid the use of parenteral narcotics.[28]

SUMATRIPTAN. Recent studies have demonstrated the efficacy of subcutaneous sumatriptan in the palliation of acute migraine. Sumatriptan succinate is a specific serotonin agonist that selectively vasoconstricts cranial blood vessels. At a dose of 6 mg, 70% of patients with acute migraine experienced marked pain relief; however, its short half-life may necessitate repeated injections to sustain relief. This drug should be used with care in patients with coronary artery disease and peripheral vascular insufficiency.[29]

Prophylactic treatment of migraine

BETA BLOCKERS. The efficacy of this class of drugs in the prophylaxis of migraine headache was discovered quite by accident, when Rabkin prescribed a beta blocker for a patient with cardiac disease who also suffered from severe migraine headache.[2] Several studies have confirmed the ability of this unique group of drugs to decrease the frequency and severity of migraine attacks.[30] Beta blockers are now viewed as first-line therapy for migraine prophylaxis.

I recommend starting patients with propranolol at 20 mg four times daily, and increasing to a total daily dose of 240 mg. A trial of at least 2 months is indicated. A long-acting form of the drug is available and may be used to increase patient compliance. Other more "selective" beta blockers such as nadolol (40 to 80 mg daily) or metoprolol (50 to 100 mg twice daily) may be considered if the patient experiences side effects with propranolol, such as somnolence, decreased libido, nightmares, or fatigue.

This class of drugs is contraindicated in patients with congestive heart failure, asthma, and chronic obstructive pulmonary disease. They should be used with caution in poorly controlled diabetics and patients taking monoamine oxidase inhibitors. Do not stop the beta blockers abruptly; rather, taper them over 2 weeks, especially in those patients with coexistent hypertension or angina.[31]

ANTIDEPRESSANTS. The use of antidepressants in the prophylaxis of migraine is somewhat controversial. Some clinical studies have demonstrated the efficacy of this class of drugs in decreasing the frequency and severity of episodic migraine headache.[2] Choice of drugs and dosage is similar to that when using these drugs to treat tension-type headache.

CALCIUM CHANNEL BLOCKERS. Some migraine sufferers who do not experience diminution of headaches with beta blockers will find the calcium channel blockers to be of value.[1] I recommend verapamil, at a starting dose of 80 mg three times daily, as the calcium blocker of first choice. Monitor patients for side effects, which include hypotension, flushing, and gastrointestinal problems. The use of sustained-release formulations will markedly decrease these side effects.

METHYSERGIDE. Methysergide is an antiserotonergic compound closely related to the ergot alkaloids.[15] It is useful in the prophylaxis of intractable migraine headaches that fail to respond to the above-mentioned therapies. This drug is given in divided daily doses of 4 to 6 mg. Unfortunately, methysergide must be used with extreme caution because of the life-threatening side effects of retroperitoneal and cardiac fibrosis. Therefore, use the drug at the lowest effective dose and never for more than 6 months without a 2-month drug-free period. Monitoring should include IV pyelography and an electrocardiogram (ECG) every 6 months.

OTHER PROPHYLACTIC MEDICATIONS. Clonidine given at a starting dose of 0.1 mg twice a day is a central alpha agonist that has been effective in prophylaxis of migraine.[32] This drug may be especially useful in patients whose headaches appear to be induced by tyramine. Hypotension as a side effect greatly limits the efficacy of this drug.

The monoamine oxidase inhibitors effectively decrease the frequency and severity of migraine headaches in the small group of patients who fail all other treatment modalities. Phenelzine is probably the first drug of choice, and a dose of 15 mg three times daily is usually effective in controlling headaches. After 2 to 3 weeks, taper the dosage to a maintenance dose of 5 to 10 mg three times daily.

Monoamine inhibitors can cause life-threatening hypertensive crisis if special diets are not followed or if they are combined with certain other medications. Therefore, their use should be limited to highly reliable and compliant patients.

Coexisting migraine and tension-type headache

The coexisting migraine and tension-type headache, previously called mixed headache syndrome, occurs much more frequently than commonly recognized.[15] Careful questioning will help identify this subset of patients. If a patient can identify more than one type of headache, ask which type he or she finds most problematic. This may not necessarily be the headache that occurs most frequently. Occasionally it is necessary to use medications for both types of headaches to control the symptoms. The physician should recognize that analgesic rebound may trigger both migraine and tension-type headache, and discontinuation of abortive headache medications and analgesics may be necessary to relieve the patient's headache symptomatology.

Cluster Headache

Characteristics. Cluster headache derives its name from its occurrence in time "clusters," which are followed by headache-free remission periods. Unlike other common headache disorders, cluster headache is more common in men, by a ratio of 5:1. It afflicts 0.4% to 1.0% of the male population.[2] The condition is often confused with migraine, but there are several differences (Table 39-1). Cluster headache ususally develops when the patient is in his or her 30s, approximately 10 years later than migraine.[4] Unlike migraine headache, cluster headache does not appear to be familial. There is no prodrome or aura, and the attacks are most likely to occur 90 minutes after the patient falls asleep.[4,33]

The clusters follow a chronobiologic pattern that appears to coincide with the seasonal change in the length of day. This results in an increase in the frequency of cluster headache in the spring and fall.

During a cluster period, attacks generally occur two or three times a day and last for 45 minutes to an hour. Cluster periods usually last 8 to 10 weeks, interrupted by remissions averaging less than 2 years.[2] Sometimes the remission period is markedly diminished, and the frequency of attacks increases up to tenfold. This situation is termed *chronic cluster headache,* which differs from the more common episodic cluster headache described above.[33,34]

Other headache syndromes besides migraine may be confused with cluster headache, and it is imperative to distinguish between these types of disorders before administering treatment (Table 39-2).[33] The use of a targeted history and physical examination allow an accurate clinical diagnosis of cluster headache to be made with a reasonable degree of certainty.[35,36]

A rare headache disorder, chronic paroxysmal hemicrania, is thought to be a variant of cluster headache. Chronic paroxysmal hemicrania is similar to cluster headache only in the type of pain that is produced. Chronic paroxysmal hemicrania occurs more commonly in women and is characterized by short attacks occurring 8 to 16 times a day without periods of remission. It invariably responds to treatment with indomethacin at a dose of 25 to 50 mg three times daily.[4,33]

Physiologic and psychologic effects. Cluster headache pain is characterized as unilateral, retroorbital, and temporal in location, with a deep burning or drilling quality. Horner's syndrome, consisting of ptosis, abnormal pupil contraction, facial flushing, conjunctival injection, and profuse lacrimation and rhinorrhea, is often present. These ocular changes may become permanent with repeated attacks. Peau d'orange skin over the malar region, deeply furrowed forehead and glabellar folds, and telangiectasia may be observed.

Table 39-1 Clinical differences between cluster and migraine headache

Cluster headache	Migraine headache
Male predominance (M:F = 8:1)	Female predominance (M:F = 2:3)
No aura	Visual/sensory aura of classic migraine present in 25%
Unilateral distribution of pain	Pain often bilateral or hemicranial on either side
Pain duration usually 30-120 min	Pain duration of 12-48 h
No family history in most cases	Family history of migraine in 70%
Headache occurs in daily attacks for 4-12 wks	Single attacks with intervals of remission
One to three attacks occur per day, often during sleep	Attacks last 1-2 days, often start on waking
Total remission after a cluster, often 6-18 mos	Shorter remission

From Pearce JMS: Cluster headache and its variants. *Headache Quarterly* 2:187, 1991.

Table 39-2 Features of syndromes misdiagnosed as cluster headache

Features	Syndrome
Long duration; vomiting; occurs periodically	Common migraine
Aura; long duration; vomiting; occurs periodically	Classic migraine
Jabs; triggers; rarely nocturnal	Trigeminal neuralgia
Progressive course; fits focal signs; raised intracranial pressure	Brain tumor
Affects the middle aged or elderly; precipitated by neck movement; restricts neck movement; no eye signs	Cervicogenic pain
Affects elderly; produces malaise, myalgia, inflamed arteries, high erythrocyte sedimentation rate	Cranial arteritis
Attack of shingles; postherpetic scarring and pigment; attacks throughout day and night	Postherpetic neuralgia

From Pearce JMS: Cluster headache and its variants. *Headache Quarterly* 2:187, 1991.

Attacks of cluster headache may be provoked by small amounts of alcohol, nitrates, histamines, and other vasoactive substances, and, occasionally, high altitude.[15] When the attack is in progress the patient may not be able to lie still and may pace or rock back and forth in a chair. This behavior contrasts with other headache syndromes, during which patients seeking relief will lie down in a dark, quiet room.[2,4,33,34]

Suicides have been associated with prolonged, unrelieved attacks of cluster headaches.[2] Therefore hospitalization is recommended in cases of uncontrollable pain. Because of the severity of cluster headache pain, the physician should watch for medication overuse or misuse by patients attempting to obtain relief.

Therapy. As with any disease characterized by unpredictable and rapid onset of symptoms, long periods of remissions, and exacerbations, prophylaxis and evaluation of treatment are difficult. However, the physician must recognize that, because of the severity of symptoms and potential for suicide, this disorder must be viewed as a true pain emergency and treated actively and aggressively. The following are accepted treatments for cluster headache.

Oxygen inhalation. This remains the safest and most effective means to abort the acute cluster headache.[2] Administer 10L of oxygen with a close-fitting mask at the first sign of headache. Instruct patients about the safe use of compressed gases and to avoid cigarette smoking or other open flames when using oxygen.

Sphenopalatine ganglion nerve block. Daily use of sphenopalatine ganglion nerve block with 2% viscous lidocaine or 10% cocaine are highly effective in aborting the acute cluster headache.[25,37] This treatment may be used in combination with oxygen inhalation and the medications listed below.

Methysergide. This antiserotonergic compound is the medication of choice for episodic cluster headache. It is closely related to the ergot alkaloids. Give this drug in doses of 2 mg three times daily. Use methysergide with extreme caution because of the life-threatening side effects of retroperitoneal and cardiac fibrosis.[2] In order to avoid these complications of methysergide therapy, use the drug at the lowest effective dose and never for more than 6 months without a 2-month drug-free period. Intravenous pyelography and an ECG should be administered every 6 months to patients taking this drug. Methysergide may be used in combination with oxygen inhalation and sphenopalatine ganglion block.

Steroids. A short, tapering course of steroids may be effective in patients that fail to respond to the above mentioned treatment modalities.[38] A starting dose of 80 mg (20 mg four times daily), tapered by 10 mg per dose per day, is usually adequate. Because there may be an increased incidence of peptic ulcer disease in patients suffering from cluster headache, gastric cytoprotective agents should be considered.

Lithium carbonate. This drug is the treatment of choice for chronic cluster headache and can be useful in a small number of episodic cluster patients who fail to respond to methysergide or steroids.[33] It has a small therapeutic window and should be used with caution. The starting dose should be 300 mg at bedtime. Increase the drug to 300 mg twice a day after 48 hours if no adverse side effects such as fatigue, polyuria, rash, nausea, and thirst are observed. In most adult patients with normal renal function, 300 mg three times a day can be used safely without routine monitoring of serum lithium levels. The concomitant use of diuretics may increase the risk of toxicity.

Surgical treatment of cluster headache. In rare instances cluster headache may become refractory to all treatment modalities. In this setting, consideration may be given to destruction of the gasserian ganglion either by retrogasserian injection of glycerol or by radiofrequency lesion.[25,39] These treatments have significant risks and should be performed only by those well versed in the techniques and potential complications.

As in other chronic headache syndromes, the use of addicting substances, including ergotamines, should be avoided.

Trigeminal neuralgia

Trigeminal neuralgia occurs in many patients because tortuous or aberrant blood vessels compress the trigeminal root.[34] Acoustic neuromas, cholesteatomas, aneurysms, angiomas, and bony abnormalities may also lead to the compression of nerve roots. About 2% to 3% of patients experiencing trigeminal neuralgia also have MS.[34]

Characteristics. Trigeminal neuralgia is an episodic pain afflicting the areas of the face supplied by the trigeminal nerve. The pain is unilateral in 97% of cases reported.[40] When it does occur bilaterally, it is in the same division of the nerve. The second or third division of the nerve is affected in the majority of patients, with the first division affected less than 5% of the time.[40] The pain develops on the right side of the face in unilateral disease 57% of the time.[5,37]

The pain is characterized by paroxysms of electric shock-like pain lasting from several seconds to less than 2 minutes. The progression from onset to peak is essentially instantaneous. Daily activities involving contact with trigger areas, such as eating, brushing the teeth, shaving, or washing the face, often provoke attacks. Avoidance of eating and drinking can cause severe dehydration, sometimes requiring hospitalization. The pain usually causes spasms of the facial muscles on the affected side; this is why this condition is also called *tic douloureux.* The patient with trigeminal neuralgia may try to avoid any contact with trigger areas. Persons with other types of facial pain, such as TMJ dysfunction, tend to constantly rub the affected area or apply heat or cold to it. Patients with uncontrolled trigeminal neuralgia frequently require hospitalization for rapid control of pain.

Between attacks the patient is relatively pain free. A dull ache remaining after the intense pain subsides may indicate a persistent compression of the nerve by a structural lesion. This disease is almost never seen in people under 30 unless it is associated with MS.

The patient with trigeminal neuralgia often has severe and, at times, even suicidal depression with high levels of superimposed anxiety during acute attacks. Both of these problems may be exacerbated by the sleep deprivation that often occurs during episodes of pain. Patients with coexisting MS may exhibit the euphoric dementia characteristic of that disease. Physicians should assure patients with trigeminal neuralgia that the pain can almost always be controlled.

Drug therapy

Carbamazepine. Carbamazepine is considered first-line treatment for trigeminal neuralgia. In fact, rapid response to this drug essentially confirms a clinical diagnosis of trigeminal neuralgia. Some investigators feel that if a patient does not respond to this medication after 48 hours of treatment with the optimal dosage, other causes of the pain need to be considered.

In spite of carbamazepine's safety and efficacy as compared with other treatments for trigeminal neuralgia, much confusion and unfounded anxiety surround its use. This medication, which may be the patient's best chance for pain control, is sometimes discontinued because of lab abnormalities erroneously attributed to it. Therefore the protocol in my practice states that baseline screening labs, consisting of a CBC, urinalysis, and Sequential Multiple Analyzer (SMA 12/60), should be obtained before starting the drug.

Start carbamazepine slowly if the patient is not suffering from uncontrolled pain. We prescribe a 100 to 200 mg dose at bedtime for two nights and caution the patient regarding side effects, including dizziness, sedation, confusion, and rash. The drug is administered in equally divided doses over 2 days, as side effects allow, until pain relief is obtained or a total dose of 1200 mg daily is reached. Careful monitoring of laboratory parameters is mandatory to avoid the rare possibility of life-threatening blood dyscrasia. At the first sign of blood count abnormality or rash discontinue this drug. Failure to monitor patients started on carbamazepine can be disastrous because aplastic anemia can occur.

When pain relief is obtained keep the patient at that dosage of carbamazepine for at least 6 months before considering tapering of this medication. Inform the patient that the drug dosage should not be changed nor should the drug be refilled or discontinued without the physician's knowledge. Routine hematologic monitoring after reaching stable dosage is unnecessary.[40] Obtain carbamazepine blood levels when noncompliance is suspected, when side effects occur at doses under 1200 mg, and when it is desirable to establish a baseline if a dose of 1200 mg per day is reached, allowing the physician to safely titrate the dosage upward.

Phenytoin. In the uncommon event that carbamazepine does not adequately control a patient's pain, phenytoin may be considered.[34] As with carbamazepine, obtain baseline blood tests before starting therapy.

We prescribe a 100 mg dose of phenytoin at bedtime for 2 nights and caution the patient about potential side effects, including dizziness, sedation, confusion, and rash. The drug is increased in 100 mg increments, given in equally divided doses over 2 days, as side effects allow, until pain relief is obtained or a total dose of 300 mg daily is reached. At this point, if the patient has experienced partial pain relief, blood values are measured and the drug is carefully titrated upward. Because this drug has a small therapeutic window, it is best to use pediatric tablets for titration. Rarely will more than 400 mg daily be required.

Baclofen. This drug has been reported to be of value in some patients who fail to obtain relief from the above-mentioned medications.[41] Obtain baseline lab tests. We prescribe a 10 mg dose at bedtime for 2 nights and caution the patient about potential adverse effects, which are the same as those of carbamazepine and phenytoin. The drug is increased in 10 mg increments, given in equally divided doses over 7 days as side effects allow, until pain relief is obtained or a total dose of 80 mg daily is reached. This drug has significant hepatic and CNS side effects, including weakness and sedation. Although some specialists feel that baclofen can be used as first-line therapy for trigeminal neuralgia, in our experience it is poorly tolerated by most patients. As with carbamazepine, careful monitoring of lab values is indicated during the initial use of this drug.

In treating individuals with any of the above-mentioned drugs, the physician should make the patient aware that premature tapering or discontinuation of the medication may lead to the recurrence of pain and that it will be more difficult to control pain thereafter.

Invasive therapy

Trigeminal nerve block. The use of trigeminal nerve block with local anesthetic and a steroid serves as an excellent adjunct to drug treatment of trigeminal neuralgia.[25,39] This technique rapidly relieves pain while oral medications are being titrated to effective levels. Carry out the initial block with preservative-free bupivacaine combined with methylprednisolone. Carry out subsequent daily nerve blocks in a similar manner substituting a lower dose of methylprednisolone. This approach may also be utilized to obtain control of breakthrough pain.

Retrogasserian injection of glycerol. The injection of small quantities of glycerol into the area of the gasserian ganglion provides long-term relief for patients suffering from trigeminal neuralgia who have not responded to optimal trials of the above-mentioned therapies.[39]

Radiofrequency destruction of the gasserian ganglion. The destruction of the gasserian ganglion can be carried out by creating a radiofrequency lesion under biplanar fluoroscopic guidance.[7] This procedure is reserved for patients who have failed all of the above-mentioned treatments for intractable trigeminal neuralgia.

Microvascular decompression of the trigeminal root. This technique, which is also called *Jannetta's procedure,* is the major neurosurgical procedure of choice for intractable trigeminal neuralgia.[42] It is based on the theory that trigeminal neuralgia is in fact a compressive mononeuropathy. The operation consists of identifying the trigeminal root close to the brainstem and isolating the offending compressing blood vessel. A sponge is then interposed between the vessel and nerve, relieving the compression and thus the pain.

SUMMARY

Headache is the most common medical complaint encountered in clinical practice. The targeted history and physical examination should allow the physician to make an accurate diagnosis and design an effective treatment plan. The rational use of adjuvant drugs combined with neural blockade results in pain relief in the vast majority of patients suffering from headache and facial pain.

REFERENCES

1. Diamond S: Diagnosis and treatment of migraine. *Clin J Pain* 5:3-9, 1989.
2. Diamond S, Dalessio DJ: *The Practicing Physician's Approach to Headache,* ed 3. Baltimore, Williams & Wilkins, 1982.
3. Russell RW, Graham EM: Trigeminal neuralgia. In Hopkins A, ed: *Headache.* Philadelphia, WB Saunders, 1988.
4. Kudrow L: Management of cluster headache. In *Cluster Headache: Mechanisms and Management.* New York, Oxford University Press, 1980.
5. Dalessio DJ: Management of the cranial neuralgias and atypical facial pain. *Clin J Pain* 5:55-59, 1989.
6. Freitag FG: Migraine headache variants. *Clin J Pain* 5:11-17, 1989.
7. Sweet WH: The treatment of trigeminal neuralgia. *N Engl J Med* 315:174, 1986.
8. Epstein MT, Hockaday JM, Hockaday TDR: Migraine and reproductive hormones. *Lancet* 1:543-547, 1975.
9. Bannister R: The examination of the patient. In *Brain's Clinical Neurology.* New York, Oxford University Press, 1985.
10. Waldman SD, Waldman K: Reflex sympathetic dystrophy of the face and neck. *Reg Anesth* 12:8-12, 1987.
11. Robinson CA: Cervical spondylosis and muscle contraction headache. In Dalessio DJ, ed: *Wolff's Headache.* New York, Oxford University Press, 1980.
12. Dalessio DJ: Headache associated with anemia. In Dalessio DJ, ed: *Wolff's Headache.* New York, Oxford University Press, 1980.
13. Russell RW, Graham EM: Giant cell arteritis. In Hopkins A, ed: *Headache.* Philadelphia, WB Saunders, 1988.
14. Bannister R: Ancillary investigations. In *Brain's Clinical Neurology.* New York, Oxford University Press, 1985.
15. Saper JR: *Headache disorders: Current concepts and treatment strategies.* Boston, John Wright, 1983.
16. Headache Classification Committee of the International Headache Society: Classification and diagnostic criteria for headache disorders, cranial neuralgias and facial pain. *Cephalalgia* 8 (Suppl 7):19-34, 1988.
17. Dalessio D: *Wolff's Headache.* New York, Oxford University Press, 1980.
18. Miller DS et al: A comparison of naproxen sodium, acetaminophen, and placebo in the treatment of headache. *Headache* 27:392-396, 1987.
19. Kunkel RS: Tension headache. *Clin J Pain* 5:42, 1989.
20. Marcer D: Biofeedback and pain. In Marcer D, editor: *Biofeedback and Related Therapies in Clinical Practice.* Rockville, Md, Aspen, 1986.
21. Cronen MC, Waldman SD: Cervical epidural blocks in the treatment of tension-type headache. *Headache* 28:314, 1988.
22. Cronen MC, Waldman SD: Cervical steroid epidural nerve block in the palliation of pain secondary to intractable tension-type headache. *J Pain Symptom Manage* 5:379-381, 1990.
23. Waldman SD: Complications of cervical epidural nerve blocks. *Reg Anesth* 14:149-151, 1989.
24. Phero J, Robbins G: Sphenopalatine ganglion block. In Raj PP, editor: *Handbook of Regional Anesthesia.* New York, Churchill Livingstone, 1985.
25. Waldman SD: The role of neural blockade in pain management. In Weiner RS, editor: *Innovations in Pain Management.* Winter Park, Fla, PMD Publishers Group, 1990.
26. Saper JR: Emergency management of headache. *Topics in Pain Management* 4:29-30, 1989.
27. Ziegler DK, Ellis DJ: Naproxen in the prophylaxis of migraine. *Arch Neurol* 42:582-584, 1985.
28. Waldman SD: Ketorolac and Dezocine. *Pain Digest* 316:220, 1991.
29. Waldman SD: Sumatriptan. *Pain Digest* 3:260-263, 1993.
30. Diamond S, Medina JL: The treatment of migraine headache. *Headache* 16:24-27, 1976.
31. Shand DG, Wool AJJ: Beta blockers in clinical practice. *Circulation* 58:202-203, 1978.
32. Ryan RE Sr, Ryan RE Jr: Clonidine: Its use in migraine therapy. *Headache* 14:190-192, 1975.
33. Pearce JMS: Cluster headache and its variants. *Headache Quarterly* 2:187, 1991.
34. Graham JG: Cluster headache and pain in the face. In Hopkins A, editor: *Headache.* Philadelphia, WB Saunders, 1988.
35. Waldman SD: Headache and facial pain: Obtaining the targeted history. *IM—Internal Medicine* April 1991, 12:20.
36. Donohoe CP, Waldman SD: Headache and facial pain: The targeted physical exam. *IM—Internal Medicine* May 1991, 12:43.
37. Kitrell JP, Grouse DS, Seybold M: Cluster headache: Local anesthetic abortive agents. *Arch Neurol* 42:496, 1985.
38. Jammes JL: The treatment of cluster headache with prednisone. *Diseases of the Nervous System* 12:275, 1975.
39. Feldstein GS: Percutaneous retrogasserian glycerol rhizotomy in the treatment of trigeminal neuralgia. In Racz GB, editor: *Techniques of Neurolysis.* Boston, Kluwer Academic Publishers, 1989.
40. Waldman SD: Evaluation of common headaches and facial pain syndromes. In Raj PP, editor: *Practical Management of Pain.* St Louis, Mosby, 1992.
41. Fromm GH, Terrence CF, Chatta AS: Baclofen in the treatment of face pain. *Ann Neurol* 15:240, 1984.
42. Jannetta PJ: Trigeminal neuralgia: Treatment by microvascular decompression. In Wilkins RH, Rengachary SS, editors: *Neurosurgery.* New York, McGraw-Hill, 1985.

QUESTIONS: HEADACHE AND FACIAL PAIN

1. The most important assessment procedure to include in
    a headache evaluation is:
    A. An MRI
    B. A CT scan
    C. An erythrocyte sedimentation rate
    D. A targeted history
    For questions 2-4, choose from the following:
    A. 1, 2, and 3
    B. 1 and 3
    C. 2 and 4
    D. 4
    E. All the answers are correct
2. Which of the following types of headaches is (are) char-
    acterized by a rapid onset-to-peak?
    1. Cluster
    2. Tension-type
    3. Increased intracranial pressure
    4. Migraine with aura
3. Which of the following premonitory symptoms and/or
    auras is (are) associated with migraine headache?
    1. Visual disturbances
    2. Photophobia
    3. Sonophobia
    4. Nausea and vomiting

4. Which of the following statement(s) regarding tension-
    type headaches is (are) true?
    1. It was previously referred to as muscle contraction
        headache.
    2. It is characterized as bandlike pressure or pain.
    3. It may be associated with cervical spine symptoms.
    4. It has a rapid onset-to-peak.
5. Side effects of methylsergide include which of the fol-
    lowing?
    A. Anemia
    B. Hyperglycemia
    C. Retroperitoneal fibrosis
    D. Photosensitivity

ANSWERS

1. D
2. B
3. E
4. A
5. C

40 Neck and Shoulder Pain

Nicolas E. Walsh and *Somayaji Ramamurthy*

The patient complaining of neck, shoulder, and arm pain should be examined for anatomic location of the pain, derangement of mechanical structures, and underlying pathologic conditions. A careful history and examination are needed to reach a diagnosis. Laboratory tests and x-rays may be necessary but may have limited diagnostic value.

The neck and upper extremity are composed of numerous pain-sensitive tissues including nerves, vessels, muscles, ligaments, and joints. Pain may result from irritation, injury, inflammation, or infection of any of these tissues.[1] Conditions causing pain in this region are those of neurogenic, musculoskeletal, soft tissue, referred, and autonomic origin (Box 40-1).

PAIN OF NEUROGENIC ORIGIN

Neurogenic pain in the neck and upper extremities may commonly be caused by spinal cord/nerve root compression, myelopathy, postherpetic neuralgia, neuritis, peripheral nerve compression, and peripheral neuropathy.

Pain caused by spinal cord/nerve root compression

Compression at the cervical level characteristically produces spinal and radicular signs in the upper limbs and long tract signs in the lower extremities. Also, the muscles of the shoulder girdle and arms lose power and bulk.

When cord or nerve root compression produces only pain, localization by clinical examination alone is difficult. Myelography, electromyography (EMG), computed tomography (CT) scan, magnetic resonance imaging (MRI), or surgical exploration are often more accurate. Pain alone in the neck, shoulder, upper arm, scapula, or interscapular area is nonlocalizing. Most of the lesions in this area involve C_5, C_6, C_7, and C_8 nerve roots (Table 40-1). Pain in the posterior aspect of the arm may be due to C_7 root lesion, whereas medial anterior or lateral arm pain may be due to C_6 or C_7 nerve roots. Forearm pain usually is caused by C_6 or C_7 nerve root lesion. Hand pain is more accurately localized to a particular nerve root. Radiating pain in the thumb is usually due to C_6 nerve root compression. Index and middle finger pain is often caused by C_7 nerve root compression, and pain in ring and little fingers is due to C_8 nerve root compression (Figs. 40-1 through 40-6).

Objective weakness[2] is much more specific for localizing root level lesions. A C_5 nerve root lesion is best located by weakness in the deltoid, supraspinatus, and infraspinatus muscles. This may be tested by abduction and external arm rotation. Weakness of the brachialis and biceps muscle is a result of a C_6 nerve root lesion. A C_7 nerve root lesion is localized by eliciting weakness primarily in the triceps

and to a lesser degree in the flexor carpi ulnaris and radialis, pronator teres, and extensor pollicis longus (see Figs. 40-1 through 40-6).

Objective hypoesthesia and hypoalgesia in the appropriate dermatomal patterns are useful in localizing nerve root lesions. The deep tendon reflexes mainly depend on the integrity of the reflex arcs; however, testing deep tendon reflexes must be done properly. A diminished triceps jerk indicates a C_7 or possibly a C_8 nerve root lesion. The brachioradialis reflex may be diminished in C_7 root lesions, but its absence indicates a C_6 root lesion. In addition, there may be inversion of the brachioradialis reflex: tapping the tendon of this muscle elicits a brisk reflex contraction of the hand and finger flexor muscles and not the usual flexion and supination of the forearm. This unusual response is due to efferent interruption of the segmental reflex arc; the spread of the response and hyperreflexia at lower spinal levels results from pyramidal tract involvement (see Figs. 40-1 through 40-6). Lesions at the cervicothoracic junction may cause unilateral Horner's syndrome, which may be associated with wasting of the small muscles of the hand and a sensory deficit on the ulnar border of the hand and forearm (C_8, T_1).

Differential diagnosis. The most common causes of cervical nerve compression are cervical spondylosis, disk degeneration, and acute disk herniation; however, there are numerous other causes. Radicular pain is a shooting, radiating type of pain that is accompanied by objective neurologic signs such as loss of sensation and changes in the reflex and muscle strength. Radiculopathy itself may be caused by other etiologic factors such as primary or secondary malignancy of the bone, involvement of the nerve root by carcinoma of the lung, and the degenerative changes of the cervical spine itself. Compression of the spinal cord from a herniated disk may produce symptoms very similar to those of nerve root compression.

Compression of the spinal cord in the neck may result in cervical myelopathy, which produces radicular symptoms in the upper extremities and long tract signs in the lower extremities. Sensory impairment, muscle weakness, and loss of tendon reflexes may be found in the upper extremities. In the lower extremities, spastic weakness, hyperreflexia, clonus, extensor plantar reflexes, and impaired vibratory and position sense may be observed. Bowel and bladder function are not usually impaired.

Pain associated with degenerative disk disease may be local and limit neck movement. Pain referred to the upper back, shoulders, and upper extremity suggests that the pathology lies in the intervertebral foramina and the adjacent

---

Box 40-1 COMMON ORIGINS OF NECK AND UPPER EXTREMITY PAIN

Neurogenic pain

Cervical spinal cord compression
Nerve root compression
Neuritis
Peripheral nerve compression
Peripheral neuropathy
Torticollis
Herpetic neuralgia
Cervical myelopathy
Neoplasm
Meningitis
Neuroma

Soft tissue pain

Acute cervical strain
Myofascial pain
Fibromyalgia

Referred pain

Cardiac
Neoplasm
Myofascial pain
Viscera

Musculoskeletal pain

Degenerative joint disease
Tendinitis and bursitis
Cervical spondylosis
Degenerative disk disease
Rheumatoid arthritis
Fracture
Neoplasm
Osteomyelitis

Sympathetic pain

Reflex sympathetic dystrophy
Causalgia

---

tissues. Myofascial pain may also produce pain in the neck and arm, but the character of the pain is different.

Investigation. Diagnostic tests may be helpful in differentiating the causes of neck and arm pain, but a thorough neurologic examination is one of the most important ways of making a diagnosis. To localize and establish the nature of lesions causing intraspinal compression, several diagnostic tests may be used. Roentgenographic investigations are the most useful, but electrophysiologic techniques, radioisotope scanning, and cerebrospinal fluid (CSF) examination may also be helpful.

Roentgenographic investigation should begin with the suspected site of spinal cord or root compression. Frontal, lateral, and oblique views are required for examination of the cervical spine; frontal and lateral views are generally satisfactory for examination of the thoracic and lumbosacral spine. Lateral films of the cervical spine in flexion and extension are needed if subluxation is suspected. In certain situations tomography may be necessary to define a bone lesion more precisely.

Films of the spine should be systematically examined: the examiner should note the number, shape, density, and alignment of the vertebrae and the contour of the pedicles; the size of the intervertebral foramen; the size and shape of the spinal canal; the width of the disk spaces; and whether abnormal soft tissue shadows or calcifications are present. The anteroposterior depth of the spinal canal is a particularly important measurement. Sagittal diameters of less than 10 mm at any level of the cervical spine usually indicate spinal cord compression; bony compression of the cord is also possible if the canal measures 10 to 13 mm but is improbable if canals are greater than 13 mm. Increases in the transverse diameter of the spinal canal may be associated with thinning of the pedicles and are characteristic of syringomyelia or intramedullary tumors. Narrowing of the spinal canal with compression of the spinal cord or roots may occur in spondylosis, achondroplasia, and Paget's disease.

X-ray films of the cervical spine, especially lateral and oblique views, are helpful in evaluating for spinal abnormalities. Dumbbell-shaped neurofibromas that enlarge the intervertebral foramen are readily apparent in x-ray films. Congenital anomalies of the vertebral bodies are at times associated with intraspinal teratomas or lipomas. Bone caries suggest an infectious process such as tuberculosis, typhoidal infection, or brucellosis. Vertebral bone destruction from infection often involves the intervertebral disk; conversely, tumor metastases to the vertebral column spare the disks. Degenerative changes in the spine are frequently seen in asymptomatic individuals, but may be normal in patients with a herniated disk.

An EMG may not be diagnostic in the acute stage, since it takes approximately 3 weeks to detect the denervation in the involved muscles. After that period, an EMG may be helpful in localizing the level of the lesions and in differentiating shoulder pain from radiculopathy and muscle disease. CT scanning and MRI are now being employed routinely and have been helpful in differentiating the various causes of nerve root compression. Myelography, especially with the water-soluble contrast medium, is helpful in differentiating the causes of the radiculopathy and in differentiating or detecting myelopathy. Not every patient with neck pain requires myelography, and most physicians request myelography only when the surgery is contemplated or a tumor is suspected.

Bone scanning after radioisotope injection may be helpful if metastases are suspected as the cause of bone destruction. However, fractures, infection, and ankylosing spondylitis may also cause increased radioisotope uptake. CSF examination rarely provides specific diagnostic information about compressive spinal cord or root lesions. However, CSF examination may suggest certain diagnostic possibilities. The presence of xanthochromic fluid indicates intraspinal hemorrhage or block of CSF circulation. Intraspinal bleeding may originate from vascular malformations, ependymomas, or melanomas. Inflammatory cells indicate an infection or chemical meningitis caused by a ruptured teratoma or dermoid cyst. Tumor cells may be identified in the CSF of patients with carcinomatous infiltration of the

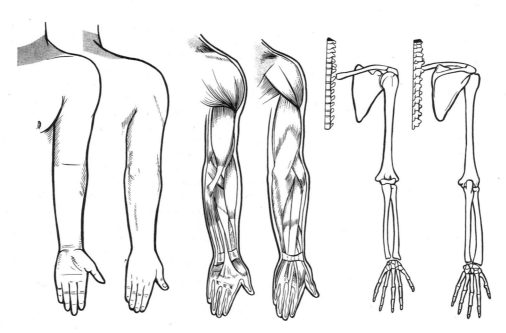

Fig. 40-1 Dermatome, myotome, and sclerotome distribution for C₃. Dermatome: neck. Myotome: paraspinals, trapezius, diaphragm. Sclerotome: bones—vertebra and periosteum: joints—facet; ligaments—longitudinal, ligamentum flavum, interspinous.(From Walsh NE, Ramamurthy S: Neck and upper extremity pain. In Raj PP, editor: *Practical Management of Pain,* ed 2. St Louis, Mosby, 1992.)

Table 40-1 Signs and symptoms of nerve root compression of the cervical region

Location of lesion	Referred pain	Motor dysfunction	Sensory dysfunction	Reflex changes
C₅	Shoulder and upper arm	Shoulder muscles (deltoid-supraspinatus-infraspinatus) abduction and external rotation	Upper and lateral aspect of the shoulder	Biceps reflex
C₆	Radial aspect of forearm	Biceps and brachialis muscles flexion of the elbow and supination wrist extensors	Radial aspect of forearm and thumb	Thumb reflex and brachioradialis reflex
C₇	Dorsal aspect of forearm	Triceps muscle extension of the elbow	Index and middle digits	Triceps reflex
C₈	Ulnar aspect of forearm	Intrinsics of the hand adduction and abduction	Ring and little digits	No change

meninges. In the absence of a block in the circulation of CSF, CSF protein levels above 60 mg/dl suggest intraspinal lesions other than an intervertebral disk protrusion or spondylosis. Spinal fluid blocks are best established by myelography.

Management of suspected nerve root or spinal cord compression. A careful history and physical examination are essential for effective physiologic treatment of pain. The examination should ascertain the extent of the pathology and the mechanism of pain. In the acute injury, x-rays should be carefully reviewed for fracture, subluxation, or dislocation. Once fracture or dislocation has been ruled out, treat the patient conservatively. The specific management

of intraspinal compression of nerve roots of the cord depends on the suspected diagnosis, the severity of the symptoms, and the extent of the neurologic signs.

Conservative management. Patients who should be treated conservatively are those with acute localized pain in the spinal or paraspinal region with or without peripheral radicular radiation. These patients do not have neurologic deficits indicative of spinal cord or severe nerve root compression. The most likely diagnosis is an acute intervertebral disk protrusion, and with time complete recovery can usually be anticipated.

Acute disk herniation is managed conservatively (most commonly with rest) using a soft collar to minimize the

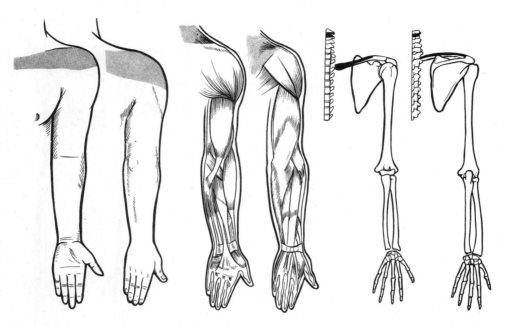

Fig. 40-2 Dermatome, myotome, and sclerotome distribution for C_4. Dermatome: shoulder. Myotome: paraspinals, trapezius, diaphragm, scapular abductors. Sclerotome: bones—vertebra and periosteum, clavicle: joints—facet; ligaments—longitudinal, ligamentum flavum, interspinous. (From Walsh NE, Ramamurthy S: Neck and upper extremity pain. In Raj PP, editor: *Practical Management of Pain,* ed 2. St Louis, Mosby, 1992.)

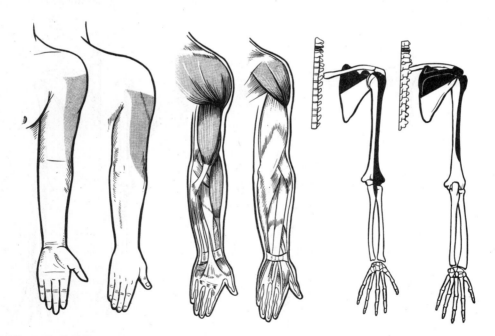

Fig. 40-3 Dermatome, myotome, and sclerotome distribution for C_5. Dermatome: lateral arm. Myotome: paraspinals, scapular abductors, scapular elevators, shoulder extensors, shoulder rotators, level flexors. Sclerotome: bones—vertebra and periosteum, scapula, humerus: joints—facet: ligaments—rotator cuff, longitudinal, ligamentum flavum, interspinous. (From Walsh NE, Ramamurthy S: Neck and upper extremity pain. In Raj PP, editor: *Practical Management of Pain,* ed 2. St Louis, Mosby, 1992.)

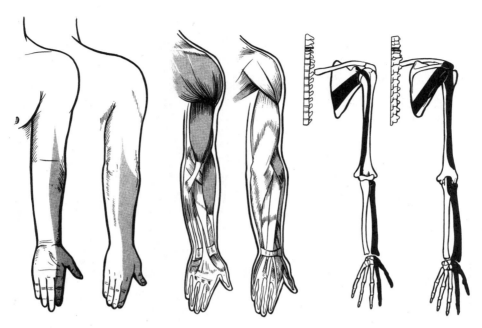

Fig. 40-4 Dermatome, myotome, and sclerotome distribution for C$_6$. Dermatome: lateral forearm, lateral hand. Myotome: paraspinals, level flexors, wrist flexors, pronators, supinators. Sclerotome: bones—scapula, humerus, radius, lateral fingers: joints—facet, shoulder, elbow: ligaments—longitudinal, ligamentum flavum, interspinous. (From Walsh NE, Ramamurthy S: Neck and upper extremity pain. In Raj PP, editor: *Practical Management of Pain,* ed 2. St Louis, Mosby, 1992.)

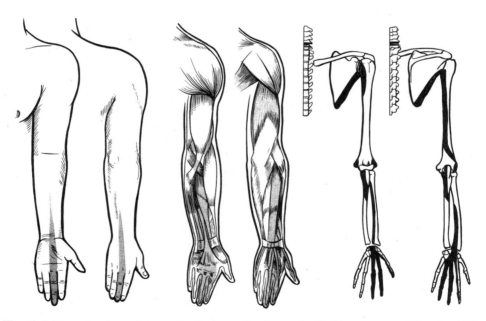

Fig. 40-5 Dermatome, myotome, and sclerotome distribution for C$_7$. Dermatome: mid-hand, middle finger. Myotome: paraspinals, pronators, elbow, extensor, wrist extensor. Sclerotome: bones—scapula, humerus, radius, ulna, middle fingers: joints—facet, wrist: ligaments—longitudinal, ligamentum flavum, interspinous. (From Walsh NE, Ramamurthy S: Neck and upper extremity pain. In Raj PP, editor: *Practical Management of Pain,* ed 2. St Louis, Mosby, 1992.)

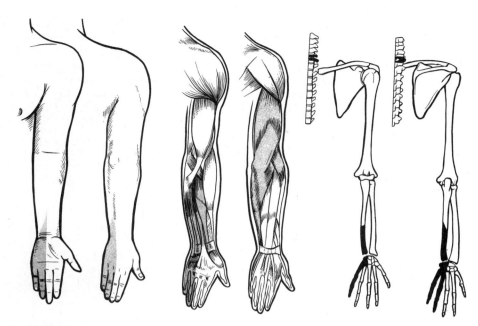

Fig. 40-6 Dermatome, myotome, and sclerotome distribution for C_8. Dermatome: medial hand. Myotome: paraspinals, elbow extensors, wrist flexors, grip, finger abduction, finger flexion, finger adduction, finger opposition, finger extension. Sclerotome: bones—vertebra and periosteum, ulna, medial fingers: joints—facet, wrist: ligaments—longitudinal, ligamentum flavum interspinous. (From Walsh NE, Ramamurthy S: Neck and upper extremity pain. In Raj PP, editor: *Practical Management of Pain,* ed 2. St Louis, Mosby, 1992.)

movements of the cervical spine. Keeping the muscles relaxed during the acute stage may be beneficial, and drugs such as cyclobenzaprine and diazepam may be useful during this stage. Nonsteroidal antiinflammatory drugs, in addition to decreasing the inflammation, are likely to reduce the pain and swelling. Muscle spasm associated with acute disk herniation may be reduced by ice massage or spray of a vapocoolant such as ethyl chloride or fluromethane. Cervical traction could be applied in the hospital or home. Heat followed by gentle limbering movements of the neck and arm may also reduce the pain and muscle spasm.

If symptoms persist despite conservative treatment, an epidural steroid injection should be considered. Inject methylprednisolone (Depo-Medrol) 80 mg or triamcinolone 25 to 50 mg at the level of the disk herniation. Improvement is likely to be seen in 24 to 48 hours. If so, give no further epidural injections. If there is partial or negligible improvement after 10 to 14 days, give a second injection of steroid. Lidocaine (2 to 5 ml of 1%) or bupivacaine (0.5%) may be injected before or during steroid injection to confirm the correct placement of the drugs in the epidural space. If two injections of steroids placed epidurally do not produce any improvement, further injections are unlikely to be useful. There is no rationale for giving a series of injections if the patient is free of pain after the first injection. If neurologic deficits and pain continue or worsen despite the conservative treatment, surgical treatment is indicated. The most commonly performed surgery is anterior cervical diskectomy.

Acute pain may be accompanied by signs of moderate sensory or motor deficit in a root distribution. Such signs are represented by some loss of strength, paresthesia, and mild sensory impairment or loss of muscle stretch reflexes. If these signs worsen or do not subside after a trial of conservative treatment, the patient should be admitted to the hospital to ensure immobilization and rest and to allow further investigation. Epidural steroids or chemonucleolysis have been used at this stage to halt the progress of the nerve compression.

Even if the patient's symptoms completely subside with any of the modalities, the patient should be given appropriate exercises to stretch and strengthen the muscles. Continued observation is required to evaluate the precipitating factors and to prevent any recurrence by early evaluation and treatment.

Management aimed at possible surgical decompression. Surgical decompression is indicated for patients showing signs of spinal cord compression. This is also advisable for patients with nerve root compression if there is intractable or severe progressive recurrent pain or if there are signs of severe neurologic deficit, particularly marked weakness and muscle atrophy with long tract signs attributable to cervical pathology. If there are no contraindications to surgery, perform myelography to establish a diagnosis and determine the site and extent of compression. If indicated, operative treatment should soon follow.

Patients in whom spinal cord compression rapidly develops require prompt investigation and surgical decompression. Impaired bladder or rectal control constitutes an emergency. Such investigations usually include plain films of the spine and an emergency myelogram. During the course of these investigations, keep patients fasting to allow the immediate institution of anesthesia if surgical intervention is required.

Physical therapy program. The physical therapy depends on past medical intervention, the extent of the lesion, and the stage of recovery. During the acute stage the patient may be treated with bed rest and immobilization. Ice massage and transcutaneous electrical nerve stimulation may be used at this stage. When the condition reaches the subacute stage, the patient should begin an exercise program suited to the level and direction of the protrusion. Aggressive physical therapy may begin in the chronic stage; if the patient is still using a cervical collar for pain relief, gradually reduce wearing time. Immobilization at this stage will increase muscle weakness, promote poor postural habits, and lead to tightening of soft tissue structures. The therapy techniques used include flexion-extension, strengthening, and mobilization.

QUESTIONS: NECK AND SHOULDER PAIN

1. Acute disk herniation is NOT managed by:
   A. Muscle relaxation by cyclobenzaprine
   B. Nonsteroidal antiinflammatory agents
   C. Gentle limbering exercises
   D. Cervical laminectomy and fusion
2. If symptoms persist after conservative management of acute cervical disk herniation, the next step is to perform:
   A. Cervical laminectomy and fusion
   B. Cervical epidural injection
   C. Chemonucleolysis
   D. Cervical facet injection
3. Neurogenic pain originating from the neck and shoulder region can be due to:
   A. Degenerative disk disease
   B. Myofascial pain
   C. Fibromyalgia
   D. Herpetic neuralgia
4. A diminished triceps jerk indicates lesion of the:
   A. C_4 nerve root
   B. C_5 nerve root
   C. C_6 nerve root
   D. C_7 nerve root

5. In a patient complaining of pain in the neck and right arm, laminectomy is indicated if the patient has:
   A. Facet arthropathy
   B. Arachnoiditis
   C. Spinal cord compression
   D. Brachial plexus entrapment

ANSWERS

1. D
2. B
3. D
4. D
5. C

41 Low Back Pain

Terrence M. Calder and John C. Rowlingson

Most adults have had at least one episode of back pain in their lifetime. Its vast potential for physical, emotional, and economic impact requires that health care professionals have an understanding of acute and chronic back pain. The differential diagnosis of back pain is large, physical findings can vary markedly from one exam to the next, no laboratory test can quantify the severity of the pain, and many causes of back pain cannot be proven by laboratory studies. Furthermore, the musculoskeletal structures of the back rarely operate alone in producing pain. Therefore the evaluation of the patient with low back pain must be thorough and systematic. In addition to the physical condition, the impact on self-perception, life-style, social relationships, and the ability to work must be considered before directing attention to treatment. Primary treatment options include medications, nerve blocks, counterstimulation techniques, and surgery. The goal is to decrease the pain enough so that the patient can cooperate with corrective/restorative physical therapy. The detrimental effects of the pain on the patient's life-style, the potential for vocational restoration, the need for helping the patient to cope with residual pain, and the mutual dealing with the compensation/disability system also need to be addressed. Patients with low back pain receiving compensation are more likely to have work-related events causing pain, pending litigation, vague diagnoses, inconsistent objective findings, more resistance to conservative treatment, greater medical and compensation costs, and a lower likelihood of returning to work.[1]

PREVALENCE

Low back pain is second only to the common cold as a cause for absence from work in people under age 55, and second only to headache as a cause of chronic pain. The cost of patient evaluation and treatment, as well as the price tag for compensation payments and time lost from work, is enormous. In one survey 56% of Americans reported back pain in the preceding year.[2] The incidence of low back pain decreased with advancing age, but the percentage of those with more than 100 days of backache was higher in those over 50. Extrapolating from their data, the authors estimated that 14% of Americans (25 million) could not work 1 or more days annually because of back pain. Three types of cost generally considered are wage replacement, wages lost, and health care costs. A small group of patients accounts for a large percentage of the expenditure. Only 7.5% of patients with low back pain who did not improve with therapy accounted for 75% of the money spent on back pain, according to the Quebec Task Force on Spinal Disorders.[3]

That study group also showed that, despite its high prevalence, most low back pain resolves in less than 2 months.[4,5] The problem seems to be worsening, with costs of long-term disability in the United States increasing 163% from 1970 to 1981.[6] Back pain is the leading cause of disability in people under 45.[7] The overall incidence of claims for low back pain covered by industrial health insurance is 1% to 2%, and those claims are disproportionately expensive compared with other claims.[8,9] Social factors have also been associated with variations on claims for disability. For instance, claims were found to vary by county in Washington according to the unemployment rate, food stamp usage, and per capita income.[10]

ETIOLOGY

Low back pain usually involves changes in the musculoskeletal structures of the lumbosacral area. Less frequent causes must be excluded in the workup.[11] Keim and Kirkaldy-Willis reviewed the extensive causes of back pain.[12] Sullivan presents a more functional approach to diagnosis, as shown in Box 41-1.[13]

Although there are many causes, several will have the same mechanism for pain. For instance, failed back syndrome, herniated disk, and pain related to cancer-cell infiltration of the nerve root have to varying extent the common pathologic denominator of inflammation of the nerve roots. This can be due to mechanical compression of the nerve root by disk material, irritation thereof by phospholipase A_2 leaked or released from the nucleus pulposus, abnormal contact of the nerve root with bone related to altered anatomy (spinal stenosis) or poor posture, or swelling induced by the invasion of tumor cells. Scarred, swollen, inflamed nerves exhibit altered electrophysiologic function, lowered threshold, sensitization to mechanical stimulation, enhanced pain transmission, altered vascular permeability (causing venous congestion and intraneural edema), and compromised movement through the intervertebral foramina.

EVALUATION OF THE PATIENT WITH BACK PAIN

Given the number of possible causes for low back pain, the evaluation protocol must be thorough and comprehensive (Box 41-2). The initial workup may be done by the primary care physician and a reasonable diagnosis established, or the patient may be referred to a specialty center for expert and extensive evaluation. The pain specialist should scrutinize the relevant records to validate the patient's history, become familiar with past physical findings, review the results of

Vertebral and paravertebral causes of back pain (+/- radiculopathy)

Herniated nucleus pulposus: cervical, thoracic, and most commonly lumbar

Degenerative joint disease: disk space narrowing, spinal stenosis, facet abnormality

Arachnoiditis: postsurgical, postradiographic contrast-material study

Musculoskeletal disorder: strain, sprain, spasm

Neoplastic: metastatic, multiple myeloma, other primary spinal tumors

Infectious: epidural abscess, vertebral osteomyelitis, Pott's disease, herpes zoster

Rheumatic conditions: ankylosing spondylitis, Reiter's syndrome, fibromyalgia

Referred causes of back pain (usually without radiculopathy)

Vascular origin: abdominal aortic aneurysm, arterial occlusive disease

Biliary origin: obstructed bile ducts, distended gallbladder

Gastrointestinal: perforated viscus

Pancreatic origin: pancreatic carcinoma, pancreatitis

Uterine origin: ovarian carcinoma, endometrial carcinoma

Renal origin: renal carcinoma, kidney stones, ureteral stones, pyelonephritis, bladder carcinoma

Modified from Sullivan JGB: The anesthesiologist's approach to back pain. In Nothman RH, Simeone FA, editors: *The Spine,* ed 3. Philadelphia, WB Saunders, 1992.

Box 41-2 **EVALUATION PROTOCOL USING A SYSTEMS APPROACH**

1. Pertinent record review
2. Questionnaire to elicit pain history, drug history, medical history, psychosocial history
3. Pain scaling: draw-your-pain, visual analog scale (VAS), verbal rating
4. Formal psychologic evaluation for selected patients
5. Physical examination: walk, bend, lift, stand, sit, lie down; and the more formal neurologic, musculoskeletal, and functional capacity evaluations
6. Ergonomic assessment
7. Laboratory studies
8. Team conference to document diagnosis and for treatment planning

---

diagnostic laboratory tests, and acknowledge past treatments and outcomes.

A complete diagnosis considers both the physical and nonphysical aspects of pain because appropriate treatment cannot be comprehensive without this understanding. History includes the onset, site, character, and quality of the pain, as well as an appreciation for what makes the pain better or worse, the degree of interference with desired and necessary activity, the response to past treatment (medical, surgical, rest, etc.), coexisting complaints, and medical diseases that may be causing the back pain (e.g., cancer with metastasis) or influencing the back pain (e.g., lower-extremity injury with a subsequent change in posture). It is important to differentiate between acute and chronic pain, since the management is quite different, and to consider the psychosocial aspects (nonphysical factors). Use of a standardized questionnaire helps to get an organized history in a consistent, systematic fashion in a format that becomes very familiar to the examiner. The outline of the patient's problem as presented allows the evaluator time to hear the patient's story in his or her words. Patients feel tremendous satisfaction in getting to relay their history; this increases the likelihood of their cooperation with the prescribed therapy.

Physical examination includes evaluation of the nervous, musculoskeletal, and vascular systems, and a search for bone disorders. In chronic pain patients the examination may not substantiate earlier assessments because of progression or regression of disease with and without treatment. Findings and physical changes may vary over time (e.g., cumulative trauma to the low back secondary to stressful posture). Furthermore, serial examinations help to determine if treatment is resulting in improvement. Neurologic appraisal elicits changes in vascular, sensory, motor, and reflex function in the lower extremity. Musculoskeletal examination evaluates range of motion (flexion and extension of the low back, straight leg raise in the supine and seated positions), range of motion of hip and leg joints, muscle shortening, spasm in muscles, the presence of trigger points, and postural changes (e.g., scoliosis or change in lumbar lordosis). The evaluation also includes a functional review: the patient's ability to walk, stand, sit, and bend. The more sophisticated functional capacity assessment of patients includes aerobic capacity, trunk strength, lifting power, mobility, elasticity, and endurance.[14] This should be obtained in selected patients for whom these data have direct implications for compensation, employment, and realistic retraining.

There is no diagnostic laboratory test that reveals every cause of low back pain.[11,14] The main sites of origin of low back pain are the posterior longitudinal ligament, the interspinous ligaments, the nerve roots and dural coverings, the facet joints, and the deep muscles.[15] Since only two of these are really evaluated by routine laboratory studies, it is easy to explain the many false negatives. A negative laboratory test does not necessarily mean there is no "real" pain, nor does it indicate a predominance of psychosocial pain. Up to 85% of patients with low back pain cannot be given a definitive diagnosis because of the poor association among symptoms, pathologic findings, and imaging results.[16] Frymoyer emphasizes the need to correlate laboratory findings with clinical findings, since 30% to 40% of computed tomography (CT) scans, myelograms, and discograms can show abnormalities in asymptomatic individuals. In patients with prior surgery, findings must be interpreted in light of postsurgical alterations in anatomy.

Plain posteroanterior and lateral x-rays of the lumbosacral spine can reveal anatomic changes (i.e., transitional vertebrae occur in 5% to 7% of the population), bony tumors, compression fractures, scoliosis, and disk space narrowing.[12,17,18] Oblique views can show spondylosis, which is a defect in the lamina that may separate the anterior body from the posterior elements, and spondylolisthesis, the sliding of one vertebral body anteriorly relative to the one inferior. Myelography, most appropriate preoperatively, will show disk herniation, nerve root compression (which can be falsely positive or negative depending on the clinical correlation) and space-occupying lesions. CT and magnetic resonance imaging (MRI) scans can reveal much of the same information noninvasively while assessing the relationship of the lumbosacral structures to neural elements.[19] A CT scan has more sensitivity for bone pathology, whereas the MRI is better at picking up soft-tissue abnormalities. Electromyography can help to determine acute versus chronic neurologic alteration and document nerve injury. Electromyographic changes are picked up in the paraspinous muscles when the posterior primary division of the lumbar nerve root is affected and in the peripheral nervous system when the anterior root is involved. Thermography use has not been scientifically clarified, so its application is not universal. It is noninvasive, though, and has only a 5% to 8% false-negative rate.[20]

In persistent or chronic pain, nonphysical and psychosocial aspects should be evaluated. It must be determined whether psychologic conflicts are being expressed through physical complaints. Waddell and colleagues suggested the following nonorganic physical signs that intimate that psychosocial factors are playing a significant role in the patient's complaints: superficial, nonanatomic tenderness (i.e., skin rolling), positive simulation response (i.e., light axial loading), discrepancy between supine and seated straight leg raising, nonphysiologic regional disturbances of sensation and/or weakness or pain distribution, and responses out of proportion to the test stimulus.[21]

Chronic pain can affect the quality of life for the entire family, both socially and economically. The relationship with the patient's employer also frequently deteriorates because of absenteeism, a mutual loss of confidence, and the questions of eventual return to work and the ability to tolerate the demands of the job. Ergonomic evaluation considers human factors in the interactions with equipment and the total work environment. This can be used to assess specific physical limitations in relationship to job requirements and to determine what activities the patient can actually do. Thus realistic decisions about employment become possible.

ANATOMIC CONSIDERATIONS

In normal posture the anterior vertebral column carries most of the weight in the low back, and the disks absorb shocks and allow flexion yet limit motion. The disks comprise one third of the height of the vertebral column in the lumbar region, and one fifth of the height in other regions.[22] Disks are composed of a viscous gel-like center of mucopolysaccharides, including phospholipase A_2, surrounded by a tough fibrous annulus. The thinnest part of the annulus is posterior, which may explain herniation in that direction with sudden or uneven loads on the spine. With age the disks become less resilient and lose the ability to distribute mechanical forces evenly.[23] The posterior longitudinal liga-

ment narrows from L_2-L_5 and is thus less of a barrier to posterolateral disk protrusion. It is not surprising that 85% of herniated disks occur at L_4-L_5 or L_5-S_1. Whereas the cervical nerves exit the foramina *above* the corresponding vertebrae, the thoracic, lumbar and sacral nerves exit *below* the corresponding vertebrae (i.e., the L_5 root exits below the L_5 vertebral body and between L_5 and S_1) The nerve roots run from the spinal cord caudally along the posterior portion of the body and disk of the vertebrae before exiting through the intervertebral foramina. Therefore when the L_4-L_5 disk herniates, it impinges on the L_5 nerve root, which leaves the vertebral column between L_5 and S_1. Only 1% to 2% of patients with low back pain have a herniated disk.

The posterior elements of the spine include the lamina, pedicles, and facet joints, which together encircle and protect the spinal cord and emerging nerve roots. The purpose of the posterior elements is to restrict range of motion and anchor muscles, ligaments, and tendons. The intervertebral foramina are formed by the pedicles and apposing articular surfaces of the facet joints. The nerve root fills 35% to 50% of the foramina. The facet joint is innervated at least by articular filaments from the medial branch of the posterior primary division of the spinal nerve at and from the level above the joint (and occasionally from three levels) (Fig. 41-1). The posterior ramus arises from the spinal nerve outside the intervertebral foramen and then divides into medial and lateral branches. The medial branch descends in a groove posterior to the medial transverse process to innervate the joint.[23] Paraspinous muscles (semispinalis, multifidus, quadratus lumborum) serve posture, motion, and support. If the spine is not in optimal position because of a disruption in coordination of the musculoskeletal system, lifting, bending, or twisting can result in injury.

COMMON LOW BACK PAIN SYNDROMES

The most common cause of low back pain is postural change associated with primary or secondary injury to supporting muscles and ligaments. Of all low back pain, 80% to 90% is postural. Cailliet[15] proposes that the lumbar lordotic curve increases secondary to pain-initiated reflex muscle spasm. Then weight bearing is transferred from the anterior structures of the spine to the posterior structures; the facet joint is maximally loaded; sheer forces on the disks increase (especially in the posterior axis); and the intervertebral foramina may be compressed, causing nerve root impingement. Most people do not have adequate tone in their abdominal muscles to counterbalance the musculoskeletal changes, so the posterior elements are stressed, leading to more muscle spasm and a vicious cycle of pain, reflex muscle spasm, and altered posture. Eventually, *postural pain* may lead to herniated disks, facet joint pain, and myofascial pain. Diffuse lumbosacral pain is described by the patient as dull and aching with no radiation except perhaps into the buttocks or hips. Pain at rest suggests causes other than mechanical low back pain.[11] The physical examination is largely nonfocal with the exceptions of possible sacroiliac joint tenderness or paraspinous spasm associated with subsequent stiffness found by testing range of motion. Laboratory findings are unrevealing. Patients with *degenerative joint disease* may have similar symptoms, but their

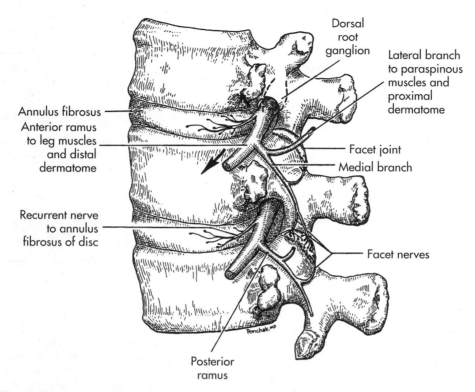

Fig. 41-1 Anatomic features of a typical lumbar nerve root. Branches to the spinal facet joints, disk annulus, and back muscles are present and may be sources of pain referred to as sciatica. (Adapted from illustration by Stephen Ponchak, M.D.)

diagnosis suggests some baseline disorder of the facet joints in addition to the postural changes.

Facet syndrome (zygapophyseal joint)[24] is related to physical stress on the facet joint or an anatomic derangement of the facet joint and is associated with pain that is most frequently referred to the gluteal region or thigh, but it can be felt anywhere in the leg. Facet syndrome[25,26] may accompany degenerative joint disease and spinal stenosis, presenting with unilateral back pain that radiates from a site off the (lumbar) midline down the back of the thigh to the knee. Pain is aggravated by hyperextension or lateral flexion. Lateral bending with extension of the spine often causes the most intense pain. Further findings may include tenderness over the facet joint, and deep tendon reflexes may be depressed and straight leg raising limited. Laboratory findings are nonspecific. Diagnosis is confirmed by relief of pain by facet injection[27] (adjacent segments will need to be blocked because of the overlap in innervation).

Acute disk syndromes frequently are associated with a history of a specific initiating event such as lifting in a bent and twisted stance. The pain is sharp and stabbing and shoots in a dermatomal fashion into the lower extremity but decreases when the patient lies down. Increasing intraabdominal pressure, as with straining during bowel movement or coughing, may exacerbate pain because the pressure increase is transmitted to the spine and the already bulging disk. Typical changes in neurologic examination include decreased deep tendon reflex, decreased sensation, paresthesias, positive straight leg raise when supine and/or seated,

and the indication that sitting causes radicular symptoms (Table 41-1). The positive straight leg raise, crossed straight leg raise (i.e., lifting the contralateral leg and causing pain in the affected side), and the bowstring sign (i.e., at the level of pain in the straight leg raise test, the leg is flexed at the knee and the tibial nerve is forcefully palpated in the popliteal fossa) are the three signs most indicative of radicular low back pain.[11] Irritation of the nerve root causes pain in its distribution; the straight leg lift duplicates this and is considered positive if radicular pain is produced when the leg is lifted more than 40°. Crossed straight leg lift also can distort the anatomy enough to irritate the affected root. The common findings are presented in Table 41-1. Reactive paraspinous muscle spasm may be marked and spine range of motion decreased. Laboratory studies may show nerve root impingement and acute denervation. Other causes of radicular pain include hypertrophic changes of vertebral margins and facet joints (osteoarthritis of spine) and spinal stenosis (fibrous and bony proliferation of the protective bony arch of the spine on a chronic basis).

Disk injury can result in the release of even small amounts of phospholipase A_2, causing marked nerve root inflammation without obvious structural changes. Homogenized autologous nucleus pulposus material was injected into the epidural space of dogs and tissue reaction compared to controls given only saline injections.[28] Experimental dogs had intensive inflammatory response in the dural sac, the spinal cord, and nerve roots. The clinical correlation is that back pain may be due to leaks of small amounts of

Table 41-1 Differentiation of level of disk herniation by physical examination and history

Level of herniation	Pain	Numbness	Weakness	Atrophy	Reflexes
L$_3$-L$_4$ disk (fourth lumbar nerve root)	Lower back, hip, posterolateral thigh, anterior leg	Anteromedial thigh and knee	Quadriceps	Quadriceps	Knee jerk diminished
L$_4$-L$_5$ disk (L$_5$ nerve root)	Over sacroiliac joint, hip, lateral thigh, and leg	Lateral leg, first three toes	Dorsiflexion of great toe and foot; difficulty walking on heels, foot drop possible	Minor	Uncommon in knee and ankle (internal hamstring diminished or absent)
L$_5$-S$_1$ disk (first sacral nerve root)	Sacroiliac joint, hip, and posterior and lateral thigh and leg to heel	Back of calf, lateral heel, foot, and toe	Plantar flexion of foot and great toe may be affected; difficulty walking on toes	Gastrocnemius and soleus	Ankle jerk diminished or absent

Adapted from Keim HA, Kirklady-Willis WH: Low back pain, *CIBA Clin Symp* 32(6), 1980.

nucleus pulposus material, which triggers intense inflammatory neuropathology in which the usual diagnostic tests would not be positive. Saal and colleagues found an increase of phospholipase-A$_2$ of 20 to 10,000 times normal in the disks removed at surgery.[29] Phospholipase-A$_2$ is an enzyme that releases arachidonic acid from cell membranes. Its action is blocked by steroids and *not* antiprostaglandin agents such as nonsteroidal antiinflammatory drugs.

After lumbar laminectomy (with or without fusion) some patients continue to have pain (i.e., *postlaminectomy syndrome* or *failed back syndrome*). Presumably this is due to scar tissue in and around the spinal nerves. Their complaints are of diffuse, ill-defined, low back pain that is dull and aching in nature, with occasional sharper pain. Pain commonly involves hips, buttocks, and upper posterior thighs. Pain may begin early in the day, as with neuropathic pain, or may worsen through the day because of progressive muscle fatigue, which imposes greater physical stress on the already compromised musculoskeletal system. The neurologic exam may be difficult to interpret because of lingering changes related to prior surgery. Frequent findings include various sensory changes, loss of reflexes, muscle weakness, decreased flexion of the lumbar spine, reduced hip motion, and straight-leg-raise testing limited by muscle spasm. Laboratory studies are problematic, since positive findings must be separated from residual effects from earlier diagnostic studies and surgery.

Both *primary* and *metastatic cancer* can cause back pain.[30] Night pain, fever, a palpable and often tender spinal mass, or a combination of these findings are the usual presenting symptoms. These can be related to bony involvement, pressure on neurologic or vascular elements, or inherent properties of the lesion (i.e., aneurysmal bone cyst). Tumor and infection must be considered in any patient who has weight loss, fever, chills, significant neurologic involvement, or atypical blood or urine tests. A specific diagnosis is made using radiologic studies with consideration to patient age (lesions in young adults, ages 21 to 50, are commonly benign, whereas in those over 50, more frequently

malignant), location (bony tumors are associated with posterior elements, whereas hemangiomas more frequently involve the vertebral body), density (increased with ivory vertebrae, decreased with multiple myeloma), type of deformity (expansion in aneurysmal bone cyst, osteoblastoma, Paget's disease), and host reaction. Malignant lesions are frequently metastatic from lung, breast, prostate, thyroid, gastrointestinal (GI) tract, kidney, and the female reproductive tract. Multiple myeloma also needs to be considered. Ivory vertebrae (a vertebral body with significantly increased opacity on radiographs) is associated with Paget's disease, prostate cancer, carcinomatosis, and Hodgkin's disease. Compression of the nerve root may indicate a need for surgical decompression unless the tumor is deemed sensitive to radiation treatment or chemotherapy.

TREATMENT ISSUES

With an acute bout of low back pain, patients expect an evaluation that readily identifies the cause for the pain and then treatment that at least reduces but hopefully eliminates the pain. Pain becomes chronic when it lasts more than 6 to 7 weeks. Treatment goals for chronic pain are necessarily different than for acute pain. There may be structural reasons such as soft tissue scarring, nerve root fibrosis, or bony derangement that explain why all pain cannot be eliminated. The presence of a number of nonphysical factors can modify the description of the patient's tolerance for and his or her ability to cope with the unending pain. Realistic goals for chronic pain management are to decrease the frequency and intensity of the patient's pain (using medications, surgery, nerve blocks, and stimulation techniques), help the patient cope with the residual pain (using psychologic strategies), and restore function (using physical therapy) (Box 41-3). Less consideration may be given to surgery than in patients with acute pain, less potent medications are desirable given the likely duration of their use, and the patient must be encouraged to participate in physical rehabilitation. The usual plan is to decrease the pain enough to allow physical therapy to strengthen muscles, improve posture, and increase activity. Psychotherapy to provide the patient with insight into the intense interaction of physical and nonphysical components may be indicated. The Quebec Task Force on Spinal Disorders recommended that, after 3 months of conservative treatment or accumulated time lost from work as a result of low back pain, the patient should be referred to a multidisciplinary pain center.[3]

Nachemson found that 70% of patients with discogenic low back pain and sciatica had relief with conservative treatment in 3 weeks; 90% had relief in 2 months.[31] Conservative treatment included decreased activity, time off work, or less strenuous physical activity. Also, the inclination for rest was reinforced by potent analgesics and indirect-acting muscle relaxants, which are mild to moderate sedatives. Physical therapy (e.g., ultrasound, diathermy, whirlpools, transcutaneous electrical nerve stimulation [TENS], massage) was used in many cases. As pain subsided, normal activity was resumed. Pain that does not resolve may need evaluation by a pain specialist. Deyo and Diehl found that the patient's satisfaction with treatment was highly correlated with the explanation given.[32] The patient is likely to be more satisfied with therapy because he or she had a say in the decision process; the physician is reassured at having presented to the patient a balanced analysis of the risks and benefits of, and rationale for, treatment.

TREATMENT OPTIONS
Medications

Proper compliance on the patient's part is needed to assume an adequate trial with any drugs. Medications need to be used purposefully; if the pain is from an inflammatory process within the musculoskeletal system, then aspirin or another nonsteroidal antiinflammatory drug should be used. Ketorolac is a moderate nonsteroidal antiinflammatory drug with good central, nonnarcotic analgesic actions. If nonsteroidal antiinflammatory drugs are contraindicated (GI upset, fluid retention, renal insufficiency, decreased platelet adhesiveness), then acetaminophen is an alternative; how-

ever, it does not have potent antiinflammatory actions, so it may offer less pain relief. In general these medications are low in cost, lack synergistic physiologic depressive effects, are readily available, and are nonaddictive.

Indirect muscle relaxants (e.g., cyclobenzaprine, methocarbamol, baclofen) can relieve reflex muscle spasm and allow increased range of motion and activity, but many have sedative side effects. They should be used only for relatively short periods of time.

Narcotics should be used for moderate to severe acute pain and in patients with acute flare-ups above and beyond their usual chronic pain. It is important to prescribe adequate amounts for up to 7 to 21 days. If the patient improves, the drug can be tapered and eliminated; if pain persists, additional workup is required to explain the persistence of severe pain. If the workup does not reveal obvious pathology and narcotics have not been effective after 2 to 3 weeks, substitution with less potent agents is reasonable and other treatment modalities are recommended.

Adjuncts to narcotics and nonnarcotic medications include hydroxyzine, promethazine, doxepin, amitriptyline, and trazodone. Sedative hypnotics such as the benzodiazepines are not recommended because of the potential for physical dependence and an antalgesic effect assumed to be related to central nervous system (CNS) serotonin depletion. Tricyclic antidepressants act pharmacologically by blocking the reuptake of norepinephrine and serotonin and therefore can enhance analgesic effects at doses *not* associated with (and faster than) an antidepressant effect. Anticonvulsant drugs can be of use in patients with neuralgic causes for low back pain, such as after laminectomy and/or spinal fusion.

As pain becomes chronic, a simple pharmacologic answer is less likely. Tolerance to narcotics can occur, and a ceiling effect on analgesia is seen with nonsteroidal antiinflammatory drugs. Increasing the dose to reestablish effectiveness frequently results in side effects. Treating the side effects with more medications may be ill-advised (i.e., adding sedative drugs to sedatives) or illogical (i.e., adding narcotic agonist-antagonist drugs to narcotics). If a long trial of drugs has been ineffective, the patient will benefit from gradual detoxification and reevaluation for alternative management strategies.

Surgery

Success is about 80% for the first surgery, but it is invasive, involves an interruption of normal activities, necessitates a variable period of hospitalization, and requires some recovery time. A specific diagnosis that can be corrected surgically (i.e., a structural and/or mechanical cause of pain such as herniated disk, spondylolisthesis, foraminal encroachment on the nerve root, or pseudoarthrosis) is desirable. It is still not known which herniated nucleus pulposus patients need surgery. Surgery is usually done for those who fail conservative therapy, have foraminal encroachment on the nerve root, or have progressive neurologic deficit. Saal and Saal reported success in treating patients with herniated lumbar disks and radiculopathy with an aggressive, *non-operative* approach.[33] With pain control followed by staged exercise training, they found 90% of patients had good or excellent results, with 92% returning to work in a study group of 52 patients. They suggested that surgery be reserved for those patients in whom function cannot be satisfactorily improved with a physical rehabilitation program. Those who failed the conservative program had a high degree of spinal stenosis.

Nonphysical aspects that influence the pain need to be considered preoperatively. Waddell and associates studied back pain after industrial accidents.[34] Of patients receiving compensation after laminectomy, 97% had persistent complaints of pain and 72% had continued impairment of function. As pain becomes more chronic and factors other than soft-tissue damage contribute to pain, surgery may be inadequate or even inadvisable. After a long exposure to pain, the nervous system may compensate for pain transmission interruption by the mechanisms of plasticity and neuron recruitment. This neural repair and recovery process may ultimately cause more pain after surgery.[35]

Chymopapain is not a conservative treatment but an option roughly comparable to surgery.[36-38] The workup usually does not indicate which patients would benefit from this treatment. Serious side effects including allergic reactions and life-threatening anaphylactoid reactions have occurred. There may be irregular distribution of chymopapain with a subsequently inadequate clinical result.[39] Success appears to be 59% to 90%.[36]

Nerve blocks

Nerve blocks can be used for diagnosis (differential nerve block) or therapy. The patient's workup must uncover the absolute contraindications to regional analgesia (i.e., use of major anticoagulants, septicemia, infection at the site of needle insertion, and refusal of the therapy). The anticoagulant properties of nonsteroidal antiinflammatory drugs are only a moderate deterrent to providing regional analgesia. The effectiveness of nerve blocks is diluted if they are used indiscriminately, as in patients with an incomplete database or when used with faulty technique. Yet when done appropriately and within the framework of a treatment program that provides pain relief and encourages physical and emotional rehabilitation in patients with lifestyle disruption caused by the pain, they can be quite effective. They can give a strong psychologic boost to the patient by demonstrating that something can be done about the pain—this creates a positive attitude that fosters cooperation with rehabilitation regimens and, ultimately, recovery.

Epidural steroid injections are effective in about 66% of selected patients.[40] Box 41-4 reviews the advantages and disadvantages of epidural steroid injections, which must be weighed for each patient. Box 41-5 suggests the types of patients who might benefit from epidural steroid injections. All patients who have received epidural steroid injections must be reassessed, as suggested in Box 41-6. Mechanical irritation of neurologic structures suggests inflammation as a cause for radicular low back pain. On average a patient is better in 4 to 6 days after an epidural steroid injection (if he or she is going to respond), in 2 to 4 weeks with bedrest, and in 11 days with a local anesthetic epidural. Corticosteroids provide a beneficial antiinflammatory effect.

Box 41-4 ADVANTAGES AND DISADVANTAGES OF EPIDURAL STEROID INJECTIONS

Advantages

· The technique is known to many practitioners and is widely available.
· The procedure can be done on an outpatient basis.
· The procedure is normally of low risk and can be done at all clinically necessary spinal levels.
· When the patient is given local anesthetics and steroids, this is two active treatments at once.
· The positive results change the patient's attitude about medication use, the need for surgery, and participation in rehabilitation.
· Money can be saved if surgery, long convalescence, and work interruption are avoided.

Disadvantages

· There is the potential for reaction to the local anesthetic drug or the corticosteroid drug injected.
· There is a risk of tissue trauma with the occurrence of bleeding, infection, ligamentous pain, or postdural puncture headache.
· The treatment may not help the patient, thereby increasing discouragement.
· There are not many studies that clearly define which patients are the most appropriate for this treatment.

Box 41-5 PATIENTS TO CONSIDER FOR EPIDURAL STEROID INJECTIONS

· Patients with radicular pain and a corresponding sensory change
· Patients with symptoms caused by a herniated disk who have not improved with 4 weeks of conservative therapy
· Patients with cancer in whom tumor infiltration of the nerve roots may be causing the radicular pain
· Active patients with chronic back pain who suffer an acute flare-up, manifest symptoms that have radicular-like features, and do not respond to conservative therapy
· Motivated patients with postural back pain that has radicular-like features and a poor response to conservative therapy
· Selected patients with chronic back pain for whom epidural steroid injection is but one component of a comprehensive treatment program

---

An additional mechanism for low back pain that is proposed and that may be more frequent after surgery is as follows: Persistent low back pain with subsequent injury to peripheral nerves or nerve roots can trigger changes in the nervous system, which affect the central modulation of afferent and efferent neuronal activity or encourage neuroma formation.[30] Corticosteroids can inhibit a neuroma's abnormal, spontaneous discharge.[41] Rocco and associates tested the use of narcotics in combination with local anesthetic and steroids in the epidural space of patients with failed back syndrome. They found no benefit with the combination of drugs, but only an increase in side effects, including respi-

Box 41-6 MEDICAL FOLLOW-UP AFTER EPIDURAL STEROID INJECTION

- If the patient is worse, the epidural steroid injection is not repeated and further explanation for the pain and the poor result is sought.
- If the patient has a neutral response, the epidural steroid injection is worth repeating to assure accurate anatomic placement of the original drugs because not all patients have a dramatic response with the first block.
- If the patient is better, further injections are held while other conservative therapy measures are continued. Recurrent pain is treated after reevaluation of the patient. The interval between necessary blocks is generally not shorter than 2 weeks.

There is no basis for withholding epidural steroid injection for a year in patients who develop recurrent symptoms months after a series of epidural steroid injections. Medical judgment and the physical and psychosocial status of the patient at the time of reevaluation should guide the repetition of therapy more than arbitrary standards.

Box 41-7 METHYLPREDNISOLONE AND TRIAMCINOLONE: DESCRIPTIONS

Methylprednisolone acetate suspension

An antiinflammatory glucocorticoid for intramuscular, intrasynovial, soft-tissue, or intralesional injection. Available in two strengths, 40 mg/ml and 80 mg/ml. Each ml contains:

methylprednisolone	40 mg	80 mg
polyethylene glycol 3350	29 mg	28 mg
myristyl-gamma-picolinium chloride	0.195 mg	0.189 mg

sodium chloride to adjust tonicity and pH adjusted with NaOH or HCl (pH is 3.5 to 7.0)

Triamcinolone diacetate suspension

Possesses glucocorticoid properties while being essentially devoid of mineralocorticoid activity. Supplied as a sterile suspension of 25 mg/ml, with each ml containing:

polysorbate 80 NF	0.20%
polyethylene glycol 3350 NF	3%
sodium chloride	0.85%
benzyl alcohol	0.9%
water for injection q.s.	

ratory depression, which required naloxone in 5 of 19 receiving the narcotic.[42] Neuraxial narcotics[43] are used by some but do not seem to add much to current treatment. Subarachnoid steroids have been used, but epidural placement seems more appropriate because the mechanical compression and/or irritation of the nerve roots occurs in the epidural space. Furthermore, few patients really have arachnoiditis with inflammatory changes; to be more pathologically accurate, they have scarring of nerve roots in the epidural space. Abram found a poor response among patients with low back pain while using triamcinolone in the subarachnoid space,[44] and Wilkinson recently reviewed this topic.[45]

The two commercial deposteroids used are methylprednisolone acetate (Depo-Medrol) and triamcinolone diacetate (Aristocort) (Box 41-7). The tissue safety of these compounds has been an issue of debate. Triamcinolone with 0.9% benzyl alcohol was demonstrated to be tissue safe in a cat model, with the finding of only a very minor inflammatory response not significantly different from the controls.[46] Cicala and co-workers used a rabbit model and found little if any irritation or inflammatory reaction with methylprednisolone.[47] Polyethylene glycol is another component of the commercial preparations that has raised concern.[48] Benzon and colleagues, using a rabbit, sheathed nerve model, found that concentrations up to 40% did not cause neurolysis.[49] Commercial preparations have no more than 3% polyethylene glycol, and this is diluted in clinical use with saline or local anesthetic. Unanswered questions about epidural steroid injections include the difference of effectiveness when using saline versus local in the injectate, the proper volume of the therapeutic injection, and the effects of prior surgery on the movement of the injected fluid. The terminal half-life of the deposteroids is a significant issue. Adrenal suppression and Cushing's syndrome have been reported in patients who manifested an unexpectedly long half-life for the injected steroid. Kay and co-

workers found suppression of the hypothalamic pituitary axis for up to 5 weeks in 12 patients after three epidural steroid injections (80 mg triamcinolone was given with each weekly injection).[50] If in doubt of the suppression of the hypothalamic pituitary axis, a cortisol stimulation test can be done, although this is not practical on a routine basis.

Other useful blocks may include paravertebral and transsacral blocks when pain is away from the midline or when a midline approach is precluded by past surgery or traumatic change. With the paravertebral blocks the drug is placed distal to the intervertebral foramen, and retrograde diffusion accounts for effectiveness. Facet joint nerve blocks have been proposed as being useful, at least in the diagnosis of the source of low back pain.[51,52] The facet joints undergo degenerative changes, and the anatomic distortion results in stress on the joint capsule and irritation of the synovial lining. Combinations of local anesthetics and steroids are injected at the level involved and, because of overlapping innervation, also at the levels above and below.

Trigger points are discrete areas in muscles or connective tissue that are exquisitely painful to palpation and can initiate some of the patient's pain. They are areas of focal ischemia that result when pain causes reflex muscle and vascular spasm. They may be the primary complaint, but more frequently are secondary to prolonged imbalance in posture from chronic low back pain. Pain in the sacroiliac joint and that at the sciatic notch associated with the piriformis muscle can be considered as trigger points.[15,53] Piriformis syndrome, a form of myofascial pain, can be associated with sciatic pain, since the muscle overlies the sciatic nerve, but it is not usually associated with low back pain. Myofascial pain seems to originate in a consistent area, and as the day progresses and muscles fatigue from persistent spasm, the pain spreads. Trigger points are found during physical examination. They are treated with massage and TENS, as well as trigger-point injections with local anesthetics, and occasionally corticosteroids or sarapin (a distillate of the pitcher plant and basically ammonium chloride salts), all done in conjunction with physical therapy.

Stimulation techniques

Based on Melzack and Wall's gate control theory,[54] small pain-fiber (C- or A-delta) input can be modified by faster A-alpha or beta neural input. Dorsal column stimulators or epidural stimulators can be used as a clinical application of this theory.[55] They have been found helpful in some patients who have failed conservative treatment and are poor candidates for surgery.[56] Technologic advances have improved their success and include a trial period before permanent implantation. As with many procedures, patient selection and proper technique are vital to increasing success.[57]

TENS is a noninvasive stimulation technique that is simple enough for home use, does not require a formal therapist for continued treatment, is used basically without age restriction, does not interfere with other therapy, has no systemic side effects, and is patient controlled. Use of TENS may not affect the primary cause of the pain but could relieve reflex muscle spasm, which may allow physical therapy that improves muscle tone, strength, and overall function.

Physical rehabilitation

Physical rehabilitation is fundamental to the patient's overall improvement. Enforced inactivity and disruption of routine may provoke anxiety, despair, anger, agitation, frustration and depression, and lead to loss of muscle tone and strength, decreased range of motion, inflexible posture, and weight gain. Attention must be directed to reversing the detrimental effects of inactivity. Which exercises are best is controversial. Traditionally accepted exercises include the pelvic tilt and knee to chest. Formal physical therapy assessment is highly recommended in patients with chronic low back pain because the training ensures that the patient has been shown the proper procedure for exercises. In principle all patients with musculoskeletal low back pain need regular, daily exercise to restore and/or maintain muscle tone, strength, coordination, and endurance in those muscle groups operative in the mechanical function of the lumbar spine. This includes not only the erector spinae (semispinalis, multifidus, quadratus lumborum) but also the anterior abdominal, gluteal, hamstring, iliopsoas, and rectus femoris muscles. If the workup suggests pain does not indicate ongoing soft-tissue injury, then pain is not necessarily a reason to stop or avoid activity. First using disused muscles will result in soreness, which should resolve in a few weeks. If persistent with exercise, the patient will gradually note an increased capacity for more activity, possibly with less pain or at least no increase in pain. The patient must understand that activities of daily living do not constitute exercise. Patients need to do daily exercises at home, increasing the number, frequency, and degree of difficulty. They should exercise to a number of repetitions, not to a pain

level. The satisfaction from doing favorite or necessary tasks again adds to the therapeutic effect.

Back school programs[58] teach anatomy; function of the back; proper body mechanics for lifting, bending, and sitting; and proper exercises, and foster an active, self-care philosophy (rather than a passive patient role). Whether back school programs are cost effective has not been extensively studied.

A patient can transiently use orthotics or braces. Wilensky[59] observed that orthotics decreased pain, protected from further injury, aided early in rehabilitation when muscles were weak, and corrected deformities. Detrimental effects of prolonged reliance on back braces or canes include muscle atrophy, contracture, posture abnormality, continued weakness in muscles, and loss of motivation for complete rehabilitation.

Psychologic rehabilitation

Emotional response is a part of pain, and lack of positive identification of pathology does not mean that a psychiatric cause is predominant. In acute low back pain with its associated anxiety component, anxiolytics may be temporarily indicated. Benzodiazepines (used mainly as sedatives rather than true muscle relaxants) help with bedrest and reduce reflex muscle spasm. As discussed above, they are not good for long-term use.

Psychotherapeutic techniques for selected patients with chronic low back pain include biofeedback, self-regulation skills, and hypnosis; they help to control muscle tension, anxiety, and spasm. There is less utility with these techniques in acute pain, since such episodes usually have resolved before they can be introduced, practiced, and learned. In chronic pain they can be of use for flare-ups above baseline or as coping strategies to help the patient tolerate pain, develop control over pain, and encourage daily function.

Vocational rehabilitation

Mayer and colleagues[14,60] found that return to work was based on improved physical capacity and renewal of the psychologic motivation to become productive. More attention may need to be paid to matching an employee with a specific job that is based on the physical demands, his or her functional capacity, and the psychology of the work environment (i.e., ergonomics). Simply doing home exercises is unlikely to restore the physical strength and stamina needed for work. Productive rehabilitation or work hardening can serve as a bridge back to work. Mayer[60] showed that with functional rehabilitation, 86% returned to work, compared to 40% of those not receiving rehabilitation. The former group also had less surgery, used fewer nonsurgical medical services, and had lower reinjury rates.

CONCLUSION

The majority of acute episodes of back pain resolve on their own in a limited amount of time. Not all pain can be documented by testing, and positive results do not necessarily explain the patient's complaints. Sound medical practice dictates that tests should not be duplicated needlessly. Rather, only those that would change the course of referral or treatment should be ordered (especially in chronic pain). When the pain persists, the cause can be complicated by reactive physical and psychosocial mechanisms that compound the signs and symptoms. Adding compensation, possible secondary gain, and pain behavior can further confuse the evaluation of the patient with chronic back pain. Following the Quebec Task Force on Spinal Disorders' recommendation to apply conservative measures for up to 6 weeks and then to obtain evaluation and treatment if needed at a multidisciplinary pain center seems prudent. The onus of improvement lies with the patient, since measures to alleviate the pain are usually aimed at allowing the patient to perform exercises to strengthen his or her back musculature. The role of back schools and work hardening is unproven in large studies but appears to support the idea of helping the patient take the lead in his or her own care. Finally, an understanding of the psychologic dynamics is needed in the proper evaluation and treatment of these patients.

REFERENCES

1. Strang JP: The chronic disability syndrome. In Aronoff GM, editor: *Evaluation and Treatment of Chronic Pain.* Baltimore, Urban & Schwarzenberg, 1985.
2. Taylor H, Curran NM: *The Nuprin Pain Report.* New York, Louis Harris & Associates, 1985.
3. Quebec Task Force on Spinal Disorders: Scientific approach to the assessment and management of activity-related spinal disorders. *Spine* 12(7S):S16, 1987.
4. National Institute on Disability and Rehabilitation Research: Report on workshop on low back pain. Charlottesville, Va, Rehabilitation Research and Training Center of the University of Virginia, Department of Orthopedics, 1989.
5. Roland M, Morris R: A study of the natural history of back pain. *Spine* 2:145-150, 1983.
6. Wood PHN, Badley EM: Epidemiology of back pain. In Jayson MJV, editor: *The Lumbar Spine and Back Pain.* London, Pitman Medical, 1980.
7. Waddell G: A new clinical model for the treatment of low back pain. *Spine* 12:632, 1987.
8. Klein BP, Jensen RC, Sanderson LM: Assessment of workers' compensation claims for back strains/sprains. *J Occup Med* 26:443, 1984.
9. Spengler DM: Back injuries in industry: A retrospective study. *Spine* 11:241, 1986.
10. Volinn, E: When back pain becomes disabling: A regional analysis. *Pain* 33:33, 1988.
11. McCulloch JA: Differential diagnosis of low back pain. In Tollison CD, editor: *Handbook of Chronic Pain Management.* Baltimore, Williams & Wilkins, 1989.
12. Keim HA, Kirkaldy-Willis WH: Low back pain. *CIBA Clin Symp* 32(6):6-28, 1980.
13. Sullivan JGB: The anesthesiologist's approach to back pain. In Rothman RH, Simeone FA, editors: *The Spine,* ed 3. Philadelphia, WB Saunders, 1992.
14. Frymoyer JW: Back pain and sciatica. *N Engl J Med* 318:291-299, 1988.
15. Cailliet R: Low back pain. In Cailliet R, editor: *Soft Tissue Pain and Disability.* Philadelphia, FA Davis, 1977.
16. Deyo RA: Fads in the treatment of low back pain. *N Engl J Med* 325:1039-1040, 1991.
17. Frymoyer JW et al: Spine radiographs in patients with low-back pain. *J Bone Joint Surg [Am]* 66A(7):1048-1055, 1984.
18. Lowry PA: Radiology in the diagnosis and management of pain. In Raj PP, editor: *Practical Management of Pain,* ed 2. St Louis, Mosby, 1992.
19. Thornbury JR et al: Disk-caused nerve compression in patients with acute low back pain: Diagnosis with MR, CT myelography, and plain CT. *Radiology* 186:731-738, 1993.
20. LeRoy PL, Christian CR, Filasky R: Diagnostic thermography in low back syndromes. *Clin J Pain* 20:(1):4-13, 1985.
21. Waddell G et al: Non-organic physical signs in low back pain. *Spine* 2:117-125, 1980.
22. Finneson BE: *Low Back Pain,* ed 2. Philadelphia, JB Lippincott, 1981.
23. Moore KL: *Clinically Oriented Anatomy.* Baltimore, Williams & Wilkins, 1985.
24. Bogduk N: Back pain: Zygapophyseal blocks and epidural steroids. In Cousins MJ, Bridenbaugh PO, editors: *Neural Blockade in Clinical Anesthesia and Management of Pain,* ed 2. Philadelphia, JB Lippincott, 1988.
25. Yank KH, King AI: Mechanism of facet load transmission as a hypothesis for low-back pain. *Spine* 9:557-565, 1984.
26. Namey TC: Differential diagnosis and treatment of sciatica: The nondiscogenic causes. *Advanced Clinical Updates* 1:33-40, 1985.
27. Bonica JJ, Sola AE: Other painful disorders of the low back. In Bonica JJ, editor: *The Management of Pain,* ed 2. Philadelphia, Lea & Febiger, 1989.
28. McCarron RF et al: The inflammatory effect of nucleus pulposus: A possible element in the pathogenesis of low-back pain. *Spine* 12:760-764, 1987.
29. Saal JS et al: High levels of inflammatory phospholipase A-2 activity in lumbar disc herniations. *Spine* 15:674-678, 1990.
30. Loeser JD et al: Low back pain. In Bonica JJ, editor: *The Management of Pain,* ed 2. Philadelphia, Lea & Febiger, 1989.
31. Nachemson AL: The lumbar spine. An orthopedic challenge. *Spine* 1:59-71, 1976.
32. Deyo RA, Diehl AK: Patient satisfaction with medical care in low-back pain. *Spine* 11:28-30, 1986.
33. Saal JA, Saal JS: Nonoperative treatment of herniated lumbar intervertebral disc with radiculopathy: An outcome study. *Spine* 14(4):431-437, 1989.
34. Waddell G et al: Failed lumbar disk surgery following industrial injuries. *J Bone Joint Surg [Am]* 61:201-207, 1979.
35. Loeser JD: Pain due to nerve injury. *Spine* 10:232-235, 1985.
36. Belkin S: Back pain. In Aronoff GM, editor: *Evaluation and Treatment of Chronic Pain.* Baltimore, Urban & Schwarzenberg, 1985.
37. Watts C: Spinal surgery. In Tollison CD, editor: *Handbook of Chronic Pain Management.* Baltimore, Williams & Wilkins, 1989.
38. Javid MJ et al: Safety and efficacy of chymopapain (Chymodiactin) in herniated nucleus pulposus with sciatica. *JAMA* 249:2489-2494, 1983.
39. Moss J et al: Decreased incidence and mortality of anaphylaxis to chymopapain. *Anesth Analg* 64:1197-1201, 1985.
40. Benzon HT: Epidural steroid injections for low back pain and lumbosacral radiculopathy. *Pain* 24:277-295, 1986.
41. Devor M, Govrin-Lippman R, Raber P: Corticosteroids suppress ectopic neural discharge originating in experimental neuromas. *Pain* 22:127-137, 1985.
42. Rocco AG et al: Epidural steroids, epidural morphine and epidural steroids combined with morphine in the treatment of post-laminectomy syndrome. *Pain* 36(3):297-303, 1989.
43. Auld AW, Maki-Jokela A, Murdoch M: Intraspinal narcotic analgesic in the treatment of chronic pain. *Spine* 10(8):777-781, 1985.
44. Abram SE: Subarachnoid corticosteroid injection following inadequate response to epidural steroids for sciatica. *Anesth Analg* 57:313-315, 1978.
45. Wilkinson HA: Intrathecal Depo-Medrol: A literature review. *Clin J Pain* 8:49-56, 1992.
46. Delaney TJ et al: Epidural steroid effects on nerves and meninges. *Anesth Analg* 59:610-614, 1980.
47. Cicala RS et al: Methylprednisolone acetate does not cause inflammatory changes in the epidural space. *Anesthesiology* 72:556-558, 1990.
48. Nelson DA: Further warnings from Australia concerning intraspinal steroids. *Arch Neurol* 48:259, 1991.
49. Benzon HT et al: The effect of polyethylene glycol on mammalian nerve impulses. *Anesth Analg* 66:553-559, 1987.
50. Kay J, Raff H, Findling JW: Epidural triamcinolone causes prolonged and severe depression of the pituitary-adrenal axis. *Anesthesiology* 75:A694, 1991.
51. Sauser DD, Neumann M: Facet block. In Raj PP, editor: *The Practical Management of Pain,* ed 2. St Louis, Mosby, 1992.

52. Sandrock NJG, Warfield CA: Epidural steroids and facet injections. In Warfield CA, editor: *Principles and Practice of Pain Management.* New York, McGraw-Hill, 1993.

53. Wyant GM: Chronic pain syndromes and their treatment, III: The piriformis syndrome. *Can Anaesth Soc J* 26:305-308, 1979.

54. Melzack R, Wall PD: Pain mechanisms: A new theory. *Science* 150:971-979, 1965.

55. North RB: Neural stimulation techniques. In Tollison CD, editor: *Handbook of Chronic Pain Management.* Baltimore, Williams & Wilkins, 1989.

56. North RB et al: Spinal cord stimulation for chronic, intractable pain: Superiority of "multi-channel" devices. *Pain* 44:119-130, 1991.

57. North RB: Spinal cord stimulation for intractable pain: Indications and technique. In Long DM, Decker BC, editors: *Current Therapy in Neurological Surgery,* ed 2. St Louis, Mosby, 1989.

58. Grimes D et al: Back school—teaching patients to love their backs. *Resident Staff Phys* 26:60-68, 1980.

59. Wilensky J: Physiatric approach to chronic pain. In Aronoff GM, editor: *Evaluation and Treatment of Chronic Pain.* Baltimore, Urban & Schwarzenberg, 1985.

60. Mayer TG, Gatchel RJ, Mayer H, et al: A prospective two-year study of functional restoration in industrial low-back injury. *JAMA* 258:1763-1767, 1987.

61. Jänig W: The autonomic nervous system. In Schmidt RF, Thews G, editors: *Human Physiology.* Berlin, Springer-Verlag, 1988.

APPENDIX

SACROILIAC JOINT DYSFUNCTION

A sprain or strain of the sacroiliac joint can be caused by vigorous muscular activities such as leaning forward, lifting a heavy object, lifting against resistance, or sudden deceleration. The sacroiliac joints are true joints consisting of two irregular articulations covered by hyaline cartilage. They are relatively stable but are weakest anteriorly. Lifting or other movements that involve contraction of the hamstring muscles causes them to be held tight. When lifting and using these muscles for leverage, the sacroiliac joints are most susceptible to injury. The patient frequently favors the affected extremity while leaning toward the unaffected side. Acute joint pain may radiate to the hip, back, and thigh as far as the knee. It is aggravated by all hip and twisting movements, by sitting on the ipsilateral ischial tuberosity, or by lying on the affected side. Spasms of the low back muscles and hamstring muscles may occur, and straight-leg raising may be positive.[61] Treatment includes manipulation, physical therapy to mobilize or stabilize the joint, heat, steroid or local anesthetic injection, and antiinflammatory medications. Acupuncture and TENS should be considered, as well as bracing or supports in certain cases.

QUESTIONS: LOW BACK PAIN

1. Waddell's signs of a nonorganic basis of low back pain are all of the following EXCEPT:
   A. Positive simulation as with skin rolling
   B. Pain increase with light axial loading
   C. Nonanatomic regional hypesthesia
   D. Positive straight leg raising (SLR) at 30°

2. The posterior elements of the vertebral column include all of the following EXCEPT:
   A. Lamina
   B. Pedicles
   C. Facet joints
   D. Vertebral discs

3. A 37-year-old man complains of low back pain radiating to the hips, buttocks, and upper posterior thighs. Pain gets worse at the end of the day, and the back gets stiff with poor range of spinal motion. The patient further gives a history of having had laminectomy for similar complaints 2 years previously. The most likely diagnosis of the low back pain is:
   A. Facet syndrome
   B. Post-laminectomy (failed back) syndrome
   C. Myofascial lumbosacral strain
   D. Arachnoiditis

4. Muscle relaxants (cyclobenzaprine, methocarbamol) are indicated for low back pain patients when the pain is due to acute myofascial pain because they:
   A. Relieve reflex muscle spasm
   B. Provide sedation
   C. Decrease range of motion
   D. Break the pain cycle

5. In appropriately selected patients, epidural steroid injection is effective in:
   A. 15% of patients
   B. 33% of patients
   C. 66% of patients
   D. 99% of patients

ANSWERS

1. D
2. D
3. B
4. A
5. C

42 Musculoskeletal Pain

Robert J. Burton, Jr.

The musculoskeletal system consists of the bones and articulations of the skeleton and the ligaments, muscles, and tendons that connect and manipulate them. These are diverse tissues with radically different characteristics. Injuries or disorders may directly affect any of these component tissues or may indirectly affect the overlying integument, musculature, or neural elements associated with or contained within the skeletal framework. All of these tissues are represented in the spinal column, and all are richly innervated.

Myofascial and skeletal pain are common pain syndromes. Although many forms of skeletal pain have an identifiable cause, myofascial pain often lacks a pathologic definition. It is typically grouped under the umbrella of myofascial pain syndrome and is also referred to as myositis, fibromyalgic pain syndrome, fibrositis, fibromyalgia, myalgia, idiopathic myalgia, myelosis, and myofascitis.[1] Skeletal pain is considered any pain emanating from the bony or supporting connective tissue, including synovium, ligaments, or cartilage.

PATHOPHYSIOLOGY OF PAIN IN PARASPINOUS MUSCLES AND TENDONS

Muscular pain may be the result of a direct injury such as a blow or puncture, which disrupts or damages the muscle tissue and its intrafascicular nerve fibers, or a result of the distention and pressure produced by the ensuing hematoma and edema. Pain also results from indirect injuries such as athletic injuries, where the muscle is torn or ruptured as it strains against an excessive resistance force. Inflammation and edema, components of the normal healing process, play a role in the mediation of pain symptoms. In major musculoskeletal injuries persistent spasm may result in severe muscle pain and further trauma to the muscle and other tissues of the soft-tissue envelope.

The primary nociceptive endings in muscle are unencapsulated free nerve endings similar to those seen in periarticular tissues, which transmit their impulses centrally by way of Type III and IV afferent fibers. Intramuscular mechanoreceptors may also produce pain impulses when exposed to noxious stimuli. In all, muscular pain receptors may be either chemonociceptive or mechanonociceptive and may respond to stimuli as either specific or polymodal receptors. Chemonociceptive endings may respond to metabolites that accumulate during anaerobic metabolism, the products of cell injury produced by injury or ischaemia, or to chemical irritants such as bradykinin, serotonin, or potassium. Mechanonociceptive units may respond to stretch, pressure, or disruption. Some receptors may also respond to thermal stimuli.[2,3] Recent studies have demonstrated that intramuscular injection of calcitonin gene-related peptide in combination with either substance P or neurokinin A elicits a significant pain sensation, though none of the neuropeptides produce muscular pain when injected alone.[4,5] It is thought that the neurogenic inflammatory response produced by calcitonin gene-related peptide, which results in persistent vasodilatation, erythema, and edema formation, may also serve to sensitize nociceptors to the presence of other pain-related neuropeptides.[6,7] This receptor sensitization, as well as increases in intramuscular blood flow and interstitial edema, may represent a primary cause of muscular pain.

A more ominous type of muscle pain occurs when excessive pressure in or around the muscle results in ischemia. Compartment syndromes occur in patients with bleeding disorders, vascular injuries, musculoskeletal trauma, systemic infections, and constrictive dressings or casts, and, though rare, have been reported in the paraspinous muscular compartments.[8] Pain in compartment syndrome is severe and unremitting and out of proportion to any injury the patient may have sustained. The clinical condition mimics the symptoms produced by experimental tourniquet pain, and it is likely that the pathophysiology of the two conditions is the same.[9,10] Like tourniquet pain, compartment syndrome pain is progressive in intensity and rapidly resolves when pressure is released, either by removing the constricting dressing or by performing a surgical release of the compartmental fascia.[11,12]

PATHOPHYSIOLOGY OF INTERVERTEBRAL DISK PAIN

A considerable controversy exists concerning if and how the intervertebral disk might produce back pain. The confusion arises, at least in part, from difficulties in separating out disk tissues from peridiscal tissues in some studies and frank differences of opinion as to the innervation of the disk itself. Some authors have failed to find any nerve fibers in the annulus fibrosis, contending that endings reported by others were actually residing in adherent portions of the posterior longitudinal ligament.[13-15] Other authors have reported finding nerve endings within the layers of the outer annulus, but only in limited areas.[16] More recent studies, however, have consistently demonstrated fine nerve endings in the outer one third of the annulus.[17,18] Using histochemical techniques, Weinstein et al. demonstrated fine nerve fibers in the annulus fibrosis of the rat disk, which were immunoreactive for a variety of pain-related neuropeptides: substance P, calcitonin gene-related peptide, and vasoactive intestinal peptide.[19] The presence of free nerve endings in the outer annulus and the adjacent longitudinal ligaments suggests a mechanism by which intradiscal pathology may directly produce pain.

PATHOPHYSIOLOGY OF BONE AND PERIOSTEAL PAIN

Bone is a dynamic composite tissue involved in a variety of physiologic processes and capable of a number of biologic responses to injury or stress. Bjurholm and co-workers demonstrated nerves containing both substance P and calcitonin gene-related peptides in the marrow, periosteum, and cortex of long bones, as well as the associated muscles and ligaments.[20] They noted a higher density of substance P and calcitonin gene-related peptide immunoreactive fibers in epiphyseal rather than diaphyseal marrow, and some fibers from the abundantly innervated periosteum penetrated the cortex and entered the marrow space by way of the Volkmann's canals. As previously noted, these two neuropeptides have been associated with nociception and may accelerate and aggravate experimental arthritis after local infusion.[21,22] Vasoactive intestinal peptide and a number of other pain-related neuropeptides have also been localized to fine nerve fibers predominantly found in cancellous bone of the epiphysis and in the periosteum.[23] Vasoactive intestinal peptide is a vasodilator,[24] whereas neuropeptide Y is a powerful vasoconstrictor.[25] Fibers containing these neuropeptides congregate at the osteochondral junction of the epiphyseal plate; vasoactive intestinal peptide fibers run in the marrow spaces, and neuropeptide Y fibers follow the small vessels nourishing the epiphysis. The primary role of these peptides is likely related to the regulation of growth, but these or similar peptides may also play a role in the production of intraosseous hypertension, another proposed cause of bone pain.

Hence bone is a tissue capable of responding to both internal and external pressure changes, physical distortion, inflammation, and periosteal injury by transmitting pain signals proximally. Bone pain may be produced by microfracture and subsidence in osteoarthritis, by periosteal elevation and distortion in infection or tumor, by vascular congestion and infarction in sickle-cell crisis, and by mechanical disruption in traumatic conditions. In the fractured vertebra, pain is initially produced by the distortion or disruption of intramedullary nerve fibers and receptors in the broken bone, by stretched or disrupted receptors in the torn periosteum, and by injury or pressure on receptors in the muscle and soft tissue overlying the fracture (Fig. 42-1). A hematoma rapidly accumulates and expands until the pressure within the compartment is significantly elevated; distention of the fascia and soft tissue triggers further pain receptors.

The tough fibrous periosteal sheath that adheres to the outer cortex of the vertebral body is highly vascular and copiously supplied with both free and encapsulated nerve endings; the complex free nerve endings are thought to generate painful discharges, and the encapsulated endings are thought to be sensitive to pressure.[26,27] The nerves found in periosteal tissues are immunoreactive to a wide variety of pain-related and vasoactive neuropeptides.[28] Gronblad and colleagues demonstrated an extensive ramification of substance-P–reactive nerve fibers in both the superficial and deep layers of the periosteal sheath.[29] They also reported the presence of substance P immunoreactivity in some encapsulated, glomerular types of receptors from the same tissue. Encapsulated substance-P–reactive nerve endings have

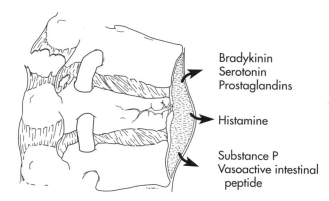

Fig. 42-1 Injury to vertebral column generates a series of inflammatory reactions which, along with mechanical disruption of tissues, may generate acute and persistent pain. With a burst fracture, for instance, disruption of nerve fibers in damaged muscle and capsular tissues results in acute pain, as will disruption of nerve endings in fractured cancellous bone, periosteum, and overlying ligaments. Expansion of fracture hematoma may elevate or distort surrounding soft tissues and may even cause cord compression if it occurs within the canal. Even after injury stabilizes, elaboration of inflammatory mediators and pain-related neuropeptides may continue to generate persistent localized pain. (From McLain, RF: Neural mechanisms of musculoskeletal pain. *Pain Digest* 3(2):82-88, Spring 1993.)

also been reported in the posterior longitudinal ligament of the spine, implicating the structure as a source of low back pain.[30]

Facet joints

Facet joints are specialized to meet specific demands of function: Articular cartilage absorbs and distributes loads; subchondral bone resists deformation and supports and nourishes the cartilage; ligaments maintain alignment and constrain joint excursion; and musculotendinous units flex, extend, and stabilize the joint. Derangement of the joint may result in destruction of the articular cartilage, fracture of the subchondral bone, attenuation or disruption of the ligaments, and excessive strains and inflammation of the muscles. Nerve endings in these or other tissues may signal the presence of ongoing or incipient tissue damage, producing the sensation of pain.

Synovial joints enjoy a dual pattern of innervation: *Primary articular nerves* are independent branches from larger peripheral nerves, which specifically supply the joint capsule and ligaments; *accessory articular nerves* reach the joint after passing through muscular or cutaneous tissues, to which they provide primary innervation.[31-33] Both primary and accessory articular nerves are mixed afferents, containing both proprioceptive and nociceptive nerve fibers. Freeman and Wyke described four basic types of afferent nerve endings in articular tissues and documented the presence of those endings in a variety of joints.[34] Although the Type 4 receptors (free nerve endings) are the only ones thought to be exclusively nociceptive, the proprioceptive endings of Types 1-3 are capable of responding to excessive joint excursion as a noxious stimulus and they play an

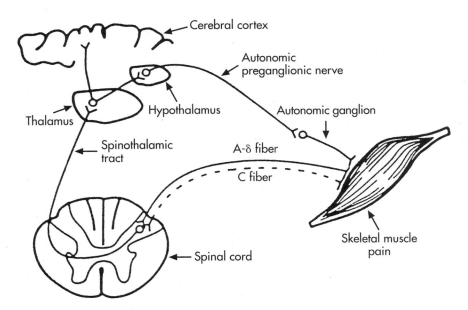

Fig. 42-2 Speculative model of mechanisms of continuing pain cycles after a skeletal muscle insult. (From Warfield CA, editor: *Principles and Practice of Pain Management.* New York, McGraw Hill, 1993.)

important role in mediating protective muscular reflexes that maintain joint stability.[35,36]

It was previously thought that the synovium was a relatively insensitive tissue[37] and that the pain of synovitis was produced by distortion of the capsule and the elaboration of inflammatory factors. Using antisera against specific neuronal markers, investigators reexamining synovial tissue found vastly greater numbers of small-diameter nerve fibers than were previously reported using standard histologic methods.[38,39] Substance P, a neuropeptide strongly associated with pain perception and transmission, was shown to accumulate in synovial fluid after intraarticular capsaicin injection and is known to produce plasma extravasation and vasodilatation in surrounding tissues.[40-42] Substance P levels are higher in arthritic joints, and infusion of the neuropeptide into joints with mild disease was shown to accelerate the degenerative process.[21] Calcitonin gene-related peptide, another pain-related neuropeptide, was also implicated as a mediator in the early stages of arthritis.[43] Whether substance P plays a direct role in the stimulation or sensitization of intraarticular pain receptors is not established, but it is now recognized that sensitization plays a role in pain production and several mechanisms of sensitization have been confirmed. Acute inflammation liberates chemical pain mediators that sensitize receptors in the fat pads and joint capsule and directly stimulate chemonociceptors.[44,45] Irritation of the synovium results in edema, synovial hypertrophy, and an effusion, all of which stretch and distort the capsule. Any motion of the joint serves to increase the tension on the capsule and mechanically distort the inflamed tissues, resulting in increased pain. Joint motion may also cause the release of noxious neuropeptides, kinins, and inflammatory agents that act on receptors in the capsule and periosteum. Inflammation results in the appearance or increase in spontaneous activity in fine joint afferents and an increase in sensitivity to movement.[46] By immobilizing the patient in a brace, these mechanisms are attenuated. Whether all of these same reactions occur within the spinal facet joints is unclear, but they are synovial joints and most likely respond in a way similar to the larger-extremity articulations.

MYOFASCIAL PAIN

In the muscular system the muscle fibers are classified as skeletal, cardiac, and smooth. This review focuses specifically on muscles of the skeletal origin. These fibers are long multinucleated cells having a characteristic cross-striated appearance under a microscope. Muscles are supplied by adjacent vessels, and each muscle is supplied by one or more nerves containing motor and sensory fibers that are usually derived from several spinal groups. Histologically, muscle nociceptors are presumably free nerve endings that are connected to the spinal cord by fine afferent fibers. Clinical and experimental evidence indicates that small-diameter afferent fibers from muscle have to be activated in order to elicit pain.[47,48] These fibers conduct action potentials at a slow velocity (below 30 m/sec in the cat). Histologically, they are either thin myelinated (A-delta or group III fibers) or nonmyelinated (C fibers or group IV fibers) (Fig. 42-2).[49]

More recent data suggest that free nerve endings are not free in the strict sense because they are almost completely ensheathed by Schwann cells. Only small areas of the axonal membrane remain uncovered by Schwann cell processes and are directly exposed to the interstitial fluid.[50] The exposed membrane areas are supplied with mitochondria and vesicles and show other structural specializations characteristic of receptive areas. They are assumed to be the site where external stimuli act.[50]

Causes of myofascial pain

Myofascial pain can be primary or secondary. Primary myofascial pain is considered to be caused by traumatic disease of the muscle, whereas secondary myofascial pain exhibits painful foci in the skeletal muscle, but the disorder arises outside the skeletal muscle. The hallmark of identification of both syndromes is the trigger point.[1] These trigger points are characterized by a discrete circumscribed painful area in the skeletal muscle. Although histologic evidence is debatable, trigger point areas appear to have structural changes observable by electron microscopy.[1] These areas show morphologic alterations that include myofibrillar degeneration, hyalin formation in the muscle fibers, and deposition of nonspecific inflammatory residue in the interstices of the skeletal muscle.[51]

It is believed that an initial muscle injury or overload results in rupture of sarcoplasmic reticulum and release of ionized calcium, which results in sustained vigorous contraction of a small band of muscles in the region involved.[52] This sustained sarcomere contractile state results in depletion of adenosine triphosphate (ATP) to a critical level, leading to local contraction and electrical silence, as observed in McArdle's disease or rigor mortis. Local ischemia and hypoxia are produced in these areas, along with the release of algogenic substances such as histamine, kinin, serotonin, and prostaglandin, which sensitizes nociceptors (Box 42-1).[53] Nociceptive impulses are carried to the central nervous system (CNS), resulting in increased muscle tension, sympathetic activity, and local ischemia. A vicious cycle is produced and the event becomes self-sustaining, eventually resulting in localized fibrosis (Box 42-2).[1]

Trigger points may be either latent or active. They are exquisitely tender points within the muscle, bone tendon junction, or associated fascia. On palpation, trigger points feel like a firm nodule or band (Fig. 42-3). The trigger points have several characteristics. They are constant anatomically, and compression can refer pain to an area far from their original site. This pain is radicular in nature, although not radicular in anatomy.[52] The precise nature of the neural pathways involved remains speculative, but normal muscle contains nociceptors that are capable of mediating a pain response. These receptors can be stimulated by a variety of algogenic substances, with the resulting impulses being transmitted over small myelinated and unmyelinated fibers to several tracts to the spinal cord.[52] Few of the fibers have a direct cortical projection, so the muscle pain is generally not well localized but diffusely represented along sclerotomal or myotomal distributions. The secondary neuron receiving input from the initial sensory neuron is also stimulated by many other nociceptive neurons, which may account for local as well as referred pain in myofascial pain complaints.[54]

Diagnosis

The diagnosis of primary or secondary myofascial pain syndrome is established by demonstrating painful trigger

---

Box 42-1 PATHOPHYSIOLOGY OF A TRIGGER POINT: FIRST MECHANISM

Acute muscle strain
damages sarcoplastic reticulum
↓
Calcium ion release and accumulation;
presence of ATP and excess calcium
↓
Initiates and maintains sustained contracture;
produces a region of uncontrolled metabolism
↓
Local vasoconstriction responses;
there is now a region of increased metabolism,
decreased circulation, and shortened muscle fiber
↓
Taut and palpable band in the muscle
↓
Trigger point

Modified from Perl ER: Pain and nociception, In Smith D, editor: *Handbook of Physiology, Section 1: The Nervous System, vol 3.* Bethesda, Md, American Physiology Society, 1984.

Box 42-2 PATHOPHYSIOLOGY OF A TRIGGER POINT: SECOND MECHANISM

Tissue injury
↓
Releases histamine, serotonin, kinins, prostaglandins
↓
Further ischemia;
increased metabolism with reduced circulation
↓
Accumulates metabolic products
↓
Increases further sensitizing products
↓
Active trigger point

Modified from Perl ER: Pain and nociception. In Smith D, editor: *Handbook of Physiology, Section 1: The Nervous System, vol 3.* Bethesda, Md, American Physiology Society, 1984.

---

points.[1,55,56] Because of their remarkable consistency in anatomic location and referred pain pattern, the most important diagnostic tool for their evaluation is a thorough history and physical examination.[57] The physical examination should include systematic palpation for these trigger point areas.

Although myofascial pain has no distinct laboratory findings, many perpetuating factors may be identified by abnormal laboratory values.[1] Trigger points can be demonstrated with the help of an algometer or by electrical stimulation. Thermography, a noninvasive technique, uses the infrared radiation from the body for diagnostic purposes. It is useful for revealing dysfunction in microcirculation from autonomic response to disease or trauma. Trigger points

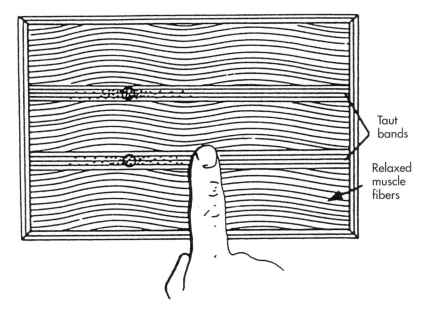

Taut bands

Relaxed muscle fibers

Fig. 42-3 Taut band in the muscle. (From Travell JG, Simons DG: Myofascial pain and dysfunction. In Travell JG, Simons DG, editors: *The Trigger Point Manual, Vol 1.* Baltimore, Williams & Wilkins, 1983.)

may cause dysfunction of microcirculation with overlying skin showing an increase in temperature, but it alone is not sufficient to make the diagnosis of myofascial trigger points.[58] Clinical electromyographic (EMG) studies have also failed to show significant abnormalities associated with trigger points, except in cases where a solitary specialized EMG study reports a burst of electrical activity when a needle is inserted into the trigger point but not into adjacent muscle.[52] EMG studies have consistently shown that the trigger point is essentially silent at rest.[52]

Clinical management

The goals of therapy in patients with myofascial pain are similar whether the syndrome is primary or secondary. They are structured to alleviate the patient's pain and enhance the patient's functional capabilities. Management of myofascial pain is empirical and should include education and psychologic intervention, which help the patient to understand and decrease the exacerbating factors that increase muscle tone, such as emotional stress, sudden overloading, or repetitive use. Patients' knowledge of proper body mechanics, work habits, and daily activities, as well as environmental contributors such as litigation, disability, and learned pain behaviors, need to be addressed. Biofeedback, cognitive behavioral therapy, hypnosis, sedatives, antidepressants, and relaxation training have all been reported to be of benefit with this syndrome.[51] Anesthetic procedures include injection therapy, which is the mainstay of treatment. Trigger-point injections, nerve blocks, and dry needling represent the most frequent methods used to interrupt the pain cycle by inactivation of the trigger point. Most commonly, the solution injected is a local anesthetic. Nonsteroidal antiinflammatory medications, long-acting steroid agents, and isotonic saline have also been used, but they show no increased efficiency when compared with local anesthetics.[51]

Modalities for management of myofascial pain

The physical modalities frequently used are heat and cryotherapy, with more recent acceptance of transcutaneous electrical nerve stimulation (TENS), acupuncture, cold laser, iontophoresis, and H-wave as valuable adjuncts to the management of the syndrome.[59,60]

Cryotherapy. Cryotherapy is useful in myofascial pain syndromes because it alleviates pain by direct and indirect mechanisms. The direct effect is a decrease in temperature of the painful area, whereas reduced pain sensation is felt to result through an indirect effect on the fibers and sensory organs. It is speculated that activation of A-delta fibers helps to close the spinal cord gate and reduces C-fiber activity.[59] Cryotherapy is usually used in addition to stretching and passive manipulation of the sore muscle groups. The application of cold as a vapocoolant spray using the stretch-and-spray method was popularized by Travell.[57]

Heat. Heat application is commonly used to treat myofascial pain. Its beneficial effect is secondary to increased collagen extensibility, blood flow, metabolic rate, and inflammation resolution. The pain threshold is believed to be raised by the direct and indirect actions of heat. Heat provided via ultrasound can increase blood flow and overcome autonomic stimulation seen in painful syndromes, whereas the medcosonolar sinusoidal current (ultrasound plus sinusoidal electric current) produces passive contraction of the muscle, which increases blood flow and reduces secondary muscle spasm.

Stimulation techniques. TENS, H-wave, and vibratory stimulation modalities are felt to suppress pain by similar mechanisms. This is believed to be via activation of large-diameter afferent nerve fibers, thereby inhibiting transmission of small-diameter pain fibers at the dorsal horn on the spinal cord. It has also been postulated that through peripheral and central mechanisms these methods increase circulating intrinsic opioids and modulating autonomic responses.[61] Physiologically, these units also increase vascularity to the areas of stimulation by producing localized vasodilation. H-wave may also decrease pain from inflammation by increasing lymphatic drainage in the affected area.[60,62,63]

Iontophoresis. Iontophoresis is a modality treatment that involves transfer of ionized substances through intact skin by the passage of direct-current (DC) electrical current between two electrodes. This method can concentrate an anesthetic solution in a localized area, which avoids the trauma that may be associated with a hypodermic needle.

Physical therapy. Physical therapy plays an important role in the treatment of primary, secondary, acute, and chronic myofascial pain. In physical therapy, patients are educated regarding their functional goals with exercise programs, postural corrections, and training in body mechanics. Patients following and maintaining a sensible regime can attain lasting results. Therapeutic exercise, modality therapy, medication management, and injection therapy directed at relieving trigger points to break the spasm-pain-autonomic reflex characteristic of this disease are the primary objectives in returning patients to normal function with myofascial pain.[64]

FIBROMYALGIA

Fibromyalgia is a syndrome of chronic, diffuse musculoskeletal pain with associated widespread discrete tender points. It occurs predominantly in women (10:1) between the ages of 20 and 60 years. Approximately 75% of patients have associated fatigue, nonrestorative sleep, and widespread stiffness. Other common features in approximately 25% of patients include irritable bowel syndrome, subjective swelling, paresthesias, symptoms of anxiety or depression, and functional disability.[65]

The physical examination of a patient with fibromyalgia is notable only for the presence of specific areas of focal tenderness. These diagnostic tender points occur at characteristic muscle-tendon junctions, with digital palpation of a tender point resulting in local pain only. A large multicenter study resulting in the American College of Rheumatology 1990 criteria for the classification of fibromyalgia highlights the importance of this tender point examination in a patient with widespread pain (Box 42-3). This study also found no difference in *primary fibromyalgia* versus fibromyalgia concomitant with another medical disorder, often termed *secondary fibromyalgia,* and therefore recommended no classification distinction.[66]

The sensitivity of the criteria suggests that it may be useful for diagnosis and classification.[66] However, on an individual basis it may be useful to exclude other conditions such as polymyalgia rheumatica and endocrine myopathies, which can also present with widespread musculoskeletal pain and stiffness. Accordingly, a complete blood count, erythrocyte sedimentation rate, and thyroid function tests should be performed. Because fibromyalgia can occur in the setting of other rheumatic disorders (e.g., systemic lupus erythematosus, Sjögren's syndrome, myositis, and rheumatoid arthritis) that would require disease-specific therapy, analysis of muscle enzymes, antinuclear antibody, and rheumatoid factor are indicated in select patients. These labora-

---

Box 42-3 THE AMERICAN COLLEGE OF RHEUMATOLOGY 1990 CRITERIA FOR THE CLASSIFICATION OF FIBROMYALGIA

1. History of widespread pain
   Definition: Pain is considered widespread when all of the following are present: pain in the left side of the body, pain in the right side of the body, pain above the waist, and pain below the waist. In addition, axial skeletal pain (cervical spine or anterior chest or thoracic spine or low back) must be present. In this definition, shoulder and buttock pain is considered as pain for each involved side. "Low back" pain is considered lower segment pain.
2. Pain in 11 of 18 tender point sites on digital palpation
   Definition: Pain, on digital palpation, must be present in at least 11 of the following 18 tender point sites:
   Occiput: bilateral, at the suboccipital muscle insertions
   Lom, cervical: bilateral, at the anterior aspects of the intertransverse spaces at C_5-C_7
   Trapezium: bilateral, at the midpoint of the upper border
   Supraspinatus: bilateral, at origins, above the scapula spine near the medial border
   Second rib: bilateral, at the second costochondral junctions, just lateral to the junctions on upper surfaces
   Lateral condyle: bilateral, 2 cm distant to the epicondyles
   Gluteal: bilateral, in upper outer quadrants of buttocks in anterior fold of muscle
   Greater trochanter: bilateral, posterior to the trochanteric prominence
   Knee: bilateral, at the medial fat pad proximal to the joint line
   Digital palpation should be performed with an approximate force of 4 kg. For a tender point to be considered "positive," the subject must state that the palpation was painful. "Tender" is not to be considered "painful."

For classification purposes, patients will be said to have fibromyalgia if both criteria are satisfied. Widespread pain must have been present for at least 3 months. The presence of a second clinical disorder does not exclude the diagnosis of fibromyalgia.
From Wolfe F et al: The American College of Rheumatology 1990 criteria for the classification of fibromyalgia, *Arthritis Rheum* 33:160-172, 1990.

---

tory tests may be considered exclusionary in the sense that fibromyalgia has no specific laboratory abnormality. Finally, on an individual diagnostic basis it must be emphasized that a patient may have fibromyalgia without having all 11 of the specified tender points of the classification criteria.[66]

The etiology of fibromyalgia is unknown. It was originally termed *fibrositis* because of a presumed inflammatory cause of the diffuse muscle pain; however, analysis of muscle biopsy specimens showed only nonspecific or normal findings.[67] Moreover, electromyograms are electrically silent, blood flow to resting muscle is normal, and exercised muscle does not demonstrate elevated lactic acid production.[68-70] However, fibromyalgia patients have been shown to have aerobically unfit muscle with diminished exercise blood flow, which may be of importance in the pathophysiology of the pain and fatigue complaints.[70] The finding of an alpha electroencephalogram (EEG) nonrapid-eye-movement sleep anomaly in some fibromyalgia patients has been proposed to represent an arousal disturbance and account for the common symptoms of nonrestorative sleep with concomitant chronic fatigue and diffuse ache.[71] Bennett postulated that this slow-wave sleep disturbance leads to fatigue with subsequent inactivity causing aerobically unfit muscle, which is then susceptible to pain from muscle microtrauma.[72]

Study regarding psychopathology in fibromyalgia has been complicated by the use of psychologic tests such as the Minnesota Multiphasic Personality Inventory (MMPI), which do not control for symptoms related to chronic pain and associated medical conditions.[73] Although there appears to be a greater prevalence of symptoms reflecting depression, anxiety, and somatoform disorders, the majority of patients with fibromyalgia do not have an active psychiatric disorder.[74,75] Moreover, the stereotypic and stable pattern of symptoms and tender points speaks against a hysteric disorder. Yunus et al. recently showed no correlation of pain sites, number of tender points, fatigue, or poor sleep with the MMPI in fibromyalgia patients and therefore postulated that these features were intrinsic to fibromyalgia per se. However, the severity of pain did appear to be influenced by psychologic factors.[76]

A potential neuroendocrinologic factor for pain-mediated pathways in fibromyalgia is under investigation by many centers with attention focused on the serotonin pathway, substance P, and the hypothalamic-pituitary-adrenal axis.[77,78] An autoimmune disturbance has not been supported.[79]

In the few controlled therapeutic trials in fibromyalgia, beneficial results were reported with low-dose amitriptyline, cyclobenzaprine, and cardiovascular fitness training.[80-83] It is interesting to speculate that their benefit relates to the sleep disturbance and aerobically unfit muscles previously reported in fibromyalgia.[70,71] The 25- to 50-mg amitriptyline dose range employed makes it unlikely that any beneficial effect is due to treatment of an associated depression. A major cornerstone in therapy is patient education. It is emphasized that fibromyalgia is common, that the symptoms are "real" but intensified by emotional upset, and that the patient has to be an active participant in the treatment process. This last factor is especially important because patients with complaints of tender, stiff muscles tend to balk at the treatment recommendation of aerobic fitness training.

Although nonsteroidal antiinflammatory agents are the most commonly used medication in these patients, there is little evidence for efficacy.[83] There is no role for corticosteroids.[84] A small, controlled study showed some potential benefit to biofeedback training.[85] This has prompted a call to employ a cognitive-behavioral therapy program in fibromyalgia patients to teach skills helpful in control of pain and disability.[86] Tender-point injections with local anesthetics, heat, and massage have been used on an individual basis with variable results.

The prevalence of fibromyalgia in an unselected population is estimated at 1%.[87] Fibromyalgia was found in approximately 5% of patients presenting to general internists and up to 20% of rheumatology clinic patients.[65] The natural history of fibromyalgia appears to be that of a chronic

Table 42-1 Characteristic features of fibromyalgia and myofascial pain syndrome

	Fibromyalgia	Myofascial pain syndrome
Demographics	Female (10:1)	Female (3:1)
Examination	Widespread tender points with local pain	Regional tender points with referred pain
Stiffness	Widespread	Regional
Fatigue	Pronounced	Usually absent
Treatment	Aerobic conditioning, tricyclics	Local injections, spray and stretch
Prognosis	Chronic	Usually good

disease with occasional, transient remissions.[88] Although symptoms have been improved by treatment, the syndrome nevertheless appears to persist for years. In fact, continued symptomatology led to patient perception of disability in 12% of 260 fibromyalgia patients in a rheumatologic practice setting.[89] In Canada fibromyalgia was responsible for 9% of disability payments awarded by a single insurance company.[90]

This common chronic pain syndrome will obviously be a continuing source of medical and economic problems until the pathophysiology is better delineated and subsequent improved treatment methods are formulated. Furthermore, understanding the neuropathophysiologic basis of fibromyalgia may have broader applicability towards an understanding of chronic pain per se.[91]

Although both fibromyalgia and myofascial pain syndrome are soft-tissue pain syndromes with overlapping features of tender muscles in the setting of otherwise normal laboratory and radiographic studies, there are many distinctive characteristics (Table 42-1). Whether they represent two ends of the same spectrum remains to be proven.

SKELETAL PAIN

The skeleton consists of bones and cartilage. Bones provide a framework of levers, protect organs from damage, and their marrow forms certain cells that substance provides for storage and exchange of calcium and phosphate ions. Cartilage is a tough, resilient connective tissue composed of cells and fibers embedded in a firm, gel-like intercellular matrix. Cartilage is an integral part of many bones, and some skeletal elements are entirely cartilaginous. Joints vary widely in structure and arrangement and are often specialized for particular functions. They are typically classified on the basis of their most characteristic structural features into three main types: fibrous, cartilaginous, and synovial.[92]

Bones are richly supplied with blood vessels (Fig. 42-4). This supply typically consists of a nutrient artery that pierces the compact bone of the shaft and divides into branches that supply the marrow and compact bone as far as the metaphysis. Metaphysis and epiphysial vessels, which arise mainly from arteries that supply the joint, pierce the compact bone and supply the spongy bone and marrow of the ends of the bone. Many nerve fibers accompany these

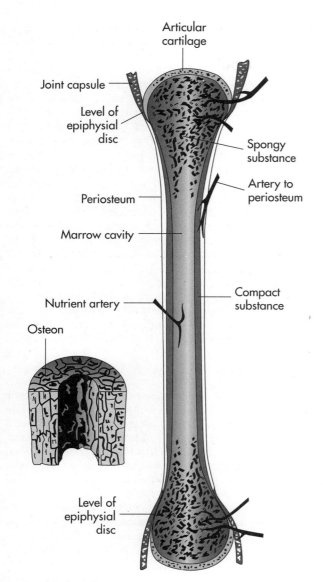

Fig. 42-4 Schematic diagram of a long bone and its blood supply. Inset shows lamellae of compacta arranged into osteons. (From Gardner E: Skeleton. In Gardner E, editor: *Anatomy: A Regional Study of Human Structure,* ed 3. Philadelphia, WB Saunders, 1993.)

blood vessels. Most such fibers are vasomotor (C fibers), but some are sensory and end in the periosteum and in the adventitia of blood vessels. Some of these sensory fibers are pain fibers that are typically of the A-delta fiber origin.[92] Pain arising in a bone may be felt locally at the site of stimulation; however, it often spreads or is referred. Epiphysial vessels are the major blood supply, and the principal distribution of nerves are the same trunks of nerves whose branches supply the groups of muscles moving the joint. They also furnish a distribution of nerves to the skin over the insertions of the same muscle. They are known as articular nerves and contain sensory autonomic fibers. Joint pain is commonly diffuse and poorly localized and usually

leads to reflex contraction of muscle, especially those that flex or adduct. Widespread plexus of A-delta fibers form pain endings, which are most numerous in the joint capsules, fatpad, and ligaments, whereas the synovial membrane is relatively insensitive.[92]

Conditions causing skeletal pain

Patients with skeletal pain are a common clinical challenge to physicians and require a systematic approach to provide the best treatment. They usually complain of pain coming from the joints, surrounding soft tissue, or bone. The vast majority of pain presenting as skeletal pain emanates from the joints, since it is the area most richly endowed with nerve fibers. In evaluating joint pain, determine whether the cause of the pain is a result of intrinsic or extrinsic disorder. Intrinsic disorders involve the structure itself (intraarticular surface, periarticular soft tissue, or adjacent bone), whereas extrinsic disorders involve pain arising outside of the structure.

The three intrinsic locations where pain arises occasionally have some overlap between anatomic regions, but a distinct location can usually be made by physical examination. Intraarticular diseases cause joint effusion and synovial or joint-line tenderness. Although periarticular conditions may also cause tenderness around the joint, they usually lack joint effusions. Lesions in the bone can be identified either by plain x-ray or with bone scan. Intraarticular causes of skeletal pain may be divided into three broad categories: inflammatory joint diseases, intraarticular derangement, and osteoarthritis.

Inflammatory conditions often have a pernicious or nontraumatic origin. The patients typically have pain and stiffness that is more severe in the morning. Pain usually improves with minor activity. The joints are usually tender, but weight-bearing activities do not necessarily worsen the symptoms. The involvement can be a monarticular or polyarticular joint pattern. Inflammatory pain includes conditions of immunologic, crystal-induced, and infectious causes.[93]

Inflammatory causes. The major immunologic disorders causing intraarticular pain are rheumatoid arthritis, psoriatic arthritis, and systemic lupus erythematosus. Rheumatoid arthritis is by far the most common, afflicting an estimated 5 million Americans. Immunologic conditions are usually polyarticular and in the case of rheumatoid arthritis pursue a relentless course with multiple remissions and recurrences until the articular cartilage is destroyed. Diagnosis is usually made with clinical examination and immunologic analysis. Mild conditions are usually treated with nonsteroidal antiinflammatory drugs (NSAIDs) and corticosteroids. More intensive therapy can include cytotoxic agents, which delay progression of the disease and decrease damage to the articular surface.[93]

Inflammatory joint pain is caused by deposits of crystalline substances, including gout and pseudogout. Uric acid and calcium pyrophosphate crystals that precipitate into the joint space cause an inflammatory response. The symptoms are usually monarticular severe joint pain and swelling. The diagnosis is confirmed by identification of crystals in the joint fluid. Treatment consists of colchicine as an initial therapy for gout, with allopurinol and probenecid to decrease production of urate and increase excretion of uric acid. Pseudogout is also known as chondrocalcinosis, and its attacks are less severe than gout. X-rays aid in the diagnosis, showing punctate or linear calcification in the fibrocartilage of the menisci and articular cartilage. The diagnosis is confirmed by identifying calcium crystals in the joint fluid.[93] Treatment is symptomatic and consists of NSAID therapy.[93]

Joint infections causing inflammation and pain occur either through direct contact or hematogenously. The clinical course of the disease depends on the infectious agent. Symptoms can be indolent or fulminant, with a swollen, painful joint and systemic signs of fever. Fluid aspirated from an infected joint is turbid and has a low glucose level. The white blood cell count consists predominantly of polymorphonuclear leukocytes. Treatment consists of identifying the correct organisms and starting the appropriate antibiotic therapy. Pyogenic joints constitute a medical emergency because lysosomal enzymes released by the leukocytes can destroy the articular cartilage within 24 hours.[94]

Intraarticular causes. Intraarticular derangement is mechanical blocking of the joint by a foreign body or abnormal joint structure. A history of episodic locking, giving way, and associated effusion is usually given; this is an indication for arthroscopy.[95] Loose bodies, torn menisci, and in rare cases, tumor can be causative factors. Osteoarthritis, also known as degenerative joint disease, is the most common form of arthritis. It is characterized by progressive loss of articular cartilage, subchondral bony sclerosis, and cartilage, as well as proliferation at the joint margin and eventual osteophyte formation. Although the cause of osteoarthritis is not clear, it usually develops in joints previously injured by inflammatory conditions or intraarticular derangement and in those joints frequently exposed to injury or stress (such as those in sports professionals and obese patients). It disproportionately involves weight-bearing joints (e.g., hips and knees) and occurs in middle-age or older people. In contrast to inflammatory arthritis, the pain usually worsens with activity and the symptoms are relieved by unloading the joints.[93] Diagnosis is made by history and clinical findings. Intermittent effusion may occur, and the joint fluid is essentially normal. X-rays may reveal a narrowing of the joint space, osteophyte, subchondral sclerosis, and cyst formation. Radiographs need to be taken while the patient is bearing weight on the suspected area to assess the extent of space narrowing. No drugs have been shown to retard the disease process; however, NSAIDs, tricyclic antidepressants, and modalities have been helpful in controlling the pain.[59] Prosthetic joint replacement is an option for patients with severe pain and disability; however, this option is usually reserved for older, less active patients. Younger patients are inappropriate candidates because higher activity levels accelerate the loosening process and component failure. Osteotomy, a procedure in which the bone is cut and realigned, is an option for younger patients; however, this procedure has not received as wide acceptance in the United States as in Europe.[94]

Periarticular causes. Joint pain from periarticular soft-tissue disorders are caused by acute inflammatory conditions (e.g., bursitis and tendinitis) or mechanical instability (e.g., dislocations). Overuse, unusual excessive activity, or trauma are the primary precipitating causes. Therapy for inflammatory conditions requires rest and antiinflammatory medications, and if symptoms persist, water-soluble glucocorticoid medication is sufficient.[94] Diseases and trauma to the bone itself can cause adjacent joint and skeletal pain. Most fractures of the bone are obvious; x-ray makes the diagnosis. Stress fractures resulting from repetitive loading produce microfractures in bone. The body's reaction to this process is to reabsorb bone in preparation for a secondary bone-forming phase to heal the fractures. Pain signals are elicited by this process; however, if ignored, it can lead to fracture because of the temporary weakness of the bone. Stress fractures occur through weakened bones caused by metabolic diseases. Treatment of the underlying medical condition should be considered first, but often stabilization through surgery may be necessary to relieve pain. Primary neoplasms, although rare, have to be considered in complaints of skeletal pain. More often, neoplasms in bone are of metastatic origin and are the first manifestation of an occult primary lesion.

SUMMARY

This chapter focused on the management of two commonly encountered pain syndromes. The clinical assessment of these problems requires a completed history and physical examination. Myofascial pain syndrome is directed at identifying trigger-point areas and directing intervention toward alleviating them with the techniques discussed. Although their etiologies are poorly understood, all forms need a coordinated approach in their regulation. Treatment of skeletal pain requires an understanding of the anatomic regions from which it arises for effective management. With a clear understanding of anatomy and physiology of these entities, the physician is able to play a role in their alleviation.

REFERENCES

1. Sola AE, Bonica JJ: Myofascial pain syndromes. In Bonica JJ, editor: *The Management of Pain,* ed 2. Philadelphia, Lea & Febiger, 1990.
2. Kumazawa T, Mizumura K: Thin fiber receptors responding to mechanical, chemical and thermal stimulation in the skeletal muscle of the dog. *J Physiol (Lond)* 273:179-194, 1977.
3. Mense S, Schmidt RF: Muscle pain: Which receptors are responsible for the transmission of noxious stimuli? In Rose CF, editor: *Physiological Aspects of Clinical Neurology.* Oxford, Blackwell Scientific Publications, 1977.
4. Pedersen-Bjergaard U et al: Algesia and local responses induced by neurokinin A and substance P in human skin and temporal muscle. *Peptides* 10:1147-1152, 1989.
5. Pedersen-Bjergaard U et al: Calcitonin gene-related peptide, neurokinin A, and substance P: Effects on nociception and neurogenic inflammation in human skin and temporal muscle. *Peptides* 12:333-337, 1991.
6. Fuller RW et al: Sensory neuropeptide effects in human skin. *Br J Pharmacol* 92:781-788, 1987.
7. Piotrowski W, Foreman JC: Some effects of calcitonin gene-related peptide in human skin and on histamine release. *Br J Dermatol* 114:37-46, 1986.
8. Carr D, Gilbertson L, Frymoyer J: Lumbar paraspinal compartment syndrome: A case report with physiologic and anatomic studies. *Spine* 10:816-820, 1985.

9. Smith GM et al: An experimental pain method sensitive to morphine in man: The submaximal effort tourniquet technique. *J Pharmacol Exp Ther* 154:324-332, 1966.

10. Sternbach RA et al: Measuring the severity of clinical pain. In Bonica JJ, editor: *Advances in Neurology*. New York, Raven Press, 1974.

11. Matsen FA: Compartmental syndrome: A unifying concept. *Clin Orthop* 113:8-14, 1975.

12. Mubarak SJ, Owen CA: Double incision fasciotomy of the leg for decompression of compartment syndromes. *J Bone Joint Surg* 59A:184-187, 1977.

13. Pedersen HE, Blunk CFJ, Gardner E: The anatomy of the lumbosacral posterior rami and meningeal branches of spinal nerves (sinu-vertebral nerves). *J Bone Joint Surg* 38A:377-391, 1956.

14. Stillwell DL: The nerve supply of the vertebral column and its associated structures in the monkey. *Anat Rec* 125:139-169, 1956.

15. Parke WW: *The innervation of connective tissues of the spinal motion segment*. Paper presented at the International Symposium on Percutaneous Lumbar Discectomy, Philadelphia, Pa, 1987.

16. Hirsch C: Studies on the mechanism of low back pain. *Acta Orthop Scand* 20:261-274, 1951.

17. Bogduk N, Tynan W, Wilson AS: The innervation of the human lumbar intervertebral discs. *J Anat* 132:39-56, 1981.

18. Yoshizawa H, O'Brien JP, Smith WT: Neuropathology of the intervertebral disc removed for low back pain. *J Pathol* 132:95-104, 1980.

19. Weinstein JN, Pope M, Schmidt R et al: Neuropharmacologic effects of vibration on the dorsal root ganglion: An animal model. *Spine* 13:521-525, 1988.

20. Bjurholm A: Substance P and CGRP immunoreactive nerves in bone. *Peptides* 9:165-171, 1988.

21. Levine JD et al: Interneuronal substance P contributes to the severity of experimental arthritis. *Science* 226:547-549, 1984.

22. Colpaert FC, Donnerer J, Lembeck F: Effects of capsaicin on inflammation and on the substance P content of nervous tissues in rats with adjuvant arthritis. *Life Sci* 32:1827-1834, 1983.

23. Bjurholm A et al: Neuropeptide Y-, tyrosine hydroxylase-, and vasoactive intestinal peptide-immunoreactive nerves in bone and surrounding tissues. *J Auton Nerv Syst* 25:119-125, 1988.

24. Said SI, Mutt V: Polypeptide with broad biological activity: Isolation from small intestine. *Science* 169:1217-1218, 1970.

25. Lundberg JM et al: Neuropeptide Y (NPY)-like immunoreactivity in peripheral noradrenergic neurons and effects of NPY on sympathetic function. *Acta Physiol Scand* 116:477-480, 1982.

26. Cooper RR: Nerves in cortical bone. *Science* 160:327-328, 1968.

27. Ralston HJ, Miller MR, Kasahara M: Nerve endings in human fasciae, tendons, ligaments, periosteum, and joint synovial membrane. *Anat Rec* 136:137-148, 1960.

28. Hill EL, Elde R: Distribution of CGRP-, VIP-, DβH-, SP-, and NPY-immunoreactive nerves in the periosteum of the rat. *Cell Tissue Res* 264:469-480, 1991.

29. Gronblad M et al: Innervation of human bone periosteum by peptidergic nerves. *Anat Rec* 209:297-299, 1984.

30. Liesi P et al: Substance P: A neuropeptide involved in low back pain? *Lancet* 1:1328-1329, 1983.

31. Wyke B: Articular neurology—A review. *Physiotherapy* 58:94-99, 1972.

32. Gardner E: The distribution and termination of nerves in the knee joint of the cat. *J Comp Neurol* 80:11-32, 1944.

33. Gardner E: The innervation of the knee joint. *Anat Rec* 101:109-130, 1948.

34. Freeman MAR, Wyke BD: The innervation of the knee joint: An anatomical and histological study in the cat. *J Anat* 101:505-532, 1967.

35. Palmer I: Pathophysiology of the medial ligament of the knee joint. *Acta Chirurgica Scandinavica* 115:312-318, 1958.

36. Eckholm J, Eklund G, Skoglund S: On the reflex effects from the knee joint of the cat. *Acta Physiol Scand* 50:167-174, 1960.

37. Kellgren JH, Samuel EP: Sensitivity and innervation of the articular cartilage. *J Bone Joint Surg* 32B:84-92, 1950.

38. Gronblad M et al: Neuropeptides in synovium of patients with rheumatoid arthritis and osteoarthritis. *J Rheumatol* 15:1807-1810, 1988.

39. Kidd BL et al: Neurogenic influences in arthritis. *Ann Rheum Dis* 49:649-652, 1990.

40. Lam FY, Ferrell WR: Inhibition of carrageenan induced inflammation in the rat knee joint. *Ann Rheum Dis* 48:928-932, 1989.

41. Lam FY, Ferrell WR: Neurogenic component of different models of acute inflammation in the rat knee model. *Ann Rheum Dis* 50:747-751, 1991.

42. Yaksh TL: Substance P release from knee joint afferent terminals: Modulation by opioids. *Brain Res* 458:319-324, 1988.

43. Konttinen Y et al: Nerves in inflammatory synovium: Immunohistochemical observations on the adjuvant arthritic rat model. *J Rheumatol* 17:1586-1591, 1990.

44. Heppelmann B, Schaible HG, Schmidt RF: Effects of prostaglandin E1 and E2 on the mechanosensitivity of Group III afferents from normal and inflamed cat knee joints. In Fields HL, Dubner R, Cerverof F, editors: *Advances in Pain Research and Therapy*. New York, Raven Press, 1985.

45. Heppelmann B et al: Effects of acetylsalicylic acid and indomethacin on single Group III and IV sensory units from acutely inflamed joints. *Pain* 26:337-351, 1986.

46. Schaible HG, Schmidt RF: Effects of an experimental arthritis on the sensory properties of fine articular afferent nerves. *J Physiol* 54:1109-1122, 1985.

47. Foreman RD, Schmidt RF, Weber RN: Viscerosomatic convergence onto T2-T4 spinorecticular, spinoreticular-spinothalamic and spinothalamic tract neurons in cat. *Exp Neurol* 85:597, 1984.

48. Foreman RD, Schmidt RF, Willis WD: Effects of mechanical and chemical stimulation on fine muscle afferents upon primate spinothalamic tract cells. *J Physiol (Lond)* 286:215, 1979.

49. Gasser HS, Grundfest H: Axon diameter in relation to the spike dimensions and the conduction velocity in mammalian A fibers. *Am J Physiol* 127:393-414, 1939.

50. Andres KH, von During M, Schmidt RF: Sensory innervation of the Achilles tendon by Group III and IV afferent fibers. *Anat Embryol (Berl)* 172:145-156, 1854.

51. Zohn DA, Mennell J: *Musculoskeletal pain: Diagnosis and physical treatment*. Boston, Little, Brown, & Co, 1976.

52. Simons DG: Electrogenic nature of palpable bands and "jump sign" associated with myofascial trigger points. In Bonica JJ, Albe Fessard D, editors: *Advances in Pain Research and Therapy*. New York, Raven Press, 1976.

53. Mense S: Peripheral mechanisms of muscle nociception and local muscle pain. *Journal of Musculoskeletal Pain* 1:1, 1993.

54. Perl ER: Pain and nociception. In Darian-Smith, editor: *Handbook of Physiology, vol 3*. Bethesda, Md, American Physiology Society, 1984.

55. Travell JG, Simons DG: Myofascial pain and dysfunction. In *The Trigger Point Manual*. Baltimore, Williams & Wilkins, 1983.

56. Simons DG: Myofascial pain syndromes due to trigger points. In Goodgold J: *Rehabilitation Medicine*. St Louis, Mosby, 1987.

57. Travell JG, Simons DG: Myofascial pain and dysfunction. In *The Trigger Point Manual*. Baltimore, Williams & Wilkins, 1983.

58. Edeiken J, Shaber G: Thermography: A reevaluation. *Skeletal Radiol* 15:545-548, 1986.

59. Lehmann JF, deLateur RJ: *Therapeutic Heat and Cold,* ed 3. Baltimore, Williams & Wilkins, 1982.

60. Lorenz KY: A neuromodulation technique for pain control. In Aronoff GM, editor: *Evaluation and Treatment in Chronic Pain*. Baltimore, Urban & Schwarzenberg, 1985.

61. Phero JC, Raj TP, McDonald JS: Transcutaneous electrical nerve stimulation and myoneural injection therapy for the management of chronic myofascial pain. *Dent Clin North Am* 31:703-723, 1987.

62. Oliveri, Lynn, Hong: Increase skin temperature after vibratory stimulation. *Pain* 20:25-44, 1984.

63. Learndri M, Brunetti O, Parodi CI: Telethermographic findings after transcutaneous electrical nerve stimulation. *Physical Therapy* 66:210-213, 1986.

64. Vasudevan S et al: Physical methods of pain management. In Raj PP, ed: *Practical Management of Pain*, ed 2. St Louis, Mosby, 1992.

65. Wolfe F: Fibromyalgia: The clinical syndrome. *Rheum Dis Clin North Am* 15:1-18, 1989.

66. Wolfe F et al: The American College of Rheumatology 1990 criteria for the classification of fibromyalgia. *Arthritis Rheum* 33:160-172, 1990.

67. Kalyan-Raman UP et al: Muscle pathology in primary fibromyalgia syndrome: A little microscopic, histochemical and ultrastructural study. *J Rheumatol* 11:808-813, 1984.

68. Zidar J et al: Quantitative EMG and muscle tension in painful muscle in fibromyalgia. *Pain* 40:249-254, 1990.

69. Klemp P et al: Blood flow in fibromystic muscles. *Scand J Rehabil Med* 14:81-85, 1982.

70. Bennett RM et al: Aerobic fitness in patients with fibrositis: A controlled study of respiratory gas exchange and Xenon clearance from exercising muscle. *Arthritis Rheum* 32:454-460, 1989.

71. Moldofsky H et al: Musculoskeletal symptoms and non REM sleep disturbance in patients with "fibrositis" syndrome and health subjects. *Psychosom Med* 37:341-351, 1975.

72. Bennett RM: Beyond fibromyalgia: Ideas on etiology and treatment. *J Rheumatol Suppl* 19:185-191, 1989.

73. Smythe HA: Problems with the MMPI. *J Rheumatol* 11:417-418, 1984.

74. Ahles TA et al: Psychological factors associated with primary fibromyalgia syndrome. *Arthritis Rheum* 27:1101-1105, 1984.

75. Goldenberg DL: Psychological symptoms and psychiatric diagnosis in patients with fibromyalgia. *J Rheumatol Suppl* 19:127-130, 1989.

76. Yunus MB et al: Relationship of clinical features with psychological status in primary fibromyalgia. *Arthritis Rheum* 34:15-21, 1991.

77. Russell IJ: Neurohormonal aspects of fibromyalgia syndrome. *Rheum Dis Clin North Am* 15(1):73-90, 1989.

78. Ferraccioli G et al: Neuroendocrinologic findings in primary fibromyalgia (soft tissue chronic pain syndrome) and in other chronic rheumatic conditions (rheumatoid arthritis, low back pain). *J Rheumatol* 17:869-873, 1990.

79. Bengtsson A et al: Absence of autoantibodies in primary fibromyalgia. *J Rheumatol* 17:1682-1683, 1990.

80. Carette S et al: Evaluation of amitriptyline in primary fibrositis: A double blind, placebo-controlled study. *Arthritis Rheum* 29:655-659, 1986.

81. Goldenberg DL, Felson DT, Dinerman H: A randomized controlled trial of amitriptyline and naproxen in the treatment of patients with fibromyalgia *Arthritis Rheum* 29:1371-1377, 1986.

82. Bennett RM et al: A comparison of cyclobenzaprine and placebo in the management of fibrositis: A double-blind controlled study. *Arthritis Rheum* 31:1535-1542, 1988.

83. McCain GA et al: A controlled study of the effect of a supervised cardiovascular fitness training program on the manifestations of primary fibromyalgia. *Arthritis Rheum* 31:1135-1141, 1988.

84. Clark S, Tindall E, Bennett RM: A double-blind crossover trial of prednisone versus placebo in the treatment of fibrositis. *J Rheumatol* 12:980-983, 1985.

85. Ferraccioli G et al: EMG-biofeedback training in fibromyalgia syndrome. *J Rheumatol* 14:820-825, 1987.

86. Bradley LA: Cognitive-behavioral therapy for fibromyalgia. *J Rheumatol Suppl* 19:131-136, 1989.

87. Jacobsson L, Lindgarde F, Manthorpe R: The commonest rheumatic complaints of over six weeks duration in a twelve-month period in a defined Swedish population. *Scand J Rheumatol* 18:353-360, 1989.

88. Felson DT, Goldenberg DL: The natural history of fibromyalgia. *Arthritis Rheum* 29:1522-1526, 1986.

89. Cathey MA et al: Demographic, work disability, service utilization, and treatment characteristics of 260 fibromyalgia patients in rheumatologic practice. *Arthritis Rheum* 33(Suppl):510, 1990.

90. McCain GA, Cameron R, Kennedy JC: The problem of long-term disability payments and litigation in primary fibromyalgia. The Canadian perspective. *J Rheumatol Suppl* 19:174-176, 1989.

91. Reilly PA, Littlejohn GO: Fibrositis/fibromyalgia syndrome: The key to the puzzle of chronic pain. *Med J Aust* 152:226-228, 1990.

92. Gardner E: Skeleton. In Gardner, editor: *Anatomy: A Regional Study of Human Structure,* ed 3. Philadelphia, WB Saunders.

93. Altman RD: Osteoarthritis. Differentiation from Rheumatoid arthritis, causes of pain treatment. *Postgrad Med* 87(3):66-72, 77-78, 1990.

94. Gerhart T, Dohlman: Joint pain. In Warfield CA, editor: *Principles and Practice of Pain Management.* New York, McGraw-Hill.

95. Zuckerman JD et al: The painful shoulder: Part II. Intrinsic disorders and impingement syndrome. *Am Fam Physician* 43(2):497-512, 1991.

96. Warfield CA, editor: *Principles and Practice of Pain Management.* New York, McGraw-Hill.

97. Jänig W: The autonomic nervous system. In Schmidt RF, Thews G, editors: *Human Physiology.* Berlin, Springer-Verlag, 1988.

98. Owitz S, Koppolu S: Sympathetic blockade as a diagnostic and therapeutic technique. *Mt Sinai J Med* (NY) 49:282-288, 1982.

99. Cannon WB: Organization for physiological homeostasis. *Physiol Rev* 9:399-431, 1929.

APPENDIX

RECTUS ABDOMINIS SYNDROME

Pain involving the muscles of the abdominal wall can mimic that of an acute abdomen. The pain can range from mild to severe and may precipitate surgical interventions for an undetermined cause yielding essentially no positive findings. The pain is found chiefly in the rectus abdominis muscle that attaches superiorly to the fifth, sixth, and seventh ribs and from below to the crest of the pelvis.[97,98] Some of the fibers connect with the costoxiphoid ligaments on the side of the xiphoid process. The pain usually starts from a localized point and may become diffuse, involving most of the abdominal wall in the quadrant where pain is primarily located. The trigger areas are identified by having the patient lift the head and feet simultaneously, tightening the rectus abdominis muscles. A pointed blunt object (e.g., a ballpoint pen with the tip retracted) can then be used to localize the specific trigger spot. The specific trigger area is then infiltrated with a local anesthetic steroid solution. These injections should be given in a series for more long-lasting relief. If they are beneficial, the use of neurolytic agents such as absolute alcohol, 50% alcohol, or phenol may be employed. Ramamurthy suggests that a spray-and-stretch procedure and a home-exercise program may be used to relieve these trigger areas. The patient proceeds to do slow back sit-ups (sit-ups in reverse) to aid in lengthening the contractures of the abdominal muscles. The pain can be particularly disabling, especially when treated with surgical intervention.[99]

QUESTIONS: MUSCULOSKELETAL PAIN

1. Trigger points:
   A. Are exquisitely tender points within muscle only
   B. Feel like firm nodules or bands within muscle
   C. Have direct cortical projections and pain is well localized
   D. Show distinct laboratory findings
   For questions 2-5, choose from the following:
   A. 1, 2, and 3
   B. 1 and 3
   C. 2 and 4
   D. 4
   E. All of the above

2. Which of the following statements is (are) true concerning thermography?
   1. It is useful in localizing trigger points in myofascial pain syndrome.
   2. It uses infrared radiation from the body for diagnostic purposes.
   3. It is useful for revealing dysfunction in microcirculation.
   4. It is usually associated with abnormal laboratory studies.

3. Cryotherapy is useful in myofascial pain syndromes because it can:
   1. Act by direct and indirect mechanism to relieve pain
   2. Stimulate A-delta fibers and reduce C-fiber activity
   3. Directly reduce pain to the affected area
   4. Increase blood flow to the muscle

4. Which of the following statements regarding pyogenic joints is (are) true?
   1. They occur when uric acid precipitates into the joint space.
   2. They are associated with systemic signs.
   3. They should be treated empirically.
   4. They constitute a medical emergency.

5. Which of the following statements concerning osteoarthritis is (are) true?
   1. A history of episodic locking, giving way, and associated effusion is common.
   2. It usually develops in joints injured by inflammatory or intraarticular derangement.
   3. Non–weight-bearing radiographs should be taken to confirm the diagnosis.
   4. Pain is relieved by unloading of the joint.

ANSWERS

1. B
2. C
3. B
4. C
5. C

43 Visceral Pain

Richard H. Docherty

Visceral pain is defined as pain emanating from soft organs in the thorax, abdomen, or pelvis. True visceral pain is a deep, dull, vague, poorly defined, difficult-to-locate pain that radiates away from the affected organ. It is usually accompanied by an increase in sympathetic outflow and spasm of adjacent musculature. The nonspecific features are probably due to a wide divergence and small number of visceral afferents activating a large area with extensive ramifications. Better localization of visceral pain occurs through facilitation referral and viscerosomatic convergence. Only when somatic structures are involved does the pain pattern become specific.

The main factors capable of inducing pain in visceral structures[1] are as follows:

1. Abnormal distention and contraction of hollow visceral walls
2. Rapid stretching of the capsule of solid visceral organs
3. Ischemia of visceral musculature
4. Formation and accumulation of algogenic substances
5. Direct action of chemical stimuli on compromised mucosa
6. Traction or compression of ligaments, vessels, or mesentery

Cutting or burning normal viscera does not induce pain. Slow distention of hollow viscera associated with tissue pathology is not painful; and visceral pleura, peritoneum, and parenchyma are sensitive to handling.

The visceral pain pathway is initiated by tissue damage activating visceral nociceptors, which can be of high or low (silent) threshold.[2] No primary algogenic substance has been proven, but bradykinin may act as a modulator.[3] Nociceptive, primary neurons travel with sympathetic, parasympathetic, and sensory afferents (mainly with sympathetic afferents) to the dorsal root ganglia and terminate in the spinal cord at laminas I, V, and IX. Neurotransmission at this point is affected by substance P, calcitonin gene-related peptide, and vasoactive intestinal polypeptide.[3] Second-order neurons then travel via spinothalamic tracts to the thalamus and are relayed to the postcentral gyrus in the parietal lobe of the cortex. Modulation of nociception by descending inhibition from the periaqueductal gray and nucleus raphe magnus inhibits nociception.[4,5]

Localizing visceral pain is difficult. Afferent nerves from viscera to spinal cord are few in number and comprise only 2% to 15% of all afferents to the spinal cord.[3,6] Visceral afferents converge onto the same second-order spinal neurons as the cutaneous afferent terminals (viscerocutaneous). Input from joints and muscles also converges with visceral input into second-order neurons (viscerosomatic).[7] Viscerovisceral convergence also occurs (e.g., visceral pain arising from biliary tract distention can be confused with cardiac pain as sympathetic afferents from cardiac and upper abdominal viscera synapse near each other at the spinothalamic tract).[8]

Theories explaining visceral pain are divided into two groups: centralist and peripheralist. The centralist theories are further subdivided. The first subdivision is the convergence projection theory,[9] which states visceral afferent fibers with nociceptive input converge onto somatosensory spinal cord neurons, and the viscerosomatic cells project through nociceptive pathways. The second subdivision is the convergence facilitation theory, which implies visceral afferent activation changes the excitation of multiple spinal units (including pain pathways) without direct activation of spinal neurons. A patient's inability to distinguish cardiac from esophageal pain may be due to convergence.[10] Peripheralist theories[11] of visceral pain propose that vasoactive factors are released into cutaneous and deep tissues, leading to hyperalgesia and referred pain from these structures. Dichotomizing fibers projecting to both somatic and visceral structures or increased sympathetic motor activity may be responsible for release of these factors. Research supports components of the above theories, but each theory alone is insufficient to account for all aspects of visceral pain.

Visceral pain is examined more closely under the headings of chest, abdominal, biliary, pancreatic, and genitourinary pain. Pelvic pain is discussed in Chapter 44. Anatomy is covered in some detail and the reader is referred to additional texts.[12-14]

CHEST PAIN OF VISCERAL ORIGIN

Fewer symptoms in medicine carry the potential gravity of chest pain. Most physicians focus on ruling out coronary artery disease, which is the safe but expensive route—there is a 50% false-negative rate among patients admitted to critical care units.[15]

Cardiac causes

Innervation. For cardiac structures, innervation is comprised of afferent and efferent sympathetic and parasympathetic fibers (Fig. 43-1). Sympathetic fibers to the heart contain preganglionic fibers for the intermediolateral cell column at T_1-T_4 (T_5). They exit the spinal cord via ventral roots to the white rami and paravertebral sympathetic chain to the inferior, middle, or superior cervical ganglia. Sympathetic fibers from the superior and middle cervical gan-

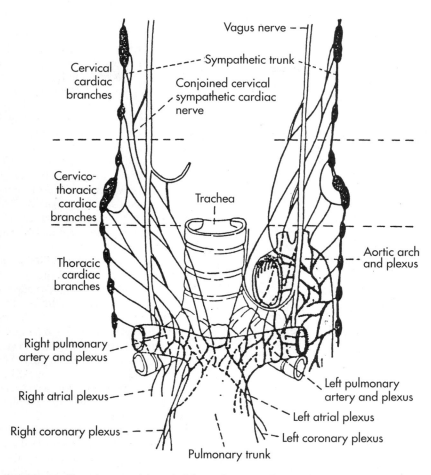

Fig. 43-1 The cardiac plexus and its subsidiary plexuses. (From Mizeres NJ: The cardiac plexus of man. *American Journal of Anatomy* 112:143, 1963.)

glion form a conjoined nerve that supplies pharyngeal, laryngeal, thyroid, carotid, and cardiac plexuses. Inferior cervical sympathetic fibers arise from inferior cervical ganglia and ansa subclavia and contribute to the aortic arch, pulmonary, and cardiac plexuses. Thoracic cardiac sympathetic fibers originate from T_2-T_5 (rarely T_6) and pass directly from the sympathetic trunk to the cardiac plexus. Parasympathetic supply arises from cell bodies in the dorsal motor nucleus of the vagus and coalesces with sympathetics subdividing into vagal cardiac nerves ending in the cardiac plexus, epicardium, and myocardium. Afferent (sensory) supply from heart and great vessels passes with sympathetic fibers through the cardiac plexus via spinal nerves T_1-T_4 to the dorsal horn of the spinal cord. Vagal afferents proceed to the medulla (nucleus tractus solitarius) and carry impulses controlling subconscious reflexes. Nociception from the heart is conveyed mainly with sympathetic afferents. Interrupting these afferents relieves cardiac pain in the chest, arms, and neck.[16] Residual pain remains in the jaw.

The pericardial nerve supply arrives via the sympathetic, parasympathetic, and afferent fibers from the cardiac and coronary plexuses. Nociception is carried with phrenic and intercostal nerves.

The thoracic aorta sustains a complex innervation (Fig. 43-2) from sympathetic and parasympathetic nerves. Nociceptive information from ascending aortic arch and descending aorta travels with sympathetic pathways. Injecting upper thoracic ganglia with procaine relieves pain from aortic aneurysm.[17] Pain from the ascending aorta can be diminished by right-sided thoracic sympathetic ganglion block, and pain from the arch or descending aorta can be blocked via left-sided thoracic sympathetic block.[18]

Clinical presentation. Obtaining a detailed pain history is essential. A sudden, severe onset may suggest dissecting aneurysm; less abrupt onset may suggest acute myocardial infarction (AMI). Retrosternal location may indicate angina. Radiation from the chest to the left arm is usually myocardial; dissecting aneurysm radiates to the back. Aggravating factors such as exertion and stress-inducing pain suggest myocardial origin. "Heartburn" can be cardiac in origin. Nitroglycerine relieves the pain of stable angina. Associated factors such as dyspnea or shock can be pericardial, myocardial, or aortic.

Physical examination for chest pain should include general, cardiovascular, respiratory, and abdominal examinations. Jugular venous distention suggests AMI or pericardial tamponade; Kussmaul's sign, pulses paradoxus, dys-

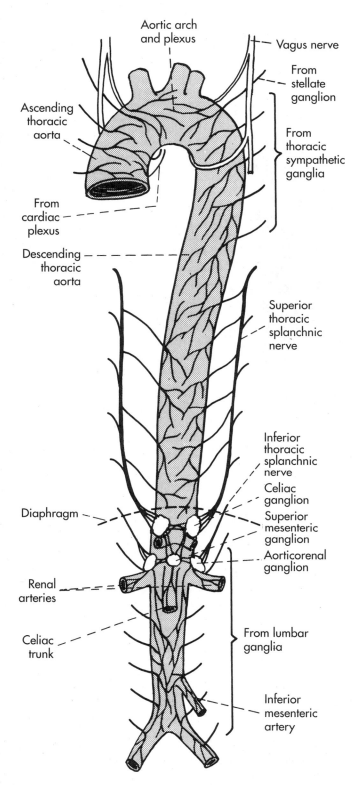

Fig. 43-2 Innervation of thoracic aorta. (From Bonica JJ: Applied anatomy relevant to pain. In Bonica JJ, editor: *The Management of Pain,* ed 2. Philadelphia, Lea & Febiger, 1990.)

rhythmias, and heart murmurs suggest cardiac causes. Mitral regurgitation is usually more consistent with AMI, and aortic regurgitation is consistent with dissecting aneurysm of aorta. Pericardial friction rub indicates pericarditis.

Investigations. Exclude anemia, and check renal function (angiography or surgical consideration). Resting electrocardiogram (ECG) is cost effective in evaluating coronary artery disease (CAD). Normal ECG does not rule out problems. Chest x-ray assesses heart failure and left ventricular enlargement, and chronic left ventricular enlargement is usually associated with chronic left ventricular dysfunction. Wide mediastinum suggests dissection. Stress ECG can assess probability of significant CAD. Thallium imaging establishes diagnosis of CAD and is helpful prognostically. Multiple gated acquisition calculates ejection fraction and assesses segmental wall motion of ventricles. Echocardiography-ultrasound image of the heart can diagnose wall-motion abnormalities, presence of masses in chambers, and pericardial fluid. Two-dimensional echocardiography is better than M-mode, which can miss abnormal segments. Cardiac catheterization is the gold standard for accurately defining CAD. Computed tomography (CT) scan can be useful for diagnosing dissecting aneurysm.

Diagnosis. Diagnosis can be straightforward after detailed history but is occasionally difficult because afferents from the heart, aorta, esophagus, lungs, and sternum share a common pathway to the spinal cord. Diagnosis can usually be made, and the main problem resides with a negative evaluation.

Management. Good medical management seeks to improve the supply and decrease the demand of the myocardium. Nitroglycerine improves the blood supply by dilating coronary arteries and decreases myocardial oxygen demand by decreasing ventricular wall stress and afterload. β-blockers decrease myocardial oxygen demand by decreasing heart rate but can exacerbate congestive heart failure and cause bronchoconstriction. β-blockers improve exercise tolerance and decrease the frequency of angina attacks. Surgery (angioplasty or coronary artery bypass graft) is reserved for proven CAD. Stellate ganglion block (left) has been used for cardiac chest pain[13] but has not been properly studied. The mainstay of pain management is still morphine, which is an excellent analgesic for visceral pain of cardiac origin and lessens myocardial oxygen demand by decreasing preload.

Noncardiac causes

The esophagus, with allusion to lungs and pleura is mainly considered. Esophageal pain can be indistinguishable from myocardial ischemia and is invariably diagnosed after an extensive cardiac evaluation concomitant with the ongoing patient anxiety and expensive hospitalization. There are two painful esophageal disorders—mucosal and motor.

Innervation. The esophagus arises from sympathetic and parasympathetic, as well as afferent and efferent, innervation. The sympathetic nerve supply extends from T_2-T_8, and parasympathetic nerve supply extends from the vagus. Sensory afferents accompany sympathetics; nociception from the upper esophagus is conducted via the vagus, and lower esophagus nociception via the greater splanchnic nerve.

Lung innervation arises from T_2-T_6 and the vagus via the pulmonary plexus. There are two types of pain receptors in the lung: *J* receptors (lining interstitial space) and *lung irritant* receptors found in epithelial lining. Mechanical or chemical damage is mediated through these receptors accommodated by the vagus nerve. Lung parenchyma is not nociceptive. Pleural innervation is by sympathetics and parasympathetics traversing the pulmonary plexus. Visceral pleura is insensate. Parietal pleura, which transmits pain via the intercostal nerve on the lateral aspects and the phrenic nerve on the diaphragm surface, is sensitive to noxious stimuli.

Clinical presentation. Pain history is important, and a slower onset occurs with reflux esophagitis. Sudden onset may suggest esophageal rupture. Retrosternal location is common with esophagitis and esophageal spasm. Lateral location suggests pulmonary embolus or pneumothorax. Radiation to the back occurs with esophagitis and esophageal spasm. Aggravating factors such as food suggest esophageal problems. Aggravation of pain by deep breathing is seen with pleurisy and pneumonia. Changes in posture producing pain signal gastroesophageal reflux. Pain relief is seen with antacids if there is an esophageal problem, and nitroglycerine gives partial relief of esophageal spasm. Associated factors such as dysphagia (esophageal cause), productive sputum (bronchopulmonary infection), or bloody sputum (pulmonary embolism) can be helpful. Pain after vomiting implicates esophageal cause, and postoperative immobilization can result in chest pain from pulmonary embolus.

Physical examination may reveal changes in percussion, (e.g., dullness [effusion or consolidation] or hyperresonance [pneumothorax]). Auscultation revealing a pleural rub, rhonchi, or rales suggests underlying infection.

Investigations. Chest x-ray is useful for lung pathology. Esophageal mucosa can be evaluated by radiography, endoscopy, or acid perfusion test.[19] Esophageal manometry demonstrates presence and correlates temporally with esophageal motor causes of chest pain. Contrast studies and esophagoscopy are useful for diagnosing esophageal cancer and esophageal lacerations. CT scan defines the extent of extraesophageal or mediastinal involvement. Ventilation/perfusion scan and pulmonary angiography are useful tools for evaluating pulmonary embolism.

Diagnosis. Make diagnosis after history, physical examination, and investigations. If cardiac and noncardiac workup are negative, a mental status evaluation with psychometric testing may be appropriate.

Management. Esophageal motor disorders with pain respond to nitroglycerin (50%). Calcium channel blockers offer little benefit. Tricyclics may be helpful.[20] Surgical myotomy can be performed if medical treatment fails. Esophageal lacerations are treated with vasopressin, tamponade, and, possibly, surgery. Esophageal cancer is treated with surgery and radiation therapy. Pain control can be achieved with opiates and interpleural and epidural analgesia, as well as neurolytic blockade. There exist a multitude of nonvisceral causes of chest pain arising from thoracic and extrathoracic causes. Psychologic causes should be considered if the chest pain is atypical in location, quality, and duration and coupled with anxiety, depression, and hypochondriasis.

ABDOMINAL PAIN
General considerations

Abdominal pain is usually caused by viscera in the abdominal cavity. Thoracic referral complicates the differential diagnosis because they both share a common somatic and visceral nerve supply. Pathology in these adjacent structures can refer pain to a similar location. One study reviewed 64 patients with abdominal pain of unknown cause, and only 15% were given a diagnosis.[21] Physicians diagnosing abdominal pain had initial accuracy of 50%.[22] This section deals with the most common painful disorders affecting viscera but does not address splenic, vascular, systemic, or extraabdominal causes of abdominal pain.

Innervation. The sympathetic supply is via thoracic and lumbar splanchnic nerves synapsing in subsidiary plexuses (i.e., celiac, aorticorenal, superior mesenteric, hepatic, splenic, adrenal, and renal plexuses). Parasympathetic innervation is via efferent (motor) and afferent (sensory) innervation conducted by the vagus and nervi erigentes (S_2-S_4). Pain travels with sympathetic and parasympathetic nerve fibers.

Clinical presentation. The pain history should be detailed and specific. The site of pain origin, alteration in location, and exact point of maximal pain should be obtained. Onset, if instantaneous, suggests perforation, rupture, or infarct of viscera. Rapid onset (i.e., minutes) includes acute inflammatory conditions (e.g., appendicitis, cholecystitis), visceral colic, or intestinal obstruction. Gradual onset suggests chronic inflammatory conditions (e.g., Crohn's disease, ulcerative colitis, diverticulitis). Burning pain in the epigastrium warns of peptic ulcer or gastritis. Severe, sudden onset of pain indicates obstruction, perforation, or infarction. Temporal relation to meals occurs with peptic ulcer. Food irritants can increase gastric acidity and aggravate ulcers, gastritis, or reflux. Fatty foods enhance biliary colic. Food and antacids relieve peptic ulcers, and avoiding food can relieve painful lower intestinal problems (e.g., Crohn's disease).

Abdominal, visceral pain presents in the midline, and parietal pain occurs secondary to inflammation of the involved viscus, referring pain to the lateral regions. Inspection of respiratory movements can help to differentiate between thoracic and abdominal causes. Chest, neurologic, and orthopedic examinations can rule out extraabdominal causes. The abdominal examination should be thorough, gentle, and specific to quadrants. Rebound can be elicited by gentle percussion and deep palpation. Local masses or tenderness can limit the differential diagnosis. Auscultation can be misleading, but a quiet abdomen suggests peritonitis and loud sounds may indicate intestinal obstruction.

Investigations. Urinalysis can diagnose presence of renal disease or infection. A complete blood count (CBC) with differential assesses anemia, infection, and sickling. Liver function tests assess liver and biliary involvement. Elevated serum amylase is seen in acute pancreatitis and intestinal obstruction. Supine and upright films can diagnose intestinal obstruction, pneumoperitoneum, or calculi. Contrast radiography, endoscopy, ultrasound, and CT scan can aid in diagnosing intestinal causes of abdominal pain.

Diagnosis. Diagnosis is less confusing if the history and physical examination are paired with a specific site in the abdomen. Visceral pain arising from the stomach, duodenum, intestine, and liver are examined in more detail.

Stomach and duodenum

Little is known of gut pain receptors. Nociception is probably via sympathetic fibers to the celiac plexus and spinal cord through splanchnic nerves T_5-T_9. Nociception from the distal duodenum occurs via T_8-T_{11} splanchnic nerves. Common disorders affecting the stomach and duodenum are gastritis, peptic ulcer disease, and neoplasm.

Gastritis

Gastritis can be erosive or nonerosive, differentiated by endoscopy and histology. Erosive gastritis is associated with stress, trauma, sepsis, burns, and drugs (e.g., aspirin, nonsteroidal antiinflammatory drugs). Nonerosive gastritis is associated with *Heliobactor pylori,* pernicious anemia, and postgastrectomy and is usually asymptomatic; erosive gastritis presents with epigastric burning pain that is intermittent and relieved with antacids and meals and associated with bleeding, nausea, vomiting, and anorexia. Diagnosis is made by therapeutic trial, contrast studies, or endoscopy. Treatment involves antacids, H_2 blockers, and sucralfate. Specific analgesics are not needed.

Peptic ulcer disease

Gastric and duodenal ulcer display similarities in presentation, evaluation, and management. Both cause significant pain and morbidity. Pathophysiology exhibits localized loss of mucosa resulting from an imbalance between acid production and mucosal protective factors. General factors (e.g., stress, smoking, drugs, tumor) and regional influences (e.g., blood flow, mucous, HCO_3, prostaglandins) are involved in the pathogenesis.

Clinical presentation entails epigastric pain, burning in character and gradual in onset, which radiates to the back, is aggravated by general factors, and is relieved by food and antacids. It is associated with nausea, vomiting, heartburn, and belching. Physical examination may demonstrate epigastric tenderness.

Diagnosis is easily made by radiographic study or endoscopy. Serum amylase elevation suggests pancreatic involvement. Serum gastrin levels should be measured if ulcers are recurrent, multiple, or refractory to therapy. If lesions persist, rule out neoplasm or Zollinger-Ellison syndrome (gastrinoma from non-β islet cells of the pancreas, which secrete gastrin, causing ulceration).

Neoplasm

Gastric cancer sustains a high mortality rate; adenocarcinoma predominates. Clinical presentation can be asymptomatic or with abdominal pain. Pain is epigastric and vague and associated with fullness, weight loss, vomiting, hematemesis, or occult blood. Examination may find an epigastric mass or lymphadenopathy, which can be axillary, supraclavicular (Virchow's node), or periumbilical (Sister Joseph's nodule). Ascites, pleural effusion, or jaundice can herald metastatic disease.

Diagnosis can be made by upper gastrointestinal studies or endoscopy with biopsy. Open biopsy is often necessary for diffuse carcinomatous involvement such as linitus plastica. CT scan documents local infiltration and possible metastases.

Treatment includes surgery (e.g., subtotal gastrectomy with node dissection) or chemotherapy (e.g., 5-FU and nitrosourea compounds). Radiation therapy is not useful. Pain can be controlled with opiates and nonsteroidal antiinflammatory drugs if bony metastases are present. Neurolytic blocks are indicated for severe pain. Alcohol celiac plexus block provided significant pain relief in 90% of patients (Table 43-1).[23] Intercostal neurolytic blocks,

Table 43-1 Effectiveness of alcohol celiac plexus block

Indications	Number of patients	Pain relief (% of patients treated)		
		Good	Fair	Poor
Pancreatic cancer*	15	73	27	0
Other abdominal cancer*	35	71	17	12
Chronic pancreatitis*	15	67	5	28
Pancreatic cancer†	25	88	8	4
Other abdominal cancer†	16	94	6	0
Pancreatic cancer‡	36	44	44	12
Pancreatitis‡	9	33	22	45
Abdominal cancer§	100	48	43	0
Abdominal cancer‖	97	62	35	3

*Black A, Dwyer B: Coeliac plexus block. *Anesth Intensive Care* 1:15, 1973.
†Bridenbaugh LD, Moore DC, Campbell DP: Management of upper abdominal cancer pain. Treatment with celiac plexus block with alcohol. *JAMA* 190:877, 1964.
‡Hegedus V: Relief of pancreatic pain by radiography-guided block. *American Journal of Radiology* 133:1101, 1979.
§Jones J, Gough D: Coeliac plexus block with alcohol for relief of upper abdominal pain due to cancer. *Am R Coll Surg Engl* 59:46, 1977.
‖Thompson GE et al: Abdominal pain and alcoholic celiac plexus nerve block. *Anesth Analg* 56:1, 1977.

neurostimulation, and neuroablative procedures have been used.

Small and large intestine

Pain fibers arising from the jejunum to the ileum travel with sympathetic afferents via splanchnic nerves through the superior mesenteric plexus to the spinal cord at T_8-T_{12}. Large bowel nociception is conducted through sympathetic afferents via the superior and inferior mesenteric plexus to the spinal cord at T_{10}-L_2 and via parasympathetic afferents to the pelvic plexus and spinal cord at S_2-S_4. Examples of visceral pathology involving the large and small intestines are addressed.

Crohn's disease. Crohn's disease is an idiopathic, inflammatory disease of the small or large intestine involving a transmural inflammatory process. Abnormal mucosa (skip lesions) are interspersed between normal bowel. Autoimmune, infectious, and psychologic factors are implicated. The clinical presentation is abdominal pain in the periumbilical or right lower quadrant. It is a continuous dull ache, aggravated by eating and relieved by starvation and bowel movements. It is associated with nausea, vomiting, bloody diarrhea, fever, and weight loss. It can present with anal or rectal involvement or extraintestinal complications (in the joint, skin, eye, and liver).

Diagnosis is made by clinical presentation, barium contrast studies, and endoscopy with biopsies. Stool cultures and serology rule out infectious cause.

Treatment should be interdisciplinary, involving the gastroenterologist, surgeon, psychologist, and nutritionist. Diet can be controlled with low-residue foods, stress control with psychotherapy, and pain control with systemic corticosteroids and sulfasalazine for flare-ups; Azathioprine and 6-mercaptopurine can prevent relapse. Potent opiates can induce spasm, increase pain, and precipitate toxic megacolon; they should not be used. Surgery is indicated for intestinal obstruction, fistulas, abscess drainage, perforation, and hemorrhage.

Ulcerative colitis. Ulcerative colitis is an idiopathic, inflammatory bowel disease limited to the mucosal surface of the large bowel. It presents with left lower quadrant pain, bloody diarrhea, cramping, and perianal fissures. It is associated with tenesmus; defecation relieves pain. Extraintestinal manifestations are similar to Crohn's disease.

Diagnosis is made clinically with sigmoidoscopy stool cultures, and serology rules out infection. Colonoscopy with multiple biopsies should be undertaken for long-standing disease because incidence of colonic carcinoma is markedly increased. Treatment parallels that for Crohn's disease. Colectomy is indicated for toxic megacolon and prevention of colonic carcinoma.

Liver

Pain transmission is probably via afferent sympathetics from distention of the liver capsule (Glisson's capsule).

The clinical presentation is dependent on the etiologic agent. Inflammatory processes can present as pain in the right upper quadrant if the parietal peritoneum is involved. Pain can be referred to the right shoulder and scapula and is sharp, intense, and well localized. Pain can also present in the epigastrium and can be vague and nonspecific. It is associated with fever, anorexia, and increased temperature. The presence of a mass, weight loss, ascites, or jaundice suggests tumor.

Diagnosis is made by elevated serum transaminases in viral hepatitis. A CT scan helps differentiate between hepatic masses (e.g., abscess or tumor).

Treatment is supportive for viral hepatitis, involving nutrition and analgesics (watch dose with liver compromise). Abscess requires incision and drainage. Hepatic carcinoma is unresponsive to chemotherapy; surgery is indicated in less than 30%.[24] Pain control is achieved with opiates, segmental analgesia (epidural), neurolytic celiac plexus block, or intrathecal opiates.

BILIARY PAIN
Innervation

Nociception travels via sympathetic fibers and right splanchnic nerves to the T_6-T_{10} level at the spinal cord. Since vagotomy does not alter pain transmission, vagal fibers play no role in pain transmission. Inflammatory disease of the biliary system stimulates afferent nerve fibers of the parietal peritoneum, causing somatic pain in the T_6-T_9 distribution, well localized to the right upper quadrant.

Acute cholecystitis

Clinical presentation reveals pain well localized to the right upper quadrant secondary to gallstones. Inflammation contacts the parietal peritoneum and refers pain to the infrascapular region and right shoulder. Palpation reproduces the discomfort, and a mass (i.e., gallbladder and adherent omentum) is palpable in 30% of patients. Pain is aggravated by deep inspiration during right upper quadrant palpation (i.e., Murphy's sign). Anorexia, nausea, vomiting, leukocytosis, fever, rebound, localized spasm, or paralytic ileus can be found on examination.

Diagnosis is made by ultrasound, although cholangiography is useful preoperatively and intraoperatively. Radionuclide scan demonstrates cystic duct obstruction. White blood cell count, serum bilirubin, and alkaline phosphatase may all be elevated.

Treatment is cholecystectomy, which relieves visceral pain in almost all patients. Segmental epidural analgesia in T_5-T_{10} can be useful for controlling biliary colic.

Postcholecystectomy pain

Postcholecystectomy pain is found in 5% or more patients. It can be caused by retained stones, postoperative biliary stricture, or common bile duct obstruction. It may be a functional disorder of biliary emptying causing biliary dyskinesia.

Clinical presentation is usually pain in the right upper quadrant after brief hiatus of postcholecystectomy pain relief. The pain is colicky, diurnal, aggravated by eating, and associated with nausea and vomiting. Examination reveals tenderness in the right upper quadrant.

Diagnosis is made by biliary manometry, which records pressures in the common bile duct, Oddi's sphincter, and the duodenum and confirms biliary dyskinesia. Endoscopic of retrograde cholangiopancreatography is useful for ruling out stones, biliary stricture, and neoplasm as potential causes.

Treatment is medical and surgical. Nitrates can relax Oddi's sphincter. All opioid agonists increase biliary duct pressure and increase tone in Oddi's sphincter in a dose-dependent fashion through opiate-receptor–mediated mechanisms.[25] An increase in duct pressure by opiates can be reversed by naloxone or glucagon.

PANCREAS
Innervation

Sympathetic afferents travel with thoracic splanchnic nerves T_5-T_9, then pass through the celiac plexus and ganglion to the spinal cord, transmitting nociception. Vagal afferents do not appear to mediate pancreatic pain.

Acute pancreatitis

Chronic alcohol abuse remains the most common cause of acute pancreatitis. Ethanol and acetaldehyde are toxic to pancreatic acinar cells. Gallstones are the most common cause in nonalcoholic patients. Hypercalcemia, postoperative viral infections, and drugs (e.g., steroids, thiazides, estrogens) are causative.

The clinical presentation is usually abdominal pain, which is constant, epigastric and boring, radiates to the back, and can last for days. It is aggravated by lying down and relieved by sitting forward.

Acute pancreatitis is associated with nausea, vomiting, abdominal distention, ileus, peritonitis, and fever. It can present with shock. Pain can impair ventilation secondary to muscle spasm and severe guarding, which could lead to respiratory insufficiency.

Diagnosis is made by clinical presentation and investigations. CT scan demonstrates pancreatic abnormality in a majority of patients (i.e., diffuse enlargement). Ultrasound is not as effective. Serum amylase is used to determine pancreatic inflammation and does not always correlate with damage. Normal values are found in 10% to 15% of patients with acute pancreatitis. Hypocalcemia is usually present.

Treatment should be aggressive because this is a medical emergency. Resuscitate by restoring intravascular volume, and support respiration. Limit inflammation and complications by prescribing nothing by mouth, nasogastric suction, steroids, trypsin inhibitors, anticholinergics, H_2 blockers, and antibiotics. Treat pain aggressively with segmental epidural analgesia[26] or celiac ganglion blockade.[27] Avoid opiates, although meperidine, which is less spasmogenic than other opiates, can be used judiciously.

Chronic pancreatitis

The cause of chronic pancreatitis in most patients is chronic alcoholism. Biliary calculus is a rare cause. Alcohol ingestion secretes protein by pancreatic cells, which precipitates into pancreatic ducts, causing obstruction, inflammation, and fibrosis.

The clinical presentation is a constant, epigastric "gnawing" pain that radiates to the back and is aggravated by food and alcohol. It is associated with chronic weight loss, mal-absorption, abdominal tenderness, endocrine insufficiency (exhibited by an abnormal glucose tolerance test), and exocrine insufficiency (i.e., steatorrhea).

Diagnosis is made by clinical presentation; serum enzymes are of little value. CT scan recognizes ductal abnormalities half of the time. An abdominal x-ray with pancreatic calcification is virtually pathognomonic.

Treatment includes abstinence from alcohol, support of endocrine and exocrine insufficiency, and palliation of pain. Diet control, anticholinergics, and H_2 blockers suppress pancreatic secretion but do not relieve pain. Pain control can be achieved with opiates. Neurolytic celiac plexus block has been used with good short-term relief, but its usefulness is not clearly demonstrated[28,29] (see Table 43-1). Intrapleural block can be useful.[30] Surgical treatment with longitudinal pancreaticojejunostomy significantly relieves pain in 70% to 80%, although complications of the surgery include operative mortality (4%) and postoperative diabetes (20%).[31]

Pancreatic cancer

Pancreatic cancer is a lethal disease, with less than 2% survival over 5 years. Clinical presentation is an epigastric, "gnawing," dull ache radiating to the back in 25% of patients. It is associated with anorexia, weight loss, nausea, vomiting, palpable mass, and jaundice.

Diagnosis is made by CT scan, endoscopic retrograde cholangiopancreatography, or percutaneous biopsy. Treatment is eligible, with 15% having 3-year survival.[32] Radiation and chemotherapy are somewhat palliative. Pain control can be achieved with opiates. If the cancer is not adequately controlled, neurolytic celiac plexus block provides significant pain relief in 80% to 90%[18,23,28,33,34] (see Table 43-1).

GENITOURINARY PAIN
Innervation

Innervation of the kidney is comprised of sympathetic, parasympathetic, and sensory contributions. Preganglionic sympathetic fibers from T_{10}-L_1(L_2) convey afferent information via the white rami and paravertebral ganglia and synapse in celiac and aorticorenal ganglia. Postganglionic fibers pass to the renal plexus. Parasympathetic fibers from the vagus traverse the celiac plexus and synapse in the renal plexus.

Sensory afferent fibers convey pain and travel with kidney sympathetic fibers via thoracic spinal nerves T_{10}-T_{12} to the dorsal horn neurons. Some afferent sensory fibers follow the vagus and may account for the nausea, vomiting, and decreased peristalsis associated with renal colic.

Ureter

The upper half of the ureter receives the same nerve supply as the kidney. The lower half is innervated by traveling with lumbar splanchnic nerves via the aortic, then superior hypogastric plexus. Sympathetic fibers from the sacral trunk also contribute to the ureter from the sacral trunk. Parasympathetics from S_2-S_4 travel with pelvic splanchnic nerves via the inferior hypogastric plexus to the ureter. Sensory fibers travel with sympathetics to T_{12}, L_1 (L_2) to the spinal cord.

Nausea and vomiting precede pain of genitourinary origin, which can be referred from the renal pelvis to the costovertebral angle and ipsilateral testicle (ovary). Midureter pain refers to the inguinal region, and distal ureter pain refers to the suprapubic region.

Renal and ureteric calculi

Clinical presentation is consistent with an acute onset of severe colicky, flank pain caused by passing the calculus. Pain referral is dependent on the position of the stone and is not relieved by position changes. It is associated with ipsilateral costovertebral angle tenderness, nausea, vomiting, urgency, extreme restlessness, and mild shock.

The diagnosis is made by clinical presentation, presence of hematuria, and radiography showing renal calculi (90% radiopaque). Intravenous pyelogram and radioisotope venography demonstrate obstruction by calculi.

Treatment depends on the size of the stone, the presence of sepsis, and pain control. Stones less than 5 mm pass spontaneously; stones greater than 10 mm are unlikely to pass. Sepsis should be treated as a medical emergency, with intravenous fluids, electrolytes, and antibiotics. Stone removal is effected by lithotripsy, endoscopy, or open surgery. Pain control by opioids can aggravate muscle spasm; meperidine may be the best choice. Continuous epidural analgesia at T_{10}-L_1 provides excellent pain control with elimination of reflex spasm and may allow spontaneous passing of the calculus.

Vascular lesions

Renal vein thrombosis involves clot-obstructing venous outflow causing capsular distention and pain. Dehydration, infection, coagulopathy, or pulmonary emboli may contribute. The clinical presentation can be acute or chronic flank pain with hematuria and proteinuria. An ultrasound detects diminished function.

The treatment is anticoagulation. Pain control is easily achieved with antiinflammatories and opiate agonists.

Renal tumor

Renal cell (clear cell) carcinoma has an unknown etiology and predominates in older men. Metastases can be widespread to the lung, liver, and bone and lymph nodes.

A clinical presentation of flank pain, palpable mass, and hematuria should alert the physician. Hypertension, weight loss, fever, anemia, or erythrocythemia (i.e., increased production of erythropoietin) are useful diagnostic signs. Confirm the diagnosis by CT scan and angiography.

Treatment involves nephrectomy if the tumor is confined to the kidney. If it is metastatic, surgery, radiation, chemotherapy, and hormonal manipulation may be added. At this stage, pain control becomes the important issue; use oral or intraspinal opiates, epidural analgesia, or neuroablative procedures if indicated.

CONCLUSION

Limited knowledge of visceral pain intensifies the difficulties in diagnosis and management. Not defining an adequate noxious stimulus for quantifying visceral nociception and lack of a good research model have hampered clinical studies. The utility of opiates in managing visceral pain has been clearly demonstrated in research[35] and in clinical practice.

Newer approaches such as intrathecal clonidine may improve visceral pain control.[36] The expression of c-fos like protein in the spinal cord may be used as a marker to elucidate nociceptive transmission of visceral pain.[37,38] Expanding our knowledge of neurotransmitters and neural processing can only enhance clinical knowledge and lead to improvements in pain control.

REFERENCES

1. Procacci P, Maresca M, Cersosimo R: Visceral pain: Pathophysiology and clinical aspects. In Costa M, editor: *Sensory Nerves and Neuropeptides in Gastroenterology.* New York, Plenum Press, 1991.
2. Cervero F: Mechanisms of acute visceral pain. *Br Med Bull* 47:549-560, 1991.
3. Ness TJ, Gebhart GF: Visceral pain: A review of experimental studies. *Pain* 41:167-234, 1990.
4. Iggo A, McMillen JA, Mokha SS: Spinal pathways for inhibition of multireceptive dorsal horn neurons by locus coeruleus and nucleus raphe magnus. *J Physiol (Lond)*32:86, 1981.
5. Yaksh T, Wilson P: Spinal serotonin terminal system mediates antinociception. *J Pharmacol Exp Ther* 208:446-453, 1979.
6. Cervero F, Connell LA: Distribution of somatic and visceral primary afferents fibers within the spinal cord of the cat. *J Comp Neurol* 230:88-98, 1984.
7. Mense S, Craig AD: Spinal and supraspinal terminations of primary afferent fibers from the gastrocnemius-soleus muscle in the cat. *Neuroscience* 26:1023-1035, 1988.
8. Foreman RD: Organization of the spinothalamic tract as a relay for cardiopulmonary sympathetic afferent fiber activity. *Proj Sens Physiol* 9:1-51, 1989.
9. Ruch TC: Pathophysiology of pain. In Costa M, editor: *Neurophysiology.* Philadelphia, WB Saunders, 1961.
10. MacKenzie J: *Symptoms and their interpretation.* London, Shaw, 1909.
11. Davis L, Pollock LJ: The peripheral pathway for painful sensations. *Arch Neurol Psychiat* 24:883-899, 1930.
12. Last RF: *Anatomy—Regional and Applied,* ed 7. New York, Churchill Livingstone, 1984.
13. Bonica JJ: Applied anatomy relevant to pain. In Bonica JJ, editor: *The Management of Pain,* ed 2. Philadelphia, Lea & Febiger, 1990.
14. Kuntz A: *The Autonomic Nervous System,* ed 4. Philadelphia, Lea & Febiger, 1953.
15. Benjamin S: Microvascular angina and the sensitive heart: Historical perspective. *Am J Med* 92:52-55, 1992.
16. White JC: Cardiac pain. Anatomic pathways and physiologic mechanisms. *Circulation* 16:644, 1957.
17. Rasmussen TB, Farr WJ: Paravertebral injection of procaine for pain produced by aortic aneurysm. *J Neurosurg* 3:267, 1946.
18. Bonica JJ: General considerations of pain in the chest. In Bonica JJ, editor: *The Management of Pain,* ed 1. Philadelphia, Lea & Febiger, 1953.
19. Bernstein LM, Fruin RC, Pacini R: Differentiation of esophageal pain from angina pectoris: Role of the esophageal acid perfusion test. *Medicine (Baltimore)* 41:143-162, 1962.
20. Clouse R: Psychopharmacologic approaches to therapy for chest pain of presumed esophageal origin. *Am J Med* 92:106-112, 1992.
21. Sarfeh IJ: Abdominal pain of unknown etiology. *Am J Surg* 132:22-25, 1976.
22. Hickey M, Kiernan G, Weaver K: Evaluation of abdominal pain. *Emerg Med Clin North Am* 7:437-451, 1989.
23. Bridenbaugh LD, Moore DC, Campbell DP: Management of upper abdominal cancer pain. Treatment with celiac plexus block with alcohol. *JAMA* 190:877, 1964.
24. Mulholland MW, Debas H: Diseases of the liver, biliary system and pancreas. In Bonica JJ, editor: *The Management of Pain, vol 2,* ed 2. Philadelphia, Lea & Febiger, 1990.
25. Radnay PA et al: Common bile duct pressure changes after morphine, meperidine, butorphanol and naloxone. *Anesth Analg* 63:444, 1984.

26. Walker T, Pembleton WE: Continuous epidural block in the treatment of pancreatitis. *Anesthesiology* 14:33, 1953.

27. Gage IM: Treatment of acute pancreatitis. *Surgery* 23:723, 1948.

28. Black A, Dwyer B: Coeliac plexus block. *Anesth Intensive Care* 1:15, 1973.

29. Hegedus V: Relief of pancreatic pain by radiography-guided block. *American Journal of Radiology* 133:1101, 1979.

30. Sihota MD et al: Successful management of chronic pancreatitis and post-herpetic neuralgia with intrapleural technique. *Reg Anesth* 13(suppl 2):40, 1988.

31. Prinz RA, Kaufman BJ, Folk FA: Pancreatico-jejunostomy of chronic pancreatitis. *Am J Surg* 141:28, 1981.

32. Kalser MH, Leite CA, Warren WD: Fat assimilation after distal pancreatectomy. *N Engl J Med* 279:570, 1978.

33. Thompson GE et al: Abdominal pain and alcoholic celiac plexus nerve block. *Anesth Analg* 56:1, 1977.

34. Jones J, Gough D: Coeliac plexus block with alcohol for relief of upper abdominal pain due to cancer. *Am R Coll Surg Engl* 59:46, 1977.

35. Gebhart GF, Ness TJ: Central mechanisms of visceral pain. *Can J Physiol Pharmacol* 69:627-634, 1991.

36. Danzebrink RM, Gebhart GF: Intrathecal coadministration of clonidine with serotonin receptor agonists produces supra-additive visceral antinociception in the rat. *Brain Res* 555: 35-42, 1991.

37. DeLeo J, Coombs D, McCarthy L: Differential c-fos like protein expression in mechanically versus chemically induced visceral nociception. *Molecular Brain Research* 11:167-170, 1991.

38. Hammond D, Presley K, Basbaum A: Morphine or U-50, 488 suppresses fos protein-like immunoreactivity in the spinal cord and nucleus tractus solitarius evoked by a noxious visceral stimulus in the rat. *J Comp Neurol* 315:244-253, 1992.

39. Mizeres NJ: The cardiac plexus of man. *American Journal of Anatomy* 112:143, 1963.

QUESTIONS: VISCERAL PAIN

For questions 1-5, choose from the following:
- A. 1, 2, and 3
- B. 1 and 3
- C. 2 and 4
- D. 4
- E. All of the above

1. Neurotransmission of nociception from lamina of the dorsal root ganglia to the second-order neurons is affected by which of the following substances?
   1. Vasoactive
   2. Calcitonin gene-related peptide
   3. Substance P
   4. 5-hydroxytryptamine

2. Visceral afferents reach the spinal cord through which of the following nerve pathways?
   1. Sympathetic
   2. Parasympathetic
   3. Splanchnic
   4. Ventral roots

3. Which of the following medications is (are) generally effective in treating esophageal pain?
   1. Nitroglycerine
   2. Calcium channel blockers
   3. Antidepressants
   4. Interleukins

4. Which of the following medications should not be used in Crohn's disease?
   1. Systemic corticosteroids
   2. Azathioprine
   3. Sulfasalazine
   4. Meperidine

5. Which of the following pain management techniques is (are) most appropriate for patients with hepatic carcinoma?
   1. Chemotherapy
   2. Celiac plexus block
   3. Abdominal surgery
   4. Segmental analgesia

ANSWERS

1. A
2. E
3. B
4. D
5. C

44 Pelvic Pain

Richard B. Patt and Ricardo S. Plancarte

Although a specific definition has not been widely accepted, chronic pelvic pain may be said to exist when there is nonmenstrual pelvic pain with or without pain in the abdomen, hips, thighs, buttocks, and rectum that has persisted for 3 or more months and is sufficiently severe to cause functional disability and require medical or surgical treatment.[1] In contrast to chronic conditions, acute pelvic pain is of more rapid onset, usually developing over the course of days when caused by infection or quite suddenly in the case of torsion or rupture of intrapelvic structures.

Chronic pelvic pain may occur in the presence of known or suspected organic pathology or in the absence of evidence of an underlying physical cause. The latter entity has been recognized for over a century and has variously been termed "chronic pelvic pain without obvious pathology" (CPPWOP), pelvic congestion, pelvic fibrosis, pelvic sympathetic syndrome, pelvic neurodystonia, pelvalgia, and irritable uterus syndrome. The high incidence of CPPWOP contributes to much of the controversy surrounding diagnosis and management. Physician selection is a further source of confusion: Patients may be treated by a variety of physicians including primary care providers; gynecologic, urologic, or endocrinologic specialists; mental health workers; and pain specialists. The specialist's approach to chronic pelvic pain will naturally be biased based on training, treatment armamentarium, and patient self-selection. Other factors that contribute to controversy include confusion among descriptive terms and uncertainty about the significance of observations of a high incidence of physical and/or sexual abuse among patients with pelvic pain.

Regardless of the setting in which care is rendered, when considered overall, the outcome of treatment for chronic pelvic pain is often poor. Despite interest by physicians from so many specialties, research regarding the natural history of pelvic pain and treatment outcomes has been sparse historically.[2] Although controlled reports are lacking, favorable results have been reported in patients completing a multidisciplinary pain program.[2,3]

EPIDEMIOLOGY

In one survey, chronic pelvic pain (CPP) accounted for 10% of patients referred to a new gynecologic clinic[4] and was observed to account for 10% to 19% of hysterectomies[5] and 40% of laparoscopies.[6] Estimates of the proportion of CPP patients with identifiable pelvic pathology range between 8% and 80%,[2] with most authorities citing the frequency of CPPWOP as being about one-third to one-half.[7] Of patients with chronic pelvic pain, a somatic cause may be more likely to be disclosed in older women.[2]

In one study 30% of patients whose symptoms indicated CPP had already undergone total hysterectomy,[8] and in another, pelvic pain persisted despite hysterectomy in 25% of pelvic pain patients,[9] confirming that extirpative surgery is not a panacea. Pooled studies of patients who have undergone laparoscopy for CPP[2] revealed the presence of endometriosis in one third of patients, adhesions in another one third, and an absence of identifiable pathology in the remaining one third of patients. The results of such studies should be interpreted cautiously, since (1) the absence of apparent pathology may reflect a lack of specificity (false negatives)[10] and (2) the presence of apparent pathology may not correlate with a given patient's symptoms (false positives).[11,12] Although one study attempting to correlate laparoscopic findings with clinical complaints determined that patients with identifiable pathology reported more severe pain and greater concomitant interference, it also noted that patients in whom pathologic conditions can be visualized often fail to complain of pain at all.[13]

PELVIC PAIN AND PRIOR ABUSE

Studies have noted a history of sexual and/or physical abuse in 50% or more of patients with CPP,[14-17] although the significance of such findings is controversial. Although actual descriptions of pelvic pain may not differ in abused versus nonabused patients, when compared to nonabused controls, patients with a history of abuse may have higher incidences of psychologic findings such as reduced perception of control, suffering, distress, and somatization.[11,12,18] In addition to higher incidences of pelvic pain, individuals with a history of being abused are more likely to have other medically unexplained symptoms (especially gastrointestinal), psychiatric diagnoses, and more surgical procedures.[19] There is preliminary evidence that these correlations are multicultural.[20]

Despite the apparent strength of the data linking childhood sexual abuse and otherwise unexplained pelvic pain, its significance must still be interpreted cautiously. It is difficult to obtain an accurate history of abuse, as is evidenced by one study in which one third of abused patients had never discussed such events with anyone and only 17% had previously admitted them to their physician.[14]

ETIOLOGY

The pelvis is a complex structure that contains the genital organs and portions of the urinary and gastrointestinal tracts, all protected and supported by a complex array of soft-tissue structures. Each of these components is a potential source of acute and chronic pain that may arise from a variety of mechanisms, and in addition pain may be referred from distant locations such as the abdomen or lower extremities. Nongynecologic pelvic pain may arise from gastrointestinal conditions (e.g., appendicitis; diverticulitis; inflammatory, functional bowel disorders such as ulcerative colitis and spastic colon), urologic conditions (e.g., urinary tract infections, ureteral stones, cystitis), and musculoskeletal dysfunction. The skeletal pelvis functions to protect the pelvic viscera; but as part of the lower extremity, it also acts as a surface for the attachment of the muscles of the trunk and lower limb and a means to mechanically transmit the weight of the upper body to the lower extremities.[21] Ordinarily the pelvis is a relatively rigid structure because of the sacroiliac, lumbar, and pubic ligaments. However, hormonal and mechanical changes during pregnancy, trauma, and obesity may all contribute to laxity and dysfunction that may produce pain. Likewise, the internal pelvic viscera are supported by a complex array of internal ligamentous and muscular structures that when deranged may produce pain.

Pain originating in gynecologic tissues per se may be due to acute processes (e.g., ectopic pregnancy, ruptured ovarian cyst, pelvic abscess) or chronic problems related to the uterus, ovaries, or ectopic endometrial implants. Such chronic problems may be infectious, neoplastic, traumatic, or postsurgical in nature. Complaints may further be influenced to variable degrees by intercurrent psychologic factors.

HISTORY

The history should be orderly, systematic, and well documented. Depending on the setting in which assessment occurs, it may be complemented by a variety of standardized questionnaires intended to assess patients with chronic pain. Given that CPP often correlates with psychosocial disturbances and a history of developmental or sexual trauma, the use of appropriate psychologic questionnaires is recommended. The history should elicit detailed information about the onset and nature of the pain and a general medical, psychologic, social, and family history.

A standard pain history should include inquiry into the pattern of onset, the presence or absence of an inciting event, the temporal pattern of pain, its quality, its severity (on average, at best, and at worst), factors that alleviate or worsen pain, drug history (e.g., efficacy and toxicity), and associated vasomotor or neurologic disturbances. Patients with pelvic pain should specifically be asked how symptoms are affected by specific activities such as standing, lying, bending, eating, swallowing, coughing, straining, the release of flatus, defecation, urination, menstruation, lateral and forward flexion of the trunk, and other movements.[18] Specific associated problems that should be sought include the presence of nausea, vomiting, melena, and urinary and menstrual disturbances.

Urinary habit may provide valuable clues as to the source of pain. Most adults void 4 to 6 times daily. Urinary frequency in the absence of increased urinary volumes may reflect reductions in the bladder's effective filling capacity that may be due to extrinsic factors (e.g., foreign body, stones, tumor, or infection) or intrinsic factors (e.g., muco-

sal inflammation, infiltration, or edema).[16] Dysuria, nocturia, hesitancy, alterations in the force and caliber of the flow of urine, and dribbling may indicate obstruction distal to the bladder, as is common with prostatic hypertrophy or infection. Incontinence may be due to bladder exstrophy, vesicovaginal fistula, congenital anatomic abnormalities, neurologic dysfunction, or injury resulting from surgery or childbirth. Stress incontinence is often due to a cystocele as a result of pelvic diaphragmatic laxity that occurs after childbirth and with aging.

Other important data include that related to menstruation (e.g., age of menarche, temporal and flow patterns, dysmenorrhea, etc.), pregnancy (e.g., number, dates, outcome, difficulty in conceiving), and sexual activity (e.g., sexual orientation, frequency of partners and activity, prior infections). Questioning should also elicit history of radiation therapy, diethylstilbestrol use (in women pregnant or born from 1947 to 1971),[16] breast and endocrinologic problems, and a family history of ovarian, uterine, and breast cancer.

PHYSICAL EXAMINATION

A thorough physical examination is of the utmost importance but may be neglected in the setting of the pain clinic for cultural reasons and because, unless referral for pelvic pain is common, clinical skills may be lacking. In addition to a standard neurologic and musculoskeletal examination, an abdominal examination should be carried out to localize the pain and exclude objective signs of an acute process. A pelvic examination should be performed to evaluate for cervical tenderness that may indicate infection and to characterize uterine and adnexal architecture, which may be abnormal in other chronic processes. An alternate approach involves employing a consultant with specific gynecologic training or ensuring close and careful communication with the referring gynecologist. Regardless of the extent of the patient's prior evaluation, the presence of trigger points must be sought, ideally with a bimanual examination, since such findings are frequently overlooked outside the confines of a pain clinic. The examination should endeavor to distinguish tenderness emanating from the abdominal wall versus deeper tissues. Surgical scars should be carefully examined to assess for the presence of nerve entrapment, adhesions, and trigger points.

DIAGNOSTIC STUDIES

Diagnostic studies will have generally been performed before pain-clinic referral. Recent results of a complete blood count, erythrocyte sedimentation rate, urinalysis and culture, and cervical culture should be available to help evaluate for chronic infection, bleeding, inflammation, and ischemia. When appropriate, a pregnancy test should be performed to exclude intrauterine or ectopic pregnancy. Ultrasonography or computed tomography (CT) scanning is frequently performed to evaluate a suspected mass, to detect the presence of free fluid or air, or in the case of pain that has persisted without an adequate explanation. As with other chronic pain conditions, the potential for a diagnostic study to suggest new treatment alternatives must be weighed against its cost and likelihood of contributing to the patient's illness conviction.

Laparoscopy is an important diagnostic tool that also has a variety of therapeutic applications, the discussion of which are beyond the scope of this chapter. Though invasive, it is generally safe, effective, and well accepted.[4] Diagnostic laparoscopy is most useful to detect or confirm the presence of endometriosis, adhesions, ovarian cysts, and uterine malformations. Even negative laparoscopy may be valuable by providing reassurance, as was apparently the case in one series of adolescents, of whom 74% experienced symptomatic improvement after negative laparoscopy.[22]

As in other chronic pain conditions, the value of neural blockade as a diagnostic tool is underrecognized. Before considering neural blockade, it should be ascertained that an evaluation has been undertaken to exclude identifiable underlying pathology. If such studies are negative or if the cause of pain is known but cannot be corrected, a trial of diagnostic neural blockade may be undertaken. The two basic approaches to such a trial are the institution of a differential spinal or epidural block and the sequential administration of more specific procedures aimed at discrete interruption of sympathetic versus somatic nerve impulses (Table 44-1).[23]

MYOFASCIAL PAIN

The concept that undetected myofascial dysfunction and spasm may explain the high incidence of CPPWOP has recently gained considerable popularity.[13] Whereas a muscular cause for otherwise obscure pelvic pain has been considered for decades,[24] the concept of underdiagnosis of muscular pain based on absence of radiologic and laboratory data parallels current opinion on the causation of other painful disorders.[25] Sustained muscular tension and resultant pain has been hypothesized to be related to stress and autonomic hyperactivity;[26] prolonged sitting;[27] and trauma resulting from parturition, sexual activity, and surgery.[19] Authorities recommend careful attention to physical examination, including bimanual examination. Reproduction of

Table 44-1 Diagnostic neural blockade for pelvic pain

Type of nerve block	Alternatives
Central	Differential epidural block, differential subarachnoid block
Sympathetic	Celiac plexus block, superior hypogastric plexus block, paracervical (inferior hypogastric plexus) block, ganglion impar block
Somatic	Pudendal nerve block, paravertebral nerve root block, intercostal nerve block, ilioinguinal nerve block, iliohypogastric nerve block, genitofemoral nerve block, trigger-point injection

pain when focal pressure is applied to periabdominal muscles, muscles of the pelvic floor and the parametrial region, and trigger points, even when located distant to the site of pain, is characteristic of a myofascial cause for pain. Slocumb[3] has recommended modifications in standard examination practices. In a sample of 35 patients with CPP-WOP, Milano and colleagues[13] detected abdominal wall and pelvic floor trigger points in 90% of patients. In another clinical series,[26] three quarters of 122 patients had very favorable responses to trigger-point therapy provided in the context of a comprehensive pain program.

SPECIFIC SYNDROMES
Endometriosis

Endometriosis, the presence of endometrial tissue located outside the uterine cavity, is estimated to affect up to 5 million women in the United States alone, or 1 in 15 (7%) of women of reproductive age.[28] Ectopic endometrial implants most frequently arise in the pelvis; and of pelvic implants, the ovary is the most common site. Implantation may occur on any peritoneal surface, especially the uterosacral ligaments, fallopian tubes, round ligaments, and broad ligaments of the uterus.[29] Causation is uncertain and has alternately been postulated to be due to retrograde menstruation and lymphatic and hematogenic spread. Maintenance by hormonal mechanisms is, however, well accepted. Pain may be due to the local release of prostaglandins, irritation from the products of menstruation, local distention, and nerve damage caused by scarring.[30]

Common symptoms include pelvic pain, dysmenorrhea, and dyspareunia. Infertility and abnormal uterine bleeding are commonly associated problems, occurring in one third or more of affected patients.[18] Although symptoms are variable, pain is commonly cyclical, initially increasing during the course of menstruation and only subsiding days after the cease of flow. Disease progression may be associated with worsening of pain and disassociation from the menses. Symptoms often resolve with the onset of menopause or after oophorectomy.

A diagnosis of endometriosis is often suggested by the above clinical picture but requires confirmation by direct visualization of lesions during laparoscopy or laparotomy. Histologic diagnosis may be difficult to obtain. Since endometriosis may be asymptomatic, its mere presence by no means confirms the cause of pelvic pain.[7,9,31]

There is substantial evidence that symptoms and actual implant volume are dependent on circulating estrogen levels.[18] The selection of treatment strategies depends on factors that include age, desire for childbirth, and severity of disease. Medical therapy includes a wide range of hormonal manipulation, mostly aimed at inducing a hypoestrogenic state. Other hormones may be added in order to ameliorate the adverse effects of primary hormone therapy. The most common medical therapy is with danazol, a mildly androgenic substance that reduces the pituitary gonadotropin production, thereby inducing endometrial atrophy. A 6-month trial is usually initiated, after which more than two thirds of women with mild to moderate symptoms improve significantly both symptomatically and at laparoscopy.[19] Symptomatic improvement after danazol therapy is often maintained with the chronic administration of low-dose oral contraceptives. Other hormonal therapies have been developed, including treatment with various gonadotropin-releasing hormone/luteinizing hormone-releasing hormone agonists and analogues, progestogens, and their combinations.

The role of surgery is more controversial. Conservative surgery consists of surgical, thermal, or laser extirpation of endometrial implants at laparoscopy or laparotomy, with careful attention to avoiding injury to adjacent structures.[32] Such therapy may be effective, particularly when fertility is desired. When performed for women who desire childbirth, the subsequent average conception rate is 45% to 65%. Subsequent pregnancy may delay recurrence of endometriosis. Total abdominal hysterectomy is considered for severe, intractable endometriosis, particularly in postmenopausal patients or individuals who do not desire childbirth. Preservation of the ovaries may be considered if evidence of parovarian involvement is absent. Adjuncts to the surgical therapies mentioned may include uterine suspension, uterosacral ligament amputation, open or laparoscopic laser presacral neurectomy, and uterine nerve ablation.[33-37] Presacral neurectomy seems to be more effective for midline pain than for lateral pain.[23,26]

Endometritis

Infection is a frequent cause of recurring or chronic pelvic pain, as well as ectopic pregnancy and infertility. Acute endometritis refers to infection that is localized to the uterus. The cervix ordinarily protects against uterine infection. Endometritis is therefore more common when the cervical barrier has been breached by surgical events (e.g., dilatation and curettage) or passage of the products of conception (e.g., spontaneous abortion or term pregnancy). The causative organism may be normal vaginal flora or sexually transmitted disease. Endometritis is usually heralded by crampy suprapubic pain and uterine tenderness, with relative sparing of the adnexa. Pain may be accompanied by foul-smelling discharge or bleeding, urinary frequency, low-grade fever, and leukocytosis. Cultures and a Gram's stain of the cervical discharge should be performed, and if a diagnosis is confirmed, treatment with appropriate oral or parenteral antibiotics should be instituted. Endometritis should be distinguished from normal uterine cramping and cystitis. The former condition is distinguished by the absence of foul-smelling discharge and fever and the latter by the presence of urinary red and white blood cells and bacteria.[24]

Pelvic inflammatory disease

Acute pelvic inflammatory disease (PID), an ascending infection involving the pelvic organs and contiguous structures, affects an estimated one million U.S. women annually.[38] If it is unrecognized or inadequately treated, patients may go on to experience infertility, adhesions, and chronic pain.[39] The causative organisms may be aerobic or anaerobic and originate in normal vaginal or cervical flora and/or may be sexually transmitted. Alterations in the cervical integrity resulting from surgical instrumentation or menstruation-mediated loss of the cervix's mucous plug may predispose patients to infection. The incidence of infection is increased with a history of multiple sexual partners, sex with an infected partner, a prior episode of PID, and the use of intrauterine devices, particularly the Dalkon shield.[23] Symptoms tend to vary with the causative organism, of which *Neisseria gonorrhoeae* and *Chlamydia trachomatis* are the most common. Acute gonorrhea usually produces severe postmenstrual pain. Mixed and anaerobic organisms often result in fever and a septic appearance; whereas other than mild pain, chlamydial infection is usually otherwise asymptomatic (so-called "silent PID"). Dysuria and dyspareunia are common findings, and nausea and diarrhea may be present. Physical signs of acute PID usually include generalized abdominopelvic pain and tenderness, rebound tenderness, and pain associated with manipulation of the cervix. Complications may be early or late and commonly include abscess formation, recurrent infection, chronic pain, infertility, and ectopic pregnancy. The differential diagnosis and treatment of PID is beyond the scope of this chapter and is discussed elsewhere.[40] It is a serious problem, however, because about one half of affected women are likely to go on to experience chronic pelvic pain, and in about one third, infertility will occur.[32]

Uterine pain

Pain of uterine origin is usually temporally associated with menstruation and is termed primary dysmenorrhea when no obvious cause can be discerned and secondary dysmenorrhea when causality has been established. In primary dysmenorrhea, pain typically begins with the onset of menstruation, builds progressively, and tapers off as flow diminishes. Findings of increased titers of prostaglandins in the endometrium and menstrual discharge in women with dysmenorrhea provides a rationale for the use of prostaglandin synthetase inhibitors (nonsteroidal antiinflammatory drugs, or NSAIDs).[41] Primary dysmenorrhea often responds to a trial of NSAIDs, to which an oral contraceptive may be added to reduce menstrual flow and intrauterine pressure.

Secondary dysmenorrhea is most often due to benign uterine growths, of which leiomyomata and adenomyosis are most common. The presentation is initially with perimenstrual pain and increased flow, which may progress to more constant or frequent pain. Adenomyosis is most common in patients in their late 30s and early 40s and tends to be associated with a tender, boggy, symmetrically enlarged uterus. Leiomyomata or fibroids may occur at any time in the reproductive years but are more common towards the end of the fourth decade. Most are asymptomatic and recede with the onset of menopause. In addition to pain, pressure, and a dragging sensation, uterine fibroids may produce heavy, irregular bleeding that is often sufficient to result in anemia. Sudden, sharp pain may result from degeneration of a fibroid tumor, a process thought to be related to rapid growth and ischemia that is especially common during pregnancy. Hysterectomy may be required for severe, persistent uterine pain, heavy bleeding, or compression of the adjacent ureter; however, it is not routinely considered because of high failure rates of 25% or more, even when surgery is for pain of presumed uterine cause.[7]

Uterine prolapse, even when severe, does not generally result in pain, although patients may complain of pressure or heaviness. Treatment is with suspension or hysterectomy, depending on child-bearing status.

Pelvic congestion

Pelvic venous congestion (so-called "female varicocele") has been proposed as a possible cause for unexplained pain. Venous stasis and reflux in dilated, incompetent ovarian varices has been proposed as a causative factor.[42] Indirect support for this hypothesis is derived from observations of an absence of venodilation and exacerbations of pain with the administration of vasoactive compounds in women with pelvic congestion compared to controls.[43] Further support may be gleaned from observations of reduced pain in patients with venographic evidence of reduced congestion after hormonal treatment.[44] Associated findings in patients diagnosed with pelvic congestion include an increased incidence of uterine enlargement, endometrial thickening, and polycystic ovaries,[45] although it is uncertain how these findings relate to venous changes.

Proponents of venous congestion as a cause for pelvic pain emphasize that this condition may be underdiagnosed because of the inability of standard diagnostic measures to detect venous abnormalities; these proponents endorse venography, ultrasound, and Doppler studies as important adjunctive diagnostic interventions.[7] Both hormonal and surgical therapy (e.g., hysterectomy,[46] ovarian vein ligation, bilateral venous embolization[29]) have been carried out with claims of success.

Pelvic adhesions

Adhesions have been observed in 30% to 50% of laparoscopies performed for unexplained pelvic pain,[48] although their significance is controversial. The most important predictor for the presence of adhesions is prior pelvic surgery.[48] The results of a recent randomized trial suggest that surgical adhesiolysis is beneficial for women with dense, vascularized (Stage IV) adhesions, especially when involving the gastrointestinal tract, but is ineffective for patients with light or moderate adhesions.[49] Another trial of surgical intervention, which stratified subjects based on the presence or absence of a "chronic pain profile" (e.g., vegetative signs of depression, impaired physical function, altered family roles), suggested that a lasting beneficial outcome was more likely in patients lacking cardinal features of the chronic pain patient.

Ovarian remnant syndrome

The ovarian remnant syndrome is an obscure, probably underdiagnosed cause of CPP that should be considered in patients with pain after bilateral oophorectomy. It should not be confused with residual ovary syndrome, another potential cause of CPP, in which a portion of an ovary is deliberately left at surgery to maintain hormonal function in premenopausal patients.[50] A diagnosis of an ovarian remnant may be suggested by elevated levels of follicle-stimulating hormone (FSH) and luteinizing hormone (LH) in premenopausal patients and a palpable or radiologically imaged adnexal mass, but it must ultimately be confirmed histologically. Pain often improves with surgical resection.[51]

Oncologic pelvic pain

Pain is usually not an early sign of pelvic neoplasm but is associated with advanced pelvic cancer in about 75% of cases,[52] presumably because of its tendency to spread locally by direct invasion or metastases to regional lymph nodes.[53] In one series,[47] pain was most commonly referred to the rectum, where it tended to be characterized either as "fullness" or "shooting like a red-hot poker," suggesting an underlying visceral versus neuropathic mechanism. Pain may also be experienced in the low back, hypogastrium, and perineum and may be most troublesome when it is associated with destruction of the sacrum.[54] Pain may be due to pressure or traction on pain-sensitive structures, obstruction of lymphatic and vascular channels, distention of hollow organs, and localized edema, inflammation, and necrosis.

Assessment of pelvic pain caused by neoplasm is often difficult because it is characteristically vague and poorly localized. Primary treatment involves modifying the source of pain with surgery, chemotherapy, and ionizing radiation. When further antitumor therapy is not feasible, pharmacotherapy with combinations of NSAIDs, opioids, and adjuvant analgesics is instituted to raise the pain threshold.[55] Invasive approaches to controlling oncologic pelvic pain are usually considered if dose-limiting side effects arise and cannot be reversed.[56]

NEUROLYTIC BLOCKADE
Sympathetic nerve interruption

Presacral neurectomy and superior hypogastric plexus block. Surgical interruption of the hypogastric plexus (presacral neurectomy) is a well-accepted procedure that has been demonstrated to relieve a variety of painful pelvic conditions, predominantly of nononcologic origin (i.e., dysmenorrhea[57,58]), and which was recently performed with a laparoscope.[27-30] Superior hypogastric plexus block, a percutaneous procedure that is analogous to presacral neurectomy, has recently emerged as an important option in the management of intractable pelvic pain of neoplastic origin.[59,60]

The superior hypogastric plexus (SHGP), also called the presacral nerve, is a retroperitoneal structure located bilaterally at the level of the lower third of the fifth lumbar vertebral body and upper third of the first sacral vertebral body at the sacral promontory and near the bifurcation of the common iliac vessels.[61-63] The SHGP is in continuity with the celiac plexus and lumbar sympathetic chains above. Via the hypogastric nerves, the SHGP innervates the following pelvic viscera: descending colon and rectum, vaginal fundus and bladder, prostate and prostatic urethra, testes, seminal vesicles, uterus, and ovary. In the first published study, SHGP block was shown to reduce pelvic pain by a mean of 70% in patients with cervical, prostate, and testicular cancer, as well as radiation injury. No complications were reported and residual pain of somatic character was amenable to other interventions.

Technique. The patient assumes the prone position with padding placed beneath the pelvis to flatten the lumbar lordosis, and the lumbosacral region is cleansed aseptically. Raise skin wheals 5 to 7 cm bilateral to the midline at the level of the L_4-L_5 interspace (verified fluoroscopically). Insert 7-inch, 22-gauge short-beveled needles with a 30° caudad and 45° mesiad orientation so that their tips are directed toward the anterolateral aspect of the bottom of the L_5 vertebral body. The iliac crest and the transverse process of L_5 are potential barriers to needle passage and may require that the needle be redirected slightly caudad or cephalad. If the body of the L_5 or S_1 vertebra is encountered, redirect the needles until their tips are fluoroscopically observed to lie about 1 cm anterior to the column, at which point a loss resistance or "pop" may be felt, indicating that the needle tip has traversed the psoas muscle and lies in the retroperitoneal space. Inject 3 to 4 ml of water-soluble contrast medium through each needle to confirm that spread is confined to the midline region on anteroposterior views and that a smooth posterior contour corresponding to the psoas fascia is observed on lateral views. After careful aspiration and the use of test doses, institute treatment with either 6 to 8 ml of 0.25% bupivacaine or 6 to 8 ml of 10% aqueous phenol through each needle.

Other techniques. Kent et al reported their results modifying this technique to include transvascular and transdiscal[64] and a single-needle CT-guided approach.[65]

Ganglion impar (ganglion of Walther). This procedure was recently proposed for sympathetically mediated pain involving the perineum and genitals, specifically of a burning or urgent nature.[66] The ganglion impar is a solitary retroperitoneal structure located at the level of the sacrococcygeal junction that marks the termination of the paired paravertebral sympathetic chains. Good results and an absence of complications have been reported for perineal pain in patients with cancer of the cervix, colon, bladder, rectum, and endometrium.

Position the patient in the lateral decubitus position, and raise a skin wheal in the midline at the superior aspect of the intergluteal crease, over the anococcygeal ligament and just above the anus. Remove the stylet from a standard 22-gauge, 3½-inch spinal needle. Then manually bend the needle about 1 inch from its hub to form a 25° to 30° angle to facilitate positioning the needle tip anterior to the concave curvature of the sacrum and coccyx. Insert the needle through the skin wheal with its concavity oriented posteriorly, and, under fluoroscopic guidance, direct it anterior to the coccyx, closely approximating the anterior surface of the bone, until its tip is observed to have reached the sacrococcygeal junction. Verify retroperitoneal location of the needle by observation of the spread of 2 ml of water-soluble contrast medium, which in the lateral view typically assumes a smooth-margined configuration resembling an apostrophe. Inject 4 ml of 1% lidocaine or 0.25% bupivacaine for diagnostic and prognostic purposes, or alternatively, inject 4 to 6 ml of 10% phenol for therapeutic neurolytic blockade.

Lumbar sympathetic block. Although no published studies exist, bilateral lumbar sympathetic block was reported anecdotally to be an effective management tool for some patients with pelvic pain.[35,56] The lumbar sympathetic chain does not directly innervate pelvic structures, but because of its continuity with the superior hypogastric plexus, large volumes of injected solutions probably diffuse caudally. As noted, however, lumbar sympathetic block has yet to be studied systematically for this indication and may be subject to a high rate of failure in patients with large masses or retroperitoneal invasion that restrict the caudal flow of neurolytic solution.

Peripheral nerve block

Peripheral neurolysis[67] cannot be considered an important option, since pain usually emanates from internal pelvic structures that are innervated by sympathetic nerves. Blockade of the intercostal or paravertebral nerves may, however, be considered when pain is referred from the bony pelvis. Adjacent segments may need to be blocked because of the potential for overlapping distribution, and local anesthetic block should ideally precede neurolysis to confirm pain relief and an absence of undesirable neurologic deficit.

Subarachnoid and epidural block

Except in patients with preexisting colostomy and urinary diversions, neuroaxial blocks[68] should be considered only as last resorts, and even then great care must be taken to avoid limb paresis. When the above conditions are met, the subarachnoid route may be preferred to epidural administration because with the former, the spread of the neurolytic substance and consequent effect is more predictable. Epidural injection warrants consideration when pain is bilateral; if available, combined unilateral cordotomy (see below) with contralateral subarachnoid neurolysis may be considered.[69] Subarachnoid phenol saddleblock is a particularly appropriate option for intractable perineal pain in the presence of urinary diversion and colostomy. It is performed with a large bore spinal needle at the L_5-S_1 interspace with the patient seated and inclined backwards 45°.[54]

Intraspinal opioid therapy

Continued administration of opioids intrathecally[70] or epidurally with[71] or without[72,73] dilute concentrations of local anesthetic is an important option for patients with pelvic pain that is refractory to conventional pharmacologic management. Administration can be carried out using a variety of drug-delivery systems ranging from a temporary percutaneous epidural catheter to a totally implanted system.[74] The effectiveness of preimplantation procedure and reversibility of effect makes this an attractive treatment option. Applications for chronic intraspinal opioid therapy are potentially limited, however, by factors that include uneven availability of the technology required for its institution and maintenance, high cost, the development of tolerance, and ineffectiveness in a proportion of patients.

NEUROSURGICAL APPROACHES

A cautious approach to the use of ablative techniques for controlling pelvic pain is dictated by the proximity of the nervous outflow to the pelvis and fibers subserving bladder, bowel, and lower extremity function. Further, many ablative approaches are effective only for unilateral pain, limiting their application for pelvic pain based on its tendency to cross the midline. Percutaneous cordotomy,[75] although effective for truncal pain, induces analgesia that is strictly unilateral. Bilateral cordotomy is infrequently considered because of risks of fatal sleep apnea (i.e., Ondine's curse) and bladder dysfunction. The combination of unilateral subarachnoid neurolysis and unilateral cordotomy has already been mentioned.[54] Midline myelotomy (i.e., commissurotomy)[76] may provide adequate pain relief but requires extensive laminectomy and an experienced team; even then, it is unreliable.

CONCLUSION

Chronic pelvic pain is a common and poorly understood complaint that is the common end point of a heterogeneous group of disorders. Pain is often multifactorial and requires careful multidisciplinary assessment to avoid overtreatment and undertreatment. There is an unfortunate tendency for patients with pain of an undetermined cause to be stigmatized with a purely psychiatric illness. Pilot studies of multidisciplinary pain treatment, particularly inclusive of psychotherapy, medications, and trigger-point therapy, show promising results,[2,3] which, when carefully integrated with more invasive treatments such as laparoscopic surgery and nerve blocks, may be helpful even in the most enigmatic of circumstances. Decision-making for pelvic pain of neoplastic origin is more linear and involves the successive and complementary application of antitumor therapy, medications, and, in selected cases, nerve blocks or spinal opioid therapy.

REFERENCES

1. Howard FM: The role of laparoscopy in chronic pelvic pain: Promise and pitfalls. *Obstet Gynecol Surv* 48:357-387, 1993.
2. Kames LD et al: Effectiveness of an interdisciplinary pain management program for the treatment of chronic pelvic pain. *Pain* 41:41-46, 1990.
3. Slocumb JC: Neurologic factors in chronic pelvic pain. Trigger points and the abdominal pelvic pain syndrome. *Am J Obstet Gynecol* 149:543, 1984.
4. Reiter RC, Gambone JC: Demographic and historic variables in women with idiopathic chronic pelvic pain. *Obstet Gynecol* 75:428-432, 1990.
5. Lee NC et al: Confirmation of the preoperative diagnosis of hysterectomy. *Am J Obstet Gynecol* 150:283-287, 1984.
6. Peterson HB, Hulka JF, Phillips JM: American Association of Gynecologic Laparoscopists' 1988 membership survey on operative laparoscopy. *J Reprod Med* 35:587-589, 1990.
7. Reiter RC, Gambone JC: Nongynecologic somatic pathology in women with chronic pelvic pain and negative laparoscopy. *J Reprod Med* 36:253-259, 1991.
8. Chamberlain A, Laferla J: The gynecologist's approach to chronic pelvic pain. In Burrows GD, Elton D, Stanley GV, editors: *Handbook of Chronic Pain Management, vol 33.* Amsterdam, Elsevier, 1987.
9. Stovall TG, Ling FW, Crawford DA: Hysterectomy for chronic pelvic pain of presumed uterine etiology. *Obstet Gynecol* 75:676-679, 1990.
10. Hodgson TJ et al: Case report: The ultrasound and Doppler appearances of pelvic varices. *Clin Radiol* 44(3):208-209, 1991.
11. Marana R et al: Evaluation of the correlation between endometriosis extent, age of the patients and associated symptomatology. *Acta Eur Fertil* 22:209-212, 1991.
12. Kresch AJ et al: Laparoscopy in 100 women with chronic pelvic pain. *Am J Obstet Gynecol* 64:672-674, 1984.
13. Stout AL et al: Relationship of laparoscopic findings to self-report of pelvic pain. *Am J Obstet Gynecol* 164:73-79, 1991.
14. Rapkin AJ et al: History of physical and sexual abuse in women with chronic pelvic pain. *Obstet Gynecol* 76:92-96, 1990.
15. Milano R: Pelvic pain: problems in diagnosis and treatment. In Bond MR, Charlton JE, Woolf CJ, editors: *Proceedings of the VI World Congress on Pain.* Amsterdam, Elsevier, 1991.
16. Walker E et al: Relationship of chronic pelvic pain to psychiatric diagnoses and childhood sexual abuse. *Am J Psychiatry* 145:75-80, 1988.
17. Toomey TC et al: Relationship of sexual and physical abuse to pain and psychological assessment variables in chronic pelvic pain patients. *Pain* 53:105-109, 1993.
18. Walker EA et al: Medical and psychiatric symptoms in women with childhood sexual abuse. *Psychosom Med* 54:658-664, 1992.
19. Drossman DA et al: Sexual and physical abuse in women with functional or organic gastrointestinal disorders. *Ann Intern Med* 113:828-833, 1990.
20. Abiodun OA, Adetoro OO, Ogunbode OO: Psychiatric morbidity in a gynaecology clinic in Nigeria. *J Psychosom Res* 36:485-490, 1992.
21. Bonica JJ: General considerations of pain in the pelvis and perineum. In Bonica JJ, editor: *Management of Pain,* ed 2. Philadelphia, Lea & Febiger, 1990.
22. Goldstein DP et al: Laparoscopy in the diagnosis and management of pelvic pain in adolescents. *J Reprod Med* 24:251, 1980.
23. Raj PP: Local anesthetic blockade. In Patt RB, editor: *Cancer Pain.* Philadelphia, JB Lippincott, 1993.
24. Thiele GH: Coccygodynia and pain in the superior gluteal region. *JAMA* 109:1271-1275, 1937.
25. Bennett RM: Fibromylagia. *JAMA* 257:2802-2803, 1987.
26. Duncan CH, Taylor MC: A psychosomatic study of pelvic congestion. *Am J Obstet Gynecol* 64:1-1, 1952.
27. McGivney JQ, Cleveland BR: The levator syndrome and its treatment. *South Med J* 58:505-510, 1965.
28. Damewood MD: Pathophysiology and management of endometriosis. *J Fam Pract* 37:68-75, 1993.
29. Johnson JG: Gynecologic pain: Locating its source. *Pain Management* 143-152, May/Jun 1990.
30. Guzinski GM, Bonica JJ, McDonald JS: Gynecologic pain. In Bonica JJ, editor: *Management of Pain,* ed 2. Philadelphia, Lea & Febiger, 1990.
31. Vercellini P, Bocciolone L, Crosignani PG: Is mild endometriosis always a disease? *Hum Reprod* 7:627-629, 1992.
32. Donnez J, Nisolle M: CO$_2$ laser laparoscopic surgery: Adhesiolysis, salpingostomy, laser uterine nerve ablation and tubal pregnancy. *Baillieres Clin Obstet Gynaecol* 3:525-543, 1989.
33. Perez JJ: Laparoscopic presacral neurectomy. Results of the first 25 cases. *J Reprod Med* 35:625-630, 1990.
34. Fliegner JR, Umstad MP: Presacral neurectomy: A reappraisal. *Aust N Z J Obstet Gynaecol* 31:76-79, 1991.
35. Nezhat C, Nezhat F: A simplified method of laparoscopic presacral neurectomy for the treatment of central pelvic pain due to endometriosis. *Br J Obstet Gynaecol* 99:659-663, 1992.
36. Candiani GB et al: Presacral neurectomy for the treatment of pelvic pain associated with endometriosis: A controlled study. *Am J Obstet Gynecol* 167:100-103, 1992.
37. Ivey JL: Laparoscopic uterine suspension as an adjunctive procedure at the time of laser laparoscopy for the treatment of endometriosis. *J Reprod Med* 37:757-765, 1992.
38. Westrom L: Effect of acute pelvic inflammatory disease on fertility. *Am J Obstet Gynecol* 121:707, 1975.
39. Stacey CM et al: A longitudinal study of pelvic inflammatory disease. *Br J Obstet Gynaecol* 99:994-999, 1992.
40. Ault KA, Faro S: Pelvic inflammatory disease: Current diagnostic criteria and treatment guidelines. *Postgrad Med* 93:85-91, 1993.
41. Picles VR et al: Prostaglandins in endometrium and menstrual flow from normal and dysmenorrheic subjects. *Br J Obstet Gynaecol* 72:185, 1965.
42. Edwards RD et al: Case report: Pelvic pain syndrome—successful treatment of a case by ovarian vein embolization. *Clin Radiol* 47:429-431, 1993.
43. Stones RW, Thomas DC, Beard RW: Suprasensitivity to calcitonin gene-related peptide but not vasoactive intestinal peptide in women with chronic pelvic pain. *Clin Auton Res* 2:343-348, 1992.
44. Reginald PW et al: Medroxyprogesterone acetate in the treatment of pelvic pain due to venous congestion. *Br J Obstet Gynaecol* 96:1148-1152, 1989.
45. Adams J et al: Uterine size and endometrial thickness and the significance of cystic ovaries in women with pelvic pain due to congestion. *Br J Obstet Gynaecol* 97:583-587, 1990.

46. Beard RW et al: Bilateral oophorectomy and hysterectomy in the treatment of intractable pelvic pain associated with pelvic congestion. *Br J Obstet Gynaecol* 98:988-992, 1991.

47. Steege JF, Stout: Resolution of chronic pelvic pain after laparoscopic lysis of adhesions. *Am J Obstet Gynecol* 165:278-283, 1991.

48. Stovall TG, Elder RF, Ling FW: Predictors of pelvic adhesions. *J Reprod Med* 34:345-348, 1989.

49. Peters AA et al: A randomized clinical trial on the benefit of adhesiolysis in patients with intraperitoneal adhesions and chronic pelvic pain. *Br J Obstet Gynaecol* 99:59-62, 1992.

50. Webb MJ: Ovarian remnant syndrome. *Aust N Z J Obstet Gynaecol* 29:433-435, 1989.

51. Pettit PD, Lee RA: Ovarian remnant syndrome: diagnostic dilemma and surgical challenge. *Obstet Gynecol* 71:580-583, 1988.

52. Bonica JJ: Cancer pain. In Bonica JJ, editor: *Management of Pain,* ed 2. Philadelphia, Lea & Febiger, 1990.

53. Baines M: Cancer pain. In Wall PD, Melzack R, editors: *Textbook of Pain,* ed 2. Edinburgh, Churchill Livingstone, 1989.

54. Patt RB, Payne R: Unpublished data, 1993.

55. World Health Organization: *Cancer Pain Relief.* Geneva, WHO, 1986.

56. Patt RB, Jain S: Therapeutic decision making for invasive procedures. In Patt RB, editor: *Cancer Pain.* Philadelphia, JB Lippincott, 1993.

57. Lee RB et al: Presacral neurotomy for chronic pelvic pain. *Obstet Gynecol* 68:517-521, 1986.

58. Frier A: Pelvic neurectomy in gynecology. *Obstet Gynecol* 25:48, 1965.

59. Plancarte R et al: Superior hypogastric plexus block for pelvic cancer pain. *Anesthesiology* 73:236, 1990.

60. Kent E, de Leon-Cassasola OA, Lema M: Neurolytic superior hypogastric plexus block for cancer related pelvic pain. *Reg Anesth* 17(suppl):19, 1992.

61. Pitkin G: Southworth JL, Hingson RA, Pitkin WM, editors: *Conduction Anesthesia,* ed 2. Philadelphia, JB Lippincott, 1953.

62. Snell RS, Katz J: *Clinical Anatomy for Anesthesiologists.* Norwalk, Conn, Appleton & Lange, 1988.

63. Brass A: Anatomy and physiology: Autonomic nerves and ganglia in pelvis. In Netter FH, editor: *The Ciba Collection of Medical Illustrations, vol 1: Nervous System.* USA Ciba Pharmaceutical Co, 1983.

64. Plancarte R, Lema M, Patt RB: unpublished data, 1993.

65. Waldman SD, Wislon WL, Kreps RD: Superior hypogastric plexus block using a single needle and computed tomography guidance: Description of a modified technique. *Reg Anesth* 16:286-7, 1991.

66. Plancarte R et al: Presacral blockade of the ganglion of Walther (ganglion impar). *Anesthesiology* 73:A751, 1990.

67. Patt RB: Peripheral neurolysis and the management of cancer pain. *Pain Digest* 2:30-42, 1992.

68. Swerdlow M: Neurolytic blocks of the neuroaxis. In Patt RB, editor: *Cancer Pain.* Philadelphia, JB Lippincott, 1993.

69. Ischia S, Luzzani A: Subarachnoid neurolytic block (L5-S1) and unilateral percutaneous cervical cordotomy in the treatment of pain secondary to pelvic malignant disease. *Pain* 20:139, 1984.

70. Wang JK: Intrathecal morphine for intractable pain secondary to pelvic cancer of pelvic organs. *Pain* 21:99, 1985.

71. Du Pen S et al: Chronic epidural bupivacaine-opioid infusion in intractable cancer pain. *Pain* 49:293-300, 1992.

72. Hamar O et al: Epidural morphine analgesia by means of a subcutaneously tunneled catheter in patients with gynecologic cancer. *Anesth Analg* 65:531-532, 1986.

73. Shaves M et al: Indwelling epidural catheters for pain control in gynecologic cancer patients. *Obstet Gynecol* 77:642-644, 1991.

74. Waldman SD et al: Intraspinal opioid therapy. In Patt RB, editor: *Cancer Pain.* Philadelphia, JB Lippincott, 1993.

75. Patt RB: Neurosurgical intervention for chronic pain problems. In Frost EAM, editor: *Clinical Anesthesia in Neurosurgery.* Boston, Butterworth-Heinemann, 1991.

76. Patt RB: Neurosurgical interventions for chronic pain problems. *Anesth Clin NA* 5:609-638, 1987.

QUESTIONS: PELVIC PAIN

1. Chronic pelvic pain without obvious pathology is found in what percentage of patients with a history of physical or sexual abuse?
   A. 10%
   B. 25%
   C. 50%
   D. 80%
2. Laparoscopy detects the presence of all of the following conditions EXCEPT:
   A. Endometriosis
   B. Ovarian cyst
   C. Uterine malformations
   D. Pelvic venous congestion
   For question 3, choose from the following:
   A. 1, 2, and 3
   B. 1 and 3
   C. 2 and 4
   D. 4
   E. All of the above
3. Which of the following is (are) the most common causative organism(s) implicated in the genesis of pelvic inflammatory disease?
   1. *Neisseria gonorrhoea*
   2. *Staphylococcus epidermitis*
   3. *Chlamydia trachomatis*
   4. *Herpes simplex*

4. Sudden, sharp abdominal pain in a 44-year-old patient with a history of abnormal bleeding is most likely to be due to:
   A. Uterine prolapse
   B. Ovarian remnant syndrome
   C. Degeneration of a fibroid tumor
   D. Ovarian cancer
5. A terminal patient is experiencing intractable cancer pain that is well localized to one side of the pelvis. Which of the following invasive procedures would be most appropriate for treating the pain?
   1. Percutaneous cordotomy
   2. Midline myelotomy
   3. Epidural block
   4. Subarachnoid phenol saddle block

ANSWERS

1. C
2. D
3. B
4. C
5. A

B. NEUROPATHIC PAIN SYNDROMES

45 Central Nervous System Pain

Christopher M. Loar

Central pain is produced by lesions of the central nervous system (CNS); however, not all CNS lesions produce a central pain syndrome. Lesions can occur in the spinal cord, brainstem, and brain. Most cases of central pain are associated with spinal cord lesions.[1] Central pain syndromes often occur with complete or partial lesions of the somatosensory pathways, especially the spinothalamic tract, which carries pain and temperature sense. When central pain occurs with a lesion in the spinothalamic tract, it may be associated with all or part of the affected sensory deficit. Central pain states, however, have been observed in patients without clinically detectable somatosensory impairment.[2]

The clinical features of central pain are similar whether the lesion is located in the spinal cord, brainstem, or brain. There are generally two types of central pain: spontaneous pain and hyperesthesia. Spontaneous pain is constant but may vary in intensity over time. It may be exacerbated by minor activity, changes in the weather, or emotional stress. The pain is often described as the sensation of tingling, burning, numbness, twisting, or pressing. A patient may even complain of bizarre symptoms such as the sensation of flesh being ripped or torn.[2]

Hyperesthesia occurs when sensory stimuli in an area of partial sensory deficit produce discomfort. The sensation is often poorly localized and unpleasant. There are two types of hyperesthesia: hyperpathia and allodynia. Hyperpathia is intense discomfort produced by mild or moderately painful stimuli, whereas allodynia is an unpleasant sensation produced by a normally nonpainful stimulus. Hyperesthetic sensations may occur in volleys or paroxysms that can be excruciating. Often the sensations will appear sometime after the eliciting stimulus, and they may last much longer than the original stimulus.[1,2]

There have been many proposed theories to explain central pain. Of the many different theories that have been advanced, three theories are more accepted. One theory is that central pain is the result of an abnormal firing pattern of sensory neurons that have lost their sensory input or have become deafferented. Another theory proposes that it is the result of hyperactivity of reticulothalamic pathways that have lost their sensory afferent input. A third common theory is the theory of denervation neuronal hypersensitivity.[2,3] This theory hypothesizes that spinothalamic neurons lose their afferent input and become oversensitive, causing overstimulation of other as yet unidentified neurons that produce pain.

SPINAL-CORD LESIONS

Spinal-cord lesions are responsible for most central pain states. The approximate percentage of spinal-cord lesions that produce central pain is debated and may vary from 7.5% to 40.0%.[1,4] Lesions at any level and of varying pathology can produce a central pain state. Pain is usually produced in an area of sensory impairment resulting from interruption of the spinothalamic tract.

There are numerous types of pathology that may produce a spinal-cord lesion and cause central pain. Traumatic lesions are the most frequent cause; however, disk disease and vascular disease, including infarction and arteriovenous malformations (AVMs), have been reported to cause central pain of spinal-cord origin.[2]

In evaluating central pain, obtain a magnetic resonance imaging study of the affected level of the spinal cord to exclude posttraumatic syringomyelia. If undetected, this process may advance and produce new neurologic deficits and pain.

The treatment of central pain of spinal-cord origin is often frustrating and difficult. There is, unfortunately, no totally effective treatment. At best, treatment focuses on lessening the discomfort. Of primary importance is the prevention and treatment of skin breakdown and skin infections; prevention and treatment of problems associated with loss of bowel and bladder control; and promotion of proper nutrition. Pay particular attention to the patient's psychologic state because this may amplify and exacerbate the discomfort.[2,4,6]

BRAIN AND BRAINSTEM LESIONS

Brain and brainstem lesions may produce central pain states. They may be produced by many different pathologies and at any level of the brain or brainstem. Central pain states may occur with lesions that produce alteration in sensory function, especially in those areas where there has been spinothalamic sensory loss.

Characteristics of central pain from brain and brainstem lesions are the same as pain from spinal-cord lesions. There is both a spontaneous pain and a hyperpathic pain that may affect all or part of the distribution of sensory loss. The sensory signs referable to lesions of the ipsilateral trigeminothalamic tract and the spinothalamic tract are most frequently associated with the development of central pain.

Brainstem lesions

Most brainstem lesions that produce pain are vascular in origin. The most common vascular cause of central pain is Wallenberg's syndrome, also called the *lateral medullary syndrome*.[5,7] The neurologic presentation in this syndrome may be variable, but the syndrome characteristically presents with crossed sensory findings. There is ipsilateral facial sensory loss and contralateral body impairment of pain and temperature sense. Other neurologic signs include an ipsilateral loss of taste (cranial nerves IX, X) and a Horner's syndrome (i.e., ptosis, miosis, or anhidrosis). There can also be ipsilateral diminished gag reflex with weakness of the palate resulting in dysphagia and vocal cord weakness producing hoarseness (cranial nerves IX, X). A lesion of the inferior cerebellar peduncle produces ipsilateral clumsiness and ataxia. This feature sometimes gives the false impression of a hemiparesis.

Other lesions besides a Wallenberg's syndrome may cause brainstem origin central pain, including syringobulbia or hematobulbia, neoplasms in the brainstem, and tuberculomas in the pontine region. Occasionally, surgically induced lesions performed for the relief of chronic pain in other areas of the nervous system may themselves produce central pain. Multiple sclerosis (MS) lesions may also cause central pain.[2,5] The symptoms reported are numbness, tingling, or prickly sensations. Lhermitte described an uncomfortable sensation frequently observed in MS with lesions in the brainstem and spinal cord. The discomfort, termed *Lhermitte's sign,* resembles an electric shock to all four extremities that is produced by flexion of the neck.[8] Multiple sclerosis may also cause trigeminal neuralgia, a different form of pain in which the anatomic lesion has been found to be at the dorsal-root entry zone of the trigeminal nerve.

Brain lesions

One of the first central pain syndromes recognized was the thalamic pain syndrome, also referred to as *Dejerine-Roussy syndrome*.[8] Dejerine and Roussy described stroke patients with a very mild hemiplegia, a hemibody analgesia or hypalgesia, hemiataxia, and choreoathetosis contralateral to the infarct. These patients experienced delayed onset of a central pain state several weeks or months after the stroke. Patients developed spontaneous intractable pain and hypesthesia in all or part of the affected sensory distribution.[2,9] Since then the thalamic pain syndrome has been considered the typical example of a central pain syndrome.

There are many lesions in the thalamus that may produce central pain. Among these, infarctions are the most common. It is reported that very few strokes develop central pain, perhaps approaching a frequency of 1:1500.[10] Other lesions in the thalamus that may cause central pain include arteriovenous malformations, neoplasms, abscesses, MS plaques, traumatic injury, nonspecific degenerations, and certain surgical lesions. There is some debate as to the area of the thalamus most responsible for central pain; however, there is the greatest acceptance for the somatosensory relay nuclei: ventral posterior medial and ventral posterior lateral.[2,11,12]

The thalamic pain syndrome may also be mimicked by nonthalamic lesions. Since the development of neuroimaging techniques, many patients with central pain have been studied. The results show that there are a wide variety of brain lesions that may produce central pain. Less than half of these lesions appeared to involve the thalamus.[13,14] Cortical lesions that mimic thalamic pain syndrome often involve the parietal cortex.[2,15] Causes of these lesions include infarct, neoplasm, and head trauma.

MEDICAL TREATMENT OF CENTRAL PAIN

Central pain is partially relieved by barbiturates but not by opiates. Anticonvulsants such as diphenylhydantoin, carbamazepine, and clonazepam may be effective. Amitriptyline in combination with anticonvulsants may also have some effect. Barbiturates, anticonvulsants, and antidepressants are generally started at low doses and gradually titrated to symptom relief. Unfortunately, the medications may reach sedative doses before pain relief is noticed.[2,5,16] Many pain physicians feel that these drugs are not clinically useful in a large percentage of patients with central pain.[16]

Mexiletine was recently studied in patients with thalamic pain syndrome[17] and was found to be effective in 8 out of 9 patients. The recommended dose is 10 mg/kg/day in two or three divided doses. Side effects are not significant. When plasma concentrations are greater than 2 μg/ml, side effects such as nausea, vomiting, tremor, dizziness, and blurred vision can occur. Do not use mexiletine in patients with intracardiac conduction disease.[18]

The use of anesthetic nerve blocks is of considerable debate. Some authors reported pain relief with repeated local anesthetic blocks.[2,19] Others have noted that peripheral nerve blocks and sympathetic nerve blocks are of limited value.

SURGICAL TREATMENT OF CENTRAL PAIN

There are two types of surgical therapy: those directed at interrupting the pain pathways and those directed at modulating sensory input.

Surgical procedures that interrupt pain pathways include rhizotomy (nerve root section), cordotomy (division of spinal-cord tracts), cordectomy (excision of spinal cord), dorsal-root entry zone procedures (producing dorsal-root entry zone lesions by surgical section of Lissauer's tract), and stereotactic surgery.[2,5,20] Unfortunately, these procedures rarely produce a long-lasting, pain-free state. They may produce some abatement of pain, but they do so by creating additional permanent neurologic lesions. These new lesions may eventually lead to the return of pain, which can be even more intense. The results of these surgical procedures were reviewed by Pagni, who concluded, "very few really persistent and complete successes have been obtained with stereotactic operations in both specific and nonspecific pain pathways at thalamic or mesencephalic levels in central pain."[5] Pagni further stated, "In cases of pain of non-malignant origin [stereotactic surgery] is still a unique way to relieve, at least temporarily, the atrocious suffering of pain due to CNS lesions after every other procedure has failed."[21]

Neuromodulation techniques are more hopeful than surgical procedures that interrupt pain pathways. The technique involves chronic electrical stimulation of the dorsal columns or the medial lemniscal pathway, both of which carry light touch, joint position sense, and vibration sensation. The exact mechanism by which chronic electrical stimulation suppresses central pain and induces paresthesias in the painful body part is unknown. Before deciding to proceed with chronic neurostimulation, a period of test stimulation is often performed and the clinical results observed.

Brain stimulation in the medial lemniscal pathway produced good results in the hands of some authors,[22-28] but it was not supported by other authors.[29,30] The risks of the procedure also appear to be considerable, with approximately 10% infection rate and 10% of patients suffering from allergic or foreign-body reaction.[31]

REFERENCES

1. White JC, Sweet WH: *Pain and the Neurosurgeon. A Forty-year Experience.* Springfield, Ill, Charles C Thomas, 1969.
2. Tasker RR: Pain resulting from central nervous system pathology (central pain). In Bonica JJ, editor: *Pain.* New York, Raven Press, 1980.
3. DeJong RH: Central pain mechanisms. *JAMA* 239:2784, 1978.
4. Richardson RR, Meyer PR, Cerullo LJ: Neurostimulation in the modulation of intractable paraplegic and traumatic neuroma pains. *Pain* 8:76, 1980.
5. Pagni CA: Central pain due to spinal cord and brainstem damage. In Wall PD, Melzack R, editors: *Textbook of Pain.* Edinburgh, Churchill Livingstone, 1984.
6. Likavec MJ: Pain secondary to paraplegia or quadriplegia. In Raj PP, editor: *Practical Management of Pain.* St Louis, Mosby, 1986.
7. Cassinari V, Pagni CA: *Central Pain: A Neurosurgical Survey.* Cambridge, Mass, Harvard University Press, 1969.
8. Lhermitte J, Levy G, Nicolas M: Les sensations de dechanges electriques, symptome precoce de la scleroser en plaque. Clinique et Pathogenie. *Presse Medicale* 39:610, 1927.
9. Dejerine J, Roussy G: La syndrome thalamique. *Rev Neurol* 12:521, 1906.
10. Gildenberg PL: Stereotactic treatment of head and neck pain. *Res Clin Stud Headache* 5:102, 1978.
11. Walker AE: Normal and pathological physiology of the thalamus. In Schaltenbrand G, Walker AE, editors: *Stereotaxy of the Human Brain.* Stuttgart, Germany, Thieme Verlag, 1982.
12. Walker AE: The anatomical basis of the thalamic syndrome. *Journal Belge de Neurologie et de Psychiatrie* 38:69, 1938.
13. Agnew DC et al: Thalamic pain. In Bonica JJ, Lindblom U, Iggo A, editors: *Advances in Pain Research and Therapy, vol 5.* New York, Raven Press, 1983.
14. Bowsher D, Lahuerta J, Brock L: Twelve cases of central pain, only three with thalamic lesions. *Pain* (suppl 2):S83, 1984.
15. Schmahmann JP, Leifer D: Parietal pseudothalamic pain syndrome: Clinical features and anatomic correlates. *Arch Neurol* 49:1032, 1992.
16. Likavec MJ: Central pain. In Raj PP, editor: *Practical Management of Pain.* St Louis, Mosby, 1986.
17. Awerbuch GI, Sandyk R: Mexiletine for thalamic pain syndrome. *Int J Neurosci* 55:129, 1990.
18. Ackerman WE et al: The management of oral mexiletine and intravenous lidocaine to treat chronic painful symmetrical distal diabetic neuropathy. *Kentucky Medical Association Journal* 89:500, 1991.
19. Livingston WK: *Pain Mechanisms: A Physiologic Interpretation of Causalgia and its Related States,* ed 2. New York, Plenum Press, 1976.
20. Bullitt E, Friedman A: Neurosurgical procedures. In Raj PP, editor: *Practical Management of Pain.* St Louis, Mosby, 1986.
21. Pagni CA: Place of stereotactic technique in surgery for pain. In Bonica JJ, editor: *Advances in Neurology, vol 4.* New York, Raven Press, 1974.
22. Hosobuchi Y, Adams JE, Rutkin B: Chronic thalamic and internal capsule stimulation for the control of central pain. *Surg Neurol* 4:91, 1975.
23. Hosobuchi Y: The current status of analgesic brain stimulation. *Acta Neurochir Suppl* 30:129, 1980.
24. Hosobuchi Y, Adams JE, Fields HL: Chronic thalamic and internal capsular stimulation for the control of facial anesthesia dolorosa and the dysesthesia of thalamic syndrome. In Bonica JJ, editor: *Advances in Neurology, vol 4.* New York, Raven Press, 1974.
25. Mundinger F, Neumueller H: Programmed stimulation for control of chronic pain and motor disease. *Applied Neurophysiology* 45:102, 1982.
26. Mundinger F, Salomao JF: Deep brain stimulation in mesencephalic lemniscus medialis for chronic pain. *Acta Neurochir Suppl* 30:245, 1980.
27. Siegfried J, Demierre B: Thalamic electrostimulation in the treatment of thalamic pain syndrome. *Pain* (suppl 2):S116, 1984.
28. Levy RM, Lamb S, Adams JE: Deep brain stimulation for chronic pain: Long-term follow up in 145 patients from 1972-1984. *Pain* (suppl 2):S115, 1984.
29. Mazars G, Merienne L, Cioloca C: Traitment de certains types de douleurs par les stimulateurs thalamiques implantables. *Neurochirurgie* 20:117, 1974.
30. Turnbull IM: Brain stimulation. In Wall PD, Melzack R, editors: *Textbook of Pain.* Edinburgh, Churchill Livingstone, 1984.
31. Adams JE: Technique and technical problems associated with implantation of neuroaugmentative devices. *Applied Neurophysiology* 40:111, 1977-1978.

QUESTIONS: CENTRAL NERVOUS SYSTEM PAIN

1. Central pain states are often associated with lesions of which central nervous system pathways?
   A. Corticospinal tracts
   B. Dorsal columns—medial lemniscal pathways
   C. Reticulospinal tracts
   D. Spinothalamic tracts
2. Brain and brain stem lesions that produce central pain are most commonly the result of:
   A. Vascular incidents
   B. Trauma
   C. Multiple sclerosis
   D. Neoplasm
3. Anatomical structures believed to be involved in thalamic pain syndrome include:
   A. VL and VA
   B. VPL and VPM
   C. VNA and VP
   D. Dorsomedial and pulvinar
4. Which of the following surgical techniques is most appropriate for treatment of central pain?
   A. Pain pathway destruction and neuromodulation
   B. Pain pathway destruction, neuromodulation, and neuroattenuation
   C. Neuromodulation and neuroattenuation
   D. Cryotherapy
   For question 5, choose from the following:
   A. 1, 2, and 3
   B. 1 and 3
   C. 2 and 4
   D. 4
   E. All of the above

5. Which of the following statement(s) is (are) true of symptoms of allodynia present in central pain?
   1. The appearance of symptoms may be delayed after the introduction of the eliciting stimulus.
   2. The symptoms may be produced by nonpainful stimuli.
   3. The symptoms may be excruciating.
   4. The symptoms can be produced by mild stimuli.

ANSWERS

1. D
2. A
3. B
4. A
5. E

46 Peripheral Nervous System Pain

Christopher M. Loar

Peripheral nervous system pain results from peripheral nerve lesions. The peripheral nervous system is composed of the cranial nerves and spinal nerves that originate from the cervical, thoracic, lumbar, and sacral nerves. The peripheral nervous system is outside of the central nervous system (CNS).

SPINAL AND PERIPHERAL NERVE PAIN

Pain may be produced by many different types of lesions of the peripheral nervous system. Peripheral nerve pain may occur because of reflex sympathetic dystrophy or causalgia, herpes zoster, polyneuropathy, radiculopathy, plexopathy, and multiple entrapment neuropathies. Many of these topics are discussed elsewhere in this book.

Polyneuropathy

Polyneuropathy, or peripheral neuropathy, is a common clinical syndrome and cause of peripheral nerve pain. It is clinically characterized by ascending and symmetric paresthesia and impairment of sensation distally more than proximally. It results in a common presentation of sensory and motor abnormalities termed *stocking/glove dysesthesia.* Polyneuropathies may present with primary sensory and primary motor abnormalities. Distally, at the level of hands and feet, sensation may be impaired but may be normal proximally. A flaccid weakness and wasting of muscle bulk is also a common occurrence in polyneuropathy, as well as the loss of distal muscle stretch reflexes.[1,2]

The pathophysiology of peripheral neuropathy relates to the two major components of the peripheral nerve: the axon and the myelin sheath. In diseases where the axon is primarily affected, there is axonal degeneration but perhaps intact myelin sheaths in the nerve. The myelin sheath may also be the primary site of pathology, and there may be a demyelination of the nerve axon. Demyelinating lesions can occur at multiple sites along the individual nerve in a pattern that is termed *segmental demyelination.* The majority of peripheral neuropathies can be classified into demyelinating, axonal, or a mixed pattern of both axonal and demyelinating abnormalities.[1,2]

Although the patient with peripheral neuropathy has a characteristic clinical appearance of stocking/glove distribution of motor and sensory abnormalities, a similar appearance may also occur in some forms of myelopathy where the lesion is in the spinal cord and affecting the posterior-column sensory tracts. These individuals may have preserved or brisk deep-tendon reflexes distally, as well as the presence of Babinski's signs. These findings may be a vital clinical clue to distinguish myelopathy from peripheral neuropathy. Cauda equina lesions may mimic a peripheral neuropathy because the distal lower extremities are involved with loss of reflexes, atrophy, and both sensory and motor abnormalities. The individual with a cauda equina lesion commonly has loss of rectal and urinary sphincter control. This sphincter involvement is rare in peripheral neuropathy. Peripheral vascular insufficiency is also in the differential diagnosis of peripheral neuropathy. It may cause paresthesias in the lower extremities but otherwise does not affect the deep-tendon reflexes or lower-extremity muscle strength.

The individual with polyneuropathy or peripheral neuropathy may have a wide variety of underlying causes. History, physical examination, and workup may be important in determining the underlying causes.

There are several important historical facts to be determined in the evaluation of the peripheral neuropathy patient. It is important to determine the tempo of the illness: Is the disorder rapidly progressive over days or weeks, or is it progressive over months to years? Family history, the presence of underlying systemic illnesses, deficiency states, toxin exposure, and drug use are also important.

On physical examination, peripheral neuropathy may become evident. There are typically absent distal deep-tendon reflexes. Sensory and motor abnormalities are distributed in a gradient from proximal to distal in the lower extremities. There may be atrophy or loss of muscle bulk.

Perform electromyographic and nerve-conduction studies as the next diagnostic review; they may confirm the presence of a peripheral neuropathy. Electromyography may also yield information that may subcategorize the type of neuropathy into either axonal, demyelinating, or mixed pattern.

Perform laboratory studies after the electromyographic examination to determine the cause of the neuropathy. Peripheral neuropathy evaluations can be costly and extensive because of the multiple possibilities in the differential. For this reason it is vital to obtain neurologic consultation.

The differential diagnosis of peripheral neuropathies includes many possibilities. The pain physician who sees patients with chronic painful symmetric symptoms will likely see peripheral neuropathy resulting from diabetes mellitus, chronic alcoholism, nutritional deficiencies, amyloidosis, paraneoplastic conditions, uremia, and arsenic ingestion. Despite a thorough investigation into the cause of peripheral neuropathy, the cause often remains unknown in 25% to 50% of cases.[2]

In situations where the cause of the peripheral neuropathy can be determined, treatment of the underlying condition supersedes the treatment of the discomfort. In those situations where the cause of the peripheral neuropathy cannot be determined, treatment of the painful state is primarily symptomatic.

Diabetic peripheral neuropathy. Diabetes mellitus may cause multiple peripheral nerve disorders. There may be mononeuropathies of the cranial nerves and a proximal amyotrophy affecting the femoral and lumbar roots, with pain and symmetric weakness of the proximal lower limb. Peripheral neuropathy or polyneuropathy is the most common peripheral nerve disease with longstanding diabetes mellitus.

Diabetic peripheral neuropathy is symmetric and involves both the sensory and motor nerves. Diabetic peripheral neuropathy can be quite disabling. The symptoms are usually gradually progressive and may begin with mild numbness, tingling, or a burning sensation in the feet. The discomfort progresses in a proximal direction over months or years, and pain may occur later in the course of the disease. Patients may describe hypersensitivity to touch of the feet or ankles. In other individuals the feet may have lost sensibility; for this reason, diabetic patients are subject to injury of the feet and development of poorly healing ulcerative lesions.[3]

The pain of diabetic neuropathy has been treated with various medications including carbamazepine and phenytoin,[3] as well as antidepressants such as amitriptyline and desipramine.[4] The pain of diabetic neuropathy is relieved with equal efficacy by desipramine and amitriptyline. The use of fluphenazine with amitriptyline was not proven effective in a double-blind, placebo-controlled, crossover study using a small group of patients.[5]

There have been several reports of promising effects by mexiletine for the treatment of painful diabetic neuropathy. The dosage regimen appears to range from 5 to 10 mg/kg/day in two or three divided doses. However, in some studies pain relief was achieved at very low dosages, as low as 75 mg/day.[6-9] The response to oral mexiletine may be anticipated by the response to intravenous (IV) lidocaine. Patients treated with IV lidocaine may notice temporary relief of discomfort with relatively low infusion rates of 3 mg/kg/min and loading doses of 65 mg. If those patients are placed on oral mexiletine, they may continue to have relief of discomfort.[6] Side effects of mexiletine appear to be few, especially when low dosages are used. When mexiletine serum concentrations are greater than 2 μg/ml, side effects such as nausea, vomiting, tremor, dizziness, or blurred vision may occur. The physician should be cautious of using mexiletine in patients with intracardiac conduction disease.[6,9]

Results of a multicenter, controlled trial suggest that topical capsaicin cream 0.075% may produce more relief of the pain of diabetic neuropathy than placebo.[10] Approximately 75% of patients obtained relief with the topical ointment, compared with 45% of placebo patients; and a significant difference was noted between placebo and study patients within 4 weeks of treatment. Significant side effects included a burning sensation at the application site, particularly when more than a thin film was applied to the skin.[10]

Alcoholic neuropathy. Alcoholic neuropathy is probably the second most common type of peripheral neuropathy in North America. It is estimated that about 20% of chronic alcoholics have peripheral neuropathy. Clinical manifestations consist of a mixed sensory and motor disorder that involves primarily the distal segments of the lower extremities. In mild cases there may be sensory symptoms only, with complaints of burning feet or painful paresthesias. With more advanced cases, motor weakness is present. In this condition the legs are always more affected than the arms. In advanced cases the arms may also become involved. Sensory ataxia may occur as a result of the loss of joint position sense in advance cases. Cerebellar ataxia resulting from cerebellar degeneration may occur simultaneously with sensory ataxia in chronic alcoholics. The neuropathy develops slowly with continued alcohol abuse, and if abstinence is achieved, recovery is generally slow.

The pathologic process is primarily axonal degeneration of the peripheral nerve. The disorder is thought to be due to deficiency of thiamine and other B vitamins. The deficiency state may be due to inadequate dietary intake and decreased absorption of vitamins, as well as greater metabolic need for thiamine. There is also indication that alcohol itself may exert a direct toxic effect on the peripheral nerve.[2]

Treatment of these individuals consists primarily of abstinence from alcohol and nutritional supplements containing thiamine and vitamin B complex. Symptomatic treatment includes the use of carbamazepine, tricyclic antidepressants, and common analgesics.[1,2]

Uremic neuropathy. Uremic neuropathy is a complication of chronic renal failure that may be present in 20% to 50% of patients with uremia. The disease may be becoming less frequent because of more effective treatment of chronic renal failure, including chronic hemodialysis and renal transplantation.

Like other peripheral neuropathies, it presents clinically with a slowly progressive, predominantly sensory neuropathy. Cramps and unpleasant dysesthesias and paresthesias often occur primarily at rest; they appear to be relieved by moving around or walking. Muscle weakness may involve the distal foot muscles, toe extensors, or flexors.

The neuropathy usually stabilizes or improves with dialysis. If the disorder worsens during dialysis, then the frequency and duration of dialysis is often increased. After renal transplantation, a rapid initial improvement is often seen within 1 to 6 months. This improvement often appears to diminish with time.[1,2]

CRANIAL NERVE PAIN

There are several disorders of the cranial nerves that may cause pain. These disorders may be caused by vascular compression, infection, or trauma, usually at one specific site on the nerve. They are not usually caused by metabolic disorders.

Trigeminal neuralgia

Trigeminal neuralgia has been traditionally described as having five fundamental features.[11] These criteria, although they have been modified, are still useful today:

1. There are paroxysmal pains with pain-free intervals. The pain is described as "sharp," "stabbing," or "electric-

shock–like" and lasts for only seconds. A burst of multiple shocks may even last up to 1 minute. In between flashes the patient is pain free. The pain is so impressive that patients can often date precisely when the attacks began and ended. Spontaneous remissions may occur for 6 months or more.

2. There are no objective clinical or neurologic findings. This traditionally held view used to divide trigeminal neuralgia into structural (with neurologic abnormalities) or idiopathic (without neurologic abnormalities). However, many surgical series of posterior fossa exploration demonstrated that up to 45% of patients have structural causes of trigeminal neuralgia that were previously thought to be idiopathic. These data led to the recommendation that a search for structural causes of trigeminal neuralgia be performed independent of the presence of abnormalities on neurologic examination.

3. There are no pathologic findings postmortem. This view is largely untenable because of reasons mentioned above.

4. Trigger zones are present. Studies of large groups of patients report that trigger zones are present in 91% of cases. Trigger zones may even be present in more than one division of the trigeminal nerve. Light touch and vibration are the best stimuli for triggering paroxysms of pain. Patients commonly report that talking, chewing, shaving, or even blowing the nose precipitate attacks of trigeminal neuralgia. The mandibular and maxillary distributions are reported to be the most commonly involved, and the right side is reported to be involved in approximately 60%.

5. Pain is restricted to the area of the trigeminal nerve. Rarely, radiation outside the trigeminal distribution has been reported in trigeminal neuralgia. The examiner should be alert for other disorders if the patient complains of pain that spreads to areas outside of the trigeminal distribution.

Medical treatment of trigeminal neuralgia

Baclofen. Baclofen is currently considered the drug of choice for trigeminal neuralgia because of its favorable side-effect profile and therapeutic efficacy. The medication should generally be begun at doses of 5 mg orally three times a day. Then increase the dose by 10 mg every other day until the patient is pain free or side effects occur. Usual maintenance dose is 50 to 60 mg/day. The most common side effects of baclofen are drowsiness, dizziness, and gastrointestinal distress. Side effects can be minimized by starting at a low dose. When the patient has been pain free for 4 to 6 weeks, taper and discontinue the drug. Baclofen may be used in conjunction with carbamazepine or phenytoin.[12]

Carbamazepine. Carbamazepine is currently the drug of second choice for trigeminal neuralgia. The effectiveness of this agent was proven in several double-blinded and controlled trials. Start the drug at doses of 100 to 200 mg twice daily, then increase it by 200 mg/day, every other day, until the patient is pain free. The onset of effect is fairly rapid, and symptoms are reported to be controlled within 24 to 48 hours. Maintenance dose is 600 to 1200 mg/day or therapeutic levels of 5 to 10 µg/ml. Side effects are most commonly drowsiness, dizziness, unsteadiness, nausea, and an-

orexia; they occur more commonly if the drug is started at high doses. Leukopenia, aplastic anemia, and agranulocytosis are other, though rare, side effects of carbamazepine and other antiepileptic drugs. Because of the very low incidence of these complications, it is unlikely that hematologic monitoring of patients on carbamazepine will signal these side effects. The patient on carbamazepine should, however, receive complete pretreatment hematologic testing as a baseline. Monitor hematologic abnormalities that occur during treatment closely; they may require discontinuation of medication should evidence of significant bone-marrow depression occur. These side effects must be balanced against the need to stop the pain of trigeminal neuralgia as soon as possible. As with baclofen, once the patient has been pain free for 4 to 6 weeks, taper and discontinue the medication.[11,12]

Phenytoin. Phenytoin is now less commonly used for medical treatment of trigeminal neuralgia. It is estimated that only 25% of patients obtain sustained relief with this medication. For this reason it is only used in patients who cannot tolerate baclofen or carbamazepine. It has an advantage over the other drugs used for control of trigeminal neuralgia in that it can be given IV, especially for the patient in severe pain. The usual loading dose is 15 mg/kg infused in normal saline and given no faster than 40 mg/min. The usual oral maintenance dose of phenytoin is 300 to 400 mg daily or 5 mg/kg. Serum levels of 10 to 20 µg/ml are recommended to avoid toxicity. Symptoms of toxicity may occur above 20 µg/ml and may include dizziness, nausea, vomiting, nystagmus, diplopia, and ataxia.[11,12,13]

Surgical and regional anesthetic treatment. Blocks of the trigeminal nerve branches of the trigeminal ganglion (gasserian ganglion) are often necessary in patients who are refractory to oral medication. There are several reasons for using this form of treatment:

1. It may allow the patient to experience the kind of numbness obtained after a destructive procedure on the nerve ganglion.

2. The rare debilitated patient may be allowed a period of oral intake and thus become a better surgical risk through a period of better nutrition.

3. It may have diagnostic significance by differentiating some forms of atypical facial pain that have a ticlike presentation.

4. It may help to relieve severe debilitating acute pain until medication can be started and become effective.

5. Some patients obtain prolonged or permanent relief. The procedures may be repeated when necessary.[11,12,14]

The second and third branches of the trigeminal nerve are the most often affected, and the blocking procedure must therefore be modified to selectively block those affected branches (Fig. 46-1). Maxillary nerve block is usually performed in the pterygopalatine fossa. Insert the needle in the coronoid fossa of the mandible, and advance it medially across the infratemporal fossa to the lateral pterygoid plate. Then "walk" the needle anteriorly until it is felt to "drop off" into the pterygopalatine fossa, then advance it slowly into this fossa containing numerous emissary veins from the

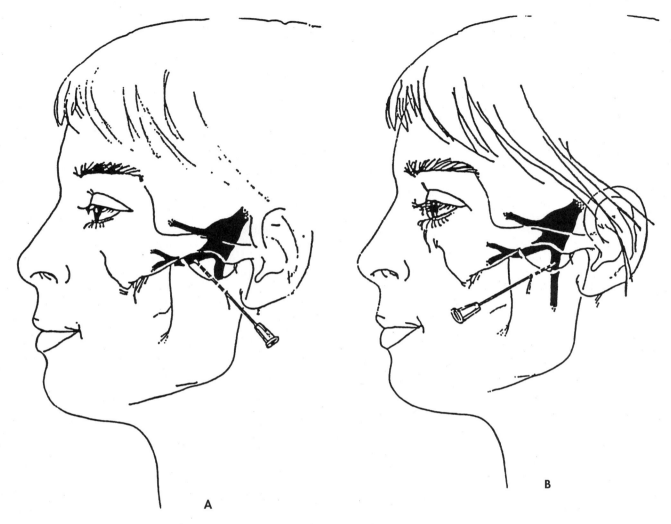

Fig. 46-1 A, Technique of maxillary nerve block by the extra oral route. **B,** Technique of mandibular nerve block by the extra oral route. (From Raj PP, editor: *Handbook of Regional Anesthesia,* ed 1. New York, Churchill Livingstone, 1985.)

orbit and the maxillary nerve. Aspirate before injection to prevent IV injection of anesthetics or neurolytics. Injection of anesthetics into these venous structures may cause blindness. If reversible agents are used, the symptoms will be transient; but more permanent complications may occur with neurolytic agents.[11,12,14]

The mandibular branch may also be blocked through the pterygopalatine fossa. Advance the needle through the coracoid notch of the mandible and across the infratemporal fossa to the lateral pterygoid plate. Then "walk" it posteriorly off the bony plate where the mandibular nerve is encountered. The superior constrictor muscle of the pharynx is nearby; if the needle is advanced too far, it may penetrate the pharynx. The middle meningeal artery may pass nearby, and intraarterial injection of anesthetic may occur if the needle position is not localized by frequent aspiration during placement.[11,12,14]

Glycerol gangliolysis is a common and useful technique for sustained relief of trigeminal neuralgia. This procedure is generally performed under fluoroscopic or computerized tomography (CT) guidance (Fig. 46-2). Place the patient in a supine position, and extend and turn the head away from the side of the block. Then turn the x-ray tube down to a 45° angle, thus visualizing the foramen ovale.[14,15,16] Maintaining this position, obtain anteroposterior and lateral views of the skull to verify the position of the needle. Then introduce a spinal needle (20-gauge, 3½ inch) into the cheek at a point drawn from a line extending inferiorly from the medial border of the pupil and beneath the malar eminence. Advance the needle in the "occlusal plane" between the coronoid process of the mandible and the lateral maxilla to the foramen ovale. The external landmarks for guiding the needle are the medial border of the pupil and a point 2.5 cm anterior to the tragus of the ear. Once in the foramen ovale, advance the needle slowly until free-flowing cerebrospinal fluid (CSF) is obtained. At this point the needle has penetrated the ganglion into the cisternal space at Meckel's cave. Inject metrizamide (Amipaque) under fluoros-

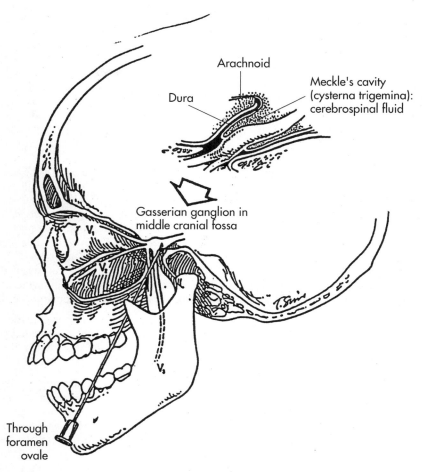

Arachnoid

Dura

Meckle's cavity
(cysterna trigemina):
cerebrospinal fluid

Gasserian ganglion in
middle cranial fossa

Through
foramen
ovale

Fig. 46-2 Technique of trigeminal ganglionolysis. (From Raj PP, editor: *Handbook of Regional Anesthesia,* ed 1. New York, Churchill Livingstone, 1985.)

copy, and visualize the region of Meckel's cave to opacify with 0.3 to 0.5 ml before the contrast spills into the posterior fossa. Once the cistern is visualized, allow the contrast to flow back out of the needle. Then draw the glycerol into a 1-ml syringe, and inject it into the area of Meckel's cave to a total of about 0.3 to 0.5 ml. The injection of this substance may produce facial dysesthesias. After injection the patient should sit with the head tipped forward for 2 hours. There may be facial pain associated with the injection, but it will resolve rapidly within minutes and disappear over a period of about 2 hours. Patients may be discharged on the first postoperative day. Approximately 89% to 96% of patients can expect complete relief of their pain. Recurrence of pain may be experienced in 7% to 10% of patients within 6 months of injection, and 7% to 21% of patients may develop recurrent pain in the first 24 months. Thus, long-term success with glycerol injection ranges from 67% to 80% without medication. Another 19% to 23% may become pain free with supplemental drug therapy. This technique is believed to work well in multiple sclerosis patients but poorly in patients with mass lesions in the posterior fossa such as tumor or arteriovenous malformation. Almost all patients report some subjective loss of sensation, including corneal hypesthesia. Reported rates of facial hypesthesia range from

24% to 84%. Usually, the extent of hypesthesia is minor and may even subside in the months after injection. In some cases there may be a brief eruption of herpes simplex in the affected area.[11,12,14]

Posterior fossa microvascular decompression of the trigeminal nerve is a procedure that is performed with the assumption that trigeminal neuralgia is caused by vascular compression of the nerve-root entry zone. Several surgical series[17-20] showed that, excluding patients with multiple sclerosis, 62% to 64% have an artery compressing the trigeminal nerve (usually the superior cerebellar or anterior cerebellar artery), 12% to 24% have a vein, 13% to 14% have a combination of artery and vein, and another 8% have a tumor or an arteriovenous malformation impinging on the trigeminal nerve. Use the posterior fossa approach; visualize the vessel at the trigeminal nerve root entry zone by magnification, and dissect it away from the nerve. Then insert a piece of padding or muscle between the vessel and the nerve to prevent further nerve compression. This procedure carries the morbidity and mortality associated with an open procedure, but because it is not a neurodestructive procedure, there are no complications of facial anesthesia or "anesthesia dolorosa." Good results are reported in more than 90% of patients.[17,19,20]

Glossopharyngeal neuralgia

Glossopharyngeal neuralgia is a disease of adults; it is more common in patients older than 50 years of age. Glossopharyngeal neuralgia is similar to trigeminal neuralgia but is much less common, occurring at ratios of 1/70th to 1/100th that of trigeminal neuralgia.[11,21] The pain of glossopharyngeal neuralgia is also shocklike in nature with spontaneous remissions. Areas that are affected include the ear, tonsils, larynx, and tongue. Trigger stimuli include swallowing, chewing, coughing, and talking. Glossopharyngeal neuralgia may be associated with trigeminal neuralgia in 10% of cases. It is rarely seen in multiple sclerosis. Medical evaluation is similar to that for trigeminal neuralgia in that magnetic resonance imaging and CT are performed to evaluate for structural causes of the disorder. Carbamazepine and phenytoin have been reported to be effective in controlling the pain initially. The benefit of the medication appears to wane after a period of weeks or months. Surgical treatment has produced good long-term results with suboccipital craniectomy and either microvascular decompression or surgical section of the glossopharyngeal nerve.[21]

Herpes zoster

Herpes zoster may produce two painful conditions: acute herpes zoster, also known as *shingles,* and postherpetic neuralgia.

Acute herpes zoster. Acute herpes zoster most commonly occurs in adults who have previously been infected with the chicken-pox virus. An outbreak of the rash may be due to an infection or a malignancy, especially lymphoma, or the immunosuppressed state. The majority of cases occur without known cause. It is believed that the virus remains dormant in the dorsal root ganglion and then later becomes reactivated. It multiplies in the dorsal root ganglion and then is transported down the sensory nerve to the nerve endings, where the zoster lesions erupt on the skin, producing the vesicular rash. The lesions are generally more widespread in the immunocompromised patient than in the immunocompetent patient. Acute herpes zoster is usually localized to a dermatomal distribution of the spinal nerve. The lesions may be distributed to the thoracic, cervical, or lumbar nerves and in the ophthalmic division of the trigeminal nerve. The discomfort is generally described as a dull, burning, aching, or shooting pain. When the trigeminal ganglia is affected, there is pain in the affected distribution and headache. There may also be weakness of the eyelid muscles, and an irregular pupil that accommodates but does not react to light (Argyll-Robertson pupil) may develop. Lesions can occur on the face, cornea, mouth, and tongue, and scarring of the cornea may be significant. There may be an associated Bell's palsy on the ipsilateral side, and symptoms of vertigo, hearing deficits, and vesicular rash in the external ear canal may occur.[13,22]

The management of acute herpes zoster today consists primarily of the use of acyclovir. Acyclovir is effective in reducing the length of time of the acute outbreak of lesions and in decreasing the pain and promoting healing.[23,24] The medication is recommended in a dose of 10 mg/kg every 8 hours. The discomfort may also be treated with analgesic medications and antiinflammatory medications. The use of corticosteroids is unclear but may help to reduce the risk of subsequent postherpetic neuralgia. It is generally recommended in a dose of 60 mg/day for 1 week and then tapered over the subsequent 2 weeks. Antidepressants and tranquilizers may relieve pain and associated depression.[25] A widely used combination is amitriptyline and fluphenazine.[11,12,22] Nerve blocks may also be effective, and local infiltration of areas of eruption using triamcinolone 0.2% solution in normal saline have been used with excellent relief of discomfort. Results were reported approaching 100% efficacy.[26]

Epidural blocks may also be effective in the treatment of acute herpes zoster of the trunk and extremities. Blocks using local anesthetics without corticosteroids have been effective: some authors reported 70% to 100% immediate relief, persisting for 1 to 5 months in follow-up.[22]

Postherpetic neuralgia. The pain of postherpetic neuralgia follows an acute outbreak of herpes zoster. Postherpetic neuralgia is said to occur when the discomfort of herpes zoster persists 1 month after the rash has healed. There are three primary components to the discomfort:

1. A constant burning or gnawing pain
2. Paroxysmal shooting or shocking pain
3. Sharp, radiating pain that is elicited by very light stimulation

There may also be scarring in the area of the healed rash, with altered touch or pinprick sensation.[13,22] Postherpetic pain is present for days to weeks after the acute outbreak of herpes zoster lesions, and the discomfort diminishes with time. The diagnosis of postherpetic neuralgia is established by the presence of pain approximately 1 month after an outbreak of acute herpes zoster with pigmentary changes of the skin.

The pain of postherpetic neuralgia is more likely to occur in the immunosuppressed and elderly patient. These patients are also at higher risk for developing acute herpes zoster.

The discomfort itself may be the result of a central pathogenesis with peripheral pathology. It is believed that there may be impairment of segmental or afferent inhibition with overreaction of wide-dynamic-range neurons.[25]

The treatment of postherpetic neuralgia is difficult. Corticosteroids may decrease the risk of developing postherpetic neuralgia. This finding, however, was not substantiated in patients treated with acyclovir during the acute phase of herpes zoster.[23,24] Acyclovir promotes healing and a resolution of the acute herpes zoster lesions. When prednisone is used, it is recommended at 60 mg/day, with a gradual dose reduction over 2 weeks. Treatment of postherpetic neuralgia includes amitriptyline or other tricyclic antidepressants. Amitriptyline is generally begun at a dose of 10 to 25 mg at bedtime and may then be increased by 10- to 25-mg increments each week. The lower starting dose is of benefit for the elderly patient who may have more sedative and anticholinergic side effects.[13,22]

Capsaicin may also be of benefit in the treatment of postherpetic neuralgia. This topical agent is applied four to five times per day for several weeks.

Atypical facial pain

Atypical facial pain is a vague, ill-defined disorder. It is characterized by a steady, diffuse, aching discomfort that may last hours or days. The pain does not occur in paroxysms or in short lancinating bursts. There are no associated trigger zones or known precipitating factors of this discomfort. In addition, the pain is not limited to the distribution of the fifth cranial nerve. It may spread over a wide area of the face and also areas supplied by the upper cervical roots.[12,13] The discomfort of atypical facial pain is not improved by surgical section of cranial nerves V or IX.

Atypical facial pain may clinically resemble a form of migraine headache. Clinical symptoms with a throbbing pain are typical. Treatment is similar to that of migraine.

In atypical facial pain the patient's symptoms may not resemble other facial neuralgias, but the patient may have similar presenting features to many other pathologies of the face and sinuses. Perform a detailed evaluation to evaluate for chronic sinusitis, allergic rhinitis, or possible occult carcinoma, particularly of the nasopharynx. Pathologic conditions of the teeth and jaw, especially the temporomandibular joint, should also be considered in the differential diagnosis.

The treatment of atypical facial pain includes antidepressants or other nonsteroidal antiinflammatory drugs. Mild analgesics or sedatives can be used. Also, nerve blocks, electrical stimulation, or biofeedback can be helpful. Occasionally, treatment of atypical facial pain appears to resemble a trial-and-error approach.[12,13]

Posttraumatic facial neuralgia

Chronic facial pain may follow trauma to the head and face. More characteristic than the discomfort is the presence of anesthesia, paresthesias, dysesthesias, or a burning discomfort. The cause of the abnormal sensation is nerve injury to the branches of the fifth cranial nerve or to the ganglion. This is based on the history, the presence of sensory deficits involving the trigeminal nerve, and the absence of other structural abnormalities.

Treatment of this form of facial pain is often unsatisfying because this discomfort typically does not respond to opiates or other analgesics. Tricyclic antidepressants and electrical nerve stimulation may be helpful.[12] Occasionally, stellate ganglion blocks or psychologic and behavioral approaches may be helpful.

REFERENCES

1. Bosch EP, Mitsumoto H: Disorders of peripheral nerves, plexuses and nerve roots. In Bradley WG et al, editors: *Neurology in Clinical Practice*. Boston, Butterworth-Heinemann 1991.
2. Oh SJ: *Clinical Electromyography: Nerve Conduction Studies*. Baltimore, University Park Press, 1984.
3. Brown MJ, Asbury AK: Diabetic neuropathy. *Ann Neurol* 15:2, 1984.
4. Max MB et al: Affects of desipramine, amitriptyline and fluoxetine on pain in diabetic neuropathy. *N Engl J Med* 326:1250, 1992.
5. Mendell CM, Klein RF, Chapell DA: A trial of amitriptyline, fluphenazine in the treatment of painful diabetic neuropathy. *JAMA* 255:637, 1986.
6. Ackerman WE et al: The management of oral mexiletine and intravenous lidocaine to treat chronic painful symmetrical distal diabetic neuropathy. *Kentucky Medical Association Journal* 89:500, 1991.
7. Chabal C et al: The use of oral mexiletine for the treatment of pain after peripheral nerve injury. *Anesthesiology* 76:513, 1992.
8. Dejgard DA, Petersen P, Kastrup J: Mexiletine for the treatment of chronic painful diabetic neuropathy. *Lancet* 1:9, 1988.
9. Stracke H et al: Mexiletine in the treatment of diabetic neuropathy. *Diabetes Care* 15:1550, 1992.
10. Tandan R et al: Topical capsaicin in painful diabetic polyneuropathy. *Neurology* 40(suppl 1):380, 1990.
11. Fromm GH: *Medical and Surgical Management of Trigeminal Neuralgia*. Mount Kisco, NY, Futura Publishing, 1987.
12. Fromm GH: Neuralgias of the face and oral cavity. *Pain Digest* 1:67, 1991.
13. Dalessio DJ: Diagnosis and treatment of cranial neuralgias. *Med Clin North Am* 75:605, 1991.
14. Raj PP et al: Nerve blocks. In Raj PP, editor: *Practical Management of Pain*. St Louis, Mosby, 1986.
15. Young RF: Glycerol rhizolysis for treatment of trigeminal neuralgia. *J Neurosurg* 69:39, 1988.
16. Calodney A, Loar C: Clinical case conference: Trigeminal neuralgia. *Pain Digest* 1:128, 1991.
17. Jannetta PJ, Rand RW: Arterial compression of the trigeminal nerve at the pons in patients with trigeminal neuralgia. *J Neurosurg* 26(suppl):159-162, 1967.
18. Jannetta PJ: Observations on the etiology of trigeminal neuralgia, hemifacial spasm, acoustic nerve dysfunction, and glossopharyngeal neuralgia: Definitive microsurgical treatment and results in 117 patients. *Neurochirurgie* 20:145, 1977.
19. Jannetta PJ: Trigeminal neuralgia: Treatment by microvascular decompression. In Wilkins RH, Rengachary SS, editors: *Neurosurgery, vol 3*. New York, McGraw-Hill, 1985.
20. Jannetta PJ, Bissonette DJ: Management of the failed patient with trigeminal neuralgia. *Clin Neurosurg* 32:334, 1985.
21. Rushton JG, Stevens JC, Miller RH: Glossopharyngeal neuralgia. *Arch Neurol* 38:201, 1981.
22. Mayne GE et al: Pain of herpes zoster and postherpetic neuralgia. In Raj PP, editor: *Practical Management of Pain*. St Louis, Mosby, 1986.
23. Peterslund NA et al: Acyclovir in herpes zoster. *Lancet* 2:8127, 1981.
24. McKendick MW et al: Oral acyclovir in acute herpes zoster. *BMJ* 293:1529, 1986.
25. Fromm GH et al: How does amitriptyline alleviate neuralgic pain? *Neurology* 39(suppl 1):327, 1989.
26. Epstein E: Treatment of zoster and post-zoster neuralgia by subcutaneous injection of triamcinolone. *Int J Dermatol* 20:65, 1981.

QUESTIONS: PERIPHERAL NERVOUS SYSTEM PAIN

For question 1, choose from the following:
- A. 1, 2, and 3
- B. 1 and 3
- C. 2 and 4
- D. 4
- E. All of the above

1. Which of the following medications is (are) appropriate for treatment of diabetic peripheral neuropathy?
   1. Carbamazepine
   2. Amitriptyline
   3. Desipramine
   4. Phenytoin

2. The healing of acute herpes zoster lesions is promoted by which of the following medications?
   - A. Acyclovir
   - B. Augmentin
   - C. Ascriptin
   - D. Amitriptyline

3. Which of the following statements about posterior microvascular decompression of the trigeminal nerve is true?
   - A. It has a significant incidence of "anesthesia dolorosa."
   - B. It may produce good results 50% of the time.
   - C. It is not indicated in multiple sclerosis with trigeminal neuralgia.
   - D. It is indicated for tumor in the anterior cranial fossa.

4. Glossopharyngeal neuralgia:
   - A. Can be diagnosed by finding trigger points
   - B. Affects the abdominal viscera
   - C. Is rarely seen in multiple sclerosis
   - D. Occurs about as often as trigeminal neuralgia

5. Atypical facial pain may present with:
   - A. Symptoms similar to nasopharyngeal carcinoma
   - B. Lancinating pains or paroxysms
   - C. Symptoms confined to the trigeminal neuralgia distribution
   - D. Muscle spasms in the neck

ANSWERS

1. E
2. A
3. C
4. C
5. A

47 The Autonomic Nervous System

Gary W. Jay

The autonomic nervous system (ANS) is divided into two general divisions, the sympathetic and parasympathetic nervous systems. The thoracolumbar sympathetic division arises for the most part from neurons in the thoracic and upper lumbar regions of the spinal cord. The craniosacral parasympathetic division arises from neurons in the midbrain, brainstem, and sacral aspects of the spinal cord.

Both the sympathetic and parasympathetic divisions of the ANS use two neurons to reach from the central nervous system (CNS) to the peripheral organ or tissue being supplied. The preganglionic neuron begins in the CNS and extends peripherally, where it synapses with the postganglionic neuron, which proceeds to the end organ. These two neurons synapse in one of the autonomic ganglia.

ANS preganglionic fibers are myelinated B-type fibers; the postganglionic fibers are small, unmyelinated C fibers.

Sympathetic preganglionic cell bodies arise from the intermediolateral gray columns of the thoracic and upper lumbar spinal cord. The preganglionic fibers leave the spinal cord through the ventral root of the spinal nerve and end in a sympathetic ganglion. There the preganglionic fibers synapse with postganglionic fibers (in a 1:20 ratio). The postganglionic fibers leave the ganglion and converge on the effector tissue they supply.

The parasympathetic preganglionic neurons originate in the midbrain, the cranial portion of the brainstem, and the sacral region of the spinal cord. The cranial portion of the parasympathetic neurons exit via cranial nerves III, VII, IX, and X. The vagus nerve (X) contains almost 75% of the efferent aspects of the entire parasympathetic system. The pelvic splanchnic nerves carry the fibers of the neurons composing the preganglionic fibers of the sacral part of the parasympathetic division. The parasympathetic preganglionic neurons synapse with the postganglionic fibers in terminal ganglia, which are usually imbedded directly in the tissue or organ that they innervate.

Almost all tissues in the body are innervated to some degree by the ANS. Some organs such as the heart are innervated by both branches of the ANS. Other tissues such as the peripheral arterioles are supplied only by the sympathetic division. Sympathetic activity is more generalized than parasympathetic activity, which is more discrete and may effect only one organ.

The sympathetically innervated adrenal medulla synthesizes and secretes epinephrine and norepinephrine directly into the blood stream, usually in an 80:20 ratio. This neurotransmitter release acts to prolong the effect of central sympathetic action.

Autonomic reflexes enable physiologic regulation by the ANS to be used in the hemostatic control of involuntary functions. This control involves peripheral monitoring, central integration, and altered autonomic regulation. The complex integration of autonomic responses may occur at several levels of the CNS, including the hypothalamus. Limbic system and cortical information may also influence the ANS via interactions with the hypothalamus, brainstem, and spinal cord.

The neurotransmitter at the preganglionic-postganglionic synapse in both divisions of the ANS is acetylcholine (ACh). Acetylcholine is also the neurotransmitter at the parasympathetic postganglionic-effector cell synapse. The active neurotransmitter at the sympathetic postganglionic-effector cell synapse is usually norepinephrine. A small number of the sympathetic postganglionic fibers also use ACh.

All preganglionic neurons and parasympathetic postganglionic neurons are considered cholinergic in nature, and most sympathetic postganglionic neurons are felt to be adrenergic. An exception to this is the use of ACh at specific sympathetic postganglionic fibers that innervate sweat glands and some blood vessels in the face, neck, and lower extremities.

Other types of neurotransmitters may also be present in the ANS. It is uncertain if these substances act as true autonomic neurotransmitters or cotransmitters that are released from the synapse along with ACh or norepinephrine. These include purinergic substances such as adenosine and adenosine triphosphate (ATP), which are possibly active in the gastrointestinal tract, and substance P and vasoactive intestinal polypeptide (VIP), which may participate in the autonomic control of respiratory and intestinal function.

AUTONOMIC RECEPTORS

The two primary neurotransmitters in the ANS, ACh and norepinephrine, are associated with specific types of postsynaptic receptors. Cholinergic receptors are found at synapses that use ACh, and adrenergic receptors are found at synapses utilizing norepinephrine. Each type of receptor has several subclassifications, which are further responsible for mediating appropriate tissue responses.

Cholinergic receptors are divided into two categories, nicotinic and muscarinic receptors. Nicotinic cholinergic receptors are found at the junction between preganglionic and postganglionic neurons in both the sympathetic and parasympathetic divisions of the ANS. The type I nicotinic receptor is located in the ANS; the type II nicotinic receptors are found at the skeletal neuromuscular junction.

The muscarinic cholinergic receptors are found at all synapses between the cholinergic postganglionic neurons and the terminal effector cells, including the parasympathetic terminal synapses and the sympathetic postganglionic cholinergic fibers, which innervate sweat glands and some blood vessels. There appear to be two types of muscarinic receptors, M_1 and M_2, which appear for now to be functionally similar. The cholinergic muscarinic receptors functionally mediate the effects of the ANS on tissue.

Adrenergic receptors are divided into two divisions, α- and β-adrenergic receptors. Each division is further divided into two further types, α_1 and α_2 receptors and β_1 and β_2 receptors. These receptors are located at the end or terminal synapse between the sympathetic postganglionic adrenergic neurons and the tissues they supply.

α_1 Receptors are found in the smooth muscle located in various tissues throughout the body, including the peripheral vasculature, the intestinal wall, and iris.

α_2 Receptors are found on the presynaptic terminal of specific adrenergic synapses. They are involved in the modulation of norepinephrine release from the presynaptic terminal in a negative feedback loop that limits the amount of norepinephrine that is released from the presynaptic terminal. Centrally located α_2 receptors are involved in the control of sympathetic discharge by promoting inhibition of sympathetic discharge from the brainstem.

β_1 Receptors are found in the heart and kidneys, whereas β_2 receptors are found in the smooth muscle of specific blood vessels, the bronchioles, the gallbladder, and uterus. Both of these receptors also function in the metabolism of liver cells and skeletal muscle.

Some organs or tissues may have two or more different adrenergic receptor subtypes, such as the arterioles in skeletal muscle that appear to have both α_1 and β_2 receptors.

In the short synopsis to follow, various neurotransmitters and medications that interact within the ANS are described, along with some of their general uses. More complete information may be found in a number of excellent texts.[1-3] A more complete neuroanatomic discussion of the ANS may be found in Manter and Gatz[4] and in any complete neuroanatomy text.

CHOLINERGIC DRUGS

ACh is one of the primary neurotransmitters in the ANS, particularly in the parasympathetic branch. ACh is also found at the skeletal neuromuscular junction. Cholinergic receptors are also found in specific areas of the brain; their effects on several neurologic disorders are discussed below.

Cholinergic medications are broadly separated into two different categories: cholinergic stimulants and anticholinergic medications.

Muscarinic cholinergic receptors are found in specific areas of the brain and the parasympathetic postganglionic neurons in effector organs. The nicotinic cholinergic receptors are found in the autonomic ganglia (type I) and the skeletal neuromuscular junction (type II).

The direct-acting cholinergic stimulants bind directly to the cholinergic receptors and act to increase the activity at the ACh synapses. Indirect-acting cholinergic stimulants act by inhibiting acetylcholinesterase at the synapse and increase ACh activity by preventing its metabolism.

The most appropriate direct-acting muscarinic cholinergic stimulants are those that affect peripheral tissues primarily and realize only minimal effects on the cholinergic receptors found in the autonomic ganglia and the neuromuscular junction. Bethanechol (Urecholine) is the primary direct-acting muscarinic cholinergic stimulant appropriate at this time for systemic usage. Pilocarpine and carbachol are used topically for the treatment of glaucoma. They have too many systemic side effects to be used nontopically.

Indirect-acting stimulants are also referred to as cholinesterase inhibitors or anticholinesterase medications. These nonspecific drugs may induce a stimulation of the peripheral cholinergic receptors and the cholinergic receptors located at the autonomic ganglia, the skeletal neuromuscular junction, and in specific areas of the CNS. These medications are used primarily to affect the skeletal neuromuscular junction and peripheral tissues with muscarinic cholinergic receptors. Neostigmine and pyridostigmine are the primary agents used. Other agents are used topically for the treatment of glaucoma.

Both direct- and indirect-acting cholinergic stimulants are used to treat the posttraumatic or postsurgical decrease in gastrointestinal tract and urinary bladder smooth muscle tone. Indirect-acting stimulants are also used in the treatment of glaucoma and myasthenia gravis. They are also used to reverse the effects of an overdose of neuromuscular blocking agents or anticholinergic medications.

The adverse effects of both the direct- and indirect-acting cholinergic stimulants include gastrointestinal distress (e.g., nausea, vomiting, diarrhea, abdominal cramping), increased salivation, bradycardia, constriction of the bronchi, increased sweating, facial flushing, and problems with visual accommodation.

Anticholinergic medications are typically competitive antagonists of the postsynaptic cholinergic receptors. They act to decrease the synaptic response to cholinergic stimulation. They may be classified as either antimuscarinic or antinicotinic medications, depending on their specificity.

Atropine is the most frequently used antimuscarinic anticholinergic medication. This group of medications is generally used to treat specific gastrointestinal difficulties (e.g., peptic ulcer), Parkinson's disease, motion sickness, irritable bowel syndrome, neurogenic bladder, and cardiac arrhythmias. Scopolamine is most frequently used for treating motion sickness.

High blood pressure is treated with various antinicotinic (type I) agents. The type II nicotinic antagonists are used to block the skeletal neuromuscular junction and induce skeletal muscle paralysis before surgery.

The most frequent side effects of the antimuscarinic anticholinergic medications include blurred vision, urinary retention, dry mouth, constipation, tachycardia, and sedation. At higher doses, confusion, dizziness, and anxiety may be seen.

ADRENERGIC DRUGS

Adrenergic agonists, or sympathomimetics, augment sympathetic activity, whereas adrenergic antagonists, also known as sympatholytics, are used to decrease sympathetic responses.

The major neurotransmitter at the ganglionic synapse in both the sympathetic and parasympathetic nervous systems is ACh, as discussed earlier. At the postganglionic synapse, the parasympathetic neurotransmitter is ACh. The sympathetic neurotransmitter is usually norepinephrine, but ACh is found at sweat glands and some blood vessels.

Adrenergic receptors are divided into several types. α-Adrenergic receptors may precede the synapse between the nerve terminal and effector cells; others may be postsynaptic. The α_1 adrenergic receptors are postsynaptic; they are located on blood vessels, the radial muscle of the eye, on the splenic capsule, and in the gastrointestinal tract.

α_2-Adrenergic receptors are either presynaptic or postsynaptic. They all serve an inhibitory function. The presynaptic α_2 receptors, when activated, inhibit the release of neurotransmitter. They are found at both adrenergic and cholinergic nerve terminals. Postsynaptic α_2 receptors are located in the CNS and in blood vessels.

Agonists for the α-adrenergic receptors include epinephrine and norepinephrine. Antagonists include phentolamine and phenoxybenzamine.

β-Adrenergic receptors are also stimulated by epinephrine and norepinephrine. Propranolol is an antagonist. β_1 Adrenergic receptors are mostly found on cells in the heart and the intestine. β_2 Adrenergic receptors are found on bronchial and vascular smooth muscle.

Adrenergic agonists, or sympathomimetic drugs include the catecholamines norepinephrine and epinephrine. These agents mimic or enhance the sympathetic nervous system. It should be remembered that in the biochemical transformation of tyrosine to norepinephrine and then epinephrine, the formation of dopamine is an intermediate step.

Norepinephrine strongly interacts with β_1 receptors and is less potent on the α-adrenergic receptors. It has minimal effect on β_2 receptors. It is used to treat hypotension during anesthesia if associated with good tissue perfusion.

Epinephrine interacts with both α and β receptors. At low concentrations, β effects predominate, whereas α effects are manifested with high concentrations of epinephrine.

Epinephrine is used to treat bronchospasm and allergic or hypersensitivity reactions, to increase duration of infiltrative anesthetics, and to treat chronic (open-angle) glaucoma. It may also be used to restore cardiac function during cardiac arrest.

The adverse effects of both epinephrine and norepinephrine include headache, anxiety, cardiac arrhythmias, pulmonary edema, and cerebral hemorrhage (from vasopressor effects).

Dopamine is a direct β_1 receptor agonist and releases norepinephrine from adrenergic terminals. At high doses, it causes vasoconstriction by its stimulation of α receptors. It is used in the treatment of septic and cardiogenic shock, as well as in chronic congestive heart failure.

Phenylephrine, a direct-acting sympathomimetic, has effects similar to norepinephrine. It is used as a nasal decongestant, to provide local vasoconstriction, and as a pressor agent.

Amphetamine indirectly increases release of norepinephrine. It is also a CNS stimulant and is used in the treatment of narcolepsy. Methamphetamine is related to amphetamine and is a mixed-acting sympathomimetic.

β_2 Agonists including metaproterenol, albuterol, and terbutaline cause relaxation (dilatation) of bronchial smooth muscle and do not effect the β_1 receptors in the heart.

Sympathetic antagonists (or sympatholytics) include phenoxybenzamine, which antagonizes the α-adrenergic sympathetic responses mediated by α-adrenergic receptors. It is used in the treatment of reflex sympathetic dystrophy, to relieve vasoconstriction in Raynaud's syndrome, and to control autonomic hyperreflexia secondary to spinal cord transection.

Phentolamine, which produces a reversible α-adrenergic blockade, produces vasodilatation. It may be used to control acute hypertensive events secondary to sympathomimetics.

The ergot alkaloids are weak α-adrenergic blockers and serotonin antagonists. They also provide partial agonistic action at α-adrenergic receptors and act as agonists at the dopamine receptors. These drugs provide vasoconstrictive actions, with ergotamine tartrate being used effectively in the treatment of migraine. Methysergide is also used for the prophylactic treatment of migraine.

Propranolol is a nonselective β-blocking agent (β-antagonist). It competes for both the β_1 and β_2 receptors. It is used for migraine prophylaxis, as well as the treatment of hypertension, cardiac arrhythmias, and the management of anxiety. There are a number of other medications that are similar to propranolol (nonselective β-antagonists), including timolol and nadolol. Atenolol and metoprolol are selective β_1 adrenergic antagonists but function similarly.

Other medications act to inhibit the activity of adrenergic nerves, including reserpine, which acts via catecholamine depletion, both centrally and peripherally. Reserpine also inhibits the presynaptic synthesis of norepinephrine, epinephrine, and serotonin. It may be used in the treatment of hypertension.

Guanethidine inhibits the release of neurotransmitters (including norepinephrine) from peripheral adrenergic neurons, therefore impairing sympathetic response to stimulation. Its direct usefulness (via Bier's block) in patients with reflex sympathetic dystrophy continues to be studied. Bretylium also blocks the releases of norepinephrine from adrenergic neurons. It produces a brief sympathomimetic effect before it blocks the neurons. It may be directly infused into the vessels via Bier's block in patients with reflex sympathetic dystrophy.

Various medications may effect neurotransmitters in different ways. They can effect the release, storage, or synthesis of a neurotransmitter; the enzymatic breakdown of a neurotransmitter; its transport into cells; and the interaction between the neurotransmitter and its receptor.

When dealing with a sympathetically mediated pain problem, the manner in which a particular drug creates its effect may be as important as the effect it produces. The importance of specific tissue receptors and receptor subtypes is immeasurable. These facts enable the use of drugs that affect specific tissues and organs with relative specificity;

no drug, however, is entirely specific for a particular receptor subtype. Even the specific β_1 agonist atenolol, which has a very high specificity or affinity to the β_1 receptors, has 10 to 20 times less affinity to β_2 receptors. If used at great enough concentrations, β_2 receptors can be affected.[5] Sumatriptan, a specific serotonin agonist that works relatively specifically at the 5-HT1D receptor subtype, also has some minor affinity to the 5-HT1A receptor.[6]

It should also be remembered that the majority of organs and tissues in the body contain more than one specific receptor subtype. A drug may therefore perform its primary effect, but also cause several other effects distinct and even distant to its primary effect.

REFERENCES

1. Ciccone CD, Wolf SL: *Pharmacology in Rehabilitation.* Philadelphia, FA Davis, 1990.
2. Jacob LS: *Pharmacology,* ed 3. Baltimore, Williams & Wilkins, 1992.
3. Gillman AG et al, editors: *The Pharmacological Basis of Therapeutics,* ed 7. New York, Macmillan, 1985.
4. Gilman S, Newman SW: *Manter and Gatz's Essentials of Clinical Neuroanatomy and Neurophysiology,* ed 8. Philadelphia, F A Davis, 1992.
5. Gerber JC, Nies AS: Beta-adrenergic blocking drugs. *Annu Rev Med* 36:135, 1985.
6. McCarthy BG, Peroutka SJ: Comparative neuropharmacology of dihydroergotamine and sumatriptan (GR 43175). *Headache* 29:420-422, 1989.

QUESTIONS: THE AUTONOMIC NERVOUS SYSTEM

1. Autonomic reflexes enable physiologic regulation by the ANS to be used in hemostatic control of involuntary functions via all the following EXCEPT:
   A. Central integration
   B. Peripheral monitoring
   C. Increased venous pressure
   D. Altered autonomic regulation
2. The primary neurotransmitter at the preganglionic-postganglionic synapses in both divisions of the ANS is:
   A. Serotonin
   B. Acetylcholine
   C. Vasoactive intestinal peptide
   D. Norepinephrine
3. Cholinergic receptors are divided into the following two categories:
   A. Nicotinic and adrenergic
   B. Adrenergic and muscarinic
   C. Cholinergic and adrenergic
   D. Nicotinic and muscarinic
4. The most common side effects of antimuscarinic anticholinergic medications include all the following EXCEPT:
   A. Bradycardia
   B. Sedation
   C. Confusion
   D. Urinary retention

5. Sympathomimetics, or adrenergic agonists, include all the following EXCEPT:
   A. Phenylephrine
   B. Ritalin
   C. Methamphetamine
   D. Phentolamine

ANSWERS

1. C
2. B
3. D
4. A
5. D

48 Reflex Sympathetic Dystrophy

P. Prithvi Raj

Reflex sympathetic dystrophy (RSD), or complex regional pain syndrome—CPRS I, applies to a variety of seemingly unrelated disorders having similar clinical features and manifesting the same fundamental disturbed physiology. The term *reflex* indicates a response to a primary exciting stimulus that is traumatic, medical, infectious, or vascular; the term *sympathetic* indicates the neurologic pathway subserving the development and maintenance of these syndromes; and the term *dystrophy* indicates that, if untreated, these syndromes uniformly result in trophic changes as a result of the persistent sympathetic stimulation.

Box 48-1 lists the many terms used to describe the syndrome that is now termed RSD. *Causalgia,* which means burning pain, is a historical term describing a reflex sympathetic dystrophy that follows partial or, rarely, complete injury to a peripheral nerve trunk.[1] It is also called complex regional pain syndrome—CPRS II. It is characterized by constant, spontaneous, severe, burning pain and is usually associated with hypoesthesia and hyperesthesia, hyperpathia, and allodynia, along with vasomotor and sudomotor disturbances that, if persistent, result in trophic changes. RSD need not be initiated by damage to a major peripheral nerve trunk. Other causes, listed in Box 48-2, are characterized by similar though perhaps less severe symptomatology. Regardless of the cause RSD can be defined[2] as a syndrome of diffuse limb pain often burning in nature and usually consequent to injury or noxious stimulus with variable sensory, motor, autonomic, and trophic changes.[3] The syndrome may spread independently of the source or site of the precipitating event and often presents in a pattern inconsistent with dermatomal or peripheral nerve distributions. Clinical findings usually include autonomic dysregulation (e.g., alterations in blood flow, hyperhidrosis, edema), sensory abnormalities (e.g., hypoesthesia, hyperesthesia, allodynia to cold and mechanical stimulation), motor dysfunction (e.g., weakness, tremor, joint stiffness), reactive psychologic disturbances (e.g., anxiety, hopelessness, depression), and trophic changes (e.g., muscle atrophy, osteopenia arthropathy, glossy skin, brittle nails, altered hair growth) (Fig. 48-1).

Regardless of cause or severity of presentation, the underlying pathophysiologic mechanism is extremely similar, if not identical, in all of these disorders. The common denominator appears to be local tissue damage, which apparently initiates a reflex response involving the sympathetic nervous system. Pain and vasomotor disturbances, with minor exceptions, are improved, cured, or otherwise modified by interruption of the involved sympathetic pathways.

The diagnosis of severe RSD is rarely difficult to make because the initiating mechanism is usually related to obvious trauma to major nerve trunks or tissues in close proximity and because the resultant syndrome and burning pain are characteristic. However, a less severe RSD, without obvious injury or cause, is frequently misdiagnosed and thus often mismanaged or neglected.

HISTORICAL REVIEW

Among the earliest descriptions of severe burning pain following peripheral nerve injury is that by the surgeon Ambroise Paré in the seventeenth century.[4] King Charles IX, ill with smallpox, was subjected to current treatment of the day: bleeding induced by lancet wound to the arm. After this therapy, the king suffered from persistent pain, muscle contracture, and inability to flex or extend his arm. Paré was called on to treat the king, whose symptoms finally disappeared.

Severe burning pain in an extremity after nerve injuries in soldiers was described in 1864 by Mitchell et al.[5] Mitchell subsequently introduced the term *causalgia* to describe the syndrome.[1] In the 1920s Leriche demonstrated that the pain of causalgia was often relieved by sympathetic blockade and that sympathectomy could effect permanent relief.[6] It later became apparent that similar types of pain occurred after trauma or surgery in nonmilitary patients, many of whom had no obvious nerve injury. Vasomotor and sudomotor disturbances and dystrophic changes were reported in patients with and without nerve lesions.

The literature on causalgic pain is confusing not only because the pathophysiology is poorly understood but also because the terminology is far from uniform. The International Association for the Study of Pain (IASP)[7] proposed a definition of RSD as "continuous pain in a portion of an extremity after trauma which may include fracture but does not involve a major nerve, associated with sympathetic hyperactivity." The IASP regards causalgia as a similar but separate entity defined as "burning pain, allodynia, and hyperpathia, usually in the hand or foot, after partial injury of a nerve or one of its major branches." Recently the Subcommittee on Taxonomy of the IASP has replaced the terms RSD and causalgia with CPRS I and CPRS II, respectively.

MECHANISM

The pathogenesis of RSD has been the subject of much attention. Many theories have been proposed to explain this disease, although none has proved conclusive, and it is likely that the explanation may involve mechanisms from several of the current theories. In 1864 Mitchell[5] suggested

---

Box 48-1 TERMS USED TO DESCRIBE RSD

Acute atrophy of bone
Algodystrophy mineures
Algodystrophy reflexes
Algodystrophy
Causalgia
Chronic traumatic edema
Mimo-causalgia
Minor causalgia
Neurodystrophy
Pain-dysfunction syndrome
Posttraumatic dystrophy
Posttraumatic pain syndrome
Posttraumatic osteoperosis
Reflex neurovascular dystrophy
Reflex sympathetic dystrophy
Shoulder hand syndrome
Sudeck's atrophy
Sympathalgia
Sympathetic overdrive syndrome
Traumatic vasospasm

Box 48-2 CAUSES OF RSD

I. Trauma
  A. Accidental injury
    1. Sprain, dislocations, fracture (usually of the hands, feet, or wrists)
    2. Minor cuts or pricks, lacerations, contusions
    3. Crush injury of fingers, hands, or wrists; traumatic amputation of fingers
    4. Burns
  B. Surgical
    1. Procedures in the extremities
    2. Excision of small tumors, ganglia of wrist
    3. Forceful manipulation, tight casts
    4. Surgical scars
    5. Damage to small peripheral nerves with a needle (e.g., during its insertion for infusion, transfusion, injection therapy, or analgesic block)
    6. Injections or irritants
II. Diseases
  A. Visceral diseases (e.g., myocardial infarction)
  B. Neurologic diseases
    1. Cerebral: vascular accidents (posthemiplegic dystrophy), tumors, syringomyelia, and others
    2. Spinal cord: poliomyelitis, combined degeneration, tumors, syringomyelia, and others
    3. Spinal nerves or their roots: herpes zoster, radiculitis
    4. Brachial plexus
    5. Infiltrating carcinoma from the breast, apex of the lung (upper extremity), or pelvis (lower extremity)
    6. Glomus tumor
  C. Infections
    1. Extremity skin and other soft tissues
    2. Periarticular
  D. Vascular disease
    1. Generalized: periarthritis nodosa, diffuse arteritis, arteriosclerosis
    2. Peripheral: thrombophlebitis, tissues
  E. Musculoskeletal disorders
    1. Postural defects
    2. Myofascial syndromes
III. Idiopathic

---

that the syndrome he would later name causalgia was the result of an ascending neuritis affecting a damaged peripheral nerve. The frequently observed failure of peripheral nerve block or surgery to abolish the pain indicates that more than a simple irritating peripheral lesion is involved. Section of the peripheral nerve at successively higher levels and even cutting the sensory pathway at a multitude of sites from the peripheral receptors to the somatosensory cortex has been attempted in the treatment of RSD with initially encouraging results but with a frustrating tendency for the pain to return.[8-10]

Any proposed explanation for the pathophysiology of RSD must be able to explain the character of the pain, the relief of pain by sympathetic block in the early phases of the disease, and the tendency for sympathectomy to fail to relieve pain in the later phases.

RSD may be thought of as prolonging the normal sympathetic response to injury (Fig. 48-2).[11] A sympathetic reflex arc is the normal response to any traumatic injury. Painful afferent impulses from the periphery travel along A-delta and C fibers through the peripheral nerves to enter the spinal cord through the dorsal roots and synapse in the dorsal horn with interneurons carrying the impulses to (1) ascending tracts, where they are then projected further to the thalamus and finally to the somatosensory cortex; (2) the anterior horn, where a motor reflex may be initiated by efferent motor fibers causing muscle contraction; or (3) the intermediolateral cell column, where the painful message is relayed to the sympathetic nerve cell bodies. A sympathetic reflex (Fig. 48-3) is activated by efferent sympathetic impulses sent out of the spinal cord through the ventral roots to a ramus communicans albus and then into the sympathetic chain to synapse in a sympathetic ganglion. The postganglionic sympathetic fiber leaves the ganglia by way of the ramus communicans griseus, where it travels with the peripheral nerve to the extremity, producing vasoconstriction. This is a normal reflex, which normally gives way to vasodilatation as part of the orderly progression toward healing.[11-13] If this sympathetic reflex arc does not shut down but continues to function and accelerate, a sympathetic hyperdynamic state ensues. This results in increased vasoconstriction and tissue ischemia, causing more pain and thus increasing the barrage of afferent pain impulses traveling to the spinal cord and reactivating the sympathetic reflex. This sympathetic efferent stimulation enhances the sensitivity of the nociceptor by causing vasoconstriction and ischemia, changes in vascular permeability, and smooth muscle contraction around the nociceptor; sensitivity is also enhanced by the direct action of locally released substances, including norepinephrine, substance P, prostaglandins, and bradykinin.

The motor arc described previously can also lead to a self-sustained reflex, producing muscle spasm and pain and

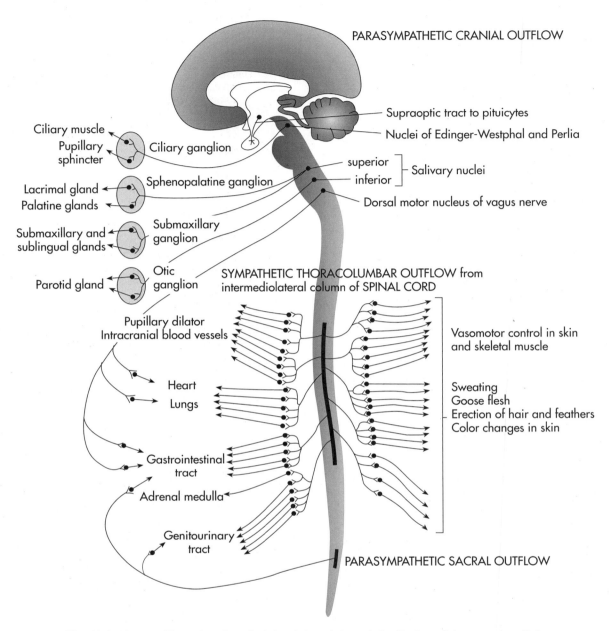

PARASYMPATHETIC CRANIAL OUTFLOW

Supraoptic tract to pituicytes

Nuclei of Edinger-Westphal and Perlia

Ciliary muscle

Pupillary sphincter

Ciliary ganglion

superior
inferior

Salivary nuclei

Sphenopalatine ganglion

Lacrimal gland

Palatine glands

Dorsal motor nucleus of vagus nerve

Submaxillary and sublingual glands

Submaxillary ganglion

Parotid gland

Otic ganglion

SYMPATHETIC THORACOLUMBAR OUTFLOW from intermediolateral column of SPINAL CORD

Pupillary dilator
Intracranial blood vessels

Vasomotor control in skin and skeletal muscle

Heart

Lungs

Sweating
Goose flesh
Erection of hair and feathers
Color changes in skin

Gastrointestinal tract

Adrenal medulla

Genitourinary tract

PARASYMPATHETIC SACRAL OUTFLOW

Fig. 48-1 Diagram illustrating the principle of the origin and distribution of the two great divisions of the autonomic nervous system. (Redrawn from Pick J: *The Autonomic Nervous System: Morphological, Clinical and Surgical Aspects.* Philadelphia, JB Lippincott, 1970.)

further reinforcing the now afferent response. Why the hyperdynamic sympathetic state continues after the initial tissue injury has healed and why the critical pathophysiologic process seems to progress from the periphery to the central nervous system in the later phases of the disease[14-16] is not known, although many theories have been proposed to explain these phenomena. These theories may be conveniently divided, according to the site of origin of the pain impulses, into peripheral tissue, peripheral nerve, and central nervous system abnormalities.[14,17,18]

PERIPHERAL TISSUE ABNORMALITIES
Vasoconstriction and vasodilatation

Changes at the peripheral tissue level have been implicated by several authors as the cause of this persistent painful state. Both vasodilated and vasoconstricted states have been suggested.[3,14,19,20]

Leriche[21] felt that vasoconstriction at the site of injury led to tissue ischemia and pain. Abnormal vasomotor reflexes were stated to be the cause of the vasospasm. Lewis[20] postulated that causalgia was a state of painful vasodilata-

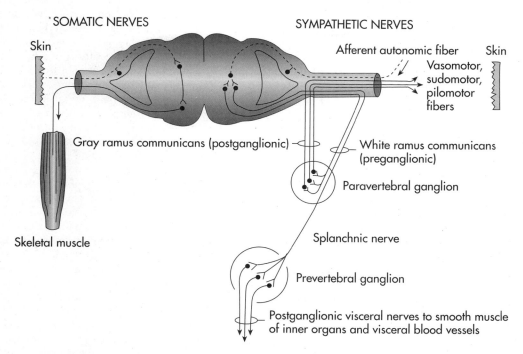

Fig. 48-2 Diagram illustrating the sympathetic outflow tract. (Modified from Pick J: *The Autonomic Nervous System: Morphological, Clinical and Surgical Aspects.* Philadelphia, JB Lippincott, 1970.)

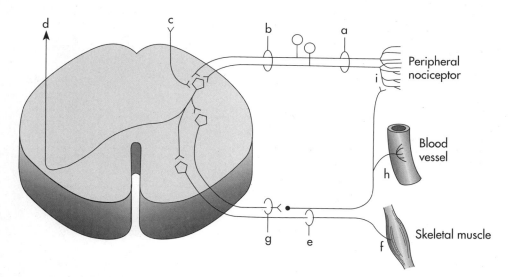

Fig. 48-3 A reflex arc is set into motion with any painful stimulus. The afferent impulses can ascend in the spinal thalamic tract and initiate an efferent sympathetic reflex or an efferent motor reflex. This is a normal response to injury but should it persist beyond the acute phase, it becomes abnormal and may set up a reflex sympathetic dystrophy. *a,* Painful afferents (A-delta and C fibers); *b,* dorsal root; *c,* descending inhibitory pathway; *d,* ascending tracts (spinothalamic); *e,* motor reflex (motoaxon); *f,* increased skeletal muscle tone and spasm; *g,* sympathetic reflex (sympathetic efferent); *h,* vasoconstriction and microcirculatory changes; and *i,* sensitization of peripheral nociceptor.

tion caused by the liberation of pain-producing vasodilator substances in response to antidromic impulses arising from the area of nerve injury.

PERIPHERAL NERVE ABNORMALITIES
Role of sympathetic afferents

There is anatomic and physiologic evidence from animal studies that some afferent fibers from the affected limb travel through the sympathetic chain before entering the dorsal horn of the spinal cord.[17,22-24] Several clinical observations suggest that some types of pain may be mediated by afferent fibers in the sympathetic chain. Echlin[25] described a patient with phantom limb pain who underwent lumbar sympathectomy under local infiltration anesthesia. After removal of a segment of the chain, mechanical or electrical stimulation of the proximal stump produced severe hip and phantom foot pain.[26] Further clinical evidence of sympathetic afferent contributions to pain is provided by a patient in whom sympathectomy relieved postamputation arm pain after extensive rhizotomy had failed to produce analgesia.[27] Stimulation of arteries in patients under regional anesthesia or with somatic nerve damage has been shown to cause burning pain, which suggests that sympathetic afferents may innervate vessel walls.[3,28]

Artificial synapse

Doupe and colleagues ascribed the "peculiar" qualities of causalgic pain to stimulation of sensory fibers by efferent impulses in the sympathetic fibers (Fig. 48-4).[29] This theory states that an artificial synapse or ephapse is created at the damaged segment of the nerve by a breakdown in the normal insulation between adjacent fibers. Efferent sympathetic impulses that are tonically active can cross over to sensory fibers in the area of injury. This artificial synapse could produce several types of nerve impulses, which could account for many of the features of the disease. Impulses that cross over to the afferent pain fibers could be directed orthodromically (toward the central nervous system) and would be interpreted as pain. Impulses crossing to afferent pain fibers directed antidromically (toward the periphery) can also cause pain by sensitizing the peripheral nociceptor, possibly through the release of a vasodilating substance, neurokinin.[30] Direct stimulation of the distal segment of a severed nerve produces pain referred to the adjacent uncut nerves.[31] Thus antidromic impulses in the afferent pain fibers may decrease the threshold of peripheral nociceptor and may initiate the generation of painful impulses in adjacent fibers. This results in impulses directed back toward the central nervous system in the damaged fibers themselves or in neighboring fibers. This would explain the spontaneous and constant pain, aggravated by emotional stress and anxiety, that is characteristic of causalgia and RSD. It would also account for the dramatic relief observed after sympathetic blockade. Trophic and vasomotor changes of the skin could be attributed to antidromic stimulation of sympathetic fibers by crossover of afferent pain impulses in a similar manner.[12,32] Experimental support for this theory unfortunately is thin, although Granit and colleagues demonstrated that motor impulses can be "short-circuited" to sensory fibers in damaged nerve segments in cats.[33]

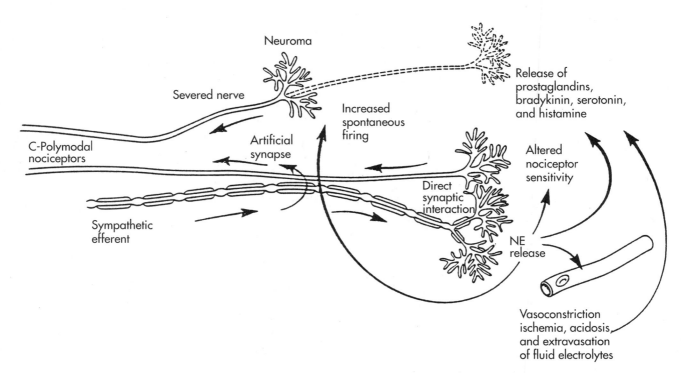

Fig. 48-4 Some proposed mechanisms of interaction between sympathetic efferent and nociceptive afferent fibers in causalgia. (Redrawn from Raj PP, editor: *Practical Management of Pain.* St Louis, Mosby, 1986.)

Fiber dissociation

An imbalance between fiber types that results from damage to a peripheral nerve is the basis for the "fiber dissociation" theory of Wall and Melzack.

Noordenbos[34] proposed that within a nerve, the fast-conducting, richly myelinated fibers are subject to proportionally more damage from high-velocity missile wounds than are the poorly myelinated or unmyelinated slower fiber types. This produces an imbalance between the slowly conducted painful impulses and the now decreased inhibitor myelinated fiber activity. The result is a facilitation of the slowly conducted painful impulses and, finally, an abnormal central response to this afferent barrage, which is felt to be the basis of causalgia.

Gate theory

In 1965, Melzack and Wall[15] introduced the "gate theory" of pain, which is a refinement of the fiber dissociation theory (Fig. 48-5).[9,13] This theory proposed a balance of input by large A-beta and small A-delta and C-fibers to the CNS. This balance could be upset by any number of pathologic processes, including soft tissue or peripheral nerve injury as in the RSDs. According to this theory, large fiber input inhibits, while small fiber input facilitates, the spinal cord transmission of afferent impulses. Causalgia is felt to be a result of selective damage of these large myelinated fibers, allowing the balance to favor small fiber activity, thus "opening" the gate and increasing the central transmission of the painful afferent impulses. Large fiber stimulation, which may form the basis for the use of transcutaneous electrical nerve stimulation (TENS), would "close" the gate and afford pain relief. Further investigation has not supported all components of this theory. Large fiber inhibition of afferent impulses has been confirmed by many other physiologists, although stimulation of small fibers has not been shown to facilitate and may in fact inhibit the transmission in the spinal cord of afferent information.[8,13,35]

Neuroma formation and sprout growth

The observation that properties of nerves change markedly after various types of nerve injury has spawned several theories based on neuroma formation and sprout outgrowth.[14,36-38]

The sensory fibers have their cell bodies in the dorsal root ganglia, just outside the spinal cord. When a nerve fiber is transected, the distal portion degenerates completely, for it is now separated from its cell body. The endoneural tube and Schwann cells surrounding the fiber remain intact, except at the point of injury. As the distal fiber degenerates, it is absorbed by neighboring cells. At the same time, the proximal portion of the fiber begins its regeneration of about 3 mm of growth daily until the fibers reach their original destination. If, however, the architecture is such that the sprouts do not find intact tubes nearby, they are surrounded by an area of tissue injury and inflammatory response. Multiple sprouts are sent out by each axon in an unsuccessful attempt to find the familiar endoneural structures. The end result of failed regeneration is called a neuroma and includes fibrous tissue and fine nerve sprouts trapped therein.[37]

Wall and Gutnick have investigated the properties of these regenerating sprouts.[38] Several unusual properties were observed that may play a role in the pathogenesis of RSD. First, these sprouts are extremely sensitive, even to light pressure stimulation. This is the basis for Tinel's sign, in which gentle tapping over a neuroma or sprouts will produce a strong, shocklike pain. Second, some of these fibers originating in the neuroma were capable of generating impulses in the absence of any obvious stimulation. Third, these fibers were found to be easily excited by small amounts of epinephrine and norepinephrine. Norepinephrine is the neurotransmitter released by the sympathetic nerve fibers. Sympathetic fibers will grow into the neuroma along with the other nerve fibers that were contained in the peripheral nerve. The proximity of these sprouts and the lack of an intact endoneural sheath provide an opportunity for cross talk or ephaptic transmission between fibers as described earlier.

CENTRAL NERVOUS SYSTEM ABNORMALITIES
Vicious circle hypothesis

Livingston proposed a central mechanism for causalgia and related states.[39] He stated that distorted information processing in the spinal cord caused by abnormal firing patterns in the internuncial pool of neurons set up a "vicious circle" of reflexes responsible for causalgia. deNo[40] wrote an elegant treatise on the activity of these internuncial neuronal chains and clarified the term as follows:

Impulses are conducted into a pool by afferent fibers and out of the pool by efferent fibers, which are axons of some cells of the pool. The cells of origin of the efferent fibers transmit the effect of the activity of the pool and may be called "effector neurons"; all the other nerve cells in the pool are internuncial neurons.

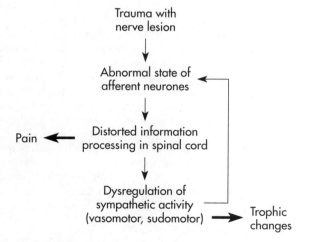

REFLEX SYMPATHETIC DYSTROPHY
(ALGODYSTROPHY)

Trauma with
nerve lesion

Abnormal state of
afferent neurones

Pain

Distorted information
processing in spinal cord

Dysregulation of
sympathetic activity
(vasomotor, sudomotor)

Trophic
changes

Fig. 48-5 Schematic expression of Livingston's hypothesis about the mechanism of generation of the syndrome of RSD. Note the cyclic response. (Redrawn from Blumberg H, Janig W: *J Auton Nerv Syst* 7:399-411, 1983.)

Livingston suggested that a partial nerve injury to a large nerve or to small nerves or nerve endings creates an irritative focus. This focus then presents the spinal cord with a constant bombardment of noxious impulses that overwhelm and upset the normal functioning of the internuncial pool. This initiates abnormal firing patterns and spawns closed, self-exciting neuronal loops in the dorsal horn of the spinal cord. Reverberating activity sends nerve impulses to the brain that are recognized as pain, and continued pool activity spreads to neurons in the anterior and lateral horns, giving rise to skeletal muscle spasm and sympathetic hyperdysfunction with vasoconstriction and tissue ischemia. This increases the noxious stimulation in the periphery, which added to the original injury or trigger point sustains and augments the abnormal central activity. In time, this process becomes self-sustaining and may spread to involve adjacent neuron pools and higher centers of the nervous system. Livingston recognized three components to this hypothesis. The first component is the abnormal afferent barrage of impulses from the periphery, the second is the internuncial pool activity in the spinal cord, and the third is the sympathetic and motor efferent activity, which in turn creates additional peripheral painful stimuli and completes this vicious circle.

Turbulence hypothesis

Sunderland[9,41] supported Livingston's theory of self-sustaining abnormal internuncial pool activity. He felt, however, that the pathologic basis of this abnormal activity was left unexplained and proposed the "turbulence hypothesis" to provide this missing link. Sunderland stated that causalgia is the "functional expression of the intensity of the retrograde neuronal reaction which follows nerve damage." When a peripheral nerve is damaged, the distal portion that is then separate from its cell body degenerates completely, as discussed previously in the section on neuroma formation. The proximal portion may also undergo retrograde changes that can affect the structure and function of parent cell bodies. Section of an axon does not invariably result in retrograde changes in the parent cell body, and the end result may be complete recovery, complete necrosis, or persistent functional impairment of the cell. The greater the violence causing the injury, the greater the retrograde reaction; thus an avulsion injury causes a more intense reaction than does surgical section of a nerve. Sunderland argued that the retrograde reaction can in fact cross a synapse and effect changes in neurons with which the initial damaged neuron communicates. This transsynaptic reaction may cause depression and failure of synaptic transmission or abnormalities in the pattern of synaptic activity and may account for the derangement in internuncial pool activity. Thus causalgia may be the result of peripheral nerve damage leading to retrograde neuronal reaction with injury or death of the parent sensory ganglion cells and further transsynaptic damage to dorsal horn cells with which they are connected. This can create hyperactive foci of abnormal spinal cord activity that become self-sustaining. These disturbances can induce similar changes along pathways as far centrally as the cortex itself, with causalgia the terminal effect of this abnormal activity. Self-sustaining activity would explain the spontaneous pain in causalgia. The ability of this reaction to spread to adjacent and higher centers would explain the extension of pain beyond the territory of the injured nerve and the difficulty in obtaining pain relief by interrupting the pain pathway at any level in the later phases of the disease.

Present status

It is known that injured tissue results in spontaneous pain, hyperalgesia, and allodynia. More recently, it has become evident that tissue injury is followed by increased responsiveness of nociceptive neurons of the spinal cord. Under some pathologic conditions, especially after nerve injury, A-beta input gains access to, and triggers, the NMDA receptor that is normally activated by C-afferent stimulation. Mechanical allodynia and slow temporal summation of allodynia may well be integrally related to the patient's ongoing "spontaneous pain."[41a]

CLINICAL PRESENTATION

RSD can be produced following any one of the causes listed in Box 48-2. Trauma secondary to accidental injury is probably the most common cause. Peculiar to sympathetic dystrophy is the lack of correlation among severity of injury, incidence, and subsequent severity of the resultant syndrome. In fact, severe trauma causing fractures of long bones and transection of nerves and blood vessels is less likely to be followed by RSD than are minor injuries to regions rich in nerve endings, such as the skin and pulp of fingertips, the skin of hands, and the periarticular structures of the interphalangeal, wrist, and ankle joints. In the majority of cases, the precipitating injury may be so minor and to the patient so insignificant that he or she may forget the incident until questioned by the physician.

In recent years it has become obvious that although injury is the most common cause, many visceral, neurologic, vascular, and musculoskeletal disorders may also produce RSD, presumably by producing injury to nerves that initiates a physiopathologic mechanism similar if not identical to that produced by external trauma. Perhaps the most notable disease process that produces RSD is myocardial infarction, although other thoracic disorders such as pneumonitis, carcinoma, and embolism may be followed several months later by RSD of the upper extremity. RSD may develop in patients with lesions of the central nervous system. Of these, vascular accidents involving the brain, and more particularly the thalamic region, with consequent hemiplegia, are the most common, but the same syndrome may be produced by tumors and diseases involving the brain, brainstem, or spinal cord. Infectious processes may incite RSD almost without respect to the system involved in the infection, and certain peripheral vascular diseases such thrombophlebitis often produce pain, edema, and vasomotor phenomena typical of RSD.

Signs and symptoms

RSD is manifested by pain, hyperesthesia, vasomotor and sudomotor disturbances, and increased muscular tone, followed by weakness, atrophy, and trophic changes involving the skin, and its appendages, muscles, bones, and joints.

Pain is certainly the most prominent and characteristic feature. Although it usually has a burning quality, not infrequently the patient describes it as an aching pain. It may vary in severity from mild discomfort to excruciating and intolerable pain, such as occurs with classical causalgia. The pain is usually constant but with recurrent paroxysmal aggravations. Initially the pain is localized to the site of injury, but typically with time it spreads to involve the entire extremity; in certain cases, the pain even spreads beyond the affected extremity to the contralateral limb, and sometimes even to the ipsilateral extremity or the entire side of the body. Hyperesthesia is almost invariably a part of the syndrome, and the patient characteristically protects the involved extremity in one way or another. Not infrequently, a patient will appear for treatment with the involved extremity wrapped in a protective cloth. If the examining physician attempts to touch the affected extremity, the patient characteristically withdraws and refuses to allow anything to make contact with it.

Disturbance of vasomotor function is the common denominator of all of the various types of sympathetic dystrophy and may manifest either as vasoconstriction, which produces cyanosis and coldness of the skin, or as vasodilatation, which results in a warm and erythematous extremity. Not infrequently, edema and sudomotor disturbances, usually hyperhidrosis, are also evident. As the disease progresses, trophic changes develop insidiously and include thin, glossy skin; atrophy of muscle; decalcification of bones; and usually loss of hair.

The severity of the signs and symptoms varies among patients and in the same patient in different phases of the disease. However, common to all cases of sympathetic dystrophy is the fact that the pain and physical signs do not conform to known patterns of nerve distribution, either segmental (dermatomes, myotomes, and sclerotomes) or peripheral. Moreover, they have a tendency to spread proximally to involve the contralateral and ipsilateral extremity. Once RSD has become established, the entire syndrome will continue even after the causal mechanism has healed or disappeared. An important characteristic common to all of the sympathetic dystrophies is the fact that the symptoms can be abol-

ished by sympathetic block at an appropriate level; if carried out before the point at which the syndrome becomes irreversible, repetitive interruption of the involved sympathetic pathways can result in resolution of the entire syndrome.

COURSE

Sympathetic dystrophy has three phases, and the presenting signs and symptoms will vary somewhat depending on the stage at the time the patient is first seen (Table 48-1).

Acute (hyperemic) stage

The acute, or hyperemic, stage commences at the time of injury or may be delayed for several weeks. It is characterized by constant pain, usually of a burning quality, of moderate severity, and localized to the area of injury. The pain is aggravated by movement and is associated with hyperpathia (delayed overreaction and aftersensation to a stimulus, particularly a repetitive one) and allodynia (pain elicited by a normally non-noxious stimulus, particularly if repetitive or prolonged). Hyperesthesia (increased sensitivity) and hypesthesia (decreased sensitivity) may also be present. The results are localized edema, muscle spasm, and tenderness. At this stage the skin is usually warm, red, and dry because of vasodilatation, although signs of vasoconstriction sometimes predominate late in this stage. Toward the end of this phase, the skin becomes smooth and taut, with decrease or loss of normal wrinkles and creases. Radiographs taken in this phase usually show slight, if any, osteoporosis. In mild cases the first stage lasts only a few weeks, but in severe cases this stage may last as long as 6 months. During this stage, the syndrome can be completely reversed by sympathetic blockade.

Dystrophic (ischemic) stage

If the acute stage is untreated, it can be expected to progress to the second, or dystrophic, stage. This stage is characterized by spreading of the edema, increasing stiffness of the joints, and muscular wasting. Pain remains the major symptom and is usually spontaneous and burning in nature. It may radiate proximally or distally from the site of injury

Table 48-1 Stages and characteristics of RSD

| Characteristic | Stage | | |
	I: Acute	II: Dystrophic	III: Atrophic
Pain	Burning/neuralgia+++	Burning/throbbing+++	Burning/throbbing++
Dysthesia	++	+++	+
Function	Minimal impairment	Restricted	Severely restricted
Autonomic dysfunction	Increased blood flow	NI or decreased flow	Decreased blood flow
Temperature	Increased	Decreased	Decreased
Discoloration	Erythematous	Mottled/dusky	Cyanotic
Sudomotor dysfunction	Minimal	++	+++
Edema	++	+++	+
Trophic changes	0	++	++++
3-phase bone scan	Increased activity, all images	Normal uptake, all phases except increased static phase	Decreased activity, all phases except NI static
Osteoporosis	—	+	+++

and may involve the whole extremity. Hyperpathia and allodynia are usually more pronounced than in the first stage. The skin is moist, cyanotic, and cold; the hair is coarse, and the nails show ridges and are brittle. Signs of atrophy become more prominent, and radiographs usually reveal patchy osteoporosis. During this stage, sympathetic blocks may still be effective in reversing the process, although the response to blockade may be short-lived and less pronounced. A larger series of blocks or prolonged sympathetic blockade may be necessary to afford permanent relief.

Atrophic stage

The third stage is characterized by marked trophic changes that eventually become irreversible. Pain is a less prominent feature. The skin becomes smooth, glossy, and tight; its temperature is lowered; and it appears pale or cyanotic in color. Although the hair is long at the beginning of this stage, by the end of the stage, the hair usually has fallen out. The subcutaneous tissues are atrophic, as are the muscles, particularly the interossei. There is extreme weakness and limitation of motion at virtually all of the involved joints, which finally become ankylosed. Contractions of the flexor tendons often occur at this stage; osteoporosis is more advanced, and the pain continues, aggravated by weight bearing, movement, and frequently by exposure to cold. At this point many of the trophic changes produced by the syndrome become irreversible, and although interruption of sympathetic pathways by blocks may still provide temporary relief, repetitive sympathetic blocks alone are no longer effective in terminating the process permanently. An aggressive approach including physical therapy, psychologic counseling, and sympathetic and somatic nerve blockade is needed to reverse the process as much as possible. No longer is the pathophysiology confined to an aberrant sympathetic reflex arc. Other nerve fiber types are now involved, including A-beta (mechanoreceptors) and A-delta (sharp pain) fibers. At this point the process may not respond to neural blockade, either chemical or surgical, performed at any point in the neuraxis because the self-sustaining mechanism may have moved to higher central nervous system centers, out of reach of these measures.

Diagnosis

A diagnosis of RSD may be obvious if (1) there is a history of recent or remote trauma, infection, or disease; (2) there is persistent, spontaneous pain that is burning, aching, or throbbing in character; (3) there are vasomotor or sudomotor disturbances; and (4) there are obvious trophic changes. However, although the "typical" case of RSD can be diagnosed without difficulty, many cases do not present with classic signs and symptoms but with vague and confusing symptomatology that not infrequently simulates other diseases. A number of diagnostic RSD scales have been proposed.[22,42,43] Current criteria under investigation by Wilson are shown in Box 48-3. A slightly different scheme using nine criteria has been proposed by Gibbons et al.[42] No weighting was given to these criteria, which include allodynia or hyperpathia, burning pain, edema, color changes or hair growth changes, sweating changes, temperature changes, radiographic demineralization, bone scan

---

Box 48-3 PUTATIVE DIAGNOSTIC CRITERIA FOR RSD

Clinical symptoms and signs
  Burning pain
  Hyperpathia/allodynia
  Temperature/color changes
  Edema
  Hair/nail growth changes
Laboratory results
  Thermography/thermometry
  Bone x-ray
  3-Phase bone scan
  Quantitative sweat test
  Response to sympathetic blockade
Interpretation based on number of criteria present
  >6, probable RSD
  3-5, possible RSD
  <3, unlikely RSD

---

consistent with RSD, and a positive response to the Quantitative Sudomotor Axon Reflex Test (Q-SART) or to sympathetic block.

A score of 0 is assigned if the criteria is absent, ½ if it is equivocal, and 1 if it is present. These scores are tabulated, and the following categories are arbitrarily determined:

0 to 2½	RSD absent
3 to 4½	Possible RSD
5 to 9	Probable RSD

As noted by Wilson,[43] these RSD scores attempt to imply presence or absence of RSD and not the severity grade (mild, moderate, or severe) or the phase (acute, dystrophic, or atrophic).

A more complicated and extensive matrix could be devised to include diagnosis, phase and grade, with possible and probable categories in each.

Differential diagnosis

Several postoperative or posttraumatic conditions have symptoms in common with causalgia and RSD. Peripheral nerve injuries may produce burning dysesthetic pain without a sympathetic nervous system component. Hyperpathia is frequently encountered within the distribution of transected or entrapped nerves. Pain is limited to the distribution of the involved nerve, and a positive Tinel's sign is often elicited over the site of nerve injury.

Inflammatory lesions such as tenosynovitis or bursitis may produce posttraumatic pain which may be burning in quality and may persist for months. Myofascial pain often develops after injury or surgery. It is nondermatomal in distribution, may be burning in nature, and is characterized by sensitive trigger points in affected muscles.[44] Although the truncal musculature is most often affected, such problems may also involve the extremities.

Raynaud's disease produces vasospasm of the extremities associated with cold skin, pallor, and often cyanosis. The condition is bilateral, involving the hands and sometimes all four extremities. The vasospasm may be relieved

Table 48-2 Retrograde differential epidural block*

Time (min)	Blood pressure (mmHg)	Pulse (beats/min)	Subjective feelings	Motor power			Sensation on pinprick	Temperature (° F)	
				Leg	Knee bend	Toes		R Leg	L Leg
Control	134/84	60	Burning pain in left foot	—	—	—		91	86
0	148/80	64	Burning pain in left foot	✓	✓	✓	✓	90	86
10	120/80	88	75% pain relief	25%	✓	✓	T_{10}	95	90
20	114/82	76	Total pain relief	—	—	—	T_8	95	92
60	140/96	64	Total pain relief	✓	✓	✓	T_{12}	95	92
70	140/96	64	Total pain relief	✓	✓	✓	✓	94	92
80	138/94	64	Total pain relief	✓	✓	✓	✓	92	90

* The results of a differential epidural block (20 ml of 3% 2-chloroprocaine) in a 22-year-old man with pain in the left foot. At first evaluation at the pain control center, patient gave the history of motor vehicle accident 6 months previously. He sustained a medial malleolar fracture at the ankle, which was surgically corrected and put in a cast. The fracture healed normally, but the patient complained of burning pain in his left foot, especially after weight bearing. A diagnosis of RSD of the left leg was made, and retrograde differential epidural block was done to confirm the diagnosis. Findings seen above show that total relief of pain was obtained by blocking the C-fibers only. A-delta and A-alpha nerve fibers did not transmit the nociceptive impulses. A series of six lumbar sympathetic blocks (left) were done at 2-week intervals with adjuvant physical therapy. The patient recovered completely.

by sympathetic blocks, but most patients are not helped by such treatment. Patients who experience transient vasodilatation with sympathetic blocks may benefit from sympathectomy or systemic α-adrenergic blocking agents.

Raynaud's phenomenon, a similar vasospastic disorder, is associated with an underlying pathologic process, frequently one of the connective tissue diseases such as scleroderma, and is often unilateral. As in Raynaud's disease, sympathetic blocks are helpful in a minority of patients.

Establishing an absolute diagnosis for a chronic pain problem is usually difficult, as multiple pain mechanisms often exist. It is often possible, however, to assess the importance of sympathetic mechanisms by comparing the degree and duration of pain relief achieved by sympathetic blocks with those produced by somatic blocks and placebo injections.

The response to a placebo injection (e.g., intramuscular saline) is often helpful diagnostically. A true placebo response, which is elicited in about one third of chronic pain patients, is usually brief (10 to 30 minutes). Pain relief persisting for days or weeks probably signifies a psychogenic pain mechanism. A very transitory response to the placebo and a prolonged analgesic effect from a sympathetic block (hours or days) provides some assurance that sympathetic pathways are involved in the pathogenesis of the pain. If no analgesia occurs after sympathetic block and pain is relieved by blocking the appropriate somatic nerves, then a somatic pain mechanism, such as neuralgia, myofascial syndrome, or radiculopathy, is likely. Failure of both sympathetic and somatic blocks to produce analgesia points to a central pain mechanism, which may be psychogenic or may result from neuronal activity within the CNS that is independent of peripheral input.

For the lower extremity pain, a differential spinal block may be used to distinguish among sympathetic, somatic, and central pain mechanisms. Following introduction of a needle into the subarachnoid space and with the patient positioned laterally, 10 ml of normal saline is injected. Relief

of pain is interpreted as a placebo response. If no analgesia occurs, 10 ml of 0.25% procaine is injected, which should block preganglionic sympathetic fibers while sparing somatic fibers. If signs of sympathetic blockade develop and pain relief ensues, a sympathetic pain mechanism is likely. If no analgesia occurs, 10 ml of 0.5% procaine is injected, and pain is reassessed after the onset of somatic blockade. Analgesia is interpreted as evidence of a somatic mechanism. Lack of pain relief points to a central or psychogenic mechanism.

Retrograde differential study can also be done as an epidural block, with less chance of postlumbar puncture headache.[45] Table 48-2 shows data from a retrograde differential epidural block in a 22-year-old man who developed RSD following a traumatic medial malleolar fracture.

Clinical investigations

Several clinical measurements and laboratory investigations are helpful in a diagnosis and treatment of patients with RSD. These studies can aid in confirmation of diagnosis and determination of phase and severity of the disease and provide objective baseline information that can then be used to monitor the patient's response to therapy.

Temperature measurement

Temperature changes in the affected extremity are a simple but important observation to record during examination of the patient with suspected RSD. Skin temperature depends on cutaneous blood flow, which is under the control of the sympathetic nervous system. Early in the course of RSD (hyperemic phase), the affected extremity may be warmer than other tissues, whereas later in the course, skin blood flow and temperature may be reduced. Although the examiner's tactile perception of temperature difference between the two extremities offers only a gross qualitative temperature measurement, surface thermistors and hand-held infrared thermometers allow for quantification and baseline recordings.

Thermography

Thermography is a noninvasive procedure that images the temperature distribution of the body surface. In contrast to radiographs, computed tomography (CT) scans, and myelography, which show only anatomic changes, thermography demonstrates functional changes in circulation following damage to nerves, ligaments, muscles, or joints.[43,46-48]

Fine detail radiography

The earliest radiographic evidence of sympathetic hyperdysfunction includes patchy demineralization of the epiphyses and short bones of the hands and feet. Subperiosteal resorption, striation, and tunneling of the cortex may occur. However, these unilateral changes are not diagnostic of RSD and may occur in any condition producing disuse of one limb. This patchy osteopenia is generally not appreciated until the disease advances to the second phase.[43,49]

Triple phase scintigraphy

Triple phase radionuclide bone scanning is helpful in both confirming the diagnosis of RSD and excluding other conditions that could be a cause of symptoms.[50] Sensitivity and specificity of this technique has varied, largely because of a lack of common diagnostic criteria.[25,51,52] The scan pattern most commonly associated with RSD is that of increased flow to the involved extremity and delayed static images that show diffusely increased activity throughout the involved extremity, usually in a periarticular distribution.

Based on more recent refinement of bone scan criteria, grading of RSD was accomplished by evaluating both early (flow and blood pool) images and delayed (static) images according to a system of bone scan interpretation and bone density measurement.[53]

Interpretation of bone scans

Differential diagnosis is not usually a problem, as few conditions mimic this scan appearance, and clinical information provides specificity. However, somewhat similar scan appearances may occur in several conditions, as noted by Lowry, including disuse osteoporosis, cellulitis, degenerative joint disease, recent trauma, and osteomyelitis. Clinical presentation, time course of the disease, and scan appearance should help differentiate these conditions.

False-negative bone scans may be fairly common.[53] Many "normal" scans correspond to phase 2 RSD as determined on clinical grounds. The most likely explanation is that as the condition progresses, the initial state of hyperemia becomes, in later stages, that of decreased flow. As this change occurs gradually, the disease passes through an intermediate stage of "normal" perfusion, at which time the bone scan appearance may be entirely normal as well. In these cases, diagnosis remains an entirely clinical one, and the bone scan is helpful only in ruling out other causes of the patient's pain (e.g., occult fracture or infection).

Bone density measurement

Nuclear bone density measurements provide a quantitative baseline measure of bone density and later provide a way to follow long-term progress of the patient.

Electromyogram

There is no evidence that peripheral neuromuscular function is abnormal in sympathetic pain states. Abnormalities seen on electromyogram (EMG) may reflect the initial injury, although evidence for EMG changes as reflex sympathetic dystrophy develops is lacking.[36,43]

Tests of sudomotor function

Sympathetic cholinergics control sweating, but an estimate of sweat production can be made by a variety of methods. Surface moisture can be demonstrated by application of triketohydrindene hydrate (Ninhydrin), cobalt blue, or starch-iodide to the skin. In the Q-SART, a perspex capsule is placed on the skin and the increase in humidity of air blown through the capsule is measured. Sweat output can then be stimulated by iontophoresis of acetylcholine into the skin, and stimulated sweat output can be measured. The stimulated output is greater and prolonged when sympathetic hyperfunction is present.[43,54]

Psychologic evaluation

The psychologic assessment is conducted to obtain understanding of the psychosocial stressors that may adversely affect treatment and to obtain information about the psychologic distress patients may be experiencing as a result of the pain and subsequent loss of function. The evaluation should consist of a structured clinical interview and personality measures such as the Minnesota Multiphasic Personality Inventory (MMPI) and the Hopelessness Index.

Previous pilot research indicates that as the RSD progresses, patients' MMPI profiles tend to resemble those of patients experiencing chronic pain, as revealed by the increasing elevations on the hypochondriasis, depression, and hysteria scales. Phase 1 patients also report more pessimism than do patients in the second and third phases of the disorder, which suggests that patients have more difficulty adjusting to the disorder in the early phases. Younger patients with RSD tend to report more pessimism and symptoms of depression than do older patients.[50]

CURRENT TREATMENT

Because the pathophysiology of RSD is predominantly a hyperactivity of the regional sympathetic nervous system, pain management in such patients should focus on interrupting the activity of the sympathetic nervous system. This interruption can be produced by different modalities classified as pharmacologic, nerve blocks, surgical or chemical sympathectomy, physical therapy, and psychology. In addition, a serious effort has to be made toward maintaining function and alleviating the stresses produced by the syndrome on the central nervous system.

Reports of treatment efficacy in RSD are plagued by the lack of uniform quantification of treatment outcome as defined by change in pain or improvement in function. This nonuniformity of outcome measurement as well as inconsistent diagnostic criteria make it difficult to draw hard inferences from many published therapeutic trials in RSD patients.[55]

PHARMACOLOGIC TREATMENT

Many drugs have been used in the treatment of RSD (Box 48-4). A wide variety of unrelated agents have been used in treating RSD because a patient suffering from this syndrome can go through phases of severe pain, limited function, and depression and eventually develop a full-blown chronic pain syndrome. For example, a patient with RSD may have severe pain requiring analgesics, often opiates, which are particularly habit-forming in these patients. As the disease progresses, anxiety increases concerning the chronicity of the illness, loss of work, and social and familial dysfunction, requiring anxiolytics. Sleep is lost to pain and worry, prompting the use of a sedative hypnotic. Exhaustion develops both physically and emotionally. The situation magnifies, and depression increases. Tricyclic antidepressants may then be prescribed. Sympathetic hyperdysfunction causes vasoconstriction, pain, and swelling as detailed previously, necessitating sympathetic blockade with local anesthetics, sympathetic blocking drugs, or vasodilatation with vasodilatating drugs. A myofascial pain component is common in reflex sympathetic dystrophy, thus a nonsteroidal antiinflammatory agent or a muscle relaxant is often utilized. At this time, anticonvulsants are used to quiet a painful peripheral or central epileptogenic focus. Rarely, neurolytic agents are used to destroy the sympathetic pathways.

Antidepressants

Three effects of tricyclic antidepressants make this class of drugs valuable in the treatment of RSD: sedation, analgesia, and mood elevation. The analgesic action of the tricyclics may be related to inhibition of serotonin reuptake at nerve terminals of neurons that act to suppress pain transmission, with resultant prolongation of serotonin activity at the receptor.[56] If that indeed is the mechanism, then amitriptyline, which has the most potent effect on the amine production, should be the most effective of the tricyclics. It is used most commonly in a dose of 50 to 100 mg orally at bedtime. Others, however, are used for their varying anti-

---

Box 48-4 DRUGS USED IN THE TREATMENT OF RSD

Antidepressants
Sedative-hypnotics
Anxiolytics
Anticonvulsants
Muscle relaxants
Narcotic analgesics
Nonnarcotic analgesics
Nonsteroidal antiinflammatory agents
Corticosteroids
Local anesthetics
Sympathetic blocking agents
Vasodilators
Neurolytics

---

cholinergic properties as well as their promotion of weight gain and effectiveness in treating sexual dysfunction.[57,58]

Narcotic analgesics

Systemic narcotics are often abused by those with chronic pain. Eventually they do little to treat sympathetic pain because tolerance develops and alternate pathways may be used by nociceptive impulses. However, when given epidurally in combination with local anesthetics in an acute inpatient setting, narcotics are extremely effective analgesics. This route also allows maximum narcotic effect in the dorsal horn with very low plasma concentrations, thus minimizing toxicity. Both morphine and fentanyl have been used by continuous infusion in doses of 0.5 mg/hour and 0.03 to 0.05 mg/hour, respectively. For chronic oral therapy, narcotics are used sparingly and only if nonnarcotic agents have been tried without success. However, in an inpatient setting, a carefully ordered narcotic regimen may be necessary to promote an effective physical therapy program. Morphine and methadone have both been used in this setting with success.

Oral nifedipine

Following a report of the use of oral nifedipine in the treatment of Raynaud's phenomenon[59] and a report by Prough and McLesky[60] of the use of oral nifedipine in the treatment of RSD, we have begun using orally administered nifedipine to relieve symptoms. Nifedipine, a calcium channel blocker, relaxes smooth muscle, increases peripheral blood flow, and antagonizes the effect of norepinephrine on arterial and venous smooth muscle. Thus it induces peripheral vasodilatation. Experience with this technique suggests that nifedipine in a dose of 10 to 30 mg TID PO may be an effective therapeutic option for the treatment of patients with RSD. In a series of thirteen patients, seven developed complete relief of symptoms, two had partial relief, and one patient failed to obtain any degree of relief. Nifedipine was withdrawn from three of the patients because of the side effect of headache.

Systemic corticosteroids

Kozin et al.[52] advocate a several-day course of high-dose systemic corticosteroids. They reported an 82% success rate in patients with "definite" RSD. Their criteria, however, were not very rigid, and three of the most important ones (burning pain, hyperpathia, and response to sympathetic block) were not among them. Many of the patients who responded to steroids had chronic pain (mean duration of pain for the group was 25 weeks). A trial of steroids might be a reasonable form of treatment for patients with longstanding pain who have failed to respond to blocks.

Adrenergic blocking agents

The use of systemic adrenergic blocking agents has met with only limited success. Several patients treated by McLesky, all of whom had pain for more than six months, experienced moderate improvement in pain, swelling, and vasoconstriction with oral prazosin treatment; the most gratifying response was in a patient with recurrent foot pain after sympathectomy. Intravenous phentolamine appears to be useful in predicting favorable responses to prazosin, as only those patients who experienced pain relief and increased skin temperature in the affected limb responded to the oral medication. Orthostatic dizziness was seen occasionally with prazosin and precluded its continued use in a few patients. As with causalgia, propranolol has been reported to be effective in the management of reflex sympathetic dystrophy.[61,62]

Nerve blocks

Although the causal mechanisms of RSD are not limited purely to sympathetic hyperactivity, sympathetic blockade and physical therapy are the mainstays of current therapeutic management. Most patients respond in an impressive manner to sympathetic blockade, and permanent resolution is possible if therapy is instituted before irreversible changes have occurred.

A series of sympathetic blocks should be performed and continued until minimal discomfort persists. If repeat injections in this manner are not possible (e.g., patient's reluctance for multiple needle sticks or inability of the patient to travel because of injury or distance), then admission to the hospital for continuous infusion of local anesthetic at the appropriate site is an alternative. For upper extremity RSD, the site of block is either at the stellate ganglion level or on the brachial plexus. Continuous stellate ganglion blockade has been reported with the use of an indwelling catheter. In a series of 29 patients with upper extremity RSD, improvement was seen in all but two patients with regard to pain. Long-term follow-up demonstrated a relapse rate of 25%, but marked improvement persisted in the rest of the patients.[63] There are numerous approaches available for blockade of the brachial plexus. For repetitive blocks, the axillary approach is the most convenient. The infraclavicular approach is excellent for continuous infusion techniques. The thoracic sympathetic chain is not a convenient site for repeated injections, is technically difficult, and requires the use of radiographic guidance. For lower extremity disease, the lumbar sympathetic chain or epidural space is the preferred site for sympathetic blockade. Either of these sites can be used with repetitive injection and continuous infusion techniques. Wang et al.[64] treated 71 patients with lower extremity RSD; of the 27 patients treated by conservative means, 41% showed improvement at 3-years' follow-up. Of the 43 patients treated with sympathetic blockade, 65% experienced progress at the 3-year evaluation. Conduction of nerve impulses through the various size nerves can be controlled by the concentration of local anesthetic injected. Low concentration lidocaine (1%) or bupivacaine (0.25%) blocks C fibers, which conduct visceral afferent impulses and dull, aching somatic pain impulses. Moderate concentration lidocaine (1.5%) or bupivacaine (0.5%) blocks A-delta fibers, which conduct sharp somatic pain impulses.

Neurolytic sympathetic blockade is not commonly performed for treatment of RSD of the upper extremity because of the close proximity of the cervical nerve roots to the cervical sympathetic chain. However, lumbar sympathetics are very amenable to neurolytic block and may be chosen as an alternative to surgical sympathectomy for persistent lower extremity involvement.

Treatment methods gaining popularity include the intravenous regional block technique (Bier block) employing reserpine, guanethidine, and bretylium, as well as nifedipine, a calcium channel blocker, as a vasodilator.[65-71]

Intravenous regional block (Bier block)

Intravenous or intraarterial infusion of ganglionic blocking agents into the affected extremity have recently gained prominence in the treatment of RSD.[65,67,69] There are two reasons why intravenous administration of ganglionic blockers is superior to intraarterial injection for treatment of RSD. First, the likelihood of systemic side effects from an injection of these vasodilating agents is significantly greater if administered intraarterially than if administered in an intravenous regional block (Bier block) technique. Second, it has been proposed that when these drugs are administered by an intravenous regional anesthetic, they are permitted to have more protracted contact with the affected extremity, allowing them to fix to the tissue and hopefully produce more significant and prolonged improvement in symptomatology. Experience with intravenous regional reserpine techniques is controversial. Abrams[3] and Brown[67] have found the results of this technique to be sporadic, and side effects including postural hypotension, facial flushing, and burning on injection are relatively common.

In an attempt to improve results and lessen side effects during treatment of patients with RSD, guanethidine has been substituted for reserpine in the intravenous regional block format. Results with the intravenous regional guanethidine technique from Europe and selected North American centers appear to be more consistent and more reliable than those with intravenous regional reserpine.[52,70,72] For upper extremity blocks, 20 mg guanethidine is diluted in 40 ml 0.25% lidocaine or 50 cc 0.25% lidocaine for lower extremity blocks. The solution is injected into an exsanguinated extremity with drug contact permitted for 30 to 45 minutes by tourniquet inflation. McLeskey et al.[74] found partial or complete success in the treatment of painful symptoms in 25 of 35 patients treated in this manner. Repeat block was required in four of these patients. The average duration of improvement of symptomatology was 17 days, with complete, permanent relief of symptoms in three patients. Side effects following intravenous regional guanethidine block are fewer than are often seen with intravenous regional reserpine block. However, patients frequently complain of burning pain of the extremity during injection of the drug, which lasts for approximately 4 to 5 minutes. Orthostatic hypotension was not seen, although precaution should still be taken to lessen the likelihood of this problem. Guanethidine is for investigational use in the United States and is not clinically available.

Intravenous regional bretylium has also been used because of its ability to accumulate in adrenergic nerves and block norepinephrine release. In a report of four patients with RSD, Ford[73] noted good to excellent pain relief in all of the patients for up to 7 months after treatment. In addition, bretylium produced objective signs of prolonged sympatholytic activity and improved function in all four patients, and side effects were minimal. Thus bretylium appears to be an attractive alternative to guanethidine or reserpine as an adrenergic blocking agent.[73]

Surgical sympathectomy

Surgical sympathectomy has been advocated for patients who do not experience permanent relief from blocks or other conservative measures. Kleinert et al.[74] reported on a series of 183 patients with upper extremity sympathetic dystrophy who were initially treated with sympathetic blocks. No demonstrable improvement was seen in 39 patients, but permanent improvement was achieved in 121 patients. In the remaining 23 patients, who experienced only transient relief from blocks, surgical sympathectomy was performed, producing permanent relief in all but four patients.

A study by Mockus et al.[75] of 34 patients who underwent sympathectomy for causalgia pain showed that satisfactory relief of pain was achieved in 97% of patients immediately postoperatively. Postsympathectomy neuralgia was seen in 40% of patients, lasting just over 1 month on average, and a 10% wound complication rate was seen. Extended follow-up showed satisfactory pain relief in 94% of the patients, with 84% reporting the same degree of relief than they experienced immediately postoperatively.

Immediate or delayed failure of sympathectomy to relieve pain in RSD may be a result of reinnervation from the contralateral lumbar sympathetic chain.[76,77] Anatomic studies of the lumbar sympathetic chain have displayed cross communications of fibers.[79]

Before electing sympathectomy, the following criteria should be met:

1. The patient should experience pain relief from sympathetic blocks on several occasions.
2. Pain relief should last at least as long as the vascular effects of the block.
3. Placebo injection should produce no pain relief, or the relief should be less pronounced and of shorter duration than that achieved with local anesthetic sympathetic blocks.
4. Possible secondary gain motives and significant psychopathology should be ruled out as possible causes of pain complaints.

Chemical sympathectomy

Neurolytic lumbar sympathetic block may be chosen as an alternative to surgical sympathectomy for lower extremity dystrophy. Boas et al.[80] cite 100% success in five patients treated with phenol sympathectomy (i.e., permanent). However, because of the proximity of the roots of the brachial plexus to the cervical sympathetic chain, neurolytic sympathectomy for upper extremity pain is too hazardous.

Sympathectomy is not without potential problems. Patients are occasionally bothered by dermatologic problems associated with skin dryness. A painful condition, sometimes termed *sympathalgia,* may begin in the second or third postoperative week.[81] Patients experience muscle fatigue, heaviness, deep pain, and tenderness in the limb that may continue for weeks. When sympathectomy includes ablation of the stellate ganglion, the resultant ptosis, conjunctival injection, and nasal congestion may be distressing but can usually be controlled with the use of 10% phenylephrine eye drops.

Physical therapy

Physical therapy is an important adjunct to sympathetic blocks and may be effective alone for the treatment of mild cases of reflex sympathetic dystrophy.[82] For longstanding cases, extensive physical rehabilitation may be necessary. Active and active assisted range-of-motion exercises, muscle strengthening and conditioning, massage, and heat (whirlpool, paraffin, or radiant heat) are particularly useful. Low-dose ultrasound (0.5 W/cm^2 $\times$ 5 minutes) has been used by Portwood et al.[83] in three patients with RSD of the lower extremity. Two of the three patients had been refractory to pharmacologic therapy, and all three preferred a conservative approach to surgical sympathectomy. All three patients were symptom free, and no complications were observed at the end of the study period. It is hypothesized that ultrasound may affect the peripheral sympathetic nerve fibers in addition to increasing blood flow to the limb.

Vigorous passive range-of-motion exercises and the use of heavy weights may retrigger symptoms. Exercises are best performed during analgesic periods following sympathetic blocks. Frequently pain is severe enough to interfere with the patient's ability to do meaningful physical therapy. These patients may require hospital admission and aggressive analgesia by way of the epidural, intravenous, or oral routes in order to participate in an effective physical therapy program.

Transcutaneous electrical nerve stimulation (TENS)

TENS has been effective as the sole treatment[84] and as an adjunctive therapy for sympathetic dystrophy. Pain control may be achieved with the regular use of TENS in some patients with longstanding sympathetic dystrophy who have not responded to sympathetic blocks. Increased skin temperature has been documented during TENS therapy.[85]

Psychology

Psychologic intervention in RSD patients should have the following three purposes:

1. Help patients deal with the psychologic distress (e.g., depression, anxiety) that results from the prolonged pain experience
2. Address psychosocial factors that may adversely affect the patient's response to treatment
3. Teach effective coping strategies

The various interventions include psychotherapy, family therapy, stress management training, biofeedback, and relaxation training. Psychotherapy and family therapy are aimed at helping patients deal with the adverse effects of pain on functioning as well as with the factors that could have a negative impact on response to treatment. Stress management training, which may include biofeedback and relaxation training, helps the patient learn effective methods of dealing with the pain or with factors that cause the pain symptomatology to exacerbate (i.e., stress).[50,86,87]

Even though a small number of patients with RSD get better spontaneously or with minimal medical procedures, the majority of them suffer for 1 to 1½ years before they begin to approach a normal and productive state. Patients in the second and third phase of the syndrome require a multidisciplinary approach to manage pain, depression, functional disability, and possible drug abuse.

REFERENCES

1. Mitchell SW: On the diseases of nerves resulting from injuries. In Flint A, editors: *Contributions Relating to the Causation and Prevention of Disease, and to Camp Disease.* United States Sanitary Commission Memoirs. New York, The Commission, 1867.
2. International Symposium on Reflex Sympathetic Dystrophy. Mainz, Germany, 1988.
3. Abrams SE: Intravenous reserpine. *Anesth Analg* 59:889-890, 1980.
4. Paré A: Of the cure of wounds of the nervous parts. In *The Collected Works of Ambroise Paré.* Pound Ridge, Milford House, Book 10:400-402, 1634 (Translated by T. Johnson).
5. Mitchell SW, Morehouse GR, Keen WW: Gunshot wounds and other injuries of nerves. Philadelphia, JB Lippincott, 1864.
6. Abrams SE: Intra-arterial reserpine. *Anesth Analg* 59:889-890, 1980.
7. IASP Subcommittee on Taxonomy. Reflex sympathetic dystrophy (I-5). *Pain* (suppl 3):S29-S30, 1986.
8. Melzack R, Wall PD: Pain mechanisms. A new theory. *Science* 150:971-978, 1965.
9. Sunderland S: Pain mechanisms in causalgia. *J Neurol Neurosurg Psychiatry* 39:471-480, 1976.
10. Sweet W: Deafferentation pain. *Man Appl Neurophysiol* 51:117-127, 1988.
11. Bonica JJ: Causalgia and other reflex sympathetic dystrophies. *Postgrad Med* 53:143-148, 1973.
12. Lankford LL: Reflex sympathetic dystrophy. In Hunter JM et al, editors: *Rehabilitation of the Hand.* St Louis, Mosby, 1984.
13. Zimmermann M: Peripheral and central nervous mechanisms of nociception, pain, and pain therapy. Facts and hypotheses. In Bonica J, editor: *Advances in Pain Research and Therapy, vol 3.* New York, Raven Press, 1979.
14. Bonica JJ: Causalgia and other reflex sympathetic dystrophies. In Bonica J, editor: *Advances in Pain Research and Therapy, vol 3.* New York, Raven Press, 1979.
15. Melzack R: Clinical aspects of pain. In *The puzzle of pain.* New York, Basic Books, 1973.
16. Wall PD: The prevention of postoperative pain. *Pain* 33:289-290, 1988.
17. Kuntz A, Farnsworth D: Distribution of afferent fibers via the sympathetic trunks and gray communication rami to the brachial and lumbosacral plexuses. *Comp Neurol* 53:389-399, 1973.
18. Tahmoush AJ: Causalgia. Redefinition as a clinical pain syndrome. *Pain* 10:187-197, 1981.
19. de Takats G: Causalgia states in peace and war. *JAMA* 128:699-704, 1945.
20. Lewis D, Gatewood W: Treatment of causalgia: Results of intraneural injections of 60% alcohol. *JAMA* 74:1-4, 1920.
21. Leriche R: Causalgia envisage comme une neurite du sympathique et son traitement par la denudation et l'excision de plexus nerveux periarteriels. *Presse Med* 23:184, 1916.
22. Kuntz A: Afferent innervation of peripheral blood vessels through sympathetic trunks. *J South Med Assoc* 44:673-678, 1951.
23. Kuntz A, Saccomanno G: Afferent conduction from extremities through dorsal root fibers via sympathetic trunks. *Arch Surg* 14:606-612, 1942.
24. Threadgill FD, Solnitzky O: Anatomical studies of afferency within the lumbosacral sympathetic ganglia. *Anat Rec* 103:96, 1949.
25. Greyson ND, Tepperman PS: Three-phase bone studies in hemiplegia with reflex sympathetic dystrophy and the effect of disuse. *J Nucl Med* 25:423-429, 1984.
26. Reference deleted in proofs.
27. White JD, Smithwick RH: *The Autonomic Nervous System.* New York, Macmillan, 1941.
28. Foerster O: *Die Leitungsbahnen des Schmerzgefuhls und die chirurgische Behandlung der Schmerzzustande.* Berlin, Urban & Schwartzenberg, 1927.
29. Doupe J, Cullen CR, Chance GQ: Post-traumatic pain and the causalgia syndromes. *J Neurol Neurosurg Psychiatry* 7:33-48, 1944.
30. Chapman LF, et al: Neurohumoral features of afferent fibers in man. *Arch Neurol* 49:82, 1961.
31. Pool. *Neurosurg* 3:468-473, 1946.
32. Bonica JJ: Causalgia and other reflex sympathetic dystrophies. In *The Management of Pain.* Philadelphia, Lea & Febiger, 1953.
33. Granit R, Leksell L, Skoglund CR: Fibre interaction in injured or compressed region of nerve. *Brain* 67:125-140, 1944.
34. Noordenbos W: *1955 Pain: Problems Pertaining to the Transmission of Nervous Impulses Which Give Rise to Pain; Preliminary Statements.* Amsterdam, Elsevier, 1959.
35. Nathan PW: The gate control theory and pain: A critical review. *Brain* 99:123-158, 1976.
36. Devor M: Nerve pathophysiology and mechanisms of pain in causalgia. *J Auton Nerv Sys* 7:371-384, 1983.
37. Melzack R, Wall PD: Pain after injuries of the nervous system. In *The Challenge of Pain.* New York, Basic Books, 1983.
38. Wall PD, Gutnick M: Ongoing activity in peripheral nerves. The physiology and pharmacology of impulses originating from a neuroma by stimulation of the sympathetic supply in the rat. *Neurosci Lett* 24:43-47, 1981.
39. Livingston WK: *Pain Mechanisms. A Physiologic Interpretation of Causalgia and Its Related States.* New York, MacMillan, 1944.
40. Reference deleted in proofs.
41. Sunderland S, Kelly M: The painful sequelae to peripheral nerves. *Aust NZJ Surg* 18:75-118, 1948.
41a. Price DD, Mao J, Mayer DJ: Neural mechanisms of normal and abnormal pain states. In Raj PP, editor: *Current Review of Pain.* Philadelphia, Current Medicine, 1994.
42. Peretti G: Pain as the cause of limitation of joint movement in degenerative lesions of arthrosis. In Tiengo M, et al, editors: *Advances in Pain Research and Therapy.* New York, Raven Press, 1987.
43. Wilson P: Sympathetically maintained pain. In Stanton-Hicks M, editor: *Sympathetic Pain.* Boston, Kluwer Academic Publishers, 1989.
44. McCain G, Scudds R: The concept of primary fibromyalgia. *Pain* 33:273-287, 1988.
45. Raj PP: *Case histories (2): Nesacaine for retrograde differential blocking. Nesacaine in case studies in obstetrical and surgical regional anesthesia.* New York, Pennwalt Corporation, 1979.
46. Pochaczevsky R et al: Liquid crystal thermography of the spine and extremities. *J Neurosurg* 56:386-395, 1982.
47. Pochaczevsky R: Thermography in skeletal and soft tissue trauma. In Traverss J et al, editors: *Radiology.* Philadelphia, JB Lippincott, 1987.
48. Thomas PS, Zauder HL: Thermography. In Raj PP, editor: *The Practical Management of Pain.* St Louis, Mosby, 1986.
49. Fahr LM, Sauser DD: Imaging of peripheral nerve lesions. *Orthop Clin North Am* 19:27-41, 1988.
50. Raj PP et al: Management protocol of reflex sympathetic dystrophy. In Stanton-Hicks M, editor: *Sympathetic Pain.* Boston, Kluwer Academic Publications, 1989.
51. Constantinesco A et al: Three-phase bone scanning as an aid to early diagnosis in reflex sympathetic dystrophy of the hand: A study of eighty-nine cases. *Ann Chir Pain* 5(2):93-104, 1986.
52. Kozin F et al: The reflex sympathetic dystrophy syndrome (RSDS). III Scintigraphic studies, further evidence for the therapeutic efficacy of systemic corticosteroids, and proposed diagnostic criteria. *Am J Med* 70:23-30, 1981.
53. Raj PP et al: Multidisciplinary management of reflex sympathetic dystrophy. In Stanton-Hicks M, editor: *Current Management of Pain.* Boston, Kluwer Academic Publications, 1990.
54. Low PA et al: Quantitative sudomotor axon reflex test in normal and neuropathic subjects. *Ann Neurol* 14:573-580, 1983.
55. Davidoff G, Morey K, Stamps J: Pain measurement in reflex sympathetic dystrophy syndrome. *Pain* 32:27-34, 1988.
56. Hollister L: Tricyclic antidepressants. *N Engl J Med* 99, 1978.
57. Abrams SE: Pain of sympathetic origin. In Raj PP, editor: *The Practical Management of Pain.* St Louis, Mosby, 1986.
58. Oxman T, Denson D: Antidepressants and adjunctive psychotropic

drugs. In Raj PP, editor: *The Practical Management of Pain.* St Louis, Mosby, 1986.

59. Rodeheffer RJ et al: Controlled double-blind trial of nifedipine in the treatment of Raynaud's phenomenon. *N Engl J Med* 308:880-883, 1983.

60. Prough DS et al: Efficacy of oral nifedipine in the treatment of reflex sympathetic dystrophy. *Anesthesiol* 61:3A, September 1984.

61. Sison G: Propranolol for causalgia and Sudek's atrophy. *JAMA* 227-327, 1974.

62. Visitunthorn U, Prete P: Reflex sympathetic dystrophy of the lower extremity. A complication of herpes zoster with dramatic response to propranolol. *West J Med* 135:62-66, 1981.

63. Linson M, Leffort R, Todd D: The treatment of upper extremity reflex syspathetic dystrophy with prolonged continuous stellate ganglion blockade. *J Hand Surg* 8(2):153-159, 1983.

64. Wang J, Johnson K, Ilstrup D: Sympathetic blocks for reflex sympathetic dystrophy. *Pain* 23:13-17, 1985.

65. Benzon HT, Chomka CM, Brenner EA: Treatment of reflex sympathetic dystrophy with regional intravenous reserpine. *Anesth Analg* 59:500-502, 1980.

66. Bonelli S et al: Regional intravenous guanethidine vs. stellate ganglion block in reflex sympathetic dystrophies: A randomized trial. *Pain* 16:297-307, 1983.

67. Brown BR: Intra-arterial reserpine. *Anesth Analg* 59:889, 1980.

68. Davies JAH, Beswick T, Dickson G: Ketanserin and guanethidine in the treatment of causalgia. *Anesth Analg* 66:575-576, 1987.

69. Kepes ER et al: Regional intravenous guanethidine for sympathetic blockade. Report of 10 cases. *Reg Anaesth* 7:52-54, 1982.

70. Sonneveld GJ, Vander Muelen JC, Smith AR: Quantitative oxygen measurements before and after intravascular guanethidine blocks. *J Hand Surg* 8:435-442, 1983.

71. Thomsen MB et al: Changes in human forearm blood flow after intravenous regional sympathetic blockade with guanethidine. *Acta Chir* (Scand) 48:657-661, 1982.

72. Hannington-Kiff JG: Intravenous regional sympathetic block with guanethidine. *Lancet* 1:1019-1020, 1974.

73. McLeskey CH et al: Use of cold-stress test and IV regional reserpine block to diagnose and treat reflex sympathetic dystrophy. *Anesthesiol* 59(A):199, 1983.

74. Ford S, Forrest W, Eltherington L: The treatment of reflex sympathetic dystrophy with intravenous regional guanethidine. *Anesthesiol* 68:137-140, 1988.

75. Kleinert HE et al: Post-traumatic sympathetic dystrophy. *Orthop Clin North Am* 4:917-927.

76. Mockus MM et al: Sympathectomy for causalgia. *Arch Surg* 12:668-672, 1987.

77. Kleinman A: Evidence of the existence of crossed sensory sympathetic fibers. *Am J Surg* 87:839-841, 1954.

78. Munn J, Baker W: Recurrent sympathetic dystrophy: Successful treatment by contralateral sympathectomy. *Surgery* 102:102-105.

79. Lowenberg R, Morton D: The anatomic and surgical significance of the lumbar sympathetic nervous system. *Ann Surg* 133:525-532, 1951.

80. Boas RA, Hatangdi VS, Richards EG: Lumbar sympathectomy—A percutaneous technique. In Bonica JJ, Albe-Fessard D, editors: *Advances in Pain Research and Therapy.* New York, Raven Press, 1976.

81. Hermann LG, Reineke HG, Caldwell JA: Post-traumatic painful osteoporosis: A clinical and roentgenological entity. *Am J Radiol* 47:353-361, 1942.

82. Pak TJ et al: Reflex sympathetic dystrophy: Review of 140 cases. *Minn Med* 53:507-512, 1970.

83. Portwood M, Lieberman JS, Taylor RG: Ultrasound treatment of reflex sympathetic dystrophy. *Arch Phys Med Rehab* 68(2):116-118, 1987.

84. Stilz RJ, Carron H, Sanders DB: Reflex sympathetic dystrophy in a 6-year-old. Successful treatment by transcutaneous nerve stimulation. *Anesth Analg* 56:438-443, 1977.

85. Abrams SE, Asiddao CB, Reynolds AC: Increased skin temperature during transcutaneous electrical simulation. *Anesth Analg* 59:22-25, 1980.

86. Barowsky E, Zweig J, Moskowitz J: Thermal biofeedback in the treatment of symptoms associated with reflex sympathetic dystrophy. *J Child Neurol* 2(3):229-232, 1987.

87. Sherry D, Weisman R: Psychologic aspects of childhood reflex neurovascular dystrophy. *Pediatrics* 88(4):572-578, 1988.

APPENDIX

REPETITIVE STRAIN INJURY

Repetitive strain injury has also been called cumulative trauma disorder, regional pain syndrome, and overuse syndrome. All have features of sympathetically maintained pain: impairment of function, allodynia, paresthesia, numbness, and hyperesthesia throughout the entire extremity. Autonomic disturbances including Raynaud's phenomenon may be present. Frank reflex sympathetic dystrophy can occur. There is usually no history of trauma, and although these symptoms may arise de novo, they may also take many weeks to appear.

Characteristically, none of these states responds to pure sympathetic blocks, either with or without physical therapy.

However, to enable the restoration of function without pain, somatic blocks are often helpful. This would suggest that such conditions are not primary disorders of the autonomic nervous system. As with conditions of the lower limb, determination of the response to sympathetic or somatic block may be the crux of making a differential diagnosis between a somatic pain mechanism (e.g., neuralgia, myofascial syndrome, or radiculopathy) and a sympathetically maintained pain condition. A prolonged response to a sympathetic block would obviously support a diagnosis of sympathetic dysfunction as being a prominent component, if not the cause, of the patient's symptoms.

QUESTIONS: REFLEX SYMPATHETIC DYSTROPHY

1. In reflex sympathetic dystrophy there is:
   A. Correlation between pain and known dermatomal distribution
   B. Abnormality in EMG studies
   C. Abnormality in peripheral angiograms
   D. Abnormality in triple-phase bone scan
2. When considering psychotherapy for longstanding reflex sympathetic dystrophy patients, one should not plan for:
   A. Management of depression
   B. Psychologic factors that affect compliance with treatment
   C. Teaching of effective coping strategies
   D. Learning new skills at work
3. One of the reasons for failure of surgical sympathectomy has been:
   A. Reinnervation of contralateral sympathetic chain
   B. Permanent destruction of the cut sympathetic chain
   C. Inability of myelinated A fibers to take over the function of sympathetic fibers
   D. Increased vascularity of the region effected by sympathectomy

4. Appropriate medications for chronic reflex sympathetic dystrophy are all of the following EXCEPT:
   A. Tricyclic antidepressants
   B. Anticonvulsants
   C. Narcotics
   D. Calcium channel blockers
5. Several clinical measurements and investigations are available for the diagnosis of reflex sympathetic dystrophy. These tests include the following EXCEPT:
   A. Temperature measurements
   B. Triple-phase bone scan
   C. Q-SART test
   D. MRI

ANSWERS

1. D
2. D
3. A
4. C
5. D

49 Phantom Pain

Allen H. Hord

Phantom limb sensation was first described in 1551 by the French military surgeon, Ambroise Paré.[1] Weir Mitchell later popularized the concept of phantom limb pain when he published a long-term study on the fate of Civil War amputees.[2] Phantom sensations may occur in any appendage but are most often described in the extremities. Phantom sensation of the tongue, penis, breast, and nose have been reported.[3-5]

It is important first to clarify the terms used to describe postamputation phenomena. Phantom limb *sensation* is the perception of the continued presence of the amputated limb. By definition, this sensation is nonpainful. Phantom limb *pain* describes painful sensations that are perceived to originate in the amputated portion of the extremity. In addition, patients may have localized pain following amputation, which originates from the stump itself.

PHANTOM LIMB SENSATION
Epidemiology

Phantom limb sensation is an almost universal occurrence at some time during the first month following surgery. Patients may have the perception of the amputated limb in the recovery room and wonder why the amputation was not carried out as planned. The limb is described in terms of definite volume and length. Patients may try to reach out with, or stand on, the phantom limb.[6] Phantom limb sensation is strongest in above-elbow amputations and weakest in below-knee amputations[7] and is more frequent in the dominant limb of double amputees.[8] Children who are born without limbs apparently do not experience phantom limb sensation.[9] The incidence of phantom limb sensation increases with the age of the amputee. For infants who have amputations before 2 years of age, the incidence of phantom limb sensation is 20%, the incidence of phantom limb sensation is nearly 100% when amputation occurs after 8 years of age.[10] Although 85% to 98% of phantom limb sensation begins in the first 3 weeks after amputation, Gillis has reported that phantom limb sensation does not occur until 1 to 12 months after amputation in up to 8% of patients.[11,12] These sensations generally resolve after 2 to 3 years if they are not associated with pain.[5]

Spinal or epidural anesthesia may be associated with phantom sensations in the anesthetized limbs. Prevoznik and Eckenhoff reported a 24% incidence of phantom limb sensation that corresponded to the onset of proprioceptive blockade during spinal anesthesia.[13] The phantom lower limbs were perceived to be raised (lithotomy position) even when the patient was supine. A later study proved that the position of rest, with all joints at the midpoints of their range

of motion, was universally present in patients with phantom limb sensation during regional anesthesia, regardless of the limb involved or position before blockade.[14]

Symptoms and signs

Patients generally describe the sensations in their phantom limb either as normal in character, or as pleasant warmth or tingling. The strongest sensations come from body parts with the highest brain cortical representation, such as the fingers and toes.[5,15] The phantom limb may undergo the phenomenon known as *telescoping* (Fig. 49-1), where the patient loses sensations from the midportion of the limb, with subsequent shortening of the phantom.[16] Telescoping is most common in the upper extremity. During telescoping, the last body parts to disappear are those with the highest representation in the cortex, such as the thumb, index finger, and big toe. Only painless phantoms undergo telescoping, and lengthening of the phantom may occur if pain returns.

Treatment

Phantom limb sensations are a natural result of amputation and should not require treatment. However, before amputation, a patient should be prepared to expect these sensations so that the psychologic impact of their presence will be minimized.

PHANTOM LIMB PAIN
Epidemiology

Early literature reported the incidence of phantom limb pain in amputees to be less than 10%.[17] It is now felt that this figure is artificially low, because of the reluctance of patients to report phantom limb pain. Patients fear that they will lose credibility with their physician by complaining of pain in a limb that is no longer there! Recent large studies have shown the incidence of phantom limb pain to be 60% to 85%.[11,16,18,19] Twenty-seven percent of these patients have phantom limb pain more than 20 days out of the month and longer than 15 hours per day.[19] Civilian amputations are generally related to systemic diseases, such as vascular occlusive disease or diabetes.[16] However, there does not appear to be a difference with respect to the incidence, time course, or intensity of phantom limb pain in amputations of military origin, which are largely traumatic.

The incidence of phantom limb pain increases with more proximal amputations. Wall reported phantom limb pain in 88% of patients after hemipelvectomy or hip disarticulation for cancer.[20] Severe pain was present in 36% of these patients. Roth and Sugarbaker reported a 68% incidence of phantom limb pain after hemipelvectomy and 40% after hip

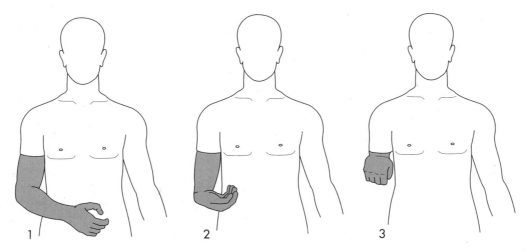

Fig. 49-1 During telescoping of the phantom limb, the original phantom *(1)* begins to shorten *(2)*. The most highly innervated areas (hands) remain, while the midportion of the phantom limb shortens in length. The phantom limb may continue to shorten until the phantom hand is perceived to be directly attached to the stump *(3)*. (From Jensen TS, Rasmussen P: Amputation. In Wall PD, Melzack R, editors: *Textbook of Pain*. New York, Churchill Livingstone, 1984.)

disarticulation, while above-knee and below-knee amputations were associated with 19% and 0% incidence, respectively.[21]

In the first month after amputation, 85% to 97% of patients experience phantom limb pain.[11,21,22] At one year after amputation, approximately 60% of patients continue to have phantom limb pain.[11,23] Phantom limb pain may begin months to years after an amputation, but pain beginning over 1 year after amputation occurs in less than 10% of patients.

Symptoms and signs

Phantom limb pain is usually described as burning, aching, or cramping.[22,24] It is sometimes described as crushing, twisting, grinding, tingling, drawing, or like being stabbed with needles.[22] Jensen reports that the descriptors "knife-like" and "sticking" are commonly used early after amputation, while "burning" or "squeezing" are used when pain persists beyond the immediate postoperative period.[23] Up to one third of patients may report sharp, shocklike pains in the phantom limb, which are excruciating but brief. Four percent of patients report unusual positions of their phantom limb, while 10% complain of spasms or jerking in the phantom.[22,25] Abnormal positions may include extreme flexion or vivid descriptions of a tightly clenched fist with fingernails digging into the palm. Phantom limb pain is often described as similar in character and location to pain that was present in the limb preoperatively, but in 82% of cases it is present below the ankle or wrist.[19]

Exacerbations of pain may be produced by trivial physical or emotional stimuli.[26] Fifty percent of patients have phantom limb pain that is provoked by emotional distress, urination, cough, defecation, or sexual activity.[16,20,23,26] Frazier speculates that autonomic input increases internuncial neuron activity and thereby precipitates phantom limb pain.[26] Pain may vary with emotional stimulation or depression, just as it may with other chronic-pain syndromes.[27]

Sunderland has suggested that patients can be divided into four groups based on the frequency and severity of pain and the degree to which it interferes with the patient's lifestyle.[28] Patients in Group I have mild, intermittent paresthesias that do not interfere with normal activity, work, or sleep. Group II is characterized by paresthesias that are uncomfortable and annoying but do not interfere with activities or sleep. Patients with pain that is of sufficient intensity, frequency, or duration to cause stress comprise Group III. However, patients in Group III have pain that is bearable, intermittently interferes with their lifestyle, and may respond to conservative treatment. Group IV patients complain of nearly constant severe pain that interferes with normal activity and sleep. The incidence of phantom limb pain may depend on whether patients in Groups I and II interpret their abnormal sensations as painful.

The usual course of phantom limb pain is to remain unchanged or to improve.[19,23] Up to 56% of patients report improvement or complete resolution.[19] Therefore when symptoms of phantom limb pain increase in severity or begin later than 1 month after amputation, the reasons should be investigated. There have been two reports of angina that presented as pain referred to the phantom left arm.[29,30] Radicular pain in the phantom limb may be associated with disc herniation.[31] Phantom limb pain may be triggered by reactivation of herpes zoster or by recurrence of cancer.[32,33] Any patient who has undergone amputation due to cancer should have an evaluation for metastatic disease if phantom limb pain significantly increases.

Pain may recur long after resolution of phantom limb pain if the patient undergoes regional anesthesia. There have been numerous case reports of phantom limb pain during spinal or epidural anesthesia.[34-38] The pain usually begins following loss of sensation or proprioception and resolves as the block wears off.

Physical examination is generally unrevealing, although the stump should be examined for the presence of trigger areas that reproduce the phantom limb pain. Neuromas are found in only 20% of patients. Thermography may be a useful diagnostic test if symptoms consistent with reflex sympathetic dystrophy (RSD) are present. Sherman has shown an inverse relationship between pain intensity and skin temperature in patients who describe burning, throbbing, or tingling in the phantom limb or stump.[27]

Cause

Theories involving peripheral, central, and psychologic mechanisms have all been proposed. None of the theories, however, fully explains the clinical characteristics of this condition.

Peripheral theories. Early investigators theorized that phantom pains originate from the cut end of nerves that previously innervated the extremity.[26] Studies support this "neuroma theory." Wall has shown that spontaneous firing occurs from neuromas that are experimentally produced in animals.[39,40] These discharges occur in small myelinated fibers.[40] Nyström placed microelectrodes into cutaneous sensory, motor, and sympathetic nerves of patients with phantom limb pain.[41] He recorded irregular spontaneous discharges and bursts of impulses conducted by cutaneous sensory nerves. Nyström also found that early discharges occur in A-delta fibers followed by late volleys of impulses in C fibers after tapping over neuromas in the stump. Blocking the neuromas with lidocaine abolished responses to tapping but did not alter the rate of spontaneous discharge.

The role of the sympathetic nervous system in phantom limb pain is unknown. An increase in the rate of spontaneous discharges originating in the neuroma occurs with stimulation of the sympathetic trunk or with intravenous (IV) injection of epinephrine.[42] Therefore decreasing sympathetic activity may decrease pain originating from a neuroma. Experimental neuromas exposed to cooling show decreased A-fiber activity and increased C-fiber activity.[43] This may explain the worsening of phantom limb pain on exposure to cold, since decreased A-fiber input to the spinal cord will lead to decreased inhibition of dorsal horn neurons in the presence of increased spontaneous C-fiber activity.

Peripheral theories do not fully explain phantom limb pain because complete sensory blockade does not provide pain relief in most patients. Neuromas have been found in only 20% of patients with phantom limb pain.[22]

Central theories. The "gate control theory" of pain is commonly used to explain phantom limb pain. Following significant destruction of sensory axons by amputation, wide-dynamic-range neurons are freed from inhibitory control.[44] Self-sustaining neuronal activity may then occur in spinal cord neurons.[44,45] If the spontaneous spinal cord neuronal activity exceeds a critical level, then pain may occur in the phantom limb. This loss of inhibitory control may lead to spontaneous discharges at any level in the CNS and explains the lack of analgesia in paraplegics with phantom body pain following complete cordectomy.[46] Increases in pain following conduction blockade are consistent with the theory, as further loss of peripheral sensory input would lead to further disinhibition. Sodium thiopental increases inhibi-

tion in the CNS and has been reported to terminate phantom limb pain during spinal anesthesia.[37]

It seems likely that peripheral painful stimulation is necessary in the early period following amputation; but, once the abnormal firing patterns in the internuncial neurons of the spinal cord are established, they become self-sustaining.[47] The initial need for peripheral input explains the rarity of phantom limb pain in paraplegics. It also makes possible the prediction that patients with preoperative or postoperative pain should be more likely to develop pain in the phantom limb after amputation.

Psychological theories. No consistent personality defect has been shown in patients with phantom limb pain, and there does not appear to be an increased incidence of neurosis or other psychologic disorders in amputees with phantom limb pain.[43,48-50] However, psychologic disturbances related to the loss of a limb or feelings of dependence may occur in any amputee. Therefore patients should be individually evaluated, since Lindesay has shown that many late psychologic problems in amputees go undetected.[51]

Patients reporting phantom limb pain have been shown to be more rigid, compulsive, and self-reliant than their cohorts.[11] Patients with this personality type tend to suppress emotions and grief response and to maintain self-esteem by denial.

It is possible that phantom limb pain exists only as the psychopathic interpretation of phantom limb sensation.[52] Phantom limb pain is usually described using the same adjectives used for description of normal phantom limb sensation.[53] Therefore phantom limb pain may result from interpretation of normal phantom limb sensation as being uncomfortable.

Treatment

Physical therapy. Since phantom limb pain occurs more frequently in patients who are unable to use a prosthesis within 6 months after amputation,[18,54] attention must be paid to the conditioning of the stump and preparation for prosthesis use. Although some success may be obtained with ultrasonic or vibratory stimulation, the failure rate with stimulation and conditioning of the stump alone is very high.[55,56] Application of heat or cold, massage therapy, or stump percussion may be tried but is rarely effective.

Transcutaneous electrical nerve stimulation. Investigators have reported excellent results with the use of transcutaneous electrical nerve stimulation (TENS) (Fig. 49-2). Long reported success in five of six patients with phantom limb pain following treatment with TENS.[57] However, in another study, Shealy found good to excellent results in only 25% of patients treated with TENS.[58]

Acupuncture. Acupuncture has been used for treatment of phantom limb, but there are few reports in the English literature. Relief from phantom limb pain of the arm has been reported with electroacupuncture,[59] and relief was also obtained with the application of TENS over the same acupuncture points. Levine reported short-term relief with the first few acupuncture treatments but found no long-term improvement in patients with a history of nerve damage, including phantom limb pain.[60]

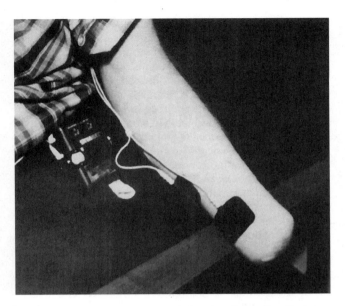

Fig. 49-2 Patient had phantom limb pain after traumatic injury and amputation of the wrist and hand. Pain was relieved with the use of TENS. (From Raj PP, editor: *Practical Management of Pain,* ed 2. St Louis, Mosby, 1992.)

Psychologic therapies. There are very few prospective studies of the use of a specific type of therapy in patients with phantom limb pain. However, Kolb has retrospectively reported good results with psychotherapy in some patients,[48] and relaxation training has also been reported to benefit patients with phantom limb pain. Relaxation can be assisted by the use of electromyogram biofeedback recorded from either muscles in the stump or the forehead.[61,62] Sherman has reported relief in two patients with acute phantom limb pain and significant improvement in 12 of 14 patients with chronic phantom limb pain. Patients required an average of six treatments to produce a lessening of pain. There was also a significant correlation between decreases in anxiety level and increase in pain relief. Hypnotic suggestion of stocking/glove anesthesia may lead to a reduction in phantom limb pain.[63,64] Cedercreutz found that 45% of patients were successfully hypnotized, and 35% had successful treatment of phantom limb pain. Relapses in pain occurred when therapy was discontinued in 34% of patients who had initially successful treatment.

Medications. Various medications have been used for the treatment of phantom limb pain, generally on the basis of anecdotal reports of success. The most commonly used classes of medications are antidepressants and anticonvulsants.[55] Tricyclic antidepressants have been thoroughly studied in other denervation syndromes such as postherpetic neuralgia and diabetic neuropathy.[65] However, there have been no studies of their specific use in the treatment of phantom limb pain. Of the anticonvulsants, carbamazepine is most commonly used. Elliott and Patterson reported cases of lancinating phantom limb pains that improved with oral carbamazepine (400 to 600 mg daily).[66,67] Logan reports a case of a patient with a 30-year history of phantom limb pain who had incomplete relief with carbamazepine but

complete relief with chlorpromazine 500 mg per day.[68] Unfortunately, the patient was unable to work as an accountant because of impaired ability to calculate, a side effect of the chlorpromazine.

β-Blockers have also been suggested for treatment of phantom limb pain, based on three cases reported by Marsland.[69] Two patients were completely relieved of pain with 80 mg of propranolol daily, whereas one patient had significant improvement with metoprolol. In a double-blind crossover trial of propranolol (up to 240 mg daily), Scadding was unable to show significant improvement in posttraumatic neuralgias.[70] The efficacy of β-blockers in the treatment of phantom limb pain is still unknown.

Kessel reported immediate short-term analgesia from IV salmon calcitonin (100 IU) in patients with phantom limb pain, whereas no relief was obtained in patients with other sources of chronic pain.[71] Although the mechanism of action is unknown, calcitonin has previously been reported to have analgesic properties.[72]

Narcotic analgesics are generally ineffective in producing long-term pain relief in patients with phantom limb pain.[19] Narcotics are therefore not currently recommended for the treatment of phantom limb pain because of the risk of addiction with long-term use.[22] In a review of five patients, Urban reported a 50% to 90% reduction in pain at 12 to 26 months follow-up of patients taking a tricyclic antidepressant and methadone (10 to 20 mg daily).[73] All five patients were additionally treated with physical therapy and behavioral management, and none of the patients had a history of substance abuse of psychologic illness. Select patients may be considered for chronic opioid therapy.

Nerve blocks. Nerve blocks are commonly used in the treatment of phantom limb pain, and the physicians performing these blocks report a high success rate.[55] Triggerpoint or direct stump injections and sympathetic, peripheral nerve, and major conduction blocks have all been used in the treatment of pain (Fig. 49-3). Most amputees report either no effect or minor temporary changes with nerve blocks.[19] Only 14% of amputees report even a significant temporary change, while less than 5% report a large permanent change or complete cure.[19] The use of neural blockade in the treatment of phantom limb pain is based on anecdotal reports in the literature. Blankenbaker reported his experience in the treatment of phantom limb pain with sympathetic blockade[74] and concluded that sympathetic blocks are successful if amputees are treated soon after the onset of phantom limb pain. Many feel that a diagnostic sympathetic block should be performed in amputees who describe throbbing pain in the phantom limb or stump.

Phantom limb pain has also been associated with trigger points in the contralateral limb.[75,76] These contralateral trigger areas can be confirmed by measuring skin conductance,[76] and injection of local anesthetics may provide pain relief. The mechanism of pain relief is unknown.

Although intraspinal narcotics may be useful in the treatment of acute postoperative pain, there is no evidence that significant long-term improvement of phantom limb pain can be obtained with single injections of intraspinal opioids.

Resolution of the acute symptoms of phantom limb pain has been reported following epidural blockade (Fig. 49-4).[77]

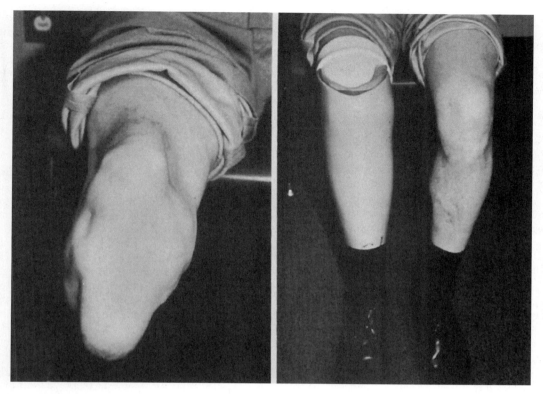

Fig. 49-3 A 78-year-old man had phantom limb sensation and pain following amputation 2 years earlier. Cramping pain radiated to the foot and increased with the use of a prosthesis and with weight-bearing. The patient was treated with a series of lumbar sympathetic blocks, local infiltration of the stump with neurolytic agents, and readjustment of the prosthesis. Six months after treatment he was able to cope with the pain and was functional. *Left,* amputated right leg 2 years earlier. *Right,* the prosthesis in use by the patient. (From Raj PP, editor: *Practical Management of Pain.* ed 2. St Louis, Mosby, 1992.)

Surgical treatment. Phantom limb pain does not respond to surgical treatment. Sherman found that neither surgeons nor patients reported good success rates with currently recommended surgical procedures.[19,55]

Stump revision. In patients who have phantom limb pain, the stump should be surgically revised when infection or vascular insufficiency is present. Otherwise, revision of the stump has poor results. Even in the 20% of patients who have palpable neuromas in the stump, only 50% have significant pain reduction following neuroma excision.[22]

Neurostimulation. Stimulation of posterior columns of the spinal cord is the most common neurosurgical technique used for treatment of phantom limb pain. To improve success rates, it is important that patients are selected who have no evidence of drug dependence or psychologic disturbances. Response to cutaneous stimulation by TENS, abrasion, or percutaneous electrical stimulation may predict a response to dorsal column stimulation,[78] but even when properly selected only 65% of patients receive a greater than 25% reduction in pain immediately after surgical implantation.[79] Nielson reported good-to-excellent results in five patients, as judged by decreased pain and increased activity. Medication use was decreased, and no patient required opioid analgesics.[80] The success rate of dorsal column stimulation steadily declines over time, and greater than 50% long-term pain reduction is present in only one third of patients originally showing improvement.[81,82]

Wester reported that dorsal column stimulation provides minimal pain relief in patients with phantom limb pain.[83] Hunt reported that only one of five patients had excellent results with dorsal column stimulation.[84]

Intracranial neurostimulation has also been attempted to relieve phantom limb pain. Levy found that 80% of patients had initial pain relief with sensory thalamic stimulation, and Mundinger reported that 86% of patients had significant relief with deep brain stimulation.[85,86] However, only 20% of patients continued to have long-term pain relief.

Neuroablation. Lesions of the dorsal root entry zone have been reported to provide long-term pain relief in patients with phantom limb pain following avulsion of nerve roots or amputation.[24,87] Saris reported that 36% of patients had pain relief on follow-up 6 months to 4 years following dorsal root entry zone lesions.[24,88] Poor relief was obtained in those patients who had only stump pain. Saris also reported that results were improved with amperage-controlled lesions rather than with the older techniques using temperature control. Nashold has reported success in three of five patients with phantom limb pain in the upper extremity, when treated with stereotaxic thermocoagulation lesions in the dorsal lateral midbrain.[89]

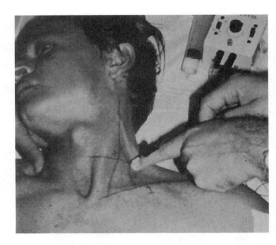

Fig. 49-4 A 32-year-old man had phantom limb pain of the left hand one day after surgery following traumatic amputation of the left upper arm. An interscalene block was done with the use of a nerve stimulator to relieve the pain in the early postoperative period. After prolonged bupivacaine infusion for 1 week, the phantom limb pain was relieved, although the phantom limb sensation remained for 3 months thereafter. (From Raj PP, editor: *Practical Management of Pain.* ed 2. St Louis, Mosby, 1992.)

Complications are common with neuroablation techniques. Saris reported that 9 of 22 patients undergoing dorsal root entry zone lesions had minor persistent neurologic deficits, while one patient was hemiplegic and incontinent postoperatively. Over 50% of patients may exhibit transient neurologic deficits following dorsal root entry zone lesions.[90] In addition to surgical complications, the failure of neuroablative procedures to cure phantom limb pain is common. Loss of inhibitory control above the level of nerve section may lead to persistent and even more severe pain. Even cordectomy has failed to improve the phantom body pain that occurs in paraplegics.[46]

STUMP PAIN
Epidemiology

Stump pain is a significant clinical problem, since it occurs in up to 50% of amputees and results in disuse of the limb prosthesis in more than half of the patients who experience it.[25,91] The incidence does not appear to depend on the presence of phantom limb pain, since tenderness or hyperesthesia in the stump also occurs in 50% of the patients with phantom limb pain.[22] Stump pain improves with time and is found in only 13% of patients after amputation.[11]

Symptoms and signs

Pain in the stump may be spontaneous or may result from pressure by the prosthesis. It is varying in nature, character, and frequency. It may be described as sharp, stabbing, or burning.

The stump should be inspected for signs of trauma from the prosthesis or the presence of a neuroma or stitch abscess. Signs of increased sympathetic activity, such as sweating, decreased skin temperature, or allodynia, may be present. X-rays may show cortical atrophy of bone in the stump, but there is no correlation with pain.[92]

Cause

Stump pain is often due to a poorly fitting prosthesis, which may cause ulceration or blistering of the skin and may lead to infection. Pain may be due to the development of bone spurs, osteomyelitis, or myofascial trigger points. Neuromas may form at the cut end of the nerves, or the nerves may become entrapped in scar tissue at the stump. Vascular insufficiency may remain at the stump site resulting from arterial obstruction or increased sympathetic activity.

Treatment

Local injuries or infection should be appropriately treated, and the prosthesis fit should be carefully examined and adjusted as necessary. Desensitization of the stump with application of repetitive cutaneous stimulation may decrease pain and allow the use of a prosthesis. If there are symptoms of sympathetic overactivity or vascular compromise, sympathetic blockade to the extremity may be useful for both diagnosis and treatment of the pain. Trigger areas may be injected with local anesthetics, such as lidocaine 1% or bupivacaine 0.5%. Although local anesthetics provide only temporary relief in most patients, some obtain prolonged relief of pain.

Surgical treatment of stump pain may be necessary if vascular insufficiency is present or if a bone spur or neuroma is repeatedly traumatized by weight bearing.

TENS, used for treatment or prevention of acute stump pain after amputation, has been reported to improve stump healing in the first 6 to 9 weeks after amputation.[93] The authors speculate that low-frequency TENS produces vasodilatation, which improves stump healing postoperatively.

PREVENTION

Some pain after amputation may be prevented by appropriate psychologic preparation of the patient. Patients may have strong feelings as to the disposition of the limb, and this should be discussed preoperatively. Psychologic support in the grieving process should be part of the preoperative preparation.

A prosthesis may be immediately fitted to the stump, and may decrease the psychologic trauma associated with the amputation by decreasing the patient's feelings of loss and dependence. Cummings has shown that the immediate fitting of a temporary prosthesis shortens the time to permanent prosthesis use by approximately 3 months.[94]

Controversy exists as to whether the prevention of preoperative pain will decrease the incidence of phantom limb pain.[11] In one study, patients with long-term pain before amputation had phantom limb pain more frequently during the first 6 months after amputation.[23] In the study, 75% of amputees had pain for over 1 month before amputation. However, Wall found no difference in the incidence of phantom limb pain in relation to preoperative pain.[20] Riddoch has suggested that long-standing anesthesia before amputation prevents phantom limb pain by altering the central body image.[5] Only one clinical study has been carried out to determine whether preoperative analgesia influences the incidence of pain after amputation. Analgesia was provided for 72 hours preoperatively by lumbar epidural bupivacaine or morphine. Patients who had preoperative lumbar epidural analgesia had less phantom limb pain after amputation, but the difference was statistically significant only at 6 months after amputation.[95]

REFERENCES

1. Keynes G: *The apologie and Treatise of Ambroise Paré*. Chicago, University of Chicago Press, 1952.
2. Mitchell SW: *Injuries of Nerves and Their Consequences*. London, Smith, Elder, 1872.
3. Hanowell ST, Kennedy SF: Phantom tongue pain and causalgia: Case presentation and treatment. *Anesth Analg* 58:436-438, 1979.
4. Jamison K et al: Phantom breast syndrome. *Arch Surg* 114:93-95, 1979.
5. Riddoch G: Phantom limbs and body shape. *Brain* 64:197-222, 1941.
6. Simmel ML: Phantoms in patients with leprosy and in elderly digital amputees. *Am J Psychol* 69:529-545, 1956.
7. Weiss SA, Fishman S: Extended and telescoped phantom limb in unilateral amputees. *J Abnorm Soc Psychol* 66:489-497, 1963.
8. Almagor M, Jaffe Y, Lomranz J: The relation between limb dominance, acceptance of disability, and the phantom limb phenomenon. *J Abnorm Psychol* 87:377-379, 1978.
9. Simmel ML: The reality of phantom sensation. *Social Research* 29:337-356, 1962.
10. Simmel ML: Phantom experiences following amputation in childhood. *J Neurol Neurosurg Psychiatry* 25:69-78, 1962.
11. Parkes CM: Factors determining the persistence of phantom pain in the amputee. *J Psychosom Res* 17:97-108, 1973.
12. Gillis L: The management of the painful amputation stump and a new theory for the phantom phenomena. *Br J Surg* 51:87-95, 1964.
13. Prevoznik SJ, Eckenhoff JE: Phantom sensations during spinal anesthesia. *Anesthesiology* 25:767-770, 1964.
14. Bromage PR, Melzack R: Phantom limbs and the body schema. *Can Anaesth Soc J* 21:267-274, 1974.
15. Miles JE: Phantom limb syndrome occurring during spinal anesthesia: Relationship to etiology. *J Nerv Ment Dis* 123:365-368, 1956.
16. Jensen TS et al: Phantom limb, phantom pain and stump pain in amputees during the first 6 months following limb amputation. *Pain* 17:243-256, 1983.
17. Sternbach T, Nadvorna H, Arazi D: A five year follow-up study of phantom limb pain in post-traumatic amputees. *Scand J Rehab Med* 14:203-207, 1982.
18. Sherman RA, Sherman CJ: Prevalence and characteristics of chronic phantom limb pain among American veterans. Results of a trial survey. *Am J Phys Med* 62:227-238, 1983.
19. Sherman RA, Sherman CJ, Parker L: Chronic phantom and stump pain among American veterans: Results of a survey. *Pain* 18:83-95, 1984.
20. Wall R, Novotny-Joseph P, MacNamara TE: Does preamputation pain influence phantom limb pain in cancer patients? *South Med J* 78:34-36, 1985.
21. Roth YF, Sugarbaker PH: Pains and sensations after amputation: Character and clinical significance. *Arch Phys Med Rehabil* 61:490, 1980.
22. Bailey AA, Moersch FP: Phantom limb. *Can Med Assoc J* 45:37-42, 1941.
23. Jensen TS et al: Immediate and long-term phantom limb pain in amputees: Incidence, clinical characteristics and relationship to preamputation limb pain. *Pain* 21:267-278, 1985.
24. Saris SC, Iacono RP, Nashold BS Jr: Dorsal root entry zone lesions for post-amputation pain. *J Neurosurg* 62:72-76, 1985.
25. Sherman RA, Sherman CJ: A comparison of phantom sensations among amputees whose amputations were of civilian and military origins. *Pain* 21:91-97, 1985.
26. Frazier SH: Psychiatric aspects of causalgia, the phantom limb, and phantom pain. *Dis Nerv Syst* 27:441-450, 1966.
27. Sherman RA, Barja RH, Bruno GM: Thermographic correlates of chronic pain: Analysis of 125 patients incorporating evaluations by a blind panel. *Arch Phys Med Rehabil* 68:273-279, 1987.
28. Sunderland S (editor): *Nerves and Nerve Injuries*. New York, Churchill Livingstone, 1978.
29. Cohen H: Anginal pain in a phantom limb. *Br Med J* 2:475, 1976.
30. Mester SW, Cintron GB, Long C: Phantom angina. *Am Heart J* 116:1627-1628, 1988.
31. Finneson BE, Haft H, Krueger EG: Phantom limb syndrome associated with herniated nucleus pulposus. *J Neurosurg* 14:344-346, 1957.
32. Wilson PR et al: Herpes zoster reactivation of phantom limb pain. *Mayo Clin Proc* 53:336-338, 1978.
33. Sugarbaker PH et al: Increasing phantom limb pain as a symptom of cancer recurrence. *Cancer* 54:373-375, 1984.
34. Carrie LE, Glynn CJ: Phantom limb pain and epidural anesthesia for Cesarean section. *Anesthesiology* 65:220-221, 1986.
35. Murphy JP, Anandaciva S: Phantom limb pain and spinal anaesthesia. *Anaesthesia* 39:188, 1984.
36. Sellick BC: Phantom limb pain and spinal anesthesia. *Anesthesiology* 62:801-802, 1985.
37. Koyama K et al: Thiopental for phantom limb pain during spinal anesthesia. *Anesthesiology* 69:598-600, 1988.
38. Mackenzie N: Phantom limb pain during spinal anaesthesia. Recurrence in amputees. *Anaesthesia* 38:886-887, 1983.
39. Wall PD, Gutnick M: Properties of afferent nerve impulses originating from a neuroma. *Nature* 248:740-743, 1974.
40. Wall PD, Gutnick M: Ongoing activity in peripheral nerves: The physiology and pharmacology of impulses originating from a neuroma. *Exp Neurol* 45:576-589, 1974.
41. Nyström B, Hagbarth K-E: Microelectrode recordings from transected nerves in amputees with phantom limb pain. *Neurosci Lett* 27:211-216, 1981.
42. Devor M, Jänig W: Activation of myelinated efferents ending in a neuroma by stimulation of the sympathetic supply in the rat. *Neurosci Lett* 24:43-47, 1981.
43. Matzner O, Devor M: Contrasting thermal sensitivity of spontaneously active A- and C-fibers in experimental nerve-end neuromas. *Pain* 30:373-384, 1987.
44. Omer GE Jr: Nerve, neuroma, and pain problems related to upper limb amputations. *Orthop Clin North Am* 12:751-762, 1981.
45. Livingston WK: *Pain Mechanism: A Physiologic Interpretation of Causalgia and its Related States*. New York, MacMillan Publishers, 1944.
46. Melzack R, Loeser JD: Phantom body pain in paraplegics: Evidence for a central "pattern generating mechanism" for pain. *Pain* 4:195-210, 1978.
47. Carlen PL et al: Phantom limbs and related phenomena in recent traumatic amputations. *Neurology* 28:211-217, 1978.
48. Kolb LC: *The painful phantom*. Springfield, Ill, Charles C Thomas, 1954.
49. University of California: *Progress Report to the Advisory Committee on Artificial Limbs*, ed 2. Berkeley, Calif, University of California Press, 1952.
50. Ewalt JR, Randall GC, Morris H: The phantom limb. *Psychosom Med* 9:118-123, 1947.
51. Lindesay J: Validity of the general health questionnaire (GHQ) in detecting psychiatric disturbance in amputees with phantom pain. *J Psychosom Res* 30:277-281, 1986.
52. Frazier SH, Kolb LC: Psychiatric aspects of pain and the phantom limb. *Orthop Clin North Am* 1:481-495, 1970.
53. Ewalt JR: The phantom limb. *Ann Intern Med* 44:668-677, 1956.
54. Steinbach TV, Nadvorna H, Arazi D: A five year follow-up study of phantom limb pain in posttraumatic amputees. *Scand J Rehabil Med* 14:203-207, 1982.
55. Sherman RA, Sherman CA, Call NG: A survey of current phantom limb pain treatment in the United States. *Pain* 8:85-99, 1980.
56. Lundeberg T: Relief of pain from a phantom limb by peripheral stimulation. *J Neurol* 232:79-82, 1985.
57. Long DM: Cutaneous afferent stimulation for relief of chronic pain. *Clin Neurosurg* 21:257-268, 1974.
58. Shealy CN: Transcutaneous electrical stimulation for control of pain. *Clin Neurosurg* 21:269-277, 1974.
59. Monga TN, Jaksic T: Acupuncture in phantom limb pain. *Arch Phys Med Rehabil* 62:229-231, 1981.
60. Levine JD, Gormley J, Fields HL: Observations on the analgesic effects of needle puncture (acupuncture). *Pain* 2:149-159, 1976.
61. Dougherty J: Relief of phantom limb pain after EMG biofeedback-assisted relaxation: A case report. *Behav Res Ther* 18:355-357, 1980.
62. Sherman RA, Gall N, Gormley J: Treatment of phantom limb pain with muscular relaxation training to disrupt the pain-anxiety-tension cycle. *Pain* 6:47-55, 1979.

63. Siegel EF: Control of phantom limb pain by hypnosis. *Am J Clin Hypnosis* 21:285-286, 1979.
64. Cedercreutz C: Hypnotic treatment of phantom sensations in 100 amputees. *Acta Chir Scand* 107:158-162, 1954.
65. Getto CJ, Sorkness CA, Howell T: Antidepressants and chronic nonmalignant pain: A review. *J Pain Sympt Manag* 2:9-18, 1987.
66. Elliott F, Little A, Millbrandt W: Carbamazepine for phantom-limb phenomena. *N Engl J Med* 295:678, 1976.
67. Patterson JF: Carbamazepine in the treatment of phantom limb pain. *South Med J* 81:1100-1102, 1988.
68. Logan TP: Persistent phantom limb pain: Dramatic response to chlorpromazine. *South Med J* 76:1585, 1983.
69. Marsland AR et al: Phantom limb pain: A case for beta blockers? *Pain* 12:295-297, 1982.
70. Scadding JW et al: Clinical trial of propranolol in post-traumatic neuralgia. *Pain* 14:283-292, 1982.
71. Kessel C, Wörz R: Clinical note: Immediate response of phantom limb pain to calcitonin. *Pain* 30:79-87, 1987.
72. Gennari C et al: Dolore osseo, endofine e calcitonine. In Gennari C, Segre C, editor: *The Effects of Calcitonin in Man.* Milano, Italy, Masson Publishers, 1983.
73. Urban BJ et al: Long-term use of narcotic/antidepressant medication in the management of phantom limb pain. *Pain* 24:191-196, 1986.
74. Blankenbaker WL: The care of patients with phantom limb pain in a pain clinic. *Anesth Analg* 56:842-846, 1977.
75. Flöter T: Pain management by contralateral local anaesthesia. *Acupunct Electrother Res* 8:139-142, 1983.
76. Gross D: Contralateral local anaesthesia in the treatment of phantom limb and stump pain. *Pain* 13:313-320, 1982.
77. Rosenblatt RM: Phantom limb pain. In Raj PP, editor: *Practical Management of Pain.* St Louis, Mosby, 1986.
78. Miles J, Lipton S: Phantom limb pain treated by electrical stimulation. *Pain* 5:373-382, 1978.
79. Krainick JU, Thoden U, Riechert T: Spinal cord stimulation in post-amputation pain. *Surg Neurol* 4:167-170, 1975.
80. Nielson KD, Adams JE, Hosobuchi Y: Phantom limb pain: Treatment with dorsal column stimulation. *J Neurosurg* 42:301-307, 1975.
81. Krainick JU, Thoden U, Riechert T: Pain reduction in amputees by long-term spinal cord stimulation. Long-term follow-up study over 5 years. *J Neurosurg* 52:346-350, 1980.
82. Krainick JU, Thoden U: Spinal cord stimulation in post-amputation pain. In Siegfriend J, Zimmerman M, editors: *Phantom and Stump Pain.* New York, Springer Publishers, 1981.
83. Wester K: Dorsal column stimulation in pain treatment. *Acta Neurol Scand* 75:151-155, 1987.
84. Hunt WE, Goodman JH: Dorsal column stimulation for phantom limb pain. *J Neurosurg* 43:250-251, 1975.
85. Levy RM, Lamb S, Adams JE: Treatment of chronic pain by deep brain stimulation: Long term follow-up and review of the literature. *Neurosurgery* 21:885-893, 1987.
86. Mundinger F, Nermuller H: Programmed transcutaneous (TNS) and central (DBS) stimulation for control of phantom limb pain and causalgia: A new method for treatment. In Siegfriend J, Zimmerman M, editors: *Phantom and Stump Pain.* New York, Springer Publishers, 1981.
87. Moossy JJ et al: Conus medullaris nerve root avulsions. *J Neurosurg* 66:835-841, 1987.
88. Saris SC, Iacono RP, Nashold BS Jr: Successful treatment of phantom pain with dorsal root entry zone coagulation. *Appl Neurophysiol* 51:188-197, 1988.
89. Nashold BS Jr, Wilson WP, Slaughter DG: Stereotaxic midbrain lesions for central dysesthesia and phantom pain: Preliminary report. *J Neurosurg* 30:116-126, 1969.
90. Samii M, Moringlane JR: Thermocoagulation of the dorsal root entry zone for the treatment of intractable pain. *Neurosurgery* 15:935-955, 1984.
91. Helm P et al: Function after lower limb amputation. *Acta Orthop Scand* 57:154-157, 1986.
92. Sevastikoglou JA, Eriksson U, Larsson SE: Skeletal changes of the amputation stump and the femur on the amputated side. A clinical investigation. *Acta Orthop Scand* 40:624-633, 1969.
93. Finsen V et al: Transcutaneous electrical nerve stimulation after major amputation. *J Bone J Surg* (Br) 70:109-112, 1988.
94. Cummings GS, Girling J: Case report: A clinical assessment of immediate postoperative fitting of prosthesis for amputee rehabilitation. *Phys Ther* 51:1007-1012, 1971.
95. Bach S, Noreng MF, Tjéllden NU: Phantom limb pain in amputees during the first 12 months following limb amputation, after preoperative lumbar epidural blockade. *Pain* 33:297-301, 1988.

QUESTIONS: PHANTOM PAIN

1. The most commonly presented medications for phantom limb pain are all of the following EXCEPT:
   A. Antidepressants
   B. Anticonvulsants
   C. Narcotics
   D. Benzodiazepines

2. Nerve blocks commonly used in the treatment of phantom limb pain are all of the following EXCEPT:
   A. Sympathetic blocks
   B. Direct stump injections
   C. Epidural block
   D. Subarachnoid block

3. Phantom limb sensation was first described in 1551 by:
   A. Weir Mitchell
   B. Ambroise Paré
   C. Hippocrates
   D. Damas

4. Phantom limb pain is usually described as all of the following EXCEPT:
   A. Burning, aching, shooting
   B. Cold and dull
   C. Sharp, shocklike
   D. Knifelike

5. Early treatment modalities for phantom limb pain are all of the following EXCEPT:
   A. Physical therapy
   B. Transcutaneous electrical nerve stimulation
   C. Acupuncture
   D. Dorsal column stimulation

ANSWERS

1. D
2. D
3. B
4. B
5. D

50 Miscellaneous Pain Disorders

P. Prithvi Raj

PSYCHOGENIC PAIN*

Criteria listed for psychogenic pain in the *Diagnostic and Statistical Manual of Disorders,* ed 3, revised (DSM-III-R) require preoccupation with pain for at least 6 months and either (1) no organic pathology or pathophysiologic mechanism is found to account for the pain, or (2) the complaint of pain or resulting impairment grossly exceeds what would be expected from the physical findings.

This condition is difficult to diagnose with confidence, in part because it depends on the assumption that medical diagnosis is accurate. It is similar to conversion disorder, in which a loss of physical function occurs without organic cause; however, 13% to 30% of those diagnosed with this condition are later found to have an organic disease causing their symptoms. Several pain syndromes (e.g., phantom pain) now known to be explicable on a neurophysiologic basis were previously thought to be psychogenic.

These patients may be dramatic, extreme in their denial of nonmedical problems, and cheerful despite a distressing degree of disability. They commonly display nonphysiologic signs on examination and demonstrate behaviors that are incompatible with the degree of impairment they describe. Waddell's signs in back patients are examples of common 'functional' findings: (1) inordinate skin tenderness; (2) pain increase by axial loading (pressing on the head) or axial rotation (pelvic rotation); (3) straight-leg raising positive while supine but negative while sitting; (4) nonphysiologic regional weakness, sensory loss, or pain; and (5) overreaction—pain behavior out of proportion to the stimulus or to the findings.

The term *central pain* is occasionally heard in casual use to denote somatoform pain disorder. It is important that "hardware" malfunctions—neuropathologic conditions in the brain and cord—not be confused with disturbances of "software" and behavior.

There is no evidence that placebo responsiveness is greater in psychogenic pains, and there is excellent evidence that organic pains often respond to placebo. This should never be considered a sign of somatoform pain.

Somatization disorder

This condition is characterized by an extensive history of multiple somatic symptoms that are psychologically caused.

In addition to many physical complaints or a belief that one is sickly, beginning before the age of 30 and persisting for several years, the criteria require at least 13 symptoms from a list of 41. The symptom list includes six gastrointestinal (GI) symptoms, seven pains, four cardiopulmonary symptoms, twelve conversion/pseudoneurologic symptoms, four sexual symptoms, and four female reproductive symptoms. A screen is provided by the following: vomiting (other than during pregnancy), pain in extremities, shortness of breath when not exerting oneself, amnesia, difficulty swallowing, burning sensation in sexual organs or rectum (other than during intercourse), and painful menstruation.

Hypochondriasis

DSM-III-R criteria for hypochondriasis require at least 6 months of preoccupation with the fear or belief that one has a serious disease, based on the interpretation of physical signs or sensations as evidence of illness. Evaluation does not reveal any physical disorder to account for the signs or sensations or the person's interpretation of them, and the symptoms are not just those of panic attacks. The fear or belief persists despite medical reassurance but is not of delusional intensity.

Delusional pain

Delusional pain is rare and usually associated with schizophrenia or psychotic depression. Somatic-type delusional disorder also occurs.

Malingering and factitious disorders

There can be physical or psychologic symptoms of malingering and factitious disorders. In these conditions the patient willfully produces or feigns symptoms of illness or injury. In the factitious disorders the goal of the behavior is the patient's "need" to be in the sick role—a need not understood by the patient. Placing drops of blood into urine specimens and pretending to have posttraumatic stress disorder (PTSD) are examples. There is no apparent external goal such as to obtain money or drugs. It is always a psychiatric illness.

This contrasts with malingering, in which the goal is a clearly defined external one. Malingering is not a psychiatric illness; it could be a healthy behavior if the person feigns amnesia to withhold information from the enemy. More commonly, malingering is intended to avoid prison or combat, or to obtain drugs, monetary compensation, or a better living situation. An example is the person who rushes to

---

*Excerpted from Covington EC: *Behavioral Medicine in Pain Management.* Comprehensive pain medicine/management certification examination review course, Dallas, Tex, Jan 14-16, 1994.

board a bus after an accident in order to litigate as an injured passenger.

Psychiatric diagnoses

Criteria for diagnosing psychiatric illnesses are provided by DSM-III-R. Psychiatric illnesses can be causes or consequences of pain and sick role behavior. Commonly nociception and psychopathology interact so that each exacerbates the other. Estimates of the prevalence of psychiatric illnesses vary tremendously with setting (e.g., the rate of depression in a behavioral-pain rehabilitation center is many times that in an outpatient rheumatology clinic). The most frequent psychiatric disorders in pain-center patients have been found to be anxiety disorders, depressions, and alcohol abuse. In 200 chronic low-back pain patients entering a functional restoration program, Polatin found that (excluding somatoform pain disorder) 77% of patients met lifetime diagnostic criteria and 59% had current symptoms for at least one psychiatric diagnosis. The most common were major depression, substance abuse, and anxiety disorders. In addition, 51% met criteria for at least one personality disorder. Of the patients with a positive lifetime history, 54% of those with depression, 94% of those with substance abuse, and 95% of those with anxiety disorders had experienced these syndromes before the onset of their back pain. Thus substance abuse and anxiety disorders preceded chronic low-back pain, whereas major depression could precede or follow it.

COCCYGODYNIA*

The term *coccygodynia*, first used by Simpson[1] in 1859 to describe a painful coccyx, is more properly identified as a symptom than a syndrome. A painful coccyx may represent any of a wide variety of disease processes (Table 50-1). Those actually related to the coccyx itself are most commonly strained coccygeal ligaments, coccygeal dislocation (Fig. 50-1) or fracture, and osteoarthritis of the sacrococcygeal joint.

Pelvic, anorectal, and spinal cord diseases are the leading sources for referred coccygeal pain.[2] In the case of pelvic pain, this may be related to the sharing of the fourth sacral nerve by both the pelvic splanchnics and the coccygeal plexus.

Although the vast majority of coccygeal pain is related to benign underlying causes, some rare tumors of the sacrum and spinal cord can cause coccygodynia. Chordoma of the sacrococcygeal region, glomus tumor of Luschka body, and metastatic carcinoma to the lower sacrum and coccyx have all been described.[3] In infants, meningiomas and teratomas of the coccygeal region are usually more obvious presentations.[1]

Adjacent structures are associated with the symptom complex of coccygodynia. The levator syndrome[4]—a symptom complex consisting of pain and pressure in the rectum, sacrum, and coccyx—is often misdiagnosed as coccygodynia. This syndrome is related to muscular spasms of the

---

*Excerpted from Gold MD: Coccygodynia. In Raj PP, editor: *Practical Management of Pain,* ed 2. St Louis, Mosby, 1992.

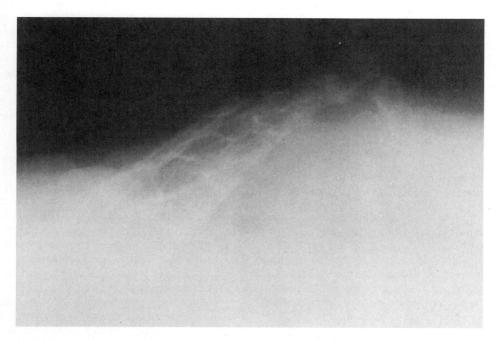

Fig. 50-1 Anteriorly dislocated coccyx in a 28-year-old female with coccygodynia who ultimately required coccygectomy for pain relief. (From Raj PP, editor: *Practical Management of Pain,* ed. 2. St Louis, Mosby, 1992.)

Table 50-1 Causes of coccygeal pain

Cause		Structure causing coccygeal pain
Primary	Acute trauma	Sprained ligaments
		Dislocation
		Fracture
		Childbirth[a]
	Chronic trauma	Osteoarthritis of the sacrococcygeal or first intercoccygeal joint[b]
	Idiopathic	Coccygeal subluxation[b]
		Subacute trauma
Secondary	Cancer	Metastatic involvement
		External compression
Referred	Spinal cord disease	Lumbar disk disease
		Cauda equina syndrome
		Arachnoiditis[c]
		Spinal cord tumor[b]
	Anorectal disease	Perirectal abscess[d]
		Perirectal fistula[d]
		Pilonidal cyst
		Rectal carcinoma
	Pelvic disease	Pelvic inflammatory disease[e]
		Pelvic tumor
	Gynecologic disease	Vaginismus
	Muscular spasm	Levator syndrome[f]
	Psychiatric	Psychoneurosis[g]

[a]Traycoff RB, Crayton H, Dodson R: Sacrococcygeal pain syndromes: Diagnosis and treatment. *Orthopedics* 12:1373-1377, 1980.
[b]Holworth B: The painful coccyx. *Clin Orthop* 14:145-160, 1959.
[c]Bohn E: Late results of sacral rhizotomy in coccygodynia. *Acta Chir Scand* 123:6-8, 1962.
[d]Gold MD, Bienasz SM, Jordan WM: The treatment of coccygodynia with radiofrequency lesions: A case report. *Pain Clin* 3:91-93, 1990.
[e]Thiele GH: Coccygodynia: Cause and treatment. *Dis Colon Rectum* 6:422-435, 1963.
[f]Grant SR, Salvati EP, Rubin RJ: Levator syndrome—An analysis of 316 cases. *Dis Colon Rectum* 18:161-163, 1975.
[g]Wein AB: Coccygodynia: Operative on non-operative management as related to the proctologist. *Am J Proctol* 8:433-438, 1957.

levator ani muscles that insert on the anterior aspect of the coccyx. On physical examination, the tip of the coccyx is usually not tender. Treatment for this problem is directed toward massage therapy and muscle relaxants.

Anatomy

The coccyx consists of three to five segments that are attached inferiorly to the sacrum by the sacrococcygeal joint. The joint represents a synarthrosis, complete with an intervertebral disk. A disk is also present between the first and second coccygeal segments. Lower segments generally undergo bony fusion with aging. The coccyx serves as the insertion site for the levator ani and coccygeus muscles on its ventral surface and for the gluteus maximus on the lateral aspect of the dorsal side. These muscles work together to flex the coccyx anteriorly. There are no corresponding coccygeal extensors, which leads to an anterior angulation of the coccyx off of the sacrum. The actual angle and morphology of the coccyx vary considerably within the normal population. There is some evidence, however, to suggest

that more acutely angled coccyxes represent a risk factor for coccygeal injury.[5] The innervation of the coccyx is supplied by the coccygeal sacral nerves in conjunction with the coccygeal nerve. Occasionally, the third sacral nerve also makes a contribution.[6]

Acute coccygodynia

Acute coccygodynia is usually related to a fall that exposes the coccyx to direct trauma. Less commonly, it may also occur during childbirth at the time of delivery. This may result in a sprain, dislocation, or fracture of the coccyx.[3] There may be swelling or ecchymosis to the area. Acute coccygodynia is far more common in women than men, possibly because of a wider distance between female ischial tuberosities, thereby affording less protection to the coccygeal area.[10,11] The complaint is relentless aching and, occasionally, stabbing pain. This discomfort may be limited to the coccyx or may radiate to the buttock. Invariably, the pain is aggravated by sustained sitting, and many patients prefer to stand during the history-taking interview. Physical examination will demonstrate impressive tenderness from the coccyx by either rectal or external palpation. X-ray examinations of the coccyx are of limited value when the history of coccygeal trauma is elicited. Frequently, x-ray films are entirely normal.[5] They may be of benefit, however, when the cause of the coccygeal pain is unclear. In this case a proctosigmoidoscopic examination will also be helpful.

Idiopathic coccygodynia

Although the pain pattern and physical examination findings of idiopathic coccygodynia are identical to those of acute coccygodynia, the history of trauma is notably absent. It is currently believed that idiopathic coccygodynia may be related to a series of subacute coccygeal injuries or a normal variation in coccygeal structure that lends itself more susceptible to injury.[5] Subacute injuries of the coccyx can be generated from poor sitting posture for extended periods. This is often related to slouching forward, which adds a weight-bearing responsibility to the coccyx.[2]

Other possibilities include posttraumatic osteoarthritis and subluxation of coccygeal vertebrae, both of which have been found in asymptomatic patients as well.[3]

Treatment

Treatment for acute or chronic coccygodynia is directed toward minimizing pressure on the coccyx. The use of cushions or rubber donuts when sitting redistributes weight-bearing away from the coccyx. Sitz baths and heating pads are often helpful in relaxing the traction of the pelvic musculature. A sitting posture that maintains lumbar lordosis minimizes the exposure of the coccyx to weight-bearing in favor of the thighs. Mild analgesics, antiinflammatory drugs, and muscle relaxants may be required. In most cases, resolution of symptoms occurs within 3 months.

When coccygeal symptoms fail to resolve spontaneously, a more aggressive approach is warranted. Digital manipulation of the coccyx, usually requiring an anesthetic, may prove helpful if the underlying problem is related to dislocation.[12] Injections of local anesthetics and steroids into and around the sacrococcygeal joint may offer significant relief when osteoarthritis is present.[12,13]

The use of caudal epidural steroids for coccygodynia has been reported by Stern.[12] In his series 41 of 50 patients gained long-term relief with this method. Repeat injections were used as needed, and treatment failures were referred for coccygectomy.

If injections or manipulations fail to provide any relief, a cause outside the coccyx must be considered. However, if the period of relief is consistent only with the duration of the local anesthetic and other conservative therapies have failed, neurolytic and surgical options should be considered.[7,8,11-23]

Neurolytic techniques for coccygeal pain are directed toward the fourth and fifth sacral and the coccygeal nerves. Transsacral injections of ammonium chloride,[23] caudal cryoanalgesia,[18] and caudal radiofrequency lesions[8] have been reported in the treatment of coccygodynia.

Wright[23] evaluated ammonium chloride in concentrations between 7% and 10% in 12 patients with intractable coccygodynia. Conservative treatments were exhausted, and three diagnostic transsacral blocks at S_4 and S_5 were performed before neurolysis. Ten patients (83%) were without pain for periods ranging from 1 month to 2 years. Repeat injections were required in 8 (80%) of the successfully treated patients. No complications were attributed to this technique. A similar approach was described by Robertson[20] using aqueous phenol for intractable perineal pain.

Evans et al.[18] described the use of cryoanalgesia via the caudal canal in 40 patients with intractable perineal pain, 12 of whom were diagnosed with coccygodynia. Although 78% of these patients showed improvement from this treatment, the mean duration of effectiveness was only 39 days and repeat treatments were necessary to sustain relief.

Gold et al.[8] also used a percutaneous approach through the caudal canal and described a case using radiofrequency lesions to create more extensive nerve injury than that achieved by cryoanalgesia. At the time of the report, the patient was without pain for 13 months and no repeat procedure was necessary. Subsequent work using his technique suggests that a good outcome can be achieved when the patient's exact pain can be produced by electrical stimulation within the caudal canal (MD Gold, personal communication, 1990).

The surgical alternatives consist of coccygectomy and surgical rhizotomy of the lower sacral roots. Albrektsson[14] described 24 cases of S_4 and S_5 bilateral rhizotomies for anococcygeal pain unresponsive to conservative management. Initially, 20 patients obtained relief from their pain. In most cases, however, the duration of relief was less than 6 months. At 2-year follow-up, only 11 patients (46%) were satisfied with the result.

Saris et al.[21] evaluated sacrococcygeal rhizotomy for persons with intractable perineal pain, including four patients with coccygodynia. Although relief was obtained in 53% of patients with cancer pain, none of the coccygodynia patients obtained a good result. In this study, diagnostic root blocks performed preoperatively did not predict the outcome from rhizotomies.

Coccygectomy is the definitive surgical procedure when conservative measures fail and the origin of the pain is believed to be confined to the coccyx. Bayne et al.[15] reviewed 48 cases of coccygectomy to assess the influence of different causes of pain on patient outcome. Those patients with a history of direct trauma or postpartum coccygodynia obtained good results in 22 of 29 (76%) cases. Those patients with idiopathic coccygodynia obtained relief in 7 of 12 (58%) cases, whereas 7 patients with coccygodynia related to previous spinal surgeries gained no relief at all. Wray and Templeton[22] and Eng et al.[17] reviewed a combined 64 coccygectomies with similar findings to those of Bayne et al. All of the investigators emphasize the need to rule out lumbar disk disease as a cause of coccygodynia before the consideration of coccygectomy.

In summary, coccygodynia represents a symptom of variable causes. When the pain is related to the coccyx, conservative approaches that emphasize minimizing pressure to the painful area are often sufficient to allow spontaneous recovery. When this plan is ineffective, more aggressive approaches—potentially leading to coccygectomy—need to be considered.

OROFACIAL PAIN*

Pain of dental origin

Diagnosis of tooth-related pain. Tooth-related pain has been described as one of the most extreme kinds of pain to endure. Frequently, the patient can precisely point to the affected tooth. The practitioner can then confirm the diagnosis by a positive painful or tender reaction to the tests of percussion or palpation adjacent to the tooth apex. To further confirm that the cause of pain is an offending tooth, the practitioner should examine for adjacent swelling, a previous history of pain in the offending tooth, caries, or intraalveolar tooth fracture. Using dental radiology, an area of rarefaction at the tooth apex can often be identified. An extreme sustained thermal reaction to the application of cold with ice or CO_2 crystals is frequently observed.

Typically, tooth-related pain is easy to identify. However, when the pain is diffuse and spread over a region of several teeth, diagnosis becomes a challenge. If the patient and practitioner are willing to delay diagnosis and treatment of this diffuse odontologic pain, the pain may localize and the offending tooth can be identified and treated.

In those instances of persistent diffuse pain often progressing from one tooth to another and back again, the diagnosis of atypical odontalgia must be considered. Often these patients have a history of root-canal therapy or extraction without remission of pain.

---

*Excerpted from Phero JC et al: Orofacial pain and other related syndromes. In Raj PP, editor: *Practical Management of Pain,* ed 2. St Louis, Mosby, 1992.

One of the most difficult conditions to evaluate is the cracked tooth syndrome. The pain occurs with chewing, and clinically the split cannot be seen radiographically or through diagnostic testing of the teeth. The practitioner can become suspicious if the pain is reproduced when the patient bites on a hard object. A split tooth can refer pain to the head and neck and be a continual source of pain.

Referred pain of dental origin. Tooth-related pain can be referred along the pathway of the trigeminal nerve. For example, affected mandibular molars can refer pain to upper molar and premolar teeth and often in the direction of the temporomandibular joint (TMJ) and ear. Pain is rarely referred across the midline.

Pain may be referred to the jaw as a result of angina pectoris and myocardial infarction (usually lower left jaw). Sinusitis can result in referred pain to the apexes of upper molar and premolar teeth. When sharp electric-like spasmodic pain acts to trigger referred pain, the diagnosis of neuralgia should be considered.

Treatment of tooth-related pain. Endodontic therapy or extraction is usually successful in relieving pain of pulpal origin. Occasionally these procedures are complemented by the selective use of incision and drainage of the swelling, antibiotics, opioid and/or nonopioid analgesics, and nonsteroidal antiinflammatory agents.

Chronic atypical odontalgia may require the use of antidepressant medications combined with a series of sympathetic blocks (stellate) for the patient to achieve pain relief.

Temporomandibular joint disorders

A differential diagnosis is the first step in the workup of a patient with pain that may be of craniomandibular origin and is related to the dental apparatus. Besides looking for obvious odontologic or periodontal disease, the practitioner evaluates the patient to see if a relationship exists among the functioning movements of the jaw, TMJ muscles, ligaments, and the tooth occlusion. If the pain appears related to the TMJ, the examiner must ascertain whether the problem is extracapsular or intracapsular, since the treatment differs. Extracapsular problems of the masticatory apparatus are mainly muscular in origin. Also, the dentition plays a role in causing referred pain to facial structures (i.e., a third molar referring pain to the ear). Intracapsular problems such as an arthritic condition, ankylosis, or displacement or dislocation of the TMJ disk, could result in inflammation or

dysfunction of the jaw and result in pain. In addition, there are other multiple diagnostic possibilities in the evaluation of facial pain that the physician must consider.

Most disorders of the masticatory system manifest either as pain or as dysfunction with jaw movement. The majority of patients treated for TMJ disorders have multifactorial problems including malocclusion, psychologic stress, joint disease, pain, dysfunction, poor body mechanics, and myofascial pain. These chronic conditions respond best to an interdisciplinary management program.

Causes of TMJ dysfunction. Extracapsular problems suggested as causes of TMJ dysfunction include possible trigger areas in masticatory muscles, psychophysiologic causes, and occlusal mechanisms.

Trigger areas in masticatory muscles. Travell[24] observed areas in muscles called trigger zones, which are responsible for referred pain patterns. She suggests that these trigger areas "are a small zone of hypersensitivity located within the muscle in spasm or in fascia. Deep pressure on the trigger area, or touching it with a needle, reproduces a spontaneous pain at a distance, and infiltrating it locally with procaine eliminates the related reference of pain." Travell showed that different parts of a skeletal muscle have a specific referred pain pattern that is consistent from one person to another. She mapped these referred-pain patterns of the head, illustrated in Figs. 50-2 to 50-6, by experimentally injecting hypertonic saline intramuscularly (IM) in

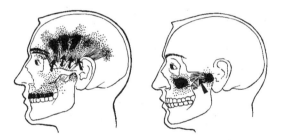

Fig. 50-2 Left: Composite pain reference pattern of the temporalis muscle. Trigger areas are indicated by arrows; their reference zones are indicated by the stippled and black regions. Right: Composite pain reference pattern of the external pterygoid muscle. (From Travell JJ: Temporomandibular joint pain referred from the head and neck. *Prosthetic Dentistry* 10:745-763, 1960.)

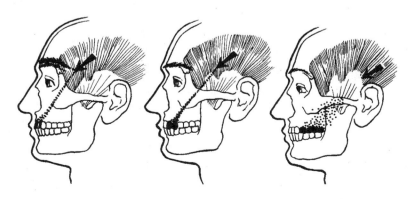

Fig. 50-3 Specific trigger areas at three sites in the temporalis muscle, as observed in a case of facial neuralgia. Trigger areas were located at arrows, and pain was referred to the black and stippled zones. (From Travell JJ: Temporomandibular joint pain referred from the head and neck. *Prosthetic Dentistry* 10:745-763, 1960.)

these areas and observing referred-pain patterns from the injection sites. She classified these areas located within the masticatory muscles as follows:

1. *Masseter muscle.* Superficial layer refers pain to the jaws, molar teeth, and surrounding gingiva. From the anterior border of the masseter muscle and upper part of this division of the muscle, pain is referred to the upper teeth; from the lower part, pain is referred to the lower molars. From trigger areas at the angle of the mandible, pain travels upward in and over the temporalis and around the outer portion of the eyebrow. Trigger areas in the deep layer of the masseter refer to the TMJ and deep in the ear.

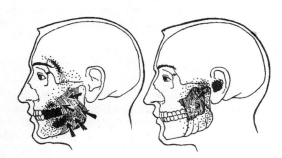

Fig. 50-4 Left: Composite pain reference pattern of the trapezius muscle, suprascapular region. Trigger areas are indicated by arrow; pain reference zones are indicated by stippled and black regions. Right: Composite pain reference patterns of the clavicular and sternal divisions of the sternomastoid. The sternal division refers pain mainly to the cheek, eyebrow, pharynx, tongue, chin, throat, and sternum. The clavicular division refers pain mainly to the forehead bilaterally, to the posterior auricular region and deep in the ear, and infrequently to the teeth. Trigger areas are indicated by arrow; pain reference zones are indicated by the stippled and black regions. (From Travell JJ: Temporomandibular joint pain referred from the head and neck. *Prosthetic Dentistry* 10:745-763, 1960.)

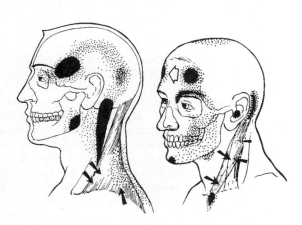

Fig. 50-5 Pain reference patterns of the masseter muscle. Left, superficial layer; right, deep layer. Trigger areas are indicated by arrows; their pain reference zones are indicated by black and stippled regions. (From Travell JJ: Temporomandibular joint pain referred from the head and neck. *Prosthetic Dentistry* 10:745-763, 1960.)

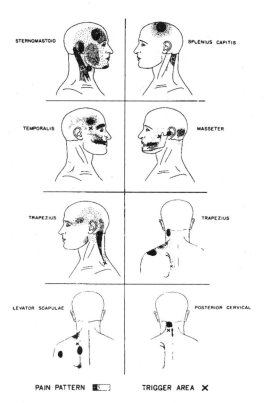

Fig. 50-6 Zones of reference in the head and neck. Solid black areas indicate so-called essentials zones, while stippled areas indicate spillover zones. The heavier the stippling, the more frequently this area is a zone of reference. (From Travell J, Rinzler SH: *Postgrad Med* 11:425-427, 1952.)

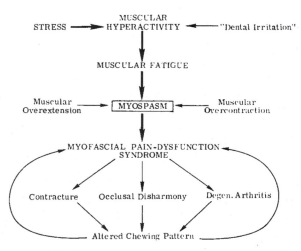

Fig. 50-7 Etiology of the myofascial pain-dysfunction syndrome. Although three means of entry into the syndrome are shown, the broad arrow indicate the most common path. The mechanism whereby stress leads to myospasm is termed the psychophysiological theory of the myofascial pain-dysfunction syndrome. (Modified from Laskin DM: Etiology of the pain-dysfunction syndrome. In Sarnat BG, Laskin DM, editors: *The Temporomandibular Joint.* Springfield, Ill, Charles C Thomas, 1979.)

2. *Temporalis muscle.* This muscle refers pain to the side of the head and to the maxillary teeth, depending on which area of the temporalis is injected. The anterior temporalis refers pain to the supraorbital ridge and maxillary incisors. The medial temporalis refers pain to the bicuspid area. The posterior temporalis refers pain to the upper molars and occiput.
3. *External pterygoid muscle* refers pain deep into the TMJ and maxillary region.
4. *Internal pterygoid muscle* refers pain mainly to structures within the mouth, tongue, and hard palate, and the TMJ and neck muscles.
5. *Trapezius muscle.* The suprascapular portion refers pain to the angle of the mandible, posterolateral neck, and mastoid process, temporal area, and back of orbit. Spasms of the trapezius muscle cause "stiff neck," with limitation of motion on the contralateral side.
6. *Sternocleidomastoid muscle* refers pain to the forehead, supraorbital ridge, inner angle of the eye, middle ear, posterior auricular region, the point of the chin, and the pharynx, with diffuse pain in the neck.

Psychophysiologic causes. Laskin et al. suggest a psychophysiologic theory of TMJ dysfunction, according to which stress and dental irritation may cause muscle hyperactivity leading to muscle fatigue and myospasm (Fig. 50-7). The four clinical signs present are pain, muscle dysfunction, clicking of the TMJ, and deviation or limited motion on opening.

To confirm joint discomfort, pain in the TMJ may be elicited by palpating the external auditory meatus. Patients with psychologic stress may exhibit teeth-clenching and/or bruxism, which may increase the intracapsular pressure in the TMJ, leading to improper joint movement.

THORACIC PAIN OF MUSCULOSKELETAL ORIGIN*

Thoracic musculoskeletal pain is a frequent complaint. It may be related to trauma, postsurgical changes, infectious processes, degenerative changes, overuse phenomenon, and inflammatory processes. The site of the pain may involve the vertebrae, the bony thorax, and the soft tissue or musculoligamentous structures.

Costochondritis (Tietze's syndrome)

Pain of the costochondral junctions along the anterior chest wall may follow blunt chest trauma; persistent coughing as with chronic obstructive pulmonary disease or acute respiratory infections; overuse of the upper extremity (from activities such as washing windows or painting); or chest surgery. True Tietze's syndrome is most frequently unilateral, involving the second and third costal cartilages (Fig. 50-8). The pain is described as mild to moderate over the anterior chest wall and, if severe enough, the patient may confuse the pain with a myocardial infarction. Differential diagnosis includes underlying malignancy and sepsis. Tietze's syndrome, which is often a diagnosis of exclusion, occurs in all age groups (including children) but is most frequently found in persons under the age of 40. Bulbous swellings that may persist for several months and point tenderness over the costochondral junction(s) are characteristic of Tietze's syndrome. Exacerbations and remissions of the pain can remain localized or radiate to the arm and shoulder. Treatment may include local heat, nonsteroidal antiinflammatory medications, local infiltration with local anesthetic solution/steroid combination, intercostal nerve blocks (Fig. 50-9), and electroacupuncture therapy. Transcutaneous electrical nerve stimulation (TENS) may be useful until the irritative process or inflammatory reaction subsides.

Costochondritis presents as inflammation of multiple costochondral or costosternal articulations. It may radiate widely and mimic intrathoracic and intraabdominal disease. Since multiple articulations are usually involved, local tenderness is elicited with palpation, which may reproduce the symptoms of the radiating pain. Costochondritis most frequently occurs in adults 40 years of age and older. Treatment is similar to that of Tietze's syndrome once the diagnosis is made, and other underlying causes of cardiac, gastrointestinal, and arthritic processes and myofascial strain have been ruled out.

Additional costochondral pain problems include trauma to the sternum and ribs, with subsequent fractures, dislocations, and separation of the ribs, cartilage, and sternum. Costochondral arthritis, osteoporosis, infection, and trauma or delayed healing after thoracic surgery can challenge therapeutic interventions. TENS therapy can be very helpful when using the electrical signal in a crossed fashion over the area of pain. Electroacupuncture therapy is a useful adjunct. Periodic intercostal nerve blocks and thoracic epidural or intrapleural catheter techniques have been described. If permissible, local infiltration near the site of pain may be beneficial.

Vertebrae

Painful disorders of the thoracic vertebrae may involve osteoporosis (Fig. 50-10), compression fractures (Fig. 50-11), thoracic facet syndrome, ankylosing spondylitis, postural abnormalities (e.g., scoliosis), and injuries involving forced or violent flexion or extension movement of the spine. Pain associated with fractures, infections, degenerative arthritic processes, metabolic bone disease, or primary or metastatic malignancies is also frequently encountered (Figs. 50-12, 50-13). Compression fractures of the thoracic vertebrae resulting from trauma, osteoporosis secondary to aging or corticosteroid use, and degenerative changes are frequently encountered. The patients complain of encircling pain along the intercostal nerves, aggravated by twisting motions, coughing, or postural changes. In the acute setting fractured vertebrae and ribs produce severe, constricting pain of the thorax, which may inhibit respiration. The pain is generally accompanied by severe muscle spasms of the intercostal and

---

*Excerpted from Neumann M: Trunk pain. In Raj PP, editor: *Practical Management of Pain,* ed 2. St Louis, Mosby, 1992.

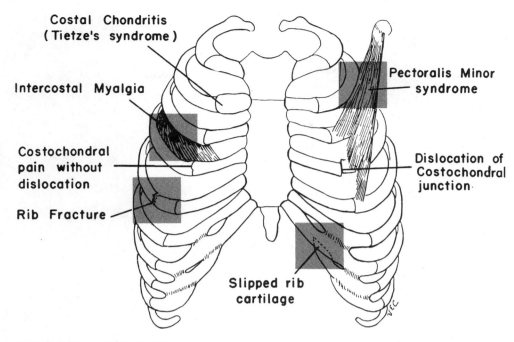

Fig. 50-8 Costochondritis (Tietze's syndrome). (From Raj PP, editor: *Practical Management of Pain,* ed 2. St Louis, Mosby, 1992.)

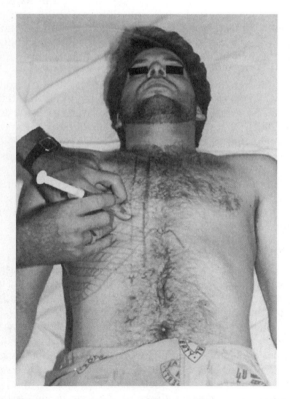

Fig. 50-9 Treatment of costochondritis. (From Raj PP, editor: *Practical Management of Pain,* ed 2. St Louis, Mosby, 1992.)

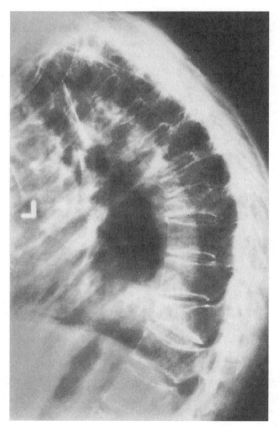

Fig. 50-10 Vertebra osteoporosis. (From Raj PP, editor: *Practical Management of Pain,* ed 2. St Louis, Mosby, 1992.)

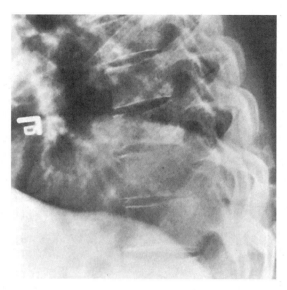

Fig. 50-11 Pathologic compression fracture. (From Raj PP, editor: *Practical Management of Pain,* ed 2. St Louis, Mosby, 1992.)

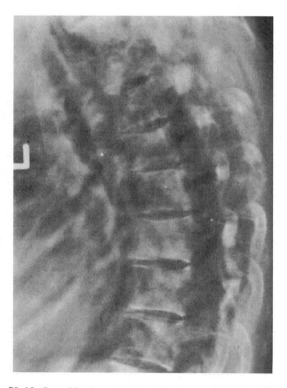

Fig. 50-12 Osteoblastic metastases from prostate. (From Raj PP, editor: *Practical Management of Pain,* ed 2. St Louis, Mosby, 1992.)

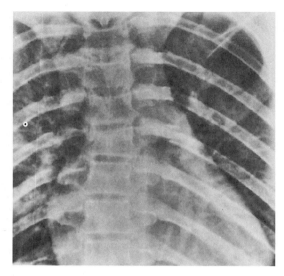

Fig. 50-13 Traumatic compression fracture of a midthoracic vertebrae with associated left rib fractures. (From Raj PP, editor: *Practical Management of Pain,* ed 2. St Louis, Mosby, 1992.)

paraspinous muscles, inhibiting the patient from obtaining adequate sleep or movement. Treatment consists of local heat or ice, TENS, nonsteroidal antiinflammatory medications, and nonopioid and opioid analgesics. Nerve-blocking techniques such as single-shot or continuous epidural blocks, single- or multiple-level intercostal blocks, paraver-

tebral somatic nerve blocks, and intrapleural catheter techniques can also be used.

Myofascial pain

Pain arising from paravertebral muscles (e.g., in longissimus thoracis and iliocostalis muscles) is a frequent cause of thoracic pain. Pain can be reproduced by pressure on the trigger area and is often relieved by massage, vapocoolant spray, or by the injection of a local anesthetic/steroid mixture.

Tender trigger points located in the pectoral and serratus anterior muscles and accompanied by spasm in those muscles are a frequent cause of anterior chest pain (see Fig. 50-8). Pain is reproduced by pressure on the trigger point and relieved by local anesthetic injection or vapocoolant spray technique. The pain is not relieved by intercostal block, since the pectoral muscles are innervated by the branches of the brachial plexus. TENS and physical therapy involving stretching exercises, deep massage, and passive then active range-of-motion techniques are helpful in preventing recurrence.

Postthoracotomy pain

Chronic pain after thoracotomy can be due to various causes. Some authors suggest that surgical excision of intercostal nerves, designed to relieve pain, may result in late postoperative pain because of neuroma formation. This technique is condemned. Complications of chemically induced intercostal neuritis with the use of absolute alcohol or other agents have given rise to recommendation against their use. Many of the common causes of postthoracotomy pain are amenable to therapeutic interventions.

Entrapment of nerve fibers in the scar tissue. A light touch on the scar produces intense radiating pain, sometimes accompanied by burning pain from associated reflex sympathetic dystrophy. Injection of the scar with a local anesthetic agent is diagnostic. Repeated injections of a local anesthetic mixed with a steroid are likely to provide long-term relief. Nelson, Glynn, and Maiwand recommend cryoanalgesia of involved intercostal nerves at the time of surgery to prevent postthoracotomy pain and pulmonary complications. However, cryoanalgesia has possible complications, since secondary neuralgias may occur. Others have suggested the use of TENS for treatment of postthoracotomy pain. For acute postthoracotomy pain management, epidural narcotic infusions may be more effective than cryoanalgesic measures of TENS.

Neuroma. A palpable neuroma in the scar, loss of pinprick sensation over the skin, and elicitation of pain on palpation are diagnostic. Repeated injection of a local anesthetic/steroid mixture may relieve the pain. Persistent pain from a localized neuroma may respond well to neurolytic injection of phenol or to cryolysis.

Sympathetic dystrophy. Burning pain associated with hyperpathia, decreased skin temperature over the area, and increased sweating characterize this syndrome. Pain is relieved by blocking the sympathetic fibers with a paravertebral sympathetic block, nerve root block, or epidural block. This pain may also respond to calcium channel-blocking drugs, β-blocking drugs, antidepressants, antiinflammatory medications, and neural stabilizing agents such as fluphenazine.

Myofascial trigger points. These points can also be the source of postthoracotomy pain. They can be located by careful palpation of the paravertebral tissues. Local injections, TENS, and epidural blocks may be helpful, as well as local heat/ice, physical therapy, and antiinflammatory agents.

Neurogenic pain

When reviewing pain syndromes of the thorax, acute herpes zoster and chronic postherpetic neuralgia should be included. Additional pain syndromes in the thoracic region involving nerve tissue or damage to nerve tissue include causalgia and intercostal neuropathies after trauma, surgical intervention, or intraneural injection. Irritation of the intercostal nerves can also occur after osteoarthritis of the joint space and destruction of or tumor invasion of the intercostal nerve with resultant mechanical compression. Hematoma or infiltration neuritis and postinjection neuritis can affect the intercostal nerves. Lesions of the spinal cord including myelopathies, demyelination, and spinal cord traumatic injuries may also contribute to thoracic pain. Causalgia involving any of the thoracic somatic nerves, thoracic intercostal nerves, or the spinal cord itself may be present.

Cutaneous pain

Scars. In the thoracoabdominal region, one can encounter noxious input from cutaneous receptors of a mild-to-severe degree secondary to scar tissue formation or nerve entrapment in the scar tissue. The pain is described as dull and aching, with frequent bouts of sharp, shooting pain associated with particular movement. Localized pain can be aggravated by direct pressure on the scar itself, and one might find referred pain to areas more closely associated with the scar tissue or more remote. The patients will complain of exquisite tenderness over areas of the scar, hyper-

algesia, and incapacitation, as the case may be. Infiltration of the scar with local anesthetic agents and steroid combinations frequently can be helpful. Cryolysis of the nerve, chemical neurolysis, excision of intercostal nerves, or thoracic dorsal-root entry-zone lesions of the spinal cord may give rise to a more "permanent," prolonged effect. Ablation of the irregular bundles of nerve element, such as neuromas, may prove beneficial. Neuroablative procedures may result in either less intense or more intense pain. It is suggested that neuromas found in scar tissue may give rise to the *viscerosensory reflex.* It is believed that the internal viscera are connected embryologically to cutaneous manifestations throughout the entire body. By pressing on or moving the various connective tissue elements of the somatosensory areas served by the same neurologic tissue, one can produce visceral or autonomic symptoms. Thus injection of a painful cutaneous scar may alleviate abdominal or thoracic visceral pain that may appear to be remote from the site itself.

REFERENCES

1. Simpson JY: On coccygodynia, the diseases and deformities of the coccyx. *M Times and Gaz* 40:1-7, 1859.
2. Thiele GH: Coccygodynia: Cause and treatment. *Dis Colon Rectum* 6:422-435, 1963.
3. Holworth B: The painful coccyx. *Clin Orthop* 14:145-160, 1959.
4. Grant SR, Salvati EP, Rubin RJ: Levator syndrome—An analysis of 316 cases. *Dis Colon Rectum* 18:161-163, 1975.
5. Postacchini F, Massobrio M: Idiopathic coccygodynia. Analysis of fifty-one cases and a radiographic study of the normal coccyx. *J Bone Joint Surg Am* 65:1116-1124, 1983.
6. Traycoff RB, Crayton H, Dodson R: Sacrococcygeal pain syndromes: Diagnosis and treatment. *Orthopedics* 12:1373-1377, 1980.
7. Bohn E: Late results of sacral rhizotomy in coccygodynia. *Acta Chir Scand* 123:6-8, 1962.
8. Gold MD, Bienasz SM, Jordan WM: The treatment of coccygodynia with radiofrequency lesions: A case report. *Pain Clinics* 3:91-93, 1990.
9. Wein AB: Coccygodynia: Operative and non-operative management as related to the proctologist. *Am J Proctol* 8:433-438, 1957.
10. Frazier LM: Coccygodynia: A tail of woe. *N C Med J* 46:209-212, 1985.
11. Johnson PH: Coccygodynia. *J Ark Med Soc* 77:421-424, 1981.
12. Stern FH: Coccygodynia among the geriatric population. *J Am Geriatr Soc* 15:100-102, 1967.
13. Kersey PJ: Non-operative management of coccygodynia. *Lancet* 1:318, 1989.
14. Albrektsson B: Sacral rhizotomy in cases of ano-coccygeal pain. A follow-up of 24 cases. *Acta Orthop Scand* 52:187-190, 1981.
15. Bayne O, Bateman JE, Cameron HU: The influence of etiology on the results of coccygectomy. *Clin Orthop* 190:266-272, 1984.
16. Borgia CA: Coccygodynia: Its diagnosis and management. *Mil Med* 129:335-338, 1964.
17. Eng JB, Rymaszewski L, Jepson K: Coccygectomy. *J R Coll Surg Edinb* 33:202-203, 1988.
18. Evans PJD, Lloyd JW, Jack TM: Cryoanalgesia for intractable perineal pain. *J R Soc Med* 74:804-809, 1981.
19. Herlin L, Del Corral-Gutiérrez JF: Neurological and neurosurgical viewpoints on proctalgias and coccygodynias. *Acta Neurol Scand* 43:189, 1967.
20. Robertson DH: Transsacral neurolytic nerve block—An alternative approach to intractable perineal pain. *Br J Anaesth* 55:873-875, 1983.
21. Saris SC et al: Sacrococcygeal rhizotomy for perineal pain. *Neurosurgery* 19:789-792, 1986.
22. Wray AR, Templeton J: Coccygectomy—A review of thirty-seven cases. *Ulster Med J* 51:121-124, 1982.
23. Wright BD: Treatment of intractable coccygodynia by transsacral ammonium chloride injection. *Anesth Analg* 50:519-525, 1971.
24. Travell JJ: Temporomandibular joint pain referred back from the head and neck. *Prosthetic Dentistry* 10:745-763, 1960.

51 Cancer Pain Syndromes

Richard B. Patt and *Sheldon A. Isaacson*

Significant pain accompanies a diagnosis of cancer in about two thirds of cases, including about 25% of patients in active treatment and up to 90% of those with advanced disease.[1] Until recently, as a result of a failure to regard pain treatment as a priority, outcome was poor, with up to 50% to 80% of patients experiencing inadequate relief.[2] Over the last decade, the concept of integrating pain and symptom management into comprehensive cancer care has been promoted by the hospice movement[3] as well as governmental and professional societies (e.g., World Health Organization,[4] American Pain Society,[5] American Society of Clinical Oncology,[6] state cancer pain initiatives).[7] This focus has resulted in a recognition that cancer pain can be controlled in more than 90% of patients,[4,8] and that undertreatment is only partially related to medical factors. A combination of knowledge deficits and cultural taboos against the medical use of the opioids is probably the most important factor limiting more effective treatment of pain in patients with cancer (Box 51-1).

THE ROLE OF PHARMACOLOGIC APPROACHES

Oral analgesics are the mainstay of therapy, and when prescribed in accordance with contemporary guidelines,[4,5,9,10] pain control can be achieved in 70% to 90% of patients.[8,11,12] When such techniques are combined with more invasive approaches and applied rigorously,[13] intractable pain should occur infrequently. These latter techniques include opioids administered by transdermal,[14] subcutaneous,[15] intravenous (IV),[15] intraspinal,[16] and intraventricular[17] routes and the provision of nerve blocks.[13]

Pharmacotherapy is preferred as the first line of treatment on the basis of its overall favorable risk-to-benefit ratio.[9] Analgesia associated with systemically administered medications is titratable and suitable for pain that is multifocal and/or progressive. Effects and side effects are reversible, and the same treatment principles can be applied safely and effectively for adults and children. Treatment is cost effective, and implementation does not depend on sophisticated technology or scarce resources and does not require special training.[18] Analgesia can usually be achieved, even in complex cases, with oral agents alone;[19] in the case of gastrointestinal (GI) dysfunction, most of the same agents can be administered intravenously or subcutaneously.[15]

THE ROLE OF INVASIVE APPROACHES

Even when pharmacologic management is applied optimally, 10% to 30% of patients experience inadequate control of pain.[8,11,12] Thus, rather than eliminating the indications for nerve blocks and other invasive procedures, the more effective and ubiquitous application of pharmacotherapy has instead resulted in a more refined role for invasive techniques. Although there is agreement that the use of such techniques should be confined primarily to those 10% to 30% of cases in which pain or side effects persist despite the judicious use of opioids, this still allows for broad application. Greater acceptance of opioid therapy has had additional positive impact on the role of neural blockade by engendering an understanding that these techniques are best viewed as complementary. Rather than judging the success or failure of an invasive technique on whether opioids could subsequently be discontinued, an opioid-sparing effect is more often sought, thus broadening indications to include cases where a reduction rather than elimination of pain is likely.

Most cancer patients have or will develop pain in multiple regions,[20] limiting the role of nerve blocks, which usually are most effective for well-localized pain. The introduction of treatment with intraspinal opioids, an invasive approach that is effective for multiple or diffuse pains, has further circumscribed the indications for neural blockade but opened a new avenue for procedurally based treatment. By providing relief at lower doses than with systemic administration, regional opioid analgesia may result in less severe side effects than systemically administered drugs.

ASSESSMENT

The assessment of pain in the cancer patient can be performed rapidly but must be integrated with a more complete history and physical examination (Boxes 51-2 to 51-4).

Purpose

Consultation accomplishes more than simply rendering a diagnosis and treatment plan.[21] It should also orient the patient, family, and referring physician to what can realistically be accomplished and serve an educational function; and, since the prognosis for controlling pain is usually good, it should ultimately be reassuring to the patient. These goals are of practical value, since patients with an improved understanding of their medical condition and confidence in their health care providers are more compliant, tend to have better outcomes, and may be less likely to use emergency services inappropriately.[22-24]

Questionnaires

Assessment may be wholly clinical in nature or supplemented by standardized pain questionnaires. The choice of a specific instrument is probably less important than it is for

Box 51-1 BARRIERS TO EFFECTIVE CANCER PAIN MANAGEMENT: MYTHS AND MISCONCEPTIONS ABOUT CANCER PAIN PREVALENT AMONG HEALTH CARE PROVIDERS*

1. **Tolerance to pain relief:** Patients need increasing doses because they inevitably become tolerant to pain relief.
2. **Intolerance to adverse symptoms:** Patients remain intolerant to side effects of analgesics
3. **Adjuvant drugs:** Relief of pain does not involve regimens of multiple classes of drugs and coanalgesics
4. **Parenteral drugs:** Severe pain calls for the administration of parenteral drugs
5. **Addiction:** Addiction is prevalent and a dangerous risk
6. **Inevitable pain:** Pain is an inevitable symptom of cancer and cannot be adequately relieved with drug treatment
7. **Ceiling dose:** There is a ceiling dose above which the opioids cannot be prescribed
8. **Physical dependence:** Patients remain physically dependent and will experience withdrawal even with gradual taper
9. **As-needed administration:** The opioids should be prescribed on an as-needed basis for cancer pain
10. **Low efficacy:** Cancer pain cannot be managed effectively with analgesics
11. **Respiratory depression:** Use of morphine to manage pain seriously depressess respiration and shortens life
12. **Prognosis:** Use of potent opioids to manage cancer pain implies "giving up" on the patient

*Adapted from Elliott TE, Elliott BA: Physician attitudes and beliefs about use of morphine for cancer pain. *J Pain Symptom Manage* 7:141-148, 1992.

Box 51-2 COMPREHENSIVE EVALUATION OF THE PATIENT WITH CANCER PAIN

Review of medical record and radiologic studies
Review of patient responses to questionnaires (if applicable)
Discussion with referring physician, primary care provider, and/or oncologist
Introduction of clinician or team, patient orientation to facility
Psychosocial history
 Marital and residential status
 Employment history and status
 Educational background
 Functional status, activities of daily living
 Recreational activities
 Support systems
 Health and capabilities of spouse/significant other
Medical history (independent of oncologic history)
 Coexisting systemic disease
 Exercise tolerance
 Allergies to medications
 Medication use
 Prior illnesses and surgery
Thorough review of systems (see Box 51-4)
Oncologic history
 Prior malignancies
 Family history
 Diagnosis and evolution of disease
 Therapy and outcome (including side effects)
 Patient's understanding of disease process and prognosis
Pain history (see Box 51-3)
Physical examination (see text)
Team meeting, if applicable
Determination of need for further studies
Formulation of clinical impression (diagnosis)
Formulation of recommendations (plan) and alternatives
Calling oncologist and/or primary care provider, if applicable
Exit interview
 Explain probable cause of symptoms
 If appropriate, discuss nature of disease
 Discuss prognosis for symptom relief
 Discuss management options
 Discuss specific recommendations
 Arrange for follow-up
 Dictate summary to referring and consulting physicians

the physician to select one that he or she feels comfortable with and will use consistently from visit to visit. Most physicians prefer to rate pain intensity on a 0-to-10 scale or 0-to-5 scale, with zero corresponding to an absence of pain and the highest number the worst pain the patient can imagine.[25] Alternatively, a categorical scale (mild-moderate-severe-intolerable) can be used.

Specific assessment tools

Two assessment tools, the Brief Pain Inventory[26,27] and the Memorial Pain Assessment Card,[28] have been specifically designed and validated for patients with cancer pain and are easy to administer, even in the presence of pain and distress. The Brief Pain Inventory requires an average of 15 minutes for completion and can be self-administered or used as an adjunct to the interview. It includes several questions about the characteristics of the pain, including its origin, prior treatments, and their efficacy. In addition, the Brief Pain Inventory incorporates two valuable features of the McGill Pain Questionnaire[29]: a graphic representation of the location of pain and groups of qualitative descriptors. Severity of pain (at best, at worst, on average) and perceived level of interference with normal function (enjoyment of life, work, mood, sleep, general activity, walking, relations with others) are quantified with visual analogue scales. A short form is available for follow-up evaluations.

The Memorial Pain Assessment Card is a simple, efficient, and valid means of facilitating rapid evaluation of the major aspects of pain experienced by cancer patients.[28] It is easy to understand and use and can be completed by experienced patients in less than 20 seconds. It consists of a two-sided 8½-inch × 11-inch card, folded to create four separate measures, and features a set of descriptive adjectives and scales for measuring pain intensity, pain relief, and mood.

One additional screening tool deserves mention because its intent and methodology are distinct from other available instruments. The Edmonton Staging System for Cancer Pain[30] is performed by the health care provider rather than the patient and was developed to prognosticate the likelihood of providing effective relief of pain in cancer patients. Patients are staged with an alphanumeric code similar to that used to characterize the clinicohistologic status of tumors.[31] It appears that treatment outcome can be predicted

---

Box 51-3 ELEMENTS OF A COMPREHENSIVE PAIN HISTORY

· Premorbid chronic pain
· Premorbid drug or alcohol use
· Pain catalogue (number and locations)
· For each pain:
  · Onset and evolution
  · Site and radiation
  · Pattern (constant, intermittent, predictable, etc)
  · Intensity (best, worst, average, current)—0 to 10 scale
  · Quality
  · Exacerbating factors
  · Relieving factors
  · How the pain interferes
  · Neurologic and motor abnormalities
  · Vasomotor changes
  · Other associated factors
  · Current analgesics (use, efficacy, side effects)
  · Prior analgesics (use, efficacy, side effects)

Box 51-4 REVIEW OF SYSTEMS (SYMPTOM LIST)

Systemic/constitutional
Anorexia
Weight loss
Cachexia
Fatigue/weakness
Insomnia

Neurologic
Sedation
Confusion
Hallucinations
Headache
Motor weakness
Altered sensation
Incontinence

Respiratory
Dyspnea
Cough
Hiccup

Gastrointestinal
Dysphagia
Nausea
Vomiting
Dehydration
Constipation
Diarrhea

Psychologic
Irritability
Anxiety
Depression
Dementia

Integument
Decubitus
Dry, sore mouth

Genitourinary
Hesitancy
Urgency

---

with some accuracy based on seven clinical features (neuropathic pain, incident pain, previous exposure to opioids, cognitive dysfunction, psychologic distress, tolerance to opioids, and a history of alcoholism or drug abuse).[30]

Pain history

The elements of a comprehensive pain history are listed in Box 51-3, and are discussed here only insofar as their application or significance differs from the assessment of the patient with chronic nonneoplastic pain.

The past medical and surgical history help determine treatability of the underlying neoplasm and the prognosis for long-term survival,[32] factors that influence the selection of antineoplastic versus palliative measures to control pain. A thorough review of systems may suggest the presence of organ-system dysfunction and systemic or regional disturbances (e.g., hypercalcemia, pleural effusion, spinal cord compression[33]) that will influence treatment. The review of systems also serves to disclose the presence of other symptoms that may be remediable or will influence the selection of analgesics.

The site(s) of localized and radiating pain helps determine its neuroanatomic source[34] and may suggest the need for further diagnostic studies. Generalized or total-body pain may indicate a system-wide problem (e.g., hypercalcemia,[33] disseminated bone metastases,[35] or the influence of psychologic distress or cognitive failure[36]). Numerous cancer pain syndromes have been described, familiarity with which can aid in diagnostics and treatment planning[1,37,38] (Box 51-5). Examples include localized pain resulting from a bone metastasis,[35] abdominal and back pain caused by retroperitoneal adenopathy,[39] and radiating pain resulting from brachial[40] or lumbosacral plexopathy.[41]

Pain intensity helps to determine whether treatment is best initiated with a nonsteroidal antiinflammatory drug (mild pain), a so-called "weak" opioid (moderate pain), or a potent opioid (severe pain).[4,5] The temporal pattern of pain helps to determine whether analgesics are best provided on a time-contingent (around-the-clock) or symptom-contingent (as-needed) basis. Most often, pain is relatively constant with intermittent exacerbations and will require treatment with an around-the-clock regimen of a long-acting opioid (e.g., controlled-release morphine, transdermal fentanyl) supplemented by the administration of a short-acting opioid (e.g., immediate- release morphine, hydromorphone, oxycodone) as needed.[42]

Patient self-report of pain descriptors may correlate with the mechanism of pain, indirectly suggesting its cause and its likelihood of responding to various interventions.[4,5,33,39] Somatic pain (i.e., emanating from bone, muscle, or ligament) is typically well localized and described as aching, sharp, or gnawing. Visceral pain is typically less well localized, more vague and deep, dull, aching, dragging, squeezing, or pressurelike. When acute it may be paroxysmal and colicky and can be associated with nausea, vomiting, diaphoresis, and alterations in vital signs. Somatic and visceral pain are subtypes of nociceptive pain (caused by activation of peripheral nociceptors and transmission along classic neuroanatomic pathways)[40] and are relatively more opioid responsive than are neuropathic disorders.[43] Neuropathic pain[35,40,44] (resulting from nerve injury) is dysesthetic in character; may be associated with objective neurologic signs or altered sensation; and is characteristically described as burning, tingling, numbing, pressing, squeezing, or itching. Examples of neuropathic cancer pain include herpes zoster, nerve impingement after mastectomy or thoracotomy, brachial or lumbosacral plexopathy caused by tumor invasion or radiation fibrosis, spinal cord injury, and leptomeningeal metastases[33,35] (see Box 51-5). As a rule, neuropathic pain is more difficult to treat than nociceptive pain, responding less favorably to opioids administered in

Box 51-5 CANCER PAIN SYNDROMES

Bone invasion: Presentation is variable; usually constant, often greatest at night and with movement or weight bearing; often a dull ache or deep, intense pain; may be associated with referred pain, muscle spasm or, when there is nerve compression, paroxysms of stabbing pain

Vertebral body invasion: Often presents as severe, localized, dull, steady, aching pain; often exacerbated by recumbency, sitting, movement, and local pressure; may be relieved by standing; localized midline tenderness may be present; associated nerve compression may produce radiating dermatomal pain and corresponding neurologic changes; may be associated with epidural-spinal cord compression

Base of skull metastases: Numerous specific syndromes described (e.g., middle fossa syndrome, jugular foramen syndrome, clivus metastases, orbital metastases, parasellar metastases, sphenoid sinus metastases, occipital condyle invasion, odontoid fractures); usually present with headache and a spectrum of neurologic findings, especially involving cranial nerves; usually a late finding; may be difficult to diagnose radiographically

Nerve invasion: Typically a constant, burning dysesthetic pain, often with an intermittent lancinating, electrical component; may be associated with neurologic deficit or diffuse hyperesthesia and localized paresthesia; muscle weakness and atrophy may be present in mixed or motor nerve syndromes

Leptomeningeal metastases, meningeal carcinomatosis: Most common with primary malignancies of breast and lung, lymphoma, and leukemia; headache is most common presenting complaint; characteristically unrelenting, may be associated with nausea, vomiting, nuchal rigidity, and mental status changes; associated neurologic abnormalities may include seizures, cranial nerve deficits, papilledema, hemiparesis, ataxia, and cauda equina syndrome; diagnosis confirmed with lumbar puncture

Spinal cord compression: Pain almost always precedes neurologic changes; urgent radiologic workup required for rapid progression of neurologic deficit, particularly motor weakness, or incontinence; early treatment may limit neurologic morbidity

Cervical plexopathy: May result from local invasion by head and neck cancers or pressure from enlarged nodes; symptoms primarily sensory, experienced as aching preauricular, postauricular, or neck pain

Brachial plexopathy: Most commonly resulting from upper-lobe lung cancer (i.e., Pancoast's syndrome), breast cancer, or lymphoma; pain is an early symptom, usually preceding neurologic findings; usually diffuse aching in shoulder girdle, radiating down arm, often to the elbow and medial (ulnar) aspect of the hand; Horner's syndrome, dysesthesias, progressive atrophy, and neurologic impairment (weakness and numbness) may occur; must differentiate from radiation fibrosis, which characteristically is less severe, less often associated with motor changes, tends to involve the upper trunks, and may be associated with lymphedema

Lumbosacral plexopathy: May be caused by local soft-tissue invasion or compression; pain is usually presenting sign; may be referred to low back, abdomen, buttock, or lower extremity

Celiac plexopathy: Usually relentless, boring, midepigastric, aching pain radiating to midback; often relieved by fetal position and worse with recumbency

Chemotherapy-induced polyneuropathy: Most common with vincristine, vinblastine and cisplatin; may include jaw pain, claudication, and dysesthetic pain in the hands or feet

Postsurgical syndromes: Most common after mastectomy, thoracotomy, radical neck dissection, nephrectomy, and amputation; usually aching, shooting, or tingling in distribution of peripheral nerves (e.g., intercostal brachial, intercostal, cervical plexus) with or without skin hypersensitivity

---

standard doses.[41] Neuropathic syndromes may be amenable to treatment with the adjuvant analgesics or coanalgesics, a heterogeneous group of drugs that includes the selected antidepressants, oral local anesthetics, and the anticonvulsants.[45]

Etiology and mechanisms

As noted above, pain may be due to an underlying nociceptive (somatic or visceral) or neuropathic mechanism and may correlate with a distinctive cancer pain syndrome (see Box 51-5). Pain may be further classified as being due directly to tumor invasion, related to treatment of the cancer, or associated with a premorbid chronic pain problem.[10]

Mechanisms by which tumors produce pain include obstruction of lymphatic and vascular channels, distention of a hollow viscus, edema and tissue inflammation, or necrosis.[40] Often unappreciated, pain is due to antineoplastic therapy in 20% or more of cases (e.g., chemotherapy-

induced polyneuritis and mucositis, osteoradionecrosis, postmastectomy and postthoractomy pain).[46] Such pain requires surveillance to distinguish it from recurrent cancer.[47] It may be challenging to treat because it is often neuropathic in nature and engenders distress in patients, who fear that it signals a recurrence.[10] In addition, because it occurs in patients with potentially long life expectancies, treatment-related pain challenges physicians, who may be reluctant to treat the pain as vigorously as they would in a dying patient.[48] Pain resulting from preexisting conditions such as arthritis or diabetic polyneuropathy may also be more difficult to manage because of the influences of learned pain behavior.[49,50]

Evaluating the person

The initial encounter should be broadly based; and rather than limiting inquiry to the pain syndrome per se, the process should encompass evaluation of the person, his or her feelings and attitudes about pain and disease, family concerns, and the premorbid psychologic history (e.g., preexisting depressive or anxiety disorders, personality disorder, substance abuse). A compassionate but objective approach to assessment serves to instill confidence in the patient and family that will be of value throughout treatment.

The philosophy underlying the hospice movement emphasizes the concept that not all pain is physical.[51,52] Attention to psychologic needs and successful treatment of underlying depression may reduce complaints of pain, whereas failure to appreciate such concomitants will render even aggressive treatment with analgesics or procedures ineffective.[53,54]

The cancer patient encounters many stressors, including fears of painful death, disability, disfigurement, and dependency.[36] In a large multicenter study,[55] although about one half (53%) of patients evaluated were adjusting normally to the stresses of cancer with no evidence of diagnosable psychiatric disorder, 47% of patients had clinically apparent psychiatric disorders. Of those with psychiatric disorders, 68% had reactive anxiety and depression (adjustment disorders with depressed or anxious mood), 13% had major depression, and 8% had an organic mental disorder (delirium). Cancer patients with pain were twice as likely to develop a psychiatric complication of cancer as their counterparts without pain. The incidence of depression and organic mental disorders (delirium) further increases in association with advancing illness.[56,57]

The presence of anxiety or depression and its relative contribution to complaints of pain should be carefully assessed in order that appropriate supportive care and/or pharmacotherapy can be instituted, a requirement that needs to be balanced against the need to limit testing that is excessively time consuming or demanding.[58] Of paramount importance is the physician's recognition that, rather than treating a disease or a pain, he or she is interacting with a unique human being in whom these events are occurring and whose needs may be complex.[59]

Review of systems

Patients with cancer tend to have multiple symptoms[60-62] (see Boxes 51-4 and 51-5 and Table 51-1). Since the ultimate goal of treatment is to enhance quality of life,[63,64] other symptoms should be carefully assessed and managed

Table 51-1 Frequency of symptoms in 275 consecutive patients with advanced cancer

Symptom	Prevalence (percent of patients)
Asthenia	90
Anorexia	85
Pain	76
Nausea	68
Constipation	65
Sedation/confusion	60
Dyspnea	12

From: Bruera E: Malnutrition and asthenia in advanced cancer. *Cancer Bull* 43:387, 1991.

with the same intensity as is applied to pain treatment.[3,65] Management is predominantly pharmacologic, and principles governing such management have been advanced in the same way as have guidelines for pain management.[3,62] Although treatment may be relatively straightforward, recent developments have suggested therapeutic alternatives for symptoms resistant to standard approaches, as well as approaches to symptoms previously viewed as irremediable, such as cognitive failure,[66] dyspnea,[67] anorexia, and weight loss.[68,69] Attention to other symptoms is particularly important for the pain specialist, since analgesic therapy may produce new symptoms or exacerbate preexisting conditions.

Physical examination

Like a careful history, the physical examination is a relatively noninvasive, cost-effective, and time-conservative means of obtaining information.[70,71] Examining patients with advanced illness is challenging to the physician and the patient because when a patient is debilitated, even a thorough examination can be demanding of his or her limited resources. A basic physical examination is important, however, especially in homebound patients whose access to routine medical care may be limited. In one study of patients referred to a cancer pain service, for example, pertinent new findings were noted in 63% of patients and in almost 20% of these cases served as the basis for the initiation of new primary antineoplastic or antibiotic therapy.[72]

The physical examination should include a determination of weight and vital signs; a thorough examination of the site of pain, surrounding sites (to check for referred pain), and sites of known tumor invasion; a complete musculoskeletal and neurologic examination; and auscultation of the heart and lungs.

Findings, particularly on examination of the neurologic and musculoskeletal systems, may be difficult to interpret when acute pain is present. Signs of simple nononcologic causes of pain such as trigger points (myofascial pain, muscle contraction headache) and positive straight-leg raising (sciatica) should not be overlooked. Compression of the spinal cord and major nerve plexuses frequently presents with pain as the first sign, and examination may reveal subtle neurologic signs that support such a diagnosis.[1,33,38,73] When integrated with data obtained from the history, findings of pain and neurologic deficit may alert the physician to the need for an urgent diagnostic workup to exclude the presence of spinal cord compression or intracranial hypertension, oncologic emergencies that require rapid specialist consultation and intervention.[33] More subtle findings may suggest the presence of neuropathic pain, which requires treatment with adjuvant analgesics[43] in addition to opioids.[41]

MANAGEMENT
The myth of addiction as a common outcome of opioid therapy

There is broad consensus that the outcome of cancer pain management should be favorable in most cases;[4,8] but that undertreatment persists, caused in large part by cultural and social factors, the most prominent of which are knowledge deficits regarding the pharmacology of chronically administered opioids[19,45,74] (see Box 51-1). Concerns regarding the potential for habituation are especially prevalent and may inappropriately impede expedient medical management.[75]

Tolerance, physical dependence, and psychologic dependence (addiction), once considered together as part of a single syndrome, are increasingly recognized as distinct phenomena.[76] Addiction is a psychobehavioral disorder with possible genetic influences that is characterized by overwhelming involvement in the acquisition and nonmedical use of drugs, despite the threat of physical and psychologic harm.[73,77] Although true addiction is a rare sequela of medical exposure, estimated to occur in less than 1% of cases,[78,79] its risk is overestimated by prescribers, which, combined with the perceived threat of sanctions by regulatory agencies, results in underprescribing, undertreatment, and poor outcome.[19]

In contrast to addiction, physical dependence and tolerance are physiologic effects of chronic opioid therapy, which, though highly prevalent, can be easily managed once identified. Physical dependence refers to the probability that a state of physical withdrawal (abstinence syndrome) will occur if drug administration is abruptly discontinued or a sufficient dose of a specific antagonist is administered. Patients on chronic opioid therapy should be assumed to be physically dependent. The sudden onset of pain associated with the administration of reversal agents (e.g., naloxone) may be followed by cardiovascular collapse in such patients[80,81] and should be avoided whenever possible. If treatment with the opioids should become unnecessary, physical dependence can be readily managed by gradually tapering opioid doses (10% to 25% each day) and avoiding the use of antagonists. Tolerance refers to the requirement for increased doses to achieve a given effect and is usually first manifested by a decrease in the observed duration of effect of each administered dose. Since there is no ceiling dose for the opioids—and because tolerance also develops to most adverse effects (notably nausea and sedation)—when suspected to be responsible for increasing pain, tolerance can usually be countered safely and effectively by simply increasing the dose.

"Pseudoaddiction" is an iatrogenic syndrome characterized by behavior that superficially appears to be addictive in nature but is actually a legitimate response of undertreated patients seeking relief from pain rather than medication per se.[82]

Concerns about addiction or perceived sanctions from regulatory agencies are not legitimate reasons to limit the prescription of opioids for cancer patients with pain. Patients who may be reluctant to take opioids because of the influence of powerful antidrug propaganda should be counseled as to their overall favorable risk-to-benefit ratio. Physicians should recognize that drug regulations are not intended to discourage appropriate medical use,[83,84] should prescribe based on medical considerations rather than the perceived threat of sanctions, and should document the rationale for therapy in the medical record.

Guidelines for pharmacologic management

The central role of pharmacologic management has already been discussed and, since the detailed pharmacology of the analgesics is described elsewhere in this text, the principles of the pharmacologic management of cancer pain are presented here.

Assessment. Careful assessment is a prerequisite for treatment. Physiologic determinants (i.e., the pain syndrome, the neoplastic process, associated symptoms, intercurrent medical conditions) and psychosocial determinants (i.e., beliefs, cultural milieu, economic status, family interactions) should be taken into account. A problem list and a set of realistic goals should be established, along with a treatment plan and contingencies.

Nonsteroidal antiinflammatory drugs. The regular (around-the-clock) administration of a nonsteroidal antiinflammatory drug (NSAID) may be instituted (1) alone for pain that is mild, or (2) in combination with stronger analgesics for moderate-to-severe pain.[4,5,85] The NSAIDS may be particularly effective for pain of inflammatory or bony metastatic origin in virtue of their ability to interfere with prostaglandin synthesis.[36] For each patient, potential benefits need to be balanced against potential toxicity (e.g., GI, renal, hematologic, and masking of fever). These are especially important considerations in the context of recent antitumor therapy and advanced age.[86] The nonacetylated salycilates (sodium salicylate, choline magnesium trisalicilate) are associated with a favorable toxicity profile (less disturbance of platelet aggregation and risk of GI bleeding, well tolerated with asthma).[87,88] A parenteral formulation of ketorolac has been introduced that has been shown to be equianalgesic to low doses of morphine in some settings but is associated with the same range of potential side effects as oral agents.[89] In contrast to the opioids, treatment with an NSAID is associated with a ceiling effect, above which dose escalations do not result in further analgesia. The ceiling dose for a given drug differs from patient to patient, though, allowing some potential for dose titration. Regular (as opposed to intermittent) use promotes both antiinflammatory and analgesic effects. Selection is based on the patient and physician's prior experience, toxicity profiles, schedule, and cost.

Weak opioids. When NSAIDs provide insufficient relief of pain or are poorly tolerated or contraindicated, the addition or substitution of a so-called "weak opioid" is usually recommended as an analgesic of intermediate potency.[4,5] These include combination preparations of acetaminophen or aspirin and propoxyphene, codeine, hydrocodone, dihydrocodeine, or oxycodone. Recently a sole-entity preparation of oxycodone was released that has been shown to be useful for even severe pain,[90] since the ceiling effect imposed by the aspirin/acetaminophen is absent. Although appropriate for mild or intermittent pain, physicians often rely excessively on codeine and its analogues, frequently continuing their use after they are no longer effective, in an ill-advised attempt to avoid prescribing more potent opioids that are also more highly regulated.[19] Propoxyphene is not usually indicated for cancer pain management because of its low potency.[19,91] Codeine preparations, though commonly prescribed, are weak analgesics relative to their capacity to

Table 51-2 Comparison of opioid agonists used in cancer pain management*

Generic name	Trade name	Route	Equivalent dose	Duration (average range)
Morphine	Various	IM	10 mg	3-4 hr
	Various	oral	20-30 mg	3-4 hr
	Various	rectal	5 mg	
Controlled Release Morphine	MS Contin Oramorph	oral	30 mg	12-8 hr
Hydromorphone	Dilaudid	oral	7.5 mg	3-4 hr
		IM	1.5 mg	3-4 hr
Oxymorphone	Numorphan	IM	1 mg	3-6 hr
		rectal	5-1 mg	4-6 hr
Meperidine	Demerol	oral	300 mg	3-6 hr
		IM	75 mg	3-4 hr
Heroin (diamorphine)		IM	5 mg	4-5 hr
		oral	60 mg	
Methadone	Dolophine	IM	20 mg	4-8 hr
		oral	10 mg	4-8 hr
Levorphanol	Levo-Dromoran	IM	2 mg	4-8 hr
		oral	2 mg	4-8 hr
Oxycodone	Various	oral	30 mg	3-6 hr
Transdermal fentanyl	Duragesic	TD	see Table 51-3	72 hr

IM, Intramuscular; TD, transdermal.
*Compared with 10 mg parenteral morphine.

induce nausea and constipation. Oxycodone is considerably more potent than codeine (up to 7.7 times)[92] and may be the most useful of the drugs in this class. The potency of hydrocodone and dihydrocodeine preparations lies between that of codeine and oxycodone.[93] These agents have the perceived advantage of not requiring triplicate prescriptions.

"Potent" opioids. When combinations of the weak opioids and NSAIDs are insufficient, therapy should progress to include more potent oral opioid analgesics in a "ladder" fashion.[4,5] That the use of the potent opioids is now considered more appropriate earlier in the course of therapy is supported by a quintupling of the U. S. consumption of morphine in the last 10 years (R. Angarola, personal communication, July 1993). Treatment with nonopioid analgesics may be continued concurrently to try to achieve an opioid-sparing effect.

Individualization and dose titration. Opioid therapy should be carefully individualized (Tables 51-2 and 51-3).[94] Dose response and side effects vary widely based on physiologic and behavioral factors (e.g., age, previous drug history, extent of disease, the presence of neuropathic pain, or pain on movement).[30,95,96] The presence of pain may antagonize the analgesic and other effects of the opioids, and as a result, effective doses often dramatically exceed guidelines recommended for acute pain in standard texts. The correct dose of an opioid for the management of cancer pain is the dose that effectively relieves the pain without inducing intolerable side effects. In this respect, treating cancer pain with an opioid is more analogous to treating diabetes mellitus than an infection, that is, a given infection can be reliably treated with an antibiotic administered in a specified dose at specified intervals for a specified duration of time; with diabetes, as much insulin is prescribed as is re-

quired to control the blood sugar. Opioids should initially be introduced in low doses, since the early appearance of side effects may reduce compliance. The starting dose is then gradually and steadily titrated upwards until either pain is controlled or side effects occur.

Adverse effects. Most side effects are manageable when patient education, identification, assessment, and management are addressed proactively. Constipation should be treated prophylactically,[97] initially with a prescription for a mild laxative when opioids are started, followed by implementation of a "sliding-scale" bowel regimen with contingencies for stronger laxatives until a regular bowel habit ensues.[98,99] Fecal impaction and bowel obstruction should be excluded when constipation and (spurious) diarrhea persist. Nausea and sedation are frequent after the start of opioid therapy or an escalation in dose, but are usually transient and resolve spontaneously over a few days as tolerance develops.[100,101] Patients should be reassured and encouraged to adhere to their prescribed regimen of analgesics. Patients may be provided with a prescription for a simple antiemetic (e.g., haloperidol, chlorpromazine) prophylactically with instructions for it to be filled if nausea occurs and then to taper its use after a few days. Refractory nausea may be treated with the neuroleptics or other agents that work by alternate mechanisms, alone or in combination.[98] Consider metoclopramide when bloating and early satiety are prominent, scopolamine if symptoms worsen when upright.[102] Other useful agents include the corticosteroids,[98] tetrahydrocannabinol (dronabinol),[103] and odansetron.[104] Sedation should not be confused with "catch-up sleep" and can be minimized by initiating opioid therapy at low doses and titrating upwards gradually. Treatment with caffeine or a psychostimulant (e.g., methylpheni-

Table 51-3 Dosage equivalency for transdermal fentanyl

| Hourly dose based on 24-hour morphine equivalents* | | |
Oral morphine† (mg/24hr)	IM morphine‡ (mg/24hr)	Transdermal fentanyl (µg/hr)
45-134	8-22	25
135-224	23-37	50
225-314	38-52	75
315-404	53-67	100
405-494	68-82	125
495-584	83-97	150
585-674	98-112	175
675-764	113-127	200
765-854	128-142	225
855-944	143-157	250
945-1034	158-172	275
1035-1124	173-187	300

*These recommendations originate from the product's package insert, supplied by Janssen Pharmaceuticals.
†*Conversion from oral morphine:* Based on a *conservative* analgesic activity ratio of 60 mg oral morphine:10 mg IM morphine (6:1 oral:parenteral conversion ratio rather than the widely accepted 3:1 ratio). As a result, converting from oral morphine to transdermal fentanyl using this chart, although generally quite safe, may result in underdosing of up to half of patients, who will then require rapid upward titration to achieve analgesia.
‡*Conversion from IV or IM morphine:* An analgesic activity ratio of 10 mg IM morphine:100 µg IV fentanyl was used to derive the equivalence of parenteral morphine to transdermal fentanyl. *These recommendations tend to be reliable.*

date 10 mg in A.M. and 5 mg with noontime meal, or dextroamphetamine)[66,105] may be considered for persistent sedation. When prescribed chronically in stable doses, the opioids are rarely responsible for sudden cognitive changes. Other potential causes of acute cognitive dysfunction (e.g., brain metastases, hypercalcemia, hypoxemia, uremia) should instead be considered.[106,107] When side effects are intractable, consideration should be given to a trial of another opioid analgesic, since side effects are often idiosyncratic and may not be triggered by agents that are in other respects quite similar (incomplete cross-tolerance).[108] Finally, the presence of intractable side effects is an indication to consider other more invasive therapeutic modalities (e.g., nerve blocks, intraspinal opioids).

Schedule. The preferred schedule depends on the tempo of the pain. Cancer pain is usually a relatively constant phenomena, punctuated by intermittent exacerbations. The continuous background pain has been referred to as "basal pain" and the peaks as "breakthrough pain," "incident pain," or "end-of-dose failure," depending on whether episodic pain occurs unpredictably in association with specific activities or just before the next scheduled dose of around-the-clock analgesic.[109] Because most patients have these two types of pain, the concurrent administration of two opioids is usually indicated: (1) maintenance therapy with a long-acting analgesic administered on a time-contingent (around-the-clock) schedule, instituted to cover basal pain, and (2) supplementation with the as-needed administration of "escape doses" or "rescue doses" of a short-acting agent. The short-acting agent initially serves to accommodate for

underestimations in the starting dose of the long-acting agent. With established use, frequent rescue doses (upwards of two to three doses/24 hr) signal the need to raise the dose of basal around-the-clock analgesic. The concurrent use of a long-acting and short-acting opioid is analogous to the simultaneous use of regular and Neutral Protamine Hagedorn (NPH) insulin for diabetes. As-needed dosing as the main means of treating pain should be avoided; the resulting fluctuations in plasma levels promote alternating intervals of pain and toxicity and serve to establish an undesirable pattern of anticipation and memory of pain.

Long-acting opioids. The preferred long-acting opioid is controlled-release morphine (MS Contin, Oramorph) administered every 12 hours or occasionally every 8 hours.[110,111] Controlled-release morphine is available in a variety of dose strengths (15, 30, 60, 100, and 200 mg) in a small tablet that should not be broken, crushed, or chewed. Transdermal fentanyl (Duragesic) is another highly acceptable means of providing basal analgesia, although its pharmacokinetics do not recommend it for unstable pain. It, too, provides relatively steady plasma levels of drug (up to 72 hours with each application of a patch that delivers 25, 50, 75 or 100 µg/hr of fentanyl), but its long latency-to-effect (consistent, near-peak plasma levels achieved within 12 to 18 hours) makes rapid titration difficult. In addition, as a result of the formation of a skin depot of drug, adverse effects may persist for 12 to 18 hours after system removal, mandating prolonged observation or, if pharmacologic reversal is required, treatment with a naloxone infusion. Methadone and levorphanol are other relatively long-acting opioids that may be considered when morphine has been poorly tolerated. Methadone is inexpensive, but it and levorphanol have long and variable half-lives that make drug accumulation and overdose a risk during the start of therapy, particularly in elderly patients and in those with renal failure.[112] They may be best started on an as-needed basis until steady state is achieved, then switched 1 to 2 weeks later to an every 4- to 8-hour around-the-clock regimen.

Short-acting opioids. Despite their relatively short duration (2 to 4 hours), immediate-release morphine and hydromorphone (Dilaudid) have the advantages of a relatively short latency of action (time-to-effect usually within 30 minutes), no accumulation, and availability in a variety of doses and formulations (e.g., liquid, tablets, parenteral, rectal). They may be used to supplement the around-the-clock administration of longer-acting agents, usually in a dose that is equivalent to 5% to 15% of the patient's 24-hour dose of long-acting drug. Alternatively, for unstable pain, the physician may wish to initiate treatment with a short-acting agent administered on an around-the-clock regimen, with allowances for extra as needed doses every hour. Patients should be instructed to maintain careful records of their analgesic use; and when breakthrough medications are used more than two to three times over a 12-hour period consistently, the dose of around-the-clock analgesic should be increased. Once stabilized, the patient can be converted to more convenient 12- or 72-hour dosing with controlled-release morphine or transdermal fentanyl.

Routes of administration and dose conversions. When possible, analgesics should be administered orally to promote independence and mobility. Transdermal administration may be associated with the same advantages as the oral route in patients with stable levels of pain. There is no evidence to suggest that superior analgesia can be achieved with parenteral administration in patients with normal GI function. Parenteral administration is therefore reserved for patients with alimentary dysfunction, (i.e., dysphagia, dehydration, malabsorption, nausea and vomiting, global weakness, obstruction) and acute unstable pain. In the case of unstable pain and intact GI function, comfort can be achieved acutely with titrated doses of IV morphine. This strategy serves a dual purpose by establishing the patient's confidence that pain can be relieved and determining baseline requirements for conversion to oral administration. Hill[19,113] recommends administering this "morphine test" with 5- to 15-mg aliquots of IV drug every 15 minutes until pain relief is achieved or side effects occur. Patients with pain that is not readily controlled by this means may require hospitalization for more protracted titration, observation, and consideration of alternate modalities. Patients with GI disturbances that are expected to persist will require prolonged parenteral therapy and a coordinated plan for home care. The pharmacokinetics and pharmacodynamics of subcutaneous and IV administration are indistinguishable,[114] and as a result, because requirements for nursing care are less, the subcutaneous route is preferred for chronic use in the home. Intravenous administration is favored in acute care settings and, when permanent venous access is already present, for chronic administration. Converting a patient to a parenteral opioid first requires summing the 24-hour dose of oral drug (including as-needed doses) and using conversion tables (see Tables 51-2 and 51-3) to determine the equianalgesic daily dose of parenteral opioid (usually morphine or hydromorphone). Most authorities recommend reducing the calculated dose by one third to account for conversion errors and then titrating upwards to effect.[10,39] The total daily dose of parenteral drug is divided by 24, and an infusion pump is set accordingly. Patients should be provided with as-needed "rescue doses" (usually equal to the hourly rate) at least every hour, the need for which serves as the basis for further titration. In suitably equipped environments, rescue doses may be initiated by the patient (patient-controlled analgesia). Rectal administration is effective but impractical over prolonged periods, so it is usually considered for the preterminal patient in whom venous access cannot be readily obtained or in whom parenteral therapy is impractical.[115]

Follow-up. A system to ensure periodic reassessment should be established, since analgesic requirements characteristically vary over time and patients may be reluctant to spontaneously initiate requests for more potent analgesics.

Adjuvants. Adjuvant drugs may enhance opioid-mediated analgesia, reduce opioid-mediated toxicity, or control other symptoms.[46] Agents from the latter two categories have been discussed briefly above and in greater detail elsewhere.[30,46,98] Numerous nonopioid agents are purported to possess analgesic properties, but only the antidepressants, anticonvulsants, corticosteroids, and oral local anesthetic agents have confirmed roles in the routine management of cancer pain. Tricyclic antidepressants may produce analgesia independent of psychologic effects,[46] a property that has been confirmed in controlled clinical trials of amitriptyline, desipramine, nortriptyline and imipramine.[116-121] Most clinicians using amitriptyline and its analogues for pain relief do so in doses inadequate to combat depression (i.e., 10 to 100 mg nightly). The tricyclics are indicated for pain of neuropathic origin, particularly when it is described as constant and dysesthetic. On the basis of well-documented efficacy of carbamazepine for the treatment of tic douloureux,[122] the anticonvulsants—carbamazepine, clonazepam, phenytoin, and valproic acid alone or in combination with the tricyclic antidepressants—have also been used successfully to treat pain of neuropathic origin,[46,123] especially when intermittent and stabbing (seizurelike). Mexiletine, an antiarrhythmic and oral local anesthetic, has been shown to be useful as a second-line agent for refractory neuropathic pain.[124-126] In addition to their role in the management of pain resulting from intracranial hypertension and spinal cord compression, the corticosteroids have been used effectively for a variety of cancer pain syndromes,[127-131] presumably because of reductions in peritumoral edema and inflammation. Despite clinical lore, there are little controlled data to support clinically important direct analgesic effects for most of the antihistamines, antipsychotics, or anxiolytics and various other drugs.

Alternate drugs and drugs to avoid. The physician should maintain familiarity with the pharmacologic profiles of a variety of drugs (see Tables 51-2 and 51-3) to facilitate conversion to an alternate route when patients lose their oral route or to convert to another drug in the presence of tolerance or adverse effects. Although extensively used to treat postoperative pain, the chronic administration of meperidine is not recommended, particularly when renal function is impaired.[4,5] Accumulation of normeperidine, an inactive metabolite with a long half-life, results in central nervous system (CNS) stimulation that may be manifested by tremors, muscle twitches, and seizures.[132] The agonist-antagonist drugs are not recommended for the treatment of cancer pain.[124] These agents are associated with ceiling doses above which further analgesia cannot be achieved and may precipitate withdrawal, and their use complicates the transition to pure agonist agents. Pentazocine (Talwin), the only oral agent currently available in the United States, is associated with a high incidence of hallucinations and confusion.

INVASIVE APPROACHES

When pain or side effects persist despite comprehensive trials of pharmacologic therapy, specialty consultation for consideration of alternative modalities including additional antitumor therapy, neural blockade, CNS opioid therapy, neurosurgery, and electrical stimulation is warranted. The general indications and considerations pertinent to these approaches have already been discussed.

Nerve blocks

A nerve block involves the injection of an anesthetic or destructive substance (neurolytic) near a nerve or nerve plexus to interrupt its function for a brief or extended period, respectively. In selected circumstances the application of intense heat or freezing (i.e., thermocoagulation and cryo-therapy) are employed for the same purposes.

General indications. Neurolytic (neurodestructive, neuroablative) blocks are considered more often than local anesthetic blocks for patients with cancer pain, since in most circumstances symptoms are due to ongoing tissue injury induced by tumor growth and pain is expected to persist.

In general, nerve blocks are most applicable for pain that (1) is well characterized, (2) is well localized, (3) is somatic or visceral in origin, and (4) that does not comprise a component of a syndrome characterized by multifocal aches and pains.

Patients with vague complaints may be poor candidates because their clinical presentation may increase the difficulty of selecting the proper procedure; in addition, those who "feel bad all over," or who volunteer that, "I can't describe it, it just hurts," may be experiencing a symptom complex defined not just by nociceptive elements, but also strongly influenced by spiritual, psychologic, and/or social factors.

Most neurolytic procedures are relatively efficacious for pain that is well localized, but—when extended to provide analgesic coverage for pain that is distributed over an extensive topographic region—are more prone to failure or are associated with increased risks of undesired neurologic deficit. Exceptions include sympathetic blockade, which often provides topographic analgesia that is ample for the visceral pain syndromes, most of which tend to be vague in character and relatively diffuse. Epidural neurolysis, although currently performed in a limited number of centers, can also often be successfully employed to manage broadly based pain without inducing unwanted neurologic deficit, although this is still a prominent risk. Finally, although its availability is even more restricted, transnasal alcohol neurolysis of the pituitary gland is applicable for widely disseminated bony metastatic pain.

Pain involving somatic or visceral structures is more likely to respond beneficially to neural blockade than is neuropathic pain, an adage that holds true for most ablative procedures and treatment with opioid analgesics.[41] Neurolytic blocks need not be summarily excluded in the management of intractable neuropathic pain, but they should be preceded by careful trials of local anesthetic blocks to determine the likelihood of efficacy.

Surveys of patients with advanced cancer have determined that pain is usually present in more than one body part simultaneously.[20] Patients may complain of one predominant source of pain only to find that when it is eliminated by a nerve block or some other procedure, other previously secondary complaints increase in severity. Nevertheless, even in patients with multiple sources of pain, a localized procedure that reduces the most severe complaint is sometimes of value, permitting control of the secondary symptoms with conservative means.

Local anesthetic blocks. Although therapeutic local anesthetic blocks are widely used in the management of pain of nonmalignant origin, they play a more limited role in the treatment of cancer pain.[133-135] The main limitation of local anesthetic blockade as a therapeutic tool in patients with cancer pain is that, with the exception of some processes involving the sympathetic nervous system, resulting pain relief tends to be transient.

Diagnostic and prognostic local anesthetic blocks. Local anesthetic injections can be broadly classified as being applicable for diagnostic, prognostic, or therapeutic purposes.[133,136,137] Diagnostic nerve blocks help to characterize the underlying mechanism of pain and define the anatomic pathways involved in pain transmission.[138] Diagnostic blocks can help to distinguish pain of somatic, sympathetic, central, or psychogenic origin. Their main use is as a preliminary step before the performance of a therapeutic nerve block or other definitive therapy. The same diagnostic nerve block may be used for prognostic purposes to affect a rough simulation of the effects expected to accompany more prolonged neuroablation.[131] Careful interpretation of the results of prognostic blocks helps to determine the potential for a subsequent neurolytic block to relieve pain and also provides an opportunity for the patient to experience in advance the side effects that sometimes accompany neurolysis. Although the results of these procedures often have good predictive value of therapeutic response and patient acceptance at least in the short term, their reliability is still incomplete.

Therapeutic local anesthetic blocks. Pain of muscular origin (i.e., cramps, myalgia, myofascial pain) is a more common cause of pain than was previously thought.[131,139,140] Underrecognition is probably due in part to the inability of standard roentgenographic techniques to document muscle injury, as well as the varied, sometimes vague and usually nonneurologic constellation of symptoms that are characteristically present. In selected cases of myofascial pain, therapeutic injections of local anesthetics into trigger points, subcutaneous foci of localized muscle spasm, in conjunction with physical therapy may provide persistent relief of pain.

Local anesthetic blocks are often administered in series for reflex sympathetic dystrophy (i.e., extremity pain of a causalgic and/or dysesthetic nature).[141,142] When similar symptoms result from tumor invasion of nervous structures (brachial or lumbosacral plexopathy), local anesthetic blockade of the stellate ganglion or lumbar sympathetic chain has been used to relieve pain for prolonged periods with some success.[143,144]

Local anesthetic injections have a potential therapeutic role in the management of painful nononcologic syndromes that occur in patients with cancer, such as herpes zoster and pain that follows thoracotomy, mastectomy, and radical neck dissection. When intralesional or perineural injections of steroids are planned, local anesthetics are often added to verify anatomic placement and to temporarily interrupt pain and muscle spasm.

Finally, local anesthetic blocks, administered either in a series or continuously via a catheter, have a potential role in the "pain emergency" to provide respite from pain and distress so that a more accurate assessment and long-term plan can be formulated.

Neurolytic blocks. Neurolytic blocks have played an important historical role in the management of intractable cancer pain and remain a primary focus of the anesthesiologist with specialized training in pain management. As has been noted, the role of neurolytic blockade is complemented by the support offered by the multidisciplinary pain management team. In general, these techniques are reserved for patients with pain of malignant origin that is severe and is expected to persist. Most techniques are appropriate for pain that is well localized and not widely disseminated or generalized. Careful selection of the proper procedure and attention to technical detail limit the incidence of side effects and unwanted neurologic deficit. The important features of patient selection are listed in Box 51-6.

Both from an historical perspective and in contemporary practice, most neurodestructive techniques involve chemical neurolysis (i.e., the injection of alcohol or phenol near a nerve or nerves for the purpose of destroying a portion of the targeted nerve to interrupt the transmission of impulses for a prolonged period of time). Cryoanalgesia is said to produce more selective destruction[145] but is generally associated with a short duration of action and may be a better choice for patients with treatment-related pain. Radiofrequency-generated thermal lesions are an effective means of inducing therapeutic nerve injury.[146] Although results are more discrete and controllable than those achieved with chemical blockade, because of the need for specialized equipment and training, chemical techniques are more commonly used.

Although well-controlled studies are lacking, large clinical series reported significant relief of pain in an average of 50% to 80% of patients, with the best results obtained when studies included patients who had received multiple blocks.[147-149] These seemingly modest outcome data can be viewed as being more meaningful when interpreted in the context of patient selection, since patients referred for treatment with nerve blocks tend to offer significant clinical challenges (by definition, their pain has been refractory to other treatment modalities). Effects tend to average 6 months in duration, an interval that is usually sufficient for most patients. There are anecdotal reports of pain relief persisting in excess of 1 to 2 years, but frequently blocks need to be repeated more often than expected, usually as a result of disease progression or the presence of tumor limiting the contact between the injected drug and the targeted nerve ("sheltering"). Overall, significant complications are reported in less than 5% of patients.[145-147] In patients with advanced disease, the relative risk-to-benefit ratio is shifted considerably in favor of invasive procedures. Optimal results are ensured by the judicious use of fluoroscopic and computed tomography (CT) guidance to verify needle localization, as well as the application of simple adjuncts such as careful aspiration, the use of a nerve stimulator, the administration of test doses of local anesthetic, and eliciting paresthesias.

Hazards of neurolysis. Nervous structures are affected indiscriminately by chemical neurolysis, and care must be exercised to relieve pain without producing unwanted motor or autonomic dysfunction. The potential for motor weakness and disturbances in autonomic function can be partly assessed in advance with local anesthetic blockade. Blockade of a purely sensory peripheral nerve will not result in motor deficit. Thorough assessment identifies patients in whom a degree of motor weakness will be well tolerated (e.g., patients already confined to bed, patients with preexisting motor deficit, and individuals with pain sufficiently severe to render an involved limb already useless).

Neither chemical nor other means of interrupting nerve function reliably produces permanent relief of pain because of axonal regrowth, CNS plasticity, and/or the development of deafferentation pain.[150,151] New deafferentation pain, usually appearing 6 to 12 months after neuroablation, is a major impediment to more widespread application. Postablative dysesthetic pain occurs infrequently after sympathetic and central blockade[134] but may follow peripheral neurolysis in a variable proportion of cases, quoted as ranging between 2% to 28%.[134,152] The incidence of neuritis after peripheral neurolysis with alcohol is widely held to be higher than when phenol is used,[134,153] although this finding has not been documented in controlled studies.[28] The significance of impermanence of effect is minimized by limiting the selection of patients to those in whom expectancy of life is unlikely to exceed the duration of pain relief and by recognizing that, in the event that effects are more short-lived than anticipated, the procedure can be repeated at the same site or more proximally. Similarly, the risk that dysesthetic pain will evolve is less of a concern in preterminal patients and those whose original pain is so severe that, by comparison, dysesthesias are unlikely to be troublesome.

The potential for overlap of sensory fields, when taken into account during the stage of diagnostic/prognostic local anesthetic blockade, is not a barrier to the success of the subsequent therapeutic nerve block. The selection of the definitive neurolytic procedure is simply guided by the results of the prognostic (local anesthetic) block.

Neurolytic drugs. Alcohol and phenol are the only agents commonly used for producing chemical neurolysis in contemporary practice, although ammonium sulfate and chlorocresol are occasionally advocated. These agents,

---

Box 51-6 PATIENT SELECTION FOR NEUROLYSIS

· Severe pain that is expected to persist
· Documented failure of aggressive trials of pharmacologic management/more conservative interventions
· Limited expectancy of life*
· Pain that is well localized†
· Pain that is not multifocal in origin‡
· Pain of somatic or visceral origin§

---

* Neurolysis may be considered for carefully selected patients in whom death is not imminent, when conservative measures have failed and the nature of the pain justifies attendant risks.
†Although true for most neurolytic procedures, sympathetic blocks, epidural neurolysis, and transnasal pituitary ablation may be appropriate for pain that is more amply distributed.
‡Neurolysis may be considered for disseminated pain when a single focus predominates.
§These syndromes are most amenable to neurolysis. Neuropathic pain is relatively less responsive.

including their histopathologic sequelae, are discussed in detail elsewhere.[154,155]

Perineural injection of alcohol is followed immediately by severe burning pain along the targeted nerve's distribution, which lasts only about 1 minute before giving way to a warm, numb sensation. Pain on injection may be blunted, indeed often eliminated, by the prior injection of a local anesthetic. The injection of phenol may also be accompanied by discomfort, but it is more often associated with a sensation of warmth and numbness.

Alcohol is commercially available in single-ml ampules as a colorless, aromatic solution that can be readily injected through small-bore needles. It is hypobaric with respect to CSF, although specific gravity is not of concern outside the theca, where injection takes place into a nonfluid medium. In the subarachnoid space and in the periphery, alcohol is generally used undiluted (100% or absolute ethyl alcohol), whereas a 50% concentration is most often used for sympathetic blockade. If left exposed to the atmosphere, highly concentrated alcohol will be diluted by absorbed moisture. Denervation and pain relief sometimes accrue over a few days after injection.

Injectable phenol requires preparation by a pharmacist.[156] Various concentrations of phenol ranging from 3% to 15% prepared with saline, water, glycerine, and different radiologic dyes have been advocated. Phenol is relatively insoluble in water: At room temperature, stable concentrations in excess of 6.7% cannot be obtained without the addition of glycerine. Phenol mixed in glycerine is hyperbaric with respect to CSF but is so viscid that, even when warmed, injection is difficult through needles smaller in caliber than 20 gauge. Shelf life is said to exceed 1 year when preparations are refrigerated and are not exposed to light. A biphasic action has been observed clinically, characterized by an initial local anesthetic effect producing subjective warmth and numbness that gives way to chronic denervation. The hypalgesia that follows phenol injection may not be as dense as after alcohol, and quality and extent of analgesia may fade slightly within the first 24 hours of administration.

Specific nerve-block procedures. Technically a nerve block can be performed at almost any site. The technical aspects of performing these individual procedures are beyond the scope of this chapter, which focuses instead on their indications and results. Selected comments on areas of special interest are provided along with references for the reader who seeks more detailed accounts of individual procedures.

Peripheral nerve blocks. Peripheral neurolysis has specific but important indications in the management of intractable cancer pain, but unfortunately it is described primarily in isolated case reports and a few small series.[135,157-160] The important differences between local anesthetic[156,161,162] and lytic blocks of the peripheral nerves lie in their (1) respective indications; (2) potential complications; (3) relative necessity for careful preliminary diagnostic and prognostic blocks; and (4) relative need for precise localization, often necessitating radiologic guidance for the latter.[163]

Specific applications
Head and neck pain. Perhaps the most frequent application for peripheral blocks is for intractable head and neck pain, as reviewed elsewhere.[155,164] Blockade of selected cranial nerves as they emerge from their foramina at the base of the skull is among the most technically demanding of nerve block procedures and usually requires radiologic guidance. Unilateral facial pain may be amenable to alcohol block of the trigeminal nerve at the foramen ovale or, if limited to the distribution of a single branch, a simpler more peripheral procedure. Lysis of the second division (maxillary nerve) or third division (mandibular nerve) is usually performed by the extraoral route, most commonly with absolute alcohol. Alcohol block of the mandibular nerve has been occasionally associated with localized gangrene and skin slough, presumably caused by vascular thrombosis. Blockade of the first division (ophthalmic nerve) is rarely employed in contemporary practice. If tumor progression is anticipated, it is preferable to prophylactically extend the field of analgesia by blocking the gasserian ganglion in its entirety. Gasserian ganglion injection is also considered for pain in the distribution of the second or third division when tumor growth or postsurgical changes prohibit access to the maxillary or mandibular nerve. When pain extends cervically or to the angle of the jaw, supplementary paravertebral blockade of the second or third cervical nerve root may be necessary for more complete relief of pain.[165]

In cases of pain that is less well localized or is concentrated near the base of the tongue, pharynx, or throat, blockade of the ninth or tenth cranial nerve may be required for complete relief.[156,166] The sensory field of the glossopharyngeal nerve includes the nasopharynx, eustachian tube, soft palate, uvula, tonsil, base of the tongue, and part of the external auditory canal. The vagus nerve subserves the larynx and contributes fibers to the ear, external auditory canal, and tympanic membrane. Bilateral destruction of the glossopharyngeal and vagus nerves is not recommended because of potential interference with swallowing mechanisms and protective airway reflexes. When available, radiofrequency coagulation is the preferred means of lesion generation.

Stellate (cervicothoracic) ganglion block (see below) may be considered for sympathetically mediated pain of the face, usually resulting from a lesion of the cervical plexus or herpes zoster.

Intractable hiccup (singultus) is also amenable to nerve block therapy. Unilateral phrenic nerve block has been used under such circumstances with excellent results, although conservative measures[167] should first be exhausted. Before performing a neurolytic phrenic nerve block, the results of a prognostic block with local anesthetic are evaluated to assure that ventilatory function will not be compromised by a more lasting procedure. Resuscitation equipment should be immediately available.

Chest wall pain. Pain originating in the thoracic wall, abdominal wall, or parietal peritoneum can be treated with peripheral nerve blocks (i.e., multiple intercostal[168-171] or paravertebral blocks[172]) or blockade of the neuraxis (i.e., subarachnoid or epidural block). Peripheral versus central blocks have not been critically compared, but an axial block may be preferred to reduce risks of neuritis, pneumothorax, and failure resulting from incomplete neurolysis and overlapping fields.

Except after pneumonectomy, the risk of pneumothorax exists for peripheral blocks performed in the thoracic region, although when proper technique is observed it should occur infrequently. For example, in a series of 50,097 intercostal blocks performed in 4333 patients, pneumothorax was detected in only four patients (0.092%).[169] The added caution is advisable when blocking the intercostal nerves of patients who have undergone complicated lung resection, as is suggested by a case report of a patient with adhesions who experienced acute bronchospasm after an unintentional presumed intrabronchial or intrapulmonary injection of a small amount (0.5 ml) of 8.0% phenol in saline.[173] Although the use of radiologic guidance has been reported for intercostal block,[166] "walking the needle off" the rib and the presence of a paresthesia are usually relied on as guides for placement.

Upper- and lower-extremity blocks. Although most patients gratefully exchange unremitting pain for numbness, iatrogenic loss of motor strength must be carefully avoided so as not to further compound the other inevitable losses associated with the experience of cancer. Since in therapeutically useful strengths alcohol and phenol produce indiscriminate destruction of neural tissue, nerves that transmit motor impulses to the limbs should not be targeted for injection unless movement is already compromised and the limb is nonfunctional or minimally functional. Neurolytic block of the brachial plexus and its branches has been described elsewhere.[155]

The sacral roots are readily accessed as they emerge from the posterior plate of the sacrum, and injections here may relieve pelvic, rectal, and lower-extremity pain. In patients with normal urinary and bowel function, selective sacral root block is preferable to spinal injections in this region because carefully executed sacral nerve blocks do not affect continence.[174] A single sacral nerve, most often one of the third[175] or sometimes fourth sacral nerves,[176] usually exerts a dominant influence on bladder musculature; as a result, blockade of the nondominant nerves, based on trials of local anesthetic injections, have little urodynamic effect. Radiologic guidance, especially lateral films, is a useful adjunct to sacral nerve block.

Sympathetic nerve blocks. Sympathetic blocks are unique in that selected patients are more likely to derive lasting benefit from a series of local injections than when somatic nerves are blocked.[139,141] If prolonged relief does not result or the patient is too ill to undergo repeated procedures, a neurolytic block may be considered. Sympathetic blockade is generally considered either for visceral pain or dysesthetic neuropathic (causalgic) pain of the limbs. Sympathetic blockade is unique in that postinjection dysesthesias are rare and neurologic deficit is unlikely, since fibers do not subserve somatic motor or sensory functions.

Blockade of the stellate (cervicothoracic) ganglion may be considered for sympathetically mediated pain of the face, neck, and upper extremity. Blockade of the lumbar sympathetic chain is likewise considered for sympathetically mediated lower-extremity pain. Celiac plexus and splanchnic nerve block are considered for upper-abdominal visceral pain, especially pain resulting from pancreatic carcinoma, and are among the most well-accepted and frequently applied nerve blocks. Blockade of the superior hypogastric plexus and the termination of the sympathetic chain (ganglion impar) have recently been introduced and are now frequently used for pelvic and perineal visceral pain syndromes, respectively.

The standard approach to celiac plexus block introduced by Kappis and modified by others is discussed elsewhere in detail.[177] A variety of alternate approaches to the celiac axis have been accepted as being safe and efficacious.[168] CT guidance[178] may be used to better visualize vascular structures and is particularly useful when regional anatomy is distorted by a bulky tumor. One of the oldest alternatives involves directing needles somewhat more cephalad (T_{11}-T_{12}) to destroy the splanchnic nerves,[179] an approach that may be particularly useful when tumor invasion interferes with classic approaches. A transaortic method[180] that involves deliberate passage of a 20- or 22-gauge needle posteriorly through the aorta may facilitate spread of the injected drug and does not seem to be associated with hemorrhagic complications. A CT-guided anterior approach,[181] similar to that used for biopsy procedures, facilitates positioning the patient, assures a wider spread of drug, and does not seem to be associated with infectious complications. Finally, although not widely practiced, the celiac axis may be infiltrated under direct vision at the time of laparotomy.[182]

Central (neuroaxial) nerve blocks. Subarachnoid (intrathecal) injections of phenol and alcohol are less commonly employed since the advent of intraspinal opioid therapy but still have important indications. They do, however, require considerable skill and specialized training and must be performed carefully to avoid unwanted neurologic deficit. They can usually be performed on an outpatient basis without radiologic guidance or special equipment and are suitable for aged or debilitated patients. Positioning may, however, be uncomfortable but is a key factor to restrict the spread of the neurolytic to targeted nerve roots. Subarachnoid neurolysis frequently needs to be repeated in order to obtain durable analgesia without unwarranted risks of undesired neurologic sequelae.[183]

Subarachnoid neurolysis produces pain relief by chemical rhizotomy at the site of injection, which may take place anywhere rostral to the midcervical region. Since alcohol and phenol destroy nervous tissue indiscriminately,[184,185] exquisite attention to selection of the injection site, volume and concentration of injectate, and selection and positioning of the patient are essential to avoid neurologic complications. Most authorities agree that neither alcohol nor phenol offers a clear advantage, except insofar as variations in baricity facilitate patient positioning in selected cases.[153,186] Because phenol sinks in CSF, patients are positioned laterally with the painful side depended and are tilted posteriorly to minimize motor block. An opposite position is adopted for alcohol, which floats in the CSF. Neurolytic saddleblock[176] using hyperbaric phenol is a relatively simple procedure that is quite effective for perineal pain, but it is usually reserved for individuals with urinary diversions and/or a colostomy.

Epidural phenol neurolysis is performed less commonly but may be considered when pain is distributed over a wider region. Because the dura limits contact between the neurolytic drug and targeted nerve roots, a catheter is usually placed and gradual neurolysis is performed serially over several days. Hospital admission and access to radiologic guidance are usually required.

Intraspinal opioids

The benefits of intraspinal anesthesia (i.e., the administration of local anesthetics into the epidural or intrathecal space) are well known for patients with acute pain related to labor, surgery, and postoperative recovery. In general, this approach to pain relief is not applicable for patients with chronic cancer pain because its effects are nonselective: reduction in pain is accompanied by motor weakness, sensory anesthesia, and interference with sympathetic activity, which can cause hypotension that would preclude routine home use. In contrast, intraspinal analgesia is achieved by the epidural or intrathecal administration of an opioid. Pain transmitted by A-delta and C fibers, which corresponds to nociceptive oncologic pain, is often dramatically relieved, but in a highly selective fashion with an absence of motor, sensory, and sympathetic effects,[187,188] making this modality highly adaptable to the home-care environment.[189,190]

The principle underlying CNS opioid therapy is that by introducing minute quantities of opioid drugs in close proximity to their receptors within the substantia gelatinosa of the spinal cord,[191] high local concentrations are achieved. As a result, in properly selected patients, analgesia is often superior to that achieved when opioids are administered by other routes, and since the absolute amount of drug administered is reduced, side effects are minimized. Not uncommonly, opioid-induced mental obtundation and so-called "narcotic bowel syndrome" (pseudoobstruction)[192] are reversed in conjunction with marked improvements in comfort at much lower overall doses.

The CNS can be accessed via an intrathecal, epidural, or intraventricular approach.[193] The intraventricular route is used infrequently for intractable head and neck pain and then usually when an access device (Ommaya reservoir) is already in place.[17] The institution of intraspinal opioid therapy requires the participation of an anesthesiologist or neurosurgeon familiar with techniques of screening, implantation, and maintenance, as well as a home-care system that is adaptable and innovative. Perhaps the most important aspect of intraspinal opioid therapy is its reversibility and the reliability and simplicity of advance screening measures for its efficacy. Screening can generally be accomplished by observing the patient's response to morphine administered through a temporary percutaneous epidural catheter. This is a simple procedure, requiring 5 to 10 minutes, is associated with minimal discomfort, and is generally well tolerated even in ill patients. Screening can be accomplished on an outpatient basis, since the side effects observed in opioid-naive patients (e.g., respiratory depression, nausea and vomiting, pruritus, urinary retention, dysphoria) are infrequent in those exposed to morphine chronically.[187] If improved

pain control and reduced side effects are sufficiently profound to warrant more prolonged therapy, temporary catheters are usually, within a period of days to weeks, replaced with a "permanent" implanted catheter in deference to concerns about infection and catheter migration.[194]

Intraspinal opioid therapy is sufficiently new so that guidelines for administration and selection of route, drug, and protocol are still emerging. A system for classifying drug-administration systems (Box 51-7) has been recommended.[195,196] A lumbar epidural catheter is the most accepted means of access to the CNS, particularly among anesthesiologists. Chronic administration of epidural opioids can be accomplished by intermittent boluses administered by the patient, family members, or nursing personnel or by continuous infusion via a standard portable infusion pump connected to the epidural port. Continuous infusion is the preferred means of administration because intervals of pain between injections are avoided and because of impressions that the development of tolerance may be delayed.[189] Preservative-free morphine, which is available commercially in a variety of concentrations or which can be made by a compounding pharmacist, is most commonly prescribed. Considerable experience has accumulated with the epidural administration of alternate, more lipid-soluble opioids (e.g., hydromorphone, diamorphine, methadone, fentanyl, sufentanil)[197] and even mixtures of dilute local anesthetic[198] for patients with refractory pain.

Subarachnoid catheter placement is a well-accepted alternative to epidural administration and usually involves the use of a subcutaneous port or totally implanted system.[188,189] Opioid requirements are about 10% of those for

---

Box 51-7 TYPES OF IMPLANTABLE DRUG-DELIVERY SYSTEMS

Type I	Percutaneous epidural or intrathecal catheter (taped)
Type II	Percutaneous epidural or subarachnoid catheter with a portion of the catheter tunneled subcutaneously from entrance site
Type IIA	Standard epidural catheter partially tunneled (usually) at bedside using another epidural needle or intrathecal catheter
Type IIB	Silastic epidural catheter more completely tunneled through paraspinal incision in operating room setting
Type III	Totally implanted epidural or intrathecal catheter attached to subcutaneous injection port
Type IV	Totally implanted epidural or intrathecal catheter attached to an implanted manually activated pump (PCA)
Type V	Totally implanted epidural or intrathecal catheter attached to implanted infusion pump (constant rate)
Type VI	Totally implanted epidural or intrathecal catheter attached to implanted infusion pump (computer programmable)

PCA, Patient-controlled analgesia.
Modified from Waldman SD, Coombs DW: Selection of implantable narcotic delivery systems. *Anesth Analg* 68:377, 1989.

epidural administration because of more direct access to the CNS and less systemic absorption. The prototype of the fully implantable systems (e.g., Shiley, Infusaid) was initially developed for intraarterial hepatic chemotherapy and uses a freon-driven pump, which is about the size and shape of a hockey puck.[199] A 50-ml reservoir is filled percutaneously every 14 to 21 days, and a constant volume of drug (2 to 4 ml/day) is infused continuously. Alterations in dosage are accomplished by replenishing the reservoir with an opioid of the appropriate concentration. A more sophisticated system has been developed that incorporates microprocessor technology to facilitate alterations in infusion rates noninvasively via a laptop computer and telemetry.[200] Because of their cost, fully implantable systems are usually reserved for patients with a life expectancy that exceeds 3 to 6 months.[201]

Neurosurgical approaches

Although ready access to neurosurgical opinion and intervention is an important component of a comprehensive cancer pain control program, only a few procedures are performed today with any frequency. The spectrum of analgesic neurosurgical operations has been extensively reviewed elsewhere.[202-204]

Percutaneous cordotomy is well suited for unilateral pain confined to the trunk or lower limb. The prototype procedure, open cordotomy, is performed under general anesthesia and involves thoracic or cervical laminectomy.[205] Percutaneous cordotomy has largely supplanted the open approach, extending this intervention to patients too ill to undergo the open procedure safely.[206-208] Usually, a probe is inserted beneath the mastoid between C_1 and C_2, and a stereotactically guided thermal lesion is generated within the lateral spinothalamic tract within the cord's anterolateral quadrant. Cordotomy is ideally suited for the treatment of intractable unilateral lower-extremity pain because preservation of proprioception, tactile sensation, and motor strength result in a minimum of dysfunction. When more extensive lesioning is performed to produce higher levels of analgesia or cordotomy is carried out in patients with pulmonary dysfunction, the incidence of both inadequate pain relief and complications increases.[202,209] Of greatest concern is the risk of Ondine's curse, a sleep apnea syndrome that, once established, has a high rate of mortality.[210]

Pituitary ablation is performed in a limited number of centers to treat intractable bilateral pain resulting from widespread bony metastases when life expectancy is moderate. Experience is greatest in patients with hormone-sensitive tumors (e.g., of the breast or prostate), but recent reports suggest efficacy in patients with other malignant neoplasms.[211] General anesthesia is induced, and a 16-gauge needle is passed through one nostril toward the pituitary fossa by the transphenoidal route. The needle tip is localized within the anterior bony margins of the pituitary fossa. A 20-gauge needle is passed through the introducer a few millimeters into the substance of the gland; and after the injection of a minute quantity of contrast medium, a total of 0.8 to 1.0 ml of absolute alcohol is injected in 0.1-ml increments over 10 to 15 minutes. During the process, anesthesia is lightened to facilitate detection of pupillary

movement or dilation that may signal damage to the optic chiasm. In addition to visual impairment, postoperative problems may include CSF leak and diabetes or addisonism that may require hormone replacement.

Electrical stimulation

Transcutaneous electrical nerve stimulation may be used as an adjunct to other more reliably effective modalities, since it rarely relieves pain entirely and is partially dependent on the placebo response.[212] It is, however, relatively innocuous, and its use may augment patients' sense of control.

The risk-to-benefit ratio of spinal cord stimulation does not seem to warrant its use in patients with cancer pain because of the expense of attendant medical hardware, the requirements for surgery, and the quality of the resulting analgesia, which is not titratable.[213]

Deep brain stimulation is a promising approach for the management of intractable pain; it has recently been redesignated as experimental and is available at only a limited number of specialized centers.[214] It may involve stimulation of areas of the brain that are densely populated with opioid receptors (e.g., periaqueductal gray),[215] in which case analgesia is generalized, apparently mediated by endorphins, and usually reversible with naloxone. Alternatively, thalamic stimulation, which produces unilateral pain that corresponds topographically to the region that is stimulated and does not appear to be mediated by endogenous opioids, is considered more frequently for nonmalignant pain.[216]

CONCLUSION

Cancer pain is comprised of a group of heterogeneous disorders characterized by variable responses to treatment. Control of pain can be achieved in most patients by the application of a carefully individualized, flexible program of analgesic drugs. Anesthetic procedures comprise an important category of complementary therapeutic options that, when carefully selected, promote improved outcome.

REFERENCES

1. Portenoy RK: Cancer pain: Epidemiology and syndromes. *Cancer* 63:2307, 1989.
2. Bonica JJ, Ekstrom JL: Systemic opioids for the management of cancer pain: An updated review. *Adv Pain Res Ther* 14:425-446, 1990.
3. Twycross RG, Lack SA: *Therapeutics in Terminal Cancer.* Edinburgh, Churchill Livingstone, 1984.
4. World Health Organization: *Cancer Pain Relief.* Geneva, WHO, 1986.
5. American Pain Society: *Principles of Analgesic Use in the Treatment of Acute Pain and Chronic Cancer Pain,* ed 3. Skokie, Ill, the Society, 1992.
6. Ad Hoc Committee on Cancer Pain: Cancer pain assessment and treatment curriculum guidelines. *J Clin Oncol* 10:1976-1982, 1992.
7. Wisconsin Pain Initiative: A report on the Wisconsin cancer pain initiative. *J Pain Symptom Manage* 3:52-55, 1988.
8. Ventafridda V et al: A validation study of the WHO method for cancer pain relief. *Cancer* 59:850, 1987.
9. Patt RB: General principles of pharmacotherapy for oncologic pain. In Patt RB, editor: *Cancer Pain.* Philadelphia, JB Lippincott, 1993.
10. Foley KM: Treatment of cancer pain. *N Engl J Med* 313:84, 1985.
11. Toscani F, Carini M: The implementation of the WHO guidelines for the treatment of advanced cancer pain in a district general hospital in Italy. *Pain Clinic* 3:37, 1989.

12. Takeda F: *Preliminary results of field-testing in Japan of the WHO draft interim guidelines for relief of cancer pain.* Geneva, WHO, 1989.
13. Patt RB, Jain S: Therapeutic decision making for invasive procedures. In Patt RB, editor: *Cancer Pain.* Philadelphia, JB Lippincott, 1993.
14. Miser AW et al: Transdermal fentanyl for pain control in patients with cancer. *Pain* 37:15-21, 1989.
15. Bruera E et al. The use of the subcutaneous route for the administration of narcotics. *Cancer* 62:407-411, 1988.
16. Ventafridda V et al: Intraspinal morphine for cancer pain. *Acta Anaesthesiol Scand* 31 (suppl 85):47, 1987.
17. Roquefeuil B et al: Intraventricular administration of morphine in patients with neoplastic intractable pain. *Surg Neurol* 21:155-158, 1984.
18. Swerdlow M, Stjernsward J: Cancer pain relief: An urgent problem. *World Health Forum* 3:325-330, 1982.
19. Hill CS: Oral opioid analgesics. In Patt RB, editor: *Cancer Pain.* Philadelphia, JB Lippincott, 1992.
20. Twycross RG: Incidence of pain. *Clin Oncol (R Coll Radiol)* 3:5, 1984.
21. Portenoy R: Management of pain in patients with advanced cancer. *Res Staff Phys* 33:59, 1987.
22. Lacroix JM: Low back pain factors of value in predicting outcomes. *Spine* 15:495, 1990.
23. Cohrn RS et al: Prospective evaluation of treatment outcome in patients referred to a cancer pain center. *Adv Pain Res Ther* 9:655, 1985.
24. Tollison CD: Patient education influences pain recovery. *Pain Management* 4:9, 1991.
25. Ahles AT, Ruckdeschel JC, Blanchard EB: Cancer-related pain II: Assessment with visual analogue scales. *J Psychosoc Res* 28:121, 1984.
26. Daut RL, Cleeland CS, Flanery RC: Development of the Wisconsin brief pain questionnaire to assess pain in cancer and other diseases. *Pain* 17:197, 1983.
27. Cleeland CS: Assessment of pain in cancer. *Adv Pain Res Ther* 16:47, 1990.
28. Fishman B et al: The Memorial pain assessment card: a valid instrument for the evaluation of cancer pain. *Cancer* 60:1151, 1987.
29. Graham C et al: Use of the McGill Pain Questionnaire in the assessment of cancer pain: Replicability and consistency. *Pain* 8:377, 1980.
30. Bruera E et al: The Edmonton staging system for cancer pain: Preliminary report. *Pain* 37:203, 1989.
31. American Joint Committee for Cancer Staging and End Result Reporting: *Manual for Staging of Cancer.* Chicago, the Committee, 1977.
32. Reuben DB, Mor V, Hiris J: Clinical sysmptoms and length of survival in patients with terminal cancer. *Arch Intern Med* 148:1586, 1988.
33. Smith JL: Oncologic emergencies. In Patt RB, editor: *Cancer Pain.* Philadelphia, JB Lippincott, 1993.
34. Payne R: Cancer pain: Anatomy, physiology and pharmacology. *Cancer* (suppl 11)63:2266, 1989.
35. Galasko CSB: *Skeletal Metastases.* London, Butterworth, 1986.
36. Breitbart W: Diagnosis and treatment of psychiatric complications. In Patt RB, editor: *Cancer Pain.* Philadelphia, JB Lippincott, 1993.
37. Patt RB: Cancer pain syndromes. In Patt RB, editor: *Cancer Pain.* Philadelphia, JB Lippincott, 1993.
38. Portenoy RK: Cancer pain: Epidemiology and symdromes. *Cancer* 63:2307, 1989.
39. Reber HA, Foley KM, editor: Pancreatic cancer pain: Presentation, pathogenesis and management. *J Pain Symptom Manage* 3:163, 1988.
40. Kori SH, Foley KM, Posner JB: Brachial plexus lesions in patients with cancer: 100 cases. *Neurology* 31:45, 1981.
41. Jaeckle KA, Young DF, Foley KM: the natural history of lumbosacral plexopathy in cancer. *Neurology* 35:8-15, 1985.
42. Portenoy R: Practical aspects of pain control in patients with cancer. *CA Cancer J Clin* 38:327, 1988.
43. Portenoy RK, Foley KM, Inturissi C: The nature of opioid responsiveness and its implications for neuropathic pain: New hypothesis derived from studies of opioid infusions. *Pain* 43:273-286, 1990.
44. Tasker RR, Dostrovsky JO: Deafferentation and central pain. In Wall PD, Melzack R, editors: *Textbook of Pain,* ed 2. Edinburgh, Churchill Livingstone, 1989.

45. Bruera E, Ripamonti C: Adjuvants to opioid analgesics. In Patt RB, editor: *Cancer Pain.* Philadelphia, JB Lippincott, 1993.
46. Campa JA, Payne R: Pain syndromes due to cancer. In Patt RB, editor: *Cancer Pain.* Philadelphia, JB Lppincott, 1993.
47. Boas RA, Schug SA, Acland RH: Perineal pain after rectal amputation: A five year followup. *Pain* 52:67-70, 1993.
48. Portenoy RK: Inadequate outcome of opioid therapy for cancer pain: Influences on practitioners and patients. In Patt RB, editor: *Cancer Pain.* Philadelphia, JB Lippincott, 1993.
49. Fordyce WE: *Behavioral Methods for Chronic Pain and Illness.* St. Louis, Mosby, 1976.
50. Pilowsky I: Pain and illness behavior. In Wall PD, Melzack R, editors: *Textbook of Pain.* Edinburgh, Churchill Livingstone, 1984.
51. Saunders C: The philosophy of terminal care. In Saunders C, editor: *The Management of Terminal Malignant Disease.* London, Arnold Edward, 1984.
52. Smith JL: Care of people who are dying: The hospice approach. In Patt RB, editor: *Cancer Pain.* Philadelphia, JB Lippincott, 1993.
53. Wand NG, Bloom VL, Friedel RO: Effectiveness of tricyclic antidepressants in treatment of coexisting pain and depression. *Pain* 7:331, 1979.
54. Spiegel D, Bloom JR: Group therapy and hypnosis reduce metastatic breast carcinoma pain. *Psychosom Med* 45:333, 1983.
55. Derogatis LR et al: the prevalence of psychiatric disorders among cancer patients. *JAMA* 249:751-757, 1983.
56. Bukberg J, Penman D, Holland J: Depression in hospitalized cancer patients. *Psychosom Med* 43:199-212, 1984.
57. Massie MJ, Holland JC, Glass E: Delirium in terminally ill cancer patients. *Am J Psychiatry* 140:1048-1050, 1983.
58. Copp LA et al: National Institutes of Health consensus panel: Integrated approach to the management of pain. *J Pain Symptom Manage* 2:35-44, 1987.
59. Mount B: Whole person care: Beyond psychosocial and physical needs. *Am J Hospic Pall Care* 10:28-37, 1993.
60. Walsh TD: Symptom control in patients with advanced cancer. *Am J Hospice Pall Care* 7:20, 1990.
61. Ventafridda V: Continuing care: A major issue in cancer pain management. *Pain* 36:137, 1989.
62. Coyle N et al: Character of terminal illness in the advanced cancer patient: Pain and other symptoms in the last four weeks of life. *J Pain Symptom Manage* 5:83, 1990.
63. Ferrell BR, Wisdon C, Wenzl C: Quality of life as an outcome variable in management of cancer pain. *Cancer* 63:2321, 1989.
64. Mor V: Cancer patients' quality of life over the disease course: Lessons from the real world. *J Chron Dis* 40:535, 1987.
65. Cummings-Ajemian I: Treatment of related symptoms. In Patt RB, editor: *Cancer Pain.* Philadelphia, JB Lippincott, 1993.
66. Bruera E, Chadwick S, Brenneis C: Methylphenidate associated with narcotics for the treatment of cancer pain. *Ca Treat Rep* 71:120, 1987.
67. Bruera E et al: Effects of morphine on the dyspnea of terminal cancer patients. *J Pain Symptom Manage* 5:341, 1990.
68. Loprinzi CL et al: Controlled trial of magestrol acetate for the treatment of cancer anorexia and cachexia. *J Nat Cancer Inst* 82:1127, 1990.
69. Wilcox JC et al: Prednisolone as an appetite stimulant in patients with cancer. *BMJ* 288:27, 1984.
70. Longmire D: The physical examination: Methods and application in the clinical evaluation of pain. *Pain Digest, 1993.*
71. Raj PP: Neurologic examination. In Raj PP, editor: *Practical Management of Pain,* ed 1. St Louis, Mosby, 1986.
72. Gonzales GR et al: The impact of a comprehensive evaluation in the management of cancer pain. *Pain* 47:141-144, 1991.
73. Gilbert RW, Kim JH, Posner JB: Epidural spinal cord compression from metastatic tumor: Diagnosis and treatment. *Ann Neurol* 3:40-51, 1978.
74. Cleeland CS: Barriers to the management of cancer pain. *Oncology* 12(suppl)19-26, 1987.
75. Foley KM: The "decriminalization" of cancer pain. *Adv Pain Res Ther* 7:11, 1989.
76. Rinaldi RC et al: Clarification and standardization of substance abuse terminology. *JAMA* 259:555, 1988.
77. Jaffe JH: Drug addiction and drug abuse. In Gilman AG et al, edi-

tors: *The Pharmacological Basis of Therapeutics,* ed 7. New York, Macmillan, 1985.

78. Perry S, Heidrich G: Management of pain during debridement: a survey of U.S. burn units. *Pain* 13:267, 1982.

79. Porter J, Jick H: Addiction rare in patients treated with narcotics. *N Engl J Med* 302:123, 1980.

80. Taff RH: Pulmonary edema following an naloxone administration in a patient without heart disease. Anesthesiology 59:576, 1983.

81. Prough BS et al: Acute pulmonary edema in healthy teenagers following conservative doses of intravenous naloxone. *Anesthesiology* 60:485, 1984.

82. Weissman DE, Haddox JD: Opioid pseudo addiction: An iatrogenic syndrome. *Pain* 36:363, 1989.

83. Jorenson DE: Federal and state regulation of opioids. *J Pain Symptom Manage* 5(suppl):12, 1990.

84. Angarola RT: Availability and regulation of opioid analgesics. *Adv Pain Res Ther* 6:513, 1990.

85. Stambaugh J: Role of nonsteroidal anti-inflammatory drugs. In Patt RB, editor: *Cancer Pain.* Philadelphia, JB Lippincott, 1993.

86. Schlegel SI, Paulus HE: Nonsteroidal and analgesic use in the elderly. *Clin Rheum Dis* 12:245, 1986.

87. Rothwell KG: Efficacy and safety of a non-acetylated salicylate, choline magnesium trisalicylate in the treatment of rheumatoid arthritis. *J Int Med Res* 11:343, 1983.

88. Leonards JR, Levy G: Gastrointestinal blood loss from aspirin and sodium salicylate tablets in man. *Clin Pharmacol Ther* 14:62, 1973.

89. Buckley MMT, Brogden RN: Ketorolac: A review of its pharmacodynamic and pharmacokinetic properties and therapeutic potential. *Drugs* 39:86-109, 1990.

90. Kalso E, Vainio A: Morphine and oxycodone hydrochloride in the management of cancer pain. *Clin Pharmacol Ther* 47:639-646, 1990.

91. Cooper SA, Beaver WT: A model to evaluate mild analgesics in oral surgery patients. *Clin Pharmacol Ther* 20:241, 1976.

92. Sunshine A, Laska EM, Olson NZ: Analgesic effects of oral oxycodone and codeine in the treatment of patients with postoperative, postfracture, or somatic pain. *Adv Pain Res Ther* 8:225, 1986.

93. Hopkinson JH III: Vicodin: A new analgesic: Clinical evaluation of efficacy and safety of repeated doses. *Curr Ther Res* 24:633-645, 1978.

94. Ferrer-Brechner T: Rational management of cancer pain. In Raj PP, editor: *Practical Management of Pain.* St Louis, Mosby, 1986.

95. Kaiko RF et al: Sources of variation in analgesic responses in cancer patients with chronic pain receiving morphine. *Pain* 15:191-200, 1983.

96. Cleeland CS, Tearnan BH: Behavioral control of cancer pain. In Holzman AD, Turk DC, editors: *Pain Management.* New York, Pergamon Press, 1986.

97. Maguire LC, Yon JL, Miller E: Prevention of narcotic-induced constipation. *N Engl J Med* 305:1651, 1981.

98. Twycross RG, Harcourt JMV: The use of laxatives at a palliative care center. *Palliat Med* 5:27, 1991.

99. Portenoy RK: Constipation in the cancer patient. *Med Clin North Am* 71:303, 1987.

100. Bruera E, Macmillan K, Hanson J: The cognitive effects of the administration of narcotic analgesics in patients with cancer pain. *Pain* 39:13, 1989.

101. Baines M: Nausea and vomiting in the patient with advanced cancer. *J Pain Symptom Manage* 3:81-85, 1988.

102. Loper KA, Ready LB, Dorman BH: Prophylactic transdermal scopolamine patches reduce nausea in postoperative patients receiving epidural morphine. *Anesth Analg* 68:144, 1989.

103. Plasse TF et al: Recent clinical experience with Dronabinol. *Pharmacol Biochem Behav* 40:695-700, 1991.

104. Cubeddu LX et al: Efficacy of odansetron (GR38032F) and the role of serotonin in cisplatin-induced nauseas and vomiting. *N Engl J Med* 322:810-816, 1990.

105. Forrest WH et al: Dextroamphetamine with morphine for the treatment of postoperative pain. *N Engl J Med* 296:712-715, 1977.

106. Bruera E et al: Delirium and severe sedation in a patient with terminal cancer. *Cancer Treat Rep* 71:787, 1987.

107. Bruera E et al: Cognitive failure in patients with terminal cancer: A prospective study. *J Pain Symptom Manage* 7:192-195, 1992.

108. Galer BS et al: Individual variability in the response to different opioids: Report of five cases. *Pain* 49:87-91, 1992.

109. Portenoy RK: Breakthrough pain: Definition and management. *Oncology* 3:25-29, 1983.

110. Hanks GW, Twycross RG, Bliss JM: Controlled release morphine tablets: a double-blind trial in patients with advanced cancer. *Anaesthesia* 42:840, 1987.

111. Hanks GW: Controlled-release morphine (MST Contin) in advanced cancer: the European experience. *Cancer* 63:2378, 1989.

112. Ettinger DS, Vitale PJ, Trump DL: Important clinical pharmacologic considerations in the use of methadone in cancer patients. *Cancer Treat Rep* 63:457, 1979.

113. Hill CS, Thorpe DM, McCrory L: A method for attaining rapid and sustained pain relief and discriminating nociceptive from neuropathic pain in cancer patients. *Pain* 5:S-498, 1990.

114. Nahata MC et al: Analgesic plasma concentrations of morphine in children with terminal malignancy receiving a continuous subcutaneous infusion of morphine sulfate to control severe pain. *Pain* 18:109-114, 1987.

115. Cole L, Hanning CD: Review of the rectal use of opioids. *J Pain Symptom Manage* 5:118-126, 1990.

116. Watson C et al: Amitriptyline versus placebo in post-herpetic neuralgia. *Neurology* 32:671-673, 1982.

117. Kishore-Kumar R et al: Desipramine relieves post-herpetic neuralgia. *Clin Pharmacol Ther* 47:305-372, 1990.

118. Panerai AE et al: A randomized, within-patient, crossover, placebo-controlled trial on the efficacy and tolerability of the tricyclic antidepressants chlorimipramine and nortriptyline in central pain. *Acta Neurol Scand Suppl* 82:34-38, 1990.

119. Sindrup SH et al: Imipramine treatment in diabetic neuropathy: relief of subjective symptoms without changes in peripheral and autonomic nerve function. *Eur J Clin Pharmacol* 37:151-153, 1989.

120. Sindrup SH et al: Clonipramine vs desipramine vs placebo in the reatement of diabetic neuropathy symptoms. A double-blind crossover study. *Br J Clin Pharmacol* 30:683-691, 1990.

121. Walsh TD: Controlled study of imipramine and morphine in chronic pain due to cancer. *Proc Am Soc Clin Oncol* 5:237, 1986.

122. Sweet WH: Treatment of trigeminal neuralgia (tic douloureux). *N Engl J Med* 315:174-177, 1986.

123. Swerdlow M: The use of anticonvulsants in the management of cancer pain. In Erdmann W, Oyamma T, Pernak MJ, editors: *The Pain Clinic.* Utrecht, Netherlands, VNU Science Press, 1985.

124. Dejgard A, Petersen P, Kstrup J: Mexiletine for treatment of chronic painful diabetic neuropathy. *Lancet* 1:9-11, 1988.

125. Lindstrom P, Lindblom U: The analgesic effect of tocainide in trigeminal neuralgia. *Pain* 28:45-50, 1987.

126. Portenoy R: Pharmacological approaches to pain control. *J Psychosoc Oncol* 8:75, 1990.

127. Shell H: Adrenal corticosteroid therapy in far-advanced cancer. *Geriatrics* 27:131-141, 1972.

128. Moertel C et al: Corticosteroid therapy in pre-terminal gastrointestinal cancer. *Cancer* 33:1607-1609, 1974.

129. Bruera E et al: Action of oral methylprednisolone in terminal cancer patients: a prospective randomized double-blind study. *Cancer Treat Rep* 69:751-754, 1985.

130. Della Luna GR, Pellegrini A, Piazzi M: Effect of methylprednisolone sodium succinate on quality of life in preterminal cancer patients: A placebo-controlled, multicenter study. *Eur J Cancer Clin Oncol* 25:1817-1821, 1981.

131. Popiela T, Lucchi R, Giongo F: Methylprednisolone as palliative therapy for female terminal cancer patients. *Eur J Cancer Clin Oncol* 25:1823-1829, 1989.

132. Kaiko RF et al: Central nervous system excitatory effects of meperidine in cancer patients. *Ann Neurol* 13:180-185, 1983.

133. Abrams SE: The role of non-neurolygic blocks in the management of cancer pain. In Abrams SE, editor: *Cancer Pain.* Boston, Kluwer, 1989.

134. Porges P: Local anesthetics in the treatment of cancer pain. *Recent Results Cancer Res* 89:127, 1984.

135. Raj PP: Local anesthetic blocks. In Patt RB, editor: *Cancer Pain.* Philadelphia, JB Lippincott, 1993.

136. Bonica JJ: *Management of Pain.* Philadelphia, Lea & Febiger, 1953.

137. Cousins MJ: Anesthetic approaches in cancer pain. *Adv Pain Res Ther* 16:249-73, 1990.

138. Raj PP, Ramamurthy S: Differential nerve bock studies. In Raj PP, editor: *Practical Management of Pain.* St Louis, Mosby, 1986.

139. Travell J: Myofascial trigger points: Clinical view. *Adv Pain Res Ther* 1:919, 1976.

140. Travell JG, Simons DG: *Mylofascial Pain and Dysfunction: The Trigger Point Manual.* Baltimore, Williams & Wilkins, 1983.

141. Payne R: Neuropathic pain syndromes, with special reference to causalgia and reflex sympathetic dystrophy. *Clin J Pain* 2:59-73, 1986.

142. Patt RB, Balter K: Posttraumatic reflex sympathetic dystrophy: Mechanisms and medical management. *J Occupational Rehab* 1:57-70, 1991.

143. Gerbershagen HU: Blocks with local anesthetics in the treatment of cancer pain. *Adv Pain Res Ther* 2311-2323, 1979.

144. Warfield CA, Crews DA: Use of stellate ganglion blocks in the treatment of intractable limb pain in lung cancer. *Clin J Pain* 3:13, 1987.

145. Evans PJD: Cryoanalgesia. *Anaesthesia* 36:1003-1013, 1981.

146. Siegfried J, Broggi G: Percutaneous thermocoagulation of the gasserian ganglion in the treatment of pain in advanced cancer. *Adv Pain Res Ther* 2:463, 1979.

147. Hay RC: Subarachnoid alcohol block in the control of intractable pain: Report of results in 252 patients. *Anesth Analg* 41:12-16, 1962.

148. Perese DM: Subarachnoid alcohol block in the management of pain of malignant disease. *Arch Surg* 76:347-354, 1958.

149. Papo I, Visca A: Phenol subarachnoid rhizotomy for the treatment of cancer pain: A personal account of 290 cases. *Adv Pain Res Ther* 2:339-346, 1979.

150. Patt R: Neurosurgical interventions for chronic pain problems. *Anesth Clin North Am* 5:609, 1987.

151. Ramamurthy S et al: Evaluation of neurolytic blocks using phenol and cryogenic block in the management of chronic pain. *J Pain Symptom Manage* 4:72, 1989.

152. Mandl F: *Paravertebral Block.* New York, Brune & Stratton, 1947.

153. Katz J: Current role of neurolytic agents. *Adv Neurol* 4:471, 1974.

154. Lipton S: Neurolytics: Pharmacology and drug selection. In Patt RB, editor: *Cancer Pain Management.* Philadelphia, JB Lippincott, 1992.

155. Swerdlow M: Neurolytic blocks of the neuraxis. In Patt RB, editor: *Cancer Pain Management.* Philadelphia, JB Lippincott, 1992.

156. Meissner W: Formulas. In Raj PP, editor: *Practical Management of Pain.* St Louis, Mosby, 1986.

157. Patt RB: Peripheral neurolysis in the management of cancer pain. *Pain Digest,* 2:30-42, 1992.

158. Patt RB, Millard RW: A role for peripheral neurolysis in the management of intractable cancer pain. *Pain* 5(suppl):S-358, 1990.

159. Bonica JJ et al: Neurolytic blockade and hypophysectomy. In Bonica JJ, editor: *Management of Pain,* ed 2. Phildelphia, Lea & Febiger, 1990.

160. Swerdlow M: Role of chemical neurolysis and local anesthetic infiltration. In Swerdlow M, Ventafridda V, editors: *Cancer Pain.* Lancaster, UK MTP Press, 1986.

161. Thompson GE, Moore DC: Celiac plexus, intercostal, and minor peripheral blockade. In Cousins MJ, Bridenbaugh PO, editors: *Neural Blockade,* ed 2. Philadelphia, JB Lippincott, 1988.

162. Pitkin GP: Blocking the trigeminal nerve. In Southworth JL, Hingson RA, Pitkin WM, editors: *Conduction Anesthesia,* ed 2. Philadelphia, JB Lippincott, 1953.

163. Pender JW, Pugh DG: Diagnostic and therapeutic nerve blocks: Necessity for roentgenograms. *JAMA* 146:798, 1951.

164. Bonica JJ: The management of pain of malignant disease with nerve blocks. *Anesthesiology* 15:280, 1954.

165. Patt R, Jain S: Management of a patient with osteroradionecrosis of the mandible with nerve blocks. *J Pain Symptom Manage* 5:59-60, 1990.

166. Montgomery W, Cousins MJ: Aspects of the management of chronic pain illustrated by ninth cranial nerve block. *Br J Anaesth* 44:383, 1972.

167. Twycross RG, Lack SA: *Therapeutics in Terminal Care.* Edinburgh, Chruchill Livingstone, 1986.

168. Moore DC: Intercostal nerve block and celiac plexus block for pain therapy. *Adv Pain Res Ther* 7:309, 1984.

169. Churcher M: Peripheral nerve blocks in the relief of intractable pain. In Swerdlow M, Charlton JE: *Relief of Intractable Pain,* ed 4. Amsterdam, Elsevier, 1989.

170. Doyle D: Nerve blocks in advanced cancer. *Practitioioner* 226:539-544, 1982.

171. Moore D, Bridenbaugh DL: Intercostal nerve block in 4333 patients: Indications, techniques, complications. *Anesth Analg* 41:1, 1962.

172. Vernon S: Paralgesia: Paravertebral block for pain relief. *Am J Surg* 21:416, 1932.

173. Atkinson GL, Supack RC: Acute bronchospasm complicating intercostal nerve block with phenol. *Anesth Analg* 68:400-401, 1989.

174. Robertson DH: Transsacral neurolytic nerve block: an alternative approach to intractable perineal pain. *Br J Anaesth* 55:873-875, 1983.

175. Clark AJ, Awad SA: Selective transsacral nerve root blocks. *Reg Anesth* 15:125, 1990.

176. Rockswold GL, Bradley WE, Chou SN: Effect of sacral nerve blocks on the function of the urinary bladder in humans. *J Neurosurg* 40:83, 1974.

177. Plancarte R, Velazquez R, Patt RB: Neurolytic blocks of the sympathetic axis. In Patt RB, editor: *Cancer Pain.* Philadelphia, JB Lippincott, 1993.

178. Singler RC: An improved technique for alcohol neurolysis of the celiac plexus. *Anesthesiology* 56:137, 1982.

179. Boas RA: Sympathetic blocks in clinical practice. *Int Anesthesiol Clin* 16:149, 1978.

180. Ischia S et al: A new approach to the neurolytic block of the celiac plexus: The transaortic technique. *Pain* 16:333, 1983.

181. Matamala AM, Lopez FV, Martinez LI: Percutaneous approach to the celiac plexus using CT guidance. *Pain* 34:285, 1988.

182. Flanigan DP, Draft R: Continuing experience with palliative chemical splanchnicectomy. *Arch Surg* 113:509-511, 1978.

183. Patt RB et al: Management of intractable cancer pain with subarachnoid neurolytic block. Abstract presented at VII World Congress on Pain, Paris, August, 1993.

184. Peyton WT, Semansky EJ, Baker AB: Subarachnoid injection of alcohol for relief of intractable pain with discussion of cord changes found at autopsy. *Am J Cancer* 30:709, 1937.

185. Smith MC: Histological findings following intrathecal injections of phenol solutions for relief of pain. *Br J Anaesth* 36:387-406, 1963.

186. Katz J: The current role of neurolytic agents. *Adv Neurol* 4:471-476, 1974.

187. Cousins MJ, Mather LE: Intrathecal and epidural administration of opioids. *Anesthesiology* 61:276-310, 1984.

188. Yaksh TL: Spinal opiates: A review of their effect on spinal function with an emphasis on pain processing. *Acta Anaesthesiol Scand* 31(suppl 85):25, 1987.

189. Smith DE: Spinal opioids in the home and hospice setting. *J Pain Symptom Manage* 5:175, 1990.

190. Crawford ME et al: Pain treatment on outpatient basis using extradural opiates: Danish multicenter study comprising 105 patients. *Pain* 16:41, 1983.

191. Snyder SH: Opiate receptors in the brain. *N Engl J Med* 296:266-271, 1977.

192. Patt RB, Jain S: Long term management of a patient with perineal pain secondary to rectal cancer. *J Pain Symptom Manage* 5:127-128, 1990.

193. Waldman SD et al: Intraspinal opioid therapy. In Patt RB, editor: *Cancer Pain Management: A Multidisciplinary Approach.* Philadelphia, JB Lippincott, 1993.

194. DuPen SL et al: A new permenent exteriorized epidural catheter for narcotic self-administration to control cancer pain. *Cancer* 59:986, 1987.

195. Waldman SD, Coombs DW: Selection of implantable narcotic delivery systems. *Anesth Analg* 68:377, 1989.

196. Waldman SD: Implantable drug delivery systems: Practical considerations. *J Pain Symptom Manage* 5:169, 1990.

197. De Castro J, Meynadier J, Zenz M: *Regional Opioid Analgesia.* Dordrecht, Kluwer, 1991.

198. Du Pen SL: After epidural narcotics: What next? *Anesth Analg* 66(suppl):S46, 1987.

199. Coombs DW et al: Relief of continuous chronic pain by intraspinal narcotics infusion via an implanted reservoir. *JAMA* 250:2336, 1983.

200. Penn RD et al: Cancer pain relief using chronic morphine infusions:

Early experience with a programmable implanted drug pump. *J Neurosurg* 61:302, 1984.

201. Bedder MD, Burchiel KJ, Larson A: Cost analysis of two implantable narcotic delivery systems. *J Pain Symptom Manage* 6:368, 1991.

202. Patt RB: Pain therapy. In Frost EAM, editor: *Clinical Anesthesia in Neurosurgery,* ed 2. Boston, Butterworth, 1990.

203. Long DM: Surgical therapy of chronic pain. *Neurosurgery* 6:317-326, 1980.

204. White JC, Sweet WH: *Pain and the Neurosurgeon: A Forty Year Experience.* Springfield, Ill, Charles C Thomas, 1969.

205. Spiller WG, Martin E: The treatment of persistent pain of organic origin in the lower part of the body by division of the antero-lateral column of the spinal cord. *JAMA* 58:1489, 1912.

206. Tasker RR: Merits of percutaneous cordotomy over the open operation. In Morley RP, editor: *Current Controversies in Neurosurgery.* Philadelphia, WB Saunders, 1976.

207. Lahuerta J, Lipton S, Wells JCD: Percutaneous cordotomy: Results and complications in a recent series of 100 patients. *Ann R Coll Surg Engl* 67:41-44, 1985.

208. Lipton S: Percutaneous cordotomy. In Wall PD, Melzack R, editors: *Textbook of Pain.* New York, Churchill Livingstone, 1984.

209. Lipton S: Percutaneous cervical cordotomy. *Adv Pain Res Ther* 2:425-437, 1979.

210. Polatty RC, Cooper KR: Respiratory failure after percutaneous cordotomy. *South Med J* 79:897-899, 1986.

211. Lahuerta J et al: Update on percutaneous cervical cordotomy and pituitary alcohol neuroadenolysis: An audit of our recent results and complications. In Lipton S, Miles J, editors: *Persistent Pain, vol 5.* New York, Grune & Stratton, 1985.

212. Ventafridda V et al. Transcutaneous nerve stimulation in cancer pain. *Adv Pain Res Ther* 2:509-515, 1979.

213. Meglio M, Cioni B: Personal experience with spinal cord stimulation in chronic pain management. *Appl Neurophysiol* 45:195-200, 1982.

214. Tasker R: Neurosurgical and neuroaugmentative intervention. In Patt RB, editor: *Cancer Pain.* Philadelphia, JB Lippincott, 1993.

215. Young RF, Brechner T: Electrical stimulation of the brain for relief of intractable pain due to cancer. *Cancer* 57:1266-1272, 1986.

216. Turnbull JM, Shulman R, Woodhurst WB: Thalamic stimulation for neuropathic pain. *J Neurosurg* 52:486-493, 1980.

QUESTIONS: CANCER PAIN SYNDROMES

For questions 1-5, choose from the following:
   A. 1, 2, and 3
   B. 1 and 3
   C. 2 and 4
   D. 4
   E. All of the above

1. Which of the following statement(s) is (are) true regarding neuropathic cancer pain syndromes?
   1. They are often due to antitumor treatment directed at the cancer.
   2. They may need to be treated with adjuvant analgesics.
   3. They are characteristically less opioid-responsive than is nociceptive pain.
   4. They are characteristically unresponsive to treatment with the opioids.

2. Which of the following statement(s) regarding opioid-mediated side effects is (are) true?
   1. They can be managed symptomatically (e.g., laxatives, antiemetics, amphetamines).
   2. They can be managed with a trial of a nonopioid adjuvant drug.
   3. They occur frequently, but with the exception of constipation most usually recede after a short period.
   4. They may serve as a rationale to institute treatment with a different opioid or a more invasive approach.

3. Which of the following statement(s) regarding the use of parenteral opioids for treating cancer pain is (are) true?
   1. They are usually more effective than treatment with oral anesthetics.
   2. They are usually administered by the intravenous rather than subcutaneous route.
   3. They are indicated based on the presence of severe pain.
   4. They are most commonly instituted because of gastrointestinal disturbances.

4. Which of the following statement(s) is (are) true regarding treatment of cancer pain with intraspinal opioid therapy?
   1. It is efficacious for pain that is present in multiple regions.
   2. The incidence of side effects is similar to that for treatment of perioperative pain.
   3. It usually is used when treatment with systemic opioids has resulted in intractable side effects.
   4. It must be administered by an expensive fully implantable infusion pump.

5. Which of the following statements is (are) true regarding subarachnoid neurolysis?
   1. The patient should be tilted 45° posteriorly when it is performed with alcohol.
   2. It usually requires radiologic guidance.
   3. The patient does not need to lie on the painful side when it is performed with phenol.
   4. It is safest when performed in the thoracic region.

ANSWERS

1. A
2. E
3. D
4. B
5. D

52 Chronic Pain Syndromes in Children

Joelle F. Desparmet and *P. Prithvi Raj*

RECURRENT ABDOMINAL PAIN

The definition of recurrent abdominal pain in childhood and adolescence is pain with no organic cause occurring on at least three occasions over a 3-month period and that is severe enough to alter the child's normal activity. This definition excludes abdominal pain caused by known medical conditions as defined by Levine and Rappaport, such as pain resulting from neurologic disorders, metabolic disease (e.g., diabetes, porphyria, hyperparathyroidism), hematologic disease (e.g., sickle cell anemia), gastrointestinal disease, gynecologic conditions, chronic infection, and pain related to congenital anomalies.[1] It also excludes acute pain caused by renal, intestinal, and gynecologic acute disorders, which can be treated surgically.

Pain for which no organic cause is found is often regarded as psychogenic and can be misdiagnosed or denied by parents or physicians and treated inadequately. Therefore recurrent abdominal pain would better be considered as psychophysiologic.[2] This implies that it is real pain triggered by stress, depression, or family-related conflicts. These stressors may be associated with physiologic disorders such as autonomic instability, lactose intolerance, and constipation. Each of these elements may sometimes benefit from specific treatment. Many of these factors can coincide, and proper diagnosis relies on physical and psychologic findings. Studies have shown that 10% to 15% of school-age children complain of nonorganic abdominal pain at some time.[3,4]

Recurrent abdominal pain seems to peak in 10- to 12-year-olds; some studies have shown a prevalence among girls. Typically, recurrent abdominal pain occurs two to four times a week and lasts ½ hour to 2 hours. The pain is often situated in the periumbilical or epigastric area and is dull, sharp, or cramplike. Half of the children have nausea, and some have vomiting with some attacks.[4] Some children have a recent history of an intestinal disorder similar to gastroenteritis or intestinal flu. The pain does not disrupt sleep but can interrupt normal activities. Some children miss school or withdraw from their family and friends. There are no physical findings other than tenderness in the periumbilical or epigastric area or over the whole abdomen. The diagnosis of recurrent abdominal pain is based on the absence of an organic cause. Laboratory tests other than complete blood cell count, urine analysis, and stool guaiac are usually not necessary if nothing is found on history and physical examination, since they rarely reveal pathology. Symptoms related to a specific psychophysiologic factor in the child's life or family's history are, on the other hand, often present.

Since this type of pain is a multifactorial phenomenon and can be related to stress in the family or school setting, treatment can be difficult to initiate. Some patients will respond to a high-fiber diet[5] or to discontinuation of intake of milk or lactose-containing foods. The most important part of the management of recurrent abdominal pain is to prepare the family and child for the diagnosis of nonorganic pain and to reassure them that the pain is not in the child's mind. Treatment includes management of stress factors if need be, through referral to behavior-medicine specialists for relaxation and biofeedback techniques and ways to change attitude toward stressors.[6] The outcome of recurrent abdominal pain is linked to the evolution of the psychophysiologic symptoms: One third of children have no pain when they are adults, whereas one third still do; leaving one third who, although free of abdominal pain, develop other psychophysiologic problems.

HEADACHE AND MIGRAINE

Headache. Headache is the most common type of pain of which children complain. It can be a benign symptom often accompanying common illness such as colds and other minor viral infections; it can then be treated with minor drugs such as aspirin and acetaminophen and disappears as the illness resolves. Headache can also be recurrent and accompany other more severe disorders. One important fact should be kept in mind when treating a child with recurrent headache: Meningitis, encephalitis, cerebral abscess, vascular malformations, trauma, tumoral masses of the meninges or cerebral structures, and degenerative cerebral disease with or without intracranial hypertension are all causes for headache.

Diagnosis of benign recurrent headache should not be reached unless a complete history and physical examination including fundoscopy are normal. Laboratory investigations can be conducted to confirm the absence of a pathologic cause to the headaches if clinically indicated. Apart from the neurologic causes of headache, other causes are sinus infections, ophthalmic and dental conditions, allergies, stress resulting in tension headaches, and psychogenic headaches that are similar to tension headaches in their clinical aspects.[7,8] Treatment starts with treatment of the ailment causing the headache. Minor analgesics such as aspirin, acetaminophen, or a combination of these drugs can be enough to relieve the headache.

Migraine. The epidemiology of childhood migraine is not well defined, but a number of reports date the start of migraine in some adults to as early as between 1 and 4 years of age[9] and, for more than 20% to 30% of sufferers, to the first decade of life.[10,11] The incidence of migraine is about 3% to 5% of prepubertal children. After puberty the incidence of migraine increases notably to reach 10% to 20% of children by age 20 (Table 52-1). Migraine in children can be defined as recurrent headache accompanied by three of the following symptoms: recurrent abdominal pain with or without nausea or vomiting; throbbing pain on one side of the cranium; relief of the pain by rest; a visual, sensory, or motor aura; and a family history of migraine.[12] It seems that childhood migraine is a vascular and neurologic disease, as evidenced by frequent association with electroencephalogram (EEG) abnormalities.[13,14] Clinically, migraine has different presentations.

Common migraine is the type of migraine seen in children before puberty. There is no aura before the headache and no unilateral focal localization of the pain. The pain is usually bifrontal or bitemporal. Only 5% of children have occipital pain. Seventy percent of the children have abdominal pain. The headache increases over 30 minutes to 2 hours and often stops when vomiting occurs. Occasionally the severity of the headache forces the child to lie down, but the headache rarely causes intense suffering. However, when it does, it can be relieved temporarily only by potent analgesics. Most children experience one or two migraines a month, but the frequency can increase along with the intensity and duration of the headache[15] and could then be related to depression.[16]

Classic migraine is different from common migraine in that the former starts with a visual aura in 30% and a sensory, sensory-motor aura, or speech impairment in 10% of children affected. These auras are followed by severe, throbbing, hemicranial, well-localized headache. An EEG shows slow activity in the affected hemisphere that can last as long

as 1 week. This type of migraine can rarely be associated with hemiplegia, coma, or confusion (familial hemiplegic migraine); in rare instances it constitutes a syndrome called alternating hemiplegia of infancy, with EEG alterations and retardation.

Ophthalmoplegic migraine is rare in children younger than 4 to 5 years, usually affects only one eye, and is often accompanied by mydriasis.

The difficult differential diagnosis of common migraine is tension (muscle-contraction) headache, which has similar symptoms. Tension headache is different clinically in that it is usually occipital and diffuse and involves the neck. It is often continuous, lasting even after sleep, but does not prevent the child from performing his or her usual daily activities. Anxiety is often present; and triggering, stressful situations are responsible for an increase in the symptoms.

Common migraine is associated with sinusitis in 15% of cases.[17] It can also be the sign of an underlying pathologic process such as arteriovenous malformations, ischemic infarction, or epilepsy.

Prophylactic treatment has classically been based on ergotamine, which causes vasoconstriction of extracranial blood vessels. Drugs such as anticonvulsants, antidepressants, antihypertensives, antihistamines, and calcium-channel blockers have been reported as successful long-term preventive treatments.

There is reason to believe that in some children migraine can be related to sensitivity to amines such as tyramine, phenylethylamine, or octopamine found in cheese, yogurt and other dairy products, chocolate, and wine. Restricting these foods is often successful in relieving the migraine in such cases.

More recently, behavioral treatments have proven very effective in pediatric migraine. Biofeedback, relaxation, and self-hypnosis are used with success in many centers. Controlled studies using relaxation techniques monitored by electromyogram (EMG) and hand temperature at Boston's

Table 52-1 Incidence of migraine

Authors	Age (years)	Percentage age with migraine
Vahlquist (1955)	10-12	4.5
Vahlquist (1955)	16-19	7.4
Brewis et al (1966)	10-14	2.4
Brewis et al (1966)	15-19	1.6
Dalsgaard-Nielsen, Engberg-Pedersen, and Holm (1970)	7- 9	3.0
Dalsgaard-Nielsen, Engberg-Pedersen, and Holm (1970)	9-11	4.5
Dalsgaard-Nielsen, Engberg-Pedersen, and Holm (1970)	11-13	6.0
Dalsgaard-Nielsen, Engberg-Pedersen, and Holm (1970)	13-15	7.5
Dalsgaard-Nielsen, Engberg-Pedersen, and Holm (1970)	15-17	8.9
Dalsgaard-Nielsen, Engberg-Pedersen, and Holm (1970)	17-19	10.3
Clarke and Waters (1974)	15-20	25.4
Mills and Waters (1974)	15-20	23.1
Sparks (1978)	10-18	3.0
Abramson, Hopp, and Epstein (1980)	15-19	9.8
Bille (1982)	7-15	3.9
Sillanpää (1983)	7-15	3.8

Children's Hospital[6] showed that the children's headaches improved and that the improvement was maintained for 1 year after treatment.

RECURRENT CHEST PAIN

Chest pain is relatively common in children. It ranks third in frequency after headache and abdominal pain and may be as common as limb pain. It is seen most often in children between 10 and 21 years of age. There is little information on etiology, evaluation, and treatment of chest pain. Costochondritis, trauma, muscle strain, "chest wall syndrome," rib anomalies, and hyperventilation have been cited as causes of the pain. Physical examination rarely finds signs of a patent disorder. Rely more on the patient's history for some indication such as a complaint of palpitations—the presence of stressful situations that trigger the pain suggesting a psychogenic cause. Nonetheless, seek a physical cause.

Costochondritis is the most common cause of chest pain in children. It often occurs after an upper respiratory infection, can radiate to the back, and can last from a few days to several months. The pain can be reproduced by palpating the painful area or by mobilizing the arm or shoulder. Tietze's syndrome is rare in children, and diagnosis requires the sine qua non presence of a visible nonsuppurative swelling near the sternoclavicular junction. Muscle spasm and strain are other common causes of chest pain and can be associated with stress fractures. Other causes are chronic cough in cystic fibrosis patients, as well as slipping rib syndrome with the eighth, ninth, or tenth rib overriding the one above it and causing a deep ache. Another cause is "stitch," a sharp, crampy pain under the costal margin that occurs while walking or running and is due to stress on the peritoneal ligaments when they are stretched between the fast-moving diaphragm and the abdomen. Asthma and other lung-, diaphragm-, or pleura-related disorders can also cause chest pain. Other intrathoracic causes are esophageal spasm or inflammation, producing retrosternal pain or referred chest pain. Vertebral column deformities can also cause referred chest pain.

Identification of the origin of the pain and reassurance of the patient and family are often the most important elements of treatment, provided specific organic causes have been investigated.[18] Since cardiac involvement is what worries the child and family most, it should be stressed that this cause is extremely rare. An ECG is only indicated as a negative, reassuring element.

SICKLE CELL ANEMIA

Sickle cell anemia is the most common hemoglobinopathy in the United States. It occurs in 0.3% to 1.3% of the American black population. Pain occurs during vasoocclusive crises, the frequency of which is unpredictable and ranges from less than one crisis a year to several times a year or month.[19] Pain occurs when and where there is occlusion of small blood vessels by sickled erythrocytes: small bones of the extremities in small children; and abdomen, chest, long bones, and low back in older ones. The painful crisis can be triggered by hypoxemia, cold, infection, and hypovolemia.

Medical treatment includes hypertransfusions (with the added risk of alloimmunization and infection) to raise the hematocrit to a higher physiologic level and treatment with hydroxyurea, which increases fetal hemoglobin without the need for transfusions. Analgesic management of painful crises is often inadequate because of the fear of inducing drug addiction if narcotics are used. Transcutaneous nerve stimulation (TENS) and acupuncture have been used with varying results.[20,21] In some cases mild analgesics such as nonsteroidal antiinflammatory drugs (NSAIDs; i.e., ibuprofen) and codeine accompanied by oral or intravenous (IV) fluid intake and rest can be enough to relieve pain during the crisis.[22]

Although the use of narcotics can lead to complications such as respiratory depression and complications resulting from atelectasis and focal pulmonary hypoxia, those grounds alone should not preclude the use of potent analgesics for patients in severe pain. These children can have excruciating pain that does not respond to nonnarcotic analgesics, and inadequate treatment of the painful crisis can lead to drug-seeking behavior and profound psychosocial problems. Morphine, hydromorphone, or methadone are used in repeated doses subcutaneously or in low-dose continuous IV infusions.[23,24] Patient-controlled analgesia (PCA) is now being used in a few centers successfully in uncomplicated sickle-cell pain crisis. Other narcotics such as shorter-acting fentanyl are given intravenously in continuous infusions with satisfying results. The short-term use of stimulants such as methylphenidate,[25] caffeine,[26] or dextroamphetamine[27] can be useful to counter significant sedation and respiratory depression. Regional anesthesia techniques using local anesthetics and narcotics have given good results in some cases for leg, hip, and chest pain.[23] Tricyclic antidepressants are not recommended for analgesia during the acute phase of a vasoocclusive crisis because they do not act quickly enough. They can, however, be useful for long-term use in patients who have very frequent crises. Behavior modification techniques such as biofeedback, self-hypnosis, and relaxation can be useful in helping children deal with the repeated painful episodes.[28-30]

HEMOPHILIA

Hemophilias are the most common inherited coagulation disorders in children and include deficiencies of factors VIII, IX, and XI. Factor VIII deficiency is the most common hemophilia; factor IX deficiency is less common. Both are X-linked recessive anomalies, affecting men and transmitted by women. Factor XI is the least common hemophilia, is present primarily in Jews, and is autosomal recessive. Factor VIII deficiency may be severe (less than 1% the normal amount of Factor VIII), moderate (1% to 5%), or mild (5% to 50%).

Hematomas can occur at any age (even in mild hemophilia), but hemarthroses usually appear when the child starts walking. Bleeding also occurs in deep soft tissues or muscles, as well as intracranially.[31] Early treatment is mandatory whenever bleeding is suspected (e.g., when discomfort is present in a joint). The benefits of early treatment include reduced tissue or joint damage and less school absence for rehabilitation. Hemarthrosis is a major problem in severe and moderate hemophilia and leads to permanent damage and pain resulting from synovial and bone changes. This can be prevented by early factor replacement therapy and joint aspiration. Synovitis occurs in the knees and elbows after recurrent hemarthroses. Treatment includes oral steroids, muscle strengthening, and in some cases synovectomy.

Analgesic therapy is an important part of the management of hemophilia, although secondary to replacement therapy. Aspirin and drugs that inhibit platelet function should be avoided; but acetaminophen, codeine, hydromorphone, and methadone can be given orally.[32] Pentazocine is never indicated, since it causes dysphoria. Steroids and nonsteroidal drugs can be used to relieve pain from arthritis, but caution should be exercised when these drugs are used because they inhibit platelet activity.

DIABETES

The epidemiology of diabetes mellitus is not well defined because studies do not characterize the disease the same way. The overall prevalence of diabetes mellitus is approximately 1%, and juvenile diabetes accounts for about one fourth of that. Juvenile diabetes is not a painful disease in itself, and children are not seen in pain clinics until they become teenagers. They then have early signs of peripheral diabetic neuropathy.

Whether the pathologic process involved in diabetic neuropathy is linked to axonal degeneration or segmental demyelination is still controversial. Both axonal loss and segmental demyelination followed by remyelination have been reported and are probably present in varying proportions. Neurologic complications do not usually occur before 15 to 20 years of the disease's evolution, so pain clinics rarely see patients under 18 to 20 years old with diabetic neuropathies. Juvenile diabetes mellitus is labile, and the first signs of neuropathy are often seen at the time of an ketoacidotic crisis. Early signs include paresthesias and hyperesthesias, absent stretch reflexes, and loss of vibratory sense. Sometimes the first presenting signs are mononeuropathic in nature, with wrist or foot drop or sensory and motor deficit of the third, fourth, or sixth cranial nerves.

Because diabetic neuropathies are more frequently seen in patients whose disease is not well regulated, the most important preventive treatment is control of the metabolic disorder. Neuropathies can occur even in patients with well-controlled diabetes. Treatment of the painful neurologic complications is often disappointing. It usually starts with the prescription of an anticonvulsant drug: Phenytoin given orally has been shown to relieve pain in as little as 3 days.[33,34] Carbamazepine and clonazepam[35] can also relieve sensory manifestations of diabetic neuropathies. The side effects caused by anticonvulsants (e.g., sleepiness, leukopenia) limit their indications in children. Tricyclic antidepressants are used with much better results in children and are commonly used in low doses to treat neuropathic pain.[36] These drugs may work by influencing descending inhibitory systems at the spinal cord level, but the relationship between their antidepressant effect and their effect on pain is unresolved. Fluphenazine should be used only as a last resort in children and can then sometimes improve depression scores and pain scores.[37]

JUVENILE RHEUMATOID ARTHRITIS

There are about 250,000 children affected by juvenile rheumatoid arthritis in the United States, proving that it is not a rare disease. It usually manifests itself before the age of 2, and 5% of all rheumatoid cases present in childhood. The disease is characterized by chronic synovitis with or without extraarticular manifestations.

The etiology of juvenile rheumatoid arthritis is still unclear. It is thought to result either from infection by a yet unknown microorganism or, more likely, from an autoimmune process. The presence of rheumatoid factor-immunoglobin complexes that would perpetuate synovial inflammation argues well for an autoimmune process in adult-onset arthritis. However, the disease can occur in the absence of rheumatoid factor (i.e., rheumatoid factor-negative polyarthritis).

Juvenile rheumatoid arthritis differs from adult-onset arthritis in that lasting damage to articular cartilage occurs later in the course of the disease, and many children never have permanent joint damage. In rheumatoid factor-positive arthritis, however, joint destruction with stiffness and pain may be present, especially when many joints are involved. Pauciarticular disease (which is not seen in adults) affects 30% of juvenile rheumatoid arthritis patients, affects mostly girls, starts before age 4, and can be associated with iridocyclitis. Systemic-onset arthritis occurs in 20% of patients and is characterized by a high intermittent fever and a rash. The evolution of the disease is marked by remissions and exacerbations. Corticosteroids are very rarely indicated except when major complications occur, such as pericarditis and severe systemic disease.[38]

Treatment of painful episodes includes NSAIDs such as naproxen, ibuprofen, fenoprofen, which should be continued at least 8 weeks,[39] and salicylates (aspirin and choline magnesium trisalicylate [Trilisate]). Intramuscular (IM) gold therapy like gold sodium thiomalate (Myochrysine) is as useful and nontoxic in children as it is in adults. Physical and occupational therapy are important to improve motion and muscular strength. Swimming and bicycling should be encouraged to the extent that they do not cause joint pain.

MUSCULOSKELETAL PAIN

Growing pains. Under the category of "growing" pains come deep pains often felt by children in the lower limbs bilaterally and for which no organic cause can be found. This type of pain occurs in school-age children in whom stress or emotional factors are sometimes found.[40,41] The pains may occur at night or during events or situations that are felt as stressful by the child (e.g., school or a particular family event). Relief of stress factors by relaxation and biofeedback techniques is the main aspect of treatment.

Myofascial pain. Myofascial pain is rare in children before their teenage years, at which time it is similar to that seen in adults. There is very little in the literature about the epidemiology of myofascial pain in smaller children. Yunus and Masi[42] described a pain syndrome in children (juvenile primary fibromyalgia syndrome) that associates depression, sleeping disorders, and problems at school or in the family setting and pain very similar to myofascial pain. This may well be a global pain/dysfunction syndrome combining myofascial pain and behavior modifications resulting from longstanding pain (chronic pain syndrome). In 1958 Bates and colleagues[43] reported 85 cases of myofascial pain in children 14 months to 17 years old. In 62 cases, trigger points were found and treated with a spray-and-stretch procedure using ethyl chloride. The response to this treatment was better in cases without underlying disease. Fine recently reported myofascial pain in the left inguinal crease in a 10-year-old boy.[44] The pain had no organic cause, was reproduced by needling of the trigger point, and was completely and lastingly relieved by injection of bupivacaine at the trigger site. Treatment of myofascial pain in children is similar to that in adults. After the recognition of trigger points, needling or injection of local anesthetic is effective, as are freeze-and-stretch techniques.[45] Ultrasonic therapy is used successfully in temporomandibular myofascial pain.[46]

REFLEX SYMPATHETIC DYSTROPHY

Reflex sympathetic dystrophy in adults has been known and abundantly described under various names such as Sudeck's atrophy, shoulder-hand syndrome, and chronic traumatic edema, as well as some others. Until recently it was rarely found in children, probably because it was not recognized. There are anecdotal case reports of reflex sympathetic dystrophy in children in the literature,[47-51] but no extensive studies have been done. Nonetheless, even though the syndrome, response to treatment, and usual outcome differ in children compared with adults, reflex sympathetic dystrophy does exist in children and is not as uncommon as was previously thought. The syndrome has been reported in children as young as 3 years.[48] Reflex sympathetic dystrophy is characterized by severe pain, often burning in quality, persisting long after what would be expected after the initial injury. The affected area, usually on a lower or upper limb (mostly hand or wrist, elbow, shoulder, or hip) is intermittently swollen, mottled, and with alternating episodes of redness or cyanosis. The extremity is at first hot and dry, then becomes cold and sweaty, and is tender to palpation. Hyperesthesia and allodynia are often present, but neurologic examination is usually normal. The pain is either diffuse or well localized over a knee or a hand and prevents normal use of the limb. In the later stages of reflex sympathetic dystrophy (usually after a few months), trophic changes such as loss of hair, brittle nails, and muscle wasting can occur. For further details, see Chapter 48.

CANCER PAIN

Cancer is the third leading cause of death in the United States in children 1 to 4 years old (18.7 childhood cancers per 100,000 children) and the second most common cause of death between 5 and 19 years of age (10.1 cancers per 100,000 children).[52] Children with cancer have pain not only from tumor compression of surrounding structures but also from the side effects and the required venous access of antimitotic drugs. Repeated small procedures such as bone marrow and organ biopsies are also painful. Fear of

treatments and of death can cause depression, thereby worsening the pain experience.

The most common tumors in children are leukemias, lymphomas, brain tumors (posterior fossa), neuroblastomas, hepatoblastomas, and bone sarcomas (Ewing's sarcoma). Pain can be visceral, resulting from stretching of abdominal structures by voluminous tumors; it may be present in bones as a consequence of bone marrow expansion, as in leukemia; or pain may be caused by nerve stretching or headache stemming from increased intracranial pressure.

The choice of drug in the treatment of pediatric oncology pain should be based on the intensity of the pain present. Fear of addiction or age-related side effects should not preclude the use of potent analgesics in children with cancer. As Twycross[53] noted, "Morphine exists to be given, not merely to be withheld. Its use is dictated by intensity of pain and failure of other methods, not by brevity of prognosis."

Gauvain-Piquard and colleagues studied children with cancer, and their assessment of pain includes not only a measure of pain but also of anxiety and depression.[54] The treatment of pain should, in the same way, address both the pain and the reaction to pain. During the early stages of the disease or during remissions, pain will respond to analgesic drugs on the lower step of the World Health Organization analgesics ladder, to transcutaneous electrical nerve stimulation (TENS), and to mild physical therapy techniques such as ice massages. Pain relief for biopsies can be provided by small doses of short-acting drugs: a benzodiazepine such as midazolam combined with a narcotic like fentanyl or alfentanil.

When pain increases, however, oral or parenteral narcotics can be used. In small children the pharmacokinetics of morphine can vary from patient to patient, and titration of the drug should be attempted while the child is hospitalized in order to obtain maximal effect with minimal side effects. Oral morphine is as efficient as IM morphine[55] and is used in increasing doses until adequate pain relief is obtained.[56] Berde uses the longer-acting methadone or morphine (MS Contin) given on a fixed schedule and, combined with shorter-acting agents such as codeine, oxycodone, or hydromorphone given as circumstances require when pain increases. Time-released morphine can also be given orally every 8 to 12 hours. Nausea is common at the beginning of the treatment and improves with prescription of phenothiazines.[57] Drowsiness can also be present at first; it responds to narcotic drug reduction. Constipation is a frequent side effect and should be treated preventively. Unfortunately, nausea and mucositis often prevent oral ingestion, and parenteral administration of narcotics becomes necessary. Continuous IV or subcutaneous infusions[58,59] of morphine, hydromorphone, methadone, or fentanyl can be used.

As the disease progresses the increasing doses required for adequate analgesia will result in respiratory depression and profound sedation. Sedation can sometimes be effectively countered with low doses of psychostimulants such as dextroamphetamines or methylphenidate. At this point, to avoid the use of higher, deleterious doses of parenteral narcotics, epidural analgesics may be invaluable in cases of intractable pelvic or thoracoabdominal pain. Epidural bupivacaine can be given in continuous infusions with minimal side effects,[60] and can be combined with low doses of narcotics (e.g., morphine or fentanyl).[61]

Disturbed sleep, fear, anxiety, and depression should be treated with behavior-modification techniques such as relaxation, biofeedback, distraction, and imagery and also small doses of tricyclics as indicated. Self-hypnosis techniques are used in children undergoing short, painful procedures such as IV line placement, biopsies, and spinal injections of antimitotic drugs. In all cases, at all stages of the disease, and during all painful procedures no matter how apparently benign, pain and fear should be treated with the same seriousness as the disease itself.

SPORTS INJURIES

The increasing participation of children in organized sports and fitness activities is the cause of a growing number and variety of sports injuries. The epidemiology of these injuries is not available yet and thus cannot be compared with those related to free-play activities.[62,63] So far there is no evidence that organized sports are more dangerous, or safer, than free play. The injuries encountered are "overuse" injuries similar to those found in the adult recreational athlete who trains incorrectly, usually doing too much over too short a period of time. The causes of these injuries also include muscle-tendon imbalance, anatomic malalignment, inadequate footwear, and growth. Growth is an important factor in these injuries for two reasons: growth cartilage is less resistant to injury than the adult-type cartilage, and growth spurts in children cause tendon and muscle tightness leading to pain and sometimes to stress fracture. These fractures are most often seen in the tibia or the fibula.

Other frequent sites of injury, tendinitis, bursitis, and joint disorders are the spine, shoulder, elbow (Little League elbow and shoulder), knee (patellofemoral stress syndrome and Osgood-Schlatter disease), hip, ankles, and feet.[64]

Treatment consists of immobilization of fractures, straight-leg strengthening exercises and use of leg braces in cases of knee injuries, rest, and use of orthotic footwear. NSAIDs and minor pain medicine such as aspirin and acetaminophen are useful when pain is present. These injuries usually respond well to these conservative measures but are best avoided through primary prevention, recognizing that they are bound to happen in young children involved in sports.

Low back pain is rare in children and shares neither the etiology nor the poor prognosis with the adult form. Most cases of low back pain in children and adolescents are sports-related and occur during the growth-spurt phase. A tendency to develop lordosis of the spine appears at that time. With overuse, low back pain may develop. Treatment consists of adapted spinal and hamstring flexibility exercises.[64] Preventive measures such as adequately supervised sports, presport muscle stretching, and safe training regimens (no more than 10%-per-week increase in training intensity) should be provided to children and adolescents involved in organized sports.

BURNS

Of the nearly 15,000 accident-related deaths in children per year, 10% are due to thermal injuries and 60,000 surviving children are hospitalized every year for the treatment of burns. Of these children, 65% are preschoolers who suffer scalds in the home from a boiling pot or from a hot-water tap.[65] Fire (17%), electrical burns often of the mouth or the hands (9%), and explosions (3%) are other causes of burns in children. Some of these injuries are intentionally inflicted on the children,[66] and this can be a factor in the psychologic management of pain.

Burns are classified according to depth: First-degree burns are characterized by epithelial involvement and minor, short-lasting pain; second-degree burns affect epithelium and dermis, and pain can be intense, particularly if the burn is superficial and blistering; and third-degree burns involve the full thickness of the skin and are said to be painless. However, when a child is burnt, different depths of burn are present at the same time, and a third-degree burn area will be painful because it is surrounded by areas of second-degree burn.

The pain related to burns and burn treatment can be tremendous, and the burned child, like any child, can be provided with appropriate pain relief without endangering him or her. The most painful and most often repeated procedure that a burned child has to endure is the dressing change. This procedure is short, lasting around 1½ hours, and requires a short-acting but potent analgesic such as fentanyl. Ketamine, which provides good "surface" analgesia, can also be used in combination with diazepam for this procedure. Other narcotics such as morphine or meperidine are of value in the initial phase of hospitalization when a long-acting IV analgesic is needed. To ensure safe use of these potent analgesics, they are best given as continuous, low-dose infusions. A codeine-acetaminophen or codeine-aspirin mixture can be used for less painful procedures later in the course of treatment.

TRAUMA

Whereas preschoolers are victims of accidents inside the home (e.g., burns, intoxication, asphyxia from inhalation of foreign bodies), school-age children fall prey to accidents occurring outside the home. Trauma is a major cause of death in that age group. In children, most accidents occur while crossing the streets on the way to or from school, whereas adolescents old enough to drive are more often victims of car accidents. The type of injury present in children hit by cars is related to the size of the child; small children will sustain head or chest trauma, and older, taller ones will have hip, abdominal, and lower limb injuries.

Except in cases of altered consciousness, potent parenteral analgesics can and should be used in severely injured children during the primary transport from the scene of the accident. Intramuscular morphine at lower analgesic doses (0.1 mg/kg) will usually provide sufficient analgesia to enable undressing and mobilization without too much pain. Simple regional techniques such as single-shot femoral nerve blocks for femoral shaft fractures and ankle blocks have been successfully used in children as small as 2 years of age at the site of the accident, before transferring the injured child from stretcher to x-ray or operating room table or before installing traction.[67] Infusions of low doses of narcotics are helpful in providing pain relief in the preoperative period before fractures are immobilized without endangering the patient, provided hemodynamic parameters are stable. One of the most important aspects of the management of trauma in children is to provide psychologic support and reassurance to minimize fear and anxiety. Even in these emergency situations, simple relaxation techniques can be applied quickly and successfully before starting painful treatments.

REFERENCES

1. Levine M, Rappaport LA: Recurrent abdominal pain in school children: The loneliness of the long distance physician. *Pediatr Clin North Am* 31:969-991, 1984.
2. Stone RT, Barbero GJ: Recurrent abdominal pain in childhood. *Pediatrics* 45:732-738, 1970.
3. Apley J: *The Child with Abdominal Pains,* ed 2. London, Blackwell, 1975.
4. Oster J: Recurrent abdominal pain, headache and limb pain in children and adolescents. *Pediatrics* 50:429-436, 1972.
5. McGrath PJ, Unruh AM: The measurement and assessment of pain. In McGrath PJ, Unruh AM, editors: *Pain in Children and Adolescents.* New York, Elsevier, 1987.
6. Masek BJ, Russo DC, Varni JW: Behavioral approaches to the management of chronic pain in children. *Pediatr Clin North Am* 31:1113-1131, 1984.
7. Passchier J, Orlebeke JF: Headaches and stress in school children: An epidemiological study. *Cephalalgia* 5:167-171, 1985.
8. Stevenson DD: Allergy, atopy, nasal disease and headache. In Dallessio DJ, editor: *Wolff's Headache and Other Head Pain,* ed 4. Oxford, Oxford University Press, 1980.
9. Vahlquist B, Hackzel G: Migraine of early onset: A study of thirty-one cases in which the disease first appeared between one and four years of age. *Acta Paediatr* 38:622-636, 1949.
10. Prensky AL, Sommer D: Diagnosis and treatment of migraine in children. *Neurology* 29:506-510, 1979.
11. Selby G, Lance JW: Observations of 500 cases of migraine and allied vascular headache. *J Neurol Neurosurg Psychiatry* 23:23-32, 1960.
12. Bille B: The prognosis of migraine in children. *Dan Med Bull* 22:112-114, 1975.
13. Lai CW et al: Hemiplegic migraine in children: Diagnostic and therapeutic aspects. *J Pediatr* 101:696-699, 1982.
14. Rossi LN et al: Benign migraine-like syndrome with CSF pleocytosis in children. *Dev Med Child Neurol* 27:192-198, 1985.
15. Prensky AL: Migraine and migrainous variants in pediatric patients. *Pediatr Clin North Am* 23:461-471, 1980.
16. Ling W, Oftedal G, Weinberg W: Depressive illness in childhood presenting as severe headache. *Am J Dis Child* 120:122-124, 1970.
17. McLean DC: Sinusitis in children: Lessons from twenty-five patients. *Clin Pediatr (Phila)* 9:342-345, 1970.
18. Coleman WLC: Recurrent chest pain in children. *Pediatr Clin North Am* 31:1007-1025, 1984.
19. Vichinski EP, Lubin BH: Sickle cell anemia and related hemoglobinopathies. *Pediatr Clin North Am* 27:429-447, 1980.
20. Wang WC et al: Transcutaneous electrical nerve stimulation [TENS] treatment of sickle cell painful crisis. *Blood* 66(suppl 1):67a, 1985.
21. Co LL et al: Acupuncture: An evaluation in the painful crisis of sickle cell anemia. *Pain* 7:181-185, 1979.
22. Greenberg J et al: Trial of low doses of aspirin as prophylaxis in sickle cell anemia. *J Pediatr* 102:781-784, 1983.
23. Berde C, Sethna N, Anand KS: Pediatric pain management. In Gregory GA, editor: *Pediatric Anesthesia,* ed 2. New York, Churchill Livingstone, 1989.
24. Cole TB et al: Intravenous narcotic therapy for children with severe sickle cell pain crisis. *Am J Dis Child* 140:1255-1259, 1986.
25. Beaver WT: Combination analgesics. *Am J Med* 77(3A):38-53, 1984.

26. Laska EM et al: Caffeine as an analgesic adjuvant. *JAMA* 251:1711-1718, 1984.
27. Forrest WH et al: Dextroamphetamine with morphine for treatment of postoperative pain. *N Engl J Med* 296:712-716, 1977.
28. Zeltzer L, Dash J, Holland JP: Hypnotically induced pain control in sickle cell anemia. *Pediatrics* 64:533-536, 1979.
29. Cozzi J, Tryon VW, Sedlacek K: The effectiveness of biofeedback-assisted relaxation in modifying sickle cell crises. *Biofeedback Self Regul* 12:51-61, 1987.
30. Thomas JE et al: Management of pain in sickle cell disease using biofeedback therapy: A preliminary study. *Biofeedback Self Regul* 9:413-420, 1984.
31. Nathan DG, Oski FA: *Hematology of Infancy and Childhood, vol 2,* ed 2. Philadelphia, WB Saunders, 1981.
32. Hilgartner M: Current therapy. In Hilgartner M, editor: *Hemophilia in Children.* Littleton, Mass, Publishing Sciences Group, 1976.
33. Ellenberg M: Treatment of diabetic neuropathy with diphenylhydantoine. *NY State J Med* 68:2653-2655, 1968.
34. Chadda VS, Mathur MS: Double blind study of the effects of diphenylhydantoine sodium on diabetic neuropathy. *J Assoc Physicians India* 26:403-406, 1978.
35. Caccia MR: Clonazepam in facial neuralgia and cluster headache. Clinical and electrophysiological study. *Eur Neurol* 13:560-563, 1975.
36. Turkington RW: Depression masquerading as diabetic neuropathy. *JAMA* 243:1147-1150, 1980.
37. Maciewicz R, Bouckoms A, Martin JB: Drug therapy of neuropathic pain. *Clin J Pain* 1:39-49, 1985.
38. Behrman RE, Vaughan VC: Juvenile rheumatoid arthritis. In Behrman RE, Vaughan VC III, Nelson WE, editors: *Nelson Textbook of Pediatrics,* ed 12. Philadelphia, WB Saunders, 1983.
39. Lovell DJ, Giannini EH, Person DA: Time course of response to nonsteroidal anti-inflammatory drugs in juvenile rheumatoid arthritis. *Arthritis Rheum* 27:1433-1437, 1984.
40. Oster J, Nielson A: Growing pains: A clinical investigation of a school population. *Acta Pediatr Scand* 61:321, 1972.
41. Naish JM, Apley J: Growing pains: A clinical study of non-arthritic limb pains in children. *Arch Dis Child* 26:134, 1951.
42. Yunus MB, Masi AT: Juvenile primary fibromyalgia syndrome. *Arthritis Rheum* 28:138-145, 1985.
43. Bates T, Grunwaldt E: Myofascial pain in childhood. *J Pediatr* 53:198-209, 1958.
44. Fine PG: Myofascial trigger point pain in children. *J Pediatr* 111:547-548, 1987.
45. Travell J: Myofascial trigger points: Clinical view. In Bonica JJ, Albe-Fessard D, editors: *Advances in Pain Research and Therapy, vol 1.* New York, Raven Press, 1976.
46. Esposito CJ, Veal SJ, Farman AG: Alleviation of myofascial pain with ultrasonic therapy. *J Prosthet Dent* 51:106-108, 1984.
47. Carron H, McHue F: Reflex sympathetic dystrophy in a ten year old child. *South Med J* 65:631-632, 1972.
48. Kozin F, Haughton V, Ryan L: The reflex sympathetic dystrophy syndrome in a child. *J Pediatr* 90:417-419, 1977.
49. Fermaglich DR: Reflex sympathetic dystrophy in children. *Pediatrics* 60:881-883, 1977.
50. Rush PJ et al: Severe reflex neurovascular dystrophy in children. *Arthritis Rheum* 28:952-956, 1985.
51. Ruggeri SB et al: Reflex sympathetic dystrophy in children. *Clin Orthop* 163:225-230, 1982.
52. Twycross RG: Strong narcotic analgesics. *Clinics in Oncology* 3:109-133, 1984.
53. First LR: Introduction to oncology. In Avery ME, First LR, editors: *Pediatric Medicine.* Baltimore, Williams & Wilkins, 1989.
54. Broadman LM, Rice LJ, Hannallah RS: Testing the validity of an objective pain scale for infants and children. *Anesthesiology* 69:A770, 1988.
55. Nahata MC et al: Variation in morphine pharmacokinetics in children with cancer. *Dev Pharmacol Ther* 8:182-188, 1985.
56. Pichard E et al: The use of opiates in children with cancer pain. In Scherpereel P, Meynadier J, Blond S, editors: *The Pain Clinic II.* Utrecht, Netherlands, VNU Science Press, 1987.
57. Berde CB: Approach to the general management of a child with cancer. In Avery ME, First LR, editors: *Pediatric Medicine.* Baltimore, Williams & Wilkins, 1989.

58. Miser AW et al: Continuous subcutaneous infusion of morphine in children with cancer. *Am J Dis Child* 137:383, 1983.

59. Miser AW, Miser JS, Clark BS: Continuous intravenous infusion of morphine sulfate for control of severe pain in children with terminal malignancy. *J Pediatr* 96:930, 1980.

60. Desparmet J et al: Continuous epidural infusion of bupivacaine for postoperative pain relief in children. *Anesthesiology* 67:108-110, 1987.

61. Berde CB et al: Caudal epidural morphine epidural analgesia for an infant with advanced neuroblastoma: Report of a case. *Pain* 36:219-223, 1989.

62. Jackson DW et al: Injury prediction in the young athlete: A preliminary report. *Am J Sports Med* 6:6-16, 1978.

63. Micheli LJ: Sports injuries in children and adolescents. In Strauss RH, editor: *Sports Medicine and Physiology.* Philadelphia, WB Saunders, 1989.

64. Micheli LJ: Overuse injuries in children's sports: The growth factor. *Orthop Clin North Am* 14:337-360, 1983.

65. Guzzetta PC, Randolph J: Burns in children: 1982. *Pediatr Rev* 4:271-278, 1983.

66. Hight DW, Bakalar HR, Lloyd JR: Inflicted burns in children: Recognition and treatment. *JAMA* 242:517, 1979.

67. Ronchi L et al: Femoral nerve blockade in children using bupivacaine. *Anesthesiology* 70:622-624, 1989.

53 Acute Pain Syndromes in Children

Joelle F. Desparmet

It is now well established that a child experiences pain very early in development. Few are those physicians who, having difficulty assessing pain in children, still doubt that they experience pain at all. The development of pain in the fetus has been extensively studied. Pain pathways and neuromodulators of pain are all present at birth (Fig 53-1). Physiologically, newborns respond to pain by demonstrating changes in heart rate and blood pressure (BP), transcutaneous PO_2, palmar sweating,[1-4] and increases in stress hormones.[5] Behavioral changes with pain have been documented in newborns. There is evidence that pain is also experienced by premature infants.[6] In preterm and full-term newborns the postoperative response to stress can be blocked or blunted by intravenous (IV)[7] or local anesthetics.[8] Having established that children indeed experience pain, the predominant problem is to assess and attempt to quantify pain and, having done that, to treat it adequately.

MEASUREMENT OF PAIN IN CHILDREN

The last decade has seen enormous progress in the measurement of children's pain and in the development of reliable tools to assess acute pain in children. Depending on the age of the child and the setting in which the pain is assessed, these tools can include one or a combination of numerical and spatial scale, behavioral, physiologic, and face scales. In the preverbal child the assessment of pain relies mostly on the measurement of physiologic parameters and the evaluation of changes in behavior.

Crying is the first vocal expression of pain or distress in the neonate. Infant cry has been analyzed,[9] showing acoustic differences between cries of pain and cries of hunger. The practicality of the spectrometric analysis of infant cries in an acute setting has yet to be demonstrated, however, but advances are being made in this field.

Facial expressions in response to sharp pain have also been studied.[10-11] Distortion of the face has been correlated with increasing degrees of pain.

Increases in heart rate, BP, palmar sweating, and changes in transcutaneous PO_2 are associated with pain in babies and are useful tools for the measurement of pain in this age group.

A combination of all these parameters is included in the Postoperative Pain Score[12] by Attia and colleagues (Table 53-1). This scoring system, used in children 1 to 8 months old, includes the quality of sleep; facial expression; cry; motor activity, including sucking; and behavioral factors such as consolability and sociability. Another scale is the Toddler-Preschooler Postoperative Pain Scale, which measures pain in children 1 to 5 years old.[13] Although this scale

has not been validated yet, it also addresses the physiologic and behavioral aspects of acute postoperative pain in small children. The Washington, D.C., pediatric Objective Pain Scale has been validated in preverbal and school-age children.[14] In this scale a verbal evaluation of pain is added. The child is asked to describe the location of the pain and whether the pain is mild or bothersome. In children older than 4 years, visual analogue scales (VAS) are still the easiest scales to use if one wants a rapid, comparative numerical score to evaluate the effect of medication, for instance.

Face scales use either representations of happy-to-sad faces or actual photographs of happy-to-sad children as in the Oucher.[15] They can be used in children 3 years and older and have been shown to have a strong correlation with behavior scores. The proliferation of pain scales is an indication of the difficulty in measuring pain in children who are unable to express their pain verbally and in those whose cognitive development does not enable them to express it in a measurable way. However, a combination of these scales provides useful information on the degree of pain and on the effect on the pain of a pharmacologic intervention.

ACUTE PAIN IN CHILDREN

Causes of acute pain in children range from sports or playground injuries to postoperative pain, major trauma, and burns. They can also be the result of an acute episode during the course of an ongoing medical condition such as sickle cell anemia and cancer. In these situations children have classically been the least medicated of patients. Fear of overdosing and a poor understanding of the manifestations of pain in children have led to the undertreatment of pain in this patient group. Certain routes of administration (intramuscular [IM] versus IV) or drugs (codeine versus morphine) are erroneously believed to be safer than others, when in fact they are often prescribed at inadequate subtherapeutic doses and intervals. New medications are always tested and approved last for pediatric use and are often available for the pediatric population years after they are available for adults, and then only in wasteful adult-dose packaging. Nonetheless, medications for all degrees of pain and all routes of administration are available for use in children; and there is no excuse to continue to undermedicate them on the basis of an increased risk in toxicity and side effects.

TREATMENT OF PAIN IN CHILDREN
Systemic

The use of pain medications in children can be grossly divided into three main categories depending on the degree

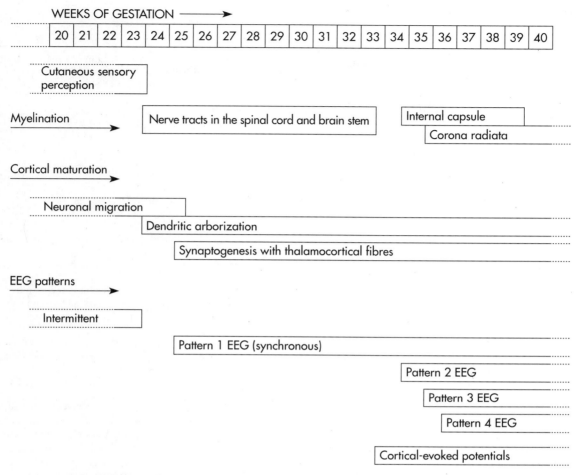

Fig. 53-1 Maturation of pain pathways in the human fetus and neonate. (From Anand KJS, Phil D, Hickey PR: Pain and its effect on the human-neonate and fetus. *N Engl J Med* 317:1321-1329, 1987.)

of pain to be relieved. Mild pain can be treated with minor analgesics, represented in children mainly by acetaminophen. Moderate pain is often relieved by the addition to acetaminophen of a minor opiate such as codeine or by nonsteroidal antiinflammatory drugs (NSAIDs). Major pain usually requires a potent opioid analgesic or the injection of local anesthetics.

NSAIDs are a large group of drugs, the oldest and best known of which is acetylsalicylic acid or aspirin. Because aspirin increases the risk of Reye's syndrome in small children, its use as a primary analgesic is not recommended in this group of patients. Acetaminophen is widely used for minor pain in children. It can be given not only orally but also by the rectal route. This makes it a valuable minor analgesic in the immediate postoperative period when the oral route cannot be used. Although it is an NSAID, it does not exhibit significant antiinflammatory effects or NSAID side effects, and this makes it a very safe analgesic when given in therapeutic doses to children. In older children codeine or oxycodone are combined with acetaminophen to provide additional pain relief.[16-17] Acetaminophen potentiates the analgesic produced by codeine, allowing a reduction in nar-

cotic dosage while achieving adequate analgesia. Codeine is prescribed in a dose of 0.5 to 1 mg/kg with acetaminophen at 10 mg/kg. Other NSAIDs are used for their analgesic properties. Diclofenac, indomethacin, and ketoprofen are widely used in Europe for children's pain after minor surgery such as dental restoration and minor ear, nose, throat, and abdominal procedures.[18-22] Diclofenac can be administered IV. Because its plasma clearance is higher in children than in adults, dosage on a mg/kg basis must be increased.[18] Ketorolac is a relatively new NSAID in North America, and its use in children is just beginning. Given IV before the start of surgery, ketorolac (0.9 mg/kg) is as effective as morphine (0.1 mg/kg) in alleviating postoperative pain and produces less postoperative emesis.[23] Oral ketorolac (1 mg/kg) was also shown to be a more effective analgesic than acetaminophen (10 mg/kg) and placebo after myringotomy.[24] In this study, however, it can be argued that 10 mg/kg of acetaminophen in children is a dose that is practically equivalent to placebo. Ketorolac (0.75 mg/kg) is also as effective as meperidine (1 mg/kg) and reduces the dose of rescue narcotics postoperatively.[25] Other NSAIDs such as ibuprofen are only available for children

Table 53-1 Postoperative pain score

	0	1	2
1. Sleep during preceding hour	None	Short naps: between 5 and 10 min	Longer naps: $\geq$ 10 min
2. Facial expression of pain	Marked, constant	Less marked, intermittent	Calm, relaxed
3. Quality of cry	Screaming, painful, high pitched	Modulated (i.e., can be distracted by normal sound)	No cry
4. Spontaneous motor activity	Thrashing around, incessant agitation	Moderate agitation	Normal
5. Spontaneous excitability and responsiveness to ambient stimulation	Tremulous, clonic movements, spontaneous Moro's reflexes	Excessive reactivity (to any stimulation)	Quiet
6. Constant and excessive flexion of fingers and toes	Very pronounced, marked and constant	Less marked, intermittent	Absent
7. Sucking	Absent or disorganized sucking	Intermittent (3 or 4) and stops with crying	Strong, rhythmic with pacifying effect
8. Global evaluation of tone	Strong hypertonicity	Moderate hypertonicity	Normal for the age
9. Consolability	None after 2 min	Quiet after 1 min or effort	Calm before 1 min
10. Sociability (eye contact); response to voice, smile, real interest in face	Absent	Difficult to obtain	Easy and prolonged

From Attia J et al: Measurement of postoperative pain and narcotic administration in infants using a new clinical scoring system. *Anesthesiology* 66:A532, 1987.

in the oral form and have limited use in the immediate postoperative period. One drawback of NSAIDs is that their onset is slow (up to 30 minutes), even when given IV. Their minimal effect on platelet aggregation and bleeding time[25,26] is not clinically significant, and there are no reports in the pediatric literature of increased postoperative bleeding.

Opiates

The use of opioid analgesics has long been denied to children based on the fact that there is an increased risk of respiratory depression in this age group. This is true in newborns, who have immature respiratory centers and in whom plasma morphine concentrations after continuous IV infusions are more than double that of older children and highly variable from one newborn to another.[27] In a study by Rosen and colleagues a maximum dose of 15 μg/kg/hr was recommended for this age group because higher doses could result in high plasma concentrations and lead to seizures. After cessation of the infusion, plasma concentration may rise even more because of enterohepatic recirculation. Another study found no age-related difference in drug disposition in children between birth and 15 years of age.[28]

Opiates can be administered by many different routes. The transmucosal route is of particular interest in children because it avoids the use of needles. The more lipid-soluble opioids (e.g., fentanyl, sufentanil, methadone, and buprenorphine) are rapidly absorbed from oral and nasal mucosa into the systemic circulation.[29] Oral transmucosal fentanyl citrate is sucked like a lollipop 30 minutes before a painful procedure[30] or before surgery.[31,32] It is still being investigated and is not currently available for clinical use.

Fentanyl can also be administered nasally. Nasally administered sufentanil (3 μg/kg) provides sedation before anesthesia and reduces postoperative analgesic requirements.[33] Opiates can be given subcutaneously in cancer patients when the oral route can no longer be used. This route is not widely used for treatment of postoperative pain, but it has been advocated in Europe to avoid repeating IM injections.[34] The dose of opiate given by this route is the same as that given IV, but the concentration should be such that not more than 0.5 to 1.0 ml/hr of the opioid solution is injected because a greater volume would lead to discomfort. In cancer patients an infusion pump with the possibility of additional boluses can be used. The IV route is the most popular route of administration of opiates in the postoperative period. Opiates can be given as repeated boluses at regular (not as-needed) 2- to 3-hour intervals or better yet as continuous infusions. Morphine, meperidine, and fentanyl are the most widely used opiates, but methadone and hydromorphone are also used by this route (Box 53-1). Continuous infusions have the advantage of avoiding the peaks and valleys of intermittent bolus injections and can be increased or decreased at will or complemented with an additional bolus when needed. Patient-controlled analgesia (PCA) has the additional advantage of letting the patients decide if and when they get the medication. PCA is now widely used in children. The pump can be programmed to deliver repeated boluses of an opioid solution or a basal infusion plus additional boluses at the patient's will. If adequately instructed preoperatively, children as young as 5 years can responsibly use PCA pumps. There is still controversy about "parent-assisted" or "nurse-assisted" PCA because this eliminates the primary safety feature of PCA,

Box 53-1 DOSAGE OF ANALGESICS IN CHILDREN

Acetaminophen	10 to 15 mg/kg orally every 4 to 6 hrs; maximum dose 60 mg/kg/day
	Infants: 25 mg/kg/orally every 6 to 8 hrs
Diclofenac	1 to 2 mg/kg IV every 6 to 8 hrs
Ibuprofen	10 mg/kg orally every 6 to 8 hrs; maximum dose 40 mg/kg/day
Ketorolac	0.5 to 1 mg/kg IV every 6 to 8 hrs
Codeine	0.5 to 1 mg/kg orally every 4 hrs
Meperidine	0.8 to 1 mg/kg IV every 2 hrs
Methadone	0.1 mg/kg IV every 4 hrs, then every 6 to 12 hrs
	0.1 mg/kg orally every 4 to 12 hrs
Morphine	0.2 to 0.4 mg/kg orally every 4 hrs
	0.1 mg IV every 1 to 2 hrs
	0.05 to 0.06 mg/kg/hr continuous IV or SC
	PCA 0.01 to 0.02 mg every 10 to 15 min boluses
	± 0.01 to 0.02 mg/hr basal infusion

which is the natural limitation of injections by the drowsiness of the patient. A variety of painful procedures including surgery, bone-marrow transplantation, cancer, or sickle cell crisis have benefited from this form of analgesic delivery.[35-40] A typical dosage of morphine for PCA is 10 to 20 µg/kg boluses every 10 to 15 minutes with or without a 10- to 20-µg/kg/hr basal infusion. This dosage can be modified after a few hours depending on the number of times the patient has triggered the machine and the occurrence of side effects.

REGIONAL BLOCKADE IN CHILDREN

Regional anesthesia is widely used in children. In some developing countries it is often the most practical and safest anesthetic to use in that age group. Central blocks differ in children compared with adults in a number of aspects.

Anatomic differences between children's and adults' spinal columns lie in the relationship of the termination of the spinal cord and the dural sac to the bony spine. The cord and dural sac rise from newborn level (respectively L_2 and S_3) to their adult level (respectively T_{12} and S_2) by the end of the first year of life.

The hemodynamic response to sympathetic block caused by intrathecally administered local anesthetics is age dependent.[41] A Doppler study showed that blood pressure and cardiac output do not vary significantly after regional anesthesia in young children[42] and that fluid loading before a regional technique in children less than 8 years old is not required in a normovolemic patient. The respiratory response to narcotics or techniques resulting in high levels of motor block can jeopardize respiration, particularly in small children.

Pharmacologic differences between children and adults lie mostly in differences in protein binding and distribution and elimination of drugs.[43-48] In children the volume of distribution for local anesthetics is up to three times that of adults, probably resulting, among other factors, from a higher water content (70% to 80% of body weight in infants) compared with adults (60% to 68% of body weight). The clearance of local anesthetics is increased in children between 1 and 3 years old but is decreased in newborns and infants who have immature oxidative pathways. The continuous infusion of local anesthetics in the epidural space has the advantage of producing low plasma concentrations at steady state. After a 48-hour infusion of 0.2 mg/kg/hr of bupivacaine in children 1 month to 15 years, mean plasma concentration does not rise beyond 1.2 µg/ml, there is no accumulation of drug, and elimination half-life is similar to that after a single-bolus injection.[49] Lidocaine has similar pharmacokinetics in children. A concentration of 1% results in moderate motor block.

Opioids are also administered epidurally in children.[50,51] Epidurally administered morphine is rapidly absorbed from the epidural space, reaches plasma peak concentration within 15 minutes, then decreases progressively with a shorter elimination half-life than in adults: 1.2 hours[52] compared with 3.5 hours in adults with comparable doses. Fentanyl is also given epidurally as repeated boluses or as a continuous infusion combined with bupivacaine. Steady-state plasma concentration remains low with clinically efficient continuous doses of 0.2 to 0.6 µg/kg/hr.[53] The main respiratory effect of epidural opioids is a progressive decrease in respiratory rate and a depressed CO_2 response. The epidural injection of 50 µg/kg of morphine in children produces a change in respiratory drive as shown by CO_2 stimulation method[52] that is maximum 3 hours after injection and lasts 14 to 22 hours. More lipid-soluble opioids such as fentanyl and sufentanil produce an earlier and shorter respiratory depression.[54]

COMMONLY USED REGIONAL TECHNIQUES

Except for premature newborns who are at risk for postanesthesia apnea, most children are put to sleep before a regional block.

A caudal block is one of the easiest to perform in children.

Epidural blocks by the lumbar approach are also commonly performed in children undergoing major surgery. Pediatric-size epidural equipment is available, and epidurals can be performed even in infants. This technique is used to provide pain relief in children not only in the operating room and postoperatively but also for medically caused pain in settings such as oncology and intensive care and for the diagnosis and treatment of sympathetically mediated pain, to name a few. The epidural technique in itself is not different in children from that in adults. For placement of long-term catheters for oncology patients, for instance, control of proper positioning by radioscopy can be valuable. Children are placed in a lateral position and an assistant holds the child's knees as close to the child's chest as possible to open up the intervertebral space. It is recommended that the person performing the epidural block be seated for the procedure with the eyes at the level of the child's spine.

Except in premature babies, spinal anesthesia is not widely practiced in children because of the incidence of headache in this age group, even though the exact incidence of postspinal anesthesia apnea up to 45 to 60 weeks

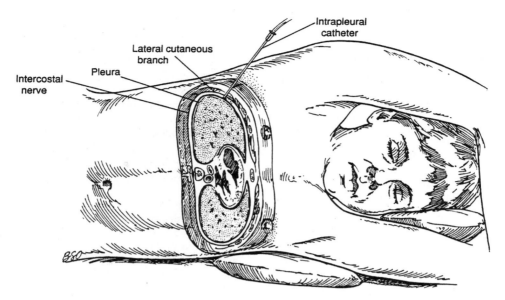

Fig. 53-2 Intrapleural catheter insertion in the closed chest. Diagram of insertion tangential to the pleural space. (From Desparmet JF: Acute pain in children. *Pain Digest* 3:3, 1993.)

postconceptual age,[55] and "awake" spinal anesthesia (i.e., without sedation or anesthesia) provides intraoperative analgesia and reduces the incidence of postoperative apnea.[56-62] The sensory block unfortunately lasts only between 60 and 110 minutes, and for procedures of longer duration a caudal block with or without insertion of a catheter might be more appropriate. The spinal block can be conducted with the child in a sitting position or lying on the side with the head slightly up.

PERIPHERAL BLOCKS

Contrary to caudal block, penile block does not involve the lower limbs and does not cause urinary retention, two reasons why in some centers it is often the preferred anesthesia technique for circumcisions.[63]

Brachial plexus block is a useful block for children with hand and arm injuries because it is easily performed in most children. The most popular techniques to block the brachial plexus in children include the interscalene, the parascalene,[64] the supraclavicular, and the axillary approach.[65] The latter approach is adequate for hand surgery but must be completed with separate blocks of the musculocutaneous and axillary nerves to anesthetize the upper arm and the lateral aspect of the forearm. Lidocaine 1% to 2% and bupivacaine 0.25% with epinephrine 1/100,000 are the most commonly used local anesthetics for brachial plexus block in children. A dose of 2 to 3 mg/kg of bupivacaine with epinephrine provides 3 to 5 hours of analgesia without resulting in toxic serum concentrations of the drug.[66]

Intrapleural anesthesia, a relatively new technique used in adults, has been performed in children after thoracotomy[67] (Fig. 53-2). It has been suggested that the anesthetic solution deposited into the pleural cavity diffuses from the pleural space through the parietal pleura and the innermost intercostal muscle to reach the intercostal space, where the

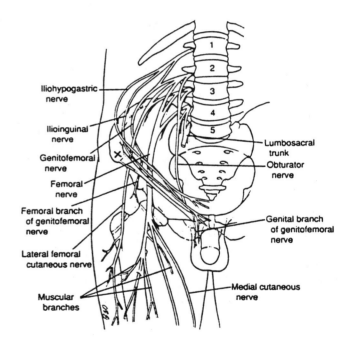

Fig. 53-3 Diagram of the major nerves of the groin—femoral, lateral femoral cutaneous, ilioinguinal, and iliohypogastric—and their relation to palpable landmarks. (From Desparmet JF: Acute pain in children. *Pain Digest* 3:3, 1993.)

intercostal nerves are blocked. It is recommended to limit dosage to 0.4 to 0.5 mg/kg/hr. It is indicated for pain relief after surgery below the diaphragm, such as liver or biliary tract surgery.

Femoral nerve block is useful preoperatively and postoperatively for patients with femoral shaft fractures or some forms of knee trauma[68] (Fig. 53-3). A dose of 5 to 7 ml of lidocaine 1% to 2% or bupivacaine 0.25% to 0.5% with epinephrine provides analgesia for 3 to 4 hours within 10 to 20 minutes of injection.

Intercostal nerve blocks are used in children for postoperative analgesia after procedures involving the thoracic and upper abdominal wall and to relieve pain after multiple rib fractures.[69,70] It is not certain that this block is beneficial in awake children because it requires large volumes of local anesthetics and involves multiple skin punctures. Bupivacaine 0.25% is usually used for its long duration of action (8 to 24 hours). Because in children blood concentration of local anesthetic can reach high peaks,[71] the total dose of local anesthetic used for the complete procedure should not exceed 3 mg/kg.

Ilioinguinal and iliohypogastric nerve blocks affect the area of the scrotum and the inner aspect of the thigh. They are used with success postoperatively after inguinal repair, varicocele, and orchiopexy in children.

CONCLUSION

After years of quasimarginalization in the pediatric press, studies on assessment, measurement, and treatment of pain in children have become prominent in journals from all specialties. Awareness is the major step toward solving the problem of adequate treatment of children's pain, and education is a major factor in increasing that awareness of everyone involved in the care of children in pain.

REFERENCES

1. Holve RL et al: Regional anesthesia during newborn circumcision: Effect on newborn pain response. *Clin Pediatr (Phila)* 22:813-818, 1983.
2. Owens ME, Todt EH: Pain in infancy: Neonatal reaction to a heel lance. *Pain* 20:77-86, 1984.
3. Johnston CC, Strada ME: Acute pain response in infants: A multidimensional description. *Pain* 24:373-382, 1986.
4. Field T, Goldson E: Pacifying effect of non-nutritive sucking on term and preterm neonates during heelstick procedure. *Pediatrics* 74:1012-1015, 1984.
5. Fiselier T et al: Influence of the stress of venipuncture on basal levels of plasma renin activity in infants and children. *Int J Pediatr Nephrol* 4:425-429, 1983.
6. Anand KJS, Phil D, Hickey PR: Pain and its effect on the human neonate and fetus. *N Engl J Med* 317:1321-1329, 1987.
7. Anand KJS, Sipell WG, Aynsley-Green A: Randomized trial of fentanyl anesthesia in preterm babies undergoing surgery: Effects on the stress response. *Lancet* 1:62-66, 243-248, 1987.
8. Williamson PS, Williamson ML: Physiologic stress reduction by a local anesthetic during newborn circumcision. *Pediatrics* 71:36-40, 1983.
9. Johnston CC, O'Shaughnessy D: Acoustical attributes of infant pain cries: Discriminating features. In Dubner R, Gebhart GF, Bond MR, editors: *Proceedings of the Vth World Congress on Pain.* New York, Elsevier, 1988.
10. Grunau RVE, Craig KD: Pain expressions in neonates: Facial action and cry. *Pain* 28:395-410, 1987.
11. Katz ER, Kellerman J, Siegel SE: Distress behavior in children with cancer undergoing medical procedures: Developmental considerations. *J Consult Clin Psychol* 48:456-465, 1980.
12. Attia J et al: Measurement of postoperative pain and narcotic administration in infants using a new clinical scoring system. *Anesthesiology* 66:A532, 1987.
13. Tarbell SE, Cohen IT, Marsh JL: The toddler-preschooler postoperative pain scale: An observational scale for measuring postoperative pain in children aged 1 to 5. A preliminary report. *Pain* 50:273-280, 1992.
14. Broadman LM, Rice LJ, Hannallah RS: Testing the validity of an objective pain scale for infants and children. *Anesthesiology* 69:102-106, 1988.
15. Beyer JE, Aradine CR: Content validity of an instrument to measure young children's perception of the intensity of their pain. *J Pediatr Nurs* 1:386-395, 1986.
16. Shannon M, Berde CB: Pharmacologic management of pain in children and adolescents. *Pediatr Clin North Am* 36:855-871, 1989.
17. Yaster M, Deshpande JK: Management of pediatric pain with opioid analgesics. *J Pediatr* 113:421-429, 1988.
18. Korpela R, Olkkola KT: Pharmacokinetics of intravenous diclofenac sodium in children. *Eur J Clin Pharmacol* 38:293-295, 1990.
19. Watters CH et al: Diclofenac sodium for post-tonsillectomy pain in children. *Anaesthesia* 43:641-643, 1988.
20. Moores MA, Wandless JG, Fell D: Pediatric postoperative analgesia. A comparison of rectal diclofenac with caudal bupivacaine after inguinal herniotomy. *Anaesthesia* 45:156-158, 1990.
21. Bone ME, Fell D: A comparison of rectal diclofenac with intramuscular papaveratum or placebo for pain relief following tonsillectomy. *Anaesthesia* 43:277-280, 1988.
22. Maunuksela E-L, Olkkola KT, Korpela R: Does prophylactic intravenous infusion of indomethacin improve the management of postoperative pain in children? *Can J Anaesth* 35:123-127, 1988.
23. Watcha M et al: A comparison of ketorolac and morphine when used during pediatric surgery. *Anesthesiology* 75:A942, 1991.
24. Watcha M et al: Perioperative effects of oral ketorolac and acetaminophen in children undergoing bilateral myringotomy. *Can J Anaesth* 39:649-654, 1992.
25. Reinhart D et al: Effects of postoperative ketorolac on coagulation as evaluated by thromboelastograph. *Anesth Analg* 74:S249, 1992.
26. Bean JD, Hunt R: Analgesic efficacy of ketorolac in postoperative pediatric patients. *Anesth Analg* 74:S20, 1992.
27. Koren G et al: Postoperative morphine infusion in newborn infants: Assessment of disposition characteristics and safety. *Pediatr Pharmacol Ther* 107:963-967, 1985.
28. Kupferberg HJ, Way EL: Pharmacologic basis for the increased sensitivity of the newborn rat to morphine. *J Pharmacol Exp Ther* 141:105-112, 1963.
29. Weinberg DS et al: Sublingual absorption of selected opioid analgesics. *Clin Pharmacol Ther* 44:335-342, 1988.
30. Schecter NL et al: Sedation for painful procedures in children with cancer using the fentanyl lollipop: A preliminary report. In Tyler DC, Krane EL, editors: *Advances in Pain Research and Therapy, vol 15.* New York, Raven Press, 1990.
31. Nelson PS et al: Comparison of oral transmucosal fentanyl citrate and an oral solution of meperidine, diazepam, and atropine for premedication in children. *Anesthesiology* 70:616-621, 1989.
32. Streisand JB et al: Oral transmucosal fentanyl citrate premedication in children. *Anesth Analg* 69:28-34, 1989.
33. Henderson JM et al: Pre-induction of anesthesia in pediatric patients with nasally administered sufentanil. *Anesthesiology* 68:671-675, 1988.
34. Lavies NG, Wandless JG: Subcutaneous morphine in children: Taking the sting out of postoperative analgesia. *Anaesthesia* 7:1903-1908, 1989.
35. Tyler DC: Patient-controlled analgesia in adolescents. *J Adolesc Health Care* 11:154-158, 1990.
36. Vetter TR: Pediatric patient-controlled analgesia with morphine versus meperidine. *J Pain Symptom Manage* 7:204-208, 1992.
37. Berde CB et al: Patient-controlled analgesia in children and adolescents: A randomized, prospective comparison with intramuscular morphine for postoperative analgesia. *J Pediatr* 118:460-466, 1991.
38. Broadman LM: Patient-controlled analgesia in children and adolescents. In Ferrante FM, Ostheimer GW, Covino BG, editors: *Patient-Controlled Analgesia.* Cambridge, UK, Blackwell, 1990.
39. Schecter N, Berrien F, Katz S: The use of patient-controlled analgesia in adolescents with sickle cell crisis: A preliminary report. *J Pain Symptom Manage* 3:109-113, 1988.
40. Gaukroger PB, Tomkins DP, van der Walt JH: Patient-controlled analgesia in children. *Anaesth Intensive Care* 17:264-268, 1989.
41. Dohi S, Naito H, Takasaki T: Age-related changes in blood pressure and duration of motor block in spinal anesthesia. *Anesthesiology* 50:319-322, 1979.
42. Payen D et al: Pulsed Doppler ascending aortic, carotid, brachial and

femoral artery blood flows during caudal anesthesia in infants. *Anesthesiology* 67:681-685, 1987.

43. Denson D et al: Alpha₁-acid glycoprotein and albumin serum bupivacaine binding. *Clin Pharmacol Ther* 35:409-412, 1984.
44. Mazoit JX, Denson DD, Samii K: Pharmacokinetics of bupivacaine in infants after caudal anesthesia. *Anesthesiology* 68:387-391, 1988.
45. DiFazio CA: Metabolism of local anesthetics in the fetus, newborn and adults. *Br J Anaesth* 51(suppl):29-32, 1979.
46. Ecoffey C et al: Pharmacokinetics of lignocaine in children following caudal anaesthesia. *Br J Anaesth* 56:1399-1442, 1984.
47. Ecoffey C et al: Bupivacaine in children: Pharmacokinetics following caudal anesthesia. *Anesthesiology* 63:447-451, 1985.
48. Eyres RL et al: Plasma bupivacaine concentrations following lumbar epidural anaesthesia in children. *Anaesth Intensive Care* 14:131-134, 1986.
49. Desparmet J et al: Continuous epidural infusion of bupivacaine for postoperative pain relief in children. *Anesthesiology* 67:108-112, 1987.
50. Jones SEF et al: Intrathecal morphine for postoperative pain relief in children. *Br J Anaesth* 56:137-139, 1984.
51. Shapiro LA et al: Epidural morphine analgesia in children. *Anesthesiology* 61:210-215, 1984.
52. Attia J et al: Epidural morphine in children: Pharmacokinetics and CO₂ sensitivity. *Anesthesiology* 65:590-594, 1986.
53. Berde CB et al: Continuous epidural bupivacaine-fentanyl infusions in children following ureteral reimplantation. *Anesth Analg* 73:A1128, 1990.
54. Benlabed M et al: Analgesia and ventilatory response to CO₂ following epidural sufentanyl in children. *Anesthesiology* 67:948-951, 1987.
55. Dalens B, Hasnaoui A: Caudal anesthesia in pediatric surgery: Success rate and adverse effects in 750 consecutive patients. *Anesth Analg* 68:83-89, 1989.
56. Satayoshi M, Kamiyama Y: Caudal anaesthesia for upper abdominal surgery in infants and children: A simple calculation of the volume of local anaesthetic. *Acta Anesthesiol Scand* 28:57-60, 1984.
57. Spear RM: Dose-response in infants receiving caudal anaesthesia with bupivacaine. *Pediatric Anaesthesia* 1:47-52, 1991.
58. Saint-Raymond S, O'Donovan F, Ecoffey C: Criteria for safe ambulation following caudal block in children. *Anesthesiology* 69:A769, 1988.
59. Warner MA et al: The effect of age, epinephrine, and operative site on duration of caudal anesthesia in pediatric patients. *Anesth Analg* 66:995-999, 1987.
60. Wolf AR et al: Bupivacaine for caudal anesthesia in children: The optimal effective concentration. *Anesthesiology* 69:102-106, 1988.
61. Kapsten JE et al: Is there an optimal concentration of bupivacaine for caudal analgesia in outpatient surgery for children? *Can J Anaesth* 33:S114, 1986.
62. Jay R et al: Epinephrine and phenylephrine increase cardiorespiratory toxicity of intravenously administered bupivacaine in rats. *Anesth Analg* 70:543-545, 1990.
63. Yoeman PM, Cooke R, Hain WR: Penile block for circumcision: A comparison for caudal blockade. *Anaesthesia* 38:862-866, 1983.
64. Dalens B, Vanneville G, Tanguy A: A new parascalene approach to the brachial plexus in children: Comparison with the supraclavicular approach. *Anesth Analg* 66:1264-1271, 1987.
65. Moore DC: Axillary approach for block of the brachial plexus. In Moore DC, editor: *Regional Block-A Handbook for Use in the Clinical Practice of Medicine and Surgery,* ed 4. Springfield, Ill, Charles C Thomas, 1981.
66. Campbell RJ, Ilett KF, Dusci L: Plasma bupivacaine concentrations after axillary block in children. *Anaesth Intensive Care* 14:343-346, 1986.
67. McIlvaine WB et al: Continuous infusion of bupivacaine via intrapleural catheter for analgesia after thoracotomy in children. *Anesthesiology* 69:261-264, 1988.
68. McNicol LR: Lower limb blocks for children. *Anaesthesia* 41:27-31, 1986.
69. Shelly MP, Park GR: Intercostal nerve blockade for children. *Anaesthesia* 42:541-544, 1987.
70. Rothtein P et al: Bupivacaine for intercostal nerve block in children: Blood concentrations and pharmacokinetics. *Anesth Analg* 65:625-632, 1986.
71. Thompson GE: Celiac plexus, intercostal, and minor peripheral blockade. In Cousins MJ, Bridenbaugh PO, editors: *Neural Blockade in Clinical Anesthesia and Management of Pain.* Philadelphia, JB Lippincott, 1980.

QUESTIONS: ACUTE PAIN SYNDROMES IN CHILDREN

1. Newborns respond to pain by demonstrating changes in the following EXCEPT:
   A. Blood pressure and heart rate
   B. Transcutaneous PO_2
   C. Stress hormones
   D. Urine output

2. Postoperative pain scoring system comprising of quality of sleep, facial expression, cry, motor activity, and sociability is used in the age group of children from age:
   A. 1 to 8 months
   B. 1 to 5 years
   C. 5 to 12 years
   D. 12 to 18 years

3. The dose of ketorolac which is comparable to 0.1 mg/kg of morphine in children is:
   A. 0.3 mg/kg
   B. 0.6 mg/kg
   C. 0.9 mg/kg
   D. 1.2 mg/kg

4. The percentage of school-age children who complain of nonorganic abdominal pain is:
   A. 0-5%
   B. 10-15%
   C. 15-20%
   D. 20-25%

5. There are pharmacologic differences between a child and an adult in terms of protein binding, distribution, and elimination of drugs. When compared to adults, the volume of distribution of local anesthetics in a child is:
   A. twice
   B. three times
   C. four times
   D. five times

ANSWERS

1. D
2. A
3. C
4. B
5. B

PART FOUR

Test Banks

The following two test banks are designed to assist readers in assessing their knowledge of content areas relevant to the field of pain medicine. The test banks cover content areas included on many pain medicine certification examinations; however, the proportion of questions devoted to each content area and the types of questions used in the tests should not be viewed as that of pain medicine certification examinations. Readers may wish to consult the candidate information bulletins of certification examinations for content areas covered and question types used on these examinations.

Test Bank I

For the following questions, choose one correct answer.

1. Dorsal root entry zone lesions are indicated for patients with:
   A. Deafferentation pain syndrome
   B. Cancer pain
   C. Benign chronic pain
   D. Reflex sympathetic dystrophy syndrome

2. In the first month after amputation, the percentage of patients who experience phantom limb pain is:
   A. 9 to 23
   B. 40 to 63
   C. 70 to 75
   D. 85 to 97

3. A terminal patient is experiencing intractable cancer pain that is well localized to one side of the pelvis. Which of the following invasive procedures would be most appropriate for treating the pain?
   A. Percutaneous cordotomy
   B. Midline myelotomy
   C. Epidural block
   D. Subarachnoid phenol saddle block

4. The mechanism of action of intravenous regional bretylium is:
   A. Accumulation and blockade of norepinephrine release from adrenergic nerves
   B. Depletion and release of norepinephrine from adrenergic nerves
   C. Blockade of the action of prostaglandins
   D. Reduction in the accumulation of substance P

5. The femoral nerve originates from which of the following roots?
   A. T_{12}, L_1, L_2
   B. L_1, L_2, L_3
   C. L_2, L_3, L_4
   D. L_3, L_4, L_5

6. If symptoms persist after appropriate management of acute cervical disk herniation, the next step is to perform:
   A. Cervical laminectomy and fusion
   B. Cervical epidural injection
   C. Chemonucleolysis
   D. Cervical facet injection

7. A 45-year-old patient with a history of chronic low back, left hip, and left thigh pain who is status post multiple lumbar laminectomy received a differential epidural block of 3% 2-chloroprocaine. Some pain resumed with return of full sensation and motor function in the lower extremities; all pain returned with return of sympathetic function. The pain was transmitted via which fibers?
   A. A alpha
   B. A delta
   C. C
   D. A delta and C

8. The cell body of the neospinothalamic tract is located in which lamina?
   A. II
   B. III
   C. IV
   D. V

9. Which of the following statements is true regarding acute systemic toxic reactions to neurolytic agents?
   A. They may involve both the central nervous system (CNS) and cardiovascular system.
   B. They are benign.
   C. They primarily involve the liver and kidneys.
   D. They are usually avoided by adding epinephrine 2.5 μg/ml to the solution.

10. The best candidates for peripheral nerve stimulation are patients with:
    A. Multiple nerve pathology
    B. Single nerve pathology
    C. Nonspecific pathology
    D. Central pain

11. The changes seen in thermographic evaluation of postherpetic neuralgia may be due to increase in the activity of what type of fiber?
    A. A alpha
    B. A delta
    C. B
    D. C

12. Second-order neurons of the nociceptive afferents are located in the:
    A. Afferent axons
    B. Dorsal root ganglion
    C. Dorsal horn of the spinal cord
    D. Sympathetic ganglion

13. Primary myofascial pain is defined as:
    A. Pain with distinct histologic evidence of hyalin formation in the muscle
    B. Deposition of nonspecific inflammatory residue in skeletal muscle
    C. Pain caused by traumatic disease of the muscle
    D. Any disorder arising outside of the muscle tissue

14. A commonly used drug for epidural steroid injection has the following ingredients EXCEPT:
    A. Methylprednisolone acetate
    B. PEG 3350
    C. Myristyl-gamma picolinium chloride
    D. Benzyl alcohol

15. The drug in question 14 is known commercially as:
    A. Depo-Medrol (methylprednisolone acetate suspension)
    B. Aristocort (triamcinolone diacetate suspension)
    C. Prednisone
    D. Solu-Medrol

16. In peripheral vascular disease, spinal cord stimulation has demonstrated which of the following physiologic responses?
    A. Unchanged tissue-oxygen pressure while tissue-carbon dioxide rises
    B. Unchanged tissue-carbon dioxide while tissue-oxygen declines
    C. Increase in tissue-oxygen pressures and decrease in tissue-carbon dioxide
    D. Decrease in tissue-oxygen and decrease in tissue-carbon dioxide

17. The α_1 acid glycoprotein is different from albumin in drug binding in that it:
    A. Has low affinity for basic drugs
    B. Has high capacity
    C. Is an acute phase reactant protein
    D. Is not present during trauma

18. Which of the following symptoms is associated with pain and should be documented in the medical history?
    A. Paresthesias
    B. Hypesthesia
    C. Weakness
    D. Loss of vibration sense

19. At what age do the spinal cord and dorsal sac rise from the newborn level to the adult level?
    A. 1 month
    B. 3 months
    C. 6 months
    D. 12 months

20. Nociceptive impulse from the periphery can be inhibited by:
    A. Increased sensitization of nociceptors
    B. Decreased threshold of nociceptors
    C. Increased segmental spinal reflex
    D. Increased counterirritation (e.g., rubbing, vibration)

21. Spinal cord lesions that produce central pain are most commonly caused by:
    A. Vascular incidents
    B. Trauma
    C. Multiple sclerosis
    D. Neoplasm

22. Baclofen acts on what type of receptor?
    A. Opiate
    B. GABA-B
    C. α-Adrenergic
    D. Benzodiazepine

23. Once a cryoprobe has frozen to equilibrium, which of the following procedures can be used to increase the size of the "freeze zone"?
    A. Increase duration of freezing.
    B. Increase nitrous oxide pressure in the cryoprobe.
    C. Repeat freeze/thaw cycles of the tissue.
    D. Rapidly cool the tissue.

24. Classic hemophilia A is associated with a deficiency of which factor?
    A. V
    B. VIII
    C. IX
    D. X

25. The mechanism of antipsychotic action of neuroleptics is due to the blockade of which type of receptor?
    A. Adrenergic
    B. Dopamine
    C. Opiate
    D. Serotonin

26. An epidural opioid infusion is preferred over patient-controlled analgesia (PCA) after major surgical procedures because:
    A. The incidence of gastrointestinal ileus is less with an infusion
    B. It provides superior analgesia with less sedation than PCA
    C. The patient cannot tamper with the infusion device
    D. Respiratory depression problems are eliminated after titration

27. Examination of a patient with neck and shoulder pain reveals referred pain in the lateral aspect of the fore-

arm, with weakness and dysfunction of the biceps and brachioradialis, and hypoesthesia in the lateral aspect of the forearm and thumb. The patient most likely has a lesion of which nerve root?
A. C_4
B. C_5
C. C_6
D. C_7

28. The most appropriate diagnostic nerve block for pain in the upper abdominal viscera is:
    A. Intercostal block
    B. Lumbar sympathetic block
    C. Celiac plexus block
    D. Hypogastric plexus block

29. Sympathetic innervation to the upper extremity is carried by which fibers of the brachial plexus?
    A. T_1-T_2 preganglionic fibers
    B. T_3-T_5 preganglionic fibers
    C. T_1-T_2 postganglionic fibers
    D. T_3-T_5 postganglionic fibers

30. When using bupivacaine for a lumbar epidural block, what concentration is most effective for producing a sympathetic block?
    A. 0.25%
    B. 0.50%
    C. 0.75%
    D. 0.125%

31. A facet joint injection of local anesthetic and steroids results in prolonged pain relief of 6 months or more in what percentage of patients?
    A. 30
    B. 50
    C. 70
    D. 90

32. Seizures produced by local anesthetics appear to arise from what area of the brain?
    A. Thalamus
    B. Geniculate bodies
    C. Reticular activating system
    D. Amygdala

33. When cervical spinal cord compression is suspected and physical examination shows radicular signs in the upper limb, the most appropriate next step in the investigation is:
    A. Surgical exploration
    B. Myelography
    C. Electromyography
    D. Magnetic resonance imaging (MRI)

34. Attempts by patients to influence the evaluation of physical abnormalities during the examination may be indicated by which of the following?
    A. Hyperactivity of patellar reflexes
    B. Increased blood pressure and heart rate

    C. Symmetric but broad-based, ataxic gait
    D. Fluctuations in eye-blink rate

35. Intense whiteness of fingers with subsequent blue coloration when cold and red coloration on rewarming is most likely due to:
    A. Frostbite
    B. Raynaud's disease
    C. Reflex sympathetic dystrophy (RSD)
    D. Acute venous thrombosis

36. Appropriate treatment of atypical facial pain includes which of the following?
    A. Antidepressants
    B. Anticonvulsants
    C. Antiemetics
    D. Cranial nerves V and IX section

37. The hypogastric plexus is composed of what type of fibers?
    A. Postganglionic sympathetic
    B. Postganglionic parasympathetic
    C. Visceral efferent
    D. A delta

38. A poorly localized, steady, dull, or boring epigastric or left upper quadrant pain that radiates to the back is most likely due to:
    A. Cholecystitis
    B. Pancreatitis
    C. Renal colic
    D. Subphrenic abscess

39. Laminectomy is indicated for a patient who complains of pain in the neck and right arm and has which of the following conditions?
    A. Facet arthropathy
    B. Arachnoiditis
    C. Spinal cord compression
    D. Brachial plexus entrapment

40. Prohormone dynorphin (Pro enk B) is a natural ligand of which receptor type?
    A. μ
    B. κ
    C. δ
    D. ϵ

41. Indications for lumbar epidural steroid injections include all of the following EXCEPT:
    A. Radicular pain with corresponding sensory change
    B. Radiculopathy due to herniated disk with failed conservative treatment
    C. Acute herpes zoster in the lumbar dermatomes
    D. Postlaminectomy (failed back) syndrome without radiculopathy

42. Which of the following is NOT a guiding principle of physical medicine and rehabilitation?
    A. Pain control

B. Functional restoration
C. Return to work and leisure activities
D. Patient dependence on prolonged physical therapy

43. All of the following are characteristic of trigeminal neuralgia EXCEPT:
A. Paroxysmal pains with pain-free intervals
B. Presence of trigger zones
C. Pain restricted to the trigeminal distribution
D. Absence of structural or pathologic findings

44. Areas innervated by the maxillary nerve include all of the following EXCEPT the:
A. Maxilla
B. Skin over the middle third of the face
C. Teeth of the upper jaw
D. Tongue

45. Which of the following nerve blocks is LEAST helpful in diagnosing sympathetically mediated pelvic pain?
A. Differential spinal
B. Pudendal nerve
C. Superior hypogastric plexus
D. Differential epidural

46. All of the following statements regarding the anatomy of the superior hypogastric plexus are true EXCEPT:
A. It lies anterior to the L_5 vertebra.
B. It lies just inferior to the aortic bifurcation.
C. It lies right of the midline.
D. It branches left and right and descends to form the inferior hypogastric plexus.

47. All of the following statements are true of red blood cell (RBC) indexes EXCEPT:
A. They define the size and hemoglobin content of the RBCs.
B. They have replaced the need for examination of the peripheral blood smear in the diagnosis of anemia.
C. Microcytic indexes with anemia may result from iron deficiency.
D. Macrocytic indexes may result from folate deficiency.

48. Which of the following statements concerning skeletal pain is NOT true?
A. Neoplasms in bone are usually metastatic.
B. The pain fibers are of A delta and C fiber origin.
C. Pain fibers accompany epiphysial vessels.
D. It is accompanied by effusion if joints are involved.

49. All of the following are indications for a stellate ganglion block EXCEPT:
A. RSD
B. Acute herpes zoster (ophthalmic division)
C. Hyperhidrosis
D. Pancreatitis

50. The acute phase of RSD includes all of the following characteristics EXCEPT:
A. Burning pain
B. Minimal functional impairment
C. Increased blood flow
D. Severe trophic changes

51. Which of the following regional anesthesia techniques is NOT commonly used with children because of its side effects?
A. Epidural block
B. Subarachnoid block
C. Caudal block
D. Brachial plexus block

52. Which of the following is NOT a characteristic of central pain?
A. Hyperesthesia
B. Spontaneous pain
C. Hypertrophia
D. Hyperpathia

53. All of the following statements are true regarding serologic testing for cancer EXCEPT:
A. CEA (carcinoembryonic antigen) is an excellent screening test for colon cancer.
B. Multiple myeloma may be diagnosed with the serum protein immunoelectrophoresis.
C. Cigarette smokers may have an elevated CEA.
D. CA 19-9 may be a useful marker for following the course of treatment in pancreatic cancer.

54. Which of the following statements is NOT true of renal cell carcinoma?
A. The etiology is unknown.
B. Metastases are widespread.
C. Erythrocythemia can provide useful diagnostic information.
D. Neuroablative procedures are rarely indicated for pain management.

55. The goals of treatment for rheumatoid arthritis include all of the following EXCEPT:
A. Relief of pain
B. Reduction of inflammation
C. Preservation of function
D. Immobilization and bed rest

56. A brachial plexus block is indicated for all of the following conditions EXCEPT:
A. Sympathetic independent pain resulting from RSD
B. Brachial plexalgia
C. Angina pectoris
D. Raynaud's disease

57. Which of the following statements regarding endometriosis is NOT true?
A. It is a common cause of pelvic pain.
B. It is hormonally maintained and hormonally responsive.

C. A diagnosis can only be made with laparoscopic histopathologic confirmation.

D. A moderate to severe condition may be associated with an absence of painful sequelae.

58. A celiac plexus block is effective in reducing pain originating from all of the following organs EXCEPT:
    A. Pancreas
    B. Transverse portion of the large colon
    C. Gall bladder
    D. Descending portion of the pelvic colon

For questions 59-75, choose from the following:
    A. 1, 2, and 3
    B. 1 and 3
    C. 2 and 4
    D. 4
    E. All of the above

59. In the comparison of biofeedback with relaxation training, which of the following statements apply?
    1. Patients usually favor the instrumentation and technology associated with biofeedback.
    2. Biofeedback and relaxation training are equally effective in the management of chronic pain.
    3. Research shows that relaxation training is more cost effective and practical than biofeedback.
    4. Biofeedback and relaxation are usually used as conjunctive treatments.

60. Which of the following neurolytic processes is (are) associated with neuritis or neuroma function?
    1. Radiofrequency thermocoagulation
    2. Phenol neurolysis
    3. Alcohol neurolysis
    4. Cryoneurolysis

61. Which of the following complications is (are) associated with tunneled epidural catheters?
    1. Infection
    2. Dislodged catheter
    3. Broken catheter
    4. Low pressure headache

62. The presence of positive sharp waves during needle electromyography of a patient who describes debilitating pain and weakness of the limb while being tested is significant because:
    1. This waveform is only found in patients with muscular dystrophy and never in pain syndromes
    2. This type of activity is an objective sign of denervation or reinnervation
    3. This pattern is an integral component of Waddell's signs of nonorganic pain behavior
    4. This pattern cannot be created fictitiously, even during reduced voluntary motor effort

63. Which of the following patients would respond best to an epidural steroid injection?
    1. A patient with back pain of less than three months' duration

2. A patient with neurologic findings that correlate with the level of the involved nerve root
    3. A patient who does not exhibit any Waddell's signs
    4. A patient who exhibits discrepancy in sitting and supine straight leg raising

64. Which of the following statements regarding local anesthetics is (are) true?
    1. The neurotoxic effects of 2-chloroprocaine are related to the substitution of a hydrogen ion with a chloride ion on its ring structure.
    2. Warming local anesthetics to 100° C has been shown to reduce the onset of epidural block.
    3. The effects of bicarbonation and carbonation of local anesthetics on the onset of nerve block are produced by the same mechanism.
    4. True allergic reaction to local anesthetics with an amino amide structure is rare and is most likely related to the preservative methylparaben.

65. When implanting a drug-delivery system, the patient should be placed in which of the following positions?
    1. Lateral
    2. Sitting
    3. Prone
    4. Supine

66. Which of the following electrodiagnostic studies is typically used to assess radicular pain involving the spine and related extremities?
    1. Selective tissue conductance tests
    2. Nerve conduction velocity studies
    3. Somatosensory evoked potentials
    4. Needle electromyographic recordings

67. A patient with renal failure on hemodialysis undergoes a small bowel resection. Postoperatively, the patient received intramuscular morphine every 3 to 4 hours for pain. The patient did well for 2 days but now is very sedated and ventilation is slow. The patient arouses quickly after receiving naloxone 0.4 mg. The most likely explanation is that:
    1. Morphine's elimination half life is greatly prolonged in renal failure
    2. Morphine 6-glucuronide is a highly lipid-soluble metabolite of morphine that accumulates quickly and easily enters the CNS
    3. Morphine 3-glucuronide is a highly lipid-soluble metabolite of morphine that quickly accumulates and easily enters the CNS
    4. Even though both morphine 6-glucuronide and morphine 3-glucuronide are less lipophilic than morphine, a sufficient amount of these metabolites is now acting on the CNS

68. Which of the following factors affect the measurement of oncologic pain?
    1. Type of pain
    2. Age of patient
    3. Physical strength of patient
    4. Pain rating scale used

69. Which of the following complications is (are) associated with percutaneous cryoneurolysis?
    1. Motor nerve damage
    2. Frostbite of the skin
    3. Vascular damage
    4. Neuroma formation

70. The McGill Pain Questionnaire is designed to measure which of the following components of pain?
    1. Societal
    2. Sensory
    3. Quantitative
    4. Evaluative

71. Data from which of the following pain assessments can be analyzed using parametric statistics?
    1. 11-point visual analogue scale
    2. Pain behavior assessment
    3. Category scale
    4. Visual analogue scale (VAS)

72. Benefits of using the Minnesota Multiphasic Personality Inventory (MMPI) with pain patients include:
    1. Assessment of emotional disorders that occur secondary to the pain experience
    2. Determination as to whether the pain is psychogenic or organic
    3. Assessment of preexisting personality factors that can adversely affect response to treatment
    4. Determination of patient's ability to go back to work

73. Which of the following complications is (are) associated with radiofrequency thermocoagulation?
    1. Neuropathic pain
    2. Carcinogenesis at lesion site
    3. Nociceptive pain
    4. Infection at lesion site

74. If stimulation at 75 Hz produces no pain during a lumbar facet radiofrequency procedure, which of the following actions should be taken?
    1. Form a lesion.
    2. Stimulate at 4 Hz.
    3. Inject 2% lidocaine.
    4. Reposition the probe.

75. Fibromyalgia differs from myofascial syndrome in that it is characterized by:
    1. Tender points that do not necessarily exhibit the "jump sign"
    2. A greater number of tender points than myofascial syndrome
    3. Frequent depression with a disturbed sleep pattern
    4. Lack of response to trigger point injections and/or antidepressants

Test Bank I   Answers

1.	A	26.	B	51.	B
2.	B	27.	C	52.	D
3.	A	28.	C	53.	A
4.	A	29.	A	54.	D
5.	B	30.	B	55.	D
6.	B	31.	A	56.	C
7.	D	32.	D	57.	C
8.	D	33.	A	58.	D
9.	A	34.	B	59.	C
10.	B	35.	A	60.	A
11.	A	36.	A	61.	A
12.	C	37.	A	62.	C
13.	C	38.	B	63.	A
14.	D	39.	C	64.	C
15.	A	40.	B	65.	B
16.	C	41.	D	66.	C
17.	C	42.	D	67.	D
18.	A	43.	D	68.	B
19.	D	44.	D	69.	A
20.	D	45.	B	70.	C
21.	B	46.	C	71.	D
22.	B	47.	B	72.	A
23.	C	48.	D	73.	B
24.	A	49.	D	74.	D
25.	B	50.	D	75.	A

Test Bank II

For the following questions, choose one correct answer.

1. Neurogenic pain originating from the neck and shoulder region is most likely due to which of the following conditions?
   A. Degenerative disk disease
   B. Myofascial pain
   C. Fibromyalgia
   D. Herpetic neuralgia

2. Which of the following tests is confirmatory in the diagnosis of carpal tunnel syndrome?
   A. Thermography
   B. Somatosensory evoked potentials
   C. Electromyography
   D. Magnetic resonance imaging (MRI)

3. A patient complains of morning stiffness and pain in multiple joints, including the joints of the hand. Subcutaneous nodules are present over the extensor surfaces, and diagnostic tests indicate abnormal amounts of HLA-DR4. The most likely diagnosis is:
   A. Osteoarthritis
   B. Rheumatoid arthritis
   C. Gout
   D. Degenerative arthritis

4. A patient is positioned prone on the fluoroscopic table, the T_1-T_4 spinous processes are identified on the ipsilateral side, and a skin wheal is raised 4 to 5 cm lateral to the spinous process. A spinal needle is directed to the lamina and "walked" laterally until there is loss of resistance. These procedures are consistent with which type of block?
   A. Stellate ganglion
   B. Thoracic sympathetic
   C. Interpleural
   D. Thoracic epidural

5. Skeletal pain generally emanates primarily from:
   A. C fibers
   B. Joints
   C. Bones
   D. Surrounding soft tissue

6. Antidepressants exert their action by:
   A. Inhibiting prostaglandin synthesis
   B. Altering synaptic monoamine transmitter activity
   C. Releasing encephalins from opiate receptors
   D. Reducing the level of substance P at nerve terminals

7. Which of the following statements is true concerning pain emanating from ureteric calculi?
   A. It is conveyed via sensory afferents from thoracic spinal nerves T_{10}-T_{12}.
   B. It is followed by nausea and vomiting.
   C. Midureteric pain radiates to the contralateral testicle.
   D. The referral pattern is independent of stone position.

8. The most common side effect from a lumbar sympathetic block is:
   A. Dizziness
   B. Backache
   C. Nausea
   D. Hypotension

9. Which of the following local anesthetics has a low potency and short duration of effect?
   A. Mepivacaine
   B. Procaine
   C. Prilocaine
   D. Lidocaine

10. The most accurate pain assessment tools for preverbal children are:
    A. Spatial scales
    B. Facial scales
    C. Numerical scales
    D. Physiologic measurements

11. The brachial plexus is formed by which rami?
    A. C_5-T_1 anterior primary
    B. C_3-T_2 anterior primary
    C. C_5-T_1 anterior and posterior
    D. C_3-T_2 anterior and posterior

12. When reflex spasm of the collateral vessels occurs because of acute vascular insufficiency, it can be promptly reversed by:
    A. Local anesthetic infiltration of the painful region
    B. A sympathetic block

C. Administration of IV narcotics

D. Oral administration of phenoxybenzamine

13. Cell bodies of preganglionic fibers of the lumbar sympathetic chain arise at which of the following sites?
    A. T_5-T_9
    B. T_{11}-L_2
    C. L_3-L_5
    D. S_1-S_4

14. Which of the following conditions mimics thalamic pain syndrome?
    A. Wallenberg's syndrome
    B. Syringomyelia
    C. Lateral medullary syndrome
    D. Parietal cortical lesion

15. The most commonly used route of administration for postoperative pain relief in children is:
    A. Subcutaneous
    B. Intramuscular
    C. Intravenous
    D. Rectal

16. Posterior rhizotomy is most effective in treating which of the following conditions?
    A. Intractable chest wall pain
    B. Sciatica after laminectomy
    C. Pelvic pain and dyspareunia
    D. Lumbar plexalgia secondary to metastatic lumbar vertebral lesion

17. The long-term effects of peripheral nerve stimulation are enhanced when the lead is in what relationship to the nerve?
    A. Wrapped directly around the nerve
    B. At least 1 cm away from the nerve
    C. Separated by muscle fascia from the nerve
    D. Placed directly against the nerve

18. Which of the following nociceptors is activated by chemical stimuli?
    A. A delta mechanoreceptor (HTM)
    B. A delta mechanothermal nociceptor (MMTN)
    C. C polymodal nociceptor (CPN)
    D. C mechanonociceptor

19. A lateral femoral cutaneous block is indicated for which of the following conditions?
    A. Meralgia paresthetica
    B. Femoral neuralgia
    C. Saphenous neuralgia
    D. Groin pain

20. Computed tomography of the head is preferred over an MRI when evaluating which of the following conditions?
    A. Multiple sclerosis
    B. Meningioma

C. Stroke

D. Glioma

21. When used as an IV contrast in MRI, gadolinium penetrates into:
    A. Edematous tissue
    B. Areas with disrupted blood-brain barriers
    C. The cerebrospinal fluid
    D. The intervertebral disks

22. Lesions producing central pain occur most commonly in the:
    A. Spinal cord
    B. Brainstem
    C. Brain
    D. Frontal cortex

23. Which of the following statements is true regarding neurolytic concentrations of less than 2% phenol?
    A. They have no effect.
    B. They selectively destroy A delta and C fibers.
    C. They have a reversible local anesthetic action when applied to nerve bundles.
    D. They destroy nerves but have no effect on blood vessels.

24. A steady state of blood drug concentration is achieved only after how many half lives?
    A. 1
    B. 3
    C. 5
    D. 7

25. Which of the following is a clinical characteristic of peripheral neuropathy?
    A. Proximal muscle weakness
    B. Absent distal deep tendon reflexes
    C. Sensory changes in a dermatomal pattern
    D. Increased muscle tone distally

26. Posttraumatic facial neuralgia is characterized by
    A. Absence of sensory deficits
    B. Trigger zones
    C. Symptoms outside the trigeminal nerve distribution
    D. Burning discomfort

27. Mydriasis, tachypnea, tachycardia, delirium, and a modest decrease in pain can be produced by agonists of which receptor type?
    A. μ
    B. κ
    C. δ
    D. σ

28. Which of the following statements regarding platelets is true?
    A. Their life span is approximately 14 days.
    B. Their function in coagulation is reversibly inhibited by acetylated salicylates.

C. Platelet count is diminished in the postsplenectomy patient.
D. The inhibition of platelets in coagulation by most nonsteroidal antiinflammatory drugs (NSAIDs) is related to elimination half-life.

29. The sciatic nerve block originally described by Labat is performed via which approach?
A. Posterior
B. Anterior
C. Lateral
D. Supine sciatic

30. A patient who sustained trauma to the right leg 6 weeks ago complains of burning pain, hyperesthesia in the leg. Vasomotor and sudomotor disturbances are present, and there is increased muscular tone. The most likely diagnosis is:
A. Peripheral neuropathy
B. Acute vascular insufficiency
C. Reflex sympathetic dystrophy (CRPS)
D. Acute osteomyelitis

31. The neurotransmitter most responsible for transmission of nociceptive impulse at the central terminals of primary afferent is:
A. Glutamate
B. Somatostatin
C. Leu-enkephalin
D. Dynorphin

32. Transcutaneous electrical nerve stimulation relieves pain by:
A. Depleting neurotransmitters in nociceptors
B. Stimulating C fibers directly
C. Activating inhibitory neurons
D. Destroying nociceptors

33. Peripheral neurectomy is most appropriate for which of the following pain syndromes?
A. "Tic" pain
B. Sciatica
C. Headache
D. Neuroma

34. Which of the following is used to assess reduction of range of motion associated with painful neuromuscular disorders?
A. Goniometry
B. Electromyography
C. Posturography
D. Inclinometry

35. What is the function of the periaqueductal gray (PAG), periventricular gray (PVG), nucleus raphe magnus (NRM), and dorsolateral funiculus (DLF) of the descending pathway?
A. Facilitation of pain transmission to the periphery
B. Modulation of pain transmission to the central nervous system (CNS)

C. Communication with the reticular formation
D. Transmission of information from the sensory cortex to the thalamus

36. A diminished triceps jerk indicates a lesion of which nerve root?
A. C_4
B. C_5
C. C_6
D. C_7

37. The peripheral theory of phantom limb pain suggests that pain is caused by:
A. Spontaneous firing of neuromas
B. Early discharges from C fibers
C. Decreased sympathetic afferent activity
D. Late discharges from A delta fibers

38. Excess stimulation of A delta fibers will result in a patient report of:
A. Motor movement in the affected area
B. Numbness in the sclerotome of the affected area
C. Contracture in the affected area
D. Unpleasant paresthesias

39. Lumbar sympathetic block has been extensively used in the diagnosis and treatment of:
A. Visceral pain of the abdomen
B. Visceral pain of the pelvis
C. Sympathetically mediated pain caused by RSD
D. Acute herpes zoster of T_6-T_8

40. Stump pain occurs in what percentage of amputees?
A. 10
B. 25
C. 50
D. 75

41. What is the medium diameter efferent fiber to the muscle spindles?
A. A alpha
B. A beta
C. A delta
D. C

42. Transdermal fentanyl is rarely used in the management of postoperative pain because:
A. Clinically available doses are too high for the intensity of postoperative pain
B. The analgesic effect is abruptly terminated when the patch is discontinued
C. There is usually a delay of 8 to 10 hours before blood analgesic concentration is reached
D. Ileus and tolerance develop faster than with morphine

43. In most studies, the incidence of chronic pain without obvious pathology is:
A. Less than 25%
B. 33% to 50%

C. 55% to 75%
D. 80% to 95%

44. To achieve sympathetic denervation of the head and neck, the best site of blocking is the:
   A. Middle cervical ganglion
   B. Superior cervical ganglion
   C. Stellate ganglion
   D. Sphenopalatine ganglion

45. The lesser splanchnic nerve is formed by which of the following sympathetic nerves?
   A. T_5-T_7
   B. T_8-T_9
   C. T_{10}-T_{11}
   D. T_{12}

46. Which of the following statements does NOT describe a characteristic of the gas expansion cryoprobe?
   A. It can cause proximal freezing if improperly insulated.
   B. It is very durable and resistant to malfunction by mechanical manipulation.
   C. It can use a variety of gases that are easily stored in pressurized tanks.
   D. It creates a freeze zone approximately two to three times the size of the probe's diameter.

47. Which of the following medications does NOT relieve central pain?
   A. Phenobarbital
   B. Morphine sulphate
   C. Carbamazepine
   D. Amitriptyline

48. Major indications for facet injection include all of the following EXCEPT:
   A. Focal tenderness over a facet joint
   B. Chronic low back pain
   C. Normal radiographic workup
   D. Arachnoiditis

49. All of the following medications are anticonvulsants EXCEPT:
   A. Phenytoin
   B. Carbamazepine
   C. Clonazepam
   D. Diazepam

50. Chronic pancreatitis is associated with all of the following features EXCEPT:
   A. History of alcohol abuse
   B. Recurrent or persistent abdominal pain
   C. Epigastric pain in underweight and malnourished individuals
   D. Back pain with radiation to T_{10} bilaterally

51. The hypogastric plexus innervates all of the following organs EXCEPT the:
   A. Vagina
   B. Bladder
   C. Prostate
   D. Descending colon

52. All of the following are contraindications to performing an MRI EXCEPT:
   A. Cerebral aneurysm clips
   B. Cardiac pacemakers
   C. Mechanical ventilation
   D. Lack of patient cooperation

53. Complications associated with a continuous epidural technique include all of the following EXCEPT:
   A. Intrathecal administration of the drug
   B. Infection
   C. Epidural hematoma
   D. Hypertension

54. All of the following statements are true of eosinophilia EXCEPT:
   A. It is defined as an eosinophil count greater than 2% of the total leukocyte count.
   B. It may be indicative of neoplasm.
   C. It may be indicative of collagen vascular disease.
   D. It may be indicative of allergy.

55. The zygapophyseal joint syndrome is characterized by all of the following features EXCEPT:
   A. Unilateral back pain
   B. Radiation of midlumbar pain to the buttocks and back of the thigh
   C. Aggravation of pain with flexion
   D. Tenderness over the facet joint

56. A work hardening program is different from a work conditioning program in that a work hardening program aims to do all of the following EXCEPT:
   A. Return an injured worker to a particular job
   B. Provide a 2- to 6-week period of specific simulated work activities
   C. Facilitate both emotional and physical reactivation
   D. Promote a gym-based personal exercise program

57. Radiofrequency thermocoagulation is NOT likely to produce ventricular arrhythmias because:
   A. Properly placed electrodes maximize transmission of cardiac current
   B. The frequency of current is very different from an electrocardiogram (ECG)
   C. Pain increases the threshold for arrhythmias
   D. No net current flows through the patient

58. Which of the following statements regarding the superior hypogastric plexus block is NOT true?
   A. It is most appropriate for pelvic pain of visceral origin.
   B. It is associated with few side effects.
   C. It must be performed with the assistance of fluoroscopy.
   D. It is most appropriate for upper abdominal pain.

59. Which of the following does NOT generally provoke visceral pain?
    A. Ischemia of visceral muscle
    B. Dividing the transverse colon
    C. Stretching of Glisson's capsule
    D. Distention of hollow viscera

60. Which of the following relationships between local anesthetics and their chemical profiles is NOT true?
    A. Prilocaine metabolites create methemoglobin.
    B. Ropivacaine racemic mixture exists almost as a pure solution of one isomer.
    C. Etidocaine creates a profound motor block that limits its usefulness for obstetric and postoperative analgesia.
    D. Mepivacaine is associated with vasodilatative activity.

61. Which of the following interventions is NOT appropriate for treating acute disk herniation?
    A. Muscle relaxation by cyclobenzapine
    B. NSAIDs
    C. Gentle limbering exercises
    D. Cervical laminectomy and fusion

For questions 62-75, choose from the following:
    A. 1, 2, and 3
    B. 1 and 3
    C. 2 and 4
    D. 4
    E. All of the above

62. Which of the following is (are) characteristic of myofascial trigger points?
    1. A firm tense band in the involved muscle
    2. A "jump sign" when the muscle band is snapped briskly
    3. A predictable referred pain pattern
    4. A pain reference zone that may exhibit autonomic changes

63. Selective tissue conductance is most appropriate in the assessment of which of the following conditions?
    1. Sudomotor dysfunction
    2. Sympathetically mediated pain
    3. Postherpetic neuralgia
    4. Ulnar neuropathy

64. Which of the following describes the process(es) by which epidural steroid injections relieve back and radicular leg pain?
    1. Inflammation in the affected nerve roots is reduced.
    2. Scar tissue surrounding the nerve roots is dissolved.
    3. Transmission of nociceptive input in C fibers is blocked.
    4. The herniated disk is realigned.

65. Which of the following electrophysiologic techniques is most appropriate for assessing chronic ocular or periorbital pain?
    1. Electrooculography
    2. Electronystagmography
    3. Electroretinography
    4. Needle electromyography

66. Which of the following opioids are partial agonists?
    1. Heroin
    2. Nalbuphine
    3. Oxycodone
    4. Buprenorphine

67. Which of the following statements regarding the Numerical Pain Scale is (are) true?
    1. It is an ordinal method of assessing pain.
    2. It requires no specialized training to administer.
    3. It can easily be adapted for use by children.
    4. It is not appropriate for assessing remembered pain.

68. Which of the following solutions is (are) used for neurolysis?
    1. Hypertonic saline
    2. Phenol
    3. Ethanol
    4. Distilled water

69. Which of the following advantages is (are) associated with a Type II (tunneled epidural catheter) drug-delivery system?
    1. Ease of insertion
    2. Ability to implant in outpatient settings
    3. Ease of removal
    4. Decreased risk of infection relative to Type I delivery systems

70. Which of the following statements is (are) correct regarding the use of hypnosis with chronic pain?
    1. The hypnotic analgesia received is mediated by the endorphin system.
    2. It can provide a cure for chronic pain.
    3. It is beneficial in treating psychogenic pain of organic pathology.
    4. It focuses on the subjective component of pain.

71. Which of the following implantable drug-delivery systems would be appropriate for a patient with a life expectancy of a few days to several weeks?
    1. Simple epidural catheter
    2. Reservoir/port
    3. Tunneled epidural catheter
    4. Implantable continuous infusion

72. When a pain patient is referred to a psychologist for evaluation, a standard assessment battery generally includes:
    1. A clinical interview
    2. A structured pain inventory

3. Objective psychometric testing
4. Projective techniques

73. The Faces pain diagrams are appropriate for use with which of the following types of patients?
    1. The elderly
    2. Children
    3. Individuals with mental retardation
    4. Postoperative patients on a ventilator

74. Which of the following statements is (are) true regarding medications that either prevent or treat NSAID gastropathy?
    1. Sucralfate works in part by reducing gastric acid secretion.
    2. Enteric coating has proven highly effective in reducing gastrointestinal toxicity.

3. Misoprostol is an inhibitor of prostaglandin E_1 and therefore reduces its damaging effect on the gastric mucosa.
4. Sucralfate promotes gastric mucous secretion via a prostaglandin-independent mechanism.

75. Which of the following procedures is (are) important when performing a cryolesion?
    1. Assuring close proximity of the cryoprobe to the site to be frozen by creating motor stimulation
    2. Infiltrating the nerve or site to be frozen with local anesthetic before lesioning
    3. Bending the cryoprobe to achieve the proper angle and proximity to the site to be frozen
    4. Using an intravenous cannula to help position the cryoprobe and provide extra insulation against inadvertent tissue freezing

Test Bank II   Answers

1.	D	26.	A	51.	D
2.	C	27.	D	52.	C
3.	D	28.	D	53.	D
4.	B	29.	A	54.	A
5.	B	30.	C	55.	C
6.	B	31.	A	56.	D
7.	A	32.	C	57.	B
8.	B	33.	D	58.	D
9.	B	34.	D	59.	B
10.	D	35.	B	60.	D
11.	A	36.	D	61.	D
12.	B	37.	D	62.	E
13.	B	38.	D	63.	A
14.	B	39.	C	64.	B
15.	C	40.	C	65.	B
16.	D	41.	C	66.	D
17.	C	42.	C	67.	A
18.	C	43.	B	68.	E
19.	A	44.	C	69.	E
20.	B	45.	C	70.	D
21.	B	46.	B	71.	B
22.	B	47.	C	72.	A
23.	C	48.	D	73.	E
24.	C	49.	D	74.	D
25.	B	50.	D	75.	D

Index